TEACHING
in NURSING
A GUIDE *for* FACULTY

Seventh Edition

TEACHING *in* NURSING
A GUIDE *for* FACULTY

Diane M. Billings, EdD, RN, ANEF, FAAN
Chancellor's Professor Emeritus
Indiana University School of Nursing
Indianapolis, Indiana

Judith A. Halstead, PhD, RN, CNE, ANEF, FAAN
Professor Emeritus
Indiana University School of Nursing
Indianapolis, Indiana

ELSEVIER

Executive Content Strategist: Lee Henderson
Content Development Specialist: Laura Fisher
Publishing Services Manager: Deepthi Unni
Project Manager: Thoufiq Mohammed
Design Direction: Margaret Reid

Printed in India

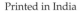

Last digit is the print number: 9   8   7   6   5   4   3   2   1

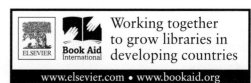

We dedicate this 25th Anniversary Edition of Teaching in Nursing: A Guide for Faculty *to our many contributors who have generously shared their expertise and wisdom with our readers to prepare them for their role as nurse educators.*

CONTRIBUTORS

Diane M. Billings, EdD, RN, ANEF, FAAN
Chancellor's Professor Emeritus
Indiana University School of Nursing
Indianapolis, Indiana
Chapters 14 and 24

Sarah M. Billings-Berg, DC, DNP, RN, CNE
Dean of Nursing and Health Science
Vermont State University
Randolph Center, Vermont
Chapter 8

Wanda Bonnel, PhD, RN, APRN, ANEF
Associate Professor Emerita
School of Nursing
University of Kansas
Kansas City, Kansas
Chapter 25

Sandy L. Carollo, PhD, MSN, ARNP
Executive Vice President and Provost
Helene Fuld College of Nursing
New York, New York
Chapter 9

Linda S. Christensen, EdD, JD, RN, CNE, FAAN
Chief Legal Officer
Legal Services
National League for Nursing
Washington, District of Columbia
Chapter 3

Jeanne R. Conner, DNP, APRN, FNP
Assistant Clinical Professor
College of Nursing
Montana State University
Bozeman, Montana
Chapter 15

Diann DeWitt, PhD, RN, CNE
Associate Professor
Nursing
Ottawa University
Phoenix, Arizona
Chapter 23

Jewel K. Diller, DNP, MSEd, RN
Assistant Vice President for Nursing (Retired)
Ivy Tech Community College
Fort Wayne, Indiana
Chapter 2

Peggy Ellis, PhD, RN
Program Director (Retired)
Nursing
Lindenwood University
St. Charles, Missouri
Chapter 26

Susan Gross Forneris, PhD, RN, CNE, CHSE-A
Associate Dean for Academic Programs
School of Nursing
University of Minnesota
Minneapolis, Minnesota
Chapter 19

Betsy Frank, PhD, RN, ANEF
Professor Emerita
School of Nursing
Indiana State University
Terre Haute, Indiana
Chapter 4

Barbara Manz Friesth, PhD, RN
Clinical Professor and Assistant Dean of Learning
    Resources
Community and Health Systems
Indiana University
School of Nursing
Indianapolis, Indiana
Chapter 21

Karen H. Frith, PhD, RN, NEA-BC, CNE
Dean and Professor
College of Nursing
The University of Alabama in Huntsville
Huntsville, Alabama
Chapter 20

Elizabeth A. Gazza, PhD, RN, LCCE, FACCE, ANEF
Professor and Associate Director for Faculty and
    Staff Development
School of Nursing
University of North Carolina Wilmington
Wilmington, North Carolina
Chapter 1

Nelda Godfrey, PhD, ACNS-BC, RN, FAAN, ANEF
Associate Dean
University of Kansas School of Nursing
Kansas City, Kansas
Chapter 6

Paula Gubrud-Howe, EdD, RN, CHSE, ANEF, FAAN
Professor Emeritus
School of Nursing
Oregon Health & Science University
Portland, Oregon
Chapter 18

Judith A. Halstead, PhD, RN, CNE, ANEF, FAAN
Professor Emeritus
School of Nursing
Indiana University
Indianapolis, Indiana
Chapter 22

Christine L. Hober, PhD, RN-BC, CNE
Professor of Nursing
Fort Hays State University
WaKeeney, Kansas
Chapter 25

Carolina G. Huerta, EdD, RN, FAAN
Professor
School of Nursing
University of Texas Rio Grande Valley
Edinburg, Texas
Chapter 17

Jane M. Kirkpatrick, PhD, RN, ANEF
Professor Emerita
School of Nursing
Purdue University
West Lafayette, Indiana
Chapter 23

Caitlin Krouse, DNP, FNP-BC, RN
Associate Professor
Division of Nursing
University of Saint Francis
Fort Wayne, Indiana
Chapter 12

Susan Luparell, PhD, RN, CNE, ANEF
Professor
Mark and Robyn Jones College of Nursing
Montana State University
Bozeman, Montana
Chapter 15

Laurie Peters, PhD, RN
Director of Regulatory Affairs
Synergis Education
Mesa, Arizona
Chapter 27

Monique Ridosh, PhD, RN
Associate Professor
Marcella Niehoff School of Nursing
Family and Community Health Nursing
    Department
Loyola University Chicago
Maywood, Illinois
Chapter 5

Mary E. Riner, PhD, RN, CNE, FAAN
Professor Emeritus
Community and Health Systems
Associate Dean for Global Affairs
Indiana University School of Nursing
Indianapolis, Indiana
Chapter 13

Gayle M. Roux, PhD, RN, NP-C, CNS, FAAN
Nursing Education Consultant
2ED LLC
Flower Mound, Texas
Chapter 5

Martha Scheckel, PhD, RN
Associate Dean for Administration and
    Associate Professor
Conway School of Nursing
The Catholic University of America
Washington, District of Columbia
Chapter 10

Elizabeth Speakman, EdD, RN, FNAP, ANEF, FAAN
Senior Associate Dean/Chief Academic Nursing
    Officer/Professor
School of Nursing
University of Delaware
Newark, Delaware
Chapter 11

Ann M. Stalter, PhD, RN, MEd
Professor
College of Nursing and Health
Wright State University
Dayton, Ohio
Chapter 16

Theresa M. "Terry" Valiga, EdD, RN, ANEF, FAAN
Professor Emerita
Duke University School of Nursing
Durham, North Carolina
Chapter 7

CONTRIBUTORS TO PREVIOUS EDITIONS

Marsha Howell Adams, PhD, RN, ANEF, FAAN
Margaret Applegate, EdD, RN, FAAN
Halina Barber, PhD, MS, RN
Donna Boland, PhD, RN
Mary P. Bourke, PhD, MSN, RN
Carole Brigham, EdD, RN
Nancy Burruss, PhD, RN, CNE
Charlene Clark, MEd, RN, FAAN
John Clochesy, PhD, RN, FCCM, FAAN
Pamela Cole, MA, RN, CS
Judie Csokasy, PhD, RN
Nancy Dillard, DNS, RN
Linda M. Finke, PhD, RN
Mary L. Fisher, PhD, RN
Natasha Flowers, PhD
Joan Frey, EdD, RN, ANEF
Nancy Gillispie, PhD
Dorothy Gomez, PhD, RN
Karen Grigsby, PhD, RN
Susan M. Hendricks, EdD, RN, CNE
Kay Hodson-Carlton, EdD, RN, FAAN
Betty J. Horton, PhD, CRNA, FAAN
Marcella Hovancsek, MSN, RN
Barbara A. Ihrke, PhD, RN
David Johnson, DNS, RN
Elizabeth Johnson, DSN, RN
Amy Knepp, MSN, RN
Gail Kost, MSN, RN
Michael Kremer, PhD, CRNA, CHESE, FNAP, FAAN
Juanita Laidig, EdD, RN

Stacy Lobozinski, MSN, RN
Julie McAfooes, MS, RN-BC, CNE, ANEF, FAAN
Terry Misener, PhD, RN, FAAN
Alexander Muehlenkord, MBA
Carla Mueller, PhD, RN
Barbara Norton, RN, MPH
Janet M. Phillips, PhD, RN, ANEF
Ann Popkess, PhD, RN, CNE
Joanne Rains, DNS, RN
Roy Ramsey, EdD
Lori Rasmussen, MSN, RN
Virginia Richardson, DNS, RN
Barbara Russo, MSN, RN
Connie Rowles, DSN, RN
Marcia Sauter, DNS, RN
Linda Siktberg, PhD, RN
Diana Speck, MSN, RN
Lillian Gatlin Stokes, PhD, RN
Dori Taylor Sullivan, PhD, RN, NE-BC, CPHQ, FAAN
Brent Thompson, PhD, RN
Prudence Twigg, MSN, RN
Melissa Vandeveer, PhD, RN
Linda Veltri, PhD, RN
Debra Wellman, MSN, RN
Pamela Worrell-Carlisle, PhD, CHPN, MA, RN
Cora Hartwell West, MSN, RN
Karen M. Whitney, PhD
Lillian Yeager, EdD, RN
Enid Zwirn, PhD, RN, MPH

REVIEWERS AND REVIEW QUESTION WRITER

REVIEWERS

Rebecca J. Bartlett Ellis, PhD, RN, ACNS-BC, FAAN
Associate Professor
Executive Associate Dean for Academic Affairs
Indiana University School of Nursing –
  Indianapolis, Bloomington, Fort Wayne
Indianapolis, Indiana

Beth L. Rodgers, PhD, RN
Professor Emerita
College of Nursing
University of Wisconsin Milwaukee
Milwaukee, Wisconsin

REVIEW QUESTION WRITER

Deborah A. DeMeester, PhD, RN, CNE
Clinical Associate Professor Emerita
Indiana University School of Nursing
Indianapolis, Indiana

Looking back on the 25 years since *Teaching in Nursing: A Guide for Faculty* was first published, we marvel at the evolution of the science of nursing education and its integration into faculty practice. While many of our teaching practices are still grounded in theories from education and the social and information sciences, we now use theoretical models and frameworks developed by nurse educators to guide the design and use of simulations, understand the stages of development of a nurse from novice to expert, and shape the caring and moral development of nursing students. Further, there is little doubt that nurse educators have embraced the shift from teaching to learning and are creating learning environments that foster civil discourse, emphasize inclusivity, respect the diverse learning needs of all students, and prepare students to provide culturally competent nursing care, assume social responsibility, and provide care based on the social determinants of health. Nurse educators are known as pioneers in distance learning and the use of high-fidelity and virtual learning experiences to prepare students for making effective clinical judgments. Nurse educators are closing the education-practice gap by collaborating with nurses in practice to design clinical electives, capstone experiences, and transition-to-practice residencies that prepare students to be an integral part of interprofessional teams. Nursing education scientists continue to produce a body of evidence for our teaching practices and have moved the results of their research from the classroom to the national stage.

Over the course of these 25 years, nurse educators established a base of practice knowledge that serves as a foundation for defining the evolving roles of the nurse educator and their related core competencies. Nursing education is now considered an advanced practice role that can be recognized in academia by promotion to full rank based on excellence in teaching and by the public through nurse educator certification for various levels of teaching expertise.

Nurse educators continue to demonstrate their resilience and innovation in the face of unexpected adversity. When faced with challenges caused by natural disasters and the COVID-19 pandemic, with the resulting closure of on-campus classrooms and lack of access to clinical learning experiences, nurse educators responded by creatively designing alternative learning experiences that allowed students to continue achieving expected learning outcomes. They drew from their teaching expertise and pivoted to online, virtual, and simulated experiences and the remote delivery of their courses, thus ensuring the safety of their students and patients. Findings from these experiences, now being reported, will add evidence that will forever change how and where we can teach our students.

This 25th Anniversary Edition of *Teaching in Nursing: A Guide for Faculty* continues our mission to prepare nurse educators throughout their career. The book is intended to be a resource for those students whose goals are to become faculty, for nurses who have recently become faculty or professional development educators and need a guide, or for those who are searching for answers to the daily challenges presented in their role as educators. This book is also written for those nurses who are combining clinical practice and teaching as preceptors or part-time or adjunct faculty and for graduate students or teaching assistants who aspire to assume a full-time teaching role. Additionally, this book is a useful resource for those nurse educators who are preparing to take an exam to become certified as a nurse educator.

In this edition, readers will find:
- All chapters updated with relevant evidence for teaching practices
- Practical strategies for teaching a diverse student body

- Information for teaching in new clinical practice environments in the home, via telehealth, and in urban and rural communities
- Redesigned chapters on curriculum development, with attention to defining program outcomes and competencies across all types of academic programs
- Strategies for responding to student diversity and ensuring equity and inclusion in classrooms and clinical settings

To help readers apply the concepts in each chapter to their own teaching practice, this edition also includes:

- Questions to facilitate reflection on the evidence and prompt integration into courses and lesson plans
- Case studies embedded in each chapter to help readers synthesize concepts of the chapter

- Two hundred seventy online practice questions to assess readers' understanding of concepts in each chapter, prepare for course tests, and study for certification exams

Twenty-five years of contributions to the practice of nursing education is a milestone achievement for us as coeditors of *Teaching in Nursing*. It is a privilege and honor for us to have this opportunity to provide a useful resource that continues to influence the preparation of nurse educators. It is our sincere wish that within the pages of this book you will find the inspiration and information you seek to guide you in your continued development as nurse educators.

Diane M. Billings
Judith A. Halstead
May, 2023

ACKNOWLEDGMENTS

We thank the continuing and new contributors to this edition of this book who shared their knowledge and experience with us, the reviewers whose feedback enhanced the development of the chapters, and the readers who continue to inspire us to serve as editors for this book. We also thank the many students and faculty who have used the book over the past 25 years.

Many thanks, as well, to those who assisted with the production process. We acknowledge the editorial support at Elsevier: Lee Henderson, Executive Content Strategist; Laura Fisher, Content Development Specialist; and Thoufiq Mohammed, Project Manager.

As always, we thank our families, colleagues, and students for their continued support and encouragement throughout the many editions of this book.

Diane M. Billings
Judith A. Halstead

CONTENTS

Teaching in Nursing
The Faculty Role[*]

Elizabeth A. Gazza, PhD, RN, LCCE, FACCE, ANEF

Nursing faculty, or academic nurse educators (ANEs), influence health outcomes by designing, implementing, and evaluating nursing education programs that prepare nurses to deliver safe, quality nursing care. ANEs educate entry-level nurses, nurse educators, clinical nurse specialists, nurse practitioners, certified registered nurse anesthetists, and certified nurse midwives in nursing programs at community and technical colleges, colleges, and universities. They use a variety of pedagogical approaches and delivery methods to facilitate learning in clinical settings, simulation laboratories, classrooms, and virtual spaces.

The ANE role has evolved over time, becoming increasingly specialized and complex. Events and trends in society, healthcare, and higher education and the advancement of nursing science influence nursing and therefore nursing education. Faculty must be equipped to use evidence-based teaching practices within the existing environment and be nimble enough to respond to abrupt changes that impact education, nursing, and healthcare such as natural disasters, public health crises, social determinants of health, structural racism, cultural racism, and discrimination (National Academies of Sciences, Engineering, and Medicine, 2021). Advancement of interprofessional collaboration and evidence-based practice; rapid advancements in health care and educational technology; the emphasis on student learning outcomes; and

limitations in financial resources in health care and education impact the ANE role and the dynamic environments in which they work.

This chapter includes an overview of the characteristics of the ANE workforce, the ANE scope of practice, a historical review of the evolution of the faculty role, roles and responsibilities, and the process of faculty appointment, promotion, and tenure (APT) within the current context of higher education. In addition, teaching as a scholarly endeavor, faculty development, and implications for changes in the faculty role needed to meet current and future expectations and demands are addressed.

CHARACTERISTICS OF THE ANE WORKFORCE

The demographic characteristics of the ANE workforce influence nursing education. An adequate supply of ANEs is necessary in order to meet projected demands for registered nurses and nurses with advanced degrees. Unfortunately, the supply of qualified ANEs has not met demand for over a decade. The Tri-Council for Nursing (2017)—made up of the American Association of Colleges of Nursing (AACN), the American Nurses Association (ANA), the American Organization of Nurse Executives (AONE), and the National League for Nursing (NLN)—reported a scarcity of prepared nursing faculty. In fact, 29% of qualified applicants were turned away from baccalaureate, 4% from RN-BSN, 9% from masters, and 15% from doctorate nursing programs because of a lack of available faculty and clinical resources (NLN, 2019).

---

[*]The author acknowledges the work of Mary L. Fisher, PhD, RN in the previous editions of the chapter.

A review of the age of ANEs reflects an aging workforce. In 2019–2020, the age range for ANEs was 23 to 85 years (Mean = 51.9 +/− 11.2; Median = 53.0; Mode = 59) (AACN, 2020a). Across faculty ranks, the average ages of doctorally prepared nurse faculty holding the ranks of professor, associate professor, and assistant professor were 62.6, 56.9, and 50.9 years, respectively. For master's degree–prepared nurse faculty, the average ages for professors, associate professors, and assistant professors were 57.1, 56.0, and 49.6 years, respectively. (*AACN, 2020b*, para. 3)

Based on projections by Fang and Kesten (2017), nearly one-third of all nursing faculty will retire by 2025. Impending retirement of aging nursing faculty will have an impact on teaching, research, mentoring, and academic leadership while providing employment opportunities for the next generation of ANEs.

According to the AACN (2020a), in 2019, nearly 80% of full-time nursing faculty were White and not of Hispanic origin, while 18.5% were underrepresented minorities. These faculty were teaching a student body of which 35.3% undergraduate, 35.4% masters, 33.6% research-focused doctoral, and 36% DNP students were racial and ethnic minorities. In AACN, 2021, the AACN reported that 11% of baccalaureate program graduates were Black/African American individuals. In addition, 12.7% of all baccalaureate graduates and 7.1% (1,455) of full-time nurse faculty were men. These data indicate that presently, the ANE workforce is predominately female (92.5%; 19,060) and limited in diversity. *The Future of Nursing: 2020 2030* report called on nursing education programs to recruit more individuals from diverse backgrounds into nursing and ANE positions (National Academies of Sciences, Engineering, and Medicine, 2021).

Career Pathway

Nurses enter faculty positions through a variety of pathways (Halstead & Frank, 2018). Having the desire to teach and experiencing the "aha moment" of making a difference in a learner through teaching motivate nurses to pursue faculty positions (Evans, 2018). Nurses often discover their interest in teaching while serving as preceptors and clinical and/or patient educators (Bond et al., 2020).

Earning a terminal degree, such as a research-focused Doctor of Philosophy (PhD) or a clinically focused Doctor of Nursing Practice (DNP), often meets the eligibility requirement to teach nursing courses at the collegiate level. In 2019, 57.6% (PhD, 27.6%; DNP, 22.7%; Nonnursing doctoral, 7.3%; and Nondoctoral, 42.4%) of the ANEs employed in baccalaureate and higher degree nursing programs had earned a terminal degree (AACN, 2020a).

Unfortunately, most PhD and DNP programs do not prepare nurses to teach. It behooves nurses with an interest in faculty work to pursue teaching-related coursework (McNelis et al., 2019). Completing graduate-level coursework in curriculum development; instructional strategies and design and assessment and evaluation; and engaging in opportunities to apply newly learned knowledge and skills during a practicum fosters the development of nurse educator competencies (Garner & Bedford, 2021). The ability to demonstrate these competencies is essential to the delivery of quality nursing education (Halstead, 2019) and improvement in nursing and health outcomes (World Health Organization, 2016).

NATIONAL LEAGUE FOR NURSING COMPETENCIES FOR NURSE EDUCATORS

Teaching in nursing is a complex activity that integrates the art and science of nursing and clinical practice into the teaching–learning process. Specifically, teaching involves a set of skills or competencies that are essential to facilitating student-learning outcomes. In 2005, the National League for Nursing (NLN) published eight core competencies of ANEs, which were reviewed and revalidated in 2012 (Halstead, 2019; NLN, 2005, 2012, 2018), that comprise the scope of practice for the ANE (Christensen & Simmons, 2020). See Box 1.1 for the Core Competencies for Academic Nurse Educators©.

In 2020, the NLN, using the ANE competencies, identified task statements for ANEs with less than 2 years of experience (NLN, 2021). The Competencies of Novice Academic Nurse Educators include "leveled down" task statements

BOX 1.1   National League for Nursing Core Competencies of Academic Nurse Educators©

Competency 1: Facilitate learning

Nurse educators are responsible for creating an environment in classroom, laboratory, and clinical settings that facilitates student learning and the achievement of desired cognitive, affective, and psychomotor outcomes. To facilitate learning effectively, the nurse educator:

- Implements a variety of teaching strategies appropriate to learner needs, desired learner outcomes, content, and context
- Grounds teaching strategies in educational theory and evidence-based teaching practices
- Recognizes multicultural, gender, and experiential influences on teaching and learning
- Engages in self-reflection and continued learning to improve teaching practices that facilitate learning
- Uses information technologies skillfully to support the teaching–learning process
- Practices skilled oral, written, and electronic communication that reflects an awareness of self and others, along with an ability to convey ideas in a variety of contexts
- Models critical and reflective thinking
- Creates opportunities for learners to develop their critical thinking and critical reasoning skills
- Shows enthusiasm for teaching, learning, and nursing that inspires and motivates students
- Demonstrates interest in and respect for learners
- Uses personal attributes (e.g., caring, confidence, patience, integrity, and flexibility) that facilitate learning
- Develops collegial working relationships with students, faculty colleagues, and clinical agency personnel to promote positive learning environments
- Maintains the professional practice knowledge base needed to help prepare learners for contemporary nursing practice
- Serves as a role model in professional nursing

Competency 2: Facilitate Learner Development and Socialization

Nurse educators recognize the responsibility for helping students develop as nurses and integrate the values and behaviors expected of those who fulfill that role. To facilitate learner development and socialization effectively, the nurse educator:

- Identifies individual learning styles and unique learning needs of international, adult, multicultural, educationally disadvantaged, physically challenged, at-risk, and second-degree learners

- Provides resources to diverse learners that help meet their individual learning needs
- Engages in effective advisement and counseling strategies that help learners meet their professional goals
- Creates learning environments that are focused on socialization to the role of the nurse and facilitate learners' self-reflection and personal goal setting
- Fosters the cognitive, psychomotor, and affective development of learners
- Recognizes the influence of teaching styles and interpersonal interactions on learner outcomes
- Assists learners to develop the ability to engage in thoughtful and constructive self and peer evaluation
- Models professional behaviors for learners, including, but not limited to, involvement in professional organizations, engagement in lifelong learning activities, dissemination of information through publications and presentations, and advocacy

Competency 3: Use Assessment and Evaluation Strategies

Nurse educators use a variety of strategies to assess and evaluate student learning in classroom, laboratory, and clinical settings, as well as in all domains of learning. To use assessment and evaluation strategies effectively, the nurse educator:

- Uses extant literature to develop evidence-based assessment and evaluation practices
- Uses a variety of strategies to assess and evaluate learning in the cognitive, psychomotor, and affective domains
- Implements evidence-based assessment and evaluation strategies that are appropriate to the learner and to learning goals
- Uses assessment and evaluation data to enhance the teaching–learning process
- Provides timely, constructive, and thoughtful feedback to learners
- Demonstrates skill in the design and use of tools for assessing clinical practice

Competency 4: Participate in Curriculum Design and Evaluation of Program Outcomes

Nurse educators are responsible for formulating program outcomes and designing curricula that reflect contemporary health care trends and prepare graduates to function effectively in the health care environment. To participate effectively in curriculum design and evaluation of program outcomes, the nurse educator:

Continued

BOX 1.1   National League for Nursing Core Competencies of Academic Nurse Educators©—cont'd

- Ensures the curriculum reflects the institutional philosophy and mission, current nursing and health care trends, and community and societal needs, so as to prepare graduates for practice in a complex, dynamic, multicultural health care environment
- Demonstrates knowledge of curriculum development, including identifying program outcomes, developing competency statements, writing learning objectives, and selecting appropriate learning activities and evaluation strategies
- Bases curriculum design and implementation decisions on sound educational principles, theory, and research
- Revises the curriculum based on assessment of program outcomes, learner needs, and societal and health care trends
- Implements curricular revisions using appropriate change theories and strategies
- Creates and maintains community and clinical partnerships that support educational goals
- Collaborates with external constituencies throughout the process of curriculum revision
- Designs and implements program assessment models that promote continuous quality improvement of all aspects of the program

Competency 5: Function as a Change Agent and Leader

Nurse educators function as change agents and leaders to create a preferred future for nursing education and nursing practice. To function effectively as a change agent and leader, the nurse educator:

- Models cultural sensitivity when advocating for change
- Integrates a long-term, innovative, and creative perspective into the nurse educator role
- Participates in interdisciplinary efforts to address health care and educational needs regionally, nationally, or internationally
- Evaluates organizational effectiveness in nursing education
- Implements strategies for organizational change
- Provides leadership in the parent institution and in the nursing program to enhance the visibility of nursing and its contributions to the academic community
- Promotes innovative practices in educational environments
- Develops leadership skills to shape and implement change

Competency 6: Pursue Continuous Quality Improvement in the Nurse Educator Role

Nurse educators recognize that their role is multidimensional and that an ongoing commitment to develop and maintain competence in the role is essential. To develop the educator role effectively, the nurse educator:

- Demonstrates commitment to lifelong learning
- Recognizes that career enhancement needs and activities change as experience is gained in the role
- Participates in professional development opportunities that increase one's effectiveness in the role
- Balances the teaching, scholarship, and service demands inherent in the role of educator and member of an academic institution
- Uses feedback gained from self, peer, student, and administrative evaluation to improve role effectiveness
- Engages in activities that promote one's socialization to the role
- Uses knowledge of the legal and ethical issues relevant to higher education and nursing education as a basis for influencing, designing, and implementing policies and procedures related to students, faculty, and the educational environment
- Mentors and supports faculty colleagues

Competency 7: Engage in Scholarship

Nurse educators acknowledge that scholarship is an integral component of the faculty role, and that teaching itself is a scholarly activity. To engage effectively in scholarship, the nurse educator:

- Draws on extant literature to design evidence-based teaching and evaluation practices
- Exhibits a spirit of inquiry about teaching and learning, student development, evaluation methods, and other aspects of the role
- Designs and implements scholarly activities in an established area of expertise
- Disseminates nursing and teaching knowledge to a variety of audiences through various means
- Demonstrates skill in proposal writing for initiatives that include, but are not limited to, research, resource acquisition, program development, and policy development
- Demonstrates the qualities of a scholar: integrity, courage, perseverance, vitality, and creativity

Competency 8: Function Within the Educational Environment

Nurse educators are knowledgeable about the educational environment within which they practice and

---

BOX 1.1 National League for Nursing Core Competencies of Academic Nurse Educators©—cont'd

recognize how political, institutional, social, and economic forces impact their role. To function as a good "citizen of the academy," the nurse educator:

- Uses knowledge of history and current trends and issues in higher education as a basis for making recommendations and decisions on educational issues
- Identifies how social, economic, political, and institutional forces influence higher education in general and nursing education in particular
- Develops networks, collaborations, and partnerships to enhance nursing's influence within the academic community
- Determines one's own professional goals within the

context of academic nursing and the mission of the parent institution and nursing program

- Integrates the values of respect, collegiality, professionalism, and caring to build an organizational climate that fosters the development of students and teachers
- Incorporates the goals of the nursing program and the mission of the parent institution when proposing a change or managing issues
- Assumes a leadership role in various levels of institutional governance
- Advocates for nursing and nursing education in the political arena

From Christensen, L. S., & Simmons, L. E. (2020). *The scope of practice for academic nurse educators and academic clinical nurse educators* (3rd ed.). National League for Nursing. Included with the permission of the National League for Nursing, Washington, DC.

---

appropriate for the novice educator. Additionally, upon recognizing the specialty practice of clinical nurse educators who facilitate learning in clinical settings, the NLN identified evidence-based clinical nurse educator competencies (Shellenbarger, 2019). See Box 1.2 for the Core Competencies of Academic Clinical Nurse Educators©. ANEs and academic clinical nurse educators develop core competencies through educational preparation, faculty orientation programs, practice, and faculty development opportunities.

CERTIFICATION FOR NURSE EDUCATORS

Engaging in continuous quality improvement fosters ongoing development in the nurse faculty role (Garner & Bedford, 2021; Halstead, 2019). Nursing faculty maintain strong clinical skills and often earn certification credentials in clinical specialties. In addition, ANEs can earn credentials as a certified academic nurse educator (CNE®), certified academic clinical nurse educator (CNE®cl), or certified academic nurse educator novice (CNE®n) through the NLN's (n.d.) Academic Nurse Educator Certification Program. As of October 2021, there were 8,448 nurse educators with CNE® certification and 402 with CNE®cl certification from these international certification programs (S. Pyle, personal communication, October 18, 2021). These certifications validate the specialized knowledge needed to teach, affirm the ANE as an advanced

practice role, and can be used to establish a formal pathway to the ANE role (Daw et al., 2021; Gazza, 2019).

HISTORICAL PERSPECTIVE OF THE FACULTY ROLE IN HIGHER EDUCATION

The role of the faculty member in academia has developed over time as the role of higher education in America has evolved. Three phases of overlapping development can be identified in the history of American higher education (Boyer, 1990).

The first phase of development occurred during colonial times. Heavily influenced by British tradition, the role of faculty in the colonial college was a singular one: that of teaching. The educational system "was expected to educate and morally uplift the coming generation" (Boyer, 1990, p. 4). Teaching was considered an honored vocation with the intended purpose of developing student character and preparing students for leadership in civic and religious roles. This focus on teaching as the central mission of the university continued well into the 19th century.

Gradually, the focus of education began to shift from development of the individual to development of a nation, signaling the beginning of the second phase of development within higher education. Legislation such as the Morrill Act

BOX 1.2   Core Competencies of Academic Clinical Nurse Educators with Task Statements

Competency I: Function Within the Education and Health Care Environments

A. Function in the Clinical Educator Role
- Bridge the gap between theory and practice by helping learners apply classroom learning to the clinical setting.
- Foster professional growth of learners.
- Use technologies to enhance clinical teaching and learning.
- Value the contributions of others in the achievement of learner outcomes.
- Act as a role model of professional nursing within the clinical learning environment.
- Demonstrate inclusive excellence.

B. Operationalize the Curriculum
- Assess congruence of the clinical agency to the curriculum, core goals, and learner needs.
- Plan meaningful and relevant clinical learning assignments and activities.
- Identify learners' goals and outcomes.
- Prepare learners for clinical experiences.
- Structure learner experiences within the learning environments to promote optimal learning.
- Implement clinical learning activities to help learner develop interprofessional collaboration and teamwork skills.
- Provide opportunities for learners to develop problem-solving and clinical reasoning skills related to learning outcomes.
- Implement assigned models for clinical learning.
- Engage in theory-based instruction.
- Provide input to the nursing program for course development and review.

C. Abide by Legal Requirements, Ethical Guidelines, Agency Policies, and Guiding Framework
- Apply the ethical and legal principles to create a safe clinical learning environment.
- Assess learner abilities and needs prior to clinical learning experiences.
- Facilitate learning activities that support the mission, goals, and values of the academic institution and the clinical agency.
- Inform others of program and clinical agency policies, procedures, and practices.
- Adhere to program and clinical agency policies, procedures, and practices when implementing clinical experiences.
- Promote learner compliance with regulations and standards of practice.
- Demonstrate ethical behaviors.

Competency II: Facilitate Learning in the Health Care Environment
- Implement a variety of clinical teaching strategies congruent with learner needs, desired learner outcomes, content, and context.
- Ground teaching strategies in educational theory and evidence-based teaching practices.
- Use technology skillfully to support the teaching-learning process.
- Create opportunities for learners to develop critical thinking and clinical reasoning skills.
- Promote a culture of safety and quality in the healthcare environment.
- Create a positive and caring learning environment.
- Develop collegial working relationships with learners, faculty colleagues, and clinical agency personnel.
- Demonstrate enthusiasm for teaching, learning, and nursing to help inspire and motivate learners.

Competency III: Demonstrate Effective Interpersonal Communication and Collaborative Interprofessional Relationships
- Value collaboration and coordination of care.
- Foster a share learning community and cooperate with other members of the health care team.
- Support and environment of frequent, respectful, civil, and open communication with all members of the healthcare team.
- Act as a role model, showing respect for all members of the health care team, professional colleagues, clients, family members, and learners.
- Use clear and effective communication in all interactions.
- Listen to learner concerns, needs, or questions in a nonthreatening way.
- Display a calm, empathetic, and supportive demeanor in all communications.
- Manage emotions effectively when communicating in challenging situations.
- Effective manage conflict.
- Maintain an approachable, nonjudgmental, and readily accessible demeanor.
- Recognize limitations in self and learners to provide opportunities for development.
- Demonstrate effective communication in clinical learning environments with diverse colleagues, clients, cultures, health care professionals, and learners.
- Communicate performance expectations to learners and agency staff.

BOX 1.2 **Core Competencies of Academic Clinical Nurse Educators with Task Statements—cont'd**

Competency IV: Applies Clinical Expertise in the Health Care Environment
- Maintain current professional competence relevant to the specialty area, practice setting, and clinical learning environment.
- Translate theory into clinical practice by applying experiential knowledge and clinical reasoning and using a client-centered approach to clinical instruction.
- Use best evidence to address client-related problems.
- Demonstrate effective leadership within the clinical learning environment.
- Demonstrate sound clinical reasoning.
- Expand knowledge and skills by integrating best practices.
- Balance client care needs and student learning needs within a culture of safety.
- Demonstrate competence with a range of technologies available in the clinical learning environment.

Competency V: Facilitate Learner Development and Socialization
- Mentor learners in the development of professional nursing behaviors, standards, and codes of ethics.
- Promote a learning climate of respect for all.
- Promote professional integrity and accountability.
- Maintain professional boundaries.
- Encourage ongoing learner professional development via format and informal venues.
- Assist learners in effective use of self-assessment and professional goals setting for ongoing self-improvement.
- Create learning environments that are focused on socialization to the role of the nurse.
- Assist learners to develop the ability to engage in constructive peer feedback.
- Inspire creativity and confidence.
- Encourage various techniques for learners to develop the ability to engage in constructive peer feedback.
- Encourage various techniques for learners to manage stress.
- Act as a role model for self-reflection, self-care, and coping skills.
- Empower learners to be successful in meeting professional and educational goals.
- Engage learners in applying best practices and quality improvement processes.

Competency VI: Implement Effective Clinical Assessment Evaluation Strategies
- Use a variety of strategies to determine achievement of learning outcomes.
- Implement both formative and summative evaluation that is appropriate to the learner and the learner outcomes.
- Engage in timely communication with course faculty regarding learner clinical performance.
- Maintain integrity in the assessment and evaluation of learners.
- Provide timely, objective, constructive, and fair feedback to learners.
- Use learner data to enhance the teaching–learning process in the clinical learning environment.
- Demonstrate skill in the use of the best practices in the assessment and evaluation of clinical performance.
- Assess and evaluate learner achievement of clinical performance expectations.
- Use performance standards to determine learner strengths and weaknesses in the clinical learning environment.
- Document learner clinical performance, feedback, and progression.
- Evaluate the quality of the clinical learning experiences and environment.

From Christensen, L. S., & Simmons, L. E. (2020). *The scope of practice for academic nurse educators and academic clinical nurse educators* (3rd ed.). National League for Nursing. Included with the permission of the National League for Nursing, Washington, DC.

of 1862 and the Hatch Act of 1887 helped create public expectations that added the responsibility of service to the traditional faculty role of teaching. This legislation provided each state with land and funding to support the education of leaders in agriculture and industry. Universities and colleges accepted the mission to educate for the common good (Boyer, 1990) and were expected to provide service to the states, businesses, and industries.

The first formal schools of nursing began to appear in the United States in the 1870s. Diploma nursing programs were established in hospitals to help meet the service needs of the hospitals. Nursing faculty were expected to provide service to the institution and to teach new nurses along the way. Nursing students were expected to learn while they helped staff the hospitals.

In the mid-19th century, a commitment to the development of science began in many universities on the East Coast (Boyer, 1990), thus beginning the third phase of development in higher education. Scholarship through research was added as an expectation to the role of faculty. This emphasis on research was greatly enhanced in later years by federal support for academic research that began during and continued after World War II.

Gradually, as expectations for faculty to seek funding for and to conduct research to advance the discipline spread throughout institutions across the nation, teaching and service began to be viewed with less importance as a measurement tool for academic prestige and productivity within institutions. Faculty found it increasingly difficult to achieve tenure without a record of funded research and publication, despite accomplishments in teaching and service. As nursing education entered the university setting, nursing faculty began to be held to the same standards of research productivity as faculty in other, more traditionally academia-based disciplines. It is important to understand that while the emphasis on research continues, institutions vary greatly in this regard based on their missions and strategic plans. Potential faculty should seek opportunities in nursing education in institutions whose missions fit their interests and credentials.

FUTURE OF THE ANE ROLE IN HIGHER EDUCATION

A rapidly changing political environment and health care reform have a dramatic effect on the role of nursing faculty. Changes in health care brought on by the Patient Protection and Affordable Care Act and subsequent ongoing political changes to how health care is organized and financed require that nursing curricula be updated to ensure that nursing graduates achieve competencies needed for the future. There is increasing emphasis on the teaching role of faculty and assessing the

outcomes of the educational process. The balance among teaching, research/scholarship, and service is being reexamined in many institutions for its congruence with the institution's mission.

A revolution in teaching strategies continues to occur as universities and colleges change the focus from teaching to learning. Sole reliance on the use of lecture is no longer an accepted teaching method. Faculty are designing and implementing innovative instructional approaches to effectively foster learning using competency-based curricula. They integrate the use of technology into their teaching and promote the active involvement of students in the learning process using a pedagogy-first approach known as "flipping the classroom" (Özbay & Çınar, 2020). Distance learning and the use of simulation technology, which accelerated rapidly in response to the COVID-19 pandemic beginning in March 2020, are commonplace in nursing and higher education as teaching and learning continues to move away from the structured classroom to the much larger learning environments of the home, community, clinical setting, and virtual space. Learning analytics, artificial intelligence and specifically, machine learning, provide new opportunities for faculty to personalize and adapt learning based on students' learning needs. Furthermore, nursing care delivery continues to shift to a community-based, consumer-driven system. The shift in emphasis from acute care to an enhanced role for primary care has an effect on the undergraduate and graduate nursing curricula, and faculty must continue to respond to this transition as well.

There also is a continuing gap in the representation of underrepresented populations in nursing education programs. There is a need to expand the number of nursing graduates from underrepresented populations and ANEs who can prepare a diverse workforce qualified to provide quality care to all individuals. Educating a diverse student body, representative of all groups and genders, results in a nursing workforce better equipped to care for a diverse population. A diverse ANE workforce helps provide perspectives that add understanding of underserved populations and assist institutions to better support and recruit a diverse student population. All nurses must increase their cultural competence skills to meet the needs of growing underserved populations in the United States. Additionally, the National Academies of Sciences, Engineering, and Medicine (2021) recommended an increase in the number of PhD-prepared nurses and to better prepare nurses to ensure health equity. The clinical movement toward advanced practice nurses holding a DNP degree creates an overwhelming need for nurses prepared with a doctorate.

FACULTY RIGHTS AND RESPONSIBILITIES IN ACADEMIA

The rights and responsibilities of academic faculty align with the "traditional triad" of the faculty role, which consists of teaching, conducting research and/or scholarship activities, and sharing their expertise through service. Faculty also have responsibilities associated with continuous improvement aimed at ongoing role development of self, colleagues, and students. Case Study 1.1 addresses faculty role responsibilities.

The professoriate in the United States has traditionally enjoyed several rights, including the right to self-governance within the university setting. In addition, the American Association of University Professors (AAUP), American Council on Education (ACE), and the Association of Governing Boards of Universities and Colleges (1966) *Statement on Government of Colleges and Universities* addresses the shared responsibility and cooperative action among governing board members, administrators, faculty, and students as a form of shared governance. Faculty participate in governance by serving on department and university committees focusing on academic and workplace issues of concern to faculty, such as faculty affairs, student affairs, curriculum and program evaluation, and providing consultation to administrators. Faculty and administrators share the responsibility for addressing issues that face the university and the community it serves. Nursing faculty also have the responsibility to expand their service beyond the university and local community to include active leadership in professional nursing organizations at local, regional, and national levels, where they often influence national public policy agendas. As a faculty member climbs the promotion and tenure ladder, service responsibilities increase and leadership at the national and international levels is expected.

The core responsibility of faculty is the teaching and learning that takes place in the institution.

CASE STUDY 1.1 Faculty Role Responsibilities

A particular faculty member began their nursing career as a full-time staff nurse and was the preceptor for numerous associate degree in nursing (ADN) students from the community college. The faculty member felt it was rewarding to prepare the next generation of nurses, so they enrolled in a Doctor of Nursing Practice (DNP) program and accepted a full-time faculty position as a clinical assistant professor at a university. The faculty member has taught classroom and clinically based courses for the last 2 years in the Bachelor of Science in Nursing (BSN) program and spent much of their time serving on various committees.

Early one semester, a natural disaster devastated the university campus. Faculty, staff, and students were not permitted on campus or at any of the clinical agencies utilized by the nursing program. In 3 days, all faculty had to teach remotely using the university's approved learning management system (LMS). This particular faculty member panicked because they never had taught online or completed an online course. The DNP program the faculty member completed did not include any courses about teaching and they never attended any professional development sessions about online teaching. The faculty member said, "I don't ever again want to feel unprepared to teach nursing."

1. In what ways was this faculty member prepared to manage this situation and how could they have been better prepared to teach nursing in the dynamic environment that exists in higher education and the world?
2. The faculty member teaches BSN courses and serves on various committees. What other role responsibilities might they have as a clinical assistant professor?
3. When the faculty member applies for promotion to clinical associate professor, how can they demonstrate continuous improvement in the teaching role?

Boards and administrators delegate decisions about most aspects of the teaching–learning process to faculty. For example, this responsibility includes not only the delivery of content but also curriculum development and evaluation, development of student evaluation methods, and graduation requirements. While engaging in these responsibilities, faculty often create new resources and use works developed by faculty, students, and others. Intellectual property, copyright, and fair-use laws govern usage and most academic settings have policies that guide the development of "works for hire," which may include course content, written works, and products. Many universities now enter into ownership agreements, with some financial split of any profits related to works developed by faculty. A wise faculty member is well informed about these institutional policies so that there is no misunderstanding about ownership of course materials and other works developed by the faculty member. Librarians and library resources can help faculty to become well informed.

TEACHING AS A SCHOLARLY ENDEAVOR

Boyer (1990) first proposed a new paradigm for scholarship that encompassed all aspects of the faculty role but placed a renewed emphasis on teaching as a scholarly endeavor. In *Scholarship Reconsidered: Priorities of the Professoriate*, Boyer called for the development of a balance between research and teaching when measuring the faculty member's success in academia. He described four types of scholarship in which faculty engage: the scholarship of discovery, the scholarship of integration, the scholarship of application, and the scholarship of teaching. In these four types of scholarship, the previously narrow view of scholarly productivity that rested only on the careful discovery of new knowledge through research has been greatly expanded. Boyer's model supports the practice model of nursing, which calls for more than the discovery of knowledge; it also calls for the application and integration of knowledge into professional practice. As Boyer stated:

We believe the time has come to move beyond the tired old "teaching versus research" debate and give the familiar and honorable term "scholarship" a broader, more capacious meaning, one that brings legitimacy to the full scope of academic work. Surely, scholarship means engaging in original research. But the work of the scholar also means stepping back from one's investigation, looking for connections, building bridges between theory and practice, and communicating one's knowledge effectively to students. Specifically, we conclude that the work of the professoriate might be thought of as having four separate, yet overlapping, functions. These are: the scholarship of discovery; the scholarship of integration; the scholarship of application; and the scholarship of teaching. (p. 16)

The Scholarship of Discovery

The scholarship of discovery is the traditional definition of original research or discovery of new knowledge (Boyer, 1990). The scholarship of discovery may be considered the foundation of the other three aspects of scholarship because new knowledge is generated for application and integration into the discipline, as well as for teaching.

It is through the scholarship of discovery that scientific methods are used to develop a strong knowledge base for the discipline and nursing education. Evidence-based practice in nursing and teaching, building on the knowledge generated by the scholarship of discovery. Most federal funding traditionally has been appropriated for the scholarship of discovery, and until recently, tenure decisions in many universities have been based primarily on the faculty member's engagement in the generation of new knowledge. The scholarship of discovery remains an important aspect of the role of many faculties, including nursing faculties. At the federal level, research efforts in nursing are supported by the National Institute of Nursing Research and content-specific institutes, such as the National Institutes of Health and the National Institute of Mental Health, and by private philanthropic foundations.

The Scholarship of Integration

The scholarship of integration involves the interpretation and synthesis of knowledge within and across discipline boundaries in a manner that provides a larger context for knowledge and the development of new insights (Boyer, 1990). The scholarship of integration requires communication among colleagues from various disciplines who work together to develop a more holistic view of a common concern in nursing practice and/or nursing education. The combined expertise of all who are involved leads to a more comprehensive understanding of the issue and results in more thorough recommendations for solutions to the phenomena of concern.

Nursing faculty have long integrated knowledge from various disciplines into their practice and have many competencies that enable them to be productive members of interdisciplinary teams that study a variety of health problems and issues. With the emphasis in today's world on the development of collaborative team-building and knowledge-sharing efforts across disciplines, the scholarship of integration assumes an ever-increasing importance for faculty who must remain at the forefront of the information age. Nursing content often builds on the knowledge students have learned from other disciplines, such as the biological and social sciences. The scholarship of integration involves designing learning models that guide students to apply their previously learned knowledge to clinical situations, such as with the use of high-amplitude patient simulation and virtual simulation. Much scholarship of integration is being published in the areas of simulation and online education at this time.

The Scholarship of Application

The scholarship of application, which connects theory and nursing practice, or nursing education, is an area of scholarship in which nursing faculty should also excel. In the scholarship of application, faculty must ask themselves, "How can knowledge be responsibly applied to consequential problems?" (Boyer, 1990, p. 21). Service activities that are directly connected to a faculty member's areas of expertise warrant consideration as application scholarship. It is in the performance of service activities that practice and theory interact, thus leading to the potential development of new knowledge.

For example, in nursing, clinical practice and expertise that result in the development of innovative instructional approaches, nursing interventions,

and positive patient care outcomes meet the definition of scholarship of application. Activities that encourage students to use critical decision making, self-reflection, and self-evaluation are examples of the scholarship of application in teaching. Faculty practice in nursing centers is another example. Faculty should disseminate the knowledge gathered through practice and service activities by publishing in professional journals.

The scholarship of application, which includes service to the profession of nursing at the local, regional, national, and international levels, also involves developing policies and practices for nursing and health care. Nursing faculty often provide leadership in professional organizations and on community or national panels and boards.

The Scholarship of Teaching

The heart of the faculty role can be found in the scholarship of teaching. An important attribute of any scholar is discovering new knowledge, disseminating and integrating evidence, and applying the best available scientific evidence to practice. "Practice," for the ANE, encompasses the scholarship of teaching, and the scholarship of teaching and learning (SoTL).

Boyer's (1990) definition of scholarship provides a model through which the special competencies and skills that are an integral part of the scholarly endeavor of teaching are acknowledged. Developing pedagogical approaches and innovative curricula, using a variety of teaching methods that actively involve students in the learning process, collaborating with students on learning projects, and exploring the most effective means of meeting the learning needs of diverse populations of students are all examples of the scholarly work of the scholarship of teaching. Systematically studying the learning outcomes associated with the implementation of evidence-based pedagogical approaches aligns with the SoTL. To produce this scholarly work, ANEs adhere to six standards: clear goals, adequate preparation, appropriate methods, significant results, effective presentation, and reflective critique (Glassick et al., 1997). Faculty have a responsibility to advance the science of nursing and nursing education through the scholarship of teaching and share their teaching expertise with their colleagues through publication and presentation of their innovative teaching methods and the outcomes of their work with students.

The scholarship of teaching brings many exciting opportunities for nursing faculty in classroom and clinical settings. It is also based on the scholarship of discovery, integration, and practice. At a time when health care practice arenas are rapidly changing, curriculum models are being designed to meet the needs of a global society. The use of technology in education is increasing, and perspectives on teaching and learning are changing. The scholarship of teaching provides nursing faculty with the opportunity to demonstrate their innovation and creativity. It also provides a means for recognizing the effort spent preparing students to be competent health care providers for the future.

Although the role of the faculty member remains complex, Boyer's (1990) broad description of scholarship continues to provide the model that legitimizes all aspects of the faculty role. Boyer has given credibility to aspects of the faculty role that extend beyond the creation of new knowledge through research to include teaching and service to the university, community, and profession. As a scholarly endeavor, teaching is the synthesis of all types of scholarship described by Boyer. Faculty can combine the role of researcher with the integration, application, and dissemination of knowledge. Boyer has provided a model for nursing faculty to use to develop their expertise in teaching as a scholarly endeavor. Nursing education has moved from the notion that there is only one way to do something to a broader perspective that recognizes the creativity and uniqueness of each student. The teacher is no longer the only expert but instead is someone who joins the student in the learning process and evaluates the results of the teaching–learning process in a scholarly manner.

APPOINTMENT, PROMOTION, AND TENURE

Faculty are appointed by the governing body of the college or university and are responsible, in cooperation with the administration of the institution, for teaching, scholarship, and service.

Faculty are appointed to fulfill various responsibilities to meet the mission and goals of the college or university and the school of nursing and are promoted and tenured or reappointed based on achievement of specified criteria and according to their degrees and experience. Criteria for promotion and tenure are based on the institution's overall mission and thus vary among institutions. In addition to considering teaching, scholarship, and service achievements for promotion and/or tenure, collegiality or civility in the workplace is considered in a growing number of institutions. This trend is in line with the Tri-Council for Nursing's proclamation outlining the critical need for civility in the workplace as essential to quality and safety (Tri-Council for Nursing, 2017).

Most institutions require full-time faculty to declare one area of excellence on which their tenure and promotion will focus. It is important that faculty choose this area carefully and early in their appointment. With careful planning and selection of activities, nursing faculty can integrate their clinical interests into teaching, scholarship, and service, thus meeting the expectations of the role in the most efficient manner. On initial appointment to a faculty position, the faculty member will be well served by the development of a 5- to 6-year career plan designed to ensure that the candidate will meet the criteria for all aspects of the role.

Some faculty work in an environment where they are represented by a union. The AAUP is probably the best-known faculty union. Faculty can also be members of AAUP as a professional organization without belonging to a union. In a setting that has a union, faculty rights and responsibilities are affected by the negotiated contract.

Appointment Tracks

Faculty may be appointed to a variety of full-time or part-time positions in higher education. At the time of hire, a full-time faculty member is appointed to a track and assigned an academic rank based on their education and experience. Each school of nursing defines the criteria for appointment. These criteria specify the responsibilities associated with teaching, scholarship, and service. The two main tracks are tenure and nontenure. Rank options, listed in ascending order, include lecturer/instructor, visiting professor, and research associate; assistant professor; associate professor; professor; and distinguished, endowed, or university professor. The criteria for appointments to tracks and ranks align with the institution's Carnegie Classification®. This classification system reflects institutional differences based on research activity, program offerings, and types of degrees awarded.

The *tenure track* was established for faculty whose primary responsibilities are teaching (60% of work effort), research (20%–30%), and service (10%–20%). A doctoral degree or near completion of the degree is required for appointment to the tenure track at most schools of nursing. Faculty appointment to this track is considered *tenure probationary* until tenure is obtained after an extensive review process, generally concluding in the 5th to 7th year of appointment. A promise of excellence and the ability to be promoted to senior ranks (associate professor and professor) is required for a tenure track appointment. Workload efforts vary by institution and if probationary or tenured. Refer to Table 1.1 for general qualifications and descriptions of each tenure track rank. Case Study 1.2 addresses tenure application.

The *nontenure track* does not offer the protection of tenure and includes the *clinical or practice* and *research scientist* tracks. The *clinical/practice track* was developed at many institutions as an educator track, clinical educator track, or educator–practitioner track, depending on the primary focus of assigned responsibilities. Workload effort in this track is primarily based on teaching (80% of workload effort), scholarship (10%), and service (10%) through clinical practice or clinical joint appointments. Joint appointments are shared between multiple departments such as a university and medical center. Workload allocations vary based on position responsibilities. Because this track allows for possible promotion through the ranks of instructor, clinical assistant, clinical associate, and clinical full professor, a doctoral degree often is required for appointment to a clinical track. Although research is not the focus of the clinical track, scholarly dissemination of clinical or educational contributions or outcomes is required for promotions within this track. The increased use of clinical track faculty is a growing trend as universities and colleges reduce their reliance on tenure. Refer to Table 1.2 for general qualifications and descriptions of each clinical track rank.

The *research scientist* track is for faculty whose primary responsibility is funded research and research dissemination through publications and presentations. Although research scientists may

TABLE 1.1	Tenure Track Qualifications and Description by Rank	
Academic Rank	**Degree Qualifications**	**Description**
Instructor/Lecturer	Minimum of Master's degree	Demonstrates effectiveness primarily as a teacher
Assistant Professor	Completed or nearing completion of doctoral degree	Demonstrates a commitment to teaching, research, and department service
Associate Professor	Doctoral Degree	Demonstrates teaching proficiency, a national reputation as a scholar, and a commitment to service beyond the department (institutional, public, professional)
Professor	Doctoral Degree	Demonstrates distinguished record of teaching, an international reputation as a scholar, and service beyond the department (institutional, public, professional)
Distinguished, Endowed, or University Professor	Doctoral Degree	Demonstrates extraordinary reputation as a scholar over the course of their careers

CASE STUDY 1.2   Applying for Tenure

A faculty member was hired 4 years ago as an assistant professor in a tenure track position at a medium-sized university. The faculty member learned about the tenure review process during new faculty orientation and often referred to the criteria as they established annual performance goals. The faculty member's mentor, a tenured professor, helped them to refine their scholarship agenda, which focused on nursing education. The faculty member secured multiple small internal grants to fund a variety of scholarship of teaching and learning (SoTL) initiatives and was very interested in designing applied learning activities and assessing their impact on student learning.

When it was time for the faculty member to prepare their tenure application, they struggled to describe their scholarship agenda and how scholarly work

influenced nursing education, and how to demonstrate teaching effectiveness. The faculty member's mentor suggested a review of Boyer's (1990) *Scholarship reconsidered: Priorities of the professoriate* and to use data where possible.

1. How could the mentor's suggestion help the faculty member to write the narrative about their scholarship agenda for the tenure application?
2. What data could the faculty member use in the tenure application to demonstrate teaching effectiveness and engagement in the scholarship of teaching?
3. How can the annual performance evaluation help to prepare an academic nurse educator for a personnel action such as promotion or tenure review?

TABLE 1.2   Clinical Track Qualifications and Description by Rank

Academic Rank	Degree Qualifications	Description
Clinical Instructor/Lecturer	Minimum of Master's degree and expertise in clinical practice	Demonstrates expertise in clinical practice, effectiveness as a teacher
Clinical Assistant Professor	Doctoral degree and national certification in clinical specialty	Demonstrates expertise in clinical specialty, a commitment to teaching, scholarship, and department service
Clinical Associate Professor	Doctoral degree and national certification in clinical specialty	Demonstrates statewide recognition as expert in clinical specialty, teaching proficiency, engages in scholarship and service
Clinical Professor	Doctoral degree and national certification in clinical specialty	Demonstrates national recognition as expert in clinical practice, teaching mastery, engages in scholarship and service

have responsibilities for working with students, serving on dissertation committees, teaching in the area of their expertise, or providing service to the school, campus, or profession, their time is protected for research through their securing of research grants from external agencies. Appointment is based on evidence of or promise of a funded program of research. A doctoral degree and at least beginning research experience are prerequisites for appointment to this track. Many Tier 1 schools in research-intensive universities hire only people with postdoctoral preparation in research into these ranks.

There are temporary positions in nursing education to which ANEs can be appointed. These are

nontenure earning positions that are less than full-time or full-time with limited terms.

Visiting positions may be appointed at any rank and designate someone who has a limited appointment (1 or 2 years), who is on leave from another institution, who is employed on a temporary basis, who is returning temporarily from retirement, or who may be under consideration for a permanent position within the school.

The *lecturer* (sometimes called *instructor*) position is considered a prerank position. Faculty who have not yet earned a terminal (doctoral) degree may be appointed to lecturer positions. Some institutions have an additional level within this track (senior lecturer), allowing for at least a small avenue for advancement. Teaching is the primary responsibility of faculty in lecturer positions.

The term *adjunct* faculty can have two meanings: In some institutions they are courtesy appointments for individuals whose primary employment is outside the nursing education program but who have responsibility as clinical preceptors or working with students on research projects. In other institutions part-time faculty are called adjunct faculty. Many institutions do not assign an academic rank to part-time faculty. Teaching is the primary responsibility of adjunct faculty who often are hired to teach courses on a semester-by-semester basis and compensated per course.

Emeritus is an honorific title that may be conferred on faculty who are retired after significant service to an institution. Faculty with emeritus status may be granted specific privileges, such as use of the library, computing services, or an office and secretarial support.

Graduate students may be employed in limited teaching positions. These appointments, such as *teaching assistant* and *associate instructor*, are temporary and usually part-time. Student employees are responsible only for teaching or assisting faculty with teaching. They do not have the same level of responsibility as full- or part-time faculty. Teaching assistants must be assigned to work with a faculty member who assumes responsibility for the quality of their work. Student employees with teaching responsibilities often receive a level of tuition waiver as part of their compensation.

Lastly, other positions, often implemented as lower-cost options, provide support to instructional faculty. *Academic coaches, instructional assistants*, and *academic specialists* are a few examples. Individuals in these positions could be employed by the institution or by an outside provider that partners with the institution to provide instructional support.

The Appointment Process

The appointment process in universities and colleges is somewhat different from positions in nursing service, and nurses who are applying for teaching positions in schools of nursing should understand the differences. A search and screen committee, appointed by the dean or another university administrator, manages the interview process. Interested individuals submit an application and curriculum vitae that are screened by this committee. Potential candidates are invited for an interview with the search committee, faculty and administrators at the school of nursing, and others at the college or university as appropriate. Depending on the requirements of the position for which they are applying, applicants may be asked to make a presentation of their research or to demonstrate their teaching skills. At the time of appointment, the applicant's records are reviewed by the appointment, promotion, and tenure (APT) committee (or another appropriately named committee) that recommends a hiring rank to the dean.

Tenure and Promotion

Tenure

Tenure is a reciprocal responsibility on the part of both the institution and the faculty. The faculty member is expected to remain competent and productive, maintaining high standards of teaching, research, service, and professional conduct. Tenure also assumes that the faculty member is promotable at the time of tenure, and typically promotion to the next level and tenure occur at the same time. Tenure, then, provides the faculty member the protection of academic freedom. Academic freedom has been affirmed since 1940 by more than 200 institutions of higher education. It guarantees protection against efforts by government, university administration, students, and even public opinion to restrain faculties' free expression in teaching or the free exercise of their research interests (AAUP, 2018).

On the other hand, academic freedom does not give faculty unbounded rights. For example, an individual faculty member does not have the right to alter the curriculum, the sequence of courses, or the content of established courses or to subject students to discussions that are irrelevant to the course. Tenure can be withdrawn for reasons of financial exigency on the part of the university and for unprofessional faculty behavior. Finally, tenure does not relieve faculty from participating in performance review. Many institutions have instituted a posttenure review process. Posttenure review policies vary greatly across institutions, so faculty should become familiar with such policies in their own institution.

Tenure is granted after an extensive review, using published criteria, of the evidence submitted by the faculty member (a curriculum vitae and dossier). The tenure or promotion review is typically held in the faculty member's 5th or 6th year, with tenure granted in the 6th or 7th year for successful candidates. Unsuccessful candidates are usually given a 1-year notice of nonappointment. Most institutions affirm excellence using additional reviewers from external peer institutions. At appointment, faculty with a record of significant achievement may be granted a specific number of years toward tenure, thus shortening the time for tenure review. Faculty who achieved tenure at a comparably ranked institution may be hired with tenure already conferred.

The tenure process is specific to each school of nursing and institution, and faculty who are appointed to a tenure track position should familiarize themselves with the criteria and process before appointment. Although the tenure and promotion process may seem mysterious, there are clear and specified criteria. The awarding of tenure results in an indefinite appointment that can be terminated only for cause or under extraordinary circumstances such as financial exigency (AAUP, 2018). Reappointment and review of continued employment in tenured positions are based on the evaluation of the teaching, research/scholarship, and service components of the faculty role; this is termed *posttenure review*. Nontenure track positions require reappointment at specific intervals (e.g., yearly or every 3–5 years).

The current attitude is to employ faculty who show high promise for attaining tenure and being promoted and to provide support and mentoring that will facilitate their developing into successful and fully capable members of the academic community. Although at one time tenure was an unquestioned right of faculty, critics are now questioning its true benefit, and some institutions of higher education have abandoned the notion altogether. Tenure is absent in many public universities, community colleges, and for-profit universities. Faculty who value tenure should seek employment in institutions committed to tenure as an ideal of academic freedom.

Promotion

Promotion refers to advancement in rank and is an option in tenure and some nontenure track positions, such as clinical track. As with the tenure review process, faculty must submit evidence, in the form of a dossier, of excellence in teaching, scholarship, and/or service, as well as other criteria established by the school, and be evaluated by a committee of peers, external reviewers, school and university administrators, and governing bodies. Criteria and processes for promotion, like those for tenure, are established by faculty committees and are made public.

Faculty should familiarize themselves with promotion criteria and processes at the time of appointment and establish a relationship with the primary APT committee and the department chair, whose role it is to inform faculty about APT policies and procedures. As noted earlier, an expectation of senior faculty is to guide and mentor junior faculty through the tenure and/or promotion process. Some schools of nursing assign mentors at the time of appointment. If a mentor is not assigned, the newly appointed faculty member should seek one.

FACULTY DEVELOPMENT

Faculty development refers to a planned course of action to develop all faculty members—not only those newly appointed—for current and future teaching positions. Faculty development is assuming new importance as faculty prepare for teaching in new and reformed health care environments and community-based settings, delivering instruction in new ways, and using new teaching and learning technologies.

Faculty development is a shared responsibility of individual faculty members, the department chair and other academic officers, and the school or university. It may include orientation, mentoring, formal and informal workshops and sessions, credit courses, "brown bag lunches," annual evaluation, and sabbatical or research leave, encouraging faculty to attend local and national conferences related to teaching and providing the financial support to do so are also important development opportunities. Because effective teaching also requires clinical competence, faculty are encouraged to maintain clinical expertise through faculty practice, by keeping abreast of changes in the field through literature review and by attending professional meetings related to the practice area.

Orientation Programs

Orientation to the teaching role for newly appointed faculty, as well as ongoing development for all faculty, is assuming renewed importance as rapid changes in higher education and health care and the use of information technologies are creating new environments for teaching and changes in the faculty role. Most schools of nursing have established orientation programs at the institutional, school, program, and/or course levels and instituted mechanisms for ongoing faculty development and renewal.

Comprehensive orientation programs are necessary to assist new faculty to acquire teaching competencies, facilitate socialization to the teaching role, and support faculty members as they develop as fully participating members of the faculty. Orientation programs should include information about the rights and responsibilities of the faculty and institution, school- and department-specific policies and procedures, an overview of the curriculum with an orientation to the instructional technologies and computer-mediated instruction used at the school, and introductions to teaching assignments and clinical facilities. Orientation is particularly important for part-time faculty members, who have fewer opportunities for contact with the school and faculty colleagues. Orientation programs are most effective when they occur over time and provide ongoing support. Comprehensive programs include institutional, school, department, program, course, and delivery method orientation programs.

Mentoring

Given the multifaceted nature of the faculty role, faculty, especially those new to the role, find that having a mentor or mentors is beneficial to establishing and succeeding in an academic career. Mentors are helpful for the career development of senior and novice faculty (Halstead & Frank, 2018) and students. Many schools of nursing have formal mentor programs in which each new faculty member is assigned to a senior faculty member who guides the new faculty member. Other mentoring relationships can occur on an informal basis, such as those that can be established through interactions with peers, course leaders, department chairs, and faculty who have specific expertise in areas that would be helpful to share with new faculty. Faculty should carefully reflect on their career development needs and seek out mentors who can help them achieve their career goals. Additionally, they are responsible for mentoring students, which includes formal academic advisement and coaching, supporting, and guiding protégés through the academic system and into their professional careers.

Providing mentoring to new faculty members is an especially important responsibility of senior and tenured faculty because nurses are not usually fully prepared in graduate nursing programs for a role in academia. Mentoring is needed to assist new faculty members as they learn to balance all aspects of their new and multifaceted role and involves coaching, supporting, and guiding them as they develop in their role as faculty. Fortunately, as the number of clinical-track faculty in nursing continues to increase, ANEs have responded by developing mentoring programs that focus on scholarship development and academic promotion (Shieh & Cullen, 2019). Regardless of appointment track, when starting at a new institution, even an experienced faculty member requires mentoring relative to specific institutional norms and processes.

Evaluation of Teaching Performance

To ensure competent teaching, the faculty members themselves, along with administrators, peers, colleagues, and students, regularly review their teaching performance. Evaluation of teaching is a critical component of annual evaluation, reappointment, promotion, and tenure review (Halstead & Frank, 2018). Results of this evaluation may also be used in making decisions about merit raises and awards that recognize and honor excellence in teaching.

Evidence for review of teaching effectiveness can be provided by several sources including student evaluations of teaching, peer and colleague observations of teaching and teaching products (e.g., syllabi, case studies, publications, videotapes, computer-mediated lessons, internet-based courses, study guides), letters from former students, the success of graduates in employment, publications of students, teaching awards, administrative review, and self-evaluation.

Peer evaluation is a vital aspect of faculty development and often is part of the documentation data considered in the decision-making process for promotion and tenure. For example, ANEs can use peer observations of teaching, which include objective assessments of teaching, to guide ongoing development of teaching competencies and enhance instructional quality

(Fletcher, 2018). Students provide feedback about faculty instruction using a standardized assessment tool. Faculty are involved in the development of fair and equitable evaluation criteria on which to base these judgments, evaluate results, and use the data to identify ways to enhance teaching effectiveness

Sabbatical Leave

Sabbatical leave provides another opportunity for tenured and research-track faculty to focus on professional growth and scholarly productivity. Leave is approved based on submission of an acceptable project plan for research or publication during the sabbatical leave. The university supports sabbatical leaves when the proposed project meets both individual and institutional goals. Specific outcome deliverables are required for sabbaticals.

CHAPTER SUMMARY: KEY POINTS

- Using specialized knowledge and skills that have evolved over time, ANEs influence health outcomes by designing, implementing, and evaluating nursing education programs that prepare entry-level and advanced practice nurses to deliver safe, quality nursing care. They teach in dynamic environments using a variety of pedagogies and delivery methods.
- Completing coursework in curriculum, teaching strategies, assessment and evaluation, and engaging in a continuous improvement process facilitates development of the ANE competencies, which can lead to specialty certification such as CNE or CNE®cl. Earning certification validates the ANE as an advanced practice role.

- Teaching is a scholarly endeavor that encompasses the discovery, application, and integration of knowledge into professional practice. Effective teaching often leads to "ah-ha" moments in which ANEs experience the rewards of making a difference.
- At the time of hire, a full-time faculty member is appointed to a track (tenure or nontenure) and assigned an academic rank (lecturer/instructor, assistant professor, associate professor, professor) based on their education and experience.
- Participating in orientation, mentoring, continuing education, and annual evaluation that includes peer review of teaching and student ratings of instruction fosters ongoing development in the ANE role.

REFLECTING ON THE EVIDENCE

1. Reflect on what interests you about teaching in nursing education and how you feel about preparing the next generation of entry-level and advanced practice nurses.
2. Interview an ANE in a tenure track position and another in a clinical track position and identify the similarities and differences between the two types of appointments.

Determine which might be the best fit for you and why.
3. Compare and contrast the faculty role expectations for tenure in a college or university that has a mission with a primary focus on research to one that has a primary focus on teaching; consider the institutional type and mission that aligns with your interest.

4. Describe a scholarly project that would fit into the Boyer model as an example of the scholarship of teaching.
5. Create an infographic that reflects the relationships between scholarly work, evidence-based teaching, the scholarship of teaching, SoTL, and building the science of nursing education.

6. Reflect on your faculty development needs and the type of mentor(s) you may need to support your growth as an ANE. Use the NLN Core Competencies of Nurse Educators to create a personalized faculty development plan for yourself.

REFERENCES

American Association of Colleges of Nursing. (2020a). *2019–2020 salaries of instructional and administrative nursing faculty in baccalaureate and grade programs in nursing.* American Association of Colleges of Nursing.

American Association of Colleges of Nursing. (2020b). *Nursing faculty shortage.* https://www.aacn-nursing.org/News-Information/Fact-Sheets/Nursing-Faculty-Shortage

American Association of Colleges of Nursing. (2021). *Data spotlight: Trends in Black/African American nursing graduates and faculty.* https://www.aacn-nursing.org/News-Information/News/View/ArticleId/25003/Data-Spotlight-Black-African-American-Nursing-Grads-and-Faculty

American Association of University Professors. (2018). *Recommended institutional regulations on academic freedom and tenure (1957, Updated 2018).* https://www.aaup.org/report/recommended-institutional-regulations-academic-freedom-and-tenure

American Association of University Professors, American Council on Education, & the Association of Governing Boards of Universities and Colleges, (1966). Statement on government of colleges and universities. *AAUP Bulletin, 52*(4), 375–379.

Bond, D. K., Peery, A. I., VanRiel, Y. M., Gazza, E. A., Phillips, B. C., Winters-Thornburg, C. E., & Swanson, M. S. (2020). RN to BSN students' intent to become faculty—A multisite study. *Nurse Educator, 45*(4), E31–E35. https://doi.org/10.1097/NNE.0000000000000732.

Boyer, E. (1990). *Scholarship reconsidered: Priorities of the professorate.* The Carnegie Foundation for the Advancement of Teaching.

Christensen, L. S., & Simmons, L. E. (2020). *The scope of practice for academic nurse educators and academic clinical nurse educators* (3rd ed.). National League for Nursing.

Daw, P. E., Seldomridge, L., Mills, M. E., & D'Aoust, R. F. (2021). The Maryland Graduate Nurse Faculty Scholarship: Program evaluation of a nurse faculty workforce initiative. *Nursing Economic$, 39*(4), 189–195. Advanced online publication.

Evans, J. D. (2018). Why we became nurse educators: Findings from a nationwide survey of current nurse educators. *Nursing Education Perspectives, 30*(2), 61–65. https://doi.org/10.1097/01.NEP.0000000000000278.

Fang, D., & Kesten, K. (2017). Retirements and succession of nursing faculty in 2016–2025. *Nursing Outlook, 65*(3), 1–10. https://doi.org/10.1016/j.outlook.2017.03.003.

Fletcher, J. A. (2018). Peer observation of teaching: A practical tool in higher education. *The Journal of Faculty Development, 23*(1), 51–64.

Garner, A., & Bedford, L. (2021). Reflecting on educational preparedness and professional development for early career nurse faculty: A phenomenological study. *Nurse Education in Practice, 53*, 1–6. https://doi.org/10.1016/j.nepr.2021.103052.

Gazza, E. A. (2019). Alleviating the nurse faculty shortage: Recognizing and preparing the academic nurse educator as an advanced practice registered nurse. *Nursing Forum, 54*(2), 144–148. https://doi.org/10.1111/nuf.12307.

Glassick, C. E., Huber, M. T., & Maeroff, G. I. (1997). *Scholarship assessed: Evaluation of the professoriate.* Wiley.

Halstead, J. A. (2019). *NLN core competencies for nurse educators: A decade of influence.* National League for Nursing.

Halstead, J. A., & Frank, B. (2018). *Pathways to a nursing education career: Transitioning from practice to academia* (2nd ed.). Springer.

McNelis, A. M., Dreifuerst, K. T., & Schwindt, R. (2019). Doctoral education and preparation for nursing faculty roles. *Nurse Educator, 44*(4), 202–206. https://doi.org/10.1097/NNE.0000000000000597.

National Academies of Sciences, Engineering, and Medicine, (2021). *The future of nursing 2020–2030: Charting a path to achieve health equity.* The National Academies Press. https://doi.org/10.17226/25982.

National League for Nursing. (2005, 2012, 2018, 2021). *Competencies for nurse educators.* http://www.nln.org/professional-development-programs/competencies-for-nursing-education/nurse-educator-core-competency

National League for Nursing. (2019). *NLN biennial survey of schools of nursing academic year 2017–2018: Executive summary.* http://www.nln.org/docs/default-source/default-document-library/executive-summary-(pdf)86d9c-95c78366c709642ff00005f0421.pdf

National League for Nursing. (n.d.). *Certification for nurse educators.* http://www.nln.org/Certification-for-Nurse-Educators

Özbay, Ö., & Çınar, S. (2020). Effectiveness of the flipped classroom teaching models in nursing education: A systematic review. *Nurse Education Today, 102*(2021), 104922. https://doi.org/10.1016/j.nedt.2021.104922.

Shellenbarger, T. S. (2019). *Clinical nurse educator competencies: Creating an evidence-based practice of academic clinical nurse educators.* National League for Nursing.

Shieh, D., & Cullen, D. L. (2019). Mentoring nurse faculty: Outcomes of a three-year clinical track faculty initiative. *Journal of Professional Nursing, 35,* 162–169. https://doi.org/10.1016/j.profnurs.2018.11.005.

Tri-Council for Nursing. (2017). *Civility considered key to promoting healthy, inclusive work environments and safeguarding patient safety.* http://tricouncilfornursing.org/documents/Tri-Council-Nursing-Civility-9-26-17.pdf

World Health Organization. (2016). *Nurse educator core competencies.* https://www.who.int/hrh/nursing_midwifery/nurse_educator050416.pdf

2

Strategies to Support Diverse Learning Needs of Students*

Jewel K. Diller, DNP, MSEd, RN

For most students, the decision to pursue a nursing degree represents a significant investment of resources in terms of effort, time, and money. They begin their nursing program with a mix of expectations, anticipation of success, and some degree of anxiety about achieving that success. Students also bring with them a wide array of diverse learning needs and life experiences, as well as multiple demands on their time. Faculty are responsible for creating a learning environment that will foster student engagement in the learning process and facilitate student success.

Student retention is a concern for many nursing programs, especially among students from underrepresented populations (Everett, 2022). Faculty must consider the many factors that can affect students' academic success and creatively design interactive learning environments that facilitate student success. This chapter presents a brief profile of today's nursing students, describes the unique demographic characteristics of students, and identifies factors that impact student success in nursing programs, including strategies for maximizing students' academic success. This chapter also addresses how understanding students' learning style preferences can help faculty assess the needs of the students in their courses and design a variety of teaching approaches that will provide meaningful and engaging learning experiences. Specific teaching and learning strategies related to students' diverse needs are presented to enable faculty to create effective learning environments for all students that will prepare them for transition into practice. Other chapters that provide related information on student learning are Chapter 16 and 18, which provide additional teaching strategies in classroom and clinical teaching, and Chapter 17, which provides an in-depth discussion on multicultural education in nursing.

NATIONAL HEALTH CARE NEEDS AND NURSING WORKFORCE DIVERSITY

The increase in older populations, combined with increasing ethnic and racial diversity, is predicted to continue in the United States until 2060 (U.S. Census Bureau, 2020). Although the actual rate of growth can only be predicated on an estimate of net international migration, census trends depict growing diversity in many regions of the country. With increasing numbers in the nation's diverse populations, there is a pressing need to address how to effectively meet the diverse health care needs of its citizens. One barrier to doing so is the continuing shortage of diversity in the nursing and health care workforce (American Association of Colleges of Nursing [AACN], 2019).

The call for increasing diversity in the health professions workforce is not new. The definitive Institute of Medicine's (IOM) extensive report, *In the Nation's Compelling Interest: Ensuring Diversity in the Health Care Workforce* (2004), and the IOM's report, *The Future of Nursing: Leading Change, Advancing Health* (2011), presented a broad and

*The author acknowledges the work of Joan L. Frey, EdD, RN, ANEF and Ann Popkess, PhD, RN, CNE, in the previous editions of the chapter.

compelling depiction of the benefits of greater diversity among health professionals and the need for strategies to increase diversity in all the health professions. Even though health care professions have made efforts, they have not kept pace with demographic changes in ethnic and racial diversity in the United States. Further, disparities in healthcare education are, in part, a result of disparities in diversity of healthcare educators (National Academy of Medicine [NAM], 2021; Wilbur et al., 2020). More recently, the National Academy of Medicine's report, *The Future of Nursing 2020–2030: Charting a Path to Achieve Health Equity* (2021), also underscored the role of the nurse in promoting health equity. The report further asserts that "a diverse workforce is one that reflects the variations in the nation's population in such characteristics as socioeconomic status, religion, sexual orientation, gender, race, ethnicity, and geographic origin" (NAM, 2021, p. 217).

With the goal of promoting health equity for all in mind, the *Future of Nursing 2020–2030* report specifically called out the need for the nursing profession to recruit and support diverse student populations of prospective nurses. While the diversity of the student populations enrolled in nursing programs has grown since the 2011 *Future of Nursing* report, the nursing workforce remains overwhelmingly White and female (NAM, 2021). By diversifying the nursing student population, it is hoped that eventually the nursing workforce will reflect a growing diversity as well. However, in order to achieve that goal, it is essential for schools of nursing to cultivate an environment that emphasizes inclusiveness. For diverse groups of students to be retained and successful in completing their nursing programs to join the workforce, barriers to academic success must be removed and supportive systems put in place. In addition to academic support, systems need to be in place to address social, economic, emotional, and academic progression needs (NAM, 2021). Professional nursing organizations have similarly adopted and published mission, vision, and/or position statements committed to diversity as an organizational and member-supported value and, specifically, promoting diversity in nursing education (AACN, 2019; ANA, 2019; National League for Nursing [NLN], 2021a).

For nurse educators to design learning environments and select teaching–learning strategies that meet the diverse learning needs of students, it is important to understand and acknowledge the implications of the United States' growing national diversity. The range of issues implicit in the discussion of diversity must be further informed with alignment to race and ethnicity, gender, the nursing profession, and, specifically, nursing education.

Racial and Ethnic Diversity in the Workforce

The number of registered nurses from underrepresented race and ethnic backgrounds has been increasing despite previous slow growth in these areas. The National Nursing Workforce Survey of Licensed Practical/Licensed Vocational Nurses and Registered Nurses conducted biennially by the National Council of State Boards of Nursing (NCSBN) and National Forum of State Nursing Workforce Centers in 2020 reported an increased number of registered nurses and licensed practical nurses from racially or ethnically diverse backgrounds. The 2020 National Nursing Workforce Survey found the percentage of registered nurses from racially or ethnically diverse backgrounds reported as 19.4%, whereas 30.5% of those licensed practical/vocational nurses responding to the survey identified as being racially or ethnically diverse (Smiley et al., 2021). As the Baby Boomer generation continues to exit the workforce through retirement, younger generations of nurses who are more ethnically diverse enter the workforce, and the landscape of the ethnicity of the nursing workforce will be changed.

A comparison of the registered nurse population versus general population diversity demonstrates the differences between the groups, especially regarding the underrepresentation of African American and Hispanic ethnic groups in nursing (Smiley et al. 2021). See Table 2.1 for a comparison of professional nursing diversity in contrast to the diversity that exists within the general population. The importance of achieving diversity in health care and the health care professions (NAM, 2021)

TABLE 2.1   Comparison of Nursing Diversity to General Population

Ethnic or Gender Group	Registered Nurse Population	General Population
African American	6.7%	12.7%
American Indian/ Alaskan Native	0.5%	0.8%
Asian	7.2%	5.6%
Caucasian	80.6%	72.3%
Hispanic	5.6%	18.1%
Native Hawaiian/ Pacific Islander	0.4%	0.2%
Female	90.5%	50.8%
Male	9.4%	49.2%

Data from National Council of State Boards of Nursing. (n.d.). *National nursing workforce study.* https://www.ncsbn.org/workforce.htm; and United States Census Bureau. (2020). https://data.census.gov/cedsci/table?q=United%20States&g=0100000US&tid=ACSDP1Y2017.DP05&vintage=2017&layer=state&cid=DP05_0001E

coupled with stark data depicting the unambiguous disparity in the nursing profession (Smiley et al. 2021) should give nursing education administrators and faculty leaders a clear focus to achieve improved diversity and inclusion in nursing education and the profession.

Gender Diversity in the Workforce

The nursing workforce remains predominately female, as does the nursing student population, which is 85% to 90% female (NAM, 2021). According to the 2020 National Nursing Workforce Survey (2021), males make up 9.4% of registered nurses working in the United States, which is a 0.3% increase from 2017 data. Males make up 8.1% of all licensed practical or licensed vocational nurses in the United States (Smiley et al. 2021). The percentage of male students varies by nursing program type with ADN (14.4%); BSN (13.6%); MSN (15.2%), PhD (9.9%), and DNP (13.1%) (NAM, 2021). There is a continued need to better understand gender-based perceptions of nursing and male student experiences in nursing schools.

PROFILE OF CONTEMPORARY NURSING STUDENTS

The profile of today's nursing students demonstrates that contemporary nursing students are becoming more representative of an increasingly diverse and global society. They have unique learning needs and expectations of their learning experiences. The differences are multifaceted and include variances in secondary education preparation for engaging in higher-order learning, student demographic differences, shifts in gender roles, life experience and generational differences, and increasing racial and ethnic diversity.

Meanwhile, student and faculty age differentials are widening, and faculty composition is less representative of the wider population demographic and the students seeking a nursing education. To adequately address the needs of a diverse student population requires a cadre of diverse nursing faculty. The characteristics of full-time nurse educators by race and ethnicity show that a wide gap exists among ethnicity of faculty, the registered nurse (RN) workforce, and general population, where only 17.3% of full-time nursing education faculty originate from minority backgrounds (NAM, 2021). The race and ethnicity backgrounds of nurse educators is depicted in Fig. 2.1 (NLN, 2021b). Planning effective learning experiences to meet the diverse learning needs of students requires faculty to embrace the diversity that exists among their students and understand how they can best support their academic success.

Enrollment Demographics

The Bureau of Labor Statistics (2021) reports that RN employment opportunities are expected to grow more than the average for all occupations at a rate of 7% from 2019 to 2029, which is faster than average projected growth for all occupations. Nursing continues to be a sought-after career, even as a second or late career choice. Nursing education programs provide the pipeline to increased diversity in the profession through the enrollment of diverse student populations (NLN, 2021c). The collective percentage of minorities enrolled in nursing programs totals 30.9% of all enrollees, and although these figures represent a decrease

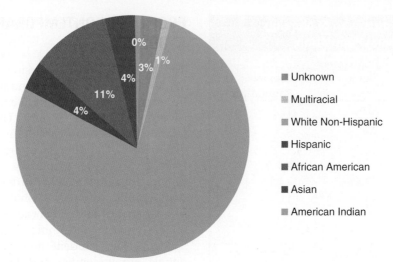

FIG. 2.1 Distribution of full-time nurse educators by race, 2020–2021. (From National League for Nursing. [2021]. Faculty census survey 2020–2021. https://www.nln.org/nln-faculty-census-survey-2020-2021)

from 32.4% as reported in 2018 (NLN, 2021c), the data depict continuing racial/ethnic disparities. Once students are enrolled, nurse educators are accountable to promote the recruitment, retention, completion, and transition to practice of all students (Maykut et al., 2021; Van Der Wege & Keil, 2019). As endorsed by the American Association of Colleges of Nursing's position paper *Diversity, Equity, and Inclusion in Academic Nursing*, "academic leadership and faculty should examine any unconscious and conscious biases that may undermine efforts to enhance diversity, inclusion, and equity, including the use of everyday verbal, nonverbal, intentional or non-intentional messages which devalue the perspectives, experiences, and/or feelings of individuals or groups These biases may restrict academic nursing's ability to attract and retain a more diverse student body and to recruit and promote diverse leaders, faculty, and academic support staff" (AACN, 2021, p. 2).

With information extrapolated from enrollment in all types of nursing programs (NLN, 2021c), it is noted that the percentages of students over 31 years of age are as follows: 22% in practical/vocational nursing (PN/VN), 18.3% in diploma, 23.7% in associate degree in nursing (ADN), 8.4% in bachelor of science in nursing (BSN), 20.3% in registered nursing (RN) to BSN, 27.4% in master of science in

nursing (MSN), and 32.6% in doctoral programs. Except for PN, diploma, and ADN programs, the percentage of students older than 31 years of age has decreased, signifying more students in younger generation cohorts engaging in BSN, RN to BSN, MSN, and doctoral nursing programs. Additionally, the (NLN, 2021c) Biennial Survey of Schools of Nursing findings indicate that prior data that reflected late entry into doctoral programs in nursing is trending to include younger age groups. This wide age diversity among nursing students offers unique challenges to nurse educators when these students are mixed in classrooms.

Admission into baccalaureate, associate, and master's degree nursing schools remains competitive, which also shifts the demographic profile of nursing students. Considerable numbers of qualified applicants are denied admission to prelicensure nursing programs across the United States each year. As reported by nursing schools, the major reasons for turning away qualified applicants include a shortage of qualified faculty, lack of qualified applicants, practice positions considered to be more appealing than faculty appointments, and lack of funds for faculty positions (NLN, 2021b). Nursing program leaders cited inability to offer competitive salaries 34.4% of the time, making it the most common deterrent to the admission of qualified applicants (NLN, 2021b).

In an attempt to address the lack of clinical sites and enroll more students, many nursing programs have utilized simulation to supplement student clinical learning in situations where clinical practice availability is limited (Lewis-Pierre, 2019; Tolarba, 2021). Use of clinical simulation in addition to face-to-face clinical experiences has enabled nursing programs to increase student enrollments (Padiha et al., 2019). However, the lack of qualified faculty, which ranks as the second most significant deterrent to the admission of qualified applicants (NLN, 2021b), remains a stumbling block to program growth. Meanwhile, faculty and administrators are challenged to continue to recruit qualified, diverse student bodies.

Generational Differences

Age and generation cohort differences can create both implicit and explicit disconnects between students and faculty. Students in education environments where generational diversity is accepted and supported will find themselves prepared to create better health care work environments. The following sections briefly summarize the generational characteristics of learners in today's classrooms and include implications for educators.

Students in nursing classrooms represent a variety of generations, each with unique perspectives and learning needs. A commitment by nursing faculty and nursing leaders to create positive and collaborative educational cultures that value inclusivity and diversity will facilitate the creation of learning and work environments to support academic success for all students (Coventry & Hays, 2021; Shepherd, 2020).

Generation X

Generation X represents a cohort of 65.2 million people born between 1965 and 1979 (Fry, 2020). Generation Xers are more diverse in race and ethnicity than previous generations but not as diverse as the generation that immediately follows them, the Millennials. Although Generation Xers are children of Baby Boomers (born 1945–1964), their work ethic and loyalties differ from those of their parents. Their characteristics can best be defined by the historical, political, and social influences of the era. As a result, they were often children

of divorced parents or working parents and were commonly referred to as *latchkey kids*. Generation Xers value inclusion and connection with others as a means to motivate their learning, although they can work equally well in teams or independently. They also demonstrate a need for immediate feedback and answers to concerns. They have learned how to manage time commitments; to be self-directed, flexible, technologically adept, and individualistic; and to value a work-life balance (Shepherd, 2020).

Implications for nurse educators. To better meet the learning challenges of generational differences, nurse educators are required to reinforce their knowledge of learning style preferences and to engage in a variety of teaching methodologies and strategies to enhance student success. Assessment of Generation Xers brings to light the group's tendency to be independent and self-sufficient and recognizes their preference for reading of assignments and guided lectures with use of technology to broaden knowledge acquisition. Generation Xers value student-faculty relationships where rules are important, and where interactive teaching techniques are limited to the student's expectation of academic success because of individualized efforts in studies and testing, supported by the long-held teaching practices of faculty (Shepherd, 2020).

Millennials or Generation Y

Millennials, or Generation Y, number 72.1 million and were born between the years 1980 and 1995 and currently make up the largest living population in the United States (Fry, 2020). Millennials are generally described as optimistic, team-oriented, high-achieving rule followers (Keener, 2020). They are the first-generational cohort that seized on Facebook as a form of social media, although they have since shifted to the use of other social media platforms (Auxier & Anderson, 2021). Millennials characteristically have good relationships with their parents and families and share their interests in music and travel. Parents of Millennials involved their children in a variety of activities from a young age to prepare them for success. Millennials are accustomed to living highly structured lives, as planned by their parents, with little free time as children. Because of these experiences, Millennials tend to feel more anxious during the transition from high school to college and need more support during that transition (Greene et al., 2019). Keener (2020) studied generational differences with regard to entitlement that is often attributed to Millennials and found that some students in this age group may present issues for educators with regard to their sense of entitlement, although other generations of students may also display entitlement. While Millennial nurses have demonstrated less interest in conventional practices, this generation of nurses engage socially and work to achieve a work–life balance for themselves as they participate in workplace activities (Coventry & Hayes, 2021).

Implications for nurse educators. Implications for nurse educators in teaching this generation include providing immediate feedback and structure in the classroom and providing opportunities for service and giving back to their communities. Millennial learners are technologically savvy and comfortable with multitasking (Coventry & Hayes, 2021; Stultzer, 2019). Shepherd (2020) noted that the learning needs of Millennials can be best met by nurse educators who develop teaching strategies that students find kinesthetically engaging while meaningful enough to sustain their participation and engagement in the learning process. Shepherd recommended that faculty use teaching–learning strategies that allow for interactive and varied learning activities.

Generation Z

The cohort of individuals born after the Millennial generation is Generation Z, or Net/Internet Generation (iGeneration), which represents those born from the middle to late 1990s to the present day. This generation has been shaped by technology and numerous societal events including wars, violence, and economic downturns (Chunta et al., 2021). Due to its sheer size of approximately 73 million persons (U.S. Census Bureau, 2019), the Generation Z cohort is considered to be a marketing target and consumer of digital technology like no other previous generation because of their continual online presence (Ford & Mosley, 2020). Generation Z students are true digital natives,

having grown up during an explosion of technology advances, and are used to interacting through the use of technology and social media (Chunta et al., 2021). Because of their constant use of technology in their daily lives, these students prefer to access information by observing through video instead of reading text. Generation Z learners also demonstrate a preference for independent learning that allows them to learn at their own pace (Medina et al., 2021).

Generation Z students are innovative and have an entrepreneurial inclination. They tend to be goal oriented and driven to address social issues. They may be prone to anxiety and require frequent one-on-one feedback (DiMattio & Hudacek, 2020). They expect the learning environment to be dynamic and like to apply what they are learning to real-life situations (Medina et al., 2021).

Implications for nurse educators. The Generation Z cohort represents yet another group of distinctly technologically focused students with contexts for learning differently from how their educators were taught (Ford & Mosley, 2020; Schlee et al., 2020). Generation Z learners prefer individual prework and reflective thought activities leading up to groupwork and collaboration with their peers (Ford & Mosely, 2020). These learners also expect greater inclusion of digital media in the classroom. With their preference for applying what they learn to real-life situations, learning experiences that provide opportunities for "hands-on" learning combined with prompt feedback appeals to them.

Addressing the Learning Needs of Generational Groups

Recognizing that each student cohort represents a mix of generational learning differences, nurse educators should proactively design learning experiences that employ active teaching strategies that nursing students, regardless of generational identification, will find engaging and meaningful (Schlee et al., 2020). The passive use of presentation software and lectures is not sufficient to capture the attention of today's students who are used to learning through interactive technology. The ability to find commonalities among the generational groups can provide stimulating and exciting opportunities for faculty to enhance classroom and online learning solutions through the use and application of technology. Today's students are avid technology users, and modern social media platforms as well as emerging learning technologies can be leveraged to promote learning and bridge generational differences.

The implications of learners' generational demographics for educators and the teaching–learning process are significant. In addition to assessing student characteristics and their collaborative abilities, teaching strategies that successfully engage Generation X, Generation Y (Millennial), and Generation Z (iGeneration) learners need to be interactive, group focused, and experiential and allow for independent learning in a supportive environment (Blevins, 2021; Ford & Mosley, 2020; Shepherd, 2020; Vizcaya-Moreno & Pérez-Cañaveras, 2020). Furthermore, multigenerational classrooms mimic the multigenerational workforce that graduates will be entering and the patient populations for which they will be caring. Developing respect for differing perspectives and the skills to work in diverse teams as students will help them become effective team members when they are delivering care in diverse work settings.

Faculty can benefit from the multigenerations of students in their classes and draw on their diverse perspectives to foster engagement in the learning process. Faculty must be attuned to the different learning needs represented among their students and ensure that student support services are adequate for all learners and that the curricula demonstrate flexibility to support achievement of student learning outcomes (Blevins, 2021; Shepherd, 2020; Dolinger et al., 2020). Students with multiple role responsibilities may require support resources such as day care and the opportunity for part-time study. Incorporating a variety of teaching–learning strategies, including interactive and web-based media, will appeal to multigenerational students who are mobile tech-savvy and self-directed learners (Dolinger et al., 2020). No matter their generation, fundamentally students learn best when the classroom environment is inclusive and collaborative, where everyone is treated equally and fairly, and the faculty are sincerely concerned for each student's success (Coleman, 2020).

Racial and Ethnic Diversity

There continues to be a lack of ethnic and racial diversity in the nursing profession as reported by the Smiley et al. (2021), which is also reflected in nursing program enrollment data. Enrollment data show that despite the concerted emphasis within the profession on recruitment of racially and ethnically diverse students, they continue to be underrepresented in nursing programs. The NLN (2021c) reported that of all nursing students enrolled in prelicensure registered nursing programs, 11.2% identified themselves as African American; 11% identified as Hispanic; 4.7% identified as Asian; 0.5% identified as American Indian; and 3.5% identified as other/unknown, meaning that approximately 30% of the students in prelicensure registered nursing programs represented racial and ethnic diversity. Graduate nursing programs reveal similar statistics, with approximately 60% of students enrolled in MSN, PhD, or DNP programs identifying as White (NAM, 2021). The nursing profession is challenged to recruit and retain students representing racial and ethnic diversity.

Implications for nurse educators. There have been numerous factors identified that are associated with the attrition of ethnically diverse students. These factors include communication barriers, cultural differences, differing learning needs, and the lack of social-emotional support (Everett, 2022).

It is important that nurse educators continue to increase their understanding of the learning needs of diverse students. Chapter 17 provides an in-depth discussion on creating an inclusive learning environment and supporting the learning needs of racially and ethnically diverse students through multicultural education.

Male Students in Nursing

As previously noted, national nursing statistics regarding the number of male students enrolled in nursing programs ranges anywhere from 9.9% to 15.2% depending upon the type of nursing program (NAM, 2021). Despite the nursing profession's efforts at recruiting increased numbers of males to a career in nursing, male nursing students continue to face challenges in their nursing program leading to their attrition from the profession (Powers et al., 2018; Younas et al., 2019) and have often experienced academic challenges related to gender discrimination in a predominately female profession. Various studies indicate that barriers exist in nursing programs that lead male students to feel marginalized and, in some cases, to abandon their career choice before graduation (Cho & Jang, 2021; Guy & van der Krogt, 2021).

It is important to note that newly graduated male nurses identify with a strong professional commitment, although many leave nursing within 3 to 4 years (Yu et al., 2021). Yu et al. noted the degree of professional commitment, social support, and resilience as factors in the retention of newly licensed male nurses. Considering the finding of strong professional commitment in male nurses, efforts need to be made to provide social support and enhance resilience in male nurses as they begin their careers, including while they are nursing students. Male nursing students report their perceptions of their experiences in nursing programs. Some of these perceptions indicate that the use of sexist language in the classroom, textbooks, and clinical areas creates a less inviting environment for male students, including the determination that curricula in nursing programs are designed for female learners (Christensen et al., 2021; Cottingham, 2019). In some instances male students are denied access to clinical experiences such as in maternity care (Powers et al., 2018). This bias can especially exist in relation to testing, classroom lecture and discussion, and course structure. A lack of male role models in the nursing program can create self-doubt and social isolation in male students, potentially contributing to increased dropout rates (Kolawole et al., 2019).

Common misconceptions of men who choose to enroll in and plan for a career in nursing include inaccurate portrayals of gay lifestyles, gender unsuitability for nursing practice and general patient care, improper labeling of men as less compassionate or caring, and other untrue opinions (Christensen et al., 2021; Jamieson et al., 2019).

Implications for nurse educators. The use of unwelcoming behaviors, sexist language, lack of role models, and biased curricula are factors preventing the successful recruitment and retention of male students in schools of nursing and, consequently, the profession. Challenges to public perceptions regarding men in nursing, dedicated initiatives to increase the number of males in all nursing programs, further research on gender diversity in nursing, and promoting mentorship opportunities in schools of nursing and workplaces are but a few of the efforts recommended to create an inclusive learning environment for men entering the nursing profession. A gender-neutral approach to the image of the nurse both within and outside the professional environment is encouraged (Kavuran & Kasikci, 2018). Avoiding sexist language in textbooks, tests, and lectures is essential. Faculty also need to be aware of any tendencies they may have to exclude male nursing students from specific clinical experiences, taking steps to ensure equal learning opportunities are afforded them (Powers et al., 2018). Male students can benefit from peer support groups and exposure to male nurse role models (Younas et al., 2019). Further research in the study of men in nursing is needed to highlight and address the issues that impact the academic success of male nursing students. Such research should also include a consideration of gender role stereotypes and cultural influences on the satisfaction of male students and their academic success in nursing programs (Cho & Jang, 2021).

Students Identifying as LGBTQ+

Students who identify as lesbian, gay, bisexual, transgender, queer, or questioning (LGBTQ+) also express encountering a unique set of challenges in the educational environment that can negatively impact their academic success, causing them to withdraw from school (Holloway et al., 2019). It is important for the nursing profession to recognize and address the diverse backgrounds of all nursing students, including individuals who are part of the LGBTQ+ communities. Studies that have focused on LGBTQ+ students in higher education have demonstrated that these students may feel isolated and experience harassment and discrimination. These students may also experience less social support, including family support, because of their sexual orientation. These experiences may become barriers to academic success and lead to higher levels of attrition among this population of learners (Holloway et al., 2019).

Implications for nurse educators. It is essential for faculty to be aware of the unique challenges and needs of learners who identify as LGBTQ+, to discourage the overt and covert discrimination of those of sexually diverse orientations. Health science students who identify as LGBTQ+ have reported that they have experienced interactions with faculty that were covertly discriminatory (Holloway et al., 2019). In such situations implicit (unconscious) bias may be a factor. Implicit bias is defined as unintentional or unconscious attitudes or viewpoints about others. Implicit bias may cause a person to dislike individuals or groups and may cause them to treat others in an unfair or negative manner (Crandlemire, 2020). Modifying the behaviors and attitudes of educators based on accurate and relevant information regarding the needs of LGBTQ+ students is an important step toward creating an inclusive environment supportive of these students. Faculty should engage in self-reflection and awareness activities to gain a better understanding of their own implicit biases toward any social group, including LGBTQ+ (Crandlemire, 2020).

Nursing curricula can be revised to include content about diverse sexual orientations to increase awareness among nursing students and support acceptance among student peer groups and equality care for patients. Incorporating implicit bias information and discussion in nursing curricula can aid in student understanding of what implicit bias consists of and also serves to diminish implicit bias. Students also can be instructed on strategies to diminish the influence that implicit bias may have in their interpersonal relationships and patient care.

Student support groups can provide benefit to students as they struggle to manage stress, improve coping skills, and work toward making connections in the college environment (McNaughton-Cassill et al., 2021). Faculty should be aware of student support services that are available on-campus to specifically serve the needs of the LGBTQ+ community (Case Study 2.1). Further research on sex and gender orientation-based information as well

---

CASE STUDY 2.1   Addressing the Needs of LGBTQ+ Students

A nurse faculty is approached by a nursing student who asks to speak with the faculty member in private. When they meet, the student informs the faculty member that they are transgender and are having issues coping with the demands of the nursing program and the "cold" environment they are greeted with by their peers. The student shares that they do not have family support and they feel like they are not "fitting in" with their peers. The student further states they are being bullied and harassed by peers because of their gender identity. After speaking with the nursing student, the nurse faculty reports the conversation to the administration and an investigative process into the reported bullying incidents is initiated following college protocol. The faculty member realizes they need to better understand the on-campus experiences of LGBTQ+ students and how these experiences impact their academic success. As the nurse faculty contemplates the student's concerns, they begin to explore available information about teaching students from diverse backgrounds such as LGBTQ+ students.

1. What research exists to provide background for nursing faculty wanting to know more about LGBTQ+ individuals in nursing education?
2. What impact can harassment and bullying have on an individual and what campus supports should be available for this student in a university or college setting?
3. How might nursing faculty work to improve equity, belonging, and inclusion within the learning environment for LGBTQ+ students, which can improve their opportunities to experience human flourishing in their nursing education program?

---

as interventions in nursing and healthcare that are sensitive to gender identity and sexual orientation is needed (Merry et al., 2021; Morris et al., 2019).

Veterans Entering Nursing

Many veterans demonstrate an interest in choosing nursing as a career following their discharge from military service. There are potential issues that confront men and women who have served in the military and faculty need to demonstrate an awareness of their special needs. Many of these veterans have received extensive medical training in their military roles, as well as serving as leaders in their military capacity (McNeal et al., 2019). They are also frequently described as being goal oriented, self-directed, adaptable, and racially/ethnically diverse (Sikes, et al., 2021). Veterans who want to apply their military occupational specialty (MOS) after completing military service have faced difficulties in transferring prior knowledge and skills to a professional nursing career. In recent years the federal government initiated efforts through the joined forces of the Veterans Administration, the Health Resources and Services Administration (HRSA), and schools of nursing to help make the transition from military service to nursing a smooth and rewarding process (HRSA, 2021).

With increased numbers of Iraq and Afghanistan war veterans being admitted into higher education institutions and programs, there has been an increased focus on the special mentoring needs of focus on and awareness of the special needs and services for student veterans entering nursing programs (McNeal et al., 2019). With improved benefits to the GI Bill added in 2018, more veterans and their family members are eligible for Veterans Administration (VA) benefits. Since implementation of the Post-9/11 GI Bill in 2009, educational assistance has been utilized by 773,000 service members, veterans, and their family members, adding up to more than $20 billion in benefits (U.S. Veterans Administration, 2021).

Regardless of improved benefits and programs focused to ease transitions, many veterans experience a culture shock as they make the transition from a regimented military culture to a less structured campus environment (Dyar, 2019; Sikes et al., 2021). Additional challenges may include administrative barriers related to transfer of academic credit, lack of campus support services for veterans, financial concerns, and academic struggles due to a lack of experience with formal education (Dyar, 2019). They can also face difficult service-to-civilian life situations that range from anxiety and depression, hypervigilance, posttraumatic stress disorder, and other mental and physical injuries to family and community readjustment issues (Chopin et al., 2020; Dyar, 2019; Sikes et al.,

2021). Prior traumatic mental and physical experiences often require veterans to recreate themselves in a civilian world that has little insight into the challenges they are facing as they enter college and forge new relationships with their peers and faculty while reacclimating to life as a civilian.

Implications for nurse educators. Faculty should familiarize themselves with the special challenges associated with veteran students and strive to develop a program culture that is inclusive of veteran students and their learning needs. Faculty can best help veteran students through availability and mentorship, willingness to listen, helpfulness in navigating an unfamiliar academic system, and guiding them to support services designed for veterans and student support services designed to facilitate academic success (Hurlbut & Revuelto, 2018; McNeal et al., 2019; Sikes et al., 2021). Faculty can also examine the curriculum and admission policies to design academic pathways for veteran students with military medical experience by considering educational transition models that award academic credit for military experiences (Hurlbut & Revuelto, 2018).

First-Generation College Students

The first year of college studies is stressful for many students. This is especially true of first-generation college students who do not have the benefit of their parent's college experiences to help them navigate college (Fry, 2021; McDonald et al., 2021; Roksa & Kinsley, 2019). Some become overwhelmed by the college environment and need support services aimed at easing the transition to college life and helping them to persist in their area of study (McDonald et al., 2021). First-generation students have higher levels of stress with lower matriculation rates and report feeling marginalized (Phillips et al., 2020).

During their first year in college, students need to establish study habits, develop time-management and test-taking skills, and generally adjust to the workload of college studies. All these challenges and more make the attainment of higher education outcomes difficult for young adults but are especially so for students who are the first in their family to seek a college degree (Farruggia et al., 2020). However, the most significant transformation for students is their change in learning, moving from dualism where students merely absorb information from faculty to relativism where thinking needs to be transformed by evidence and reasoning (see Chapter 14 for a discussion of learning theories).

Imagine the same challenges experienced by students who are the first in their family to attend college. They may be older than many of their classmates, face financial challenges, work part-time or full-time, or perceive social class differences while attending a postsecondary institution (McDonald et al., 2021). They may have no family member or role model to mentor or counsel them through these different and difficult scenarios, as they do not have family members who developed the self-confidence to navigate the college experience to relay that same confidence to them.

Implications for nurse educators. Nursing faculty can best assist first-generation students by developing student-centered environments that not only identify these students but dedicate resources and personnel to assist them in successful program completion (Bui & Rush, 2016; NCES, 2017; Yee, 2016). Mentoring relationships are one example of a student-centered environment that can support first-generation students as they adjust to the expectations of nursing education (Fruiht & Chan, 2018). Other student supports needed by first-generation students include caring faculty and readily available advisors (Ricks & Warren, 2021).

Second-Degree Seeking Students

Students who already possess a nonnursing baccalaureate degree and are returning to college for a second degree in nursing often will enroll in an accelerated program that recognizes prior learning by either granting transfer credit or evaluating prior learning for previously completed nonnursing courses. Second-degree nursing completion programs are generally 12 to 24 months in length and may include distance learning modalities (El-Banna et al., 2017; Sinacori & Williams-Gregory, 2021).

Second-degree nursing students possess life experiences that enable them to successfully engage in the nursing workforce after licensure (Sinacori & Williams-Gregory, 2021). They also have unique learning needs, which are driven, in part, by their previous education and life experiences. Second-degree students often report high levels of stress due to the fast pace of the accelerated nursing program and coping with work and family responsibilities while returning to school for a nursing degree, which can impact their success (El-Banna et al., 2017). Even though they have prior college degrees, they may not be ready for the rigor of study required for the pursuit of a nursing degree (Cantwell et al., 2020).

Implications for nurse educators. Flexible scheduling of classes, support services such as advising available outside of usual business hours, and technology support are vital to the success of adult learners seeking second degrees (Sun, 2019). Bernard et al. (2021) studied what motivates second-degree students to prepare for class. Study results indicated that the consistent use of engaging activities such as preclass preparation assignments and in-class work that highlight valuable concepts was beneficial. They also recommended the use of incentives for completion of preclass preparation as motivators for class preparation. Second-degree students may also need to fine-tune study skills and take a fresh approach to coursework to be successful. Students may struggle with the application of complex nursing concepts if their previous degree was more based on factual knowledge that could be memorized (El-Banna et al., 2017). El-Banna et al. (2017) studied second-degree nursing students' motivation in learning and recommended that faculty support student motivation to learn through the use of varied and active learning strategies in the classroom and prompt feedback on performance.

FACTORS AFFECTING ACADEMIC SUCCESS OF DIVERSE LEARNERS

Students with diverse backgrounds can face several barriers that hamper their ability to succeed in college. Cultural differences between and within student and faculty groups, the previously discussed gender and generational differences, and inexperience with a rigorous academic environment can contribute to the difficulties experienced by a diverse student body (Farruggia et al., 2020; Kilburn et al., 2019; Phillips et al., 2020). The most common factors that can affect the academic success of diverse learners are primarily related to financial resources, academic preparedness, social class differences, English language skills, and access to diverse faculty role models.

Financial Resources

Financial problems are a major stressor for many students. Rising tuition costs and other fees, coupled with a reduction in government support for higher education, affect all students. Financial concerns may be particularly difficult for racially and ethnically diverse students and first-generation students. They often come from low-income households, and therefore their families may lack the necessary financial resources to support their education. Financial aid in the form of loans or scholarships is becoming more competitive, although available grants are beginning to increase while availability of student loan amounts is decreasing (NCES, 2021). Therefore it is important for nursing programs to provide caring and responsive financial aid advisors who are knowledgeable about eligibility criteria and can assist students to navigate the often daunting and complicated financial aid processes (NCES, 2021).

Financial student aid may not be the only financial struggle students face. They may also lack access to basic needs such as food, health care, affordable housing, and child-care. Faculty should be aware of the social support services that are available within the institution and the community and how to refer the students to these other social service supports as needed.

Academic Preparation

Insufficient academic preparation and lack of support can lead to student attrition from the nursing program. Parental involvement and preparation of students before their college years has been determined by longitudinal studies to be statistically significant in the prediction of success for first-generation students, especially where the parents' constant and stable resource of encouragement in the home environment provided the impetus for future success (Bui & Rush, 2016). Many racially and ethnically diverse students may have attended elementary and secondary schools with few academic and physical resources and are thus not prepared for the academic rigor of a nursing program. Colleges often offer special enrichment programs to help students achieve basic academic skills and adjust to the college learning environment. Nursing programs may offer similar opportunities designed specifically for nursing students to help them adjust to the expectations of the nursing major. Through academic advisement, skills assessment, and assistance with developing study and testing skills, instructors can help students achieve a better academic record.

Social Class Background

For many students, social integration into the campus environment precedes academic success. The presence of social networks, including family support, can facilitate student transition into college life and promote persistence in academic studies (Reynolds & Parrish, 2018; Roksa & Kinsley, 2019). A sense of belonging for students can facilitate their adjustment to the academic environment and lead to overall performance success (Roksa & Kinsley, 2019).

Social class disparities affecting the achievement of learning outcomes were described by Phillips et al. (2020) for first-generation students, whereby higher learning education environments may serve to maintain social class disparities allowing them to persist through to graduation affecting the academic success of students. The interdependent cultural norms employed by first-generation students as they navigated the college environment were less successful than the more independent and interactive range of strategies used by middle-class students. As a result, first-generation students were found to be less likely to have a sense of belonging, express personal needs, or ask questions compared to students with one or both parents having a 4-year college degree. These types of behaviors make first-generation students less advantaged in the context of a college environment. The authors' study found that culture in the form of social class shapes the academic struggles of undergraduate students to achieve success and, consequently, leads to academic outcome disparities. Phillips et al. also noted that middle- and upper-class students often differentiate themselves from first-generation students through the use of a broader repertoire of academic engagement strategies that include self-expression and communication of personal preferences to their faculty.

Therefore it is not sufficient to assume that all students understand the importance of reaching out to faculty and the processes to use to increase understanding of course materials and assignments. It is suggested that faculty and academic support staff provide opportunities for students to engage in collaborative learning, which can help develop a sense of affirmation and belonging in all students (Hadden et al., 2020).

English as an Additional Language

For many students, English is not their primary language; rather their use of English is as an additional language (EAL). They may speak one language at home and English at school. Several studies have found that EAL students experience several barriers, such as lack of self-confidence, reading/writing and learning difficulties, isolation, prejudice, perceived inferiority, and stereotyping (Guler, 2022; Murray, 2020; Soriano & Alonso, 2020).

Lack of English language skills is often considered to be the primary determinant in the success of ethnically diverse students who succumb to learning challenges during nursing program studies (Merry et al., 2021). It is also true that even students who are reasonably proficient in the English language may need assistance with understanding discipline-specific language (Guler, 2022).

Understanding and affirmative support from faculty can be keys to building the self-confidence and academic performance of ethnically diverse students who speak English as an additional language (Everett, 2022). Choi (2019) studied the effects of student support groups on providing support to EAL students in nursing programs. Based on findings from those studies, Choi recommended developing discipline-specific student support groups that provide both academic and psychosocial support. Such support can be beneficial, as solely addressing the students' academic needs is not sufficient. EAL students also benefit academically from having a social network and sense of community to lessen their sense of isolation.

Guler (2022) also noted that many faculty report not feeling prepared to teach culturally and linguistically diverse students and need support to do so effectively. Faculty need to receive training and have access to those who have expertise in supporting EAL students so that they can meet the students' learning needs.

Diverse Faculty Role Models

A lack of racial, ethnic, and gender diversity among nursing faculty influences the profession's ability to recruit and retain diverse populations of students in undergraduate and graduate programs. Furthermore, the lack of diverse faculty can perpetuate a culture of insensitivity and lack of awareness of the learning needs of diverse students. Faculty need to embrace the cultural differences of their students and use available resources to foster a successful learning environment for all students. Faculty also need to receive training and support in learning how to best assess and meet the learning needs of the diverse students in their classrooms (Guler, 2022). Collaboration with campus ethnic student associations and organizations supporting LGBTQ+ students can assist faculty to promote learning among their culturally diverse student population. Furthermore, faculty can work to promote student success by offering access to role models, peer support and encouragement, tutoring and mentoring opportunities, and communication strategies for students of racial, ethnic, and gender diversities (Coleman et al., 2022; Holloway et al., 2019; Powers et al., 2018; Younas et al., 2019).

STRATEGIES TO INCREASE THE SUCCESS OF DIVERSE STUDENTS

Many nursing programs have created academic success initiatives that include strategies specific to course learning and learner motivation, coupled with retention and progression strategies. While recent reports (AACN, 2019;

National Academy of Medicine [NAM], 2021; NLN 2021a) continue to cite the need for increasing diversity in the nursing workforce, it is important for nurse educators to design curricula and use teaching–learning strategies that promote the success of diverse students. As previously noted, students with diverse learning needs have identified specific barriers encountered during nursing education experiences including discrimination from faculty, peers, nursing staff, and patients; feelings of isolation; and potential faculty bias in grading practices. Efforts to encourage and increase diversity in student nursing program enrollment cannot meet expected levels of achievement for retention and completion goals unless academic leaders and faculty work to create policies, environments, and practices that support equal opportunities for all students. Quality programs should consider and understand how diverse students experience nursing education so that these programs can identify strategies to overcome discriminatory practices and learning inequities (Graham et al., 2016).

Many nursing programs actively recruit a diverse, cross-cultural representation of students to provide opportunities for those called to nursing. In so doing, the programs also accept the responsibility to provide support services for these students, such as tutoring, mentoring, and campus life programs, including mixed group organizations that combine generations and/or ethnic clusters, to assist enrolled students through academic coursework and challenging campus environments. Good intentions, however, may not be effective when these services are not accessed by the students for whom the assistance is intended. Multiple demands on the students' time because of work schedules and family responsibilities create prioritization issues for many diverse students (McDonald et al., 2021).

Regardless, the three primary support areas that are most needed to enhance students' success are aligned with academic, social, and financial interventions. Clear communication of expectations, timely feedback, tutoring, planned and regular review sessions, more time for assignments, medical terminology and English preparatory courses, networking opportunities, academic advising, technical support, and financial aid information and budgeting sessions all fall under the umbrella of institutional commitment to the individual student (Ferrell & DeCrane, 2016; McNaughton-Cassill et al., 2021).

In addition to the important institutional commitment to supporting diverse and high-risk students, it is equally significant for nursing faculty to acknowledge students' perceptions of the need for emotional and moral support (van der Zanden et al., 2019). Faculty perception of students' needs can be markedly different from how students perceive their needs. Even when students meet educational goals and seemingly achieve appropriate outcomes, students may have very different perceptions of what occurred and those perceptions should be explored. Clearly, faculty support and the strategies created to support student learning are key to the retention and success of students. Support groups led by peer mentors (McNaughton-Cassill et al., 2021) and safe spaces for students from diverse backgrounds are integral to promoting diversity and inclusion, student support, and retention (Cordes, 2021). Efforts to enroll diverse, at-risk students must be actively supported with comprehensive educational practices along with sincere efforts to establish and promote meaningful and ongoing teaching–learning relationships that enhance outcomes. Strategies to support the success of diverse students can be directed toward admission processes, role model and mentoring programs, discipline-specific language support for EAL students, and creating a culture of inclusivity.

Admission Processes

The recruitment of a diverse student population in the nursing profession is an important issue, with many nursing programs directing considerable resources to recruit and admit diverse student bodies. However, equal, if not increased, efforts must be dedicated to assisting these students to achieve academic success so that they can be retained and successfully graduate (Lee et al., 2019; van der Zanden et al., 2019). It is important to acknowledge that many nursing programs continue to rely on standardized tests and grade point averages (GPAs) as criteria for admission. These types of recruitment strategies do not consider the educational experience of many minority students and constitute incomplete efforts to strategize for the success of diverse students when seeking admission to nursing school. It is painfully obvious to potential applicants who are socially or economically disadvantaged—particularly when a limited number of admission slots are available—that they may be excluded when admissions are determined by GPA alone. Such selection processes can lead to admission outcomes where only a few diversity students are admitted (Kilburn et al., 2019).

In 2017 the AACN stated that the traditional pool of nursing student applicants must be expanded to improve the quality of education, address persistent health care inequities, and enhance the potential for nursing students to become future leaders and introduced the concept of holistic admission in nursing education programs. It was recommended that nursing programs reduce their sole reliance on quantitative data for admitting students and consider additional qualitative criteria. Nonacademic factors such as motivation, leadership skills, professionalism, ability to work in teams, intercultural sensitivity, and organization ability are commonly evaluated through holistic admission (Hossler et al., 2019). Other prospective qualitative criteria to consider include the ability to overcome difficulties, life experiences, and how an applicant can contribute to the academic institution and the nursing profession (AACN, 2017). The use of holistic admission reviews for applicants is gaining support from both mainstream academic organizations and smaller colleges. For example, the American Association of Medical Colleges (AAMC, 2021) employs an integrated, holistic admission process incorporating a balance of experiences, attributes, and academic metrics (EAM) in the selection process of candidates. The AACN (2020) has published a white paper outlining promising practices that can help faculty implement holistic admissions reviews.

The adoption of holistic review processes by higher education institutions has led to positive outcomes related to increased diverse enrollments and improved graduation rates. For example, the Uniformed Services University of the Health Sciences (USU) revised admission practices in 2016 to include holistic admission review, which resulted in admission of a cohort markedly

---

CASE STUDY 2.2 Facilitating Success of Students with Diverse Backgrounds

A prelicensure nursing program has recently implemented holistic admission strategies to increase the diversity of the nursing student body. At the midpoint of the first term, a faculty member teaching fundamentals of nursing identifies that several students are not passing the course. Upon closer investigation, the faculty member identifies that the majority of the students in the course are nontraditional students and many are from diverse backgrounds. As the faculty member shares their findings in a faculty meeting, they state that they do not believe the holistic admission strategies are working out as planned. Other faculty members note that students from diverse backgrounds may need additional academic support. As the nursing faculty work to identify their role in facilitating student success, they explore the nursing literature to determine their role in facilitating success for students from diverse backgrounds.

1. What role does holistic reviews play in increasing the diversity of student populations in nursing programs?
2. What are common barriers that students from diverse backgrounds may face when studying nursing? What support strategies are available to address those issues?
3. What can faculty do to better understand the needs of students who are struggling academically? How can faculty facilitate their academic success?

---

different from previous cohorts that was more representative of the entirety of the Military Health Service in terms of demographics (Dong et al., 2020). Holistic reviews are tools to consider as first steps to add other success initiatives, such as first-year experience programs, academic early warning interventions, and other academic support programs (Case Study 2.2).

Role Models and Mentors

One means by which to support diverse students and increase retention is to identify role models and mentors who can help students be academically successful and envision a professional nursing career for themselves. Practicing nurses who are representative of racially, ethnically, and gender-diverse populations can be encouraged to serve as role models and mentors. Many nursing students plan to practice in a hospital or community setting after graduation, and matching them with a practicing nurse is a way to instill confidence in them that they can be successful. Nursing school faculty can work with their school's alumni association and with diverse nursing groups to provide role models for students.

In addition to practice role models, diverse students can also benefit from experiencing positive student–faculty relationships with faculty who are not responsible for assigning a grade to them. Using faculty mentors is one of the most important strategies that successfully aid in retention (Farruggia et al., 2020; Holloway et al., 2019; Mireles-Rios & Garcia, 2019). Other highly effective student–faculty centered strategies include faculty availability, faculty tutoring, and timely feedback on clinical performance and test performance (King et al., 2020; McNaughton-Cassill et al., 2021; Merry et al., 2021).

Faculty can also assist in the recruitment and retention of racial and ethnically diverse students by modeling a commitment to developing cultural competence among the faculty. Assessment of faculty cultural competence is an important step in gaining commitment and support for the value of working with racially and ethnically diverse students and colleagues. Cultural competence is an important concept to consider in role modeling and mentoring. See Chapter 17 for further discussion of the importance of cultural awareness and competence in multicultural education.

Faculty can also advocate for policies and procedures and support services that assist students and support an institutional faculty "mix" that is diverse. Faculty members need to remember that many diverse students feel isolated in their educational experience, and therefore faculty may need to be more assertive in establishing and maintaining open lines of communication with these students. Assisting students in accessing campus support services will help students feel more connected to the institution.

Academic Support Programs

Commitment to developing special support programs and encouraging active participation can increase the likelihood of academic success for diverse learners. The more faculty can share best practices and lessons learned about teaching and learning with diverse student populations, the more successful faculty will be in creating learning environments that promote the retention and graduation of students, allowing them to transition to active nursing practice (Freeman & All, 2017; Gubrud et al., 2017; Pritchard et al., 2020).

The implications for the development of success strategies and programs are implicit in the obligation nursing programs have for supporting the success of their enrolled students.

Pritchard et al. (2020) described a multifaceted program of resources to support the recruitment and retention of racially and ethnically diverse, underrepresented, and disadvantaged students. Freeman and All (2017) conducted a comprehensive review of research literature focused on support for at-risk students. Examples of support included in their review were academic coaching, one-on-one and group tutoring, mentoring and role modeling, review sessions by content experts, study skills, test-taking strategies, time management, psychosocial support, remediation interventions at key curriculum milestones, mandatory attendance policies, and structured learning assistance activities.

Additional support strategies for faculty to consider include early curriculum development of critical thinking skills; inclusion of academic support programs; the development of nondiscriminatory policies for the identification and coaching of at-risk students; and the adoption of supplemental materials such as tutorials and review modules. It is also important to garner student input through evaluations and direct conversations to determine what they perceive to be most helpful. (Ford & Mosley, 2020; Freeman & All, 2017).

Discipline-Specific Language Support

Support for improved English language proficiency can be provided in the form of language evaluation, academic networking, faculty interventions, and social activities to enhance students' success in nursing school (Merry et al., 2021). Perceptions regarding the link between reading comprehension and nursing student success are gaining greater attention in the evaluation of the specialized language used in nursing textbooks and applied in clinical practice.

Disciplinary literacy (DL) is the term that describes and recognizes the specialized language of nursing coursework, where early interventions are being employed to develop faculty understanding of disciplinary literacy principles. Such principles include developing teaching–learning adaptations to improve student language comprehension, employing coteaching models for nursing and science faculty to integrate disciplinary literacy principles in their course reading assignments, and using academic coaches to support student comprehension of reading materials and test-taking skills. Improvement of language skills for nursing students needs to venture beyond the traditional and fundamental applications of reading comprehension to the evaluation of general education research, such as disciplinary literacy, which has more specific applications to the science of nursing education (Elleman & Compton, 2017; Price & Fulmer, 2017).

Creating Inclusive Learning Environments

Although faculty may believe that their classrooms embrace cultural and societal neutrality, given all the discussion and research devoted to the needs of diverse learners, nurse educators need to embark on an honest assessment of institutional support for inclusive teaching and individual classroom strategies that engage in inclusive teaching, including a personal assessment of their cultural competencies (Gibbs & Culleiton, 2016; Gillson & Cherian, 2019).

Inclusive classrooms are ones in which students and educators work together to create and sustain an environment where students feel safe to express views, course content can be viewed from multiple perspectives, opinions can be expressed to the greater understanding of all concerned, and all lived experiences (student and faculty) can be shared and valued with equanimity (Gibbs & Culleiton, 2016).

To create an inclusive learning environment for student and faculty interactions, nurse educators must first recognize their own tendencies to stereotype students or hold biases and engage in activities to increase their understanding of diverse students' learning needs. Following this initial self-reflection, faculty can consider other factors that contribute to establishing an inclusive classroom. Considerations include having an understanding of to what degree class interactions can be affected by course content; prior assumptions and awareness of potential cultural issues in classroom settings; knowledge of diverse student backgrounds; and evolving issues, comments, and interactions that may occur during class sessions (Gibbs & Culleiton, 2016). Chapter 17 provides further discussion on multicultural education and promoting inclusivity in the classroom.

INFLUENCE OF STUDENT'S INDIVIDUAL CHARACTERISTICS ON ACADEMIC SUCCESS

College success is important to students because it demonstrates that they are achieving their long-term personal and career goals. Several student outcomes are associated with measuring academic success in college, including GPA, retention and degree completion, employment in fields associated with degree preparation, and attainment of life skills. An important question to be answered is what individual student characteristics are most likely to have an impact on student progress toward achieving these academic outcomes. What characteristics increase a student's likelihood of being successful in college? Individual student characteristics that can affect academic success can be categorized into three groups of variables: Academic achievement, circumstance, and personal.

Academic Achievement Variables

Academic achievement variables that can influence a student's success in the nursing curriculum are those variables that provide evidence of a history of learning achievements that demonstrate previous academic success. These variables include such data as high school GPA and scores from generalized aptitude tests like ACT and SAT. A record of successful completion of pre-requisite science courses is another academic variable that is considered to be a potential predictor of student academic success in nursing.

Circumstance Variables

Circumstance variables include socioeconomic status, geographical location, ethnicity, and other situational factors such as being a first-generation college student. The extent to which a student is engaged with or perceived to have a good fit with the institutional environment is considered to be a variable of circumstance. It is important to note that little can be done by the student to influence circumstance variables.

Personal Variables

Personal variables have also been found to be significantly linked to student outcomes. Personal variables influencing student success include motivation, self-confidence and self-efficacy, study habits, and problem solving (critical thinking and decision making). More recently, the concepts of grit and self-regulated learning and the relationship with academic achievement have been studied with varying results (Hagger & Hamilton, 2019).

Research in the past decade on self-control, grit, and other noncognitive attributes of success demonstrates that these attributes outperform talent and opportunity—though inconsistently—across age and types of achievement. It is important to recognize that self-control, grit, and self-regulation strategies can be taught (goal setting, planning) and situational strategies can make temptations less obvious, and over time these strategies can become habits (Duckworth & Seligman, 2017).

These habits can then contribute to student engagement and success as learners.

Grit

Grit is defined as the tenacious pursuit of a dominant superordinate goal in the face of setbacks over time and includes aspects of perseverance and consistency of interest (Credé et al., 2017; Duckworth & Gross, 2014). Therefore the essence of grit is the passion and determination when working toward a goal over time (Calo et al., 2019). Grit appears to represent a personal characteristic that may be associated with a student's tendency to be successful in certain academic contexts. Grit entails the use of self-discipline to pursue higher-level goals persistently over long stretches of time in the face of adversity or setbacks (Hagger & Hamilton, 2019). Grit can be measured in a variety of ways, with several questionnaires used to quantify grit, resilience, and mindset (Calo et al., 2019). A study of secondary school students demonstrated a relationship between grit, effort, and self-discipline with better grades (Hagger & Hamilton, 2019). Lam and Zhou (2021) also studied grit in relation to academic achievement and found mixed results, which may be attributable to cultural factors.

Self-Regulated Learning

Self-regulated learning is another related process through which students may take an active role in managing their motivation, engagement, and use of different cognitive learning strategies. Self-control is the capacity to regulate attention, emotion, and behavior in the presence of temptation. In contrast to grit, self-control is the resolution of conflict between two impulses to act, one corresponding to a goal that is of more immediate value and the other to a goal of more enduring value (Hagger & Hamilton, 2019). Prospective longitudinal studies have indicated that higher levels of self-control earlier in life predict later academic achievement and attainment. There was also some indication that high-school females may show higher levels of self-control than high-school males (Kuo et al., 2021; Meindl et al., 2019).

Positive Education

Positive psychology is an evidence-based approach that seeks to understand and develop human character strengths that allow people to cope better with adversity and in turn to flourish. Positive education is the application of positive psychology to all levels of education and can be used by educators to refocus on their traditional mission of character building and intellectual development. Positive education focuses on the student's academic success and well-being (Halliday et al., 2019).

LEARNING STYLE PREFERENCES

Another individual student characteristic that may influence learning is learning style. Learning styles can be defined as the ways in which learners gather and organize information, analyze and interpret it, and then store the knowledge for future use (Chick, 2010). Students have diverse learning style preferences. It has been commonly accepted that learners prefer to learn new knowledge in specific ways. Examples of individual learning style preferences include visual, aural, and kinesthetic strategies.

Competency 2, Facilitate Learner Development and Socialization, of the NLN's *Core Competencies for Academic Nurse Educators* (NLN, 2021d) states that educators have the responsibility to facilitate student development and socialization. One means by which to achieve this is by identifying students' individual learning style preferences and leveraging these preferences to meet the unique learning needs of students. However, studies that have attempted to correlate the use of learning style preferences with an increase in achieving learning outcomes have not produced strong evidence of correlation (Chick, 2010; Childs-Kean et al., 2020). Instead, researchers have suggested that faculty should put effort into matching instruction to the content they are teaching and the desired learning outcomes.

Despite the lack of consistent evidence that using learning style preferences increases learning, it is important for nurse educators to understand that students may have preferred ways of learning and that each classroom contains students with a mix of learning style preferences. Nurse educators are challenged to develop appropriate learning experiences to match content that will meet the various learning needs of their students (McMillan et al., 2020). Students may also find it helpful to understand their preferred learning style. Learning styles should be identified early in the nursing curriculum with the intent to empower individual students to understand their preferred ways of learning and use their knowledge, experience, and abilities to achieve positive learning outcomes and success on the licensure examination (Dozier et al., 2021).

There are numerous learning style frameworks and models that have been identified in the literature, along with instruments that can be used to assess a person's learning style preferences. While advocates of learning style models posit that students learn in different ways, there is a lack of evidence to support the notion that students *only* learn in those preferred ways or that learning styles differ based on gender, race, or ethnicity. Therefore the use of learning style inventories should be tempered and regarded as one guide to better understand students' learning needs. Studies have supported the idea that the use of multimodal methods of learning may help students regardless of learning style (Lee, 2019; Payaprom & Payaprom, 2020). Learning style preferences may change over time and vary according to the nature of learning taking place. An effective teacher will assist students to identify their learning style preferences and then will design learning experiences that engage students and appeal to various learning preferences.

Learning Style Frameworks and Models

Numerous theoretical frameworks, models, and instruments have been identified to describe and measure learning styles. Various models are categorized according to senses/acquiring information, such as visual, aural, read-write, kinesthetic (VARK, 2021) personality, such as Myers-Briggs Type Indicator (The Myers and Briggs Foundation, 2023); information processing and experience, such as Kolb Experiential Learning Profile (KELP) 2021; or environmental characteristics, such as the TruTalent Learning & Productivity survey, formerly known as the Productivity Environmental Preference Survey (PEPS) (Human eSources, 2022). Some of the most commonly used assessments of learning style preferences in nursing education literature are discussed further in the following paragraphs. Further explanations of other learning theories can be found in Chapter 14 and are not described here.

VARK

VARK is an acronym for visual, aural, read/write, and kinesthetic and was developed by Neil Fleming after observing more than 9,000 classes in the New Zealand education system in the 1980s. The instrument is designed to assess various ways in which an individual prefers to give and receive information while learning. Those with a strong Visual preference make best use of information in graphs, diagrams, charts, and maps. Those with a strong Aural preference use listening and speaking strategies. Those with a strong preference for Reading/Writing value handouts and notes, and those with a strong Kinesthetic preference make best use of experience and practice with simulations, models, and virtual reality (Chaudhry et al., 2020; Fleming, 2022). The 16-item instrument is available online and takes minutes to complete. Feedback on the student's preferred styles of communication is provided along with strategies derived from the student's preferences (http://vark-learn.com). Box 2.1 describes learning strategies that best correspond to the VARK learning preferences.

Myers-Briggs Type Indicator

The Myers-Briggs Type Indicator (MBTI), in use since 1962, is based on the theory of psychological types defined by C. J. Jung and defines 16 personality types via the use of 4 factors. The factors used by this model are extroversion/introversion; sensing/intuition; thinking/feeling; and judging/perceiving (http://www.myersbriggs.org/my-mbti-personality-type/mbti-basics). The factors described by the MBTI indicate preferences for the ways individuals take in or perceive and interpret information. The 93-item instrument is available online for a fee, and results are provided directly to the individual (https://www.myers-briggs.org/).

Kolb Model of Experiential Learning

The Kolb Model of Experiential Learning (Kolb, 1984) is an information-processing model that describes Kolb's learning cycle. As Kolb defines it, the learning circle includes four learning elements or modes through which learners process and learn information: Active experimentation or passive observation and concrete experiences or abstract conceptualization. An individual's preferred approach to learning (learning style) emerges through various combinations of these elements. The primary four learning styles were defined as diverging, assimilating, converging, and accommodating (Dantas & Cunha, 2020; Kolb & Kolb, 2021).

An individual's learning style can be assessed through Kolb's Learning Style Inventory (LSI). The Kolb LSI 4.0 has been one of the most commonly administered LSI's in nursing education. Kolb's LSI version 4.0 was revised in 2011 to include nine style typologies that better defined the unique patterns of individual learning styles. The nine new styles were initiating, experiencing, imagining, reflecting, analyzing, thinking, deciding, acting, and balancing. These styles were described as dynamic states that can flex to meet the demands of different learning situations. Recently, the Kolb LSI 4.0 instrument has been replaced by the Kolb Experiential Learning Profile (KELP) (Kolb & Kolb, 2021, https://learningfromexperience.com/downloads/research-library/kelp-2021-technical-specifications.pdf). The KELP is the latest version of the original LSI and is intended to be a self-reflection tool to help students better understand their own preferred approach to learning. Fig. 2.2 represents the KELP's nine learning styles corresponding to the four learning modes of experiencing, reflecting, thinking, and acting.

TruTalent Learning & Productivity Assessment

The Dunn et al. (1984, 1991, 2000) Productivity Environmental Preference Survey (PEPS), now known as the TruTalent Learning & Productivity

BOX 2.1	Learning Strategies Corresponding with VARK		
Visual	**Aural**	**Read/Write**	**Kinesthetic**
Diagrams and graphs	Debates	Books and texts	Cases
Designs	Discussions	Reading	Trial and error
Maps and charts	Stories	Note taking	Experiential exercises
	Guest speakers	All formats (online	Examples
	Chats	or print)	

Retrieved and adapted from http://vark-learn.com

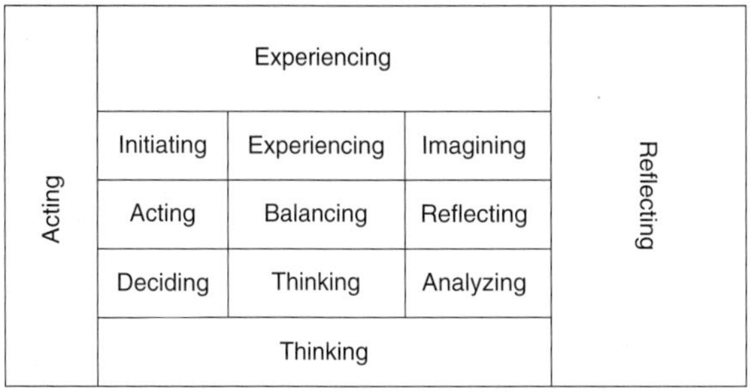

FIG. 2.2 Kolb Experiential Learning Profile (KELP). (From Institute of Experiential Learning. [2022]. Learning styles. https://experientiallearninginstitute.org/resources/learning-styles/)

BOX 2.2 TruTalent Learning & Productivity Preferences

Environment	Sensory	Mindset
Intake	Auditory	Focus
Time of day	Kinesthetic	Structure
Mobility	Tactile	Collaborative or
Sound	Visual	independent
Temperature	learning	Authority
Light		motivation
Physical setting		Self-motivation

Data from Human eSources. (2021). *TruTalent learning & productivity statistical analysis.* https://assets.humanesources.com/materials/TT-LearningProductivity-Statistical-Analysis.pdf.

Assessment (http://humanesources.com/ttlp/), provides information about patterns through which learning occurs. The theory underpinning the development of the TruTalent Learning & Productivity assessment is that students possess biologically based physical and environmental learning preferences that, along with well-established traits like emotional and sociological preferences, combine to form an individual learning style profile.

The TruTalent Learning & Productivity assessment was rebranded in 2018 to include 16 assessment factors divided into 3 preference areas: Environment, sensory, and mindset (Human eSources, 2021). See Box 2.2 for a listing of the preferences assessed in the TruTalent Learning & Productivity Assessment.

Facilitating Learning for students With Diverse Learning Styles

Faculty interested in knowing more about graduate and undergraduate nursing student learning style preferences are encouraged to assess student learning style preferences utilizing one of the many instruments available to help students develop an awareness of their preferred learning styles (Hampton et al., 2017). Using the results may also enhance the faculty's ability to select and design learning activities that appeal to a broad range of learner preferences.

Students are diverse in their experiences, cultural backgrounds, learning style preferences, and needs. A one-size-fits-all educational accommodation is likely to cause stress and discomfort for students if their individual uniqueness is not recognized and responded to instructionally. As a result of this diversity, it is unlikely that any single teaching style would be effective for all or most students in a class. Students may experience a difficult transition caused by the loss of individuality in large classes in which personal recognition is absent. To increase teaching effectiveness, faculty should employ a variety of creative and active teaching–learning approaches to engage the diversity of learners in larger classes.

It is also important for faculty to assist individual students to identify their learning style preferences, help them improve study habits, and aid them in the selection of courses or work environments that are compatible with their learning styles (Hampton et al., 2017; Piza et al., 2019). In class, simulation, and clinical settings faculty can use learning style preferences to create a learning environment where the different types of learner preferences are valued and accommodated and higher-order thinking is stimulated through the use of evidence-based teaching strategies (Piza et al., 2019).

ASSESSING THE LEARNING OUTCOMES OF DIVERSE STUDENTS

Nurse educators have a responsibility to prepare students to successfully meet program outcomes and graduate from the nursing program prepared to assume the nursing practice role for which they have been educated. To this end, it is important that faculty become adept at assessing student learning outcomes to determine if course assignments and chosen teaching–learning strategies are effectively addressing the learning needs of a diverse student population.

Faculty can use a variety of methods to assess learning outcomes, such as mind maps, simulation events and demonstration, problem-based learning and case studies, essays and reflective writing, and presentations. In undergraduate nursing programs the assessment technique most often used to measure student progress in achieving expected learning outcomes is objective and standardized testing. In some instances entire course grades, progression, and graduation are based solely on results of objective or standardized examinations, essentially creating high-stakes testing environments. These high-stakes tests are defined by the American Education Research Association (2014) as tests that have significant consequences for the test takers, curricula, or institution; the implications of their use are discussed further in Chapter 25. Strategies for assessing learning outcomes are presented in Chapter 24.

Additional types of assessments of learning outcomes include the use of high-impact educational practices, which have been described as "carefully constructed educational practices that promote myriad student outcomes" (Fassett & BrckaLorenz, 2021, p. 2). There are 11 evidence-based high-impact practices (HIPs) identified by the American Association of Colleges and Universities' (AAC&U's) Institute on High Impact Practices and Student Success that have been demonstrated to have positive impact on learning outcomes, especially for students who have been historically underserved in higher education (American Association of Colleges and Universities [AAC&U], 2022). These practices are identified in Box 2.3. Each of these practices provides students with opportunities to engage with faculty and peers while being immersed in experiential learning activities.

In a study of the quality of HIPs on student engagement and whether outcomes differed for students of diverse backgrounds, Zilvinskis (2019) notes that underserved students may benefit from high-impact educational practices, but the results were inconsistent due to inequities in how students experienced HIPs, leading the author to state that further study was warranted. This has implications for faculty and administrators who choose to implement HIPs designed to meet the learning needs of diverse student populations. Development of learning communities for health professions students, collaborative or team assignments, courses that explore cultural experiences or study/service abroad, co- or intracurricular service learning, and capstone projects to integrate and apply knowledge learned are examples of HIPs that nurse educators can design and evaluate with diverse learners to facilitate academic success among all students.

BOX 2.3 Positive Learning Practices

- First-Year Seminars or Experiences
- Common intellectual experiences
- Learning communities
- Writing intensive courses
- Collaborative assignments and projects
- Undergraduate research
- Diversity/Global learning
- Service learning/community-based learning
- ePortfolios
- Capstone courses and projects
- Internships

Data from American Association of Colleges & Universities. (2022). *High-impact educational practices.* https://www.aacu.org/trending-topics/high-impact

PREPARING DIVERSE LEARNERS FOR TRANSITION TO PRACTICE

The transition from education to practice is a stressful period for the new graduate. New graduates are faced with integrating the perceived expectations of their new role with the reality of being socialized into practice and unfamiliar organizational cultures in the practice setting. New graduates report heightened work stress caused by feelings of incompetence and anxiety (Hampton et al., 2020; Wildermuth et al., 2020). The IOM (2011) recommended that health care agencies support the transition to practice of new graduate nurses through the use of nurse residency programs (NRPs). Since that time, it has been increasingly recognized that there is a need for NRPs as a strategy to improve job satisfaction and reduce new nurse turnover (Shinners et al., 2021).

According to Meleis' (2010) transition theory, the success of transitions of any kind can be supported or hindered by a number of factors including personal, social, and community characteristics. Personal characteristics may include socioeconomic status and cultural beliefs; social characteristics may include stereotypes and stigma; and community characteristics include the presence of support from family, friends, and other influential individuals (Wildermuth et al., 2020). The influence of these various characteristics can potentially be applied to transition to nursing practice, but there is currently a lack of research identifying the variables that are most likely to contribute to the success of NRPs, especially those with diverse backgrounds. NRPs can assist in promoting novice nurses' health and wellbeing as they are mentored and supported during the transition to the role of the nurse. Surprisingly little literature exists about the transition-to-practice experience

of new graduates of diverse backgrounds. The transition needs of new graduates from diverse backgrounds, including racial, ethnic, and gender diversity, is an area that would benefit from further research. Current literature does suggest that transition programs such as NRPs, internships, and preceptorships can positively influence the transition experiences of new nurses and that academic-practice transition models should be pursued to support development of these programs (Hampton et al., 2020; Roush et al., 2021).

There is also evidence that transition programs that begin prior to graduation and continue post graduation can be effective in supporting new nurses (Roush et al., 2021). However, at this time, little consistency exists among the many different transition-to-practice programs, and further research is encouraged to identify what factors contribute to the success of transition to practice programs (Hampton et al., 2020). The responsibility of nurse educators to ensure the academic success of diverse learners extends to facilitating their success as they graduate and move into their first practice position. Chapter 6 further discusses residency programs for new graduates.

CHAPTER SUMMARY: KEY POINTS

- Disparity exists between the diversity of the general population and the diversity of nursing students and their faculty.
- Through use of holistic admission practices, the number of students with racial, ethnic, generational, and gender diversity may be admitted to schools of nursing, thus increasing the diversity among nursing students.
- As the increase in nursing student diversity is addressed, nursing education leaders are also challenged to recruit and retain a more diverse nursing faculty.
- By examining their conscious and unconscious bias as well as development of an awareness of diversity issues, nursing faculty can be better prepared to recruit, support, and retain nursing students from diverse backgrounds.
- Knowledge of the wide variety of preferred learning styles can enable nurse educators to

employ a range of teaching–learning strategies to address the various learning styles of their students and facilitate their academic success.
- Students are responsible for identifying and communicating the learning environments that will help them learn so that their individualized learning needs can be met.
- Inclusivity for students identifying as LGBTQ+ is enhanced by use of curricula that address care for LGTBQ+ individuals and also enhance health equity in nursing education.
- Understanding students' diverse learning needs will enable faculty and students to develop collaborative partnerships that foster the acquisition of the professional attitudes, knowledge, and skills necessary to transition into the nursing role for which they are being prepared.

■ REFLECTING ON THE EVIDENCE

1. Engage your colleagues and academic leaders in a discussion regarding the subject of implicit bias and its implications for nursing programs as they strive to achieve greater inclusivity within their programs and the nursing profession.

2. Assess available learning style instruments to determine which tools might best fit the needs of your students. How might you encourage students to identify their learning style preferences? How would you assist the students to use their knowledge of their preferred learning styles to align their preferences with learning strategies to support their academic success?

3. Nursing schools are beginning to adopt holistic admission processes as they strive to increase diversity within their programs. Research indicates positive gains in diversity of student body, learning environments, and student engagement with holistic admission processes. How can nursing faculty and administrators reduce barriers to the use of holistic nursing processes in schools of nursing?

REFERENCES

American Association of Colleges of Nursing. (2017). *Diversity, equity and inclusion in academic nursing.* https://www.aacnnursing.org/Portals/42/News/Position-Statements/Diversity-Inclusion.pdf

American Association of Colleges of Nursing. (AACN). (2019). Enhancing diversity in the nursing workforce. https://www.aacnnursing.org/Portals/42/News/Factsheets/Enhancing-Diversity-Factsheet.pdf

American Association of Colleges of Nursing. (2020). *Promising practices in holistic admissions review: Implementation in academic nursing.* https://www.aacnnursing.org/Portals/42/News/White-Papers/AACN-White-Paper-Promising-Practices-in-Holistic-Admissions-Review-December-2020.pdf

American Association of Medical Colleges. (2021). *Holistic admissions.* Retrieved from https://www.aamc.org/services/member-capacity-building/holistic-review

American Education Research Association. (2014). *Standards for educational and psychological testing.* American Education Research Association.

American Nurses Association. (2019). ANA position statement: The Nurse's role in addressing discrimination: Protecting and promoting inclusive strategies in practice settings, policy, and advocacy. *OJIN: The Online Journal of Issues in Nursing, 24*(3). https://doi.org/10.3912/OJIN.Vol24No03PoSCol01.

American Association of Colleges and Universities (AAC&U). (2022). *High-impact educational practices.* https://www.aacu.org/trending-topics/high-impact

Auxier, B., & Anderson, M. (2021). *Social media use in 2021.* Pew Research Center. Retrieved from https://www.pewresearch.org/internet/2021/04/07/social-media-use-in-2021/

Bernard, R., Rosales, M., & Zurcher, N. (2021). Exploring nursing students' motivation to prepare for class. *Nursing Education Perspectives, 43*(2). https://doi.org/10.1097/01.NEP.0000000000000833.

Blevins, S. (2021). Learning styles: The impact on education. *MEDSURG Nursing, 20*(4), 285–286.

Bui, K., & Rush, R. (2016). Parental involvement in middle school: Predicting college attendance for first-generation students. *Education, 136*(4), 473–489.

Bureau of Labor Statistics, U.S. Department of Labor. (2021). Occupational outlook handbook. In Registered nurses. Retrieved from http://www.bls.gov/ooh/healthcare/registered-nurses.htm

Calo, M., Peiris, C., Chipchase, L., Blackstock, F., & Judd, B. (2019). Grit, resilience and mindset in health students. *Clinical Teacher, 16*(4), 317–322.

Cantwell, E. R., Avallone, M., & Bowler, G. (2020). Using new careers in nursing research findings to develop an evidence-based pre-entry immersion program. *Journal of Professional Nursing, 36*(6), 490–496.

Chaudhry, N. A., Ashar, A., & Ahmad, S. A. (2020). Association of visual, aural, read/write, and kinesthetic (VARK) learning styles and academic performances of dental students. *Pakistan Armed Forces Medical Journal, 70*, S58–S63.

Chick, N. (2010). *Learning styles.* Vanderbilt University Center for Teaching. https://cft.vanderbilt.edu/guides-sub-pages/learning-styles-preferences/

Childs-Kean, L., Edwards, M., & Smith, M. D. (2020). Use of learning style frameworks in health science education. *American Journal of Pharmaceutical Education*, 84(7), 919–927.

Cho, S., & Jang, W. (2021). Do gender role stereotypes and patriarchal culture affect nursing students' major satisfaction? *International Journal of Environmental Research and Public Health*, 18(5), 1–9.

Choi, L. (2019). Continued influence of an English-as-an additional language nursing student support group. *Journal of Nursing Education*, 58(11), 647–652. https://doi.org/10.3928/01484834-20191021-06.

Chopin, S. M., Sheerin, C. M., & Meyer, B. L. (2020). Yoga for warriors: An intervention for veterans with comorbid chronic pain and PTSD. *Consulting Psychology Journal: Practice & Research*, 72(4), 888–896. https://doi.org/10.1037/tra0000649.

Christensen, M., Purkis, N., Morgan, R., & Allen, C. (2021). Does the nursing curriculum influence feelings of gender-role conflict in a cohort of nursing degree male students. *British Journal of Nursing*, 30(17), 1024–1030. https://doi.org/10.12968/bjon.2021.30.17.1024.

Chunta, K., Shellenbarger, T., & Chicca, J. (2021). Generation Z students in the online environment: Strategies for nurse educators. *Nurse Educator*, 46(2), 87–91. https://doi.org/10.1097/NNE.0000000000000872.

Coleman, C. (2020). Learnings through explorations of the teaching space: Creating climates of collaboration. *Teachers and Curriculum*, 20(1), 9–12.

Coleman, J., Harvey, N. R., & Pritchet, T. (2022). Factors contributing to success in nursing school: Experiences of African American BSN students. *Nursing Education Perspectives*, 43(2), 123–125. https://doi.org/10.1097/01.NEP.0000000000000854.

Cordes, C. C. (2021). Developing antiracist integrated health professionals. *Families, Systems, & Health*, 39(2), 404–407. https://doi.org/10.1037/fsh0000625.

Cottingham, M. D. (2019). The missing and needed male nurse: Discursive hybridization in professional nursing texts. *Gender, Work & Organization*, 26(2), 197–213. https://doi.org/10.1111/gwao.12333.

Coventry, T., & Hays, A. -M. (2021). Nurse manager's perceptions of mentoring in the multigenerational workplace: A qualitative descriptive study. *Australian Journal of Advanced Nursing*, 38(2), 34–43. https://doi.org/10.37464/2020.382.230.

Crandlemire, L. A. (2020). Unconscious bias and the impacts on caring: The role of the clinical nursing instructor. *International Journal for Human Caring*, 24(2), 84–91. https://doi.org/10.20467/HumanCaring-D-19-00048.

Credé, M., Tynan, M. C., & Harms, P. D. (2017). Much ado about grit: A meta-analytic synthesis of the grit literature. *Journal of Personality and Social Psychology*, 113(3), 492–511.

Dantas, L., & Cunha, A. (2020). An integrative debate on learning styles and the learning process. *Social Sciences and Humanities Open*, 2, 100017. https://doi.org/10.1016/j.ssaho.2020.100017.

DiMattio, M. J., & Hudacek, S. (2020). Educating generation Z: Psychosocial dimensions of the clinical learning environment that predict student satisfaction. *Nurse Education in Practice*, 49, 1–6. https://doi.org/10.1016/j.nepr.2020.102901.

Dong, T., Hutchinson, J., Torre, D., Durning, S. J., Artino, A. R., Schreiber-Gregory, D., Landoll, J., Pflipsen, M., Anderson, D., & Saguil, A. (2020). What influences the decision to interview a candidate for medical school? *Military Medicine*, 185(11/12), e1999–e2003. https://doi.org/10.1093/milmed/usaa237.

Dozier, A. L., Gilbert, B. G., Hughes, V. W., Mathis, D. P., & Jenkins, L. J. (2021). The use of active learning strategies during the COVID-19 pandemic to promote critical thinking. *ABNF Journal*, 32(1), 12–16.

Duckworth, A., & Gross, J. (2014). Self-control and grit: A related but separable determinants of success. *Current Directions in Psychological Science*, 23(5), 319–325.

Duckworth, A. L., & Seligman, M. E. P. (2017). The science and practice of self-control. *Perspectives on Psychological Science*, 12(5), 715–718. https://doi.org/10.1177/1745691617690880.

Dunn, R., Dunn, K., & Price, G. (1984, 1991, 2000). Productivity environmental preference survey. Price Systems.

Dyar, K. (2019). Veterans as students in higher education: A scoping review. *Nursing Education Perspectives*, 40(6), 333–337. https://doi.org/10.1097/01.

El-Banna, M., Tebbenhoff, B., Whitlow, M., & Wyche, K. F. (2017). Motivated strategies for learning in accelerated second-degree nursing students. *Nurse Educator*, 42(6), 308–312. https://doi.org/10.1097/NNE.0000000000000391.

Elleman, A., & Compton, D. (2017). Beyond comprehension strategy instruction. What's next? *Language, Speech & Services in Schools*, 48(2), 84–91.

Everett, M. C. (2022). Factors that affect the success of ethnically diverse nursing students: An integrative review of the literature. *Nursing Education Perspectives*, 43(2), 91–95.

Farruggia, S. P., Solomon, B., Back, L., & Coupet, J. (2020). Partnerships between universities and nonprofit transition coaching organizations to increase student success. *Journal of Community Psychology*, *48*(6), 1898–1912. https://doi.org/10.1002/jcop.22388.

Fassett, K., & BrckaLorenz, A. (2021). *Linking faculty involvement in high-impact practices to first-year student participation*. National Research Center for the First-Year Experience and Students in Transition, University of South Carolina. https://sc.edu/nrc/system/pub_files/1614103370_0.pdf

Ferrell, D., & DeCrane, S. (2016). S.O.S. (student/s optimal success). A model for institutional action to support minority nursing students. *Journal of Cultural Diversity*, *23*(2), 39–45.

Fleming, N. (2022). *VARK: A guide to learning styles*. http://www.vark-learn.com

Ford, C., & Mosley, L. (2020). Challenges to health professions education and strategies for moving forward. *New Directions for Teaching & Learning*, *2020*(122), 199–201. https://doi.org/10.1002/tl.20404.

Freeman, L., & All, A. (2017). Academic support programs utilized for nursing students at risk of academic failure: A review of the literature. *Nursing Education Perspective*, *38*(2), 69–74. https://doi.org/10.1097/01.NEP0000000000000089.

Fruiht, V., & Chan, T. (2018). Naturally occurring mentorship in a national sample of first-generation college goers: A promising portal for academic and developmental success. *American Journal of Community Psychology*, *61*(3/4), 386–397. https://doi.org/10.1002/ajcp.12233.

Fry, R. (2020). *Millennials overtake Baby Boomers as America's largest generation*. https://www.pewresearch.org/fact-tank/2020/04/28/millennials-overtake-baby-boomers-as-americas-largest-generation/.

Fry, R. (2021). *First-generation college graduates lag behind their peers on key economic outcomes*. https://www.pewresearch.org/social-trends/2021/05/18/first-generation-college-graduates-lag-behind-their-peers-on-key-economic-outcomes/

Graham, C., Phillips, S., Newman, S., & Atz, T. (2016). Baccalaureate minority nursing students perceived barriers and facilitators to clinical education practices: An integrative review. *Nursing Education Perspectives*, *37*(3), 130–137.

Gibbs, D., & Culleiton, A. (2016). A project to increase educator cultural competence in mentoring at-risk nursing students. *Teaching and Learning in Nursing*, *11*, 118–125.

Gillson, S., & Cherian, N. (2019). The importance of teaching cultural diversity in baccalaureate nursing education. *Journal of Cultural Diversity*, *26*(3), 85–88.

Greene, N. R., Jewell, D. E., Fuentes, J. D., & Smith, C. V. (2019). Basic need satisfaction in the parental relationship offsets millennials' worries about the transition to college. *Journal of Social Psychology*, *159*(2), 125–137. https://doi.org/10.1080/00224545.2019.1570905.

Gubrud, P., Spencer, A., & Wagner, L. (2017). From start-up to sustainability: A decade of collaboration to shape the future of nursing. *Nursing Education Perspectives*, *38*(5), 225–232. https://doi.org/10.1097/01.NEP.00000000000000212.

Guler, N. (2022). Teaching culturally and linguistically diverse students: Exploring the challenges and perceptions of nursing faculty. *Nursing Education Perspectives*, *43*(1), 11–13. https://doi.org/10.1097/01.NEP.0000000000000861.

Guy, M., & van der Krogt, S. (2021). Supporting male nursing students—What works best? *Kai Tiaki Nursing New Zealand*, *27*(2), 22–24.

Hadden, I. R., Easterbrook, M. J., Nieuwenhuis, M., Fox, K. J., & Dolan, P. (2020). Self-affirmation reduces the socioeconomic attainment gap in schools in England. *The British Journal of Educational Psychology*, *90*(2), 517–536. https://doi.org/10.1111/bjep.12291.

Hagger, M. S., & Hamilton, K. (2019). Grit and self-discipline as predictors of effort and academic attainment. *British Journal of Educational Psychology*, *89*(2), 324–342. https://doi.org/10.1111/bjep.12241.

Halliday, A., Kern, M., Garrett, D., & Turnbull, D. (2019). The student voice in well-being: A case study of participatory action research in positive education. *Educational Action Research*, *27*(2), 173–196. https://doi.org/10.1080/09650792.2018.1436079.

Hampton, D., Pearce, P. F., & Moser, D. K. (2017). Preferred methods of learning for nursing students in an on-line degree program. *Journal of Professional Nursing*, *33*(1), 27–37.

Hampton, K., Smeltzer, S., & Ross, J. (2020). Evaluating the transition from nursing student to practicing nurse: An integrative review. *Journal of Professional Nursing*, *36*(6), 551–559. https://doi.org/10.1016/j.profnurs.2020.08.002.

Health Resources and Services Administration. (2021). *Veterans*. https://www.hrsa.gov/veterans/index.html

Holloway, I. W., Ochoa, A. M., Wu, E. S. C., Himmelstein, R., Wong, J. O., Wilson, B. D. M., & Miyashita Ochoa, A. (2019). Perspectives on academic mentorship from sexual and gender minority students pursuing careers in the health sciences. *American Journal of Orthopsychiatry, 89*(3), 343–353.

Hossler, D., Chung, E., Kwon, J., Lucido, J., Bowman, N., & Bastedo, M. (2019). A study of the use of nonacademic factors in holistic undergraduate admissions reviews. *Journal of Higher Education, 90*(6), 833–859. https://doi.org/10.1080/00221546.2019.1574694.

Human eSources. (2021). *Productivity Environmental Preferences Survey (PEPS) areas*. https://www.humanesources.com/research/peps-areas/

Human eSources. (2022). *TruTalent Learning & Productivity*. https://www.humanesources.com/ttlp/

Hurlbut, J., & Revuelto, I. (2018). Transitioning veterans into a BSN pathway: Building the program from the ground up to promote diversity and inclusion. *Med-Surg Nursing, 27*(4), 266–269.

Institute of Experiential Learning. (2022). *Kolb Experiential Learning Profile (KELP)*. https://experientiallearninginstitute.org/programs/assessments/kolb-experiential-learning-profile/

Jamieson, I., Harding, T., Withington, J., & Hudson, D. (2019). Men entering nursing: Has anything changed. *Nursing Praxis in New Zealand, 35*(2), 18–29. https://doi.org/10.36951/ngpxnz.2019.007.

Kavuran, E., & Kasikci, M. (2018). Determination of nursing students' perspectives at Ataturk University Health Sciences Faculty on gender equality. *International Journal of Caring Sciences, 11*(1), 108–117.

Keener, A. (2020). An examination of psychological characteristics and their relationship to academic entitlement among millennial and nonmillenial college students. *Psychology in the Schools, 57*(4), 572–582. https://doi.org/10.1002/pits.22338.

Kilburn, F., Hill, L., Porter, M. D., & Pell, C. (2019). Inclusive recruitment and admissions strategies increase diversity in CRNA educational programs. *AANA Journal, 87*(5), 379–389.

King, R., Ryan, T., Wood, E., Tod, A., & Robertson, S. (2020). Motivations, experiences and aspirations of trainee nursing associates in England: A qualitative study. *BMC Health Services Research, 20*(1), 1–12.

Kolawole, I. O., Andrew, A., & Evelyn Olorunda, M. O. (2019). Knowledge and attitude of registered and student nurses on mentor-mentee relationship in specialist hospital, Yola. *International Journal of Caring Sciences, 12*(3), 1734–1743.

Kolb, D. (1984). *Experiential learning: Experience as the source of learning and development*. Prentice Hall.

Kolb, A., & Kolb, D. (2021). *The Kolb experiential learning profile: A guide to experiential learning theory, KELP psychometrics and research on validity*. Experience Based Learning Systems, LLC. https://learningfromexperience.com/downloads/research-library/kelp-2021-technical-specifications.pdf

Kuo, Y. -L., Casillas, A., Allen, J., & Robbins, S. (2021). The moderating effects of psychosocial factors on achievement gains: A longitudinal study. *Journal of Educational Psychology, 113*(1), 138–156. https://doi.org/10.1037/edu0000471.

Lam, K. K. L., & Zhou, M. (2021). Grit and academic achievement: A comparative cross-cultural meta-analysis. *Journal of Educational Psychology* https://doi.org/10.1037/edu0000699.supp. (Supplemental).

Lee, J., Kim, N., & Wu, Y. (2019). College readiness and engagement gaps between domestic and international students: Re-envisioning educational diversity and equity for global campus. *Higher Education, 77*(3), 505–523. https://doi.org/10.1007/s10734-018-0284-8. (00181560).

Lee, Y. (2019). Integrating multimodal technologies with VARK strategies for learning and teaching EFL presentation: Am investigation into learner' achievements and perceptions of the learning process. *Australian Journal of Applied Linguistics, 2*(1), 17–31. https://doi.org/10.29140/ajal.v2n1.118.

Lewis-Pierre, L. (2019). Preparing for the next generation of educators and nurses: Implications for recruitment and educational innovations. *ABNF Journal, 30*(2), 35–36.

Maykut, C. A., Dressler, M., & Newell-Killeen, H. (2021). Fostering successful transitioning to practice: Responding to the covid crisis. *International Journal of Caring Sciences, 14*(1), 760–766. http://www.internationaljournalofcaringsciences.org/docs/81_colleen_special_14_1-2.pdf.

McDonald, D., Baker, S., & Shulsky, D. (2021). Against the professorial odds: Barriers as building blocks for educational advancement. *Journal of Advanced Academics, 32*(1), 92–131. https://doi.org/10.1177/1932202X20966569.

McMillan, L., Johnson, T., Parker, F., Hunt, C., & Boyd, D. (2020). Improving student learning outcomes through a collaborative higher education partnership. *International Journal of Teaching and Learning in Higher Education, 32*(1), 117–124.

McNaughton-Cassill, M. E., Lopez, S., Knight, C., Perrotte, J., Mireles, N., Cassill, C. K., Silva, S., & Cassill, A. (2021). Social support, coping, life satisfaction, and academic success among college students. *Psi Chi Journal of Psychological Research, 26*(2), 150–156.

McNeal, G. J., Tontz, P. A., Smith, T. C., Reyes, J., & Parsons, A. (2019). A pilot intervention using professional nursing mentoring to engage prior corpsman and medic nursing students in academic success. *ABNF Journal*, 30(3), 74–80.

Medina, M., Pettinger, T., Niemczyk, M., & Burnworth, M. (2021). Teaching A to Z for a new generation of pharmacy learners. *American Journal of Health-System Pharmacy*, 78(14), 1273–1276. https://doi.org/10.1093/ajhp/zxab174.

Meindl, P., Yu, A., Galla, B. M., Quirk, A., Haeck, C., Goyer, J. P., Lejuez, C. W., D'Mello, S. K., & Duckworth, A. L. (2019). A brief behavioral measure of frustration tolerance predicts academic achievement immediately and two years later. *Emotion (Washington, D.C.)*, 19(6), 1081–1092.

Meleis, A. I. (2010). *Transitions theory: Middle range and situation specific theories in nursing research and practice*. Springer.

Merry, L., Vissandjée, B., & Verville-Provencher, K. (2021). Challenges, coping responses and supportive interventions for international and migrant students in academic nursing programs in major host countries: A scoping review with a gender lens. *BMC Nursing*, 20(1), 1–37. https://doi.org/10.1186/s12912-021-00678-0.

Mireles-Rios, R., & Garcia, N. M. (2019). What would your ideal graduate mentoring program look like?: Latina/o student success in higher education. *Journal of Latinos & Education*, 18(4), 376–386. https://doi.org/10.1080/15348431.2018.1447937.

Morris, M., Cooper, R. L., Ramesh, A., Tabatabai, M., Arcury, T. A., Shinn, M., Im, W., Juarez, P., & Matthews-Juarez, P. (2019). Training to reduce LGBTQ-related bias among medical, nursing, and dental students and providers: A systematic review. *BMC Medical Education*, 19(1), 325. https://doi.org/10.1186/s12909-019-1727-3.

Murray, B. P. (2020). Language and adjustment anxieties of first-year college student English language learners. *Journal of Behavioral & Social Sciences*, 7(2), 119–136.

The Myers and Briggs Foundation. (2023). Myers-Briggs Type Indicator. Retrieved from https://www.myersbriggs.org/my-mbti-personality-type/mbti-basics/

National Academy of Medicine. (2021). *The future of nursing 2020–2030: Charting a path to achieve health equity*. https://www.nationalacademies.org/our-work/the-future-of-nursing-2020-2030

National League for Nursing. (2021a). National league for nursing public policy agenda 2021–2022. https://www.nln.org/docs/default-source/uploadedfiles/advocacy-public-policy/nln-public-policy-agenda-final.pdf

National League for Nursing. (2021b). NLN faculty census survey 2020–2021. https://www.nln.org/nln-faculty-census-suvey-2020-2021

National League for Nursing (2021c). Biennial survey of schools of nursing, academic year, 2019–2020: Percentage of students in nursing program by gender and type, 2020. https://www.nln.org/news/research-statistics/newsroomnursing-education-statistics/nln-biennial-survey-of-schools-of-nursing-2019-2020-5383cd5c-7836-6c70-9642-ff00005f0421

National League for Nursing. (2021d). *NLN core competencies for academic nurse educators*. Retrieved from https://www.nln.org/education/nursing-education-competencies/core-competencies-for-academic-nurse-educators

National League for Nursing, (2020). *The scope of practice for academic nurse educators and academic clinical nurse educators (3rd ed.)*. Wolters Kluwer.

National Center for Education Statistics. (2018, February 8). *Stats in brief*. First-generation students: College access, persistence, and post bachelor's outcomes. https://nces.ed.gov/pubsearch/pubsinfo.asp?pubid=2018421

National Center for Education Statistics (NCES). (2021, May). *Loans for undergraduate students*. https://nces.ed.gov/programs/coe/indicator/cub

Padiha, J., Machado, P., Ribeiro, A., Ramos, J., & Costa, P. (2019). Clinical virtual simulation in nursing education: Randomized controlled trial. *Journal of Medical Internet Research*, 21(3). https://doi.org/10.2196/11529.

Payaprom, S., & Payaprom, Y. (2020). Identifying learning styles of language learners: A useful step in moving towards the learner-centred approach. *Journal of Language and Linguistic Studies*, 16(1), 59–72. https://10.17263/jlls.712646.

Phillips, L. T., Stephens, N. M., Townsend, S. S. M., & Goudeau, S. (2020). Access is not enough: Cultural mismatch persists to limit first-generation students' opportunities for achievement throughout college. *Journal of Personality and Social Psychology*, 119(5), 1112–1131. https://doi.org/10.1037/pspi0000234.

Piza, F., Kesselheim, J. C., Perzhinsky, J., Drowos, J., Gillis, R., Moscovici, K., Danciu, T. E., Kosowska, A., & Gooding, H. (2019). Awareness and usage of evidence-based learning strategies among health professions students and faculty. *Medical Teacher*, 41(12), 1411–1418.

Powers, K., Herron, E., Sheeler, C., & Sain, A. (2018). The lived experience of being a male nursing student: Implications for student retention and success. *Journal of Professional Nursing, 34*(6), 475–482. https://doi.org/10.1016/j.profnurs.2018.04.002.

Price, C., & Fulmer, E. (2017). Implementing a nursing literacy initiative to address the needs of students in a licensed practical nursing program. *Teaching & Learning in Nursing, 12*(4), 258–262.

Pritchard, T. J., Glazer, G., Bankston, K. D., & McGinnis, K. (2020). Leadership 2.0: Nursing's next generation: Lessons learned on increasing nursing student diversity. *Online Journal of Issues in Nursing, 25*(2).

Reynolds, J. R., & Parrish, M. (2018). Natural mentors, social class, and college success. *American Journal of Community Psychology, 61*(1–2), 179–190.

Ricks, J., & Warren, J. (2021). Transitioning to college: Experiences of successful first-generation college students. *Journal of Educational Research and Practice, 11*(1), 1–15. https://doi.org/10.5590/JERAP.2021.11.1.01.

Roksa, J., & Kinsley, P. (2019). The role of family support in facilitating academic success of low-income students. *Research in Higher Education, 60*(4), 415–436. https://doi.org/10.1007/s11162-018-9517-z.

Roush, K., Opsahl, A., & Ferren, M. (2021). Developing an internship program to support nursing student transition to clinical setting. *Journal of Professional Nursing, 37*(4), 696–701. https://doi.org/10.1016/j.profnurs.2021.04.001.

Schlee, R., Eveland, V., & Harich, K. (2020). From Millennials to Gen Z: Changes in student attitudes about group projects. *Journal of Education for Business, 95*(3), 139–147. https://doi.org/10.1080/08832323.2019.1622501.

Shepherd, J. (2020). Generational differences in learning style preferences among adult learners in the United States. *Journal of Behavioral & Social Sciences, 7*(2), 137–159.

Shinners, J., Africa, L., Mallory, C., & Durham, H. (2021). Versant's nurse residency program: A retrospective review. *Nursing Economics, 39*(5), 239–246.

Sikes, D. L., Patterson, B. J., Chargualaf, K., Elliott, B., Song, H., Boyd, J., & Armstrong, M. (2021). Predictors of student veterans progression and graduation in Veteran to Bachelor of Science in Nursing (VBSN) programs: A multisite study. *Journal of Professional Nursing, 37*(3), 632–639. https://doi.org/10.1016/j.profnurs.2021.03.008.

Sinacori, B., & Williams-Gregory, M. (2021). The effect of distance learning on knowledge acquisition in undergraduate second-degree nursing students: A systematic review. *Nursing Education Perspectives, 42*(3), 136–141.

Smiley, R., Ruttinger, C., Oliveira, C., Hudson, L., Allgeyer, R., Reneay, K., & Silvetre, J. (2021). The 2020 national nursing workforce survey. *Journal of Nursing Regulation, 12*(1), S1–S96. https://doi.org/10.1016/S2155-8256(21)00027-2.

Soriano, F. M., & Alonso, B. E. (2020). Why have I failed? Why have I passed? A comparison of students' causal attributions in second language acquisition (A1–B2 levels). *British Journal of Educational Psychology, 90*(3), 648–662. https://doi.org/10.1111/bjep.12323.

Stultzer, K. (2019). Generational differences and multigenerational teamwork. *Critical Care Nurse, 39*(1), 78–81. https://doi.org/10.4037/ccn2019163.

Sun, Q. (2019). Conspiring to change the learning environment for adult learners in higher education. *Adult Learning, 30*(2), 89–90.

Tolarba, J. (2021). Virtual simulation in nursing education: A systematic review. *International Journal of Nursing Education, 13*(3), 48–54.

U.S. Census Bureau. (2019). *Quickfacts: Population estimates, July 1, 2019.* https://www.census.gov/quickfacts/fact/table/US/PST045219

U.S. Census Bureau. (2020). Demographic turning points for the United States: Population projections for 2020 to 2060. https://www.census.gov/content/dam/Census/library/publications/2020/demo/p25-1144.pdf

U.S. Veterans Administration. (2021). Education and training: Forever GI Bill – Harry W. Colmery Veterans Educational Assistance Act. https://www.benefits.va.gov/gibill/forevergibill.asp

Van Der Wege, M., & Keil, S. (2019). Answering the call of the nursing profession. *Kansas Nurse, 94*(2), 12–14.

van der Zanden, P. J. A. C., Denessen, E., Cillessen, A. H. N., & Meijer, P. C. (2019). Patterns of success: First-year student success in multiple domains. *Studies in Higher Education, 44*(11), 2081–2095.

VARK. (2021). *The VARK questionnaire.* https://vark-learn.com/the-vark-questionnaire/

Vizcaya-Moreno, M. F., & Pérez-Cañaveras, R. M. (2020). Social media used and teaching methods preferred by Generation Z Students in the nursing clinical learning environment: A cross-sectional research study. *International Journal of Environmental Research and Public Health, 17*(21). https://doi.org/10.3390/ijerph17218267.

Wilbur, K., Snyder, C., Essary, A., Swapna, R., Will, K., & Saxon, M. (2020). Developing workforce diversity in the health professions: A social justice perspective. *Science Direct, 6*(2020), 222–229. https://doi.org/10.1016/j.hpe.2020.01.002.

Wildermuth, M. M., Weltin, A., & Simmons, A. (2020). Transition experiences of nurses as students and new graduate nurses in a collaborative nurse residency program. *Journal of Professional Nursing, 36*(1), 69–75. https://doi.org/10.1016/j.profnurs.2019.06.006.

Yee, A. (2016). The unwritten rules of engagement: Social class differences in undergraduates' academic strategies. *The Journal of Higher Education, 87*(6), 831–858.

Younas, A., Sundus, A., Zeb, H., & Sommer, J. (2019). A mixed methods review of male nursing studetns' challenges during nursing education and strategies to tackle these challenges. *Journal of Professional Nursing, 35*(4):260–276. https://doi.org/10.1016/j.profnurs.2019.01.008.

Yu, H., Huang, C., Chin, Y., Shen, Y., Chiang, Y., Chang, C., & Lou, J. (2021). The mediating effects of nursing professional commitment on the relationship between social support, resilience, and intention to stay among newly graduated male nurses: A cross-sectional questionnaire survey. *International Journal of Environmental Research and Public Health, 18*(14). https://doi.org/10.3390/ijerph18147546.

Zilvinskis, J. (2019). Measuring quality in high-impact practices. *Higher Education (00181560), 78*(4), 687–709. https://doi.org/10.1007/s10734-019-00365-9.

3

The Academic Performance of Students
Legal and Ethical Issues

Linda S. Christensen, EdD, JD, RN, CNE, FAAN

Nursing faculty have many considerations in performing their roles as academic nurse educators. Developing curriculum content, choosing teaching strategies, developing student evaluation plans, and dealing with current academic issues can be major areas of focus. However, in carrying out these functions, faculty must also consider the legal and ethical concepts that influence the process and product of nursing education.

Just as nurses in practice have legal and ethical guidelines, nurse educators also have legal and ethical guidelines. Nursing faculty are responsible for understanding the broad legal and ethical principles that apply in all circumstances and those that are specific to their own academic educator practice. Major problems can occur if faculty lack an understanding of these principles and are unable to apply them appropriately.

Many potential problems can be avoided if faculty take a proactive approach to anticipate student concerns. Faculty members who treat students with respect, provide honest and frequent communication about progress toward course goals and objectives, and are fair and considerate in evaluating performance are less likely to encounter student challenges. A learning environment that supports student growth and questioning is likely to reduce the incidence of problems, especially litigation. Nurse educators must have an awareness of the legal issues and regulations for their practice, and they must implement this knowledge within their role as an academic nurse educator. Suggestions for avoiding such problems are discussed later in this chapter.

The goal of the educational experience remains that students develop knowledge, skills, and values that will enable them to provide safe, effective nursing care. Nursing faculty who are able to apply general legal and ethical principles are much more likely to play their part in effectively meeting that goal.

This chapter provides an overview of the most common legal and ethical issues related to student academic performance that nurse educators face in the classroom and clinical setting. The chapter includes a discussion of the importance of student–faculty interactions and the legal and ethical issues related to academic performance, including the provision of due process, the student appeal process, assisting the failing student, academic dishonesty, and special issues affecting practice as an academic nurse educator.

STUDENT–FACULTY INTERACTIONS

The student–faculty relationship that is developed during the teaching and learning process is a very important one. Students have often identified student–faculty relationships as the relationships that most often affect learning. There is little doubt that a positive interaction between faculty and students is likely not only to decrease legal issues but also to promote student success.

The significance of this relationship has been well noted over many years. Mutual trust and respect have been identified as the basis for an effective relationship between the instructor and the student (Gaberson et al., 2022). Bastable (2021) noted that multiple relationship systems influence the students' motivation, and the teacher–learner interaction is one of the significant relationships that can influence learning either positively or negatively. The National League for Nursing (NLN) has identified the importance of establishing a positive relationship multiple times over the past several years. The NLN has long maintained that the focus of the faculty should be on establishing a learning environment that is "characterized by collaboration, understanding, mutual trust, respect, equality, and acceptance of differences" (NLN, 2005, p. 4). Such a learning environment fosters professional growth and development on the part of the nurse.

The NLN clearly identified the importance of the student–faculty relationship within the *Core Competencies of Nurse Educators* (NLN, 2020a). The importance of interpersonal interactions on learner outcomes is noted (Caputi, 2019) specifically in NLN Competency II, which is focused on facilitating learning development and socialization.

Faculty in the classroom and in clinical settings encounter students whose backgrounds and learning needs are extremely diverse. Faculty who are able to address the needs of students from an educational perspective and establish positive interpersonal relationships with students of varied backgrounds will make positive contributions in assisting students to meet the desired outcomes. The challenge for faculty in assisting students is to identify ways to address these varied needs. To successfully assist students, faculty must understand and appreciate cultural diversity and be able to use multiple learning strategies to assist students with varying learning styles and needs. The student role in the educational process has changed and must be one of active involvement. When faculty view students as partners or colleagues in an educational experience, they promote the development of a relationship that supports student growth and development and the attainment of educational goals and objectives.

The first step in the process of developing a learning environment that encourages collaborative and positive student–faculty interactions requires faculty to carefully examine and develop an awareness of their own beliefs and values about the teaching–learning process. Working collaboratively with students will require faculty to adopt strategies that involve active student participation and do not place faculty in the role of having sole responsibility for determining learning experiences. Activities such as cooperative group work, debate and discussion, role playing, and problem-solving exercises are examples of interactive teaching strategies that shift the focus from the faculty to the student. Such a pedagogical shift in teaching may also require faculty to leave behind the "safety" and control of the classroom lecture and develop more fully the skills necessary to successfully incorporate interactive teaching strategies in the classroom. Chapter 16 provides further discussion of teaching strategies that promote active learning.

Another important step in the process of developing a positive learning environment is examining attitudes and beliefs that students bring to the learning environment. Students may lack confidence in their abilities in the academic environment, especially those who are first-generation college students without role models who have been successful in pursuing higher education. Empowerment of students can occur when faculty demonstrate a sense of caring and commitment to students and use courtesy and respect in interactions. Having a role in developing their own learning experiences can also prove to be an empowering experience for students.

How can nursing faculty successfully incorporate this concept of empowerment and equity into student–faculty relationships? Educators can provide a variety of motivational factors that will support students in meeting their specific learning needs (Bastable, 2021). Learning activities can be designed to promote positive faculty–student interactions. For example, the use of computer-mediated communication, such as email and online discussion forums, tends to remove the elements of status and power from communication, thus allowing a freer exchange of information. The use of learning laboratories introduces realism into student learning to promote preparation for actual patient care experiences (Oermann, 2017). Integrating content and discussion about empowerment, collaboration, collegiality, and teamwork throughout the curriculum can also help nurture positive student–faculty interactions. Ongoing, open dialogue with students that results in clear communication of mutual expectations and responsibilities is an essential component of all successful student–faculty interactions, as is illustrated in the rest of this chapter.

LEGAL CONSIDERATIONS OF STUDENT PERFORMANCE

An established responsibility of faculty in nursing education programs is the evaluation of student performance in the classroom (didactic) and clinical setting. This responsibility carries with it accountability because the outcomes of such evaluation have a major effect on the student's progress in the course and even status in the program. In addition, faculty serve as the safeguard for society at large from practitioners who have not demonstrated the ability to practice safely. In a precedent-setting case, the court clearly set the standard that it will not interfere with academic decision making regarding student progress and content (*Board of Curators of the University of Missouri v. Horowitz*, 1978). Other courts continue to follow the Horowitz court by repeatedly affirming faculty members' responsibility for evaluation as long as due process has been provided and there is no finding of arbitrary or capricious facts. However, to ensure due process and avoid being viewed as arbitrary or capricious, the evaluation process must be based on principles that ensure students' rights are not violated.

Student Rights

Faculty must be aware that students enter the educational experience with rights, just as faculty have rights. A few decades ago, it would have been rare to find litigation involving a nursing student and the nursing program, but litigation involving nursing programs has dramatically increased. Many cases involving student litigation within nursing programs have their legal basis in the concepts of due process, fair treatment, contract law, and confidentiality and privacy.

Due Process

Due process is a term that is frequently used in education and may be misunderstood. The general concept of *due process* is based in fairness and is intended to ensure that certain rights are respected within the particular situation. There are two types of due process. *Substantive due process* refers to the fairness of the "outcome" in relation to the "infraction." In other words, does the punishment fit the crime? It would most likely be a breach of substantive due process to dismiss a student from a course because he or she arrived a few minutes late to class. The second type of due process is *procedural due process*. Procedural due process ensures that the accused will receive notice and an opportunity to be heard. Providing the student with a clear notice of the potential issue and providing the student with the opportunity to present his or her side of the situation is essential to meet the procedural due process requirements.

Student rights in the broadest sense are protected by the Fifth and Fourteenth Amendments of the US Constitution, which limit the restrictions that can be imposed on an individual. These amendments state that no citizen may be deprived of life, liberty, or property without due process of law and require that the federal government provide due process for all citizens (U.S. Const. amend. V & XIV).

Although the Fourteenth Amendment includes language referring to state or government actions (which includes public institutions), the principles of due process are applied by the courts to all educational settings. Within the educational setting, a 1961 case applied the principles of due process to a situation in which students were dismissed without notice and without a hearing (*Dixon v. Alabama State Board of Education*, 1961). In *Dixon*, Alabama State College, which was a segregated black college, expelled six students for unspecified reasons without a hearing, although the presumptive cause was that they participated in civil rights demonstrations. The appeals court ruled that a public college could not expel them without a public hearing. The judicial system expanded the holding of the *Dixon* case with *Goss v. Lopez* (1975), when the court clearly noted that the due process protections of *Dixon* applied to all students facing expulsion from a public institution, regardless of whether the institution is a grade school, high school, or college or university.

The legal principle of due process has been extended to cases involving private college and university settings, upholding the student's due process rights regardless of attendance at a public or private institution (Kaplin & Lee, 2020).

Student due process rights have their foundation in two types of due process: Procedural due process and substantive due process. Procedural due process refers to a step-by-step process that includes both notice and an opportunity for the student to be heard at various levels and appeal options. Procedural due process affords the student an opportunity to be heard or to present the case to parties involved in the decision-making process. Table 3.1 summarizes the key elements of procedural due process.

Substantive due process involves the basis for the decision itself (or the substance of the decision) and is based on the principle that a decision should be fair, objective, and nondiscriminatory. Students who might challenge this principle would seek to prove that a faculty decision was arbitrary or capricious. Substantive due process has often been summarized as asking, "Did the punishment fit the crime?"

There is a difference between student concerns or grievances based on academic performance and those based on disciplinary circumstances. Academic concerns are based solely on grades or clinical performance, whereas disciplinary misconduct is based on violation of rules or policies within the school or department. Academic due process includes the requirement that the student be informed of the academic issue, the requirements necessary to meet academic standards, a time frame for meeting the academic requirements, and notice of the consequences if the academic standards are not met. When disciplinary action is considered, the concept of due process is applied with a higher degree of scrutiny. In this circumstance, the individual must receive notice of the specific charge that is being made and the policy and code that has been violated. The student must have an opportunity to present a defense against the charges, usually at a formal hearing, but at least in writing. Because disciplinary dismissals may have more long-lasting effects on the individual, more complicated due process rules apply.

TABLE 3.1	Sample Student "Due Process Procedure"*	
Element	**Comment**
Notice of the charges against the student	Students must be given clear and complete notice of all charges against them.
Discovery rights and opportunity to present a defense	The time between receiving notice of the charges and the time of any hearing must be sufficient to provide the student an opportunity to investigate the matter, obtain counsel if desired, and present a defense.
Hearing and confrontation rights (right to cross-examine witnesses, right to counsel)	The student has the right to be represented by counsel, bring their own evidence and witnesses, have the opportunity to examine any evidence brought forth by the school, and cross-examine any witnesses brought by the school.
Impartial tribunal	Throughout the process, all steps by the program must be fair and impartial. The tribunal must be made up of impartial individuals who are knowledgeable of any significant rules, procedures, and guidelines of such procedures.
Right to appeal; right to obtain a record of the hearing	The student has the right to obtain a record of the hearing and appeal the hearing with a second impartial decision maker.

*Based on procedural due process guidelines

Consider the due process rights of the student illustrated in the following scenario. Jane Short is a sophomore nursing student who has completed her first nursing course with a barely passing grade. She had difficulty performing the basic nursing skills, stating that having someone watch her made her nervous. She did not come to college with a strong academic background and has struggled in making the adjustment to the required higher-level thinking and need for decision making. However, she was able to complete the course requirements in the basic nursing course, although at a minimal level. As she progresses to the next course, she is having more difficulty. Her study skills need development, and she has missed several classes. She is not doing well on tests and has been late for clinical on two occasions in the first 3 weeks of class. Her instructor has asked to meet with her to discuss these concerns. She informs Jane of the issues of concern and relates what needs to be done to address these concerns. She suggests some new study strategies and asks that Jane practice in the laboratory to become more comfortable with the procedures and skills. She also relates that continued absences and tardiness will negatively affect Jane's classroom performance and her clinical evaluation. She reminds Jane of the School of Nursing Policy that states that students who miss one-third of their clinical experiences will be automatically dismissed from the program. The faculty member tells Jane that she needs to demonstrate improvement in these areas within the next 3 weeks. The faculty member asks Jane to add her comments to the documents containing all this information and gives Jane a copy of the document explaining the concerns and including the suggestions for improvement and the consequences if no change occurs. The faculty member schedules times to provide regular feedback to Jane about her progress.

What has the faculty done to uphold Jane's due process rights in this circumstance? The faculty member has made Jane aware of the situation and what needs to be done to improve it. She has made suggestions for improvement and provided Jane with a written copy of those suggestions and the consequences if no change occurs. Jane has been informed and duly notified, and her due process rights have been addressed within the student–instructor interactions.

Fair Treatment

Students have the right to be treated fairly, consistently, and objectively. Fairness principles can be viewed from a perspective of how one student is treated as opposed to another student in the same course, or treatment inconsistencies between courses, or even expectations of students from one program to another program.

Standards of expectations for the course provide the objective guide for evaluation and must be communicated to students early and often. Course requirements should be consistent for all students, including classroom and clinical assignments. Students should receive equivalent assignments, even if they are not identical, that allow them to demonstrate progress toward meeting course objectives. In addition, students must be provided with opportunity and an appropriate time to demonstrate the outcomes required in the course. Students cannot be held accountable for end-of-course outcomes on the first day of class, and the same principle applies in the clinical setting. Students must be provided with time to learn before evaluation can take place; students must clearly understand the difference in the learning and the evaluation portion of the clinical experience.

An example of violating the principle of fair treatment might occur when a faculty member allows one student extra credit in a course but does not afford the same opportunity to all students to increase their grade. Clinically, holding students to different standards of evaluation will be considered a violation of the principle of fair treatment. If the instructor consistently gives a student less challenging assignments and then evaluates the student as not providing a complex case, the issue of fairness is again relevant.

Program policies must be applied consistently across courses within the program, or there must be a reasonable and justifiable reason why exceptions might occur. For example, if a program has a grading scale that is universally applied to all nursing courses, a faculty could not independently determine to make exceptions to the policy in their course based upon their own biases. Exceptions to program policies being applied consistently within all courses might be justified in situations where, for example, clinical agency requirements might require additional health and safety requirement that is beyond those included within the nursing program health and safety policy.

In determining appropriate standards of fairness, courts may review typical policies and expectations from similar programs to the program in question. Although program policies and practices may vary from one program to another, a significant variation might signal that the particular policy or practice is unfair to the student. For example, the likelihood of student success could be greatly impacted if their expectations for the student's clinical skills competency for an introductory clinical course would be at the level of a senior-level student who had satisfactorily performed the skill multiple times. That type of expectation could be viewed as unfair because it would most likely be inconsistent with other similar programs.

Contract Law and Student Rights

Other legal concepts that influence student rights come from principles of contract law. Students may also use these concepts in seeking action against an institution. Contract law is applied in this circumstance with the understanding that when students enter a university or college, they actually enter into a contract with the school. If students complete the degree requirements and follow the required procedures, then a degree will be awarded. The implied contract between the student and the school forms the basis for much of the student rights-oriented precedent law. Courts may view institutional documents as contracts, regardless of whether there may be a written disclaimer on the particular document that the institution does not intend the document to be a contract between the institution and the student.

A common example of a document that is often implied to be a contract is a course syllabus. The course syllabus may contain a statement that it is not intended to be a contract between the institution and the student but is often viewed by the court as being an implied contract. Even in a situation in which students agree to a proposed change in the syllabus, the original syllabus terms may govern in a dispute because the students who are voicing agreement may be viewed as unable to object without teacher reprimand or harassment from other students. Additionally, students have successfully won cases against educational institutions based on contract theory when the educational institution was determined to be in breach of implied contract because they did not follow their own policies and procedures (*Boehm v. U. of PA. School of Vet. Med*, 1990; *Schaer v. Brandeis University*, 2000).

Confidentiality and Privacy

Legislation that has been passed to protect health information and the privacy of patients should remind faculty of their obligation to protect information from and about students. The need for confidentiality in the faculty role is based in the same code of ethics and common law regarding privacy that guides all nurses. Students have a right to expect that information about their progress in the program, their academic and clinical performance, and their personal concerns will be kept confidential.

In the course of the teaching role, faculty are often privy to information about students that is of a personal and private nature. Students often confide in faculty about events that may influence their performance in the classroom or may simply seek advice from persons they feel they can trust. This can lead to a conflict for the instructor, because, as nurses, the instructors might have a tendency to respond in a therapeutic manner (Gaberson et al., 2022). It is important for the instructor to remember that their primary role is that of faculty, not health care provider. There must be a compelling purpose, such as the safety of the student or following institutional policy, for the instructor to disclose personal student information. Unless there is a need for disclosure of information to protect the student, faculty should respect the student's privacy. This guideline is consistent with the legal precedent set in *Tarasoff v. Regents of the University of California* (1976). In *Tarasoff*, the court held that the patient–provider confidentiality rule did not apply when there was a reasonable belief of impending harm to another individual caused by a patient disclosure.

It is easy for caring faculty to disclose private student information based on the belief that it is in the student's best interests. But without the student's consent or the faculty's reasonable belief that harm may come from nondisclosure, the faculty would be violating the student's right to privacy to share confidential information without student consent. Faculty are often eager to share a student's strengths and weaknesses with other faculty members who will have the student in subsequent semesters. Faculty must seriously consider the implications of such a practice as a standard approach. A student's performance or challenges in one class will not necessarily follow him or her to the next class. Informing other faculty members about an individual student's strengths or weaknesses may provide prejudicial information and could be interpreted as unjust and violate the student's right to privacy. However, alerting faculty to information that may affect patient or student safety may warrant discussion. This is a difficult concept for nurse educators and most often more information is shared than would be considered necessary, at the expense of creating bias against the student.

In addition to confidentiality, privacy—especially of student records—is essential. The Federal Educational Rights and Privacy Act of 1974 (FERPA), often referred to as the *Buckley Amendment*, provides the basis for protection of student records. This law was enacted to ensure that students older than age 18 have access to their educational records and to ensure that they have some input about who can receive the information in that record without their consent. The amendment also mandates that a procedure be in place that allows students to contest information in the record that is inaccurate or that they do not agree with. In actual practice, one of the most frequent applications of this law occurs when parents seek information about student progress or grades without student permission. Parents are often dismayed to find that they have no right to information about student progress unless the student provides permission. It is imperative that faculty understand the components of this legislation and follow it implicitly. For example, faculty cannot post grades in any form in public, leave graded materials for students to retrieve in a public place, or circulate a printed class list with student IDs or social security information as an attendance list. All of these constitute violations of FERPA and make faculty and their institutions subject to prosecution. An excellent reference of the requirements of FERPA can be obtained online through the US Department of Education website (http://www2.ed.gov/policy/gen/guid/fpco/ferpa/index.html).

Schools of nursing must follow the guidelines of the institution regarding FERPA, but they must also give particular attention to guarding student health records. These health records are usually kept in a separate file and should follow the Health Insurance Portability and Accountability Act (HIPAA, 1996) guidelines. Student records and evaluation notes maintained by faculty during the process of course evaluation must also be guarded to protect privacy.

Student privacy must be strictly guarded. Whether based in common law privacy standards, FERPA, or HIPAA, students have a legal right to have their information protected within the educational system.

Guidelines for Providing Due Process to Students

Due Process for Academic Issues

The potential for litigation always exists, even in the best of circumstances; therefore it is prudent to take actions and establish policies that decrease the likelihood that litigation will occur as a result of academic failure or dismissal. The following practices help keep students informed of faculty expectations and their progress in coursework and provide the basis for ensuring that students receive the information they need.

1. *Provide a copy of student and faculty rights and responsibilities in formal documents.* On admission to the program, students should be given a copy of rights, responsibilities, policies, and procedures that apply to students and faculty. Although institutions have the right to establish policies, they also have the responsibility to communicate those policies and guidelines to students and faculty. Policies and procedures that are in effect for all students in the institution and those that are specific to a program should be available and must be congruent. Policies should address progression, retention, graduation, dismissal, grading, and conduct. Students should also be informed of circumstances that will interfere with progression and those that would result in termination from the program. They should learn the process to follow in filing a grievance. These policies should be readily available and are usually published in faculty and student handbooks. Strategies that

ensure that students have read and understand the information contained in these documents should be a part of the orientation process. In every course, faculty should plan to reinforce this information, including providing specific expectations for the course. Written specifics of requirements should be contained in the course syllabus and discussed with students on the first day of class.

2. *Review and update policies in the handbook and catalog periodically.* Published materials given to students and faculty should contain current information about academic policies and procedures. This serves to keep students and faculty informed about the policies and procedures they are subject to, and it is a requirement of institutional and program accreditation agencies. Regular review of policies and procedures ensures that faculty are aware of current policies and increases the likelihood that they will be consistent in following them.

3. *Course requirements and expectations should be clearly established and communicated at the beginning of the course.* The course syllabus should explain course requirements, critical learning experiences, and faculty expectations of student performance to satisfactorily complete the course. Schools commonly establish guidelines for information to be included in all syllabi developed for nursing courses, and faculty should follow these criteria. A course syllabus should include the following information, at a minimum: Description of the course, course objectives, course credit hours, faculty responsible for the course, class schedule, attendance policies, teaching strategies used in the course, topical outlines, evaluation tools and methods, due dates for assignments, late work policy, and standards that must be met for students to pass the course. Many institutions also require that course syllabi include a statement about the need for students to notify faculty about desired accommodations for a disability. The syllabus for a course should be distributed on the first day of class to provide students with the opportunity to understand and clarify course requirements.

4. *Retain all tests and written work in a file until the student has successfully completed at least the*

course requirements and in some cases the program requirements. Student assignments, tests, and evaluations are invaluable, especially in cases of academic deficiency that may result in a student challenge. All evidence of a student's performance in a class should be kept at least until that course is completed. Faculty must be aware of institutional policy or standards that govern maintenance of records and should follow those. There are no universal rules for how long student files should be maintained, and the policy may vary from institution to institution. Student clinical evaluations often become a part of the student's permanent file, although in some programs, these are only retained until the student completes the program. The maintenance of files of student work and tests may also serve to decrease the likelihood of plagiarism of other students' work, because knowing that faculty keep a copy of assignments and tests may make students less likely to attempt to claim other students' work as their own. Files of student work may also serve as examples of assignments to share with evaluators during accreditation visits or to assist in outcome assessment efforts. Samples of student work may also be used to provide positive examples to other students. Faculty must obtain a student's permission to share his or her work with others. Some schools choose to have students sign a standard form granting such permission and to keep this on permanent file.

5. *Students should have the opportunity to view all evaluation data that are placed in the student file.* Students have the right to see all documentation that has been used to determine an evaluation of their performance. Students also have the right to disagree with the appraisal of their performance and should be provided with an opportunity to respond to the comments of the evaluation with comments of their own. Faculty should ask students to sign and date the evaluation form to indicate that the evaluation has been discussed with them while providing an opportunity for them to register their own comments on the form.

6. *When students are not making satisfactory progress toward course objectives and the potential for course*

failure or dismissal exists, students must receive notification of and information about their academic deficiencies. Students should receive regular feedback about the progress they have made toward meeting class and clinical objectives throughout the course. If deficiencies occur, students must receive details of what behavior is unsatisfactory, what needs to be done to improve the behavior, and the consequences if improvement does not occur. Faculty should hold formal conferences with students who are in academic jeopardy, identify the deficiencies in writing, and work with the student to determine a plan to address the deficiencies. Both the faculty member and the student should sign the document to indicate mutual involvement in and agreement to the plan. Subsequent follow-up conferences should be held to note progress or lack of progress made toward achieving the agreed-on goals and note revisions or additional strategies employed. All conferences should be documented in writing, and both parties should receive a copy of the documentation. An example of how this might occur was presented in the earlier example relating to Jane Short.

Faculty who fail to evaluate a student's unsatisfactory performance accurately, through either a reluctance to expose the student to the experience of failure or a fear of potential litigation, are guilty of misleading the student, possibly jeopardizing patient care, placing faculty peers in a difficult situation, and potentially being subject to a claim of educational malpractice. Nursing faculty and even the university are responsible for preparing safe and competent practitioners. When the faculty does not fulfill their responsibilities, they can be held liable for educational malpractice, because they are breaching their duty as an educator. Student deficiencies may eventually be identified and dealt with by subsequent faculty. Students might legitimately ask why they were not notified earlier in the educational experience of these deficiencies and accuse the "failing" faculty of prejudicial behavior. It is much fairer to inform students of their unsatisfactory behaviors when such behaviors are first identified. Informing students of deficiencies in a caring, constructive manner allows them the opportunity to improve

performance; to not inform them denies them this opportunity and right.

These procedures help ensure that students receive the due process related to academic failure that is their right by law. Maintaining open lines of communication with a student who is not progressing is a key component in resolving such situations satisfactorily and decreasing faculty liability. Students are much less likely to sue if they perceive that they have been treated in a fair and impartial manner and have been given information throughout the process.

Due Process for Disciplinary Issues

Students who are dismissed because of misconduct or for disciplinary reasons should receive additional assurances that due process has been followed. A disciplinary action occurs when a student violates a regulation or law or has engaged in activity that is not allowed. Disciplinary actions brought against the student need to include providing the student with a written copy of the accused violation. The information should include details about what policy or rule was violated, and enough information must be provided to ensure that the student can develop a defense against the charges. Procedural due process should include an impartial decision maker, notice of the charges and evidence against the student, an opportunity to appear before the decision maker, an opportunity to suggest witnesses, protection of the imposition of sanctions against the witnesses, and permitting the student to voluntarily accept discipline or the ruling of the decision maker (*A v. C. College*, 1994). If the student desires, legal counsel can be present to provide the student with advice but not to question or interview other participants in the proceedings. Legal counsel for the institution is usually available as well. No action should be taken by the faculty or university until a formal hearing has occurred. Depending on the institution, a committee usually decides the outcome of the charges. Courts may be more likely to become involved in disciplinary actions because they involve less professional judgment and evaluation.

In the example presented earlier, if Jane Short's absences continue in clinical and she misses enough clinical days that she is dismissed from the program, then the provision for due process as a disciplinary event must include more faculty action. The faculty member must provide written information about the school policy that has been violated (although one hopes she has done that at the earlier conference) and provide an opportunity for Jane to respond to the accusations. The process must provide an opportunity for Jane to present a defense for her actions or an opportunity to explain her actions to those persons who will make the final decision about the outcome of her situation. In this circumstance, because the issue is a disciplinary one, faculty must take additional steps to ensure that due process rights are protected.

Grievances and the Student Appeal Process

Even when a student has been treated in accordance with due process with a clear communication of policies and expected academic standards, it is possible that the student may wish to seek legal recourse in the face of an academic failure or dismissal. In such cases, the student may appeal to the court on the basis that faculty has acted in a capricious or arbitrary manner. Courts traditionally have not overturned academic decisions unless the student can prove that faculty did not follow "accepted academic norms so as to demonstrate the person or committee responsible did not actually exercise professional judgment" (Regents of University of Michigan v. Ewing, 1985). In this case, a student who was dismissed from medical school brought suit against the university, citing that university faculty moved to dismiss him based on circumstances that were not rational and were capricious. The court ruled that the university faculty did have cause to dismiss the student and thus a "substantive due process claim" had not occurred.

There are other reasons that students may choose to bring suit against an institution. Breach of contract, described earlier, may be charged by students who may not be provided with due process protections, particularly in private institutions. The court has generally followed the "well-steeled rule that relations between a student and a private university are a matter of contract" (Dixon v. Alabama State Board of Education, 1961). However, there is inconsistency in court cases that

address grievances of contract issues depending on the substance of the case. Students may also make charges of defamation or violation of civil rights, including discrimination. Courts generally have not hesitated to analyze cases in which discrimination based on any parameter (e.g., race, gender, age, or disability) has been charged. The best way to avoid such litigation is to maintain policies that clearly demonstrate adherence to the institution's and program's guidelines, which must be in compliance with all federal and state laws regulating civil rights.

The Student Appeal Process

Before seeking assistance from the court system, students must first use all available recourse within the institution. A well-established principle of educational law is that the courts have generally relied on academic institutions to deal with grade disputes and have intervened only when there is evidence of the violation of student rights. Institutions of higher learning have established policies for hearing student grievances and appeals. The purpose of these guidelines is to establish common procedures to ensure that students are provided due process and that faculty rights are supported. A sample appeal process that illustrates the typical steps students should initiate before filing a formal appeal is included in Table 3.2. Faculty and nursing program administrators should familiarize themselves with this "chain of command" to ensure that students are afforded due process while faculty rights are also respected.

Institutional and program policies related to student appeals and grievance procedures should be made available in writing to students and faculty. Faculty are usually given this information in the faculty handbook on orientation to the institution and should refer to them periodically as changes are made.

Likewise, students should be informed that a formal grievance process policy exists and that it is their responsibility to initiate the procedure. It is recommended that programs distribute this information to students when they are first admitted to the institution and document that students have received such notification. Students may choose

TABLE 3.2 Appeal Process Sample

Steps in the Appeal Process	Comments*
Step 1: Instructor Conference	Many issues can be resolved informally between the instructor and the student, and this should be the level at which discussions are initiated. The student should make an appointment to meet with the instructor to discuss the issue and present objective evidence supportive of the student's position. The instructor is responsible for summarizing the outcomes of the meeting, providing the student with a copy of the summary, and placing a copy of the summary in the student's file.
Step 2: Academic Advisor Conference	Some nursing programs use academic advisors as part of the appeals process; other nursing programs do not. The academic advisor can serve as an impartial third party to listen to the grievance and as facilitator to resolve the matter. A written summary of the conference should be created, a copy given to the student, and a copy placed in the student's file.
Step 3: Program Director Conference	The next level is often the program director but may be a different position dependent on how the nursing program is structured. The director can view the issue from a broad perspective. The student again has the opportunity to discuss the matter and bring supporting evidence. A written summary should be created, a copy given to the student, and a copy placed in the student's file.
Step 4: Dean of Nursing Conference	Some nursing programs may only have a program director, in which case the next step may be the formal filing of a grievance and meeting with the grievance committee. If a dean of nursing is present, this individual serves as another party to facilitate resolution of the issue. A written summary should be created, a copy given to the student, and a copy placed in the student's file. The dean of nursing would follow up with the faculty involved to the extent appropriate.
Step 5: Appeal Committee	An appeal committee may review the matter based solely on written materials presented or after a hearing in which the student presents the issue. The student should always have the opportunity to prepare for the appeal committee and present evidence for their position. The written outcome of the appeal committee will be given to the student and placed in the student's file.
Step 6: Chief Academic Officer Conference (Academic Vice President or Provost)	The institution's chief academic officer is typically the final step in the grievance process. The chief academic officer reviews all of the materials and makes a final determination of the matter.

*Each step of the appeals process should provide sufficient time for the student to prepare adequately for the next level of appeal yet ensure that the matter is dealt with in a time-effective manner. As educational institutions vary in organizational structure, so will the actual steps. For example, not all nursing programs have a dean of nursing.

not to initiate the grievance procedure that is their right, but they should always be aware of the option of doing so. Information about the appeal process should be reviewed with an individual student if the situation warrants.

When a grievance occurs and the appeal process is implemented, there are two possible outcomes. The appeals board may review the information provided and find that there are insufficient grounds for the student's charge and that the assigned grade or faculty action should stand. The other option is that a recommendation for corrective action may be made based on a review of evidence that indicates that the student's charges have merit. This may mean a change of grade or an opportunity for further evaluation.

Implementation of the recommendations may vary depending on the specific charges and circumstances. If, at the conclusion of the institutional appeal process, the student is not satisfied with the outcome, the student has the right to pursue further recourse in the court system.

Faculty Role in the Appeal Process

Being involved in the appeal process can be a stressful experience for both the faculty member and the student. When a student indicates dissatisfaction with an assigned grade or evaluation and is considering an appeal, the faculty member should give consideration to reevaluation. If the faculty member finds that the student's evidence is legitimate and that the student truly deserves a higher grade, then the grade should be changed. If the faculty member believes no changes are justified after reviewing the situation and finding that all procedures and standards have been applied consistently and justly, then the faculty member should maintain the assigned grade. However, a faculty member should not act in haste or out of fear in reaction to the threat of a grievance procedure. Changing a grade without justification sets a dangerous precedent and should be avoided. Clear, consistent use of standards for grading that are made known to students will help effectively support grades that are assigned. Planning before the implementation of a course assignment or activity and providing clearly established grading criteria may help decrease student misunderstanding.

ACADEMIC PERFORMANCE IN THE CLINICAL AND CLASSROOM SETTINGS

One major responsibility of nursing faculty is the evaluation of student academic performance. In many circumstances faculty are charged with evaluating students in both classroom (didactic) and clinical settings. Student evaluation is an expectation of faculty at all levels and requires careful consideration for many reasons.

The outcome of evaluation has a major effect on students, and faculty must always be aware of this. Student assessment is critical to evaluating student learning and determining competence to practice (Oermann & Gaberson, 2019). Faculty may have limited preparation in how to evaluate students within the classroom or the clinical setting. The outcome of an evaluation usually means that students progress in the program, but an unsatisfactory evaluation means that students may face having to repeat a course, a delay in their education, or removal from the program. These outcomes have financial, emotional, and other costs for students. In addition, faculty may also experience negative consequences, such as emotional distress, pressure from administration to maintain numbers, and a sense of personal failure when it is necessary to assign a failing grade. In the context of this stressful situation for all involved, faculty must be aware of the legal concepts important to the evaluation process.

Academic Failure in the Clinical Setting

Faculty who teach clinical nursing courses are responsible for guiding students in the development of professional nursing judgments, skills, and values. Faculty must ensure that the learning experiences chosen provide the student with the opportunity to develop those skills to ensure that they will become safe, competent practitioners. Applying a theoretical knowledge base, developing psychomotor skills, using appropriate communication techniques with patients and staff, exhibiting decision-making and organizational skills, and behaving in a professional manner are examples of the types of competencies that nursing students are expected to achieve through their clinical experiences. Faculty are also expected to make judgments and decisions about the ability of students to satisfactorily meet the objectives of the clinical experience. When students are unable to satisfactorily meet the objectives of the clinical experience, faculty have the legal and ethical responsibility to deny academic progression.

Legal and ethical grounds exist for dismissal of a student who is clinically deficient. Nurse practice acts exist in all states to regulate nursing practice and nursing education within a given state. Successful graduation from a nursing program should indicate that the student has achieved the minimum competencies required for safe practice.

When providing clinical care, nursing students will be held accountable for professionally negligent actions and are required to come pre-pared to clinical learning situations and to ask for help when needed. Although nursing practice is regulated by state law, which results in variations in practice standards between states, the prevail-ing view is that students are practicing on their own "fictitious license" and not the license of their instructor. As a result, students will be held to the same standards of practice as a reasonable, pru-dent nurse with the same education and experi-ence. Patients should expect that the care provided will be safe, quality care at the level that is needed. In addition, students and faculty are expected to follow professional standards of practice and codes of ethics that have been developed to guide the profession, even though the students' educa-tional experiences are not completed.

When engaged in clinical learning experiences, the nursing student is under the supervision of the clinical faculty with input from agency staff. The nursing staff in the facility have ultimate control over patient care that is delivered, so there must be constant and appropriate communication between staff, faculty, and students. The clinical agency contract that allows the school to use the facility for learning experiences may also contain a clause stipulating that the school of nursing will provide supervision of students. It is also common for the agency to retain the right to request removal of stu-dents and faculty if the level of performance does not meet the standard of care acceptable to the institution and could result in the loss of the clini-cal agency as a site for future clinical experiences.

Faculty must accept responsibility for ensuring that students practice with an acceptable level of competence. Each member of the health care team is liable for his or her own potential negligence related to patient care. If the student does not pro-vide care according to applicable standards, the student is liable for any resulting damage. If the nursing faculty does not adequately assign, moni-tor, and supervise the student, the nursing faculty is liable for resulting damage. And if the clinical staff, who retain ultimate responsibility for the patient's care, neglect their duties in overseeing the care, they are liable for resulting damage.

Clinical faculty have several responsibilities related to the instruction of students. First, clinical faculty must set clear expectations for student per-formance and communicate these expectations to students before the onset of any learning experi-ence. These expectations must be reasonable for students to meet and must be consistently and equitably applied to all of the faculty member's assigned students. Second, faculty must determine the amount of supervision to provide to students. When determining the appropriate level of super-vision, faculty should consider the severity and stability of the assigned patient's condition, the types of treatments required by the patient, and the student's competency and ability to adapt to changing situations in the clinical setting. Another responsibility of clinical faculty is to judge the abil-ity of the student to transfer classroom knowledge to the clinical setting.

Application of theory to nursing care is an important component of safe nursing practice, and faculty must engage in data collection to deter-mine the level of student performance in this area. Faculty may collect data in multiple ways. For example, before providing care, students may be asked to develop written care plans or care maps and provide the rationale for their proposed nurs-ing interventions. Faculty may also verbally ask students to explain the significance of patient assessment data they have gathered, or students may be asked to keep a weekly journal that pro-vides insight into their clinical decision making. Chapters 18 and 26 provide further discussion of clinical teaching and evaluation. Whatever data collection methods are used by faculty to assess student performance must be consistently applied to all students. Because faculty retain the legal lia-bility for appropriate student assignments and stu-dent monitoring to insure applicable standards of care are being followed, the faculty has the respon-sibility to remove students from providing clinical nursing care when the student is unsafe.

Fearing legal action, faculty may hesitate to fail a student who performs poorly in the clinical setting. However, federal and state courts have frequently upheld the responsibility and right of faculty to evaluate students' clinical performance and dismiss students who have failed to meet the criteria for a satisfactory performance. The courts have long indicated that faculty, as experts in their profession, are best qualified to make decisions about the academic performance of students. When teaching a clinical course, faculty must clearly establish and communicate the course and clinical objectives; they must document student performance and effectively communicate with students on an ongoing basis about their progress in the clinical area. These measures are discussed in greater depth in Chapter 18. Key to the success of any of these measures is that there has been clear communication of expectations to students.

As part of this communication, faculty should clearly identify at the beginning of the course, along with the clinical objectives, the level of clinical competence that students will be expected to achieve. These requirements should be stated in the course syllabus along with information about how the clinical grade will be determined for the course. The clinical syllabus should clearly identify all of the evaluation measures that will be used in determining the clinical grade. Chapter 26 provides more information about the process of clinical evaluation. Students must be informed about how data will be obtained and whether the clinical evaluation will be formative, summative, or a combination. Students must receive continuing input through a formative evaluation process, periodically receiving information about progress and suggestions for improvement. Students must have time to demonstrate the course competency requirements during the clinical experiences and cannot be required to master those competencies until the end of the course. The consequences of not meeting objectives should also be clearly communicated to students.

Written records of all clinical experiences and student–faculty conferences should be kept for each student during the course. Recording student observations during clinical learning experiences are very effective in assisting the faculty to recall specific objective observations (Gaberson et al., 2022).

Written records of a student's learning experiences document that the student has been provided with adequate opportunity to meet the clinical objectives. If opportunities to meet clinical objectives have not been provided, students cannot be evaluated or failed on unmet objectives.

Anecdotal records should be objectively written, describe both positive and negative aspects of a student's performance, and address the objectives of the course. Faculty should avoid commenting on the personality of the student but instead should reflect on what the student has or has not accomplished in relation to the course objectives. Notes of the student's daily and weekly assignments should be based on fact and should be nonjudgmental. Documenting both aspects of performance indicates that the student's total performance was taken into account when the final clinical grade was assigned.

Throughout the clinical experience, faculty should provide consistent, constructive feedback to students. Identifying positive aspects of a student's clinical performance and areas needing improvement will help that student develop self-esteem and confidence as a practitioner. Feedback is best conveyed in privacy, away from peers, staff, and patients, thus maintaining student confidentiality. Persistent clinical deficiencies should be addressed in conferences with the student, ideally away from the clinical setting. Written records of student–faculty conferences are used to document areas of faculty or student concern that have been discussed, along with the measures that are being taken to correct these deficiencies. Information about the progress the student makes toward correcting clinical deficiencies and any lack of progress should be included in follow-up notes. Both the faculty member and the student should sign these written records.

Communicating effectively with a student who is not performing satisfactorily can be difficult. When feedback is given to a student about deficiencies in performance, it is essential for the faculty member to convey to the student a sense of genuine concern about helping the student improve his or her performance and to convey the faculty member's responsibility for ensuring patient safety in the clinical setting. Providing feedback during clinical learning experiences should be continuous and include suggestions for students to improve their performance (Oermann & Gaberson, 2019). Students should be allowed the opportunity to clarify and respond to the feedback given by the faculty member. Sometimes an objective third party, such as a department chairperson or course coordinator, can assist by providing an objective perspective of the circumstances and serving as an impartial witness to what was said by both the faculty member and the student.

When notifying a student that course requirements are not being met and failure of the course may result, the faculty member must follow the institutional guidelines that have been established for such situations. Informing a student of unsatisfactory clinical performance can produce a stressful situation for the student, but it also provides the due process that is the student's right in cases of academic deficiency. It enables the student to understand that his or her performance is unsatisfactory and provides the student with the opportunity to correct deficiencies. It is equally important that the faculty member communicate information about the student's performance to other faculty who are administratively responsible for the course.

Assisting the Failing Student in the Clinical Setting

How do clinical faculty determine when a student's clinical performance is unsatisfactory and warrants failure of the course? How many opportunities should the student be given to learn before being evaluated? These are questions that have been debated in nursing education for decades without resolution. Faculty are responsible for evaluating the cognitive, psychomotor, and affective behaviors of students during clinical learning experiences. Even with reliable and valid evaluation tools, it can be difficult to objectively evaluate the behavior of students, especially in the affective domain.

Clinical evaluation has many inherent challenges for the nurse educator. Clinical evaluation can become subjective in nature, and evaluation criteria may be misinterpreted by faculty or students. Faculty in the clinical setting need to implement clear clinical evaluation measures and provide the student with frequent feedback as to their progress in meeting the clinical expectations. However, once having determined that a student's performance is unsatisfactory and that failure of the course is likely to occur, faculty must

implement actions to protect the student's right to due process and assist the student through what will undoubtedly be a stressful experience.

Faculty may use several guidelines when working with students whose clinical performance is unsatisfactory. For example, as previously mentioned, unsatisfactory clinical behaviors should be identified and discussed with the student as early as possible. Documentation should be maintained of the student's performance and all conferences with the student.

Working in collaboration with the student, faculty should develop a plan or "learning contract" in which the needed areas of improvement are identified along with appropriate measures to ensure the improvement of performance. The student should be made aware that isolated instances of good or inadequate performance will not lead to a passing or failing grade. Instead, it is essential that the student strive to develop a consistency of behavior that portrays continuing improvement in performance and the delivery of safe patient care. The student should also understand that successful completion of any remedial work identified in the plan may not be sufficient to ensure a passing grade for the course; satisfactory completion of the course objectives will be required. After the plan has been detailed in a document, both the student and faculty should sign and date it. The student should be given a copy of the plan for his or her own records and reference.

Frequent feedback sessions are essential during this time, as the student attempts to make an improvement in performance. The number of sessions depends on the situation, but it is often helpful to agree to meet on a regular basis, for example, weekly. The faculty member should maintain objective and factual records of all sessions held with the student, including a description of strategies for intervention that were developed. Student self-appraisal should be a part of the process.

The student should also understand that during this period of evaluation, increased supervision and observation by faculty may be necessary to continue to ensure that patient safety is maintained. The student may report feeling he or she has been treated unfairly or harassed and indicate that the increased faculty supervision is creating a stressful situation. It may be helpful at this time to refer the student to a counselor or other qualified individual for assistance with stress management. Role confusion can occur when the faculty acts in the capacity of caregiver or counselor to the student rather than maintaining the educator role. It is imperative that the nurse educator only act within the boundaries of his or her position and role. This also extends to situations when the faculty tries to assume the role of health care provider to the student, when there is no legitimate nurse–patient relationship between the faculty and the student.

At times, a clinical instructor may experience a sense of concern about a student's performance but have difficulty clearly identifying the unsatisfactory behaviors. The instructor may wish to seek input from another faculty member about the student's performance. Faculty have the right, but no legal responsibility, to obtain an objective evaluation by another faculty member. If this is done, the faculty member must make the student aware of the purpose of this observation and that the results of the objective evaluation may affect the grade awarded.

If the student continues to provide unsafe patient care despite the interventions to improve performance, faculty can withdraw the student from the course before the end of the semester. Students who might qualify for removal from the clinical setting are those who demonstrate a consistent lack of understanding of their limitations, those who clearly and repeatedly cannot anticipate the consequences of their actions or lack of action, and those who consistently fail to maintain appropriate communication with faculty and staff about patient care. If a student is dishonest with faculty and staff about the care provided to a patient, serious legal and ethical implications occur.

In all of these cases, patient care may be jeopardized and unsafe situations may be created for patients. Clinical faculty can refuse to allow a student to continue to provide care in the clinical setting, but if the student's performance is safe, the student must be allowed to complete the clinical requirements of the course, even if the student is not meeting course objectives. Students are not required to achieve course objectives until the end of the course.

Following the mentioned procedures helps ensure that a student's right to due process has been upheld. Maintaining effective communication with the student throughout the experience may be difficult but is essential to achieving a satisfactory resolution to the situation for both faculty and student. When students perceive that they have been treated fairly and objectively, most will accept that they were unable to satisfactorily meet the objectives required of the course. Faculty should avoid excessive self-blame for the clinical failure of a student.

Academic Failure in the Classroom Setting

Nursing program curricula are by necessity academically rigorous. Academic classroom failure, with a subsequent attrition from the nursing program, is not uncommon, and retention of nursing students is a familiar concern of nurse educators. However, faculty have a responsibility to uphold academic standards and must at times assign a failing grade in a course.

The reasons for academic failure in the classroom are numerous. First, students may initially underestimate the amount of time that they will need to devote to course study to be successful in the pursuit of a nursing degree. Students may be unprepared and lack the study- and time-management skills necessary to organize their schedules and study time appropriately. Students can quickly become overwhelmed by the academic demand of a nursing program, and the resulting stress serves to further increase anxiety and the inability to deal with course requirements.

Second, many of today's nursing students are attempting to fulfill numerous roles, simultaneously juggling the responsibilities and demands of work, family, and school. Role overload becomes excessive, and the students' grades are adversely affected. Students are often forced to make difficult decisions and may be ill equipped to identify appropriate priorities when addressing these issues.

Third, some students have difficulty with the level of cognitive ability required in nursing courses. Although adept at memorizing facts and information, they are not able to apply the concepts and develop the appropriate decision-making abilities. This is usually demonstrated by their inability to perform well on tests that demand application, analysis, and synthesis levels of cognition. Students who have never before been required to think on these levels may become frustrated when they spend much time memorizing information but still do not perform well on tests.

Some students may have learning disabilities that affect their ability to read with comprehension, successfully take tests, memorize information, or maintain concentration. Some students have satisfactory clinical performance but are unable to perform well in the classroom setting. See Chapter 4 for further discussion of students with learning disabilities. Students for whom English is a second language may also experience these difficulties.

Faculty have an ethical responsibility to identify students who are considered to be at high risk for academic failure in the classroom. The same examples of high-risk characteristics Donovan identified in 1989 are still pertinent today and include low grade point average, low standardized test scores, decreased critical thinking skills, and attendance at several universities without attaining a degree. Additional factors that can cause students to be at a higher risk for academic failure include having poorer reading and comprehension skills, and having English as an additional language. When students who have these characteristics are accepted into a nursing program, academic support services must be provided to increase their chances of success.

Faculty also have the responsibility for developing and providing academic support services that increase students' chances for success and thus increase student retention in the nursing program. There are many services that may be available to assist students academically, such as tutoring programs, individual course study sessions, study skills workshops, faculty–student mentoring programs, test-taking support, peer study sessions, and time and stress management training. Faculty should be aware of resources within other departments in the institution that can offer valuable assistance to students in need. They should also encourage activities that provide a support system for students, such as participation in student clubs and organizations. Many nursing programs have implemented peer mentoring programs that

have achieved positive outcomes for the students. Developing and providing support services for students with academic difficulties helps ensure that students receive the assistance they need at the earliest possible intervention point.

Assisting the Failing Student in the Classroom Setting

When designing intervention programs that will assist students to be academically successful in a nursing program, faculty must consider the academic experience from the perspective of the student, because this may have major implications for student retention and success. Faculty should obtain feedback from students in the program about their areas of concern, both academic and nonacademic. For example, if students believe that large class size is interfering with their ability to learn, strategies that provide students with access to faculty in small groups could be implemented. Student focus groups can provide much feedback, and faculty can use this information to develop interventions.

Faculty also need input about what programs or interventions are working (e.g., tutoring services, orientation programs, peer-to-peer study assistance groups) so that these can be continued or eliminated according to their success. Faculty need to know what concerns students have that can be addressed with appropriate resources. Using this information, faculty would be able to develop a retention-intervention program designed to maximize students' positive experiences and enhance academic success.

More specifically, faculty can implement several proactive strategies that support students' academic efforts in the classroom. First, faculty should remain aware of the changing student population and students' different learning styles. Nurse educators need to develop innovative, flexible programs designed to support the academic needs of the increasing numbers of nontraditional adult learners, graduate students, and culturally diverse students.

Flexible class scheduling, the use of technology to provide learning at convenient times for students, campus child care, recognition of students' life experiences, and support for students with English as a second language can all help students achieve their educational goals. The learning expectations and strategies of today's college students are likely to be different from those of students of the past. Much literature has been published that addresses the varying learning styles of the current generation, and information gained from those studies should be used to provide meaningful learning experiences for students.

Students who are successfully integrated academically and socially into the learning environment will more likely be retained in the system. Institutions must realize that students bring diverse needs to the educational process. The faculty adviser has a key role in helping students successfully adjust to their academic responsibilities. Faculty need to be informed about academic policies that affect student advisement so that they are able to provide accurate, timely information.

A typical role of the academic nurse educator often involves serving as an academic advisor for the nursing students. Faculty who understand the particular challenges of their students and the particular demands of their nursing program can promote student retention and educational success. The NLN (2017) identifies the importance of creating academic environments where diversity can flourish. Nursing associations or organizations can be a source of encouragement for students and can serve as a vehicle for socializing students into the nursing profession.

Individually, faculty members can take several steps to assist students who are doing poorly in the classroom. When a student demonstrates evidence of a lack of understanding of content of the course, such as failing a test or not completing an assignment properly, the faculty member should meet with the student to identify the student's perception of the problem. Students are often able to recognize the problem themselves, such as not enough time spent in preparation, lack of understanding of the material, or personal problems. Each of these reasons for poor performance requires the use of different intervention strategies, and the student should be involved in determining what actions are to be taken. Tests should be reviewed to assess the areas of difficulty and to determine whether the problem is potentially

related to, for example, lack of knowledge about content, reading difficulties, anxiety associated with test taking, poor study skills, or personal difficulties. Once the potential causes have been identified, intervention strategies can be designed and implemented to help correct the situation.

Faculty must realize that it is the student's responsibility to learn and to use the resources available to improve academic performance. Students must take responsibility for carrying out the plan of action developed in conjunction with the faculty member. Faculty cannot assume responsibility for ensuring that all students are successful in the course, but they must make certain that students are active participants in identifying concerns, developing strategies to address deficiencies, and improving performance. Faculty should always be willing to listen to student concerns and make referrals to available program resources when appropriate.

If, despite various efforts, a student cannot satisfactorily meet the course requirements, faculty have no alternative but to assign a failing grade. At this point, the student will require guidance and support as the available options are reviewed. If this is the first nursing course that the student has failed, it is commonly program policy to allow one retake of the course. If this is the second nursing course failure for the student, the student may be dismissed from the program. The student should receive appropriate academic advice as he or she plans future educational goals.

ETHICAL ISSUES RELATED TO ACADEMIC PERFORMANCE

Many ethical principles that influence student–faculty relationships and interactions are the same ones that guide interactions between nurses and patients. The relationship should be characterized by mutual respect and open communication. Faculty have a responsibility to conduct themselves in a manner that is exemplary, fair, nonjudgmental, and just and should serve as role models for students in demonstrating honest academic conduct. It is apparent, though, that there is the potential for student–faculty conflict to develop in these interactions. Faculty should consider the ethical implications that exist in relationships developed with students. This section addresses ethical issues that can develop in student–faculty relationships, including academic dishonesty and the nature of interactions occurring between students and faculty. Suggestions are provided for avoiding the development of unethical situations.

Academic Dishonesty

A student copies from another student during a test or uses "crib" notes; another student agrees to help an academically weaker student by providing answers to a test. Lacking the time it takes to write a term paper, a student turns in a paper written by another student, and yet another student plagiarizes portions of a term paper, taking the chance that the professor will not detect the omission of appropriate reference citations. During a clinical experience, a student forgets to administer a medication on time. Fearing the consequences of admitting the error, the student instead documents it as given. These are all examples of academic dishonesty or cheating, representing one of the most difficult situations faculty have to deal with in their interactions with students.

Unfortunately, such incidents are not uncommon, and as technology has developed and students have become more proficient, the methods of cheating have become more sophisticated, complicated, and complex (Oermann & Gaberson, 2019). As computer technology has become commonplace, students have used more sophisticated high-tech methods of cheating, such as the use of smartphones, cameras, and text messages and inappropriate computer use. Additional cheating methods may include use of tattoos, labels on drinking containers, and papers purchased online. Numerous reports detail alarming statistics that demonstrate an increasing occurrence and acceptance of cheating in schools at every level. Although nursing is consistently reported as a top-trusted profession, academic dishonesty is nearly as prevalent in nursing as in other disciplines (Aplin-Snider et al., 2021).

Oermann and Gaberson (2019) noted that both low-technology cheating and more sophisticated use of technology in cheating are widely believed to be common on US college campuses. Nursing faculty often are hesitant to deal with student cheating because of fear of consequences to themselves. After confronting students regarding cheating, faculty may encounter altered relationships with students. Faculty may also fear for their own safety from students who become confrontational and make threats. Another faculty fear may be that their administration will not support them if a student threatens legal action or retaliation against the school.

Many factors may influence a student's decision to cheat. Several authorities note that an alarming number of students do not consider their behavior to be unethical or cheating but see it as acceptable and common. Students and faculty may differ on their interpretation of what actions constitute cheating, and this often includes varying perceptions of the gradations of inappropriate actions (Ezarik, 2021). Dishonesty in the classroom setting is a concern for nursing faculty because of the potential for the student to also demonstrate dishonest behavior within the clinical setting, first as a student and later as a practicing professional (Pittman & Barker, 2020).

Numerous strategies and practices have been identified to deter cheating in nursing education. An initial strategy to address academic honesty should be a careful review of the faculty's own behaviors. For example, do faculty cite sources on materials presented to students in class? Are student contributions to research and publications appropriately acknowledged? Are faculty expectations realistic in terms of time requirements for students? Is there discussion about the importance of values and values development in students, or do these discussions occur only when a crisis situation has occurred? It is important to create a learning environment that integrates ethics into the entire curriculum and use of learning strategies that work to develop values and behaviors in students.

In 2017 the Tri-Council for Nursing (2017) issued a proclamation focused on nursing civility that identified the need to promote health and civil work environments. Nurses have the obligation to create cultures of civility and respect, as well as foster safe, inclusive work environments (Clark et al., 2022). Civility toward others must extend into the academic nurse educator role and is supported by faculty maintaining civility in student–faculty interactions. Bullying occurs in nursing education as well as in nursing practice. Faculty are in a power position with respect to the student because faculty hold the power over a student's grade and program progression. Faculty may not think that their actions would be considered bullying, but when the imbalance of power in the teacher–student relationship is considered, actions the faculty perceive as innocent or even helpful may in fact fit the definition of student bullying. It is imperative that faculty not allow an environment of incivility or bullying to occur within the nursing program.

Faculty can take a number of actions to deter cheating in their courses. One of the most common forms of academic dishonesty is cheating on classroom tests. This may be done by copying from another student's test, with or without the cooperation of the other student, concealing and bringing potential answers to the test into the classroom, or obtaining test questions from students who were previously enrolled in the course. Developing alternate test forms that can be used in subsequent semesters can help decrease the likelihood of questions being shared between classes of students. Alternative test forms can also be used among students in the same class, thus decreasing the chance that students can cheat by looking at the test of the student sitting next to them. Requiring students to leave books and other personal items at the front of the classroom or under their desks and rearranging the seating can also make it more difficult for students to cheat. Directing students to look only at their own tests can serve to remind students that their behavior is being observed and that they are responsible for not conveying the appearance of cheating.

Another common method of cheating is plagiarism of written work, through either the use of papers written by other students or the inappropriate citation of references. Students may be unclear about what constitutes plagiarism; therefore faculty should consider clarifying this at the beginning of the course, including how and when citing is to be done and what consequences will take place if plagiarism occurs. The proactive approach has been shown to be more successful, especially when tied to the development of an environment of academic honesty, often linked to an honor code or honor system. This may reduce the number of "I did not know that was wrong" excuses from students. Requesting that copies of the references cited in written work be turned in with the assignment can facilitate faculty review of the materials and reduce the likelihood that students will deliberately plagiarize. Keeping on file copies of past student papers can also decrease the likelihood that students will be able to represent a previous student's work as their own.

Sometimes students are pressured into helping another student cheat on coursework, either through a misguided sense of feeling sorry for and wanting to "help" the student or sometimes through fear. It can be helpful to periodically review the institution's policy on academic dishonesty with students in the class, especially if the faculty member suspects there may be a problem. Many students do not realize that institutional policies commonly state explicitly that a student participating in and enabling another student to cheat is also guilty of academic dishonesty and may be disciplined as well. In addition, most institutions have policies that provide guidance for students who feel that they are being verbally and otherwise harassed by another student.

A wide variety of practices are described in the literature to deter cheating (Oermann & Gaberson, 2019). Academic honor codes can be codeveloped by faculty and students. Nursing programs typically have academic honesty policies that should be used to guide situations involving both perceived and actual academic dishonesty. It is also helpful if written statements on course syllabi are used to remind students of the institution's policy on academic dishonesty and the academic code of honor, if one exists. The consequences of cheating and violating the honor code should also be clearly delineated in course syllabi. If cheating has occurred, does the student get an F for the assignment or an F for the course? Or are other options a possibility? This information can be included in the evaluation section of the syllabus and lets students know that any incidents of cheating will be taken seriously by the faculty member. It is important that these outcomes be guided by school policy and procedure; all course policies must be congruent with those of the broader school guidelines.

If a faculty member has evidence that a student has engaged in some form of academic dishonesty, it becomes necessary for him or her to confront the student about the incident.

Multiple steps should be taken by the faculty when dealing with instances of cheating. The faculty should ensure privacy with the student when initiating a discussion about the suspected cheating. This discussion often includes a third person, such as another faculty member or the department chairperson. The faculty should clearly and objectively state the observed behavior and reference it to the expected behavior. Potential consequences for the student's actions should be reviewed. The student should be informed of institutional policies and the importance of adhering to professional standards of conduct. The conference should be documented by the faculty member and the student should receive a copy of the documentation. As mentioned previously in the section regarding disciplinary action and due process, the student's right to due process should be ensured before any action is taken.

Academic Dishonesty in an Online Environment

Online education is becoming increasingly common within nursing programs. And online education brings additional challenges related to the monitoring and prevention of student academic dishonesty.

Cheating on online exams is a very common type of online issue that can occur if precautions are not taken. One of the easiest ways for a student to cheat is simply to have another person take the exam for them in a setting where the student's identity is not verified by a system such as biometrics or facial recognition. Software is available that uses sophisticated keystroke analysis, to identify a unique persona that is difficult for an imposter to replicate. Students may use remote software to connect with web sources or other students while they are taking an exam, which can be blocked by implementing a system to lock down the student's browser during exams.

Students may claim to have bathroom emergencies or bad computer connections during online testing. These types of issues allow the student to access resource material, or cheat, during the exam. Programs must have policies in place to deal with this type of testing emergency, which may include the use of subsequent alternative exams or simply ending the exam early.

Online exams can also be proctored by a real-time proctor, who observes the student while the test is being conducted. The real-time proctor typically begins the exam by having the student move a camera around the testing environment to ensure there are no forbidden items (such as sticky notes, crib sheets, additional technology sources) available for the student in the testing area. A method referred to as "record and review" videotapes the student during an exam session. The computer programs used with record and review are programmed to monitor student eye movements (is the student looking away at what could be a cheat sheet?), talking with others in the testing area, or unusual pauses during the testing session, which could indicate cheating. If activities of the tester violate the parameters preset into the record and review programs, the testing session can be terminated immediately.

Online test monitoring according to the typical monitoring standards is not considered a violation of privacy for the student. Typical standards would include that the monitoring process does not begin until the test session begins and ends at the conclusion of the test. The student may be asked to move the camera around the area where they are testing, but that is a basic environmental scan to ensure no cheating materials are present where the student is testing. Prior to commencing the test, the process is explained to the student.

With the increase in online education during the recent COVID-19 pandemic, it is speculated that there has been an increase in online cheating. A recent report of online cheating during COVID-19 identified that students are creating new methods of cheating as they think no one is watching them (Subin, 2021). Subin also reported that many students indicated they only plan to cheat in the short term during the COVID-19 pandemic (2021).

Student–Faculty Relationships

As discussed earlier in this chapter, the nature of the relationships that students develop with faculty in the classroom and clinical setting can have a profound influence on the quality of the students' education experiences. The relationship of the student with faculty in nursing may be closer than in other disciplines because of the increased amount of individual contact that occurs between students and faculty. Novice faculty often are uncertain about how to appropriately develop relationships with students. This can have a major effect on the success of faculty in the classroom and their personal satisfaction with their role as an educator. Faculty may indeed be very knowledgeable about the content they teach, but if they cannot relate in a positive manner to students, the students may not listen to the substance of the information being conveyed. Novice faculty should be encouraged to seek guidance on how to develop an effective interpersonal style with students.

Behaviors that help develop effective relationships with students are those that have been described throughout this chapter. Open, ongoing dialogue with students throughout the educational process is essential. Students have the right to expect respect from faculty for their ideas and opinions (although not necessarily agreement); constructive, helpful feedback on their academic performance; a willingness to answer questions and address concerns the student may have; and a respect for student confidentiality. Displaying an appropriate sense of humor and warmth with students is also important and allows students to see the human side of faculty.

Behaviors that are inappropriate and unethical in the teaching situation include using sarcasm or belittling the student, threatening the student with failure, criticizing the student in front of others, acting superior, discussing confidential student issues with other faculty, and displaying inappropriate sexual behavior. Standards and guidelines addressing sexual harassment are part of each institution's policies and procedures. Nursing faculty must be informed about such policies and must follow them explicitly. Faculty may also serve to assist students to access appropriate resources should students have issues with sexual harassment by other members of the university community and need such assistance.

Showing favoritism in the treatment or grading of students, refusing to answer students' questions, behaving rudely, and being authoritarian are other examples of unethical teaching behaviors. Student–faculty interactions that are based on the inappropriate use of power and control cannot result in caring, collegial relationships. In some institutions, policies govern the contact that is appropriate between students and faculty. Those policies must always guide decisions about appropriate student contact and interaction.

Faculty can foster the development of positive student–faculty relationships through the design of learning experiences that promote collaborative, collegial learning exchanges between faculty and students. Faculty need to examine their beliefs about the teaching–learning process and student–faculty relationships to gain an understanding of their own attitudes. The first step in the process of fostering a learning environment that is empowering for both faculty and students is conceptualizing the student–faculty relationship as a collaborative partnership instead of an authoritarian one.

EMERGING LEGAL ISSUES

Today's nurse educator is confronted with a variety of emerging legal issues that were not present a few years ago. Some of the most significant emerging issues deal with social media, high-stakes testing, use of criminal background checks and drug testing, and current trends in litigation with nursing programs.

Social Media Use and Misuse

Social media has emerged within nursing education because of the potential for teaching innovations. Although social media is openly used in one's personal life, use of social media within education or health care brings special legal concerns associated with confidentiality and privacy.

The National Council of State Boards of Nursing (NCSBN, 2018) created guidance for nurses on the use of social media. They caution that nurses who breach confidentiality and privacy can be held

CASE STUDY 3.1   Use of Social Media

Situation: During the COVID-19 pandemic, a nursing theory course was moved to a "remote" format because in-person classes were temporarily stopped. The nursing program did not have a formal learning management system in place, so faculty became creative and started posting course materials on various video posting and social media communication platforms. Although nursing theory courses have resumed in-person classes, many faculty continue to use a popular social media platform page for class discussions, actual patient case studies, and student messaging.

1. What issues could arise by posting videos on an open-source video platform?
   a. What type of content might be appropriate to post? What type of content would not be appropriate to post?
   b. What types of legal issues could arise by posting inappropriate content?
   c. Would your nursing program (and parent institution) have policies related to the use of externally posted video media? If so, what do those policies require or restrict?
   d. What types of policies and legal statements might be provided by the external video platform?
2. Some students do not have a social media presence and refuse to create an account. What actions would be appropriate for the nurse educator in that situation?
3. What types of content and information should and/or should not be posted on social media?
4. If a faculty is investigating the implementation of social media within a nursing course, what permissions should be obtained at the nursing program (and institution) before taking any steps to do so?
5. What guidelines does your nursing program currently have in place related to the use of social media for students? For faculty?

information posted to social media cannot be regarded as private even though the individual may have set access restrictions to the information. It is also important to realize that even if posted information is later deleted, it may still be able to be retrieved.

Nurses and students must not use social media to post private patient information on any social media site. This includes the posting of written words and images. Postings that do not include the names of patients may still be considered violations of patient privacy when the postings can lead to the identification of the patient. Postings should never include disparaging or harassing remarks about others. These principles not only apply to posting patient information but also serve as guidelines for student postings about instructors or other students, as well as instructor postings about students and other students. Professional guidelines apply to postings on social media, and the poster will be held liable.

Many faculty are unaware of how social media operates and thus are not able to provide guidelines to students as to the appropriate use of social media as a nursing professional. Students may have established practices of openly communicating on social media without any consideration of professional standards related to social media. Without appropriate guidance from faculty, students may be unaware of the significant legal and ethical concerns related to the use of social media.

Violations of social media by nursing students are making their way to the courtroom. In *Byrnes v. Johnson County Community College, et al.* (2011), three nursing students posted a picture of a placenta on social media. The clinical instructor had given permission for the picture to be taken on the condition that there were no identifying marks present in the picture. The clinical instructor was told that the students involved intended to post the picture on Facebook. The college dismissed the students. Byrnes filed suit and prevailed on the basis that she was not afforded appropriate due process before being dismissed for an "academic" matter. The court characterized this as a disciplinary matter and noted that no patient privacy rights were violated in the photograph. Byrnes was reinstated as a student and allowed

liable not only for civil and criminal privacy violations but for a variety of consequences that can lead to disciplinary actions for the licensed nurse and continued employment. For students, such privacy violations can result in dismissal from school in addition to the civil and criminal sanctions. See Case Study 3.1 related to use of social media by faculty and students to support classwork.

Students and faculty must be aware of the issues with the use of social media. For example, to continue her education. It is worth noting that the court stated there were no restrictions on this type of behavior or use of social media within the student handbook and the students had no way of knowing that posting the photograph would be an issue.

Another case involving a nursing student held in favor of a nursing program that dismissed the student for blogging about a patient who was giving birth (*Yoder v. Univ. of Louisville*, 2013). The court viewed the matter as "academic" (as the program argued) and not "disciplinary" (as the student argued). The distinction is significant, as disciplinary matters are held to considerably more due process safeguards. The court noted that the student's first amendment right was waived by the student with her signing various agreements with the nursing program related to maintaining professional confidentiality. Case law reflects the importance of clearly identifying the required standard of conduct regarding the maintenance of professional confidentiality with social media.

High-Stakes Testing

High-stakes testing refers to any test that has significant consequences for the tester. In nursing, high-stakes testing typically refers to nationally standardized examinations that are used to determine a student's progress in nursing, such as when they are used as a requirement to pass a course or graduate. The use of high-stakes testing has been debated in nursing education for several years. Court cases have been held both in support of and against the use of high-stakes testing. State boards of nursing have also weighed in on the appropriateness of using high-stakes testing in nursing. Some state boards of nursing have provided limits as to how high-stakes testing can be used in nursing programs.

The NLN (2020b) developed the document *Fair Testing Guidelines for Nursing Education*, which supports appropriate testing and evaluation measurements that provide feedback on student learning and curriculum effectiveness but advises that more than one mode of learning assessment should be used to make high-stakes decisions.

Litigation continues related to the use of high-stakes testing in nursing education. The typical case involves a nursing program requiring students to take and achieve a set score on a high-stakes test to qualify for graduation, regardless of previous academic performance in the program. Steps that nursing programs can implement to support the use of standardized testing would be to clearly provide adequate notice of the requirement and to support students who may not achieve the desired results from testing before facing disturbing consequences, as well as the use of multiple assessment methods for determining outcomes, such as graduation requirements. The nursing program must also consult with their state regulatory board for any specific state requirements regarding the use of standardized testing.

Use of Criminal Background Checks and Drug Testing

Many nursing programs require students to undergo criminal background checks and drug testing. This type of requirement has become quite common and is often required by the clinical agencies where students will be obtaining learning experiences. In determining program requirements, nursing faculty should consult with their state regulatory boards as to specific guidelines regarding the use of criminal background checks and drug testing and the educational institutional policies and the requirements of the clinical agencies used for student learning experiences.

CURRENT TRENDS IN LITIGATION WITHIN NURSING EDUCATION

Over the past decade, there has been a significant increase in the number of legal cases filed within nursing education with multiple causes of action. Some of these cases have been filed by attorneys and others have been filed by the students themselves acting in a "pro se" capacity (meaning they will represent themselves rather than retain an attorney for representation). For example, a CRNA student who was dismissed for clinical performance issues filed a suit with the following multiple causes of action: Disability discrimination, defamation, intentional infliction of emotional distress, negligent infliction of emotional distress, and breach of contract (*Walsh v. U. of Pittsburgh*, 2015).

A review of case law also identifies cases by nursing programs against their state board of nursing (ATS Institute of Technology, Associate of Applied Science in Nursing Program, v. Ohio Board of Nursing, 2012; Camtech School of Nursing and Technological Sciences v. Delaware Board of Nursing, 2014; Ohio American Health Care, Inc. Practical Nursing Program, v. Ohio Board of Nursing, 2014). Health care programs have also sued accrediting agencies for "unjust" loss of accreditation (Professional Massage Training Center, Inc. v. Accreditation Alliance of Career Schools and Colleges, 2014). Students are also filing suit against their nursing programs when they have lost professional accreditation (McCabe v. Marywood University, 2017). Overall the litigation within the nursing education arena is becoming more diverse and creative. As a result, the nurse educator must be vigilant to practice as a nurse educator according to legal principles and overall best practices. See Case Study 3.2 for an example of a possible litigation situation.

More recent cases have continued to focus on basic legal issues typically associated with nursing education. For example, in *Blevins v. Eastern Kentucky* (2020), a former student was denied readmission into a nursing program following the student's course withdrawal in lieu of receiving an unsatisfactory grade in clinical. Blevins asserted claims based on substantive due process, procedural due process, gender discrimination, First Amendment retaliation, and intentional infliction of emotional distress. Another case in which a wrong medication was administered by a student registered nurse in a graduate nurse anesthetist program focused on the issue of whether the student was acting independently or as an agent of the clinical agency where the student was receiving clinical experience (*Methodist Hospital v. Addison*, 2019). The question of whether or not the student's violation of a behavioral contract was a sufficient basis for dismissal from a nursing program was the focus of *Rolfe v. Baker College*, 2021. Although final outcomes of the above cases may not have been determined as of the time of this writing, they illustrate the types of cases being taken to court.

The legal effects following the impact of COVID-19 on nursing programs are just beginning to appear.

CASE STUDY 3.2 Grading Issue

Situation: A majority of nursing students within a particular class are failing the course. The nursing instructor wants to help the students be successful, so the instructor makes the following offer to the students.

I am willing to change the course requirements by adding an additional major writing assignment. This will give those who are failing an opportunity to raise their grade. For those who are passing, it will just provide more experience in writing scholarly papers. But, you will each have to vote on this proposal, and if the majority vote for the proposal, all students will have to abide by the new course requirements and complete the additional written assignment.

1. If the proposal to change the course requirements passes by student vote:
   a. What are the consequences to the students who are currently passing the course and do not have the time to complete another written assignment?
   b. What are the consequences to the students who were passing before the vote who receive a poor grade on the additional assignment and now are not passing the course? Would they have a cause for a grievance? A legal action?
   c. What are the consequences to the students who are not currently passing if the class does not vote to support the addition of an additional assignment? Would they have a strong case to win a grievance on the basis that "other students prevented them from passing the class?" Would there be sufficient cause for a legal action?
2. What liability is the faculty taking by changing the course grading criteria during the middle of a course? Does it matter if it was the students' decision or the faculty's decision?
3. Identify potential issues that could arise if the faculty requires a unanimous student vote, and there is one student who votes "no", thus preventing the proposal from being adopted.
   a. Could the students file a grievance against the one student who voted no?
   b. What type of liability may occur for the school and faculty if the one student who voted no became the subject of bullying by the other students?
   c. Could the students file a grievance against the faculty for not just changing the course requirements?

As court cases may not appear until toward the end of the statute of limitations filing period, two cases have appeared that represent common "Covid-related complaints" reported in the general news media. Students who were barred from attending a 3-day required clinical during their last course prior to their scheduled graduation from an Associate Degree Nursing Program brought a case for injunctive relief claiming a sincere religious objection to receiving the COVID-19 vaccination (*Thoms v. Maricopa County Community College District*, 2021). Students have also filed suit with claims of breach of contract and unjust enrichment against schools that canceled in-person classes and moved courses to online courses only during the COVID-19 pandemic (*Fedele v. Marist College et al.*, 2021).

One trend is consistent. There are consistent themes with litigation in nursing education. These are themes presented in this chapter. New case circumstances will be taken to court, but they are largely based on the same themes of breach of contract, lack of due process, disability claims, harassment and intentional infliction of emotional distress, and basic malpractice issues.

CHAPTER SUMMARY: KEY POINTS

- The faculty–student relationship should provide an environment for learning and mutual respect as guided by established ethical and legal principles.
- Students should always be provided with an effective due process to support the resolution of academic issues.
- The Federal Educational Rights and Privacy Act (FERPA) requires that privacy of student records be maintained.
- Academic failure in the classroom and clinical settings is a major reason that students seek legal action against the faculty and nursing program. Faculty can implement various best practices to provide a fair environment for student learning and performance evaluation.
- Academic dishonesty should be addressed by multiple strategies, including clarification with students on what constitutes academic dishonesty and the consequences of violating academic dishonesty policies.
- Current relevant legal and ethical issues in nursing education include issues related to social media use, high-stakes testing, criminal background checks, and drug-testing.

REFLECTING ON THE EVIDENCE

1. What are the best practices for a nurse educator to take when student dishonesty is suspected?
2. What type of student information is appropriate for faculty to share with other faculty? What type of student information is not appropriate for faculty to share with other faculty?
3. Why is due process significant for the student? Why is due process significant for the nurse educator and the nursing program?
4. What type of student rights exist within higher education?
5. How does the Federal Educational Rights and Privacy Act (FERPA) apply to nursing programs? What student records are covered by FERPA? Are there exceptions to FERPA?

REFERENCES

A. v. C. College, 863 F. Supp. 156 (S.D.N.Y. 1994).

Aplin-Snider, C., Buterakos, R., Creech, C., Schapel, S., & Feige, D. (2021). Academic integrity in online examinations in a graduate nurse practitioner program: Student perceptions and lessons for nurse educators. *Nurse Education Today, 107.* https://doi.org/10.1016/j.nedt.2021.105099.

ATS Institute of Technology. (2012). Associate of Applied Science in Nursing Program v. Ohio Board of Nursing. In *2012 Ohio 6030*. 985 N.E.2d 198, 2012 Ohio App. LEXIS 5242.

Bastable, S. (2021). *Nurse as educator: Principles of teaching and learning for nursing practice* (6th ed.). Jones & Bartlett.

Blevins v. Eastern Kentucky University, No. 5:18-CV-190-REW (E.D. Ky. 2020).

Board of Curators of the University of Missouri v. Horowitz. (1978). *435 U.S. 78*.

Boehm v. U. of PA. School of Vet. Med., 573 A.2d 575 (Pa. Super. Ct. 1990).

Byrnes v. Johnson County Community College, et al. (Civil Action No. 10-2590-EFM-DJW 2011).

Camtech School of Nursing and Technological Sciences v. Delaware Board of Nursing, N2014 Del. Super. LEXIS 40 (Del. Super. Ct. 2014).

Caputi, L. (2019). *Certified nurse educator review book: The official NLN guide to the CNE exam* (2nd ed.). National League for Nursing.

Clark, C. M., Gorton, K. L., & Bentley, A. L. (2022). Civility: A concept analysis revisited. *Nursing Outlook, 70*(2), 259–270. https://doi.org/10.1016/j.outlook.2021.11.001.

Dixon v. Alabama State Board of Education, 294 F. 2d 150 (5th Cir. 1961).

Donovan, M. (1989). The "high-risk" student: An ethical challenge for faculty. *Journal of Professional Nursing, 5*(3), 120.

Ezarik, M. (2021, December 7). Shades of gray on student cheating. Inside Higher Education

Fedele, v. Marist College, Nos. 20 CV 3559 (VB), 20 CV 3584 (VB). (S.D. N.Y. 2021).

Federal Educational Rights and Privacy Act (FERPA), 20 U.S.C. § 1232 g; 34 CRF Part 99 (1974).

Gaberson, K., Oermann, M., & Shellenbarger, T. (2022). *Clinical teaching strategies in nursing* (6th ed.). Springer.

Goss v Lopez. (1975). *419 U.S. 565*.

Health Insurance Portability and Accountability Act, Pub.L. 104–191, 110 Stat. 1936 (1996).

Kaplin, W., & Lee, B. (2020). *The law of higher education: Student version* (6th ed.). Jossey-Bass.

McCabe v. Marywood University, No. 1436 MDA 2016 (2017).

Methodist Hosp. v. Addison, No. 14-17-00917-CV (Tex. App. 2019).

National Council of State Boards of Nursing (2018). *A nurse's guide to the use of social media*. Retrieved from http://www.ncsbn.org/NCSBN_SocialMedia.pdf

National League for Nursing. (2005). *Transforming nursing education*. Author.

National League for Nursing. (2017). *NLN diversity and inclusion toolkit*. Author.

National League for Nursing. (2020a). *The scope of practice for academic nurse educators & academic clinical nurse educators* (3rd ed.). Author.

National League for Nursing. (2020b). *Fair testing guidelines for nursing education*. Author.

Oermann, M. (2017). *Teaching in nursing and the role of the educator: The complete guide to best practice in teaching: evaluation, and curriculum development* (2nd ed.). Springer.

Oermann, M., & Gaberson, K. (2019). *Evaluation and testing in nursing education* (6th ed.). Springer.

Ohio American Health Care, Inc. (2014). Practical Nursing Program, v. Ohio Board of Nursing. In *2014 Ohio 2622*. 11 N.E.3d. 1241, 2014 Ohio App. LEXIS 2329.

Pittman, O., & Barker, E. (2020). Academic dishonesty: What impact does it have and what can faculty do? *Journal of the American Association of Nurse Practitioners, 32*(9), 598–601.

Professional Massage Training Center, Inc. v. (2014). Accreditation Alliance of Career Schools and Colleges. *Civil Action* No. 1-12-cv-911.

Regents of University of Michigan v. Ewing, 474 U.S. 214 (106 S. Ct 507 1985).

Rolfe v. Baker College, No. 352005 (Mich. App. 2021).

Schaer v. Brandeis University. (2000). *432 Mass. 474*.

Subin, S. (2021, March 21). How college students learned new ways to cheat during pandemic remote schooling. *CNBC*.

Tarasoff v. Regents of the University of California, 17 Cal. 3d 425, 551 P.2d 334, 131 Cal. Rptr. 14 (Cal. 1976).

Thoms v. Maricopa County Community College District, No. CV-21-01781-PHX-SPL (D. Ariz. 2021).

Tri-Council for Nursing. (2017). *Civility considered key to promoting healthy, inclusive work environments and safeguarding patient safety*. Retrieved from http://tricouncilfornursing.org/documents/Tri-Council-Nursing-Civility-9-26-17.pdf

U.S. Const. amend. V & XIV.

Walsh v. U. of Pittsburgh, No. 13-00189, 2015 U.S. Dist. LEXIS 2563 (D. Penn. 2015).

Yoder v. Univ. of Louisville, No. 09-6008 (6th Circuit 2013).

4

Teaching Students With Disabilities

Betsy Frank, PhD, RN, ANEF

Congress passed the Rehabilitation Act in 1973. This act states that any program or activity that receives federal funding cannot deny access or participation to individuals with disabilities. Section 504 of this act specifically addresses higher education and prohibits public postsecondary institutions that receive federal funds from discriminating against individuals with disabilities. Furthermore, more than 30 years ago, Congress enacted the Americans with Disabilities Act (ADA, 1990). This act was further updated in 2008 and is now sometimes referred to as the Americans with Disabilities Act Amendments Act of 2008 (ADAAA). A summary of key provisions has been published to facilitate use of the act's provisions (Equal Employment Opportunity Commission [EEOC], 2011). Because of these two laws, colleges and universities have experienced an increased number of students with disabilities admitted to their programs, including nursing programs.

Nursing students with special needs present a challenge to nursing faculty in both the classroom and clinical settings. Students who have special needs include those who have a physical disability, such as a visual, hearing, or mobility impairment; a chronic illness; a learning disability; mental health issues; or a chemical dependency problem. Many nursing programs have had experience in meeting the needs of these students, and learning disabilities are among the most common type of disability reported. The majority of students do not disclose their disability before admission. Neal-Boylan and Miller (2017) found that some students with disabilities had to apply to multiple schools before being accepted.

This chapter addresses the issues related to the education of students with disabilities. It specifically focuses on common problems experienced by college students and nursing students: learning disabilities, physical disabilities, mental health problems, and chemical impairment issues. The Rehabilitation Act of 1973, the ADA as amended in 2008 (EEOC, 2011), and the significance of these acts to nursing education are also addressed.

LEGAL ISSUES RELATED TO STUDENTS WITH DISABILITIES

Faculty should be aware of the legal issues associated with teaching students with disabilities. The ADA protects the rights of individuals with disabilities in the arenas of education, employment, and environmental accessibility. Higher education institutions must guarantee individuals with disabilities equal access to educational opportunities. Discrimination against individuals with physical and mental disabilities is prohibited by the ADA. However, the ADA does not guarantee that an admitted student will achieve academic success—only that the student has the *opportunity* to achieve academic success. According to the law, all students should know what campus office can assist with seeking learning accommodations (Neal-Boylan et al., 2021).

The full effect of the ADA on professional education continues to be determined as more potential students with disabilities seek admission to nursing and other health professions programs. Focusing on stated program outcomes rather than on specific skills puts faculty in a better position to make decisions about what reasonable accommodations are for students who are disabled or have other special needs. The institution and faculty may be sued for failing to make reasonable accommodations. For example, a Missouri Appeals Court ruled that a nursing program had erred in dismissing a deaf nursing student because she needed accommodations in clinical practice (*Wells v. Lester E. Cox Medical Centers*, 2012). However, if the student does not request accommodation, the university is not required to provide such (*Buescher et al. v. Baldwin Wallace University*, 2015).

Implications for Nursing Education

Although many students with disabilities are enrolled in nursing programs, faculty often have reservations about their ability to deliver safe patient care. However, Philion et al. (2021) have pointed out that no evidence exists that nurses with disabilities delivered unsafe care. Furthermore, all nursing students presumably are supervised by faculty or preceptors. Therefore their practice is continually monitored for safety issues. Many students enter nursing as a second career and as a result may have disabilities not evidenced in younger students. Furthermore, as the nursing workforce ages, many changes in the work environment can be made to make the environment accessible to practitioners and students alike. Making the clinical environment more welcoming and accessible can promote retention of an experienced nursing workforce.

The *Future of Nursing 2020–2030* (National Academy of Sciences, Engineering, and Medicine, 2021) suggests that admitting nursing and other health professions students with disabilities to educational programs promotes cultural diversity. In 2016, the National League for Nursing emphasized this point in its vision statement *Achieving Diversity and Meaningful Inclusion in Nursing Education*. Admitting students that represent various groups within the population promotes a workforce that better reflects the population as a whole. Sanderson et al. (2021) stated that a diverse student population promotes equity and inclusion in the educational environment. As more students with disabilities seek admission to nursing

programs, and as those within the profession age, retaining nurses with disabilities in the workforce will be essential.

Barriers to student success may be related more to faculty and clinical partners rather than students' abilities to meet the essential functions (Calloway & Copeland, 2021; Elting et al., 2021; Epstein et al., 2020). A study by L'Ecuyer (2019) showed that with proper support from clinical faculty and preceptors, students with disabilities can be successful during clinical experiences. Faculty have the obligation to explain the legal requirements for accommodations to clinical partners. Faculty also need to be proactive, with the student's permission, in explaining what accommodations are to be made. Students also have an obligation to share what strategies they use to be successful. Education for faculty related to providing accommodations and understanding the possibilities for achievement among students with disabilities is key to students' academic success.

When a student makes known the presence of a disability and gives permission to share this information with faculty, course faculty are notified about the disability that requires accommodation. Course faculty must keep this information confidential and are not to share this information with other faculty, as it is the student's responsibility to decide when and where to disclose the presence of a disability. Students may choose not to disclose a disability in some courses. Even when student consent is given to share information with faculty and clinical faculty, the nature of the disability is the student's responsibility to share. Box 4.1 is an example of a statement of services provided for students with disabilities. To receive accommodation, the student must disclose the presence of a disability before engaging in the learning experience; it is not possible to retroactively claim the need for accommodations after the student has already unsuccessfully engaged in the experience.

Faculty are not allowed to inquire about the nature of the disability. In fact, decisions regarding whether accommodation is possible must be made after the student has been admitted, unless essential abilities are published and *all* students are asked before admission whether they possess the abilities needed for academic success. Most

---

BOX 4.1   Example of Campus Resources for Students Needing Accommodations

The Accessibility Resource Office at Indiana State University (ISU) coordinates academic and residential accommodations for ISU students with physical, neurological, and psychological needs. The goals of these services are:

- to enable students with disabilities to participate in and benefit from University programs, on-campus living, and activities by providing services, accommodations, and assistive technology
- to ensure the ISU environment is free of barriers
- to encourage students with accommodations to become as independent and self-reliant as possible and to help students secure services
- to provide information and consultation about the types of accommodations and how they address a variety of specific needs

(Courtesy Indiana State University. Retrieved from https://www.indstate.edu/services/student-success/cfss/student-support-services/disability-student-services)

---

question such requirements (American Nurses Association, 2021). Although some schools publish technical abilities that students must achieve, faculty need to consider if they are truly essential to nursing practice. Neal-Boylan and Smith (2016) stated that published essential functions were barriers for students who wish to apply to nursing programs, even though they may otherwise be qualified.

When considering the standards that students must meet, Ailey and Marks (2017, 2020) advocate for separating functional and technical standards. Functional standards for nursing include acquiring knowledge, developing communication skills, interpreting data, making clinical judgments, and using appropriate professional behaviors and attitudes (Ailey & Marks, 2017, 2020). Technical standards such as being able to stand for long periods and working 12-hour shifts are standards that are meant to be used in the employment setting, not the educational setting (Davidson et al., 2016). Such technical standards as being able to hear can be met with assistive devices (Argenyi, 2016). Not all nurses practice in all health care settings (Neal-Boylan & Miller, 2017). Faculty have the ability to

accommodate students when meeting program outcomes in a variety of ways and settings appropriate to meeting those outcomes, including simulation. Yet, faculty have noted that coordination of accommodations can be cumbersome, and education is needed on how accommodations can be made (Yarbrough & Welch, 2021). Although not all those with disabilities can successfully complete a nursing program, technological advances open the door to wider opportunities for students and practicing nurses. Faculty must remember, however, that students are not required to disclose disabilities before admission. When considering the admission of a student who has a disability, admission committees in schools of nursing must consider the following questions:

- Disregarding the disability, is the individual otherwise qualified to be admitted to the program?
- What reasonable accommodations can the school make to enable the student to be successful in the pursuit of becoming a nurse who can deliver safe patient care?

Although institutions are not expected to lower or alter academic or technical standards to accommodate a student with a disability (Neal-Boylan et al., 2021), they are expected to determine what accommodations would be reasonable for a student who is disabled. According to Neal-Boylan and Miller (2017), most accommodations are determined by the campus offices that deal with students with disabilities and the nursing programs themselves.

Examples of reasonable accommodations include altering the length of test-taking times or methods, providing proctors to read tests or write test answers, allowing additional time to complete the program of study, providing supplemental study aids such as audiotapes of texts, providing note-takers, or altering the method of course delivery, such as the use of simulation for some clinical practice. Other accommodations include closed captioning (Neal-Boylan & Miller, 2017). The same considerations must be given to students who become disabled during their enrollment in a nursing program. Questions to be asked include:

- Disregarding the disability, is the student otherwise qualified to continue in the nursing program?

- What reasonable accommodations can be made to allow the student to continue?

Using concepts of universal design accommodates a variety of learning styles for all students, not just students with disabilities (Harris, 2018). Universal design acknowledges that barriers to learning are environmental and not related to one's medical diagnosis (Carroll & Eaton, 2019). Universal design promotes course design that uses multiple ways to present course materials and multiple ways for students to demonstrate knowledge acquisition. Most learning management systems allow faculty to use universal design in presenting their course materials. Assessing all students' knowledge at the beginning of a course allows the faculty to make adjustments according to students' individual needs (Anderson et al., 2019). As a result, faculty can plan to use a cadre of universal design strategies as appropriate.

Levey's (2018) integrative literature review found that one of the biggest barriers to universal course design was lack of knowledge on the part of faculty. As a result of this integrative literature review, Levey (2018) provided an extensive list of universal design strategies. Whether one teaches online or in face-to-face environments, instructional design specialists should be part of the team that designs accessible distance courses and on-campus classes. See Box 4.2 for suggested universal design strategies.

Universal design is not just applicable to the classroom setting; it can also be applied in the clinical setting. For example, a nursing student with dyslexia could use a Livescribe pen to take legible notes. General design principles include prioritizing learning outcomes as essential and optional such as adjusting shift work to account for a student experiencing fatigue associated with a chronic illness, providing expected tasks to students ahead of the clinical experience to allow students to practice ahead of time, and using simulation for clinical experiences.

Even though many different teaching and learning strategies are a part of universal design (sometimes called inclusive teaching strategies), faculty and student attitudes toward the strategies can foster or hamper their use. Levey's (2018) integrative literature review found that one of the biggest barriers to universal course design was lack of knowledge on the part of faculty.

Levey (2016) investigated a nationwide sample of nurse educators' attitudes toward adopting inclusive teaching strategies using the Inclusive Teaching Strategies in Nursing Education (ITS-NE) instrument. Levey's results showed that more years of teaching experience negatively correlated with willingness to use inclusive teaching strategies. Social support was a positive indicator of willingness to use universal design principles in nursing courses.

All students desire success, want to communicate well with professors, and have ready access to course materials. Courses that take into account universal design promote success for all students.

Gawronski et al. (2016) compared 179 community college faculty and 449 students' perceptions of universal design strategies using the ITSI and the Inclusive Teaching Strategies Inventory-Student (ITSI-S). Faculty and students alike perceived that accommodations, accessible course materials, multiple means of presentation, and inclusive lecture strategies were important. Students thought that course modifications, such as allowing those with disabilities extra credit, and inclusive assessments, such as having alternative assessments to demonstrate knowledge, were important—but faculty did not. One should note that 13% of student respondents identified as disabled, but disability status was not identified for faculty.

Faculty should consider that just because a student has a disability, he or she is not necessarily ill, and the type of support needed is not the type needed to cure an illness but to promote positive attitudes toward and the potential for growth of students with disabilities (Neal-Boylan & Smith,

---

BOX 4.2 Universal Design Strategies

1. Have course materials available in audio and video format.
2. Design uncluttered webpages that don't rely on color alone.
3. Provide accessible JavaScript.
4. Provide access to webpages that convert text to audio and audio to text.

2016). Whether a person's limitations are viewed as a disability is defined by society rather than by the actual abilities of the person involved. Thus making the decision regarding what is a reasonable accommodation for a person with a disability is a complex process influenced as much by faculty and practice partner attitudes as by actual student abilities.

Nurse educators must keep current with legal developments related to the effect of ADA, now ADAAA, that relate to the education of individuals with disabilities who are pursuing degrees in the health professions. Some suggestions for increasing faculty awareness of the needs of students with disabilities include periodic continuing education sessions related to the legal implications of educating such students and the use of consultants who are experts in working with students with disabilities. Most institutions of higher education have an office dedicated to assisting and supporting students with disabilities who are enrolled on campus. This office can provide resources and expert advice to faculty and students. Another source of information may be individuals with disabilities who have successfully developed a career in nursing. These successful nurses can help nursing faculty understand the issues involved in educating students with disabilities, and they can serve as mentors to students with disabilities who are pursuing a nursing education. Practicing nurses with disabilities can serve as advocates for students and help nursing programs advocate for students who graduate and then seek employment.

Nursing faculty should begin to separate the truly essential components of nursing education from what has traditionally been included in nursing curricula. Nursing faculty should also use a variety of teaching strategies for all students (Harris, 2018; Scheirer, 2021). Physical and occupational therapists and engineering students could work with those who have disabilities in order to develop appropriate accommodations (Neal-Boylan & Miller, 2020). In addition, nursing faculty need to consider such philosophical issues as whether nursing education might be extended to those individuals who will never practice bedside nursing in an acute care setting. Such nursing jobs might include staff development, infection control, case management, or a variety of jobs in the community settings where nursing care is delivered.

Faculty can use a variety of clinical settings to achieve the prescribed learning outcomes. Working with preceptors in practice not only assists students in their educational process (Philion et al., 2021) but could also demonstrate that disabled students can be successful as graduates. In addition, Philion et al. (2021) noted that safety issues experienced by students with disabilities were no different from students without disabilities.

THE NURSING STUDENT WITH A LEARNING DISABILITY

Learning disabilities are the most common type of student disability reported on college campuses (National Center for Education Statistics [NCES], 2011). Despite a growing number of college students with learning disabilities, not all seek help in order to be successful in their endeavors. Exact figures regarding the number of students with learning disabilities are unclear. The 2018 survey by the American College Health Association demonstrated that 27.5% of college students surveyed reported a variety of disabilities, including 8.2% with attention deficit hyperactivity disorder (ADHD). The National Center for Educations Statistics (2019) reports that of the 19% of undergraduate students who report having a disability, 3.6% have a specific learning disability and 26.4% have an attention deficit disorder, which is a form of a learning disability. The traditional definition of a learning disability is an incurable neurological disorder interfering with learning in a variety of ways. Approximately 15% of those in the United States have some form of learning disability (LD Resources Foundation [LDRFA], n.d.). Learning disabilities include ADHD, dyslexia, problems with mathematical calculations, and autism.

Students frequently begin college with learning disabilities undetected. In nursing education learning disabilities are commonly uncovered when faculty notice striking differences between a student's classroom performance and clinical performance. The student may display an adequate knowledge base and competent skills during clinical experiences but be unable to demonstrate the same degree of knowledge when taking tests in the classroom. Such disparities in performance can lead to much frustration and stress for the student even though their reading difficulties in many instances may not hamper their ability to complete their program of study due to lack of self-confidence (Crawford et al., 2022). Because some students may need some assistance to complete their education, faculty should have an understanding of the characteristics of learning disabilities so that they can refer students to the university or college office that works with students with various disabilities.

Characteristics of Learning Disabilities

Learning disabilities may manifest as a number of characteristics, each necessitating a different treatment and accommodation, and are life-long conditions. Learning disabilities, including dyslexia, may involve reading and spelling difficulties; problems with mathematical abilities; difficulty with writing, auditory, and visual processing; and nonverbal processing such as intuition and holistic processing (LD Basics, 2021). Among those with diagnosed learning disabilities, 80% have trouble with basic reading skills (What is a learning disability, n.d.). Adult students with learning disabilities may have difficulty summarizing materials, spell incorrectly, be slow in their work, and may also either be hyper-vigilant regarding details or pay little attention to details. Abstract concepts may also present difficulties for students (Common signs of learning disabilities, n.d.). Students may also have auditory processing deficits that may have an effect on their ability to recite from memory, although the diagnosis of auditory processing is not clear-cut (Maggu & Overath, 2021). Prioritization is often a problem for those with learning disabilities (Sharfi et al., 2022). In turn, time management may become problematic for the student.

Needs of students with learning disabilities are highly individualized. Crouch (2019) interviewed 12 students with dyslexia and 22 mentors. Students and mentors revealed a variety of challenges and strategies to cope with those challenges.

Being accurately diagnosed with a learning disability means students can make adjustments in their study habits and receive support. Like all students, individualized learning support for students with learning disabilities is critical to successfully meeting the academic standards.

Many students don't want to disclose their learning disability for fear of stigma (Crawford et al., 2022). Despite fear of disclosure of learning challenges, Crawford et al.'s (2022) study of 1152 nursing students demonstrated that the GPAs and program completion did not differ between those with identified learning disabilities and those without learning disabilities. Crawford et al. (2022) concluded that appropriate learning accommodations can help those with learning disabilities to achieve program success.

Accommodating Learning Disabilities

When faculty believe that a student may have a previously undiagnosed learning disability, the initial action is to refer the student to the campus office that assists students with special needs. After the diagnosis has been made, a plan for accommodation of the disability can be developed. Counseling may also help a student with learning disabilities gain self-confidence in the learning environment. As stated earlier, if the student chooses, the faculty can be made aware of the disability and what accommodations are required. Faculty members who are made aware of a student's disability are not allowed to discuss that information with other faculty members unless the student gives permission.

Depending on the type of learning disability, a variety of accommodations may be appropriate for the student. Once diagnosed, some students may need some accommodation (Case Study 4.1). Zeng et al. (2018) conducted a literature review of studies pertaining to strategies used to promote academic success for students with learning disabilities. Strategies identified included talk-to-text software to promote writing success, one-on-one tutoring, and education on test taking strategies. Active learning strategies are also helpful (Cox et al., 2019). Crouch (2019) outlined other strategies that could be useful in both clinical and classroom settings. Audio recordings of lectures also facilitate understanding of complex materials, which can be done easily with lecture-capturing software integrated into learning management systems, making

---

CASE STUDY 4.1   Supporting Students with Learning Disabilities

A retired veteran of the Armed Forces was admitted to a nursing program. The veteran was a medic in Afghanistan. As faculty work with the student, they notice that he has trouble focusing and expressing himself in writing. Many words are frequently misspelled despite the use of a spell checker. During clinical experiences, the student has excellent technical and interpersonal skills and can orally express the care plan for the day with appropriate rationale for the care delivered. Charting in the EHR is often scattered and classroom testing is problematic. The student has failed two examinations. Faculty suspect the student has a learning disability.

1. What should faculty do if they suspect this student is having learning difficulties?
2. Where would faculty refer the student for help in overcoming a possible learning disability?
3. What teaching strategies could help this and other students with learning disabilities?
4. How should faculty respond to a clinical agency that seems unwilling to accept a student with learning disabilities? What legal protections do the program and the student have in such a situation?

---

to-do lists, and the use of colored pens when taking notes.

Helping students understand their own learning styles helps them discover strategies that promote success. Box 4.2 lists universal design strategies that can guide faculty when teaching students with learning disabilities. The use of simulation is another strategy that can help students build self-confidence in their ability to develop clinical competence (Labrague et al., 2019).

Students may also benefit from the assistance of an in-class note taker, which is a generally accepted accommodation according to ADA. This allows students to concentrate on classroom discussion without the distraction of trying to take notes. Some students have difficulty processing multiple stimuli at once. Students who have difficulty reading and, as a result, read slowly often find this disability to be the greatest barrier to their academic success. Faculty can help students overcome this difficulty by providing an audio recording of textbooks and other readings and providing them with the required reading assignments early in the semester or helping them identify the key sections of reading assignments.

Students with learning disabilities may also need accommodations for testing, because slow reading skills can affect the student's ability to complete a test within the time allowed. Questions that are grammatically complex or contain double negatives, although difficult for all students, can be particularly challenging for students with learning disabilities and should be avoided. Providing the student with an extended testing time and a quiet room free of distractions may also be necessary accommodations (Birkhead, 2018). A test proctor who either reads the test to the student or writes and records the student's dictated answers to the test questions may also be helpful.

An additional strategy that faculty can use to assist students with learning disabilities is to incorporate a multimedia approach, such as computer-assisted instruction. Again, use of universal design principles can help students with learning disabilities and the student body at large. These include providing copies of ancillary learning materials before class and placing visual cues within class notes. The use of smart phones with appropriate applications may also be helpful for all students but particularly those with learning disabilities. Another strategy that benefits all students, including those with learning disabilities, is to meet with students on a regular basis to ensure that learning goals are being set appropriately and are then being achieved.

Accommodation does not mean that academic standards are lowered, but that multiple ways to achieve those standards are provided for all students, including those with learning disabilities. All classrooms contain students with multiple learning styles. By structuring classes to account for different learning styles and providing a variety of learning aids, nurse educators also help accommodate those with diagnosed learning disabilities (Harris, 2018). When faculty consider that students have different ways of learning, they will design learning experiences that accommodate these diverse learning needs.

Campus Support Services

As previously mentioned, most institutions of higher education have established an office responsible for providing support services to students who identify themselves as learning disabled. Use of these services is voluntary, and they are usually available at little or no cost to the student. Services vary among institutions but typically include assessment and diagnosis of learning disabilities, identification of appropriate accommodations for the student, guidance counseling, and development of study and test-taking skills.

Moreover, classroom and clinical faculty need education on how to best facilitate success of students and graduates with learning disabilities (Major & Tetley, 2019). Education about students with learning disabilities is another service commonly provided by these offices. Campus teaching and learning centers can assist faculty with how to design courses in line with universal design principles.

Accommodations for the National Council Licensure Examination

Nurse educators need to be familiar with the accommodations provided to students with disabilities in their states when taking the National Council Licensure Examination (NCLEX). Accommodations are offered to individuals with learning and other disabilities in accordance with the ADA. Each state determines the degree of accommodation offered to students on a case-by-case basis. Educators should investigate and verify the accommodations offered to students in their respective state and encourage students with disabilities to seek appropriate accommodations. One of the most common accommodations has to do with time allotted for the examination. Regulations do change, and the student and faculty are encouraged to check with the National Council of State Boards of Nursing (NCSBN) website (https://www.ncsbn.org) or the individual state board of nursing for further information. The student must provide documentation as to what accommodations have been made during his or her course of study before arriving at the testing center.

THE STUDENT WITH PHYSICAL DISABILITIES

Thinking of physical disabilities as hindrances and environments that favor those without disabilities may limit opportunities for students and nurses with disabilities (Epstein et al., 2020). Required abilities that schools use to exclude students may include hearing, seeing, and lifting. Essential competencies for basic nursing programs may be different from those required in specialty graduate programs. For example, Elisha et al. (2020) developed a competency-based clinical assessment tool that demonstrated that competencies could be met with appropriate accommodations by those with disabilities. And the AACN's *The Essentials: Core Competencies for Professional Nursing Education* (2021) outlines competencies that are largely within the realm of cognitive domains including critical thinking and communication.

The US Supreme Court ruled more than 40 years ago that a prospective nursing student with a hearing impairment could be denied admission because of the potential for lowering educational standards (*Southeastern Community College v. Davis*, 442 U.S. 397, 1979). The ADA and ADAAA have clarified that such a student has the potential to succeed with reasonable accommodations. Many aids, such as sophisticated amplified stethoscopes, are now available, and an interpreter could be used for auscultation (Association of Medical Professionals With Hearing Losses, n.d.). Through the use of note takers and audio recorders, many students with hearing impairments have little difficulty participating in the classroom. Pagers and cell phones that vibrate may help students keep in contact with others in the clinical setting. Looking at the student when speaking is also helpful (Moriña & Orozco, 2020).

Much of the evidence regarding physical disabilities is case study evidence. However, Moriña and Orozco's (2020) qualitative study of 19 health professions faculty, including nursing faculty, demonstrated that faculty could work with those with visual and hearing impairments, as well as other disabilities, in order to facilitate student success (Case Study 4.2). Because nurses with visual impairments are active in the workforce, faculty

CASE STUDY 4.2   Accommodation for a Hearing Impairment

A graduate student is admitted into a BSN-DNP program. For the past 10 years, she has worked in a Visiting Nurse Association as a case manager. Her goal is to become a family nurse practitioner and work in a hospice environment. During an advanced physical assessment course, faculty notice that the student has difficulty using the stethoscope provided to her in a simulation setting. When exploring this issue with the student, she discloses that she has developed a hearing impairment in the last 5 years but was afraid to tell faculty for fear of being dismissed from the program. The faculty refer the student to the office of student support that works with students with learning impairments. The office of student support says this student needs a note taker in the classroom, closed captioning for online courses, and an interpreter in the clinical setting.

1. How should faculty accommodate this student?
2. What assistive devices might help this student? If the student is evaluated for accommodations and one of the accommodations is for the student to have a service dog, how would faculty work with clinical agencies to accommodate this student?

---

can assume that some students with impaired vision may be accommodated. Providing alternative learning environments and enabling students to work with preceptors may be accommodations that can reasonably be made. For example, a student with a visual impairment might need a magnifier to help with reading printed matter, larger font sizes on a computer, or a text-to-voice apparatus. Universal design is key to the success of those with hearing or visual impairments and others with physical disabilities (Pavlik et al., 2019).

Students in wheelchairs may also be accommodated and go on to have a successful nursing career (Neal-Boylan & Smith, 2016). Such students might need to lower a bed or overbed table to deliver care. Practicing in the learning laboratory will help the student get accustomed to the accommodation before learning in the clinical arena. Nurses with missing limbs have also functioned as staff nurses, including starting intravenous infusions (Quinn, 2018). Likewise, Neal-Boylan et al. (2021) presented a case study of a nursing student with a missing limb. Their case study outlined steps that could be used to accommodate such a student without compromising patient safety.

Lifting restrictions should not be a barrier, because many hospitals and nursing homes are striving for an environment that minimizes lifting. However, one barrier to promoting safe handling of patients could be what students observe in their clinical placements. Lee and Lee (2017) conducted a cross-sectional survey of 221 California staff nurses. Their results showed that a culture of safety in organizations included lift availability and nurses reported fewer musculoskeletal injuries when safe handling practices were promoted. If students are in clinical placements in an organization that doesn't have a strong safety culture, they may engage in unsafe handling practices. Students with chronic disabling conditions, which are not readily apparent, may also need accommodations. Agarwal and Kumar (2017) provided guidance for faculty who teach students with lupus erythematosus. Accommodations such as the use of note takers, counseling, and principles of universal design were recommended to promote student success. Although their recommendations were not specific for nursing and other health professions students, they were very appropriate.

Nursing faculty may need to afford accommodations for students with service dogs. Prior to admission, students do not need to disclose their use of a service dog (Shilling et al., 2020). Students who are hearing impaired may use a service animal to alert them to sounds such as alarms. Those with a seizure history may use a service animal to alert them to an impending seizure. Faculty will need to have knowledge of regulations related to service dogs and work with clinical partners to accommodate the service dog (Shilling et al., 2020).

Color blindness, or color vision deficiency, need not disqualify a student from clinical practice. A study of 218 physicians in India conducted by Dhaliwal et al. (2020) concluded that physicians with color vision deficiency could practice safely with good lighting and peer verification for observations where color is critical. According to Webster (2021), approximately 9695 persons registered with the British Nursing and Midwifery

Council have color vision deficiency. This figure is based on the rate of color vision deficiency in the larger population. Webster noted, similar to Dhaliwal et al. (2020), that nurses with this condition might need assistance in identifying such conditions and hematuria or blood in the stool.

Students may become disabled during their time in school, and thus reasonable accommodations for students with physical disabilities may include time extensions for assignments and the assignment of an "incomplete" grade for courses that have not been completed on time. Students may also have disabilities that are less readily apparent, such as diabetes, colitis, or chronic fatigue syndrome. Faculty can help students work in groups so that those who need it can get a rest period. Furthermore, in some instances, providing alternative clinical experiences might allow a student to achieve the clinical objectives—just in a different setting.

When students with physical disabilities graduate, their successful employment may depend on nurse managers' experience in working with nurses who are disabled. Like instructors who ask students what they need to be successful (Epstein et al., 2020), so too do employing agencies. In addition, patients with disabilities may respond positively to health care professionals with disabilities. Jarus et al. (2020) interviewed 21 patients who had visible and nonvisible disabilities and 7 nondisabled patients. Two themes were identified: positive impacts, which included perceiving that care would be more patient centered, providing role models; and the second theme was "as long as," which meant if health care professionals were licensed and could "fit in" to the clinical setting and knew their capabilities. A survey of 207 Australians revealed that 81.4% of disabled physicians would be advantageous in the clinical setting because they could be more empathetic (Mogensen & Hu, 2019).

Military Veterans with Disabilities

Disabled military veterans are a special population that may require assistance from the veteran support office or the office that handles all students with disabilities. About 26% of veterans enrolled in college have any kind of disability (NCES,

2019). Veterans enrolled in universities and colleges, including those in nursing programs, face challenges in the college environment but at the same time have strengths that are an asset to those enrolled in nursing programs (Gibbs et al., 2019). Some of the barriers that veterans face are related to long and frequent deployments. Yet, facilitating their education promotes diversity in the workforce because military veterans are diverse in gender, age, and ethnicity (Sikes et al., 2021). They may have financial issues and family problems related to their deployments. Working with peers who are not as focused as they are may also be an issue, as are negative attitudes toward the military that some teachers and students may hold (Dyar, 2016). In addition, veterans are, for the most part, used to working in hierarchal structures, and learning independently may be difficult. Some clinical situations may trigger flashbacks and PTSD (Gibbs et al., 2019).

Veterans have many strengths, however, that promote success in a nursing program. If they have been medics, their skills can transfer into the clinical arena, despite their possible frustration with having to be closely supervised as a student. Leadership skills and working in teams and the ability to focus on the task at hand are strengths.

Returning to civilian life can be a difficult transition for veterans. Therefore having a veterans office on campus may ease the transition to college life for veterans, not just those with posttraumatic stress syndrome and physical disabilities. Veterans may have invisible injuries such as traumatic brain injury (Rattray et al., 2019). Such veterans will need university staff and health care providers to partner together to promote the success of military veterans in nursing programs.

THE NURSING STUDENT WITH SUBSTANCE ABUSE

Determining the number of nursing students who may be impaired by drug or alcohol use is difficult. The college environment does provide students with easy access to alcohol and drugs, including prescription stimulants, such as Ritalin, and can expose students to situations in which alcohol and drug use is considered an acceptable activity. The results of the 2020 national survey on substance abuse and mental health indicators showed that 34.5% of those persons aged 18–25 had used marijuana in the past year (Substance Abuse and Mental Health Services Administration, 2021), and 37% admitted to any illicit drug use. This same survey showed that among persons aged 18 to 22, 4.1% had abused opioids in the past year. More than 31% reported binge drinking at least once in the past month. Binge drinking was defined as five or more drinks for males and four or more drinks for females at one time.

Arria et al. (2018) conducted a nationwide study of 6962 full-time undergraduate students who didn't have attention deficit hyperactivity disorder (ADHD). They found that 11.2% had used nonprescription stimulants in the past 6 months. Approximately 65% of this group believed the stimulants provided academic benefit. Even 63.7% of those who didn't use the stimulants either strongly agreed, agreed, or were unsure about the academic benefit of nonprescription use of stimulants. Alcohol and marijuana use were correlated with the stimulant use.

Kirkpatrick and Boyd (2018) surveyed 249 nursing students for the purpose of determining the misuse of prescribed stimulants such as Ritalin and Adderall in the past year. Out of them, 24 (9.3%) had received a prescription for stimulants for ADHD; 16 used the medications only as prescribed, and 1.2% misused their prescriptions. Over 10% used prescriptions nonmedically, that is, using medications prescribed for another person. Three students diverted their medications to others, meaning they shared with others or sold their medication. The primary reason for using stimulants was to focus better while studying and working. In addition to asking about stimulant use, Kirkpatrick and Boyd (2018) found that 117 students had two or more behaviors indicative of potential substance abuse.

Serowoky and Kwasky (2017) explored substance use and abuse among undergraduates at a small Catholic university. Out of the 2175 undergraduates, 14% responded to the survey. Of note, 46% of the survey responses came from nursing students. Mean alcohol use was 2.5 drinks per week, less than the national average of 4.4 drinks per week. Students also reported using nonprescription drugs for nonmedical reasons, including stimulants (4.2% using at least six times within the past year) and pain medications (2.8% in the past year). Alcohol and substance abuse was related to a number of negative consequences, including sexual assault, physical violence, and ethnic and racial harassment. Grades were negatively affected for 20% of those who abuse drugs and alcohol.

Tavolacci et al. (2018) surveyed health behaviors of health care professional students in 2007 and 2014. Nursing students were 28.3% (738) of the sample. Between the two time periods, binge drinking increased from 14.1% in 2007 to 16.6% in 2015. Kritsotakis et al. (2020) measured lifestyle risk behaviors in nursing and social work students in the first year of their educational programs and at the end of the last year of their studies. For the nursing students, binge drinking in the last 30 days increased from 56.3% in the first year to 64.9% in the last year. Likewise, marijuana use increased from 6.6% to 23.9% from the first to the last year of their studies.

Ponce-Blandón et al. (2021) surveyed nursing students in Spain, Belgium, France, and Brazil regarding illegal drug abuse. Of the 496 students who responded, approximately 36% had engaged in illicit drug use in their lifetime. Males had a higher use of such drugs. Cannabis was the most frequently used drug. Excess cannabis use can impair decision-making and have academic consequences such as receiving a failing grade in a subject (Tabet et al., 2020). Cannabis use is particularly problematic, as it is legal for recreational purposes in a number of states in the United States. Yet drug screens for clinical partners might exclude those students and employees with cannabis in their system. Faculty need to caution students about this possibility.

One consequence of illicit drug use, particularly prescription stimulants, is academic dishonesty. Galluci et al. (2017) found in a study of 974 undergraduate students that use of prescription stimulants for nonmedical purposes was associated with academic dishonesty, including copying homework and letting others copy off their homework and plagiarizing content from the internet.

All undergraduate college students experience academic pressures that may lead to substance abuse, but nursing students have additional stressors. Often nursing programs have retention and dismissal policies that put pressure on students to do well in their studies. Dealing with patients with a variety of complex health problems adds more stress. As a result of stress, students may resort to illicit drug use and overuse of prescribed medications, which in turn can lead to errors in patient care and course failures.

Boulton and O'Connell (2017) conducted a nationwide study of student nurses' substance misuse and level of stress. More than 4000 students nationwide answered the survey; 5% reported the use of illicit drugs and 61% reported the use of alcohol 1 to 40 times in the past year. Drugs included nonprescription stimulants, pain pills, and tranquilizers. Arria et al. (2018) found that use of stimulants was primarily to enhance academic performance. Students who reported more stress experienced more substance abuse. High levels of faculty support did not ameliorate the correlation between stress and substance abuse.

Characteristics of Students With Chemical and Alcohol Impairments

The potential for substance abuse obviously exists among nursing students. Common signs of substance abuse include slurred speech, smell of alcohol, constricted pupils, sleeping during class, and frequent absences or tardiness. In particular, binge drinking can lead to poor performance in the classroom and in clinical practice.

Students with depression are prone to substance abuse. Sainz et al. (2019) investigated the relationship between depression and substance abuse in 1176 Mexican nursing students. Depression was related to the use of sedatives but not alcohol or stimulations. Kameg et al. (2020) explored substance abuse in both graduate and undergraduate nursing students at four universities. Undergraduate students exhibited higher rates of alcohol abuse compared to graduate students. Since alcohol abuse is widespread among college-age students, this finding is not surprising, as undergraduates tend to be younger and more prone to gather at events where alcohol is served in excess.

Rattner (2021) used the phenomenological method to analyze interview data from 14 who were either enrolled in or recently graduated from their nursing program. Seven of the interviewees identified personal issues such as depression, ADHD, and PTSD that led to their substance abuse. Students identified stigma related to mental health issues, including substance abuse. But one student noted that patient safety was paramount, and caring for patients while impaired posed a risk for patients. Participants relied on peer support for identifying resources for help. They expressed a need for more information regarding resources to deal with substance abuse.

Faculty Responsibilities Related to Students With Impairments

What are the responsibilities of faculty if they suspect that a student is displaying characteristics that are indicative of chemical impairment? Faculty have ethical responsibilities toward the student and the student's patients and therefore should not ignore or make excuses for such behavior indicative of substance abuse. Faculty need to ensure that students deliver safe patient care, which includes protecting clients from the actions of a potentially unsafe student whose clinical performance has been compromised. Faculty should be aware of the characteristics of students who may be chemically dependent and monitor all students for signs of substance abuse.

Faculty need to be knowledgeable about the policies and procedures within their institution that relate to students who are chemically dependent and familiar with the support services that are available to students who have a chemical dependency problem. Active treatment for substance abuse is covered under ADA (The ADA and Opioid Use Disorder: Combating Discrimination Against People in Treatment or Recovery, 2022).

Mandatory drug testing of nursing students has become more widespread, probably in response to clinical agency requirements. What is not clear is who has the right to know whether a student has tested positive for substance abuse. According to

Nigro et al. (2020), policies should be established that protect the rights of all involved, including students, faculty, administrators, and patients. For example, policies need to address whether students can be dismissed from the nursing program for substance abuse. Written policies about chemical impairment that include the institution's definition of chemical dependency, the nursing faculty's philosophy on chemical dependency, and student and faculty responsibilities related to suspected chemical dependency should be clearly stated in the student handbook. For online students, detecting chemical impairment may fall to the preceptor. Policies for mandatory drug and alcohol testing need to be in place for online and on-campus students need to be in place when substance abuse is suspected (Indiana State University, n.d.).

A faculty member might have to take immediate action if, for example, a student appears impaired in the clinical area and remove the student from the clinical setting. In cases in which the student does not pose an immediate danger to clients but is suspected of substance abuse, an appointment might be made with the student for the purpose of taking appropriate action. In addition to the faculty, a second person, such as an administrator, should be present to ensure that the student is dealt with according to policy and that due process is not denied.

Adhering to the institution's established policies helps ensure that the student's right to due process is not denied and protects faculty from possible legal action by the student. The National Student Nurses' Association (2020) and the Emergency Nurses Association (2017) support alternative to discipline policies that promote treatment and rehabilitation for students with substance abuse problems. In addition, the NCSBN's (2021) "alternative to discipline policy" model also advocates for treatment of substance abuse. The alternative discipline model includes random drug screens and attendance at Alcoholic and Narcotics Anonymous meetings as well as peer support. However, not all states include students in their programs for helping nurses with substance abuse. Whatever a school's policy is, confidentiality in dealing with the student and promoting wellness are key. Reentry policies for students after treatment should be established (Nigro et al., 2020).

Whether a school should institute a policy for random drug testing is controversial. Knowing the signs of substance abuse may be more beneficial, as random drug testing measures substance abuse at one point in time. Constant monitoring of student behavior by faculty may be a more accurate measure of a student's substance abuse. Although athletes are subject to random testing and most agencies have preemployment drug screening, the extent to which nursing students are required to undergo random screening is unknown. Although schools may not have policies requiring drug testing, students should be made aware that clinical agency policies may require blood or urine testing of individuals, including students, suspected of chemical dependency or as a requirement for engaging in clinical experiences within the agency. Nevertheless, some schools are instituting policies for drug screening before admission because of clinical agency requirements, and schools will require a drug screen if chemical impairment is suspected. Much more research is needed to determine the extent and nature of drug screening policies within nursing programs. Strobbe and Crowley (2017). Education may raise students' awareness of substance abuse disorders in nurses. Part of that education includes recognizing the signs and symptoms of substance abuse disorders. Stewart and Mueller (2018) instituted a curriculum improvement project for 200 prelicensure students in BSN and MN programs. Learning activities included videos, case studies, and assigned readings. A pre- and posttest design was used. Posttest scores for the BSN prelicensure students increased, while posttest scores for MN students didn't increase as much as for the undergraduates. Stewart and Mueller (2018) posited that the method used for case study analysis may have made the difference. BSN students had a faculty-moderated online discussion for 1 week, whereas MN students had one in-class small group discussion, which lasted 15 to 20 minutes.

Finally, faculty need to make sure that students applying for licensure disclose any substance use that resulted in criminal action, such as driving while intoxicated (DWI). Not disclosing such events can cause an application for licensure to be denied.

NURSING STUDENTS WITH MENTAL HEALTH PROBLEMS

High-stakes testing, academic policies such as dismissal following two-course failures and the clinical learning environment are examples of academic issues that may cause students extreme anxiety. Nursing students, like many other college students, must balance multiple life priorities (Mills et al., 2020). Finding time to sleep, exercise, and eat healthy, all essential for mental well-being, may be difficult with a demanding academic schedule. Mental health issues include anxiety, depression, eating disorders, obsessive-compulsive behavior, and suicidal ideation. Mental health issues are common among college students. For example, a nationwide sample of college students revealed that 41% of all college students had depression and 34% had anxiety. Twenty-seven percent had a lifetime diagnosis of depression (*Winter/Spring The Healthy Minds Study*, 2021).

Nursing students may also have mental health problems before enrolling in nursing school, which may have led them to be attracted to a helping profession. Students who experience mental health problems may need professional assistance in identifying and addressing these problems. Adverse childhood experiences, such as abuse, may influence students' overall mental health. Hedrick et al. (2021) surveyed 409 undergraduate nursing students. Those that had experienced more childhood abuse exhibited more signs of depression.

A variety of formally diagnosed conditions such as anxiety and other mental illnesses and learning disabilities may impact nursing students' ability to learn. Brown et al. (2020) surveyed Canadian first-year nursing students three times during their first year and second through fourth-year students twice during the academic year. The total sample size in this cross-sectional study was 1327. Those who used learning accommodations had statistically significantly more anxiety related to testing

and studying. Of interest is the fact that diagnosed anxiety peaked at the end of the third year. One could surmise that as the rigor of academic courses increased, so too did anxiety.

Testing, including high-stakes testing, such as those used as NCLEX pass rate predictors, and clinical practice present many challenges for nursing students' mental health. Faculty need to be aware of the impact on students' mental health so that strategies can be implemented to mitigate adverse mental health outcomes. Wang et al. (2019) examined the level of anxiety in 93 Canadian students in the final year of their program of studies. Fear of making mistakes and being watched by instructors produced the most anxiety. Younger students reported the most anxiety. Perhaps life experiences might mitigate some of the anxiety in older students.

Yildirim and Dalcali (2020) investigated the effect of problem solving on students' anxiety in the clinical arena. Like the students in Wang et al.'s (2019) study, fear of making mistakes and fear of negative evaluation of their performance were paramount causes of anxiety. Motivation was negatively correlated with anxiety; that is, as anxiety increased, motivation decreased. Faculty need to be aware of the fact that students who have high anxiety may lack motivation to overcome the causes of their anxiety.

The recent worldwide pandemic has revealed that undergraduate and graduate nursing students have experienced special mental health challenges related to the abrupt move to online learning, adjustments to clinical experiences, changes in work for pay, and increased family responsibilities. One study in Australia (Middleton et al., 2021) compared younger students, identified as Generation Z or the iGeneration, with older students. Results showed that older students had more knowledge about COVID-19. While both age groups perceived the University gave them adequate information about COVID-19, the iGeneration received more of its information from social media. There were no differences related to attending clinicals or grades in courses, but iGeneration students had more concerns related to completing clinical requirements. The iGeneration also had more anxiety than older students. The authors noted that in general, younger students have more mental health issues than do older students.

Another Australian study by Kerbage et al. (2021) explored the resilience, coping skills, and challenges experienced by 121 undergraduate nursing students at one school. One interesting finding was that students who were employed in health care were more resilient than those students who were not. The authors posited that students received support from peers in the work setting. Like participants in the Middleton et al. (2021) study, students had mental health problems related to isolation. Daily routines helped with coping, as did online interaction with friends. More time with family was noted as a positive experience.

Graduate students also have experienced mental health challenges during the pandemic. Rosenthal et al. (2021) surveyed master's and doctoral students (n = 222). Results showed that almost 10% of students had severe or extremely severe depression. Nearly 24% had experienced trauma that may have interfered with their mental health. Those employed in hospitals were at higher risk for mental health problems. Given the working conditions during the pandemic, this finding is not surprising. But those living with their families had less problems with their mental health. Family support appears to be critical to student well-being. Given the challenges students experienced as a result of the pandemic, nursing faculty should be alert to symptoms of mental health issues such as depression and anxiety, which could impact student success. Referrals to counseling centers could be made if needed.

The findings of these and other studies, as well as anecdotal reports, should heighten faculty awareness of how changes in the learning circumstances can affect students due to pandemics and other catastrophic events. In fact, Pereira et al. (2019) suggest that faculty have a critical role in providing a learning climate that motivates students to withstand the rigors of the nursing profession no matter the challenges that may arise.

Faculty and clinical partners must work together to help alleviate nursing students' anxiety so that students' learning can be maximized. Mitigating anxiety is critical to student success. Various strategies can help alleviate overall anxiety experienced by nursing students. Mindfulness-based strategies are one way to decrease nursing student anxiety. A meta-analysis of 10 randomized control trials with nursing students demonstrated that mindfulness strategies lowered depression and anxiety and increased mindfulness in participants (Chen et al., 2021).

Young-Brice and Dreifuerst (2019) stated that mindfulness interventions seek to decrease acting in routine and rigid ways. Furthermore, mindfulness can make a person aware of automatic negative thinking. By being aware of such thinking, a person can take steps to decrease negative emotions, decrease anxiety, and improve academic performance. In a qualitative study Young-Brice and Dreifuerst (2019) used semistructured interviews to explore mindfulness in 20 ethnic minority undergraduate students. Thematic analysis showed that self-awareness helped students deal with negative feelings and overcome challenges. Another theme was described as being in the moment or not dwelling on the past but moving forward with what is at the present time. Themes of self-doubt, feeling like a robot, and struggling to focus were examples of mindlessness. The authors concluded that promoting the use of mindfulness strategies could facilitate student success and promote overall health.

Stinson et al. (2020) used a quasiexperimental study to explore whether a mindfulness meditation could decrease anxiety and increase student retention. A convenience sample of 49 junior baccalaureate students participated in an author-developed mindfulness meditation intervention. Each session was 60 minutes in length and weekly sessions were offered over an 8-week period, but 49% attended at least one session and 65% participated in two to five sessions. The control group consisted of 117 junior students. Of note is the fact that originally a total of 85 students agreed to participate in the intervention but 36 then did not participate in the intervention. Anxiety decreased over the semester for the intervention group, but retention was no different between the groups. The investigators attributed the lack of difference to the fact that remediation strategies were available to all students.

Graduate students also experience anxiety that may be alleviated by mindfulness meditation.

Foley and Lanzillota-Rangeley (2021) used a 10-day trial of guided meditation delivered via a smartphone app to graduate RN students in a nurse anesthetist program. Students who participated in the guided meditation had statistically significant reductions in stress, anxiety, and depression. The majority of participants planned to continue mindfulness meditation to improve their overall mental well-being.

Cornine (2020) reported the results of an integrative literature review concerned with alleviating student anxiety in clinical practice. Cornine noted that most of the evidence was of low quality and had inconsistent findings. However, Cornine stated that mentoring was one successful strategy used to reduce anxiety associated with clinical experiences. Tambağ (2021) small quasiexperimental study of peer support (13 students in the experimental group and 13 students in the control group) confirms Cornine's conclusion. Although Stewart et al. (2018) did not find a statistically significant difference in anxiety when peer mentors were used for evaluation of skill performance in a learning laboratory prior to faculty evaluation, students did express that peer mentoring was helpful. The small sample size might have accounted for the statistical nonsignificance as well as the small number of skills evaluated. Studies with larger sample sizes might confirm whether or not peer support reduces students' anxiety.

Other studies, albeit mostly single site, provide additional evidence for faculty on how to ameliorate anxiety associated with clinical, as well as overall coursework. Heath et al. (2021) evaluated a program called Cultivating Practices for Resilience (CPR). The program included a CPR room where students could engage in relaxation and mindfulness activities. Mental health resources were available in every course through the learning management system. In addition, a director of student mental health and wellness was appointed. An investigator-designed online survey measured the effectiveness of the CPR program, and 131 students answered the survey. Out of them, 55% felt the CPR program was helpful. Yet, only 54% felt the college had a positive environment for mental health and wellness. Providing resources for mental health and well-being is not enough. Student-to-faculty, faculty-to-faculty, and student-to-student interactions must all be within a positive and supportive environment.

High-fidelity simulation has been used to decrease anxiety and enhance self-confidence. A systematic review of research reported from 2007 to 2017 revealed that simulation affirmed that simulation was effective in decreasing anxiety and enhancing self-confidence in performing clinical skills (Labrague et al., 2019). Labrague et al. did note, however, that most studies in their review had small sample sizes and had other methodological constraints including lack of control groups for comparison and statistical power. While simulation holds much promise in decreasing students' anxiety, larger studies with stronger methodologies need to be conducted.

Other strategies used to increase students' self-confidence and decrease anxiety in their clinical courses include a clinical skills refresher course (Shahsavari et al., 2017). One hundred sixty students in their final year were a part of Shahsavari's study. The students in the intervention group engaged in a 3-day refresher course where 10 skills including intravenous therapy, wound care, and injections were reviewed prior to an internship. The control group did not participate in the refresher course. Two weeks into the internship, both groups of students completed questionnaires that measured self-efficacy and anxiety. Clinical performance ratings by faculty were analyzed for both groups. Students in the intervention group had higher self-efficacy and less anxiety than students in the control group. Clinical skills were also rated higher for the intervention group. Like simulation, short-term refresher courses may have potential to decrease anxiety, enhance self-efficacy, and improve overall clinical performance.

A small study (n = 11) by Peters et al. (2019) tested a smartphone app designed to measure and help control anxiety when students were in clinical practice. In addition to quantitative data, focus group data were also analyzed. The 11 students used the app 29 times and only 10.5% reported no anxiety, while 63.2% reported a moderate level of anxiety (Peters et al., 2019). Approximately 68% used the app during clinicals. Students in the focus group reported that the interventions suggested during the app were helpful in dealing with anxiety experienced during clinical experiences.

Considering that most, if not all, students have access to a smartphone, further development and large-scale testing of smartphone applications to alleviate stress and anxiety may be warranted.

Test Anxiety

Test anxiety is a special form of anxiety experienced by nursing students. Although test anxiety is not recognized as a disability under the Americans with Disabilities Act unless the anxiety is part of a larger mental health issue (Burke, 2017), nursing faculty should provide evidence-based interventions to alleviate test anxiety in order to promote student success. Test anxiety can occur before, during, and after tests. Poorman et al. (2019) reviewed the literature in order to summarize evidence-based strategies faculty can use to ameliorate test anxiety. Strategies recommended by Poorman et al. (2019) include cognitive restructuring, such as asking, "Are my thoughts really rational?"; snapping a rubber band on one's wrist as a form of thought suppression if negative thoughts intrude in one's mind; and using earplugs to block out noise during a test and are helpful to some. Progression relaxation techniques were also noted by Poorman et al. (2019). Having students write questions for the test helps anxious students to organize learned material as opposed to focusing on memorization of facts. Faculty can also insert test questions into lectures so that students get practice applying learned material.

Specific strategies for alleviating test anxiety in nursing students have been tested in several small studies. Anderson et al. (2021) used pet-assisted therapy to reduce test anxiety prior to a medication calculation exam. Using a convenience sample, students were randomly assigned to the pet therapy group and the control group. While there wasn't a significant difference in exam scores between the two groups, the intervention group did demonstrate less measurable anxiety posttest. Reduction in anxiety may be achieved via pet therapy, even if academic achievement was not impacted. Nevertheless, pet therapy is one potential strategy to help students cope with anxiety.

As mentioned in Poorman et al.'s (2019) literature review, relaxation techniques are beneficial in reducing stress and anxiety. Manansingh et al. (2019) offered a 6-week session of relaxation to first-year students. Various relaxation techniques such as guided imagery, aromatherapy, listening to music, and muscle relaxation were offered in 15 to 30 minute sessions, and students were instructed to use the relaxation techniques prior to all exams. Pre- and posttests were given to measure academic stress and test anxiety at the beginning and end of the semester. Paired t-tests demonstrated that test anxiety and academic stress were significantly decreased. Additional focus group data did confirm that students felt the various techniques helped to reduce test anxiety.

Aromatherapy hand massage was used in Farner et al.'s (2019) pilot study to increase self-efficacy and decrease test anxiety. All groups showed improvement in test anxiety, but no difference was observed on the self-efficacy measure. The authors attributed their findings to a small sample size.

A study in Israel compared 148 first- and 92 fourth-year Jewish and Arab students on the roles social support and academic self-efficacy play in the level of test anxiety (Warshawski et al., 2019). Results showed that first-year students used more social media for support than did fourth-year students. Fourth-year students had higher academic self-efficacy, which is not surprising given that their ability to succeed had been demonstrated. Lower test anxiety was related to higher academic self-efficacy. Jewish students had higher academic self-efficacy as compared to Arab students, but Arab students found more support from social media. Anxiety was no different between the two groups. In a stepwise regression analysis higher social support from social media and higher academic self-efficacy were related to lower test anxiety. However, more social media usage in females was related to higher test anxiety. In other words support from social media is important, but more usage in and of itself may result in higher test anxiety, particularly in females.

One interesting proposal by Birkhead (2018) has some merit. She suggested that all students should be offered extended testing time in order to relieve test anxiety. Perceived wisdom for nurse educators is to allot 1 minute per multiple choice question because of the belief that NCLEX is a timed test (Birkhead, 2018). However, this is not the case. In fact, all who take NCLEX are allotted a maximum of 5 hours for 145 possible items (National

Council of State Boards of Nursing, personal communication, December 8, 2021). With the upcoming changes in NCLEX style questions, allowing more testing time for teacher-made tests, which include the newer style questions, may be advantageous for all students. In addition, while a variety of strategies have been shown to alleviate test anxiety, more research needs to be done to demonstrate the value of these strategies in improving academic performance resulting in better student retention.

Faculty Responsibilities Related to Students With Mental Health Problems

All faculty have the obligation to provide an educational climate that promotes strategies to mitigate stress and promote student success (Alsaqri, 2017). Instituting interventions early on can help ameliorate stress and anxiety experienced by nursing students. However, when students' performance is adversely affected by stress, anxiety, or other mental issues, the process used to assist students with suspected mental health problems is similar to the approach used with any student whose academic progress is jeopardized by unsatisfactory performance. First, the ADA/ADAAA prohibits discrimination against individuals who are mentally impaired. Second, all actions taken by faculty must be congruent with existing institutional policies and afford students the due process that is their right.

When mental health issues interfere with student behavior, faculty must deal with this behavior in a manner that is consistent with institutional policy. However, many university campuses offer counseling to all students for free or for a reduced fee. If, despite interventions, the behavior does not improve and the student is unable to perform effectively or patient safety is compromised, administrative withdrawal or dismissal from the program may be necessary. As always, the student who is administratively withdrawn or dismissed has the right to pursue the grievance and appeal process in place within the institution.

In addition, faculty should consider if present policies related to classroom testing and high-stakes testing promote or hinder student success.

Aside from strategies outlined above, what other services such as structured remediation should be offered? As suggested by Heath et al. (2021), providing a positive culture within a program can contribute to students' overall mental health.

CRIMINAL BACKGROUND CHECKS

In addition to mental health issues, which can compromise patient safety, the student who has a record of criminal activity can also compromise patient safety. Patient safety is a major concern for state boards of nursing and health care accreditation agencies. The Joint Commission (2021/2016) states, "Staff, students and volunteers who work in the same capacity as staff who provide care, treatment, and services, would be expected to have criminal background checks verified when required by law and regulation and organization policy" (para 1). Therefore nursing programs often require criminal background checks prior to admission. Furthermore, almost all states require self-disclosure of past criminal convictions or a formal criminal background check for initial licensure. The NCSBN model rules for state boards of nursing include a requirement for criminal background checks as part of the application process for licensure (NCSBN, 2021). Faculty will need to make sure students are apprised of this requirement prior to application for licensure. Regardless of whether a school requires a criminal background check before admission, faculty have a duty to warn students that although they may have successfully completed the nursing program, licensure could be denied if a student has a criminal background. A search of individual state boards of nursing websites will provide students with information regarding background checks before licensure.

Additionally, as noted earlier, clinical agencies may have requirements for background checks and may refuse clinical placements based on the results of the criminal background check, even if the student has been admitted into a nursing program. An example of a criminal background check policy is found in Box 4.3.

Denying admission based on the results of a criminal background check requires careful consideration. Decisions need to be made in line with

BOX 4.3   Example of Criminal History Check Policy

At the time of application to the nursing major, students are required to purchase and submit a current national-level criminal history check, which is part of the criteria used to determine your eligibility. Criminal background information will be maintained in your nursing student file and is considered confidential. The student is responsible for notifying the Associate Director of Students of any new charges or additions to one's criminal history promptly. Failure to report new charges may result in dismissal from the Baccalaureate Nursing Campus Track that they are attempting. The Baccalaureate Nursing Campus Tracks are required to share background items with Clinical Agencies. Clinical Agencies may require additional criminal history checks at the student's expense. Clinical Agencies have the right to refuse to permit students to have patient contact due to items on the background check.
(Courtesy Indiana State University School of Nursing. Retrieved from https://www.indstate.edu/health/program/son-undergrad/campus-bsn-student-handbook)

in place for the clinical agency and results of the criminal background checks must be evaluated on a case-by-case basis. Faculty have the burden of keeping track of agency requirements and students bear the financial burden of criminal background checks and drug testing (Williamson et al., 2018). Once a student is admitted to the program, however, faculty will find it difficult to deal with students who are denied entry into clinical facilities due to a criminal background check. It is better to identify issues before admission.

Requiring criminal background checks of international students before admission necessitates special consideration. If a student is coming directly from a country outside the United States, the visa application process should have included a criminal background check.

The areas of criminal background checks and drug testing continue to evolve, and nursing faculty will need to keep apprised of changes in health care agency policies and state laws. Each clinical agency may have different requirements for student criminal background checks. Students are often located in a multitude of states. Therefore nursing programs have to keep track of the different requirements in each state and faculty who teach clinical courses will need to ensure students have met the requirements for criminal background checks, as well as drug testing, for each agency used for clinical education.

to all faculty and students. When admission decisions are made, faculty need to consider the nature of the criminal conviction and how long ago the offense occurred and afford due process for those denied admission. Faculty must follow the policy

CHAPTER SUMMARY: KEY POINTS

- Having a disability doesn't automatically disqualify a student from achieving success in a nursing program.
- Fear may prevent a student from disclosing a disability.
- By law, it is a disabled student's responsibility to request accommodations in order to achieve program learning outcomes.
- Faculty cannot decide what appropriate accommodations are. A designated campus office will work with faculty and students in order to formulate appropriate learning accommodations.
- Essential functions for the nursing profession are different from technical functions.

- All students, including those with disabilities, must maintain the required academic standards necessary to achieve program outcomes.
- Program outcomes can be met in a variety of ways in diverse clinical settings, including in simulation labs.
- Faculty must work with clinical partners in order for accommodations to be met in the clinical arena.
- Universal design principles will promote an inclusive learning environment for all students, not just students with disabilities.

REFLECTING ON THE EVIDENCE

1. To promote diversity in the workforce, accepting students with disabilities is essential to prepare a workforce that mirrors diverse patient populations. What functions are truly essential to becoming a nurse, and how can these functions be demonstrated in a variety of ways with a student in a wheelchair, a vision-impaired student, or a hearing-impaired student?
2. What policies could promote an alternative to disciplinary action for those students who have impaired practice due to substance abuse?
3. What are the characteristics of an inclusive learning climate that promotes student success and helps lessen stress for all students?

4. What universal design strategies could be implemented in nursing education classrooms and clinical placements? How might these strategies benefit disabled and nondisabled students alike?
5. What nursing education program policies that are considered to be accepted practice do not create a positive learning environment and do not promote student success?
6. Most research studies related to nursing students with special needs have small sample sizes or are reports of case studies. How can nursing education research be strengthened in this area of study?

WEB RESOURCES

The following websites contain information regarding how to accommodate students with disabilities:

- The American Associate of Colleges of Nursing (n.d.). *Accommodating students with disabilities*. Retrieved from http://www.aacnnursing.org/Education-Resources/Tool-Kits/Accommodating- Students-with-Disabilities
- American Medical Professionals with Hearing Loss, https://www.amphl.org/about-us
- Job Accommodation Network, https://askjan.org/
- National Organization of Nurses with Disabilities, http://nond.org/

REFERENCES

Agarwal, N., & Kumar, V. (2017). An invisible student population: Accommodating and serving college students with lupus. *Work*, 56(1), 165–173. https://doi.org/10.3233/WOR-162477.

Alsaqri, S. H. (2017). Stressors and coping strategies of Saudi nursing students in clinical training: A cross-sectional study. *Education Research International*, 2017, 1–8. https://doi.org/10.1155/2017/4018470.

Ailey, S. H., & Marks, B. (2020). Technical standards for nursing education programs in the 21st century. *Rehabilitation Nursing*, 45(6), 311–320.

https://doi.org/10.1097/rnj.0000000000000297. Original publication 2017.

American Association of Colleges of Nursing. (2021). *The essentials: Core competencies for professional nursing education*. https://www.aacnnursing.org/Portals/42/AcademicNursing/pdf/Essentials-2021.pdf

American Nurses Association. (2021). *Safe patient handling and mobility: Interprofessional national standards across the care continuum* (2nd ed.). Author.

Americans With Disabilities Act, 42 U.S.C. § 12111 et seq. (1990). http://www.ada.gov/pubs/ada.htm

Americans With Disabilities Act, 42 USCA § 12101 note. (2008). http://www.eeoc.gov/laws/statutes/adaaa.cfm

Anderson, D., White, S. H., Ohm, R., Brown, S., & Poggio, J. P. (2021). The effect of animal-assisted therapy on nursing student anxiety: A randomized study. *Nurse Education in Practice*, 52, 103042. https://doi.org/10.1016/j.nepr.2021.103068.

Anderson, K. M., Davis, D., & McLaughlin, M. K. (2019). Implementing universal design instruction in Doctor of Nursing Practice education. *Nurse Educator*, 44(5), 245–249. https://doi.org/10.1097/NNE.0000000000000642.

Argenyi, M. (2016). Technical standards and deaf and hard of hearing medical school applicants and students: Interrogating sensory capacity and practice capacity. *AMA Journal of Ethics*, 18(10), 1050–1059. https://doi.org/10.1001/journalofethics.2016.18.10.sect1-1610.

Arria, A. M., Geisner, I. M., Cimini, M. D., Kilmer, J. R., Caldeira, K. M., Barrall, A. L., Vincent, K. B., Fossos-Wong, N., Yeh, J-C., Rhew, I., Lee, C. M., Subramaniam, G. A., Liu, D., & Larimer, M. E. (2018). Perceived academic benefit is associated with nonmedical prescription stimulant use among college students. *Addictive Behaviors, 76*, 27–33. https://doi.org/10.1016/j.addbeh.2017.07.013.

Association of Medical Professionals With Hearing Losses. (n.d.). *Stethoscopes.* https://www.amphl.org/comparison-table/

Birkhead, S. F. (2018). Testing off the clock: Allowing extended time for all students on tests. *Journal of Nursing Education, 57*(3), 166–169. https://doi.org/10.3928/01484834-20180221-08.

Boulton, M., & O'Connell, K. A. (2017). Nursing students' perceived faculty support, stress, and substance misuse. *Journal of Nursing Education, 56*(7), 404–411. https://doi.org/10.3928/01484834-20170619-04.

Brown, J., McDonald, M., Beese, , Manson, P., McDonald, R., Rohatinsky, N., & Singh, M. (2020). Anxiety, mental illness, learning disabilities, and learning accommodation use: A cross-sectional study. *Journal of Professional Nursing, 36*(6), 579–586. https://doi.org/10.1016/j.profnurs.2020.08.007.

Burke, C. (2017). The Americans With Disabilities Act and test anxiety: When accommodations are appropriate. *Journal of Physician Assistant Education, 28*(3), 156–157. https://doi.org/10.1097/JPA.0000000000000142.

Calloway, K., & Copeland, D. (2021). Acute care nurses' attitudes toward nursing students with disabilities: A focused ethnography. *Nurse Education in Practice, 51*, Article e102960. https://doi.org/10.1016/j.nepr.2020.102960.

Carroll, S. M., & Eaton, C. (2019). Accessible simulation: A necessity in nursing education. *Journal of Nursing Education, 58*(11), 619–621. https://doi.org/10.3928/01484834-20191021-01.

Chen, X., Zhang, , Zhang, B., Jin, S. -X., Quan, Y. -X., Zhang, X. -W., & Cui, X. -S. (2021). The effects of mindfulness-based interventions on nursing students: A meta-analysis. *Nurse Education Today, 98*, e104718. https://doi.org/10.1016/j.nedt.2020.104718.

Common signs of learning disabilities. (n.d.). https://www.ldonline.org/getting-started/ld-basics/common-signs-learning-disabilities

Cornine, A. (2020). Reducing the nursing student anxiety in the clinical setting: An integrative review. *Nursing Education Perspectives, 41*(4), 229–223. https://doi.org/10.1097/01.NEP.0000000000000633.

Cox, T. D., Ogle, B., & Campbell, L. O. (2019). Investigating challenges and preferred instructional strategies in STEM. *Journal of Postsecondary Education and Disability, 32*(1), 49–61.

Crawford, C., Black, P., Melby, V., & Fitzpatrick, B. (2022). The academic journey of students with specific learning difficulties undertaking pre-registration nursing programmes in the UK: A retrospective cohort study. *Nurse Education Today, 111*, 105318. https://doi.org/10.1016/j.nedt.2022.105318.

Crouch, A. T. (2019). Perceptions of the possible impact of dyslexia on nursing and midwifery students and of the coping strategies they develop and/or use to help them cope in clinical practice. *Nurse Education in Practice, 35*, e90–e97. https://doi.org/10.1016/j.nepr.2018.12.008.

Davidson, P. M., Ruston, C. H., Dotzenrod, J., Godack, C. A., Baker, D., & Nolan, M. N. (2016). Just and realistic expectations for persons with disabilities practicing nursing. *AMA Journal of Ethics, 18*(10), 1034–1040. https://doi.org/10.1001/journalofethics.2016.18.10.msoc1-1610.

Dhaliwal, U., Singh, S., Nagpal, G., & Kakkar, A. (2020). Perceptions of specialist doctors of the ability of doctors with colour vision deficiency to practise their specialty safely. *Indian Journal of Medical Ethics, 5*(4), 1–18.

Dyar, K. L. (2016). Veterans in transition: Implications for nurse educators. *Nursing Forum, 51*(3), 173–179. https://doi.org/10.1111/nuf.12135.

Elisha, S., Bonanno, , Porche, D., Mercante, D. E., & Gerbasi, F. (2020). Development of a common clinical assessment tool for evaluation of nurse anesthesia education. *AANA Journal, 88*(1), 11–17.

Elting, J., Avit, E., & Gordon, R. (2021). Nursing faculty perceptions regarding students with physical disabilities. *Nurse Educator, 46*(4), 225–229. https://doi.org/10.1097/NNE.0000000000000940.

Emergency Nurses Association, (2017). Joint position statement: Substance use among nurses and nursing students. *Journal of Emergency Nursing, 43*(3), 259–263. https://doi.org/10.1016/S0099-1767(17)30168-X.

Epstein, I., Stephens, L., Severino, S. M., Khanlou, N., Mack, T., Barker, D., & Dadashi, N. (2020). "Ask me what I need": A call for shifting responsibility upward and creating inclusive learning environments in clinical placement. *Nurse Education Today, 92*, 104505. https://doi.org/10.1016/j.nedt.2020.104505.

Equal Employment Opportunity Commission. (2011). *Fact sheet on the EEOC's final regulations implementing the ADAAA.* https://www.eeoc.gov/laws/guidance/fact-sheet-eeocs-final-regulations-implementing-adaaa

Farner, J., Reed, M., Abbas, J., Shmina, K., & Bielawski, D. (2019). Aromatherapy hand massage for test anxiety and self-efficacy in nursing students: A pilot study. *Teaching and Learning in Nursing*, *14*(4), 225–230. https://doi.org/10.1016/j.teln.2019.04.008.

Foley, T., & Lanzillotta-Rangeley, J. (2021). Stress reduction through mindfulness meditation in student registered nurse anesthetists. *AANA Journal*, *89*(4), 284–289.

Galluci, A. R., Martin, R. J., Hackman, C., & Hutcheson, A. (2017). Exploring the relationship between the misuse of stimulant medications and academic dishonesty among a sample of college students. *Journal of Community Health*, *42*(2), 287–294. https://doi.org/10.1007/s10900-016-0254-y.

Gawronski, M., Kuk, L., & Lombardi, A. R. (2016). Inclusive instruction: Perceptions of community college faculty and students pertaining to universal design. *Journal of Post-Secondary Education and Disability*, *29*(4), 331–347.

Gibbs, C. E., Lee, C. J., & Ghanbari, H. (2019). Promoting faculty education on needs and resources for military-active and veteran students. *Journal of Nursing Education*, *68*(6), 347–353. https://doi.org/10.3928/01484834-20190521-05.

Harris, C. (2018). Reasonable adjustments for everyone: Exploring a paradigm change for nurse educators. *Nurse Education in Practice*, *33*, 178–180. https://doi.org/10.1016/j.nepr.2018.08.009.

Healthy Minds Network. *The Healthy Minds Study 2021 Winter/Spring data report*. https://healthymindsnetwork.org/wp-content/uploads/2021/09/HMS_national_winter_2021.pdf

Heath, J., Walmsley, L. A., Braido, C., Brouwer, K., Wiggins, A. T., & Butler, K. M. (2021). Cultivating Practices for Resilience with baccalaureate nursing students: A pilot study. *Perspectives in Psychiatric Care*. Advance online publication https://doi.org/10.1111/ppc.12960.

Hedrick, J., Bennett, V., Carpenter, J., Dercher, L., Grandstaff, D., Gosch, K., Grier, L., Meek, V., Poskin, M., Shotton, E., & Waterman, J. (2021). A descriptive study of adverse childhood experiences and depression, anxiety, and stress among undergraduate nursing students. *Journal of Professional Nursing*, *37*(2), 291–297. https://doi.org/10.1016/j.profnurs.2021.01.007.

Indiana State University. (n.d.). SON Graduate chemically impaired student nursing policy. indstate.edu

Jarus, T., Bezati, R., Trivett, S., Lee, M., Bulk, L. Y., Battalova, A., Mayer, Y., Murphy, S., Gerber, P., & Drynan, D. (2020). Professionalism and disabled clinicians: The client's perspective. *Disability and Society*, *35*(7), 1085–1102. https://doi.org/10.1080/09687599.2019.1669436.

Joint Commission. (2021, October 25). *Criminal background check requirements*. https://www.jointcommission.org/standards/standard-faqs/laboratory/human-resources-hr/000001355/

Kameg, B. N., Lindsay, D., Lee, , & Mitchell, A. (2020). Substance use and exposure to adverse childhood experiences in undergraduate and graduate nursing students. *Journal of the Psychiatric Nurses Association*, *26*(4), 354–363. https://doi.org/10.1177/1078390320905669.

Kerbage, S. H., Garvey, L., Willetts, G., & Olasoji, M. (2021). Undergraduate nursing students' resilience, challenges, and supports during corona virus pandemic. *International Journal of Mental Health Nursing*, *30*(Suppl. 1), 1407–1416. https://doi.org/10.1111/inm.12896.

Kirkpatrick, Z., & Boyd, C. J. (2018). Stimulant use among undergraduate nursing students. *Journal of Addictions Nursing*, *29*(2), 84–89. https://doi.org/10.1097/JAN.0000000000000219.

Kritsotakis, G., Georgiou, E. D., Karakonstandakis, G., Kaparounakis, N., Pitsouni, V., & Sarafis, P. (2020). A longitudinal study of multiple lifestyle health risk behaviours among nursing students and non-nursing peers. *International Journal of Nursing Practice*, *26*, e12852. https://doi.org/10.1111/ijn.12852.

Labrague, L. J., McEnroe-Petitte, D. M., Bowling, A. M., Nwafor, C. E., & Tsaras, K. (2019). High-fidelity simulation and nursing students' anxiety and self-confidence: A systematic review. *Nursing Forum*, *54*(3), 358–368. https://doi.org/10.1111/nuf.12337.

LDOnline. (2021). http://www.ldonline.org/ldbasics/whatisld

LD Resources Foundation. (n.d.). *Learning disability statistics*. https://www.ldrfa.org/

L'Ecuyer, K. (2019). Perceptions of nurse preceptors of students and new graduates with learning difficulties and their willingness to precept them in clinical practice (Part 2). *Nurse Education in Practice*, *34*, 210–217. https://doi.org/10.1016/j.nepr.2018.12.004.

Lee, S. J., & Lee, J. H. (2017). Safe patient handling behaviors and lift use among hospital nurses: A cross-sectional study. *International Journal of Nursing Studies*, *74*, 53–60. https://doi.org/10.1016/j.ijnurstu.2017.06.002.

Levey, J. A. (2016). Measuring nurse educators' willingness to adopt inclusive teaching strategies. *Nursing

Education Perspectives, 27(4), 215–220. https://doi.org/10.1097/01.NEP.0000000000000021.

Levey, J. A. (2018). Universal design for instruction in nursing education: An integrative review. *Nursing Education Perspectives*, 39(3), 156–161. https://doi.org/10.1097/01.NEP.0000000000000249.

Maggu, A. R., & Overath, T. (2021). An objective approach toward understanding auditory processing disorder. *American Journal of Audiology*, 30(3), 790–795. https://doi.org/10.1044/2021_AJA-21-00007.

Major, R., & Tetley, J. (2019). Recognising, managing and supporting Dyslexia beyond registration: The lived experiences of qualified nurses and nurse academics. *Nurse Education in Practice*, 37, e146–e152. https://doi.org/10.1016/j.nepr.2019.01.005.

Manansingh, S., Tatum, S. L., & Morote, E. -S. (2019). Effects of relaxation techniques on nursing students' academic stress and test anxiety. *Journal of Nursing Education*, 58(9), 534–537. https://doi.org/10.3928/01484834-20190819-07.

Middleton, R., Fernandez, R., Moxham, L., & Tapsell, A. (2021). Generational differences in psychological well-being and preventative behaviours among nursing students during COVID-19: A cross-sectional study. *Contemporary Nurse*. Advance online publication https://doi.org/10.1080/10376178.2021.1987941.

Mills, A., Ryden, J., & Knight, A. (2020). Juggling to find balance: Hearing to the voices of undergraduate nursing students. *British Journal of Nursing*, 29(15), 897–903. https://doi.org/10.12968/bjon.2020.29.15.897.

Mogensen, L., & Hu, W. (2019). "A Doctor who really knows…": A survey of community perspectives on medical students and practitioners with disability. *BMC Education*, 19(1), e288. https://doi.org/10.1186/s12909-019-1715-7.

Moriña, A., & Orozco, I. (2020). Facilitating the retention and success of students with disabilities in health sciences: Experiences and recommendations by nursing faculty members. *Nurse Education in Practice*, 49, e102902. https://doi.org/10.1016/j.nepr.2020.102902.

National Academies of Sciences, Engineering, and Medicine, (2021). *The future of nursing 2020–2030: Charting a path to achieve health equity*. The National Academies Press. https://doi.org/10.17226/25982.

National Center for Education Statistics. (2011). *Students with disabilities at degree-granting postsecondary institutions: First look*. http://nces.ed.gov/pubs2011/2011018.pdf

National Center for Education Statistics. (2019). *Profile of undergraduate students: Attendance, distance and remedial education, degree program and field of study, demographics, financial aid, financial literacy, employment, and military status: 2015–2016*. https://nces.ed.gov/pubsearch/pubsinfo.asp?pubid=2019467

National League for Nursing. (2016). *Achieving diversity and meaningful inclusion in nursing education*. http://www.nln.org/docs/default-source/about/vision-statement-achieving-diversity.pdf?sfvrsn=2

National Student Nurses' Association. (2020). *Code of ethics*. https://www.dropbox.com/s/a229ong58d-5jx4p/Code%20of%20Ethics.pdf?dl=0

Neal-Boylan, L., & Miller, M. (2017). Treat me like everyone else: The experience of nurses who had disabilities in school. *Nurse Educator*, 42(4), 176–180. https://doi.org/10.1097/NNE.0000000000000348.

Neal-Boylan, L., & Miller, M. (2020). How inclusive are we, really. *Teaching and Learning in Nursing*, 15, e237–e240. https://doi.org/10.1016/j.teln.2020.04.006.

Neal-Boylan, L., Lussier-Duynstee, P., & Serrantino-Cox, J. (2021). *The Student physical disability: Sam Stone, a nursing student with a missing limb*. In L. Neal-Boylan, L. Meeks, & L. M. Neal-Boylan (Eds.), *Disability as diversity*. Springer. https://doi.org/10.1007/978-3-030-55886-4_9.

Neal-Boylan, L., Miller, M., & Lussier-Duynstee, P. (2021). Failing to fail when disability is a factor. *Nurse Educator*, 46(4), 230–233. https://doi.org/10.1097/NNE.0000000000000965.

Neal-Boylan, L., & Smith, D. (2016). Nursing students with physical disabilities: Dispelling myths and correcting misconceptions. *Nurse Educator*, 41(1), 13–18. https://doi.org/10.1097/NNE.0000000000000191.

Nigro, T. M., Schwartz, P. S., Roche, B. T., & Tariman, J. D. (2020). Comprehensive reentry policy for student registered nurse anesthetists with substance abuse disorder. *AANA Journal*, 88(4), 319–323.

Pavlik, D. L., Melcher, B. Q., Agnew, D. M., Smith, D. A., & Marciante, K. (2019). The Americans with disabilities act, reasonable accommodations, and medical education. *The Journal of Physician Assistant Education*, 30(4), 214–218. https://doi.org/10.1097/JPA.0000000000000277.

Pereira, F. L. B., Medeiros, S. P., Salgado, R. G. F., Castro, J. N. A. C., & Oliveira, A. M. N. (2019). Anxiety signs experienced by nursing undergraduates. *Revista de Pesquisa Cuidado é Fundamental Online*, 11(4), 880–886. https://doi.org/10.9789/2175-5361.2019.v11i4.880-886.

Philion, R., St-Pierre, I., & Bourassa, M. (2021). Accommodating and supporting students with disability in the context of nursing clinical placements: A collaborative action research. *Nurse Education in Practice, 54,* e10312.

Peters, A. B., Kellogg, M., & Zhang, Y. (2019). Implementation of a smartphone app to measure and manage anxiety in undergraduate clinical nursing students. *Nursing Education Perspectives, 40*(6), 367–369. https://doi.org/10.1097/01.NEP.0000000000000403.

Ponce-Blandón, J. A., Martinez-Montilla, J. M., Pabón-Carrasco, M., Martos-García, R., Castro-Méndez, A., & Romero-Castillo, R. (2021). International multicenter study on drug consumption in nursing students. *International Journal of Environmental Research and Public Health, 18,* e9526.

Poorman, S. G., Mastorovich, M. L., & Gerwick, M. (2019). Interventions for test anxiety: How can faculty help. *Teaching and Learning in Nursing, 14*(3), 186–191. https://doi.org/10.1016/j.teln.2019.02.007.

Quinn, E. (2018, April 26). *Eileen Quinn how to insert an IV with one hand* [Video]. YouTube. https://www.youtube.com/watch?v=2NfmRXtS4xg&t=256s

Rattner, I. (2021). A phenomenological study on substance use and misuse among nursing students. *Journal of Nursing Education, 60*(11), 607–613. https://doi.org/10.3928/01484834-20210913-01.

Rattray, N. A., True, G., Natividad, D. M., Salyers, M. P., Frankel, R. M., & Kukla, M. (2019). The long and winding road to postsecondary education for U.S. veterans with invisible injuries. *Psychiatric Rehabilitation Journal, 4*(3), 284–295. https://doi.org/10.1037/prj0000375.

Rehabilitation Act, 29 U.S.C. 794 § 504 et seq. (1973). https://www.dol.gov/oasam/regs/statutes/sec504.htm

Rosenthal, L., Lee, S., Jenkins, P., Arbet, J., Carrington, S., Hoon, S., Purcell, S. K., & Nodine, P. (2021). A survey of mental health in graduate nursing students during the COVID-19 pandemic. *Nurse Educator, 46*(4), 215–220. https://doi.org/10.1097/NNE.0000000000001013.

Sainz, M. T., Nagy, G., Mohedano, G. R., Vélez, N. M., García, A. C., Cisneros, D. P., & Rey, G. N. (2019). The association between substance use and depressive symptomology in nursing university students in Mexico. *Nurse Education in Practice, 19,* e114–e120. https://doi.org/10.1016/j.nepr.2019.03.005.

Sanderson, C., Hollinger-Smith, L., & Cox, K. (2021). Developing a Social Determinants of Learning™ framework: A case study. *Nursing Education Perspectives, 42*(4), 205–211. https://doi.org/10.1097/01.NEP.0000000000000810.

Scheirer, T. F. (2021). Using universal design principles in a fundamentals course to promote student transition to nursing education. *Nursing Education Perspectives, 42*(6), e111–e113. https://doi.org/10.1097/01.NEP.0000000000000672.

Serowoky, M. L., & Kwasky, A. N. (2017). Health behaviors survey: An examination of undergraduate students' substance use. *Journal of Addictions Nursing, 28*(2), 63–70. https://doi.org/10.1097/JAN.0000000000000165.

Shahsavari, H., Ghiyasvandian, S., Houser, M. L., Zakerimoghadim, M., Kermanshahi, S. S. N., & Torabi, S. (2017). Effect of a clinical skills refresher course on the clinical performance, anxiety and self-efficacy of the final year undergraduate nursing students. *Nurse Education in Practice, 27,* 151–156. https://doi.org/10.1016/j.nepr.2017.08.006.

Sharfi, K., Rosenblum, S., & Meyer, S. (2022). Relationships between executive functions and sensory patterns among adults with specific learning disabilities as reflected in their daily functioning. *PLoS One, 17*(4), e0266385. https://doi.org/10.1371/journal.pone.0266385.

Shilling, S. D., Lucas, L., Silbert-Flagg, J., & Nolan, M. T. (2020). Federal, state, and institutional regulations regarding a nursing student with a service animal. *Journal of Professional Nursing, 36*(6), 454–457. https://doi.org/10.1016/j.profnurs.2020.03.004.

Sikes, D. L., Patterson, B. J., Chargualaf, K. A., Elliott, B., Song, H., Boyd, J., & Armstrong, M. L. (2021). Predictors of veterans progression and graduation in Veteran to Bachelor of Science in Nursing (VBSN) programs: A multisite study. *Journal of Professional Nursing, 37*(3), 632–639. https://doi.org/10.1016/j.profnurs.2021.03.008.

Southeastern Community College v. Davis, 442 U.S. 397. (1979).

Stewart, P., Greene, D., & Coke, S. (2018). Effects of peer evaluation technique on nursing students' anxiety level. *Nurse Educator, 43*(4), 219–222. https://doi.org/10.1097/NNE.0000000000000474.

Stewart, D. M., & Mueller, C. A. (2018). Substance use disorder among nurses: A curriculum initiative. *Nurse Educator, 43*(8), 132–185. https://doi.org/10.1097/NNE.0000000000000466.

Stinson, C., Curl, E. D., Hale, G., Knight, S., Pipkins, C., Hall, I., White, K., Thompson, N., & Wright, C. (2020). Mindfulness meditation and anxiety in nursing students. *Nursing Education Perspectives, 41*(4), 244–245. https://doi.org/10.1097/01.NEP.0000000000000635.

Strobbe, S., & Crowley, M. (2017). Substance use among nurses and nursing students: A joint position statement of the Emergency Nurses Association and the International Nurses Society on Addictions. *Journal of Addictions Nursing, 28*(2), 104–106. https://doi.org/10.1097/JAN.0000000000000150.

Substance Abuse and Mental Health Services Administration. (2021). *Key substance use and mental health indicators in the United States: Results from the 2020 National Survey on Drug Use and Health* (HHS Publication No. PEP21-07-01-003, NSDUH Series H-56). Center for Behavioral Health Statistics and Quality, Substance Abuse and Mental Health Services Administration. https://www.samhsa.gov/data/

Tabet, A. C., Meyer, D. G., Martinez, J., & Diaz, R. P. (2020). The consequences of cannabis use: A review of self-reported use and experiences among college students. *Journal of Doctoral Nursing Practice, 13*(3), 229–234. https://doi.org/10.1891/JDNP-D-19-00082.

Tambağ, H. (2021). Examination of nursing students' anxiety levels related to clinical practice with respect to peer support. *Perspectives in Psychiatric Care, 57*(3), 1114–1119. https://doi.org/10.1111/ppc.12664.

Tavolacci, M. P., Delay, J., Grigioni, S., Déchelotte, , & Ladner, J. (2018). Changes and specificities in health behaviors among healthcare students over an 8-year period. *PLoS One, 13*(3), e0194188. https://doi.org/10.1371/journal.pone.0194188.

The ADA and Opioid Use Disorder: Combating Discrimination Against People in Treatment or Recovery. (2022). https://www.ada.gov/resources/opioid-use-disorder/

Wang, A. H., Lee, C. T., & Espin, S. (2019). Undergraduate nursing students' experiences of anxiety-producing situations in clinical practicums: A descriptive survey study. *Nurse Education Today, 76,* e103–e108. https://doi.org/10.1016/j.nedt.2019.01.016.

Warshawski, S., Bar-Lev, O., & Barnoy, S. (2019). Role of academic self-efficacy and social support on nursing students' test anxiety. *Nurse Educator, 44*(1), e6–e10. https://doi.org/10.1097/NNE.0000000000000552.

Webster, B. (2021). Colour vision deficiency: The "unseen" disability. *British Journal of Nursing, 30*(8), 468–469. https://doi.org/10.12968/bjon.2021.30.8.468.

What is a learning disability. (n.d.). https://www.ldonline.org/getting-started/ld-basics/what-learning-disability

Williamson, T. W., Hughes, S., Flick, J. E., Burnett, K., Bradford, J. L., & Ross, L. L. (2018). Clinical experiences: Navigating the intricacies of student placement requirements. *Journal of Allied Health, 47*(4), 237–242.

Yarbrough, A. E., & Welch, S. R. (2021). Uncovering the process of reasonable academic accommodations for prelicensure nursing students with learning disabilities. *Nursing Education Perspectives, 42*(1), 5–10. https://doi.org/10.1097/01.NEP.0000000000000666.

Yildirim, T. A., & Dalcali, B. K. (2020). The effect of nursing students' problems in the clinical practice environment on anxiety level and motivation. *International Journal of Caring Sciences, 13*(3), 2054–2063.

Young-Brice, A., & Dreifuerst, K. T. (2019). Exploration of mindfulness among ethnic minority undergraduate nursing students. *Nursing Educator, 44*(6), 316–320. https://doi.org/10.1097/NNE.0000000000000629.

Zeng, W., Ju, S., & Hord, C. (2018). A literature review of academic interventions for college students with learning disabilities. *Learning Disability Quarterly, 41*(3), 159–169. https://doi.org/10.1177/0731948718760999.

5

Forces and Issues Influencing Curriculum Development*

Gayle M. Roux, PhD, RN, NP-C, CNS, FAAN and Monique Ridosh, PhD, RN

Curriculum development is a dynamic process aligned with the magnitude, pace, and patterns of change within the health care arena. Curriculum development, implementation, and evaluation ideally occur within a very planful and collaborative environment. However, faculty also need to be skilled in the fundamental process of curriculum change to provide education and support for students in an emergent, unexpected situation. Faculty are called to ensure curriculum matches the critical thinking and assessment needed to respond quickly to a natural disaster or a pandemic such as COVID-19. Many programs quickly transitioned to hybrid and online delivery during the pandemic, changing how they delivered didactic and clinical curriculum. Carolan et al. (2020) identified this change as both disruptive and transformative. An overall purpose of the role of nurse educators is to continually develop and implement relevant curricula. Curricula emphasizing critical thinking and analytical skills help prepare graduates to respond to emerging trends across their careers. Science and technology advancements, national and international events, increasing diversity and aging of the US population, merger of health systems, accreditation requirements, public health policy changes, and social justice values regarding diversity, equity, and gender identity are all common influencing issues requiring continual curriculum revisions.

The purpose of this chapter is to first discuss strategies and tools to identify influential forces and issues for nursing curriculum. Several strategies are presented to help nurse educators identify and select what is most relevant to their learning environment. Following description of identification strategies, major issues and forces influencing curriculum development will be highlighted. Some forces like the values in the mission statement are unique, and some forces like diversity and health equity are common across the nation and world. The ability to deliver a contemporary and meaningful curriculum within a dynamic and changing health care environment requires understanding of these common forces directing change. Lastly, possessing strategies for identification of issues and developing systems for curriculum change and approval can provide the map for changing the direction of professional nursing education.

This chapter focuses on the current context of curriculum development within major internal and external issues and forces across the metaparadigms. The concepts in the metaparadigm provide structure for how the nursing discipline should function. The four concepts of person, environment, health, and nursing address the patient as a whole, the patient's environment, the patient's health and well-being, and the nursing profession and responsibilities. As the metaparadigm provides an overall structure for how nursing should function, reflecting on the issues and forces in each concept is one way of examining their emphasis in curriculum development. This chapter aggregates

*The authors acknowledge the contributions of Linda Veltri, PhD, RN in previous editions of this chapter.

forces and issues within the four concepts of the metaparadigm as a way to conceptualize the overall global structure of curriculum development. This is only one of the various ways to conceptualize the strong links connecting curriculum development to the art and science of nursing.

It is important that faculty retain purpose and meaning in curriculum development. Didactic and clinical curriculum are focused on selected issues so that nurses entering the workforce are equipped with current knowledge and competencies needed to provide culturally relevant and patient-centered care. Graduates should be advocates for improved health care access and decreasing health disparities. Opportunities in the curriculum should be available to prepare graduates to assume leadership roles at the bedside and in the boardroom across their career.

STRATEGIES TO IDENTIFY INFLUENTIAL FORCES AND ISSUES

This section presents strategies that will assist nurse leaders and educators to identify meaningful influences. Thoughtful curriculum change is achieved by initially exploring these strategies to provide the "360-degree view." The current body of knowledge, direction of the strategic plan, epidemiological patterns and trends of social determinants of health, and research findings should be at the forefront of curriculum changes.

Environment—Body of Knowledge and Life-Long Learning

In health care knowledge of changes assists educators, nurses, and other health care professionals to understand the current climate. The depth and breadth of the body of knowledge provides direction to inform the work that needs to be done to shape health care delivery systems and improve the health of the nation. The goal of conducting literature reviews and assessing the current state of science is to help leaders, managers, and educators become aware of general trends and events affecting health care, nursing, and higher education. Information can be acquired in various ways, including careful review of scientific

and professional journals, updating from national and international organizations such as the World Health Organization and the Centers for Disease Control and Prevention, reading the lay literature and newspapers, and attendance and networking at professional meetings.

The American Hospital Association conducts an annual review to identify forces and trends shaping health care in the United States (US) (American Hospital Association [AHA], 2022). The scan identified forces that have created transformation in 2021, stating that COVID-19 has caused a reshaping of the health care environment. Major themes highlighted in Table 5.1 include the hospital and health system landscape; coexisting with COVID-19; workforce; health equity; behavioral health; access and affordability; and innovation and delivery transformation. Some 2022 categories were consistent with earlier strategic plans such as access and affordability, health equity, and behavioral health. Persistent forces and trends include high numbers of uninsured and underinsured Americans, skyrocketing drug prices, high total US health care spending compared to outcomes, and increasing health care disparities. However, the 2022 scan emphasized the forces shaping health care were greatly exaggerated by the pandemic. The COVID-19 pandemic has created critical challenges requiring new solutions such as the need for digital and information health literacy. Additionally, mental health and substance use disorders have reached critical peaks during the pandemic (AHA, 2022).

In academia, faculty continually practice life-long learning to explore the generation of new knowledge and advance knowledge dissemination. This body of knowledge forms the context of the forces affecting curriculum development. This allows faculty to be simultaneously reactive and proactive when developing nursing curriculum at all levels. Through awareness and acknowledgment of significant trends (reactive), faculty can more actively choose a future direction for nursing education and develop relevant curriculum (proactive). The current body of knowledge provides a broad scope of information. The evaluation of its relevance to nursing curriculum is the foundation of the other strategies that follow.

TABLE 5.1 **American Hospital Association 2022 Environmental Scan**		
Major Themes	**Impact on Health Care**	**Influence on Curriculum**
Hospital and health system landscape	Increased inpatient average length of stay, and decreased preventive services	Primary care and community health nursing to deliver chronic disease management and behavioral health
Coexisting with COVID-19	Specialty care for COVID-19 infection and aftereffects, hospitalization, and vaccination	Evidence-based models of care to address public health emergencies
Workforce	Prevalence of health care worker mental health conditions and critical staff shortages	Advanced practice nursing and strategies for resiliency
Health equity	COVID-19 disparities, rural health care access, and barriers to digital access	Quality and patient safety strategies, care delivery models in alternative settings, and address social determinants of health
Behavioral health	Increased demand for behavioral health	Mental health care across settings and lifespan
Access and affordability	High cost of health care and prescription drug prices	Leadership for value-based model of care
Innovation and delivery transformation	Use of artificial intelligence and telehealth	Telehealth, team-based care, and use of digital health technologies

From Major Themes and Impact on Healthcare sections adapted with permission from © American Hospital Association, 2022 Environmental Scan at https://www.aha.org/guidesreports/2022-12-05-2022-environmental-scan.

Strategic Planning: Giving Direction

Often nurse leaders, managers, and educators are so preoccupied with the "tyranny of the urgent" or "teaching to the test" that they lose sight of course outcomes, program outcomes, and desired national and global health goals. Content-focused curriculum leads to task-oriented nurses disregarding professional identity formation. Thus faculty can miss opportunities to make desired changes. Therefore it is important to collaboratively engage faculty in strategic planning and continuous quality improvement efforts.

Strategic planning and curriculum change is a group process that administration, faculty, students, and stakeholders use to determine direction of the desired change. When building consensus, the input of all parties involved is carefully considered. The goal of consensus building is for all parties to work cooperatively to embrace a curriculum change that meets the needs of the students, faculty, stakeholders, and public we serve.

Student surveys and the use of consultants in strategic planning processes are examples that provide an opportunity for organizations and educators to facilitate tapping the rich diversity of group wisdom related to complex curricula issues. The strategic planning process may include the use of the Strengths, Weaknesses, Opportunities, and Threats (SWOT) analytical framework to help organizations or educators become fully aware of all factors involved when making decisions. Educators charged with curriculum development or redesign can use the SWOT analysis before implementing or making new changes and to identify key curricular components that are working well. Taking time to invest in a formalized SWOT analysis can assist educators to capitalize on curricular strengths and improve student outcomes (Schooley, 2021). A faculty retreat in an environment away from the usual campus atmosphere is another strategy to generate creative and meaningful curriculum planning ideas.

Epidemiology: Factors Related to Health Patterns

Epidemiology is the scientific study of the distribution and causes or risk factors of health-related states and events in US populations and globally (Centers for Disease Control and Prevention [CDC], n.d.). According to the CDC, epidemiology provides nursing faculty with systematic ways to understand patterns of disease and injury, characteristics of people at high risk for disease, and environmental factors. Using epidemiological data with groups or populations, nurses can understand and document the need for programs and policies to reduce risk and promote health. Epidemiology can therefore be seen as a method for planned change. In the same way nursing faculty responsible for the development of curriculum can use epidemiological data and methods to understand factors affecting the health of populations and trends occurring in patterns of morbidity and mortality. Epidemiologic analysis provides faculty with methods for understanding the broad patterns of health and the impact of social determinants of health in the population. Just one example of using epidemiological data and information on social determinants of health to inform curriculum is when teaching the increasing rate of maternal morbidity and mortality in the United States, especially in comparison to rates in other developed countries (CDC, 2020). Additionally, racial and ethnic disparities persist in pregnancy-related deaths, especially in Black and Native American/Alaska Native women (CDC, 2019).

Research: State of the Science

Research priorities established by organizations such as the National Institute of Nursing Research and the World Health Organization provide clear focus on influential issues to be integrated into the curriculum. Modeling the use of the scientific process, curriculum that highlights scientific findings, and effective clinical interventions facilitate learning. The graduates are hence more readily prepared to utilize and apply research findings throughout their nursing career. In addition to using evidence based-guidelines and new evidence useful to update curriculum in the clinical areas, research findings can also be applied to the teaching and learning environment.

Integration of Strategies: An Iterative Process

The strategies of exploring the environment for the current body of knowledge, engaging in strategic planning to give direction to changes, updating on epidemiological health trends and patterns of social determinants of health, and utilizing research, all have utility in preparing for curriculum development or revision. Using some combination of these four strategies, faculty can be equipped to develop curriculum compatible with the current and future issues influencing nursing and health care. The measurement of student learning outcomes provides data to inform faculty that indeed the curriculum and teaching were effective or that refinement and change is needed (see Chapters 22, 23, and 26 on evaluation). Measurements indicating an identified need for curriculum change place these four strategies again back at the forefront of curriculum planning. Thus the process of curriculum development is circular and dynamic.

ISSUES AND FORCES UNIQUE TO THE MISSION AND REGION

The mission statement is important to curriculum as it is the declaration of values and what philosophically drives the program of nursing. While there are many values shared by programs of nursing across the nation and world such as caring, safety, and quality, each program has a unique mission statement. It is best practice for each program to periodically evaluate their mission statement for the need for revisions and to examine the relevancy of the mission in the curriculum. For example, a program in a sparsely populated state may have rural health as a primary focus in the mission statement. A program in a historically Black college and university may include a value to engage historically diverse and underserved populations and expand access to higher education (see Chapter 7).

State boards of nursing have state-specific rules and regulations specifying their requirements for nursing education curriculum. Each program of nursing must align their course curriculum, program outcomes, and the evaluation of their programs to meet their state board of nursing requirements as well as those of their specific accreditation agency. Programs of nursing devote attention to the congruence of their curriculum and outcomes to the standards of their respective college and university accreditation agencies. It is important to examine curriculum through a comprehensive lens considering dynamic forces and issues in addition to the standards of accreditation agencies (see Chapter 27).

Additionally, a shared but also unique issue of curriculum development is the student community itself. Curriculum is developed and continually revised according to the issues students bring to the learning process. For example, a major force of undergraduate curriculum is feedback from students and clinical faculty on competencies the students have mastered and ones that need further reinforcement in the didactic and simulation curriculum (see Chapter 25).

MAJOR FORCES AND ISSUES COMMON IN CURRICULUM DEVELOPMENT

Person

Changing Population Demographics

The US population continues to age and grow more racially and ethnically diverse. By 2060, it is estimated that the population 65 and older will be 55% non-Hispanic White, 13% non-Hispanic Black, 8% non-Hispanic Asian, and 21% Hispanic (Federal Interagency Forum on Aging-Related Statistics [FIFARS], 2020). Poverty rates also vary greatly by sex, race, and ethnicity, with the lowest poverty rates seen among the non-Hispanic White population and men aged 65 and over (FIFARS, 2020). Housing costs and utilities remain a major source of economic burden. Many people of diverse racial and ethnic backgrounds across the nation were greatly impacted by unemployment and economic loss during the pandemic.

Changing population demographics increase the likelihood that nurses and other health care providers will encounter growing numbers of older and diverse adults who are living with a variety of chronic health conditions and facing increased health care costs. By 2030, it is estimated that people aged 65 and older will represent almost 21% of the total US population and more than half of the population age 85 and older are women (FIFARS, 2020). Among the older population, increasing age is associated with higher rates of poverty and housing cost burdens. Many elders will enter assisted living or long-term care facilities or be cared for by their families and communities (FIFARS, 2020).

Application for curriculum development. Initiatives such as those of the Hartford Institute for Geriatric Nursing (http://hign.org) provide nurse educators with excellent examples of how to incorporate best practices and other resources to improve the quality of life and health care outcomes of older adults. End-of-life issues also loom large for the US geriatric population and nursing profession. In 2000, the Robert Wood Johnson Foundation initially funded the End-of-Life Nursing Education Consortium (ELNEC), which continues today through a partnership between the American Association of Colleges of Nursing (AACN) and the City of Hope National Medical Center. This consortium project is a national and international education initiative dedicated to educating nurses in the delivery of excellent palliative care. To date, more than 45,280 nurses and other health care professionals, from all 50 US states and 100 countries, have received ELNEC training (elnec.academy.reliaslearning.com) and are using this innovative strategy to equip the nursing workforce with needed palliative care-related skills and knowledge (American Association of Colleges of Nursing [AACN], 2021b). Nursing competencies across diverse contexts and settings at different levels of palliative care (e.g., generalist, specialist) continue to be defined (Hökkä et al. 2020), therefore requiring changes in curriculum to align competencies for provision of care. An integrative review of international literature (i.e., not restricted to publications in English) reported six main dimensions of nursing competencies for palliative care: Communication and cultural issues; collaboration with patient, family, and team; clinical; leadership; ethicolegal; and psychosocial and spiritual (Hökkä et al. 2020). The Center to Advance Palliative Care (capc.org) is a central resource for training across disciplines and settings in the United States accessible to professionals at member health organizations (e.g., participating health system membership).

Diversity, Equity, and Inclusion

The changing composition of America has turned this country into a microcosm of the world's peoples. In response, the nursing profession has long recognized the challenges this increasing diversity creates in the provision of high-quality, culturally responsive nursing care. Cultural sensitivity and cultural humility are essential curricular components of baccalaureate and graduate nursing education.

Diversity references a broad range of individual, population, and social characteristics (e.g., age; sex; gender identity; race; ethnicity; sexual orientation; language; immigrants and refugees; learning abilities; AACN, 2021a). Inclusion represents environment and organizational cultures in which all (e.g., faculty, students) thrive, environments in which multiple perspectives are respected. Equity considers the ability to recognize differences in resources or knowledge needed to fully participate (AACN, 2021a). Intentional changes to curriculum that address diversity, equity, and inclusion (DEI) in teaching and learning environments are needed to address persistent inequities in health care.

The diversification of the US population has highlighted challenging social justice issues related to inequities in housing, employment, poverty, mortality rates, and health outcomes for people of color. Over the last few years, the increased rates of police violence, murders, and disproportionate incarceration of Blacks have created a societal uprising and movement for change. Institutions of higher education have been one setting for these movements, resulting in a rise in campus activism. Nationwide, communities of students and faculty are closely examining social justice issues including discrimination, inclusivity, safe campus environments, and lack of equity within the health care system. See Chapter 17 for additional information on multicultural education in nursing.

An issue with historical roots that persists today is access to higher education (i.e., inclusion). The issue of access—regardless of gender, race, ethnic background, disability, or immigration status—is important considering society's transformation from an industrial economy to an information-based, global economy. Historically, women and other ethnic and racial groups have been a minority of the student population enrolled in institutions of higher education. The ability of all Americans to take advantage of the multiple benefits and opportunities that higher education affords requires public policies and political will that support access and higher education institutions that make those opportunities real. As administrators of nursing schools pursue robust enrollments of diverse and talented students, affordability and access are crucial considerations for the profession to develop a diverse nursing workforce.

Each of these forces promotes increased public scrutiny and higher expectations. Accountability therefore becomes a multidirectional force with multiple stakeholders. Institutions of higher education depend on the government for funding and are therefore highly accountable to the public for academic productivity and fiscal prudence. Governments, in response to their perceived accountability to the public, act to regulate and reform higher education. Schools of nursing are accountable to state legislatures, Congress, and the public regarding the workforce preparation of adequate numbers of competent nurses. This accountability includes incorporation of and adherence to regulations set forth by state boards of nursing, accrediting bodies, and others who set standards for prelicensure and graduate nursing education. Clearly accountability continues to be a significant theme in curriculum and higher education.

Application for curriculum development. Curriculum is continually revised and evaluated to inform students and promote sensitivity to the culturally diverse population of the world. Curriculum should address the subjective meaning of health and healing practices for diverse clients. Resources and web toolkits for developing and revising curriculum to enhance DEI are plentiful. Table 5.2 provides examples of resources from the major nursing accreditation organizations and American Association of Universities and Colleges. Faculty should follow strategies that guide curriculum development in DEI including networking with university and community DEI

TABLE 5.2 Diversity, Equity, and Inclusion (DEI) Resources for Curriculum and Faculty Development	
Resource	**Strategies for Curriculum and Faculty Development**
National Academy of Medicine (2021). *The Future of Nursing 2020–2030: Charting a Path to Achieve Health Equity.* A Consensus Study from the National Academy of Medicine. https://nam.edu/publications/the-future-of-nursing-2020-2030/	Podcasts and webinars discuss strategies for nursing to advance health equity. Comments from nurses working on the frontline and health experts are included.
National League for Nursing (2017). *Diversity & inclusion toolkit.* http://www.nln.org/docs/default-source/professional-development-programs/diversity_toolkit.pdf?sfvrsn=6	Addresses comprehensive DEI strategies for leadership, the academic mission, and recruitment and retention of diverse students and faculty. Extensive resources included for each topic. Reflective questions promote examination of our own biases. Honest answers to the questions provide guidance for enhancing DEI in the curriculum.
American Association of Colleges and Universities (2022). *Mission and strategic plan.* http://www.aacu.org/about/strategicplan	The strategic plan for DEI is addressed in behaviors across academic and health care systems. Action plans are recommended.
American Association of Colleges of Nursing (2022). *Diversity, equity, and inclusion.* https://www.aacnnursing.org/diversity	DEI Leadership Network is available for faculty members to join.
AACN (2021a). *DEI faculty toolkit.* https://www.aacnnursing.org/Portals/42/Diversity/Diversity-Tool-Kit.pdf	Toolkit depicts a model for DEI in schools of nursing.

experts, remaining open to our own unconscious biases, and evaluating curriculum with feedback from groups representing the DEI issue. Interactive learning strategies such as poverty simulations and case studies give faculty and students opportunities to explore their own biases before actual patient care experiences.

The rise in societal and campus unrest spreading across the United States requires administrators and educators to develop curriculum that promotes health equity and recognizes practices and microaggressions that discriminate against or exclude people based on race, ethnicity, sexual orientation, and gender identity. Additionally, it is incumbent upon institutions of higher education to assume a no-tolerance stance toward racism or discrimination of gender identity and sexual orientation exhibited by administrators, faculty, staff, or students. Institutions and nursing colleges must provide student support services and implement policies that support inclusivity and create safe campus environments for all.

Colleges of nursing should continue their efforts to create and initiate strategies aimed at attracting, recruiting, and retaining increasing numbers of students and faculty from diverse backgrounds. Doing so infuses nursing curriculum with alternative perspectives and helps establish a nursing workforce that is diverse and equipped to serve a culturally and racially diverse patient population, which is essential to meet the nation's health care needs and reduce health care disparities. One specific charge for colleges of nursing is to articulate the cost-effective contribution that nursing makes to the improved health access and decreased health disparities of the nation.

Whether the demographic shifts include age, diversity, or gender identification, there are implications for health and the resources needed to promote health. Regardless of the venue in which a culturally diverse and aging population receives care, issues surrounding diversity and geriatric health require educators to prepare nurses to promote culturally sensitive health and self-care and promote management of chronic conditions and quality of life in an aging population. Faculty should provide opportunities in the curriculum for students to develop political advocacy skills needed to influence public policy decisions related to the allocation of resources toward health and human needs. The responsibility to prepare future nurses in this manner is in keeping with a vision for quality health care explicated by the National Academy of Medicine *The Future of Nursing 2020–2030: Charting a Path to Achieve Health Equity* (National Academies of Sciences, Engineering, and Medicine [NAM], 2021), which includes discussion of accessible health care for diverse populations, disease prevention, promotion of wellness, and provision of compassionate care across the lifespan. Additionally, preparation of tomorrow's nursing practitioners requires attention to all demographic revolutions of both developed and developing areas of the globe, including patterns of growth, migration, and ethnic or racial composition.

Environment

To develop relevant curricula, faculty must have an understanding of the social context within which nurses practice and how that social context creates issues external to nursing yet critically relevant to the profession. Being knowledgeable about the social context and accompanying issues is an essential competency for faculty to build the foundation necessary to develop a contemporary and meaningful curriculum. External issues such as violence, war, immigration, and climate change are key variables in public health across the world. The increasing prevalence of natural disasters like forest fires and hurricanes provides the environmental context for the world in which nurses learn and practice. Collectively, these and other issues encompass risk factors for health and disease, contribute to the complex web of causation, and describe the current states of humanity and health.

Health issues are increasingly related to the sociopolitical and economic characteristics of the communities where people live, work, and play. The following dominant environmental trends, which capture significant developments and concerns for society, represent the broad sociopolitical and economic context of nursing education and practice. These trends include health care reform, violence, natural disasters and catastrophic events, and intensifying environmental challenges.

Health Care Reform

Health care reform efforts in the United States such as primary care and pay-for-performance initiatives—along with implementation of the federal 2010 Patient Protection and Affordable Care Act (PPACA)—have changed US health care systems. Under the PPACA, for the first time in America's history, all citizens could have access to affordable health care insurance. As a result, in 2016 the number of uninsured Americans reached a historic low. Uninsured nonelderly Americans fell from 48 million in 2010 to 28 million in 2016, before rising again to 30 million in the first half of 2020 (Assistant Secretary for Prevention and Evaluation [ASPE], 2021). Although this indicates progress in the United States, the impact of how health care is financed continues to disproportionally affect demographic groups (e.g., Black or Hispanic/Latino, young adults, individuals with low income, people who live in states that have not expanded Medicaid; ASPE). Globally, building capacity for health financing is supported by the World Health Organization (WHO, 2022). Knowledge of health care financing models which promote equitable access to high-quality health care is necessary for students at all levels.

In the United States nursing practice and education greatly benefited from the passage of the PPACA through amendments to Nursing Workforce Development programs, more familiarly known as Title VIII of the Public Health Service Act [42 U.S.C. 296 et seq.]. Annual reauthorization of funding is vital to institutions focused on educating nurses for practice in rural and medically underserved areas, enhancing workforce diversity, and providing ongoing support of nursing education at every level. It is important for nurse educators to monitor the federal funding of programs and advocate for adequate funding to sustain such programs, because they have a direct effect on the preparation of a skilled nursing workforce that is prepared to meet the health care needs of patients and decrease health inequities.

Application for curriculum development. The eva-luation of the best processes for health care delivery systems and improved access continues to be debated. Health care proposals emerge at the federal and state levels of government. It is imperative for nurse educators to consider the curricular implications for preparing nurses who are knowledgeable about the political process and able to advocate effectively for safe, quality patient care and a competent and diverse nursing workforce.

In response to a reformed and at times uncertain health care arena, nurse educators must ensure that prelicensure and graduate program nursing curric-ula prepare nurses to provide care that spans the wellness to illness continuum across diverse set-tings (i.e., care for patients in ambulatory or com-munity settings), possess skills to coordinate patient care, and provide quality and value-based care. Curriculum must emphasize techniques and com-munication skills to engage in patient care advo-cacy and work as members of interprofessional teams particularly within emerging care models (see Chapter 11). Nursing program curricula should increasingly focus curriculum on wellness, disease prevention, risk reduction, and improving health equities versus management of acute patients in acute care settings. Dolansky and Livsey (2021) stated curriculum should be expanded to include a full scope of practice in primary care, which few schools are currently doing. The integration of cur-rent knowledge and practices in telehealth across levels of the nursing curriculum is recommended (Solari-Twadell et al., 2021).

The movement of care to the community and emerging emphasis on health equities has created demand for accessible, coordinated, and cultur-ally congruent patient-centered care. Therefore it is imperative that educators prepare nurses for their essential role in community team-based care involving a spectrum of team members including patients, families, health care and allied health professionals, public health providers, and other volunteers. Nursing curricula should also seek to provide students with the opportunity to envision, create, or actively lead and participate in the rede-sign of new or revolutionary models of health care delivery systems and to advocate for policy change.

Disasters and Catastrophic Events

It has been more than 20 years since hijacked air-planes hit the World Trade Center towers in New York and the Pentagon near Washington, DC, with a fourth plane crashing in rural Pennsylvania. The rising threat of global terrorism along with the emergence of new infectious diseases like Ebola (2014) and COVID-19 (2020) and the aftermath of natural disasters such as Hurricanes Harvey and Irma (2017) and Katrina (2005), the tsunami that struck Japan (2011), the earthquake in Haiti (2021), and the drought with forest fires in California (2020–2021) have changed our nation and the world. In response to these and other events, the nation, health care systems, and universities have focused on developing and implementing disas-ter-preparedness strategies, education, and drills to prepare for unpredictable and diverse cata-strophic events.

The biggest proportion of the health workforce is composed of nurses who are ideally positioned to respond to and serve as essential caregivers during a disaster. Nurses, regardless of their workplace setting, should be informed on disaster prepared-ness activities in their organization. Historically, little time has been devoted to teaching disaster content at every level of nursing education, fac-ulty have lacked preparation to teach disaster preparedness content, and practicing nurses face similar learning deficits despite the daily occur-rence of disasters throughout the world that pose severe threats to the health of individuals and the public (International Council of Nurses, 2019).

During the COVID-19 pandemic, nurse educa-tors were challenged to pivot from undergraduate in-person learning to online learning and simu-lation in the middle of a semester. In the United States the National Council for State Boards of Nursing (NCSBN) communicated changes in education requirements to allow alternative clini-cal learning experiences (NCSBN, 2020). This shift provides opportunities to offer theory and prac-tice in parallel versus serial format (Carolan et al., 2020). E-learning is most effective for transferring clinical skills and knowledge; the application in virtual case studies combining different styles and modes promotes learning (Regmi & Jones, 2020) as opposed to instructor-centered learning (i.e., passive instructor lecture). Konrad et al. (2021) detail strategies for online clinical learning experiences that encourage students to think like a nurse, deliberate and practice communication, and experience technology-enhanced physical assessment/virtual simulation. While the pandemic was an interruption for higher education, it can be a catalyst for enduring active learning strategies in the future of nursing education (Case Study 5.1).

Application for curriculum development. It is imperative for nurse educators to ensure curricula is updated to reflect disaster preparedness nursing knowledge, skill, and judgment so that nurse graduates are prepared with leadership skills and the ability to respond to disasters, work interprofessionally, and function as a member of the disaster relief team. Educators must also prepare graduates who can fully participate in the creation of emergency response systems, work within the public health infrastructures characterized by community-wide collaboration and communication, and take their rightful place at the public policy table. Nurses must also possess clinical knowledge related to biological agents and skills to manage and support surviving individuals, families, and communities experiencing the psychosocial effects in the aftermath of disaster events.

In 2009, the International Council of Nurses' Framework for Disaster Nursing Competencies proposed educational competencies aimed at preparing the generalist nurse for all aspects of disaster nursing. These competencies are organized under the four areas of mitigation/prevention, preparedness, response, and recovery and rehabilitation. In addition, 10 domains, including risk reduction, policy development, communication, and ethical practice, were identified within these four areas. The American Nurses Association's (ANA's) (2017) issue brief *Who Will Be There? Ethics, the Law, and a Nurse's Duty to Respond in a Disaster* also identified need for nursing curricula to address nurses' ethical and legal duty to respond in a disaster and how to personally prepare for a disaster. This and the Centers for Disease Control and Prevention website (https://www.emergency.cdc.gov/) are useful resources related to responding to a disaster along with emergency and personal preparedness.

CASE STUDY 5.1   Shifting to Remote Emergency Learning During Pandemic

Students in a traditional face-to-face undergraduate nursing education program enrolled in a nursing research course shifted from a classroom to an online learning environment to mitigate the spread of COVID-19 (i.e., remote emergency learning). Students and faculty located equipment and internet access and created new learning spaces. Many students at the same time transitioned their living situations (i.e., moved out of on-campus housing, traveled, shared living spaces and/or isolated). Students and faculty simultaneously faced illness, changes in social support, and employment conditions. The design of the course changed to offer multiple modes of course delivery (i.e., text-based online course material, recorded lecture, synchronous and asynchronous online discussion) to foster a sense of community and relationships between students and faculty and provide engaging learning activities. The faculty-to-student ratio remained high given the transition from classroom to online. Content was redesigned in a text-based format within the learning management system with opportunities for online comments after asynchronous reflection to offer flexibility in review of course material. Weekly synchronous class time was offered via Zoom platform to engage in learning activities (e.g., student-generated research questions and answers supported by literature using a curated resource for coronavirus science, https://www.ncbi.nlm.nih.gov/research/coronavirus/). Other activities included presentation of articles and discussion led by students (i.e., journal club) and group research presentations based on review and critique of the literature (e.g., semester-long project culminating in prerecorded presentation and synchronous discussion). The synchronous sessions were not recorded. Weekly knowledge checks offered formative assessment; these were formatted for mastery learning, whereas students could complete assessments multiple times and the highest score would be recorded. Summative assessments transitioned to cumulative online exams.

1. What factors in this scenario pose barriers to learning?
2. What factors in the case facilitate equitable teaching and learning?
3. What resources are necessary to ensure future emergency remote teaching success?

Nurse educators can refer to the ICN Frame work as a resource for curriculum development (World Health Organization and International Council of Nurses [ICN], 2009). The second version of the ICN competencies in disaster nursing is a valuable curriculum tool found at https://www.icn.ch/sites/default/files/inline-files/ICN_Disaster-Comp-Report_WEB.pdf (ICN, 2019).

Additionally, schools of nursing are increasingly incorporating use of virtual-world reality platforms into the curriculum. Virtual-world reality can be used to authentically simulate real-world, interactive classroom and clinical nursing settings in which students can assess, intervene, and triage in various national disasters.

Intensifying Environmental Challenges

Environmental and epidemiological hazards are an intensifying issue worldwide. Besides health issues across the globe, there are growing environmental concerns regarding sustainable development, energy availability, potable water, climate change, and global warming, to name a few. Increasingly, Americans are becoming aware that the threats to public health and life are found in the frailty of our earth and our delicate interdependence. Therefore it is important for nurses to be aware of how the environment affects health.

Application for curriculum development. The curriculum must acknowledge the broad influence of the environmental context of health to prepare nurses to effectively intervene in complex problems such as bioterrorism and other mass disasters, global and domestic violence, and global warming. Nursing curricula should address environmental health content and what constitutes environmentally responsible clinical practice. Additionally, curricula should encourage and prepare nurses to factor environmental issues into the web of disease causation and to intervene to improve environmental health. The implications of climate change provide an excellent platform for students to discuss the ethics of protecting the environment and ways to conserve resources. Curriculum should address how health care agencies can make educated choices among products that are environmentally friendly. Excellent environmental

health resources are available on the ANA website (http://nursingworld.org/rnnoharm/) and the Alliance of Nurses for Healthy Environments website (http://www.envirn.org/). Another opportunity is nurses' responsibility to address gun violence, an environmental public health crisis in which nurses are called to action (American Nurses Association, 2018; Cox, 2018; Keaton, 2022). Learning experiences that engage nurses in direct care opportunities to prevent firearm injuries through health screening and develop advocacy skills to support policy change at the community level are needed. Recommendations from the American Public Health Association (APHA) include resources that address these priority issues (American Public Health Association, 2021).

Health

Globalization and Global Health

Our world continues to become more global, creating a sense of a "global village." *Globalization* is a term used to describe the increasing connectedness and interdependence of world cultures and economies (National Geographic Society. n.d.). This process, driven by international trade, investment, and information technology, affects the environment, culture, political systems, economic development, prosperity, health, and the well-being of people around the globe. As a result, national boundaries have become less relevant in an era of instantaneous telecommunications, free trade, multinational corporations, and worldwide travel. In comparison, a proposed definition of global health is collaborative transnational research and action for promoting health for all (Beaglehole & Bonita, 2010). In an important policy document the United Kingdom (UK) Government recognized that global health is determined by problems, issues, and concerns that transcend national boundaries (Primarolo et al., 2009). Over the last decade, the definition of global health has evolved to identify its role in reducing health disparities specifically: "an area of research and practice committed to the application of overtly multidisciplinary, multisectoral and culturally sensitive approaches for reducing health disparities that transcend national borders" (Salm et al., 2021, p. 11).

The consequences of globalization are significant, depending in part on a country's state of development, and have both a positive and negative effect on global health. In a positive sense globalization has resulted in new opportunities for international trade and investment. Proponents of globalization believe it allows for the improved economic status of poor countries and their citizens, thus raising their standards of living (National Geographic, 2022; Ortiz-Ospina, 2017). Opponents believe it has benefited multinational corporations more than the standard of living for people in developing countries. Globalization has also created an interconnected workforce, including nursing and health care.

Another positive and emerging health outcome of globalization is related to the unprecedented spread of mobile technologies such as mobile phones, patient monitoring devices, personal digital assistants, and other wireless devices that are being used to strengthen health systems and achieve health-related goals. In particular, the smartphone and its corresponding medical applications are an example of how mobile technology has transformed the way health information and services are retrieved, delivered, and managed. All of this is made possible by the infiltration of mobile phone networks into a multitude of low- and middle-income countries. Greater than 93% of the world's population live in an area covered by a mobile-broadband network (International Telecommunications Union, 2020, https://www.itu.int/en/ITU-D/Statistics/Documents/facts/FactsFigures2020.pdf).

However, advances in globalization have also served to affect health negatively. For example, adoption of unhealthy habits and lifestyles has resulted in increased obesity and chronic disease. Additionally, "in today's interconnected world, disease can spread from an isolated, rural village to any major city in as little as 36 hours" (Centers for Disease Control and Prevention, 2017). One major downside to globalization can be seen in the increased risk for the transmission of infectious diseases like Ebola, severe acute respiratory syndrome (SARS), and COVID-19. Globalization has been dramatically apparent throughout the COVID-19 pandemic and the resultant challenges in global health outcomes across the entire world.

Globalization has positively increased the mobility of the nursing workforce within and between states, provinces, or countries. However, increased mobility secondary to poor working or living conditions in a nurse's home country, for example, can decrease the local supply of the nurses and thus negatively affect health of the developing country or region.

Application for curriculum development. Globalization presents a challenge and ethical responsibility for educators to design and implement curricula that will introduce students to the tenets of a global society and global health and prepare competent caregivers within a global society. To this end, didactic and clinical teaching and learning strategies should be aimed at developing knowledge, skills, and attitudes nurses need to identify and influence the social determinants of health for marginalized populations worldwide. A framework to facilitate the process of curriculum development can be found in the Interprofessional Global Health Competencies identified in 2015 by a subcommittee of the Consortium of Universities for Global Health (CUGH) (Jogerst et al., 2015). A toolkit with specific teaching strategies and resources for curricular content at various levels, from global citizen to advanced levels of training can also be found at CUGH's website (https://www.cugh.org/online-tools/competencies-toolkit/).

Opportunities for virtual exchange and collaborative online international learning have proliferated in recent years. Further internationalization of curriculum accompanied by interculturality will ensure students learn from and with one another regardless of geographic boundaries. An important resource developed by the International Nursing Education Services and Accreditation joint taskforce of the National League for Nursing and the National League for Nursing Accrediting Commission for US faculty involved in global learning experiences is the NLN Faculty Preparation for Global Experiences Toolkit (https://www.nln.org/education/teaching-resources/professional-development-program steaching-resources/toolkits). See Chapter 13 for additional information related to global health.

Social Justice and Social Determinants of Health

Driven by the pursuit of social justice, nurses have a responsibility for fairness and equitable treatment to promote health and well-being of society. A commitment to identify and improve conditions that interfere with health trajectories is a way for nursing to take action. Social justice is a moral obligation that pushes society to rectify the unfair treatment of vulnerable populations that limit their development or well-being through the course of action. This action is exemplified within our practice, research, education, and policy formation at a local, national, and global scale. The Centers for Disease Control and Prevention defines the social determinants of health as "conditions in the places where people live, learn, work, and play that affect a wide range of health and quality-of-life-risks and outcomes" (https://www.cdc.gov/socialdeterminants/index.htm, para. 1).

Social determinants of health (SDH) are grouped into five domains: Economic stability, education access and quality, health care access and quality, neighborhood and built environment, and social and community context (https://health.gov/healthypeople/priority-areas/social-determinants-health). SDH are major variables in health disparities and inequities. The County Health Rankings & Roadmaps program led by the University of Wisconsin Population Health Institute is working on addressing gaps attributed to SDH; they release a report each year with a call to action (University of Wisconsin Population Health Institute, 2022). Linkages are seen across physical environment, social and economic factors, clinical care, and health behaviors. For example, people who do not have access to grocery stores or who cannot afford fresh produce are at risk for health conditions like heart disease, diabetes, and obesity.

The SDH were very apparent throughout the pandemic with higher COVID infection rates and death for people with lower income and of Black and Hispanic race/ethnicity. To address the inter-linkages of SDH and health outcomes, Healthy People 2030 has an increased and overarching focus on SDH.

Application for curriculum development. Nurse educators can use Healthy People 2030 (U.S. Department of Health and Human Services, 2020) to guide students to develop strategies that address US priorities. The site includes access to resources and benchmarking data (https://health.gov/healthypeople/tools-action/use-healthy-people-2030-your-work). Another rich source of data to inform strategies linked to social determinants of health is the County Health Rankings (https://www.countyhealthrankings.org/). Globally, the United Nations ([UN], n.d.) 2030 Agenda for Sustainable Development Goals (SDGs) is a comprehensive blueprint for the domains of social determinants of health built on years of work by countries and the UN, including the UN Department of Economics and Social Affairs. The 17 Sustainable Development Goals (SDGs) call for all developed and developing countries to join in a global partnership for change. The SDGs range from good health and well-being to climate action, gender equity, and clean energy, to name just a few. Reaching the SDGs is fully aligned with strategies that improve national and global health (https://sdgs.un.org/2030agenda). The goals and targets direct sustainable development in the dimensions of social, economic, and environmental change. Table 5.3 highlights the dimensions of the UN 2030 Agenda SDGs to transform public health organizations and communities of the world. Nursing faculty can take action to improve the conditions in people's environments by addressing the SDGs and social determinants of health across didactic courses and clinical experiences. See Chapter 12 for further reading on strategies to develop social responsibility.

Nursing

This chapter began by looking through the lens of the broad health outcomes and socioeconomic, environmental, and sociopolitical issues. These forces and issues shape the world and the United States and influence contemporary life. Hence these issues are topical changes guiding nursing curriculum and student learning. This section focuses the lens more specifically on the nursing profession and highlights issues of consideration within the profession. Included in the context of nursing care delivery is a discussion on emerging technologies, advanced nursing practice, and competencies needed for contemporary nursing practice.

TABLE 5.3 Dimensions of the UN 2030 Sustainable Development Goals (SDGs)

Dimension of Change	Agenda for SDGs to Transform Our World
People	End poverty and hunger. All humans can fulfill their potential in dignity and equality and in a healthy environment.
Planet	Protect the planet from degradation. Taking urgent action on climate change, so that it can support the needs of the present and future generations.
Prosperity	All human beings can enjoy prosperous and fulfilling lives and that economic, social and technological progress occurs in harmony with nature.
Peace	Foster peaceful, just and inclusive societies which are free from fear and violence. There can be no sustainable development without peace and no peace without sustainable development.
Partnership	Implement this Agenda through a revitalized Global Partnership for Sustainable Development, based on a spirit of strengthened global solidarity.

Data from United Nations (UN). (n.d.). *2030 agenda for sustainable development goals.* https://sdgs.un.org/2030agenda.

The nursing profession both influences and is influenced by the health care delivery system, which provides a context for nursing services. The American Hospital Association's 2022 Environmental Scan provides insight into topical driving forces affecting health care and professional nurses. Four areas describing *the way nursing is practiced* are highlighted in this section including science and technology; primary and community-based nursing care; quality, safety, and affordability; and preparing nurses across their career.

Science and Technology

The way nursing is practiced is changing as science, current and emerging technology, and information management continue to revolutionize health care possibilities at the point of care and within the academic community. *The Future of Nursing 2020–2030* (Consensus report of National Academies of Medicine) stated that nurses will be summoned to fill expanding roles, master technological tools and information systems, and collaborate and coordinate care across teams of health professionals. The report suggests that nurses practicing at their full scope of practice and achieving health equity are national priorities for the next 10 years (NAM, 2021).

Emerging technologies poised to transform nursing practice include genetics and genomics, electronic health records, telehealth, apps and wearables for symptom or disease management and wellness, and continued innovations in the management of infectious diseases such as COVID. Genetic testing is currently being used for many reasons, including identifying gene mutations that may increase risk of developing specific diseases, determining carrier status, and screening newborns (American Cancer Society, 2020). Future applications of genetics and genomics will transform the health care system even further.

Telehealth has provided multiple benefits including increasing access for those who do not have transportation or live in rural areas, less human contact to decrease transmission of infection during the pandemic, and consistent follow-up and communication for patients with chronic health conditions such as diabetes. In addition to telehealth consultation, the capacity for remote monitoring will facilitate disease management and improve care for older adults with comorbidities who can remain in the community by aging in place.

Technology continues to advance and transform the world at warp speed and has greatly affected health care and nursing practice. For example, nationwide adoption and use of electronic health record (EHR) systems has required nurses, educators, and students to use, navigate, and accurately document in the EHR. The American Recovery and Reinvestment Act of 2009, which encompassed the Health Information Technology for Economic and Clinical Health Act (HITECH), helped accelerate the adoption of standardized EHRs and the meaningful use of health information technology as a means to capture clinical information that could be used to improve health outcomes and lower health care costs. Further examples of emerging health care technologies that affect nursing practice include the use of remote monitoring technologies, telehealth to deliver care from a distance, e-health tools and resources that engage patients in their health care, and social media networks that provide patient support sites. See Case Study 5.2 related to clinical decision-making support and the EHR.

Application for curriculum development. Faculty and other nurse leaders must be aware of how emerging technologies and informatics affect nursing practice so that they can proactively create nursing curricula. Leadership programs and continuing education webinars are needed to ensure new and practicing nurses possess competencies necessary to practice safely and ethnically in a highly technical work

---

CASE STUDY 5.2 Clinical Decision-Making Support: Using the EHR for Mental Health Screening and Referral

Primary care health care providers have identified an increase in mental health and social needs in patients and their families during primary care well visits. Therefore the practice protocol was established to conduct mental health and social screenings on all patients at each visit. As a requirement of their clinical objectives, all nursing students document patient assessment data on employment, insurance, housing, transportation, and social support to identify the need for mental health and social resources. If the mental health or social screenings in the EHR show a need for follow-up, nurses in the primary care practice setting receive an alert to facilitate referral through the EHR. The nurse and student nurse further discuss feelings with the patient and explore their abilities or any barriers to accessing mental health care. The patients are offered referrals to personal or telehealth services from a mental health provider or social worker affiliated with the primary care practice. The primary care and mental or social health providers collaborate on the comprehensive parameters of the patient's progress and any suggested changes in the plan of care through the EHR.

1. What is missing from the student nurse's assessment to best coordinate referral for mental health care?
2. What resources are available to leverage technology in the provision of care?

---

environment. It is incumbent upon nursing, as a profession, to be at the forefront in planning and preparing for the challenges that have and will emerge as science and technology continue to evolve.

Nursing education must incorporate skills and competencies related to health care technology into the curriculum to stay up to date with current practice demands. Nurse educators must develop curricula that incorporate health information technology competencies so that graduates are computer and information literate and capable of applying this knowledge to the management of patient care. As nursing practice becomes increasingly higher tech and digitalized, it becomes incumbent upon nurse educators to prepare nursing students with skills and ability needed to respond appropriately to emerging and other technologies. Nurse educators must continue to incorporate concepts related to health information technology into the curriculum and develop teaching strategies requiring students to access, document, collect, and retrieve health care data and other information from electronic sources such as the EHR. As technology becomes embedded in nursing curricula and health care systems become increasingly automated and digitized, nurse educators and practitioners must remain mindful of the need to balance the essence of caring and nursing presence at the bedside and in all patient relationships.

Technological advancements have also greatly affected ways in which nursing education is delivered. For example, greater numbers of nursing programs have found that e-learning, simulation, and mobile devices offer much potential for nursing education, and web-enhanced or online learning provides opportunity for practicing nurses to pursue educational programs at times convenient for learners. As a result, technology allows for educational mobility, provides 24/7 access to education and knowledge, enhances opportunities for teaching and learning or career advancement, and contributes to the availability of a qualified nursing workforce (NAM, 2021). Barton (2020) emphasized the need for self-reflection and assessment of existing teaching activities forced by the pandemic, which can ultimately result in long-term improvements in learning experiences for students in field-based disciplines. One resource available to nurse educators is a National Telehealth Toolkit developed by Center for Telehealth Innovation, Education & Research [C-TIER] (https://teleheal-theducation-ctier.com/national-telehealth-tool-kit-for-educators/). Another resource with specific recommendations for curricula and courses based on health information and technology, developed by an international and interprofessional taskforce, provides a nursing-centric framework (TIGER International Competency Synthesis Project; https://www.himss.org/tiger-initiative-interna-tional-competency-synthesis-project). Please see Unit IV on *Technology-Empowered Learning* and Unit V on *Evaluation* for further details.

Primary Care and Community-Based Nursing Care

Nurses have been recognized as the most trusted profession by the public. Additionally, nurses serve in many community settings with opportunities to build strong, consistent relationships with the public. Thus nursing is well positioned to serve as advocate for the culture of public health. Nurses play an important role in reaching the national goals of improving primary health and achieving health equity.

The ability to effectively manage care of patients with chronic and behavioral health issues is critical to containing health care spending in the United States. It is anticipated that 54.9 million Americans will have diabetes in the year 2030, at the cost of more than $622 billion. Currently, one in five adults experiences mental illness each year, with serious mental illness costing $193.2 billion in lost earnings annually (AHA, 2022). In addition, the misuse of and addiction to opioids—including prescription pain relievers, heroin, and synthetic opioids such as fentanyl—is one of the most serious public health crises in US history (Volkow & Blanco, 2021). As the numbers of those who suffer from these and other chronic conditions increase along with the number of Americans seeking access to health care, the need for nurses to educate and care for them increases. This, along with shifting of health care away from acute, hospital-based care toward a community-based approach to care, accelerates the need for outpatient and community primary

care services with RNs engaged as partners (Josiah Macy Jr. Foundation, 2016). This new direction in how health care is delivered is timely given that community-based home health programs have been shown to provide cost-effective health care to adults with chronic diseases and decrease health care use and positively affect quality of life.

Application for curriculum development. As the venue in which health care is delivered continues to move toward a community-based approach, nurses must be prepared to coordinate collaborative interdisciplinary community-based care, act as primary care providers, and practice to the full extent of their education and training (NAM, 2021). As a result, schools of nursing must restructure their curricula and move away from their traditional focus on acute and hospital-based instruction to one that includes a team-focused, community-based practice. Innovative nurse educators will respond to the shift in health care venues by building collaborative relationships with patients "aging at home" and primary health clinics to provide nursing students with clinical experiences that demonstrate the principles of health promotion, community care, leadership, and client care in community settings (NAM, 2021). In addition, educators should seek to develop partnerships between academia and health care organizations, government entities, or foundations. These interprofessional partnerships are important delivery systems that should be modeled in the curriculum of didactic and clinical courses to prepare nursing graduates for the future. Please see Chapter 18 for more details.

The Quadruple Aim

Despite years of focus on improving the health care system and patient care, a need still exists to improve patient safety and the provision of quality care at a reasonable cost to all patients. Although some parameters of quality have slowly improved during the past decade, further improvement continues to lag. Patients and their families now have access to publicly reported quality measures (i.e., hospital performance on safety and the patient experience). This, along with increasing reporting requirements, has challenged health care organizations to collect the most accurate data possible and then improve patient care based on that data. The Centers for Medicare and Medicaid Services (CMS) (2022) launched several value-based programs that reward health care organizations and providers with incentive payments when they provide quality care to people with Medicare. Nursing has been given a call to action by several authorities, including the National Academy of Medicine, the Robert Wood Johnson Foundation, and the Agency for Healthcare Research and Quality. These agencies recognize the key role nurses play in protecting patient safety and providing high-quality, affordable health care.

More recently, the Quadruple Aim (Arnetz et al., 2020) was proposed as an addition to the previously accepted Triple Aim (Berwick et al., 2008). The Quadruple Aim framework encompasses reducing costs and improving population health and patient experience, with a new fourth domain: Health care team well-being. Creation of positive workplace environments is crucial for retaining new and experienced nurses in the workforce. The American Association of Critical Care Nurses (2016) affirmed six essential standards for establishing and maintaining healthy work environments: (1) Skilled communication, (2) true collaboration, (3) effective decision making, (4) appropriate staffing, (5) meaningful recognition, and (6) authentic leadership. Research shows that nurses are stressed and get less sleep than other Americans, which has been worsened by the pandemic (ANA, 2021). The highlight on well-being, self-nurturing, and positive personal wellness activities are a more recent and much-needed focus related to the Quadruple Aim. The American Nurses Association, ANA Enterprise, pioneered the *Healthy Nurse, Healthy Nation* program (ANA, 2022). It is an initiative to improve health of nurses and their organizations in five areas: Physical activity, nutrition, rest, quality of life, and safety (https://www.healthynursehealthynation.org).

Application for curriculum development. There exists a need to better prepare today's nurses to meet the challenges of the Quadruple Aim. Teaching strategies and concrete examples of learning activities that nurse educators can use to teach quality and safety competencies can be found on the Quality and Safety Education for Nurses (QSEN) website at http://qsen.org/competencies/. Additionally, educators should assist students to understand the proactive

steps that the nursing profession is taking within the changing health care environment to define nursing practice and educate the public on nursing's role in quality care.

Faculty and health care organizations are becoming far more attentive to curriculum outlining resilience and inner strength exercises, continued support strategies, and behavioral health resources to maintain their own health and safety so that nursing can serve to improve the health of the nation. Nurse educators should adopt the Healthy Nurse, Healthy Nation (ANA. 2021) initiative and Critical-Care Nurse standards (Ulrich et al., 2019) into their curriculum and clinical teaching environments.

Career Competencies and Workforce Demands

The mission, values, and ethics of nursing education challenge educators to prepare students for the commitment to life-long learning. A major force and issue influencing curriculum is the inclusion of skills that prepares a student for the immediate workforce demands after graduation. However, curriculum should include analytic and leadership skills that can be applied across the career span. Curriculum should emphasize leadership and management principles, civility, negotiation, and the benefit of professional organizations.

It is necessary for the nursing workforce to be informed about organizations that accredit and certify health care agencies such as The Joint Commission (https://www.jointcommission.org/). Two of the American Nurses Credentialing Center's (ANCC) most prominent programs for evaluating standards and data demonstrating improvements are the Pathway to Excellence Program, which recognizes a health care organization's commitment to creating a positive nursing practice environment, and the Magnet Recognition Program. Health care organizations achieving Magnet recognition have demonstrated and documented required nursing practices and quality patient outcomes (ANCC, https://www.nursingworld.org/ancc/).

Human capital continues to significantly affect the health care delivery system secondary to supply and demand of nurses and physicians. The United States has experienced nursing shortages periodically; the nursing shortage facing America today began long before the pandemic. However, the pandemic has been an enormous strain on nurses and the health care system. The magnitude of the current nursing shortage is persistent given the reports projecting that 1.2 million new registered nurses (RNs) will be needed in the United States and 5.7 million needed in the world by 2030 to address the current shortage (Bean, 2020).

There is an inequitable distribution of nurses per population, which has created a greater problem in some states than in others. For example, two densely populated states, California and Texas, are ranked first and second for the greatest shortages of nurses in 2030, respectively. It is projected by the year 2030 that each state's supply and demand for RNs will range from a shortage in California to a surplus in Florida (Buerhaus, 2021). The demand for advanced practice nurses and physician assistants is anticipated to rise as these practitioners are increasingly used to provide primary care services. Factors affecting the future supply and demand for both nurses and physicians include the aging US population, economics, and increased retirements and resignations of providers related to the pandemic.

Application for curriculum development. The ability to retain new nurse graduates is important given that they account for the greatest number of nurses entering and exiting the profession. Retention of new graduates begins through delivery of nursing curriculum designed to provide the academic foundation and practical skills needed to work in the real-world environment. Curriculum needs to provide clinical learning experiences that allow them to learn how to navigate across existing and emerging settings with changing health care challenges (see Chapter 18). In addition, curriculum should address and clearly explicate role expectations of new nurse graduates. Interactive exercises and case studies can prepare graduates to recognize and receive the support and mentoring they need. Many health care organizations have implemented nurse residency programs as a way to reduce new graduate nurse turnover, and many new nurse graduates seek out such programs to ease their transition into practice.

Nurses, as the largest group of health care professionals, require leadership skills to influence health care delivery, reform, and policy. The ability to lead and influence change is an essential nursing skill. Faculty can use several models of leadership to inform and guide curriculum and practice. Curriculum should give opportunities for students to discuss communication and team building necessary for nurse leaders to motivate those they lead to achieve a shared vision and make positive contributions to a climate of improved health outcomes for the patient, family, and the nation.

CHAPTER SUMMARY: KEY POINTS

- Curriculum is a nonlinear, dynamic process. Curriculum development, implementation, and evaluation are planful and based on emerging trends in health care.
- Faculty need to be skilled in the fundamental process of curriculum change to provide education and support for students in an emergent, unexpected situation such as COVID-19. The current body of knowledge, direction of the strategic plan, epidemiological patterns, and research findings should be at the forefront of curriculum changes.
- The nursing program and university mission statement is a declaration of values, and it should be relevant to the curriculum.
- Communities of students and faculty are closely examining social justice issues including discrimination, equity, inclusivity, and safe campus environments. Institutions and nursing colleges are providing services and implementing policies that embrace inclusivity.
- The nursing profession deserves and requires nurse educators to design curricula that are both compatible with contemporary health trends and flexible enough to respond quickly to unexpected natural disasters and pandemics.
- Curricula should prepare nurses to factor environmental issues into causation of illness and to intervene to improve environmental health.

- Educators sensitive to major sociopolitical and economic trends can develop curriculum that matches global health needs.
- Globalization presents a responsibility for educators to prepare competent nurses within a global society.
- Nursing education must incorporate skills and competencies related to health care technology into the curriculum to stay up to date with current practice demands.
- Faculty must remain mindful of the need to balance technology skills with the essence of caring and nursing presence at the bedside and in all patient and family relationships.
- The Quadruple Aim incorporates the well-being of the nurse and the health care team. Curriculum strategies should address sustaining the physical and mental needs of a healthy nurse.
- Curriculum should prepare nurses to coordinate interprofessional community-based care; provide high-quality, safe, and affordable care; and advocate for their own health and positive workplace environments.

REFLECTING ON THE EVIDENCE

1. What strategies can be used to keep a nursing program's curriculum relevant to its mission? How can the faculty keep the curriculum relevant to broad societal changes, issues, or health care reform?
2. How does your nursing program curriculum prepare students for nursing practice within the context of science and technology, community-based nursing care, and quality and safety?
3. How is your nursing program curriculum responding to new developments in nursing education and discipline such as genetics and gender identity?
4. In what ways do the faculty in your nursing program collaborate and share new input and acknowledge new influences on curriculum development? How do faculty respond to those voices of change?
5. How can nursing program curriculum prepare students to intervene to improve environmental health?
6. What strategies can be emphasized in the curriculum for students to sustain their own health and healthy work environment?

REFERENCES

American Association of Colleges of Nursing. (2021a, August). *DEI faculty toolkit*. https://www.aacnnursing.org/Portals/42/Diversity/Diversity-Tool-Kit.pdf

American Association of Colleges of Nursing. (2021b, August). *End of life nursing education consortium (ELNEC) fact sheet*. https://www.aacnnursing.org/Portals/42/ELNEC/PDF/ELNEC-Fact-Sheet.pdf

American Association of Colleges of Nursing. (2022, January 12). *Diversity, equity, and inclusion*. https://www.aacnnursing.org/diversity

American Association of Colleges and Universities. (2022, January 12). *Mission and strategic plan*. http://www.aacu.org/about/strategicplan

American Association of Critical Care Nurses. (2016). *Standards for establishing and sustaining healthy work environments: A journey to excellence* (2nd ed.). https://www.aacn.org/wd/hwe/docs/hwe standards.pdf

American Cancer Society (2020, June 9). *What happens in genetic testing for cancer risk?* https://www.cancer.org/cancer/cancer-causes/genetics/what-happens-during-genetic-testing-for-cancer.html

American Hospital Association (AHA). (2022, January 12). *The 2022 environmental scan*. https://www.aha.org/environmentalscan

American Nurses Association. (2017). *Who will be there: Ethics, the law, and a nurse's duty to respond in a disaster*. https://www.nursingworld.org/~4af058/globalassets/docs/ana/ethics/who-will-be-there_disaster-preparedness_2017.pdf

American Nurses Association. (2018). *Stop the madness: End the violence!* https://www.nursingworld.org/news/news-releases/2018/stop-the-madness-end-the-violence/

American Nurses Association, (2021). Healthy nurse, healthy nation. Year 4 highlights 2020–2021. *American Nurse Journal, 18*(10), 29–39.

American Nurses Association. (2022). *Healthy nurse, healthy nation.* https://www.healthynursehealthy nation.org

American Public Health Association. (2021). *Gun violence.* https://www.apha.org/Topics-and-Issues/Gun-Violence

Arnetz, B. B., Goetz, C. M., Arnetz, J. E., Sudan, S., vanSchagen, J., Piersma, K., & Reyelts, F. (2020). Enhancing healthcare efficiency to achieve the Quadruple Aim: An exploratory study. *BMC research notes, 13*(1), 362. https://doi.org/10.1186/s13104-020-05199-8.

Assistant Secretary for Prevention and Evaluation (ASPE) Office of Health Policy (2021, February 11). Trends in the U.S. uninsured population, 2010–2020. https://aspe.hhs.gov/sites/default/files/private/pdf/265041/trends-in-the-us-uninsured.pdf

Barton, D. (2020). Impacts of the COVID-19 pandemic on field instruction and remote teaching alternatives: Results from a survey of instructors. *Ecology and Evolution, 10*(22), 12499–12507. https://doi.org/10.1002/ece3.6628.

Beaglehole, R., & Bonita, R. (2010). What is global health? *Global Health Action,* 3. https://doi.org/10.3402/gha.v3i0.5142.

Bean, M. (2020, April). World may be short 5.7M nurses by 2030: 4 report takeaways. *The Journal of Nursing* https://www.asrn.org/journal-nursing/2286-world-may-be-short-57m-nurses-by-2030-4-report-takeaways.html

Berwick, D., Nolan, T., & Whittington, J. (2008). The triple aim: care, health, and cost. *Health Affairs, 27*(3), 759–769. https://doi.org/10.1377/hlthaff.27.3.759.

Buerhaus, P. I. (2021). Current nursing shortages could have long-lasting consequences: Time to change our present course. *Nursing Economics, 39*(5), 247–250.

Carolan, C., Davies, C. L., Crookes, P., McGhee, S., & Roxburgh, M. (2020). COVID 19: Disruptive impacts and transformative opportunities in undergraduate nurse education. *Nurse Education in Practice, 46,* 102807. https://doi.org/10.1016/j.nepr.2020.102807C.

Centers for Disease Control and Prevention. (n.d.). *Epidemiology-fact sheet.* https://www.cdc.gov/eis/downloads/epidemiology-factsheet.pdf.

Centers for Disease Control and Prevention. (2017). *CDC works worldwide 24/7 to protect the U.S. from disease threats.* https://www.cdc.gov/globalhealth/what/default.html

Centers for Disease Control and Prevention. (2019, September 5). *Racial and ethnic disparities continue in pregnancy-related deaths.* https://www.cdc.gov/media/releases/2019/p0905-racial-ethnic-disparities-pregnancy-deaths.html

Centers for Disease Control and Prevention. (2020, August 13). *Maternal mortality.* https://www.cdc.gov/reproductivehealth/maternal-mortality/index.html

Centers for Medicare and Medicaid Services. (2022, August 21). *Value-based programs.* https://www.cms.gov/Medicare/Quality-Initiatives-Patient-Assessment-Instruments/Value-Based-Programs/Value-Based-Programs

Cox, K. S. (2018). A public health crisis: Recommendations to reduce gun violence in America. *Council for the Advancement of Nursing Science.* https://www.nursingoutlook.org/article/S0029-6554(18)30232-X/fulltext.

Dolansky, M., & Livsey, K. (2021). Preparing RNs for emerging roles in primary care. *American Nurse Journal, 16*(10), 77–80.

Federal Interagency Forum on Aging-Related Statistics (FIFARS). (2020). *Older Americans 2020: Key indicators of well-being.* U.S. Government Printing Office. https://agingstats.gov/docs/LatestReport/OA20_508_10142020.pdf.

Hökkä, M., Martins Pereira, S., Pölkki, T., Kyngäs, H., & Hernández-Marrero, P. (2020). Nursing competencies across different levels of palliative care provision: A systematic integrative review with thematic synthesis. *Palliative Medicine, 34*(7), 851–870. https://doi.org/10.1177/0269216320918798.

International Council of Nurses. (2019). *Core competencies in disaster nursing.* Version 2. https://www.icn.ch/sites/default/files/inline-files/ICN_Disaster-Comp-Report_WEB.pdf

International Telecommunications Union. (2020). *Measuring digital development. Facts and figures 2020.* ITU Publications. https://www.itu.int/en/ITU-D/Statistics/Documents/facts/FactsFigures2020.pdf.

Jogerst, K., Callender, B., Adams, V., Evert, J., Fields, E., Hall, T., Olsen, J., Rowthorn, V., Rudy, S., Shen, J., Simon, L., Torres, H., Velji, A., & Wilson, L. L. (2015). Identifying interprofessional global health competencies for 21st-century health professionals. *Annals of Global Health, 81*(2), 239–247. https://doi.org/10.1016/j.aogh.2015.03.006.

Josiah Macy Jr. Foundation. (2016). *Registered nurses: Partners in transforming primary care.* [Conference summary]. https://macyfoundation.org/assets/reports/publications/201609_nursing_conference_exectuive_summary_final.pdf

Keaton, M. (2022). Decrying senseless gun violence, NLN issues urgent call for bold action to combat rising public health crisis. *National League for Nursing.* https://www.nln.org/detail-pages/news/2022/05/27/decrying-senseless-gun-violence-nln-issues-urgent-call-for-bold-action-to-combat-rising-public-health-crisis

Konrad, S., Fitzgerald, A., & Deckers, C. (2021). Nursing fundamentals–supporting clinical competency online during the COVID-19 pandemic. *Teaching and Learning in. Nursing, 16*(1), 53–56.

National Council for State Boards of Nursing (NCSBN) (2020). *Changes in education for nursing programs during COVID-19.* https://www.ncsbn.org/Education-Requirement-Changes_COVID-19.pdf.

National Academies of Sciences, Engineering, and Medicine. (2021). *The Future of Nursing 2020–2030: Charting a Path to Achieve Health Equity.* The National Academies Press. https://doi.org/10.17226/25982.

National Geographic Society. (n.d.). *Globalization.* https://www.nationalgeographic.org/encyclopedia/globalization/

National Geographic. (2022, August 7). *Effects of economic globalization.* https://education.nationalgeographic.org/resource/effects-economic-globalization

National League for Nursing. (2017, April 6). *Diversity & inclusion toolkit.* http://www.nln.org/docs/default-source/default-document-library/diversity-toolkit.pdf?sfvrsn=2

Ortiz-Ospina, E. (2017, August 7) *Is globalization an engine of economic development?* https://ourworldindata.org/is-globalization-an-engine-of-economic-development

Primarolo, D., Malloch-Brown, M., Lewis, I., & Interministerial Group for Global Health. (2009). Health is global: A UK government strategy for 2008–13. *Lancet (London, England), 373*(9662), 443–445. https://doi.org/10.1016/S0140-6736(08)61820-6.

Regmi, K., & Jones, L. (2020). A systematic review of the factors–enablers and barriers–affecting e-learning in health sciences education. *BMC Medical Education, 20*(1), 1–18. https://doi.org/10.1186/s12909-020-02007-6.

Salm, M., Ali, M., Minihane, M., & Conrad, P. (2021). Defining global health: Findings from a systematic review and thematic analysis of the literature. *BMJ Global Health, 6*(6). https://doi.org/10.1136/bmjgh-2021-005292.

Schooley, S. (2021, October 29). SWOT analysis: What it is and when to use it. *Business News Daily.* https://www.businessnewsdaily.com/4245-swot-analysis.html.

Solari-Twadell, P. A., Flinter, M., Rambur, B., Renda, S., Witwer, S., Vanhook, P., & Poghosyan, L. (2021). The impact of the COVID-19 pandemic on the future of telehealth in primary care. *Nursing Outlook, 70*(2), 315–322. https://doi.org/10.1016/j.outlook.2021.09.004.

United Nations (UN). (n.d.). *2030 agenda for sustainable development goals.* https://sdgs.un.org/2030agenda.

University of Wisconsin Population Health Institute. (2022). *County health rankings national findings 2022.* https://www.countyhealthrankings.org/reports/2022-county-health-rankings-national-findings-report

U.S. Department of Health and Human Service. (2020). *Healthy People 2030. Social determinants of health.* https://health.gov/healthypeople/objectives-and-data/social-determinants-health

Ulrich, B., Barden, C., Cassidy, L., & Varn-Davis, N. (2019). Critical care nurse work environments 2018: Findings and implications. *Critical Care Nurse, 39*(2), 67–84. https://doi.org/10.4037/ccn2019605.

Volkow, N., & Blanco, C. (2021). The changing opioid crisis: Development, challenges and opportunities. *Molecular Psychiatry, 26*(1), 218–233. https://doi.org/10.1038/s41380-020-0661-4.

World Health Organization and International Council of Nurses. (2009). *ICN framework of disaster nursing competencies.* International Council of Nurses.

World Health Organization. (2022). *Health financing.* https://www.who.int/health-topics/health-financing

6

An Introduction to Curriculum Development*

Nelda Godfrey, PhD, ACNS-BC, RN, FAAN, ANEF

The topic of curriculum development and redesign remains a focal point for educators in nursing and other fields. A curriculum that optimizes student and faculty performance is necessary to achieve desired education outcomes in service to society. The collective faculty has responsibility for creating an effective, efficient, and contemporary curriculum that prepares graduates to achieve professional practice standards at each level of education to improve the health and well-being of the populations served. The National League for Nursing (NLN, 2022) has outlined expected competencies for nursing faculty that include a strong focus on the role of educators in curriculum development, delivery, and evaluation.

In today's world, multiple factors affect and challenge institutions of higher education to demonstrate effectiveness in preparing graduates for entry into the workplace. At the same time, concerns regarding the cost of postsecondary education and a demonstrated shortage of nurse faculty are among other influencing factors and changes affecting the education of nurses (see Chapter 5).

As institutions of higher education reevaluate how to best achieve their stated missions and position themselves for the future, it is apparent that sweeping changes in higher education are affecting the development and delivery of curricula. Considering health professions education specifically, there is grave concern regarding both the supply and quality of graduates being educated in the United States. In June 2017, the Josiah Macy Jr. Foundation convened a conference of national health care educators with the goal of creating recommendations related to health professions education. The title of the conference report, *Achieving Competency-Based, Time-Variable Health Professions Education*, telegraphs proposed changes for higher education. Acknowledging that health professions education requires "radical transformation" to ensure a high quality of care delivery, the Macy recommendations noted that health professions education is "fragmented, time-bound, and too often disconnected from the practice of optimal pedagogies and existing health care challenges. To fulfill the social contract implicit in the provision of health care requires change that is more than evolutionary or incremental" (Lucey, 2018, p. 2).

The Macy report also identified many changes that exist in health professions education, including the information explosion, discontinuity in education, student debt burden, faculty burnout, assessment challenges, marginalization of patients, challenges to workforce diversity, inadequate preparation for transitions, and inadequate faculty development. The summary position of the Macy report is that "We are now at an important inflection point; our current, predominantly time-fixed health professions education system must accelerate the transition to a competency based, time-variable system" (Lucey, 2018, p. 4).

The Macy recommendations extend and support prior publications calling for nurse educators in academia to be actively involved in creating

*The author acknowledges the work of Dori Taylor Sullivan, PhD, RN, NE-BC, CPHQ, FAAN in the previous editions.

contemporary, cost-effective, and comprehensive curricula that produce graduates who are well prepared to assume their role (American Association of Colleges of Nursing [AACN], 2019; NLN, 2022).

The quality, effectiveness, and efficiency of a curriculum in achieving the desired outcomes for a given program of study is of increasing importance to nursing and other health professions. A number of nursing organizations and specially convened groups have called for innovation and change in nursing education in part because of the impact of the COVID-19 pandemic. The *Tri-Council for Nursing Report* (2021), AACN's Vision for Academic Nursing (2019), NLN's Nurse Educator Core Competencies for Academic Nurse Educators (2020), AACN's The Essentials: Core Competencies for Professional Nursing Education (2021), and the National Academies of Sciences, Engineering and Medicine's Future of Nursing 2020–2030 (2021) strongly advocate for nursing education reform to support evolving health care systems and patient needs. Each of these documents proposes greater attention to diversity, inclusion, and health equity, a shift to competency-based education and assessment, and a stronger emphasis on academic-practice partnerships when designing and implementing curricular change.

Curricular quality must be ensured across all curriculum elements that compose a curriculum. These elements include the institution's mission, vision, and values and those of the school of nursing; professional values and the beliefs, values, and expertise of the faculty; the school of nursing philosophy and organizing or conceptual framework; end-of-program outcomes and competencies; level competencies; curriculum design; courses, teaching strategies, and learning experiences; and resources needed to implement the curriculum. Guidelines for framing these curricular components come from state nursing board rules and regulations as well as criteria within national nursing accreditation standards. Professional nursing and health care standards are also used to guide curriculum development.

This chapter provides an overview of curriculum ideologies, a historical perspective on definitions of *curriculum* and *curriculum development*, and descriptions of the elements that compose a curriculum, including curriculum models. The process of curriculum development within a changing environment and the role of faculty are described. The influence of selected reports is addressed, along with recent evidence related to education methods and priority-related topics that require significant changes in approaches to nursing education curricula to ensure that nurses are prepared to meet current and evolving health care needs.

CURRICULUM IDEOLOGIES

A common understanding of how a discipline and a school and its faculty consider the term *curriculum* is crucial to development of a comprehensive curriculum that is current, consistent, and congruent. Understanding the underlying principles and assumptions on which a curriculum is created enhances the structure, processes, and outcomes of that curriculum plan. Schiro (2013) proposes the term *curriculum ideologies* to describe the underlying beliefs and philosophy of educators and identifies four major approaches to education. The four ideologies are scholar academic, social efficiency, learner centered, and social reconstruction. Each of these ideologies has evolved from rich traditions in the field of education, and all have the potential to enhance society, but the approaches and central values of the various ideologies are quite different. A brief description of the four ideologies reveals some of the frequently reported issues of debate that arise when faculty engage in curriculum development or curriculum revision activities.

The *scholar academic* ideology is organized around the concept of academic disciplines. Adherents believe that learning should be centered on a growing knowledge of the discipline by novices and expansion of that knowledge base by those more expert. A discipline's knowledge includes ways of thinking, conceptual frameworks, traditions, and specific content (Schiro, 2013, p. 4). A hierarchical relationship flows from the scholar to the teacher to the student, who is the discoverer, user, and consumer of new knowledge. A scholar academic approach focuses on ensuring that the curriculum reflects the essence of the discipline.

Social efficiency ideology focuses on service to society by preparing students to meet the needs of society through their knowledge-based work contributions and through productive lives that enhance societal functioning (Schiro, 2013, p. 5). A curriculum reflecting the social efficiency ideology relies on a stimulus–response model that is characterized by faculty creating terminal objectives and attending to the type and sequencing of learning experiences and to the extent to which learners are able to meet the identified priority societal needs.

The *learner-centered* ideology focuses on individuals rather than society as a whole, with the belief that talents and abilities should develop naturally and in harmony with individuals' unique characteristics and preferences. Within this ideology, individual learning goals become the desired learning outcomes, and the role of the educator is to create an environment that stimulates growth through social interactions and learner creation of meaning for themselves (Schiro, 2013, p. 6).

The final curriculum ideology is *social reconstruction*. The chief driving force of those who embrace social reconstruction thinking is that education is the major factor in addressing and changing societal issues and injustices. The goal of education within the social reconstruction frame is to facilitate creation of a new and more just society that benefits all members. As education is viewed from a social perspective, the focus is on meaning as influenced by cultural and other social experiences, with the goal of creating desired societal values that will improve society overall and thereby benefit individual members of society (Schiro, 2013, p. 6). As a profession, nursing is increasingly focused on contributions that will improve society and health for all, requiring inclusion of skill building for nurses to achieve these goals.

Influence of Curriculum Ideologies on Nursing Education

There are examples of nursing curricula that reflect all these ideologies, with the potential exception of learner-centered ideology because of the required focus on demonstrated competencies as established by the state boards of nursing to maximize the success of graduates in passing the licensing examination. However, strong and growing support for the use of learner-centered pedagogy strategies is dramatically influencing nursing education and is described later in this chapter.

The scholar academic ideology is prominent in many schools of nursing and influences both the curriculum and the hierarchy of perceived value of faculty contributions (e.g., tenure track researchers versus practice track or clinical experts as a common exemplar). Curricula within this category tend to be closely tied with medical or clinical specialties and are consistent with current practice patterns and health care organization structures (e.g., service lines). Some of the implications of this ideological stance position faculty as the knowledgeable experts who make many of the decisions regarding what is to be learned, when it is to be learned, and in what manner. Thus use of learner-centered strategies and learner engagement might be considerably lower in programs that embrace the scholar academic ideology model, compared with schools of nursing that implement other curricular ideologies. The scholar academic ideological foundation is most apparent in research-focused institutions compared with those whose mission is primarily focused on teaching and service.

In response to the increased expectations for accountability from institutions of higher education, along with other factors, the social efficiency ideology model has become more evident in many schools of nursing. How are professional curricula, such as that found in nursing and the health professions, being affected, and what are the implications of a social efficiency ideology for faculty in redesigning a content-laden curriculum? Restructuring and reforms in the health care system are rapidly changing the focus of nursing curricula, as graduates must learn to deliver care within a health care environment that is focusing more and more on transitional care and the primary health care needs of individuals. At the same time, there are calls to restructure basic tenets of various societies through education to address social, financial, and other inequities. Nursing practice must be safe and cost effective across patient-care settings, and nursing education must continue to maintain standards and meet the requirements of state boards of nursing and national accrediting agencies while meaningfully addressing these crucial considerations and expectations.

Social reconstruction ideology has implications for developing student and faculty competencies in participating in and leading health care policy and advocacy. Health care disparities, global health issues, and population health issues are increasingly important issues that nurses can and should address as global leaders. Designing learning experiences that foster competency in health policy advocacy is an example of an essential program outcome in contemporary nursing education.

DEVELOPING CONTEMPORARY NURSING CURRICULA

Faculty first need to be familiar with their state's rules and regulations about nursing education programs and outcomes. Secondly, a detailed understanding of the standards of the school's national nursing accreditation body is critical. Thirdly, faculty need to consider emerging trends in nursing and health care in addition to traditional and foundational concepts when developing contemporary nursing curricula. For example, nursing curricula need to include concepts related to patient safety, coordination of care, self-management, and health literacy, with emphasis on the burden of health problems on patient and family, strategies to decrease the gap between practice and evidence-based practice, and strategies that are generalizable across populations. Also important to nursing curricula are leadership and other skills to support achieving the stated goals from Healthy People 2020 (n.d.), including improving health care for all with a focus on reducing disparities, preventable diseases, disability, injury, and premature death. Finally, evolving opportunities for personalized nursing care and precision medicine must be integrated into the nursing curriculum (Fangonil-Gagalang & Schultz, 2021). In an example of curricula reflecting contemporary and innovative thinking, Hsieh et al. (2022) used the Delphi method for faculty experts to determine leadership competencies for a baccalaureate nursing program, then invited learners to evaluate

their ability to meet these competencies via self-report. These competencies were integrated into all semesters of the baccalaureate curriculum.

There are innumerable position statements, professional standards, recommendations, and guiding principles from various sources that faculty must be knowledgeable about and consider for inclusion in any curricula they are designing. It is important for faculty to find ways in which they can perform regular environmental scans with a goal of maintaining a curriculum that is dynamic, fluid, and contemporary. To develop relevant undergraduate and graduate nursing curricula for the future, faculty must consider the following questions:

- Are students prepared to practice in a complex and changing health care environment?
- Are students anticipating the need to be lifelong learners?
- Based on the impact of the global pandemic, are students ready to actively engage in disaster management and crisis events?
- Are students prepared to make clinical decisions based on evidence, demonstrating the requisite knowledge and skills?
- Do students have a sense that they are part of a global community, recognizing the need to treat all humans with respect and civility and practicing the principles of diversity, equity, and inclusion? Are students learning to demonstrate a professional identity in nursing and exemplify ethical decision-making and practice?
- Does the curriculum integrate a major focus on evidence-based research and practice, promoting faculty and student collaboration with interprofessional colleagues in inquiry and improvement?
- Are faculty working to design curricula, including innovative clinical models of instruction, that will most effectively prepare graduates for the workforce in a variety of settings, including ambulatory and community environments?
- Will graduates be prepared to lead care teams in advocating for improved health care outcomes and services locally, nationally, and internationally?
- Are curricula being delivered using active learning strategies, including narrative pedagogies

such as unfolding case studies, scenarios, and reflective thought, and are interactive technologies used that require students to engage with the topics and apply their knowledge?

- Does the university or college provide programs that are high quality, accessible, and of good value compared with peer institutions?
- Are the curricula meeting the needs of the programs' communities of interest and other relevant stakeholders, including formal and informal transition to practice programs?
- Do the curricula foster use of instructional and patient care technologies, and are faculty adequately prepared to integrate these new technologies into their teaching?

Additionally, the exponential expansion of knowledge, dramatically changing sociodemographics and cultural diversity, an economically and consumer-focused political environment, and increasing acts of global terrorism will continue to challenge nursing faculty to critically review current curricula and methods of instruction with the goal of preparing graduates for the future. Nursing education must address the myriad issues affecting curriculum design and implementation and transform nursing education to prepare graduates at all levels of education for an increasingly complex work environment that has greater practice expectations and a heavier reliance on the use of advanced technologies across the entire health care continuum.

DEFINITION OF CURRICULUM

The term *curriculum* was first used in Scotland as early as 1820 and became a part of the education vernacular in the United States nearly a century later. Over time, *curriculum*—derived from the Latin word *currere*, which means "to run"—has been translated to mean "course of study" (Wiles & Bondi, 1989).

In 1949 Tyler published a handbook on principles of curriculum and instruction that has been used for more than six decades (Tyler, 2013). Among other important concepts, Tyler proposed three major criteria for effective organization of a curriculum: continuity, sequence, and integration. Continuity is achieved through careful attention to

"vertical reiteration of major curriculum elements" (Tyler, 2013, p. 84). This approach has been a mainstay of nursing curriculum development since its introduction.

In addition, because of the amorphous nature of the term *curriculum*, it has had a variety of definitions. Educators prefer particular definitions based on individual philosophical beliefs and the emphasis placed on specific aspects of education. Parkay et al. (2014) conceptualized a curriculum that includes all educational experiences that learners have in an educational program to achieve broad goals and related specific objectives developed with a framework of theory and research, past and present professional practice, and the changing needs of society.

Common elements found in many definitions of curriculum include:

- Preselected goals and outcomes to be achieved
- Selected content with specific sequencing in a program of study
- Processes and experiences to facilitate learning for traditional and adult learners
- Resources required to support curriculum delivery
- Extent of responsibility for learning assumed by the teacher and the learner
- How and where learning takes place
- Interschool activities, including extracurricular activities, guidance, and interpersonal relationships
- Individual learner's experience as a result of schooling

Types of Curricula

The classic work of Bevis (2000) identified five types of curricula that may occur concurrently regardless of the ideological interpretation of curriculum. The *official (or legitimate) curriculum* includes the stated curriculum framework with philosophy and mission; recognized lists of outcomes, competencies, and learning objectives for the program and individual courses; course outlines; and syllabi. Bevis (2000) stated that the "legitimate curriculum ... [is] the one agreed on by the faculty either implicitly or explicitly" (p. 74). These written documents are distributed to faculty, students, health care practice partners, and accrediting agencies to document the planned curriculum, including what is to be taught and expected learning outcomes and competencies at program completion.

The *operational curriculum* consists of what is actually taught by the teacher and how its importance is communicated to the student. This curriculum includes knowledge, skills, and attitudes (KSAs) emphasized by faculty in the classroom and clinical settings.

The *illegitimate curriculum* is one known and actively taught by faculty yet not evaluated because descriptors of the behaviors are lacking. Such behaviors include "caring, compassion, power, and its use" (Bevis, 2000, p. 75).

The *hidden curriculum* consists of values and beliefs taught through verbal and nonverbal communication by the faculty. Faculty may be unaware of what is taught through their expressions, priorities, and interactions with students, but students are very aware of the "hidden agendas" of the curriculum, which may have a more lasting influence than the written curriculum. The hidden curriculum includes the way faculty interact with students, the teaching methods used, and the priorities set.

The *null curriculum* represents content and behaviors that are not taught. Faculty need to recognize what is not being taught and focus on the reasons for ignoring those content and behavior areas. Examples include content or skills that faculty think they are teaching but are not, such as clinical reasoning. As faculty review curricula, all components and relationships need to be evaluated.

Curriculum Development in Nursing

From a historical perspective, how nurse educators approached curriculum development was greatly influenced by the work of Bevis. Bevis defined curriculum as "those transactions and interactions that take place between students and teachers and among students with the intent that learning takes place" (2000, p. 72). Bevis challenged nurse educators to move from what she termed the *Tylerian behaviorist technical paradigm of curriculum development* to one that focuses on human interaction and active learning and incorporates a focus on students' and teachers' interactions.

A contemporary nursing curriculum is based on current practice and emerging trends, professional standards, accreditation standards, regulatory requirements, institutional values, and faculty values and interests. Because of the relative freedom faculty have to develop curricula within these standards and guidelines, each of these items may contribute to a lack of curricula standardization within the profession. New opportunities abound to foster collaborative debate and dialogue on several issues, including how to do the following:

- Enhance students' delegating, supervising, prioritizing, clinical reasoning, decision-making, and leadership skills to effect change.
- Focus on health promotion, disease prevention, and care transitions to improve outcomes in health care disparities across health care settings.
- Enhance student–faculty–preceptor interactions in the learning process.
- Design effective clinical education models that allow for student immersion in the practice setting.
- Develop learner-centered environments.
- Use evidence-based research and nursing practice to deliver efficient and effective care.
- Integrate culture of safety concepts, including care coordination and transitions, in specifically designed interprofessional education and collaborative practice experiences.
- Focus on patient-centered care within the overarching "quadruple-aim" goal of improving the patient care experience (including quality and satisfaction), improving the health of the populations, reducing the per-capita cost of health care, and care of the provider
- Expand culturally sensitive nursing practice with a focus on reducing health disparities and promoting health equity.

Valiga (2021) asserts that faculty must look carefully at the major concepts addressed throughout the curriculum in order to have a greater social impact. Curriculum, combined with designing relevant learning experiences that help students engage with vulnerable populations, will be key to making nursing education current. Further, curriculum can also help "students internalize an identity as a nurse, scholar and leader who can deal effectively with change and uncertainty" (Valiga, 2021, p. 680).

Role of Faculty in Curriculum Development

The development of curricula is the responsibility of faculty, as they are the experts in their respective disciplines and the best authorities in identifying the knowledge and competencies students need to acquire by graduation. The NLN's *Scope of Practice for Academic Nurse Educators* outlines nurse educators' responsibility for "formulating program outcomes and designing curricula that reflect contemporary health care trends and prepare graduates to function effectively in the health care environment" (NLN, 2020, p. 12).

As the emphasis on designing contemporary and cost-effective curricula continues to increase, so does the need to involve a broader community of stakeholders in the curriculum development process. Practice disciplines such as nursing are actively engaging a diverse array of stakeholders in curriculum design, development, implementation, and evaluation. The desire to increase engagement can and does add to the complexity of the development process and the ability to alter curricula in a timely manner. To address the need to create curricula that are responsive to workforce expectations requires faculty to develop curricula that are flexible in design, open to broader interpretation as expectations change, and capable of being implemented using a variety of different methodologies.

Nursing faculty have come to approach curriculum development from an outcomes perspective rather than the traditional teaching process orientation used in the delivery of nursing curricula. Focusing on learning as the product (outcome), the emphasis is placed on how students can use knowledge to practice competently in changing and often uncertain clinical situations. This approach assumes that both students and faculty have some latitude in individualizing the learning experience and related processes used in creating knowledge.

Traditionally, faculty autonomy has been closely tied to curriculum; in fact, faculty are considered to "own" the curriculum. This means faculty are accountable for designing, assessing, implementing, evaluating, and changing the curriculum to ensure quality and relevance in programs. In today's educational climate, the value of education is measured against job marketability. In the discipline of nursing, emphasis has been placed on what knowledge and competencies graduates have on completion of their programs as it relates to the expectations of the settings and roles within which they will practice.

When curriculum development is undertaken, the concepts of academic freedom versus curricular integrity inevitably arise. As suggested by the prior statements, faculty are collectively charged with using their significant expertise and diverse talents to construct curricula that will produce successful, high-quality graduates. Curricular integrity is achieved through faculty striving for—but not always arriving at—consensus decisions. Communication throughout the curriculum is a key determinant in the quality and consistency of the curriculum and the student experience.

A statement from the American Association of Colleges and Universities (AAC&U) specifically addressed this topic: "There is, however, an additional dimension of academic freedom that was not well developed in the original principles, and that has to do with the responsibilities of faculty members for educational programs. Faculty are responsible for establishing goals for student learning, for designing and implementing programs of general education and specialized study that intentionally cultivate the intended learning, and for assessing students' achievement. In these matters, faculty must work collaboratively with their colleagues in their departments, schools, and institutions, as well as with relevant administrators" (AAC&U, 2006, p. 1).

National Reports, Education Trends, and Recommendations of Significance

In addition to the Macy Foundation report recommendations discussed earlier, other seminal position statements, reports, and recommendations have been issued by prestigious organizations or groups that require substantive curricular change and in some cases disruptive innovation. Six of the most significant sources that call for substantive curricular changes are reviewed to contextualize the definitions of and processes related to curriculum in nursing.

Quality and Safety Education in Nursing Initiative

The Institute of Medicine (IOM, 2001) released a now-classic seminal report titled *Crossing the Quality Chasm*, calling for substantive reform of health professions education to enhance quality and safety practices within health care. Simply stated, the report identified five competencies as essential for health professionals of the 21st century: Patient-centered care, teamwork and collaboration, informatics, evidence-based practice, and quality improvement (including safety). It was also recommended that the disciplines develop common language in important areas, integrate learning experiences, use evidence-based curricula and teaching strategies, and offer faculty development to model these competencies. Subsequent reports have addressed a variety of related areas (IOM, 2003, 2010).

Following the IOM's *Crossing the Quality Chasm* report, the Quality and Safety Education in Nursing (QSEN) project was launched in 2005 with the overall goal of ensuring that all graduating registered nurse students had developed the relevant quality and safety competencies that would prepare them for practice.

From feedback received from nursing faculty and practice leaders of the time, it was clear there was an urgent need for faculty development to ensure that faculty were teaching contemporary and accurate information regarding quality and safety practices and that quality and safety content be integrated into all prelicensure nursing programs as quickly as possible. To provide information to nursing faculty that could be immediately incorporated into courses, the QSEN project developed a KSA curricular framework (QSEN, n.d.) that addressed each of the five competencies (separating quality and safety for a total of six) identified in the 2001 IOM report. A QSEN website (http://qsen.org/) was established to assist in the dissemination of the KSA framework and serves as a clearinghouse for teaching and learning resources.

The QSEN project was expanded to include graduate-level nursing competency development, resulting in KSAs for this level of nursing program

to advance quality and safety competency development (http://qsen.org). A partnership with the AACN and communications with the NLN have resulted in continuing faculty development opportunities related to QSEN along with a comprehensive text (Sherwood & Barnsteiner, 2017).

Essential content from the QSEN project has been integrated into nursing education program accreditation standards so that a formal review of the presence and effectiveness of QSEN content in nursing education programs is ensured. The QSEN initiative has also spurred nursing education research to develop and evaluate evidence-based QSEN teaching strategies to include in undergraduate and graduate nursing curricula (Schuler et al., 2021). There is, however, still work to do. Though the 2017 National Quality and Safety Education for Nurses Faculty Survey indicated that 36% of respondents were currently using QSEN in some manner in their teaching, the application was notably inconsistent (Altmiller & Armstrong, 2017).

Future of Nursing Report 2020–2030

On May 11, 2021, the National Academy of Medicine released another groundbreaking report on how the profession of nursing can be an integral part of the United States' long struggle for health equity. The report, *Future of Nursing 2020–2030: Charting a Path to Achieve Health Equity*, advances new goals that build on the themes of the first Future of Nursing report. "The expert committee extended the vision for the nursing profession into 2030 and charts a path for the nursing profession to help our nation create a culture of health, reduce health disparities, and improve the health and well-being of the U.S. population in the 21st century" (National Academies of Sciences, Engineering, and Medicine, 2021, p. 1). Achieving health equity will require changes in the thinking of educators and subsequent curricular change.

Carnegie Foundation for the Advancement of Teaching: Educating Nurses

The Carnegie Foundation for the Advancement of Teaching launched a multiyear comparative study titled *The Preparation for the Professions*, which focused on professional education in medicine, nursing, law, engineering, and preparation of the clergy in the United States. The goals of this significant initiative were to better understand how the various professions are prepared to practice through identification of educational approaches and how the outcomes of professional education could be strengthened and improved. The fourth volume of this series of studies on the professions was *Educating Nurses: A Call for Radical Transformation* (Benner et al., 2010). Four major recommendations emerged from this study, which have many implications for curriculum development and implementation:

1. Emphasize teaching for a sense of salience, situated cognition, and action in particular situations instead of covering decontextualized knowledge. This recommendation is often expressed as teaching students how to "think like a nurse."
2. Integrate clinical and classroom teaching instead of maintaining a separation of the two. Given the complexity and breadth of knowledge required for today's nursing practice, it is essential that faculty design strategies to better link classroom and clinical teaching to reflect the actual complexities and pace of nursing practice.
3. Emphasize clinical reasoning and multiple ways of thinking instead of critical thinking. Examples of the multiple ways of thinking include clinical reasoning, clinical imagination, and scientific reasoning.
4. Focus on formation rather than socialization and role taking. Nursing students need experiential learning environments that provide the opportunities to learn about and internalize the elements of being a professional.

These four recommendations, especially when coalesced into actual teaching practices, require educators to think very differently about how curricula are created and to acquire and effectively use many new teaching and learning strategies within the context of a health care system that is evolving rapidly to achieve the "triple aim" (now the quadruple aim) of health care. The quadruple aim seeks to improve the patient experience of care (including quality and satisfaction), improve the health of populations, reduce the per-capita cost of health care, and care for health providers (Bachynsky, 2020).

Use of Simulation

The use of simulation technology in nursing and health professions education has exploded during the past decade both in frequency of use and in efforts to measure student learning outcomes. Further, simulation has been shown to measure increases in students' clinical judgment (Klenke-Borgmann, 2020). Current students and faculty expect that simulation activities, including access to a clinical laboratory environment with equipment and simulators, will be readily available and resemble actual clinical settings. State boards of nursing and other professional nursing organizations are increasingly considering simulation as equal to or as replacement hours for direct clinical experiences in both graduate and undergraduate programs. Honkavuo (2021) reported that simulation resulted in nursing students' formation process and bridge-building between theory and clinical practice.

Interprofessional Education and Collaborative Practice

The importance of interprofessional education (IPE) and collaborative practice in achieving the quality, safety, and innovation goals of the overall health care system within the United States is supported by numerous major reports and statements previously described. The World Health Organization (WHO, 2010) and several organizations promoting interprofessional education have offered definitions of IPE that are guiding efforts in this area. These definitions describe interprofessional education as students from multiple professions learning with and about the various health professional roles so that the foundation for professional collaboration around care will more easily occur in real-world settings.

In 2009 six national education associations representing different health professions (nursing, allopathic and osteopathic medicine, dentistry, pharmacy, and public health) joined forces to create the Interprofessional Education Collaborative (IPEC) and to develop core competencies related to interprofessional collaborative practice (https://ipec.memberclicks.net/assets/2016-Update.pdf; IPEC, 2011). These organizations have the ability to influence curricular changes across the named disciplines. The goals of IPEC include the advancement of substantive IPE to prepare future clinicians for team-based patient care. Thus IPE is considered a precursor to promoting effective interprofessional collaborative practice across settings. A metanalysis of interprofessional education in health care showed a positive impact and effectiveness of educational intervention by the IPE program in various disciplines of health care (Guraya & Barr, 2018). The IPEC core competencies have been incorporated into virtually all involved health disciplines' accreditation standards, leading to more widespread adoption within the various curricula (Laverentz et al., 2020). See Chapter 11 for a discussion of interprofessional education and collaborative practice and the competencies that need to be incorporated into health professions curricula to prepare graduates for interprofessional practice.

Use of Learning Technologies

One of the most important trend reports regarding learning technology is the EDUCAUSE *Horizon Report*. This annual report details key trends, significant characteristics impeding higher education technology adoption, and important developments in educational technology for higher education. Key trends in the most recent teaching and learning report included: widespread adoption of hybrid learning models, increased use of learning technologies, widening of the digital divide, remote work/learning, learning analytics, and artificial intelligence (EDUCAUSE Horizon Report, 2021). Each of these technologies and trends impacts higher education because of the central nature of technology in today's learning environment. Students and faculty will need sophisticated learning to keep abreast of these influences. Further, faculty will need to be intentional in incorporating current technology in curriculum design and implementation.

Online learning had become an increasingly accepted mode of education in the wake of the COVID-19 pandemic when faculty had to quickly adapt to teaching online. Having an awareness of and planning for predicted changes in teaching and learning because of online course delivery is critical when developing or redesigning curricula at all levels. Easier access, convenience, adult-friendly education and services, better learning technology, and flexible programming schedules contribute to the appeal and utility of online learning. Teachers are expected to have sophisticated skills in instructional design and engaged learning using an online or hybrid delivery system. Fitzgerald and Konrad (2021) report that teachers need to create a structured learning environment, abide by the course schedule, and communicate changes in a timely fashion in times of increased student anxiety and stress, like the COVID-19 pandemic. See Chapter 21 for further information related to learning online and from a distance.

CURRICULUM DESIGN MODELS

A well-conceived curriculum is critical to the preparation of practicing nurses at all levels. Once a program's curriculum is designed, curriculum building becomes an ongoing task that is indispensable to, yet separate from, the acts of teaching and learning. Curriculum is a dynamic, evolving entity shaped by learner needs and desired achievement, faculty's beliefs about the science and art of nursing, and emerging needs of the populations served within changing health care services, delivery structures, and organization.

Creating a specific curriculum design for a given program must take into account many factors, including the mission, vision, and goals of the educational entity; the philosophy of the educational entity and that of the nursing program; and the priorities of major stakeholder groups (e.g., students, faculty, employers, and alumni). After deciding on desired program outcomes and competencies, faculty are positioned to design the curriculum. It is important to note, however, that it is helpful to create a working organizing framework to guide the development of program outcomes and competencies, as these components must become synchronized for curricular integrity.

The topic of curriculum design models is complex because of the numerous and often overlapping nomenclature or differential use of the same terms. This discussion is further complicated because nursing education programs frequently use a combination of design models. Descriptions of three of the most commonly used models for curricular design currently in use in nursing education curricula are presented.

The overall organization of a curriculum may be identified as based primarily on one of three models of design: (1) *blocks* of content (often in nursing education reflecting clinical specialties), (2) *concepts* (that often reflect subjects within nursing and from other disciplines thought to be critical for nursing practice), or (3) *competencies* (that reflect broad areas of expected graduate performance that are sequentially "leveled" throughout the curriculum by semester, year, or another time parameter to enable students to advance in knowledge and skill development and achieve desired learning outcomes).

Virtually all nursing education programs incorporate a strong focus on competencies because nursing is a practice profession and because program accreditation and professional licensing requirements incorporate expected results or competencies. Competencies can be imbedded throughout either "blocking" or concept design models. A specific challenge that nursing and other practice disciplines share is how to best plan for clinical or practice experiences. The more traditional model consists of a mostly concurrent plan, wherein didactic courses are paired with clinical experience courses with the goal of matching the two. In reality, this rarely works, and the logistical issues can be insurmountable. Many programs use a mixed approach, in which some didactic nursing courses have associated clinical experiences and others do not. Some programs are experimenting with frontloading didactic content and sometimes clinical simulation activities, after which a clinical intensive or immersion occurs with the goal of integrating the targeted knowledge, skills, and attitudes (KSAs) competencies to be achieved. Faculty should also carefully consider clinical learning sites that will provide students with exposure to clinical experiences across the care continuum and in collaboration with learners from other disciplines.

Blocked Content Curricula

Faculty who wish to design a curriculum primarily using *blocks* of content must first carefully enumerate the major blocks or clusters of information that need to be represented within the curriculum. Patterns can be built on the premise of sequencing specific courses and corresponding clinical learning experiences. This approach assumes that there is a logical order to sequencing content that will facilitate learning and requires faculty to consider what evidence exists to help them make evidence-based decisions regarding what the "logical" order might be.

Courses in a blocked curriculum are usually structured around clinical specialty areas, patient population, pathological conditions, or physical systems. Historically, nursing programs have been organized by type of patient (medical condition, specialty, or age) and sometimes by settings (predominantly acute care hospitals with some ambulatory or skilled nursing focus and clinical experiences as well as within the community). Courses with titles based on medical or clinical specialty areas such as adult medical–surgical, pediatric, maternal–child, and community nursing are examples of a blocked approach to curriculum design. Other important content or concepts are taught in separate courses, such as research- and evidence-based practice and foundations of professional nursing, among others. Additionally, some important content or concepts are placed in courses that seemed to be the best match; such examples include quality and safety, leadership, and cultural diversity topics. It is also possible to have a predominately blocked approach to curriculum design with selective integration of some content areas across the curriculum, such as pharmacology and nutrition, or some concepts such as pain or inflammation.

The idea of blocking content organizes both teaching and learning. It facilitates faculty course assignments and complements faculty expertise, allowing faculty to teach primarily in their areas of expertise in a specific location within the curriculum. It is also relatively easy to trace placement of content in the curriculum.

However, the segregation or blocking of content into specific courses can cause content to become isolated from previous or subsequent coursework and can impede the learner's ability to integrate knowledge and transfer concepts, information, and experiences from one course to another. By and large, this curriculum design model produces a curriculum that is highly structured, with little latitude for deviation and meeting individual learning needs. Faculty who design curriculum with a block design also need to guard against the tendency for a strong sense of course ownership to develop among faculty who consider a course to be "theirs" and thus become resistant to changes within their course that need to occur to maintain curricular integrity. Open, ongoing communication and shared faculty decision making around curriculum development and revision are essential to maintain curricular integrity.

Blocked curriculum design also has the potential to obscure issues with learner development and growth as a professional. When a student does not pass a course, it is not uncommon to hear faculty say that the student failed pediatrics or intensive care, for example. In reality, although the student was not able to apply the expected knowledge, skills, or behaviors to a given population, it was actually the student's inability to transfer and apply the key concepts required to demonstrate safe clinical reasoning skills that led to the failure. Faculty must look beyond the content to the concepts to gain an understanding of what has led to the failing performance.

Concept-based Curricula

Significant interest in a more conceptual approach to curriculum design continues to grow with the use of core concepts as a focal point of curriculum construction (Fletcher et al., 2019, Laverentz & Kumm, 2017). Concept-based curricula are designed to better reflect the complexity of nursing and health care while using core ideas or concepts important to nursing practice to help learners grasp the connections and master deeper learning of how these concepts explain a variety of conditions and situations they will encounter in nursing practice. These goals are in contrast to a traditional curriculum organized around medical diagnoses or patient groups that use a less flexible and encompassing schema, such as described when "blocking" curriculum.

In a concept-based curriculum, faculty identify and define concepts considered to be core to nursing practice and integral to achieving the program's established end-of-program outcomes for graduates. The concepts are integrated (threaded) throughout the curriculum in a manner that facilitates acquisition of competencies that are leveled throughout the curriculum, ultimately leading to student achievement of expected end-of-program outcomes. Faculty develop learning experiences that will guide the students' application of the concepts across a variety of patient populations and care settings.

Although there is significant variation in the concepts chosen to organize a nursing curriculum, some concepts have emerged across the majority of undergraduate nursing programs. Examples of these common concepts include oxygenation, cognition, pain, nutrition, pharmacology, and lifespan development. Additionally, nursing roles, communication and teamwork, quality and safety, and ethics and legal issues are also frequently present. Graduate curricula may also be organized by concepts relevant to advanced practice roles and settings.

An example of content integration may be seen in the following description of the concept of pain. Early in the curriculum, students first learn about the pathophysiologic causes of pain, causes and cardinal characteristics of pain, factors that shape or affect pain, and how to assess and evaluate the characteristics of pain. As students move through the curriculum, they increase their understanding of the manifestations of and treatments for pain, review research related to the concept of pain, and identify appropriate therapeutic nursing interventions related to the care of a patient with pain, thus progressing from a global understanding of pain to a more specific, in-depth understanding of the concept. Eventually, students learn about pain as it relates to acute and chronic health issues, to physical or non-disease-based causes, or to specific situations such as surgery and childbirth in various clinical populations. Additionally, the QSEN standards provide key concepts related to quality and safety that can be used to create a framework to organize curricula along with other important concepts (Sherwood & Barnsteiner, 2017).

Historically, accreditation standards and performance expectations have had a significant effect on many organizing frameworks as faculty recognize the need to directly address these expectations that include such concepts as clinical reasoning, problem solving, communication, caring, diversity, and therapeutic nursing interventions (Olds & Dolansky, 2017; Sherwood & Barnsteiner, 2017). The concepts of clinical reasoning and clinical judgment or "thinking like a nurse" is increasingly replacing the more general critical thinking concept to better focus on and measure situated knowledge development that leads to action rather than a general intellectual skill (Gonzales et al., 2021; Klenke-Borgmann, 2020).

Faculty adopting a concept-based, outcome orientation to curriculum must be able to construct the context and meaning that the outcomes will have in the curriculum structure. An outcomes focus reflects the need to achieve designated competencies that students are expected to have at the completion of the program to demonstrate expected program outcomes. Faculty must identify and integrate the curriculum concepts that will support the students' achievement of the identified competencies and outcomes. Hendricks et al. (2016) grouped curricular concepts into themes to map content to courses and major program learning outcome focus areas, which creates a clear roadmap for use by faculty, students, and other stakeholders.

In a concept-based curriculum design, there are no boundaries to knowledge development and skill acquisition, as noted in the blocking approach. The concepts that form the curriculum must be clearly and visibly explicated for students so that they can see and experience the integration of the concepts across the curriculum. Students use clinical experiences to learn the essence of identified concepts and are encouraged to transfer and expand their knowledge and skills to different settings, populations, and experiences. Active, engaged teaching and learning strategies pair naturally with this conceptual approach to nursing education. Problem-based learning, team-based learning, case studies, and reflection are just a few examples of teaching and learning strategies that can be used to facilitate student understanding of the concepts being studied and help them to become "users" of knowledge. See Chapter 16 for further discussion of active learning strategies.

Disadvantages of a more conceptual approach to curriculum design include difficulty in maintaining the integrity of the curriculum because of the lack of discrete boundaries for content and the potential for inadvertently eliminating from the curriculum key aspects of the concept. Faculty must carefully map the concepts across the curriculum to ensure that the students' knowledge of the concept will grow in depth and breadth and not become mired in repetition or omission. See the "Guiding Principles for Developing Organizing Frameworks" section of this chapter for further suggestions on how to select curricular concepts.

Another potential disadvantage is that student learning styles may favor a more traditional and less conceptual approach to learning, as that is how they have likely become accustomed to learning. Faculty need to consider the various learning styles of students in their classroom and design approaches that will facilitate students adjusting to a more conceptual approach to learning.

Competency-Based Education

The term *competency-based education* (CBE) as a curriculum approach has a specific, formal definition. "Competency-based education (CBE) is an approach to preparing [practitioners] for practice that is fundamentally oriented to graduate outcome abilities and organized around competencies derived from an analysis of societal and patient needs. It deemphasizes time-based training and promises greater accountability, flexibility, and learner centeredness" (Frank et al., 2010). Moving to a competency-based model would foster intentionality by defining competencies and associated attributes, methods for achievement, and outcome measurements (AACN Vision for Academic Nursing, 2019). See Case Study 6.1.

In contrast, traditional education programs employ learning objectives with definitions of competence that are less clear and precise and sometimes a weaker or inconsistent approach to actually testing and measuring competency achievement. Supporters of CBE cite its systematic and valid assessment of competencies and the opportunity for students to progress at their own pace rather than fit into a planned time for and sequence of learning activities. Additionally, CBE may be more resource effective than traditional education methods. A recent systematic review of CBE in the health professions suggested that, while noting the complexity of and variation among the disciplines' sets of competencies, CBE can be useful and effective in meeting learning needs across professions (ten Cate et al., 2021). Challenges to fully implementing CBE in health-related roles include identifying the health needs of the community, defining competencies, developing self-regulated and flexible learning options, and assessing learners for competence (Kavanagh & Sharpnack, 2021). A formal CBE approach also may not suit all learners' preferences and abilities.

As noted earlier, virtually all nursing and professional education programs incorporate some aspects of CBE, as it is required for accreditation and licensure, but the amount of and consistency with which CBE principles are employed varies widely across nursing education programs.

Ordering or Constructing Knowledge Within the Curriculum

Regardless of the curriculum design model chosen, faculty must still make decisions about how knowledge will be ordered or constructed within the curriculum. Wiles and Bondi (2011) describe five patterns of ordering or constructing knowledge in a curriculum. Similar to the blending of curricular design approaches, many nursing education programs use aspects of the five patterns within the overall curriculum, sometimes within the same semester or course. It is helpful that faculty be clear and guide students through how the curriculum and courses are organized to avoid confusion and provide clear expectations.

In a *building blocks design*, content and learning activities commence with foundational knowledge or skills, followed by more detailed or specialized material and, if appropriate, a higher level of depth or specialized knowledge. A *branching design* is similar to a building blocks design in that foundational knowledge or skills occur first, after which there are varied learning option pathways to achieve the desired KSAs. This pattern is typically strongly represented in the blocked curriculum design model.

In a *spiral design*, selected areas of knowledge appear repeatedly through the curriculum in greater depth or breadth. In some fields, this area is further differentiated into a spiral versus a strand design. In a spiral curriculum, many different topics are covered at designated points throughout the curriculum. The points may be at regular or intermittent intervals because of concerns that students often forget previously covered information as a result of the brief instructional time devoted to each and because students do not have time to master important foundational knowledge. To minimize these issues, some education experts advocate the use of a strand (sometimes also called a *thread*) design. In a strand design, topics are arranged into meaningful groups that are regularly repeated, thus building better achievement and retention rates. Spiral or strand designs are prominent in concept-based curricula.

A *tasks or skills design* is characterized by presentation of specific knowledge and experiences that are expected to lead learners to achieve the desired competencies. There may be varying pathways for students as individuals or by groupings that reflect learning preferences or other characteristics. This pattern is usually prominent in CBE programs, although the tasks and skills are grouped into the larger competencies for assessment purposes.

The fifth pattern of ordering knowledge is the *process* design, where the focus is on the process of learning with specific information or content-provided examples to illustrate the process. Some educators believe that the enhanced focus on narrative pedagogy and related teaching and learning strategies (e.g., the concept of learning to "think like a nurse") reflect a process design.

CURRICULUM ELEMENTS

Curriculum development is a challenging yet rewarding endeavor that ranks among the top responsibilities of a collective faculty. Although much has been written about curriculum and its associated processes, there are multiple approaches and terminologies proposed, leading to confusion and disagreements about what elements compose a curriculum. For purposes of this chapter, the following curricular elements are included and discussed: curriculum design, organizing framework, end-of-program outcomes and competencies, level competencies, course design, teaching strategies and learning experiences, and resources needed to implement the curriculum. The terminology and definitions reflect some of the most commonly used across schools of nursing. The influence of contemporary thinking and newer approaches to teaching and learning are highlighted within each element.

Organizing Frameworks

Organizing frameworks can be a means for creating access to knowledge about the phenomena of interest or importance to the discipline. Organizing frameworks do provide a logical structure for cataloging and retrieving knowledge. This structure, often depicted as a schematic conceptualization, is essential to the processes of teaching and learning as faculty guide students in the development of cognitive linkages among knowledge. This helps faculty and students understand the abstract nature of nursing. Fawcett's (1989) classic work on conceptual models and frameworks can provide readers with a discussion of theories, models, and concepts that is beyond the scope of this chapter.

Organizing frameworks have been used in curriculum development to delineate the constructs embedded in a traditional philosophy statement that reflects the collective faculty belief. It is important that organizing frameworks not be construed as a permanent feature of a program but as a kaleidoscope of complex patterns related to what students need to know and how they will best learn it.

The purpose of constructing frameworks is to systematically design a mental picture that is meaningful to the faculty and students when determining what knowledge is important and has value to nursing today and how that knowledge should be defined, categorized, and linked with other knowledge. Although the majority of nurses continue to practice in acute care settings, with the increasing emphasis on transitional care, there needs to be broader orientation to a continuum of care settings within a global context. This thinking is consistent with the widely held view that tomorrow's nurse be prepared to practice across a broad range of settings, including community-based care for individuals and populations. Organizing curriculum frameworks provide a blueprint for determining the scope of knowledge (i.e., which concepts are important to include in the teachers' and learners' mental picture) and a means of structuring that knowledge in a distinctive and meaningful way for faculty and students. As such, organizing curriculum frameworks are the educational road maps to teaching and learning. As with any road map, multiple route options are available for arriving at a given destination or outcome. A number of approaches are used in defining and shaping frameworks. However, an organizing framework must reflect the sphere of nursing practice, the phenomena of concern to nurses, and how nurses relate to others who are dealing with health concerns, often referred to as nursing's *metaparadigm* (Lee & Fawcett, 2013).

Fig. 6.1 shows one school's depiction of an organizing framework for the undergraduate program, which the faculty have titled "The Baccalaureate Big 5" (Godfrey & Martin, 2016). Concepts are presented once in the curriculum, applied in interactive classroom activities, and incorporated as interrelated concepts at other points in the curriculum. Using this organizing framework as the structural curriculum guide, faculty are expected

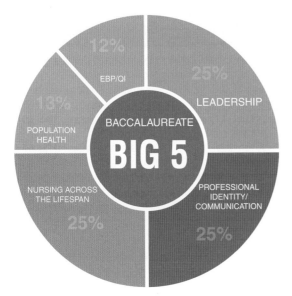

FIG. 6.1 The Baccalaureate Big 5: An organizing framework for undergraduate nursing education. Numbers represent the percentage of AACN baccalaureate essentials outcomes in each category. (© 2022, University of Kansas.)

to design learning experiences that foster students' application of these concepts in increasingly complex and contextualized clinical experiences with patients, families, communities, and populations.

As faculty embrace adoption of an outcome orientation in curriculum building, organizing frameworks or models will continue to serve the same purposes but will be driven by philosophical views and futuristic mental pictures regarding the evolving practice of nursing. For example, the role of nurses in telehealth and retail-based clinics, in both undergraduate and graduate roles, provide new and expanding career options for nurses, so competencies must reflect a wider perspective on nursing practice essentials. There is also growing support for increasing the number of registered nurses practicing in primary care settings (Alley et al., 2021; Lukewich et al., 2020). Organizing frameworks directly guide development of end-of-program outcomes and competencies that are also leveled for more detailed planning purposes.

The process of selecting or designing an organizing framework that will best serve a program or school is not an easy task, but this process is an exceptional opportunity for faculty to build

teamwork and innovation skills. Two general approaches may be used in determining the kind of organizing framework faculty wish to construct. The first approach is to select a single specific nursing theory or model on which to build the framework, a traditional approach that is used today in some schools. A second, more commonly used approach is more eclectic and blends concepts from multiple theories or models, a method that has gained in popularity as the complexity of nursing and the health care environment has increased.

Developing a Single-Theory Framework

Historically, one traditional approach to constructing an organizing framework for nursing program curricula was to use a particular nursing theory or model to help shape the visual image that is consistent with the philosophy of the faculty. For example, if faculty believe that caring is at the core of nursing, a theory of caring (Clark, 2016; Monsen et al., 2017). Pajnkihar et al. (2017) might serve as the anchoring model when explaining the discipline to students and cataloging knowledge about the discipline of nursing. The advantage of building an organizing framework on a single theory or model is the ability to use a single image with a defined vocabulary that is shared by both the learner and the teacher. Using a single theory or existing conceptual model has limitations and poses challenges, including that it may not reflect everybody's view of nursing and nursing practice. This becomes problematic when faculty have developed or been educated in curricula with a different theory or orientation to the discipline. The use of only one theory in a framework may limit the ability of faculty to pull together all elements of their curriculum, which provides a rationale for moving away from this approach, as does recognizing that the practice of nursing is being transformed by a dynamic, evolving health care system. Further, it is clear that nurse educators and practitioners may not agree on a single theory. Students educated in a curriculum driven by a single theory can benefit from a focused view of nursing and find themselves making useful connections to the strong guiding theory for the duration of their nursing education experience.

Developing an Eclectic Framework

Given the challenges and limitations of using a single theory as an organizing framework, faculty choice does not have to be constrained by a single theory or model. Those who believe that a combination of many theories or concepts is more reflective of their beliefs about nursing may use an eclectic approach to developing a curricular framework.

The use of a more eclectic approach when designing an organizing framework is not without its pitfalls. Some view this approach as an impediment to the development of a comprehensive nursing theory and the development of a body of knowledge that is uniquely nursing. The advantage of an eclectic approach is the ability to "borrow" concepts and definitions that best fit the faculty's beliefs and values from nursing and non-nursing theories. The eclectic approach may also promote incorporation of contemporary or evolving conceptualizations of nursing, health, the environment, and other key concepts and better reflect the practice of nursing across the continuum of settings and patient populations. However, if faculty develop an eclectic framework in which concepts and their definitions are "borrowed" from a number of theories, they need to ensure that in the act of borrowing they have not changed the conceptual meaning. It is important to clearly show the relationships among selected concepts. Therefore, it is important to clarify the meaning of concepts that will be used in an organizing framework so that faculty and students are clear about the phenomena being studied.

Guiding Principles for Developing Organizing Frameworks

Although there are no specific steps or "how-tos" for developing organizing frameworks for curriculum, there are some guiding principles that faculty can follow (see Box 6.1).

The first principle is to choose those concepts that most accurately reflect the faculty's beliefs about the practice and discipline of nursing and how students learn. The introduction of contemporary, student-centered approaches to learning, which stem from constructivism theory (see

> **BOX 6.1   Steps for Developing Organizing Frameworks**
>
> 1. Choose concepts that reflect faculty's beliefs about nursing and how students learn.
> 2. Clearly define major concepts underpinning the curriculum framework.
> 3. Explain linkages between and among the concepts identified.
> 4. Determine that the curriculum framework is consistent with the school's mission and values.
> 5. Assess congruence between curriculum framework and program goals and professional standards.

development (Epp et al., 2021). The concepts identified should also reflect or complement the philosophy, mission, and goals of the college or university in which the program is embedded. By creating an organizing framework that reflects concepts valued by both the discipline of nursing and the parent institution, faculty have begun to articulate the contributions their nursing program makes to all stakeholder entities.

The most important aspect of choosing the concepts that tie the curriculum together is relevancy. This means that the concepts chosen must be relevant and meaningful to the future practicing nurse, be consistent with the science and art of nursing, and address the needs of the populations served through health care delivery systems. During this phase of curriculum development, it is important to involve stakeholders in the process. Reading professional standards and recommendations; understanding regulatory and accrediting criteria; and gathering input from practice partners, students, community leaders, and other identified stakeholders can all help faculty with selecting appropriate concepts.

The selected concepts are often organized into a graphic representation to facilitate understanding and recognition of the organizing framework. The second principle is to clearly define the major concepts underpinning the curriculum framework. Consensus should be established in this process because it will fall to the faculty to articulate these concepts to the students. Consistency in terminology and definitions along with making the organizing framework visible to faculty, students, practice partners, and other program stakeholders will enhance the framework's role in mastery of the desired level of competency at program completion.

The third principle is to explain the linkages between and among the concepts identified. This is critical because the linkages are the basis for how students comprehend, apply, analyze, synthesize, and evaluate knowledge learned throughout the educational process. These principles are analogous to putting together a jigsaw puzzle in which the concepts are the puzzle pieces and the total picture is of high-quality, contemporary nursing practice. Puzzles come in various numbers of pieces. Usually, the greater the number of pieces, the greater the challenge in its construction. The outline and coloring of the pieces are the definitions of the concepts. The more clearly the puzzle pieces are defined and the sharper the color delineations, the easier it is to fit the puzzle together. It is critical that faculty and students grasp an understanding of the framework without an intensive investment of time and energy.

Faculty must decide on the major concepts that make up the organizing framework and focus on illustrating the linkages among those concepts. It is not necessary or desirable to identify each and every concept that students will be introduced to. The more faculty focus on minute concepts, the more likely it is that they are defining facts (not concepts) that will quickly become irrelevant. It is important to keep the work of concept identification, definition, and linkage at a broader level involving concepts that will retain salience with safe, quality practice.

However faculty decide to approach the work of developing a framework for their curriculum, the framework that is eventually constructed must be consistent with the school's mission and philosophy statements, faculty values and beliefs, program goals, professional standards, state and federal regulations, and current and future nursing practice trends. Faculty should have broad-based agreement on the curriculum framework because such agreement is fundamental to the consistent interpretation, implementation, and evaluation of the curriculum in meeting the expected program goals and outcomes. If there is a disconnect among philosophy, values, program expectations, professional practice expectations and outcomes, and the framework, faculty need to raise significant questions as to the utility of the created frameworks.

Once the work has been completed, faculty should share the completed framework with various stakeholders, soliciting feedback on how the organizing framework is interpreted by others. Such an exercise can help faculty determine whether they have been successful in publicly articulating their beliefs and values to others.

Outcomes and Competencies

If curriculum frameworks are the road maps to understanding the discipline of nursing, then outcomes can be equated with the trip's destination and competencies with the mileage markers seen along the way. Program outcomes (also referred to as *end-of-program outcomes, learning outcomes* or sometimes *expected outcomes*) then take the place of what was traditionally and more generally called *terminal objectives* as the outcomes represent the integrated knowledge, skills, and abilities or competencies students are expected to demonstrate at program completion.

Program outcomes, in the simplest of terms, are those characteristics students should display at a designated time, most often at the completion of the curriculum, and reflect a description of the ideal program graduate. Outcomes are also developed at the course level and are progressively designed and integrated into the curriculum to lead the learner to the achievement of the program outcomes. Competencies are sometimes described as what students can do with what they know at designated points during and at the end of the educational program. It is the demonstration of competencies as integrated throughout the curriculum that enables students to eventually achieve the program outcomes. Each broader desired outcome may be linked with multiple competencies to achieve a meaningful level of specificity for student assessment and, in the aggregate, for program evaluation. The chapters in Unit V – Evaluation provide detailed information about assessing student learning, program evaluation, and related topics.

Identifying Curriculum Outcomes

The movement to an outcomes orientation has developed over time in nursing education as it has in higher education. These changes communicate a strong focus on the quality and value of postsecondary education (K–12 has experienced a similar set of changes with a focus on competency testing). Being able to demonstrate achievement of the stated program outcomes is consistent with the social efficiency ideology of curricula presented earlier in this chapter. Regional higher education accrediting bodies have fully embraced the idea that educational outcomes should prepare graduates to serve some aspect of societal need or improvement, resulting in strong and, some argue, prescriptive approaches to the assessment of student learning and enhanced review of program evaluation metrics.

Over the past decade, the focus on outcomes in higher education and nursing education has continued to increase. The NLN first addressed the development of outcomes and competencies across the continuum of academic programs by convening an advisory group to identify the outcomes and competencies needed at each educational program level, from licensed practical nurse to the clinical doctorate. A similar effort has occurred within the AACN (2021), with the development of *The Essentials: Core Competencies for Professional Nursing Education* document. This recently approved (April 2021) document identifies the competencies of prelicensure baccalaureate education and graduate nursing education and is in the process of being introduced to nursing programs for implementation.

With the need for nursing educators to ensure that the curricula they design will keep pace with the ongoing changes in health care and higher education, more emphasis will continue to be placed on the school's ability to demonstrate success. Outcomes assessment has been seen as the key by which nursing programs can document strengths and weaknesses. A comprehensive assessment program can help faculty determine what works and what does not in achieving academic quality and producing the desired program outcomes (Oermann & Gaberson, 2019; Wittenberg et al., 2021).

This logic is a significant departure from the predominantly process-oriented Tylerian approach to curriculum and evaluation, in which the emphasis was placed on detailed course objectives, the identification of content needed to meet course objectives, and the appropriate pedagogical approaches to complement the type of content needing to be taught. Outcome assessment emphasizes assessment of competencies, that is, what students have actually learned and related skills they are able to demonstrate in their educational experiences, not merely the knowledge and experiences that were designed with the intent of achieving these results. These differences, which may seem like nuances to many, are core to the changing focus in curriculum development and student learning assessment and evaluation that continues to evolve in higher education and nursing education.

When moving to a curriculum that is more centered on the development of outcomes relevant to nursing practice, it is often easier to think about curriculum development as starting at a program's end rather than its beginning. Outcomes then become the critical focus of curriculum development. This method of curriculum development places a different emphasis on the need for organizing frameworks as a starting point for curriculum development. Approaching curriculum development beginning with the desired outcome or what the student needs to demonstrate at graduation to be a competent nurse and then working backward toward the beginning of the curriculum provides faculty with an opportunity to identify the essential outcomes and competencies that they wish to see their students demonstrate at the completion of the program.

It is important to note that development of outcomes should be significantly informed by the mission, vision, values, and philosophy of the program; an environmental scan that includes the perspectives of major external stakeholders; the use of best current evidence in nursing and health professions education; and internal stakeholder preferences from faculty, students, alumni, and appropriate others. See Box 6.2 for an example of mission and vision, philosophy, and program outcomes at a faith-based college.

BOX 6.2   Sample Curriculum for a Faith-Based Institution: Vision, Mission, Philosophical Framework, and Program Outcomes

School of Nursing Vision

We prepare highly skilled professional nurses who are culturally responsive, practice clinical excellence with ingenuity, and proactively improve whole-person healing to advance health equity and social justice.

School of Nursing Mission

Inspired by Catholic intellectual tradition, the School of Nursing embraces academic excellence by fostering a caring culture during students' preparation for entry into professional RN practice.

Our graduates will partner with others, serving as culturally responsive leaders who value intellectual inquiry to act wisely in the provision of ethical and compassionate whole-person and whole-community care that promotes human flourishing.

They will provide this care with ingenuity, dignity, and respect for diverse populations to advance health equity and social justice.

Philosophical Framework

At the St. Thomas School of Nursing, we believe that nursing occupies a unique presence amid an array of health care providers through caring for the whole person and whole community through nursing's fundamental patterns of knowing: empiric, ethical, aesthetic, personal, and emancipatory (Carper, 1978; Chinn & Kramer, 2018). These patterns of knowing provide students with the foundation to achieve our mission, vision, and program outcomes, as well as to exemplify the Morrison Family College of Health Principles. In facilitating learning about *empiric knowing*, we believe students gain the strong scientific foundation necessary to solve clinical problems through engaging in clinical reasoning, demonstrating sound clinical judgment, and developing an evidence-based practice. Under the auspices of Catholic intellectual tradition, we know that nursing is a fundamentally moral endeavor where students learn to embody *ethical knowing* as they understand their obligation to provide fair and just health care for the common good. We firmly embrace the important value of *aesthetic knowing* in all facets of nursing practice to aid in promoting health and healing. These facets include creating and engaging in interprofessional and relationship-based care milieus,

using integrative nursing care practices, and incorporating forms of art into nursing care, such as stories and poetry. We believe in educating students to have a keen sense of *personal knowing*, especially self-awareness to providing safe, quality, and respectful care, including caring for cultures other than one's own culture. And, as aligned with Chinn and Kramer, we believe in the intersection of *emancipatory knowing* with all of the patterns of knowing so that students engage in critical reflection and ingenuity as they become professional nursing leaders, advocates, and change agents to bring about health equity and social justice for all people.

Program Outcomes for BSN and MSN Curricula
BSN Program Outcomes

1. Integrates liberal education for the provision of professional nursing care for the whole person and whole community.
2. Develops person-centered plans of care through therapeutic relationship, respect, holistic assessment, prioritization, intervention, and evaluation to achieve dignified health outcomes.
3. Promotes the common good through ethical, moral, and socially just nursing care for people and populations through health promotion, disease prevention, and emancipatory praxis.
4. Demonstrates clinical decision-making, scholarship, and evidence-based nursing practice in the provision of care within complex systems.
5. Uses ingenuity, innovation, and multiple ways of knowing to proactively and continuously improve quality and safety in nursing practice and health care systems.
6. Demonstrates interprofessional teamwork that values similarities and differences to enhance and strengthen health outcomes.

MSN Program Outcomes

1. Synthesizes knowledge from liberal education for the provision of professional nursing care for the whole person and whole community.
2. Creates person-centered plans of care through therapeutic relationship, respect, holistic assessment, prioritization, intervention, and evaluation to achieve dignified health outcomes.

Continued

BOX 6.2   Sample Curriculum for a Faith-Based Institution: Vision, Mission, Philosophical Framework, and Program Outcomes—cont'd

MSN Program Outcomes—cont'd

3. Advances the common good through ethical, moral, and socially just nursing care for people and populations through health promotion, disease prevention, and emancipatory praxis.
4. Integrates clinical judgment, scholarship, and evidence-based nursing practice in the provision of care within complex systems.

5. Leads through ingenuity, innovation, and multiple ways of knowing to proactively and continuously improve quality and safety in nursing practice and health care systems.
6. Facilitates interprofessional teamwork that values similarities and differences to enhance and strengthen health outcomes.

Courtesy University of St. Thomas School of Nursing.

The interrelationship between the organizing framework and the outcomes and competencies becomes clear, with the organizing framework being shaped by the theories and concepts embedded in the outcomes and competencies. For example, if faculty believe that students need to possess clinical reasoning, communication, teamwork, and leadership skills, these concepts will be evident in the organizing framework. In an outcomes-focused curriculum the driver of faculty conversations is not what content must be taught but rather what KSAs students need to demonstrate to meet expected curriculum outcomes. Before they can think about curriculum from the outcome, or end stage, faculty first must identify the desired program outcomes using a stakeholder-informed and future-oriented picture of nursing practice (Sroczynski et al., 2017). See Box 6.3 for an example of end-of-program outcomes that reflect evolving stakeholder priorities through emphasizing interprofessionally focused, safe, evidence-based care that is culturally sensitive and occurs in all settings.

As faculty identify outcomes, it is important to embed these outcomes in actions that promote the practice of nursing. Using an outcomes perspective, it is important that faculty not only clarify and define the concepts they wish to use in the development of outcomes but also ensure that they have outcomes that are broad enough to incorporate all of the attributes desired.

A common question is how many program outcomes are needed. There is no evidence-based answer to this question, but many programs strive for no more than 8 to 10 outcomes. Keep in mind that these should be broad-based outcomes that encompass a number of competencies that will evolve with changing practice. If faculty are identifying a large number of program outcomes, it is likely that they have confused program outcomes with the knowledge, skills, or behaviors related to competencies. Program outcomes should not need to be frequently updated; they should stand the test of time. For example, consider the BSN program outcomes in Box 6.3. These outcomes are written broadly and will be contemporary for some time to come. The knowledge, skills, and behaviors (competencies) that the graduate will need to acquire to demonstrate these outcomes will likely change, but the outcomes will remain current. The faculty can review and update the competencies as needed to stay current.

Some of the criteria that will be useful in determining how many outcomes to include are ensuring that the major aspects of the organizing framework are included, that significant professional practice and accreditation standards are appropriately reflected, and that a clear picture of the major components of a practitioner who is engaged in safe, quality nursing care emerges when the outcomes are considered as a whole.

Consideration of a more ontological philosophical approach to defining outcomes adds the perspective of the learner on core characteristics. The importance of reflection and reflective practice is increasingly recognized as a crucial strategy to develop professional identity, emotionally intelligent practitioners, and a commitment to lifelong learning and development (Horton-Deutsch & Sherwood, 2017).

BOX 6.3 **Example of BSN Program Outcomes**
1. Effectively communicate with all members of the health care team, including clients and their support system. 2. Use clinical judgment to design quality, safe, evidence-based patient care. 3. Deliver safe, compassionate, culturally competent, patient-centered nursing care across the lifespan. 4. Use health care resources to effectively deliver high-quality, cost-effective patient care 5. Demonstrate leadership in the evaluation of outcomes, improvement of care, and advancement of nursing practice. 6. Provide health promotion, disease prevention, end-of-life care, and/or palliative care to individuals and populations in a variety of settings. 7. Examine the micro- and macrosystems that influence health care delivery to achieve quality patient care within economic boundaries. 8. Contribute the unique nursing perspective with the interdisciplinary health care team to achieve optimal health care outcomes. 9. Demonstrate professionalism in attitudes and behaviors.

Courtesy University of Kansas School of Nursing.

Identifying and Developing Competencies

After the expected program outcomes have been established, the next step in the curriculum development process is to identify the competencies that students need to possess to attain these outcomes. Competency statements identify the knowledge, skills, and professional attitudes and values that students need to develop if they are to achieve the program outcomes. Competency statements are behaviorally anchored and student focused. Nursing faculty must approach curriculum development from the premise that nursing knowledge and skills are built on or interwoven with general education knowledge and skills. Outcomes should include those competencies that are specific to the nursing discipline and those competencies that establish a foundation for lifelong learning. Students achieve the identified competencies through acquisition of necessary KSAs over time, leading to the achievement of the expected program outcomes whether as an undergraduate or graduate student

Competency statements are important in assessing student learning because they become the foundation that drives evaluation. When identifying competencies, faculty should give attention to determining the right student, the right behavior, the right level of behavior, and the right context of the behavior. Here, *student* refers to the level of student from whom faculty are expecting these behaviors (e.g., prenursing, nursing sophomore, nursing senior, master's, or doctoral level); *level of behavior* refers to the level of learning or performance at which the behavior is to be demonstrated (this is where learning taxonomies are helpful); and *context of the behavior* refers to the environment in which the behavior should occur. For example, if faculty believe that it is essential for students to exhibit a particular skill, knowledge, or attitude across a continuum of health care settings or with a select population of patients, then the competency statement should indicate the parameters in which the behavior should be expressed. It is equally important for faculty to remember not to be so specific as to "paint themselves into a corner" from which there is no escape (e.g., if faculty specify that a certain behavior will be demonstrated with postoperative patients in an outpatient surgical setting, all students must be guaranteed this type of experience for faculty to make an accurate and consistent assessment and evaluation of student performance).

Leveling Competencies

In leveling or specifying competencies, faculty must recognize the level at which the KSAs need to be demonstrated to obtain the outcome desired throughout the curriculum. One strategy is to divide the competencies into beginning, middle of the curriculum, and end-of-program as a means of determining where specific competencies can be most effectively learned and assessed. Regardless of the type of categorization, the learning environment will need to be designed to enable the students to acquire knowledge at the level identified. Evaluation measures also need to be consistent to ensure consistency in evaluation from the time of input of information through the time of output of the expected competency. Learning occurs at various levels, and the level of learning needs to be explicitly stated in the competencies faculty generate for each level within the curriculum. Table 6.1 shows how a specific competency can be leveled across the final four semesters of a baccalaureate nursing program.

Once competencies have been leveled to a year or semester or academic level, faculty must carefully examine these competencies and determine how courses can be designed to contribute to the ongoing development of these competencies. The behaviors embedded in each competency become the focus for writing course-level competencies. Not all competencies will or should be included in all courses that make up the curriculum. Competencies at the course level are more concrete and detail how the chosen competencies explicitly relate to the course. The faculty will then need to identify what prerequisite and requisite knowledge and skills students will need to possess to demonstrate this behavior.

If, for example, faculty believe that the individualization of a standard care map is critical to a nurse practitioner student learning experience, then a course-level competency resulting in course objectives, learning activities, and evaluation of learning will be included to reflect this behavior. This way of thinking easily leads to regular assessment of end-of-program student learning outcomes and allows for a mindset of backward design, assuring that the end-of-program outcomes are solidly situated with the rest of the curriculum and can be met by the learners. A formalized mapping process may be helpful.

Because structured learning tends to be grounded in developmental theories, students are expected to become more accomplished in applying knowledge to increasingly more complex or new situations as they move through the curriculum. Course outcomes and the accompanying competencies (course expectations) should be written to reflect the placement of the course within the curriculum; the expectations of learning for courses that precede, articulate, and follow each course; and how each course can contribute to the development of program competencies and achievement of program outcomes. Precision is needed when writing competency statements. The language of the competencies must reflect a continued sense of development. Development may take the form of increasing complexity, differentiation, delineation, or sophistication.

Strategies for Identifying and Leveling Competencies

Outcomes are typically measured through more specific competency statements that, in aggregate, provide evidence that the outcome was achieved. To maintain curricula integrity, tracking competencies associated with each program outcome is an important activity, but tracking the numerous competencies associated with all outcomes can become an onerous task. Comprehensive content

TABLE 6.1 Example of Leveled Competencies for Demonstrating One's Professional Identity in Nursing in a Four-Level Associate Degree Nursing Program

Level 1	Level 2	Level 3	Level 4	End-of-Program Outcome
Identify the definition and four domains of professional identity in nursing: values and ethics, knowledge, nurse as leader, and professional comportment.	Examine the professional identity in nursing as observed in the clinical environment through the lens of the four domains: values and ethics, knowledge, nurse as leader, and professional comportment.	Evaluate one's progress in developing and demonstrating professional identity in nursing.	Reflect on the domains of professional identity of nursing, synthesizing how the four domains can be integrated into one's own nursing practice.	Demonstrate a professional identity of nursing.

BOX 6.4   Strategies for Identifying and Leveling Competencies

- Competencies need to be observable and assessable. Therefore, focus on what students *know* and *can do*.
- Focus on necessary core knowledge and how the learner can demonstrate that knowledge (performance).
- Think about the competency as part of an overall program of assessment.
- Use multiple modes of assessment when possible.

Data from Oermann, M. H. (2022). Some principles to guide assessment of competencies. *Nurse Educator, 47*(1), 1.

---

grids are useful and necessary, but they can be so voluminous that they lose utility for depicting the building blocks of KSAs desired. Box 6.4 provides some strategies faculty can use to level competencies.

Several methods for documenting learning progression and competency achievement may be used. Each program outcome is measured through multiple derived competencies created to reflect learning achievement of that given outcome. These associated competencies can be placed in a grid that includes the program outcome, information regarding the course location, specific course outcomes and learning activities, and evaluation criteria used to assess student learning. Once these are agreed on by faculty, individual faculty may not independently change the key learning activities and evaluation methods. Additionally, selected assignment products may be used to create student portfolios as an expression of their comprehensive achievement of the desired learning outcomes.

Finally, specification of key learning activities is an effective tool to identify content duplication and gaps. In one recent example within a nursing program, it was discovered that students were asked to perform three community assessments in three different courses using almost identical criteria. Faculty agreed that one community assessment was sufficient and thus freed up precious time for other learning topics. Competency grids can be reviewed by faculty on a regular basis to incorporate new information and concepts, with the designated faculty group making decisions

regarding changes. This practice is an example of how curricular integrity can be balanced with the concept of academic freedom.

Course Design

After faculty have completed the overarching curriculum structure with the identification of the organizing framework, outcomes, and competencies, the competencies can now be organized or threaded through the courses that faculty develop. To begin this process, faculty must consider the antecedents or factors that need to be in place for the outcomes and competencies to be achieved in each course in the curriculum. *Antecedents* are defined as the prerequisite knowledge needed to develop or foster the identified attributes or characteristics. It is assumed that each course within the curriculum will make a *unique* contribution to the ability of students to meet the identified competencies at each level of the program.

The key is for faculty as curriculum developers to consciously consider and design courses and sequences that will best lead to achieving the desired learning outcomes across the diversity of students within the population. See Chapter 10 for an in-depth discussion on designing courses and learning experiences.

DEVELOPING AND REVISING CURRICULUM

Faculty are responsible for the development and revision of the curriculum. Faculty involved in updating or developing curricula should have a firm understanding of content, as well as accreditation and professional standards, regulatory requirements from licensing boards and certification bodies, and forces and trends influencing curriculum (see Chapter 5).

For many faculty, the curriculum development process may be an unfamiliar one. Developing or revising curricula requires faculty to possess content expertise, an understanding of how the various curricular elements interact, and the ability to negotiate and manage change (Case Study 6.2). Box 6.5 provides an overview of the curriculum development process, which is briefly described here.

CASE STUDY 6.2   Developing Curricula

You have been asked to be part of the six-person team to lead curriculum development for a new associate degree nursing program. Your school has had a practical nursing program for the past 6 years and administration has requested the addition of an associate degree nursing program to begin in 18 months. You have more experience with curriculum development than all but one person on the committee. In preparation for the first meeting all members of the curriculum development team have been asked to consider what questions or data will be important to consider as planning before the new program begins.

1. What questions do you think will be important for the faculty to consider in preparation for curriculum development for the new program?
2. As a faculty who has more curriculum development experience than some of the other team members, what advice can you provide the others about the curriculum development process? What should the team's first steps be in the planning process?
3. A novice faculty member asks you: "How do you know what needs to be included in an RN program?" What would your answer be?

BOX 6.5   Processes in Curriculum Development

1. Build stakeholder readiness for curricular change
   - Ensure structure exists to support effective faculty decision-making
   - Minimize competing priorities for faculty time
   - Prepare a realistic timeline for the development process
2. Create the Vision
   - Summarize and share views of stakeholders
   - Align vision with program mission
   - Identify relevant professional standards in nursing and health care
   - Explore multiple perspectives envisioning future curriculum
3. Mobilize Resources
   - Identify resources needed to develop or revise curriculum
   - Outline what and how much effort is needed
   - Consider utilizing a project management approach
   - Explore funding options

BOX 6.5   Processes in Curriculum Development

4. Choose Organizing Parameters
   - Identify curricular elements (program outcomes, competencies, concepts)
   - Determine the organizing framework for the curriculum
   - Progressively integrate outcomes, competencies, and concepts into the curriculum
5. Design the Curriculum
   - Establish end-of-program curricular outcomes
   - Define concepts or content threads for mapping
   - Identify and level competencies across curriculum
   - Create an overview of proposed courses
6. Develop the Courses
   - Develop course outcomes
   - Design learning modules (units)
   - Identify student learning outcomes
   - Select teaching/learning strategies
   - Design evaluation strategies
7. Implement and Evaluate the New Curriculum
   - Obtain required curriculum approvals
   - Communicate the plan to stakeholders
   - Implement the new curriculum
   - Plan for evaluation of new curriculum and expected outcomes
8. Disseminate Outcomes of Curriculum Change Process
   - Consider curriculum change to be a scholarly endeavor
   - Share process and outcomes of curriculum change process through publications and presentations
   - Contribute to the body of evidence-based nursing education literature

Preparing for Curriculum Change

Preparing the faculty to participate in curriculum change is an important first step to beginning the process of any major curriculum development or revision. Start by building readiness for change through securing the resources needed to support faculty engagement in curriculum development and taking steps to ensure that faculty have a basic understanding of curriculum design. Also, consider the timing of other significant institutional or program changes or commitments to minimize competing priorities. For example, faculty may want to consider timing curriculum revision to not conflict with simultaneously preparing for an upcoming accreditation visit. It is also imperative to positively prepare faculty and stakeholders for any needed curricular revisions by creating and reinforcing an awareness of the need for the revisions along with a desire to change (Pawl & Anderson, 2017). Effective planning also includes understanding the steps to any required approval processes that will be associated with the proposed changes and establishing a realistic timeline for completing the work.

Creating the Vision

The nursing curriculum that is being developed should reflect the mission, vision, and values espoused by the institution while maintaining congruence with the school's philosophy and vision. Chapter 7 provides further discussion of the relationship of mission, vision, and values to curriculum development. In addition, the faculty should carefully consider emerging trends in health care and higher education, as well as the inclusion of relevant professional nursing and health care standards.

Faculty must also consider the input of stakeholders as they design the new curriculum. For example, understanding the learning needs of the student population that will be served is essential. Involving learners in the visioning of the curriculum can provide helpful insights into their perceived needs. See Chapter 2 for further discussion about the diverse learning needs of students.

Seeking input from clinical partners and advisory committee members can also provide faculty with important insights about future health care workforce needs. Without such vision, curricula will consistently lag behind the rapidly changing health care environment and become irrelevant, to the detriment of the profession.

Assessing and Mobilizing Resources

When designing or revising curricula, it is important to consider the effects of various decisions on the resources that will be required to implement those plans in a manner that will ensure a quality outcome (AACN, 2019). This assessment and discussion requires collaboration between academic administration and the faculty leading the curriculum efforts. It is most helpful to agree on assumptions regarding resources of faculty (full-time and clinical instructors or others), simulation and related materials, clinical sites, and support services. In some cases, resources will be constrained, requiring that curricula be created with that fact in mind.

Decisions regarding many of the curricular elements have implications for resources, with three elements creating the most potent influence on resources: the organizing framework, learning outcomes, and pedagogical strategies. As an example, if a problem-based learning approach is identified as a major teaching strategy, additional faculty facilitators might be desirable for the same number of students. Or if simulation activities are to be increased in amount and level of complexity—perhaps using simulated patients—the costs of these plans must be considered and approved before the process of curriculum change is completed, not after. Academic administrators and faculty leaders would be well advised to outline the scope of the curriculum development or change project, including an assessment of and future assumptions about resources to avoid disappointment and rework.

Another aspect of resources related to curricular design and change is the amount of faculty time and effort expended to accomplish this important work. Unfortunately, in many cases, curricular change is handled according to existing processes and meetings structures, which may be onerous, time consuming, and sometimes unclear. Viewing the work of curricular change from the lens of project management and quality improvement leads to embracing tested models for data collection, assessment, and decision making within a prescribed timeframe versus an open-ended approach to completing the desired work.

Given the central importance of resources in any curriculum, a clear understanding of the assumptions and the amount and type of available resources will position a curriculum project for success.

Choosing Organizing Parameters

Planning, implementing, and evaluating the nursing curriculum should ensure that the end-of-program curriculum outcomes, competencies, and major concepts are organized in a meaningful way, integrated throughout the curriculum, and associated with course outcomes and learning modules/units. Before revising the current curriculum, faculty may want to conduct an evaluative review to determine what gaps or redundancies exist, whether current course outcomes are set at an appropriate cognitive difficulty level, and whether the assigned course credit load is realistically aligned with the expected student learning outcomes. When revising an existing curriculum, using evaluation findings to identify the strengths and challenges in the current organizational design is essential in creating a plan that improves upon the existing model.

Designing the Curriculum

The faculty should oversee the entirety of the draft curriculum elements before developing courses in detail so that courses are well suited to learners' needs and lead to learning outcomes in a meaningful way. Specifically, program outcomes, major concepts and integrated conceptual threads, competencies, and strategies for evaluation should be mapped across the curriculum for congruence and to ensure logical, progressive sequencing.

The creation of mapping documents to ensure integrity of the curriculum plan can be helpful. Furthermore, creating maps of relevant professional standards and criteria, including accreditation criteria, can be used to demonstrate to stakeholders that the curriculum is addressing required elements. Such curricular maps or "crosswalks" can also be instrumental in helping faculty retain a visual representation of the various curricular elements and how they relate. This can be particularly helpful when orienting new faculty to the curriculum and when engaging in future curriculum evaluation and revision efforts.

Developing the Courses

At the course level, curricular integrity can be best achieved if faculty follow a consistent approach to course development. For example, course outcomes (or objectives) should be able to be mapped to the established program curricular outcomes and competencies. When creating or revising course learning modules (or units), student learning outcomes, teaching strategies, and evaluation strategies for each of the modules should be created. Chapter 10 discusses designing courses and learning experiences in detail.

Implementing and Evaluating the New Curriculum

A complete and organized curriculum plan ensures that faculty have the resources needed for effective program implementation and evaluation. Besides sharing the curriculum plan with faculty and students, communicating the plan broadly to all stakeholders such as employers, clinical partners, and alumni garners support. Sharing both broad curriculum goals and course-specific outcomes assists clinical partners who will interact with students to contribute meaningfully to the educational process. The proposed curriculum changes may also require the review of licensing or certification boards and accreditation bodies

When implementing a revised curriculum plan, there will be a period of time in which faculty will need to "teach out" the old curriculum while smoothly implementing the newly revised curriculum. This period of transition places demands on faculty time and the resources, faculty, and learning experiences, including clinical sites required to successfully put the new curriculum in place while phasing out the old curriculum, should be carefully considered prior to implementation.

As faculty implement the new curriculum, some thought should be given to how to proactively evaluate the anticipated outcomes of the new curriculum. The use of formative evaluation allows for data collection that can be analyzed to help faculty adjust as needed when implementing the new curriculum. Using established mechanisms to gather, analyze, and respond to evaluation data about the new curriculum can help faculty determine whether further changes are needed. When phasing out a curriculum that is being replaced, planning for continued quality and attention to the students is important to ensure learning experiences remain meaningful. Otherwise, students in the last offering of a curriculum that is being phased out may feel devalued.

Disseminating the Work

Sharing the outcomes of the curriculum revision with stakeholders is the final step in the process. The work of curriculum development and revision can also be a scholarly activity. Faculty should consider the value that their work may have for other faculty and share their processes and outcomes through publications and presentations. By doing so, faculty are contributing to the body of literature addressing curriculum design and development.

CHAPTER SUMMARY: KEY POINTS

- Curriculum design and revision require a systematic, planned approach.
- Curriculum ideologies describe the underlying beliefs and philosophy faculty hold related to education.
- Learner-centered pedagogy strategies are major influencers in nursing education and curriculum development.
- Helping faculty become familiar with the curriculum design process will yield positive results.
- Developing the faculty's basic understanding of the curriculum design process is a necessary step before undertaking curriculum development activities.
- The most common curriculum design models used in nursing education are: (1) blocked content curriculum (typically reflecting clinical specialties), (2) concept-based curriculum, and (3) competency-based education.
- When developing or revising curriculum, faculty should have a firm understanding of content, as well as accreditation and professional standards, regulatory requirements from licensing boards and certification bodies, forces and trends influencing curriculum, and the change process.
- When creating the organizing framework for the curriculum and choosing the concepts that tie the curriculum together, the concepts chosen must be relevant and meaningful to the future practicing nurse, be consistent with the science and art of nursing, and address the needs of the populations served through the health care delivery system.
- End-of-program outcomes are those characteristics students are expected to display at the completion of the curriculum and reflect a description of the ideal program graduate.
- Course outcomes are progressively designed and integrated into the curriculum to lead the learner to the achievement of the program outcomes.
- Competencies are sometimes described as what students can do with what they know at designated points during and at the end of the educational program. It is the demonstration of competencies as integrated throughout the curriculum that enables students to eventually achieve the program outcomes.
- Each program outcome may be linked to multiple competencies to achieve a meaningful level of specificity for student assessment.
- A clear understanding of resources needed and resources available for curriculum design or revision is important before beginning the design process.

REFLECTING ON THE EVIDENCE

1. How can faculty use student and program outcome data to assess the effectiveness of the current curriculum design and determine what changes may need to occur to retain relevance of the curriculum?
2. What can faculty do to ensure the curriculum maintains integrity while adapting the design to emerging evidence and innovations?
3. How can faculty effectively solicit stakeholder input when contemplating curriculum revisions? Who would those stakeholders be?
4. What would you consider to be the major benefits and disadvantages of the most common curriculum design models used in nursing education—blocked content, concept curriculum, and competency-based curriculum?

REFERENCES

Alley, R., Carreira, E., Wilson, C., & Pickard, K. (2021). Using nurse-sensitive indicators to assess the impact of primary care RNs on quality ambulatory patient care. *Nursing Economic$, 39*(4), 200–207.

Altmiller, G., & Armstrong, G. (2017). 2017 National quality and safety education for nurses faculty survey results. *Nurse Educator, 42*(5S Suppl 1), S3–S7. https://doi.org/10.1097/NNE.0000000000000408.

American Association of Colleges and Universities. (2006). Academic freedom. http://www.aacu.org/publications-research/periodicals/academic-freedom-and-educational-responsibility

American Association of Colleges of Nursing (AACN). (2019). *AACN's vision for academic nursing.* https://www.aacnnursing.org/Portals/42/News/White-Papers/Vision-Academic-Nursing.pdf

American Association of Colleges of Nursing (AACN). (2021). *Essentials: Core competencies for professional nursing practice.* Author.

Bachynsky, N. (2020). Implications for policy: The triple aim, quadruple aim, and interprofessional collaboration. *Nursing Forum, 55*, 54–64.

Benner, P., Sutphen, M., Leonard, V., & Day, L. (2010). *Educating nurses: A call for radical transformation.* Jossey-Bass.

Bevis, E. O. (2000). Nursing curriculum as professional education. In E. O. Bevis & J. Watson (Eds.), *Toward a caring curriculum: A new pedagogy for nursing* (pp. 74–77). National League for Nursing Press.

Clark, C. S. (2016). Watson's human caring theory: Pertinent transpersonal and humanities concepts for educators. *Humanities, 5*(2), 21.

EDUCAUSE. (2021). *EDUCAUSE Horizon Report® 2021Teaching and Learning Edition.* https://library.educause.edu/-/media/files/library/2021/4/2021hrteachinglearning.pdf

Epp, S., Reekie, M., Denison, J., de Bosch Kemper, N., Willson, M., & Marck, P. (2021). Radical transformation: Embracing constructivism and pedagogy for an innovative nursing curriculum. *Journal of Professional Nursing, 37*(5), 804–809. https://doi.org./10.1016/j.profnurs.2021.06.007.

Fangonil-Gagalang, E., & Schultz, M. A. (2021). Diffusion of precision health into a baccalaureate nursing curriculum. *Journal of Nursing Education, 60*(2), 107–110. https://doi.org/10.3928/01484834-20210120-10.

Fawcett, J. (1989). Conceptual models of nursing. F. A. Davis.

Frank, J. R., Snell, L. S., Cate, O. T., Holmboe, E. S., Carraco, C., Swing, S. R., Harris, P., Glasgow, N. J., Campbell, C., Dath, D., Harden, R. M., Jobst, W., Long, D. M., Mungroo, R., Richardson, D. L., Sherbino, J., Silver, I., Taber, S., Talbot, M., & Harris, K. A. (2010). Competency-based medical education: theory to practice. *Medical Teacher, 32*(8), 638–645.

Fletcher, K. A., Hicks, V. L., Johnson, R. H., Delois, M. L., Phillips, C. J., Lynelle, N. B., Pierce, , Wilhoite, D. L., & Gay, J. E. (2019). A concept analysis of conceptual learning: A guide for educators. *Journal of Nursing Education, 58*(1), 7–15. https://doi.org/10.3928/01484834-20190103-03.

Fitzgerald, A., & Konrad, S. (2021). Transition in learning during COVID-19: Student nurse anxiety, stress, and resource support. *Nursing Forum, 56*, 298–304.

Godfrey, N., & Martin, D. (2016). Breakthrough thinking in nursing education: The Baccalaureate Big 5. *Journal of Nursing Administration, 46*(7–8), 393–399. https://doi.org/10.1097/NNA.0000000000000364. PMID: 27442902.

Gonzales, L., Nielsen, A., & Lasater, L. (2021). Developing students' clinical reasoning skills: A faculty guide. *Journal of Nursing Education, 60*(9), 485–493.

Guraya, S. Y., & Barr, H. (2018). The effectiveness of interprofessional education in healthcare: A systematic review and meta-analysis. *The Kaohsiung Journal of Medical Sciences, 34*, 160–165.

Hendricks, S. M., Taylor, C., Walker, M., & Welch, J. A. (2016). Triangulating competencies, concepts, and professional development in curriculum revisions. *Nurse Educator, 41*(1), 33–36.

Honkavuo, L. (2021). Ethics simulation in nursing education: Nursing students' experiences. *Nursing Ethics, 28*(7–8), 1269–1281. https://doi.org/10.1177/0969733021994188.

Horton-Deutsch, S., & Sherwood, G. D. (2017). Reflective practice: Transforming education and improving outcomes. *Sigma Theta Tau*

Hsieh, L., Chang, Y., & Yen, M. (2022). Improving leadership competence among undergraduate nursing students: Innovative objectives development, implementation, and evaluation. *Nursing Education Perspectives, 43*(1), 24–29. https://doi.org/10.1097/01.NEP.0000000000000866.

Institute of Medicine, (2001). *Crossing the quality chasm: A new health system for the 21st century.* The National Academies Press.

Institute of Medicine, (2003). *Health professions education: A bridge to quality.* The National Academies Press.

Institute of Medicine, (2010). *The future of nursing: Leading change, advancing health.* The National Academies Press.

Interprofessional Education Collaborative Expert Panel. (2011). Core competencies for interprofessional collaborative practice: Report of an expert panel. Retrieved from https://www.ipecollaborative.org/resources.html

Kavanagh, J. M., & Sharpnack, P. A. (2021, January 31). Crisis in competency: A defining moment in nursing education. *OJIN: Online Journal of Issues in Nursing, 26*(1). manuscript 2.

Klenke-Borgmann, L. (2020). High-fidelity simulation in the classroom for clinical judgment development in third-year baccalaureate nursing students. *Nursing Education Perspectives, 41*(3), 185–186. https://doi.org/10.1097/01.NEP.0000000000000457.

Klenke-Borgmann, L., Cantrell, M. A., & Mariani, B. (2020). Nurse educators' guide to clinical judgment: A review of conceptualization, measurement, and development. *Nursing Education Perspectives, 41*(4), 215–221. https://doi.org/10.1097/01.NEP.0000000000000669.

Laverentz, D., & Kumm, S. (2017). Concept evaluation using the PDSA cycle for continuous quality improvement. *Nursing Education Perspectives, 38*(5), 288–290. https://doi.org/10.1097/01.NEP.0000000000000161.

Laverentz, D. M., Young, E., & Cramer, E. (2020). Effect of a longitudinal IPE passport program on nursing students' attitudes toward interprofessional practice. *Nursing Education Perspectives (online ahead of print)* https://doi.org/10.1097/01.NEP.0000000000000636.

Lee, R. C., & Fawcett, J. (2013). The influence of the metaparadigm of nursing on professional identity development among RN-BSN students. *Nursing Science Quarterly, 26*(1), 96–98. https://doi.org/10.1177/0894318412466734.

Lucey, C. R. (2018). Achieving competency-based, time-variable health professions education: Conference recommendations, June 2017. Josiah Macy, Jr. Foundation.

Lukewich, J., Allard, M., Ashley, L., Aubrey-Bassler, K., Bryant-Lukosius, D., Klassen, T., Magee, T., Martin-Misener, R., Mathews, M., Poitras, M. -E., Roussel, J., Ryan, D., Schofield, R., Tranmer, J., Valaitis, R., & Wong, S. T. (2020). National competencies for registered nurses in primary care: A Delphi study. *Western Journal of Nursing Research, 42*(12), 1078–1087. https://doi.org/10.1177/0193945920935590.

Monsen, K. A., Le, S. M., Handler, H. E., & Dean, P. J. (2017). We can be more caring: A theory for enhancing the experience of being caring as an integral component of prelicensure nursing education. *International Journal for Human Caring, 21*(1), 9–14.

National Academies of Sciences, Engineering, and Medicine. (2021). *The future of nursing 2020–2030: Charting a path to achieve health equity.* The National Academies Press. https://doi.org/10.17226/25982.

National League for Nursing, (2020). *The scope of practice for academic nurse educators* (3rd ed.). National League for Nursing.

National League for Nursing. (2022). *NLN nurse educator core competencies for academic nurse educators.* Author. http://www.nln.org/professional-development-programs/competencies-for-nursing-education/nurse-educator-core-competency

Oermann, M. H. (2022). Some principles to guide assessment of competencies. *Nurse Educator, 47*(1), 1.

Oermann, M. H., & Gaberson, K. B. (2019). *Evaluation and testing in nursing education* (6th ed.). Springer Publishing Company.

Olds, D., & Dolansky, M. A. (2017). Quality and safety research: Recommendations from the Quality and Safety Education for Nursing (QSEN) Institute. *Applied Nursing Research, 35*, 126–127.

Pajnkihar, M., McKenna, H. P., Stiglic, G., & Vrbnjak, D. (2017). Fit for practice: Analysis and evaluation of Watson's theory of human caring. *Nursing Science Quarterly, 30*(3), 243–252.

Parkay, F. W., Anctil, E. J., & Hass, G. (2014). *Curriculum leadership: Readings for developing quality educational programs* (10th ed.). Prentice-Hall.

Pawl, J. D., & Anderson, L. S. (2017). The use of change theory to facilitate the consolidation of two diverse Bachelors of Science in Nursing programs. *Nursing Outlook, 65*(2), 233–239. https://doi.org/10.1016/j.outlook.2016.10.004.

Quality and Safety Education for Nurses (QSEN). (n.d.). http://qsen.org/

Schiro, M. (2013). Curriculum theory (2nd ed.). Sage.

Schuler, M., Letourneau, R., Altmiller, G., Deal, B., Vottero, B., Boyd, T., Ebersole, N., Flexner, R., Jordan, J., Jowell, V., McQuiston, L., Norris, T., Risetter, M., Szymanski, K., & Walker, D. (2021). Leadership, teamwork, and collaboration: The lived experience of conducting multisite research focused on quality and safety education for nurses competencies in academia. *Nursing Education Perspectives, 42*(2), 74–80. https://doi.org/10.1097/01.NEP.0000000000000725.

Sherwood, G., & Barnsteiner, J. (Eds.). (2017). *Quality and safety in nursing: A competency approach to improving outcomes.* John Wiley & Sons.

Sroczynski, M., Conlin, G., Costello, E., Crombie, P., Hanley, D., Tobin, M., & Welsh, D. (2017). Continuing the creativity and connections: The Massachusetts initiative to update the nurse of the future nursing core competencies. *Nursing Education Perspectives, 38*(5), 233–236.

ten Cate, O., Carraccio, C., Damodaran, A., Gofton, W., Hamstra, S. J., Hart, D. E., Richardson, D., Ross, S., Schultz, K., Warm, E. J., Whelan, A. J., & Schumacher, D. J. (2021). Entrustment decision making: Extending Miller's pyramid. *Academic Medicine, 96*(2), 199–204. https://doi.org/10.1097/ACM.0000000000003800.

Tri-Council for Nursing. (2021). Transforming together: Implications and opportunities from the COVID-19 pandemic for nursing education, practice, and regulation. https://img1.wsimg.com/blobby/go/3d-8c2b58-0c32-4b54-adbd-efe8f931b2df/downloads/Tri-Council%20COVID-19%20Report%20-%20FINAL.pdf?ver=1627563792961

Tyler, R. W. (2013). *Basic principles of curriculum and instruction*. University of Chicago Press.

Valiga, T. M. (2021). Postpandemic nursing education: Moving forward with new ideas. *Journal of Nursing Education, 60*(12), 680–685.

Wiles, J. W., & Bondi, J. C. (1989). *Curriculum development: A guide to practice* (3rd ed.). Merrill.

Wiles, J. W., & Bondi, J. C. (2011). *Curriculum development: A guide to practice* (8th ed.). Pearson Education.

Wittenberg, E., Goldsmith, J. V., Prince-Paul, M., & Beltran, E. (2021). Communication and competencies across undergraduate BSN programs and curricula. *Journal of Nursing Education, 60*(11), 618–624. https://doi.org/10.3928/01484834-20210913-03.

World Health Organization. (2010). Framework for action on interprofessional education & collaborative practice. World Health Organization. http://whqlibdoc.who.int/hq/2010/WHO_HRH_HPN_10.3_eng.pdf

7

Philosophical Foundations of the Curriculum

Theresa M. "Terry" Valiga, EdD, RN, ANEF, FAAN

Beautiful words. Admirable values. Published prominently on websites and in catalogs, student handbooks, and accreditation reports. The philosophical statement of a school of nursing is accepted by faculty as a document that must be crafted to please external reviewers, but for many, it remains little more than that. In fact, the lack of attention to the focus, purpose, or importance of philosophical statements is evident in a review of current literature, supporting, perhaps, the claim that it is a component of curriculum development and a school's overall culture that is seen as not particularly critical. Far too often, the school's philosophy remains safely tucked inside a report but is rarely seen as a living document that guides the day-to-day workings of the school.

In reality, the philosophy of a school of nursing should be referenced and reflected upon often. It should be reviewed seriously with candidates for faculty positions and with those individuals who join the community as new members. It should be discussed in a deliberate way with potential students and with enrolled students as they progress throughout the program. And it should be a strong guiding force as the school revises or sharpens its goals, outlines action steps to implement its strategic plan, and makes decisions about the allocation of resources.

This chapter explores the significance of reflecting on, articulating, and being guided by a philosophy; examines the essential components of a philosophy for a school of nursing; and points out how philosophical statements guide the design and implementation of the curriculum and the evaluation of its effectiveness, as well as how it influences the overall culture in the school. The role of faculty, administrators, and students in crafting and "living" the philosophy is discussed, and the issues and debates surrounding what educational philosopher Maxine Greene (1973) called the "doing of philosophy" are examined. Finally, suggestions are offered regarding how faculty might go about writing or revising the school's philosophy.

WHAT IS PHILOSOPHY?

Maxine Greene (1973) challenged educators to "do philosophy." By this, she meant that we need to take the risk of thinking about what we do when we teach and what we mean when we talk about enabling others to learn. It also means we need to become progressively more conscious of the choices and commitments we make in our professional lives. Greene also challenged educators to look at our presuppositions, to examine critically the principles underlying what we think and what we say as educators, and to confront the individual within us. She acknowledged that we often have to ask and answer painful questions when we "do philosophy."

In his seminal book *The Courage to Teach*, Parker Palmer (2007) asserted that "though the academy claims to value multiple modes of knowing, it honors only one—an 'objective' way of knowing that takes us into the 'real' world by taking us 'out of ourselves'" (p. 18). He encouraged educators to challenge this culture by bringing a more human, personal perspective to the teaching–learning experience. Like Greene, Palmer suggested that to do this, educators must look inside so that we can understand that "we teach who we are" (p. xi) and so that we can appreciate that such insight is critical for "authentic teaching, learning, and living" (p. ix).

Philosophy, then, is a way of framing questions that have to do with what is presupposed, perceived, intuited, believed, and known. It is a way of contemplating, examining, or thinking about what is taken to be significant, valuable, or worthy of commitment. Additionally, it is a way of becoming self-aware and thinking of everyday experiences as opportunities to reflect, contemplate, and exercise our curiosity so that questions are posed about what we do and how we do it, usual practices are challenged and not merely accepted as "the way things are," and positive change can occur. Indeed, each of us—as a fundamental practice of being—must go beyond the reality we confront, refuse to accept it as a given, and, instead, view life as a reality to be created.

These perspectives on "doing philosophy" focus primarily on individuals—as human beings in general or as teachers in particular—reflecting seriously on their beliefs and values. There is no question that such reflection is critical and is to be valued and encouraged. However, "doing philosophy" also must be a group activity when one is involved in curriculum work. In crafting a statement of philosophy for a school of nursing, the beliefs and values of all faculty must be considered, addressed, and incorporated as much as possible. In fact, the very process of talking about one's beliefs and values—although it may generate heated debates—leads to a deeper understanding of what a group truly accepts as guiding principles for all it does.

PHILOSOPHICAL STATEMENTS

A philosophy is essentially a narrative statement of values or beliefs. It reflects broad principles or fundamental "isms" that guide actions and decision making, and it expresses the assumptions we make about people, situations, or goals. As noted by Bevis (1989) in her seminal work *Curriculum Building: A Process*, the philosophy "provides the value system for ordering priorities and selecting from among various data" (p. 35).

In writing a philosophical statement we must raise questions, contemplate ideas, examine what it is we truly believe, become self-aware, and probe what might be—as well as what should be. It calls on us to think critically and deeply, forge ideas and ideals, and become highly conscious of the phenomena and events in the world in which we currently exist and, in the case of education and to the extent that we can anticipate it, the world in which our graduates will practice.

We also must reflect on the mission, vision, and values of our parent institution and of our school itself, as well as the values of our profession. Fig. 7.1 illustrates how a school's statement of philosophy is related to but differs from these other sources. A *mission statement* describes unique purposes for which an institution or nursing unit exists: to improve the health of the surrounding community, to advance scientific understanding or contribute to the development of nursing science, to prepare responsible citizens, or to graduate individuals who will influence public policy to ensure access to quality health care for all. A *vision* is an expression of what an institution or nursing unit wants to be: the institution of choice for highly qualified students wishing to make a positive difference in our world; the leader in integrating innovative technology in the preparation of nurses; or a center of synergy for teaching, research, professional practice, and public service. Institutions and schools of nursing often also articulate a set of *values* that guide their operation: honesty and transparency, serving the public good, inclusivity, respect, excellence, innovation, or constantly being open to change and transformation.

As stated, a *philosophy statement* is the narrative that reflects and integrates concepts expressed in the mission, vision, and values of the institution or profession; it serves to guide the actions and decisions of those involved in the organization. Educational philosophy is a matter of "doing philosophy" with respect to the educational enterprise as it engages the educator. It involves becoming critically conscious of what is involved in the complex teaching–learning relationship and what education truly means. The following statements about education, many by well-known

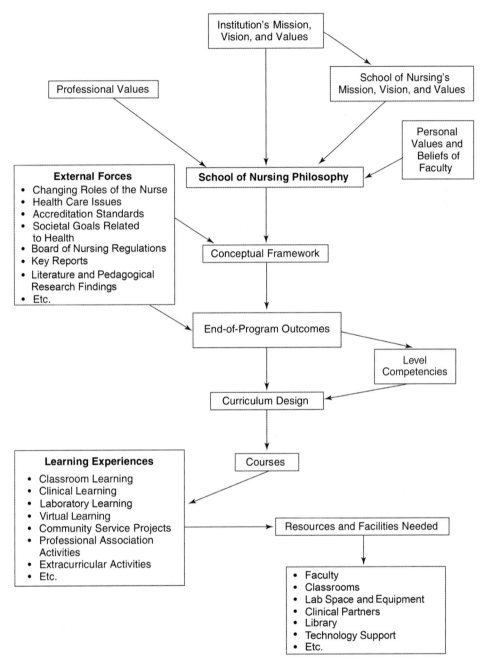

FIG. 7.1 Interrelation of curricular elements.

individuals, provide examples of different philosophical perspectives:

- *The secret of education lies in respecting the pupil.*—Ralph Waldo Emerson (1921)
- *If the student is to grow, the teacher must also grow.*—Confucius
- *I think [education] refines you. I think some of us have rough edges. Education is like sanding down a piece of wood and putting the varnish to it.*—Suzanne Gordon (1991, p. 131)
- *The whole art of teaching is only the art of awakening the natural curiosity of young minds for the purpose of satisfying it afterward.*—Anatole France (1920)
- *The teacher learns from the student just as the student learns from the teacher with their encounters as examples of mutual openness to each other's needs.*—Nili Tabak, Livne Adi, and Mali Eherenfeld (2003, p. 251)

PHILOSOPHY AS IT RELATES TO NURSING EDUCATION

As noted earlier, "doing philosophy" must move from individual work to group work when engaged in curriculum development, implementation, and evaluation. Faculty need to reflect on their own individual beliefs and values, share them with colleagues, affirm points of agreement, and discuss points of disagreement. Table 7.1 summarizes many of the philosophical perspectives expressed through the years, and faculty are encouraged to explore the meaning and implications of each as they engage in developing, reviewing, or refining the philosophical statement that guides their work. A discussion of three basic educational ideologies is presented here to point out how differences might arise if each person on a faculty were to approach education from her or his own belief system only.

TABLE 7.1 Summary of Philosophical Perspectives	
Philosophical Perspective	**Brief Description**
Behaviorism	Education focuses on developing mental discipline, particularly through memorization, drill, and recitation. Because learning is systematic, sequential building on previous learning is important.
Essentialism	Because knowledge is key, the goal of education is to transmit and uphold the cultural heritage of the past.
Existentialism	The function of education is to help individuals explore reasons for existence. Personal choice and commitment are crucial.
Hermeneutics	Because individuals are self-interpreting beings, uniquely defined by personal beliefs, concerns, and experiences of life, education must attend to the meaning of experiences for learners.
Humanism	Education must provide for learner autonomy and respect their dignity. It also must help individuals achieve self-actualization by developing their full potential.
Idealism	Individuals desire to live in a perfect world of high ideals, beauty, and art, and they search for ultimate truth. Education assists in this search.
Postmodernism	Education challenges convention, values a high tolerance for ambiguity, emphasizes diversity of culture and thought, and encourages innovation and change.
Pragmatism	Truth is relative to an individual's experience; therefore education must provide for "real-world" experiences.
Progressivism	The role of learners is to make choices about what is important, and the role of teachers is to facilitate their learning.
Realism	Education is designed to help learners understand the natural laws that regulate all of nature.
Reconstructionism	Education embraces the social ideal of a democratic life, and the school is viewed as the major vehicle for social change.

Adapted from Csokasy, J. (2009). Philosophical foundations of the curriculum. In D. M. Billings, & J. A. Halstead (Eds.), *Teaching in nursing: A guide for faculty.* Saunders.

One basic educational ideology is that of *romanticism*, a perspective espoused by Jean-Jacques Rousseau and Maria Montessori. It was a philosophical movement during the Age of Enlightenment and surfaced again in the 1960s, emphasizing emotional self-awareness and learner-centeredness. Within this ideological perspective, one would construct an educational environment that is permissive and freeing; promotes creativity and discovery; allows each student's inner abilities to unfold and grow; and stresses the unique, the novel, and the personal.

Although many nurse educators believe that current nursing education reflects this student-centered perspective, those who have acknowledged our "content-laden curricula" (Diekelmann, 2002; Diekelmann & Smythe, 2004; Giddens & Brady, 2007; Hardin & Richardson, 2012; Tanner, 2010)—an issue that persists to this day—would disagree and posit that, although a "romantic" philosophy is embraced as an ideal, it is not always evident in our day-to-day practices.

A second educational ideology, that of *cultural transmission*, is more society or culture centered. With this perspective, another significant manifest function of school—besides socialization in general or to a particular role—is the transmission of cultural norms and values to new generations with the goals of helping to mold a diverse population into one society with a shared national identity and preparing future generations for their citizenship roles. Here the emphasis is on transmitting bodies of information, rules, values, and the culturally given (i.e., the beliefs and practices that are central to our educational environments and our society in general). One would expect an educational environment that is framed within a cultural transmission perspective to be structured, rigid, and controlled, with an emphasis on the common and the already established, perhaps with a serious unwillingness to address difficult contemporary issues such as racism and social justice.

The third major educational ideology, originally espoused by Dewey (1944), has been called *progressivism*, where the focus is oriented toward the future and the goal of education is to nourish the learner's natural interaction with the world. Here the educational environment is designed to present resolvable but genuine problems or conflicts that "force" learners to think so that they can be effective later in life. A curriculum reflective of this philosophical perspective, therefore, would focus more on helping students *think* than on attempting to cover an extensive amount of content that learners need to memorize, and it would attend to the *total* development of learners, not merely their cognitive or intellectual abilities.

Increasingly, education experts agree that development must be an overarching paradigm of education, students must be central to the educational enterprise, and education must be designed to empower learners and help them fulfill their potentials. Beliefs and values such as these surely would influence expectations faculty express regarding students' and their own performance, the relationships between students and teachers, how the curriculum is designed and implemented (see Fig. 7.1), and the kind of "evidence" that is gathered to determine whether the curriculum has been successful and effective.

There is no doubt that a statement of philosophy for a school of nursing must address beliefs and values about education, teaching, and learning. However, it also must address other concepts that are critical to the practice of nursing, namely human beings, society and the environment, health, and the roles of nurses themselves (Valiga, 2018). These major concepts have been referred to as the *metaparadigm of nursing*, a concept first introduced by Fawcett in 1984.

CENTRAL CONCEPTS IN A SCHOOL OF NURSING'S PHILOSOPHY

Several central concepts are typically contained within a nursing school's statement of philosophy about which faculty communicate their beliefs and values. These concepts include beliefs about human beings, the societal or environmental context in which humans live and act, health, and nursing. Faculty may also add additional concepts about phenomena they hold to be particularly meaningful to the learning environment they are creating within their programs. Indeed, "ideas expressed in the philosophy should highlight the core concepts that faculty will integrate throughout the curriculum: concepts which then serve as the *framework* for continued curriculum work" (Valiga, 2018, p. 324).

In preparing or revising the school of nursing's statement of philosophy, faculty must articulate their beliefs and values about *human beings*, including the individual patients for whom nurses care, patients' families, the communities in which patients live and work, populations of care, students, and fellow nurses and faculty. It is inconsistent to express a belief that patients and families want to be involved in making decisions that affect them and then never give students an opportunity to make decisions that will affect them. Likewise, it is admirable to talk about respecting others, treating others with dignity, and valuing differences among people, but when faculty then treat one another in disrespectful ways, are incivil toward one another, or insist that everyone teach in the same way and do exactly the same thing, the validity of those expressed values must be questioned. Consider the following statements about human beings that might be expressed in a school's philosophy, keeping in mind that *human beings* refers to students, faculty, and administrators, as well as patients, families, communities, and populations:

- Human beings are diverse, unique, complex, holistic individuals.
- Human beings have the inherent capacity for rational thinking, self-actualization, and growth throughout the life cycle.
- Human beings engage in deliberate action to achieve goals.
- Human beings want and have the right to be involved in making decisions that affect their lives.
- All human beings have both strengths and weaknesses, and they often need support and guidance to capitalize on those strengths or to overcome or manage those weaknesses or limitations.
- All human beings are to be respected and valued.

Faculty also need to reflect on their beliefs and values related to *society and environment*, their effect on human beings, and the ways in which individuals and groups can influence their environments and society. The following statements may be ones to consider as faculty write or refine the philosophy of their school of nursing:

- Human beings interact in families, groups, and communities in an interdependent manner.
- Individuals, families, and communities reflect unique and diverse cultural, ethnic, experiential, and socioeconomic backgrounds.

- Human beings determine societal goals, values, and ethical systems.
- Human beings must collaborate to create systems of social justice.
- Society has a responsibility for providing environments conducive to maximizing the health and wellbeing of its members.
- Although human beings often must adapt to their environments, the environment also adapts to them in reciprocal ways.

Because the goal of nursing is to promote *health* and wellbeing, faculty must consider the values and beliefs they hold about health. For example, the following statements express values and beliefs about health that a faculty might consider:

- Health connotes a sense of wholeness or integrity.
- Health is a goal to be attained.
- Health is the energy that sustains life, allows an individual to participate in a variety of human experiences, and supports one's ability to set and meet life goals.
- Health is a dynamic, complex state of being that human beings use as a resource to achieve their life goals; it is therefore a means to an end rather than an end in itself.
- Health can be promoted, maintained, or regained.
- Health is impacted by where individuals live or by their race, ethnicity, or gender (i.e., social determinants of health are real and significant).
- Health is a right more than a privilege.
- All human beings must have access to quality health care.

Finally, it is critical for faculty to discuss their beliefs about *nurses* and *nursing* because this is the essence of our programs. In doing so, it may be important to reflect on the current and evolving roles of the nurse, the purpose of nursing, the ways in which nurses practice in collaboration with other health care professionals, and how one's identity as a nurse evolves. The following statements may stimulate thinking about beliefs and values related to nurses and nursing:

- Nursing is a human interactive process.
- The focus of nursing is to enhance human beings' capacity to take deliberate action for themselves and their dependent others regarding goals for optimal wellness.

- Nursing is a practice discipline that requires the deliberate use of specialized techniques and technologies as well as a broad range of scientific knowledge to design, deliver, coordinate, and manage care for complex individuals, families, groups, communities, and populations.
- Nurses are scholars who practice with scientific competence, intellectual maturity, and humanistic concern for others.
- The formation of one's identity as a nurse requires deep self-reflection, feedback from others, and a commitment to lifelong learning.
- Nurses must be prepared to provide leadership within their practice settings and for the profession as a whole.
- Nurses collaborate with patients and other professionals as equal yet unique members of the health care team.
- The practice of nursing must be based on evidence rather than tradition.
- Nurses are accountable for their own practice.

Box 7.1 provides examples of actual statements of philosophy regarding these components of the metaparadigm. The examples illustrate the beliefs of various groups of faculty in schools that have been designated by the National League for Nursing as Centers of Excellence in Nursing Education (http://www.nln.org/recognition-programs/centers-of-excellence-in-nursing-education). Some of these statements express vastly different perspectives and some express essentially the same idea but through different words.

PURPOSE OF A STATEMENT OF PHILOSOPHY

"Doing philosophy" is hard work, takes time, and may lead to substantial debates among faculty. In light of these realities, one may ask, "Why bother?" Perhaps part of the answer to that question lies in a statement made by Alexander Astin (1997), a noted educational scholar whose seminal study of more than 20,000 students, 25,000 faculty members, and 200 institutions helped educators better understand who our students are; what is important to them; what they value; what they think about teachers; how they change and develop in college; and how academic programs,

faculty, student peer groups, and other variables affect students' development and college experiences. Although Astin's original research was completed 25 years ago and focused on traditional-age students enrolled, typically, on a full-time basis—thereby not fully reflecting today's student population—the following comment has relevance for this discussion of why faculty need to "bother" with philosophy: "The problems of strengthening and reforming American higher education are fundamentally problems of *values* [emphasis added]" (Astin, 1997, p. 127).

Engaging in serious discussions about beliefs and values—about human beings, society and environment, health, nurses and nursing, and education—challenges faculty to search for points of congruence, brings to the surface points of incongruence or difference, and highlights what is truly important to the group. In a time when nursing faculty are struggling to minimize content overload and focus more on core concepts, gaining clarity about what is truly important can be helpful in deciding "what to leave in and what to leave out" of the curriculum.

Such exercises also help faculty minimize or avoid what is often referred to as the "hidden curriculum" (Mossop et al., 2013) by ensuring that faculty are fully aware of and committed to upholding certain beliefs and values in how they interact with and what they expect of students and one another. Such agreement and consistency is likely to avoid having three components to the curriculum: "what is planned for the students, what is delivered to the students, and what the students experience" (Prideaux, as cited in Ozolins et al., 2008, p. 606). For example, the *plan* may be to help students think of themselves as evolving scholars; what is *delivered* is little more than content about the research process or evidence-based practice; and what is *experienced* by students is minimal discussion by faculty of their own scholarly activities and how they think of *themselves* as scholars. When what is delivered to and experienced by students does not match what was planned for them, confusion can reign, due process can be challenged, and the relationships between students and teachers can be irreparably damaged.

Likewise, faculty and administrators are challenged to reflect on what is said in public

BOX 7.1   Examples of Statements of Philosophy From Current Schools of Nursing

Ursuline College Breen School of Nursing (Pepper Pike, OH)*

At this Catholic liberal arts institution of higher learning, "students experience a values-based, holistic, collaborative, and progressive education within a caring framework." Faculty believe that "the person is a unified whole with physical, socio-cultural, emotional, intellectual, and spiritual components. As a unique individual, each human being draws on personal resources, interaction with others, and cultural values in the pursuit of health. Individuals have the right to freedom of choice, personal dignity, and equality of opportunity for achieving their potential. As unique, complex, multi-dimensional beings that possess thoughts, feelings and values, individuals are capable of self-care and have the right to make informed choices. Each individual has dignity, value, and worth and, as reflected in the Christian view of person, is endowed with reason and the freedom to develop a personal relationship with God. ... Nurses are taught to recognize the dignity, worth, and rights of all persons within the continuum of living and dying. ... Nursing is a theory-guided, evidence-based, relationship-centered practice that facilitates health and healing [and] requires critical thinking and subsequent clinical judgments that enable the professional to provide care in an independent, collaborative, and inter-professional manner. ... The faculty views education as a life-long, dynamic, intellectual, and social process of development toward self-actualization. ..."

https://www.ursuline.edu/files/assets/bsnhandbook1-12-22revisedadacompliantupdated01132022.pdf

Duke University School of Nursing (Durham, NC)*

Duke University School of Nursing is committed to achieving distinction in research, education and patient care predicated on our beliefs regarding human beings, society and the environment, health and health care delivery, nursing and teaching and learning. ... We believe that each human being is a unique expression of attributes, behaviors, and values which are influenced by his or her environment, social norms, cultural values, physical characteristics, experiences, religious beliefs, and practices. ... As socio-cultural beings, humans are affected by and, in turn, influence the environments in which they exist—environments that are both internal (i.e., physiological, psychological,

ethical) and external (i.e., cultural, political, social, economic, professional, global). Such environments influence the health of individuals and groups and also influence health care delivery systems, access to care, and health disparities. We believe that society has a responsibility for providing environments that are conducive to maximizing the potential of its individual members and of society as a whole, for eliminating long-term inequities that contribute to health disparities, and for creating systems and roles that protect its members. ... Because health is an innate characteristic of humans, we believe that high-quality health care is a human right. ... We believe that health care must be patient-centered and that mutual trust between patients and providers is created by relationships that reflect respect for dignity, diversity, integrity, self-determination, empathy, and a capacity for grace and empowerment. ... We believe that nursing is a scholarly discipline centered on assisting people to protect, promote, and optimize their health and abilities: prevent illness and injury; and alleviate suffering. ... Nursing is committed to a holistic and evidence-based approach to human caring and compassion, respecting the dignity, self-determination, and worth of all human beings. ... We believe that nursing has a moral responsibility to the common good and an obligation to social justice and equitable access to culturally sensitive, high-quality care for all human beings. Nurses also are responsible for helping to reduce health disparities and reaching out to those, locally or abroad, who are vulnerable. ... We believe that our purpose is to develop nurse leaders in practice, education, administration, and research by focusing on students' intellectual growth and development as adults committed to high ethical standards and full participation in their communities. ... We affirm that it is the responsibility of faculty to create and nurture academic initiatives that strengthen our engagement of real-world issues by anticipating new models of knowledge formation and applying knowledge to societal issues. This, we believe, equips students with the necessary cognitive skills, clinical reasoning, clinical imagination, professional identity, and commitment to the values of the profession that are necessary to function as effective and ethical nurse leaders in situations that are under determined, contingent and changing over time.

https://nursing.duke.edu/about-us/philosophy

* Courtesy of the Ursuline College Breen School of Nursing and the Duke University School of Nursing.

documents, including the statement of philosophy, and what is done on a day-to-day basis, as noted by Valiga (2017), who questioned whether schools of nursing truly value excellence in *teaching* and whether their actions related to excellence in teaching are congruent with their words. Thus having clear statements of values to which all faculty agree to subscribe can serve a most practical and philosophical purpose.

DEVELOPING OR REFINING THE SCHOOL OF NURSING'S STATEMENT OF PHILOSOPHY

Developing or refining the school's statement of philosophy, although important and valuable, is far from easy. It takes time and effort and is not to be taken lightly. But just how does a group of faculty go about developing a philosophical statement for the school and getting "buy-in" on it? As expected, there are no formulas or step-by-step guidelines on how to go about doing this work, but some examples (Colley, 2012; Snyder, 2014; Thistlethwaite et al., 2014) and suggestions for a process may be helpful. One approach to engaging in this work may include reflecting on the nursing theories that have been developed to determine whether any of them capture the essence of faculty beliefs. For example, if faculty are in agreement that human beings are self-determining individuals who want to take responsibility for their own health and need specific knowledge, skills, and attitudes to do whatever is required to maintain, regain, or improve their health, then Orem's (1971) self-care nursing model may be evident in that school's statement of philosophy. Likewise, Roy's (1980) adaptation model may be reflected in the philosophical statement of a school where the faculty believe that a central challenge to individuals and families is to adapt to their environments and circumstances and that the role of the nurse is to facilitate that adaptation.

Finally, if the concept of caring is essential to a third group of faculty, their philosophy may clearly be congruent with Watson's (2008) theory of human caring.

Whether or not to acknowledge a single nursing theory in a school's statement of philosophy (and then use that theory to develop the school's conceptual framework, end-of-program outcomes, and other curriculum elements) has been debated in recent years. Those in favor of such an approach argue that it provides students with a way to "think nursing" and approach clinical situations in ways that clearly are nursing focused, not medical model focused, and it provides an opportunity to contribute to the ongoing development of the theory and therefore the science of nursing. Those against such an approach argue that it limits students' thinking and engages them with language and perspectives that are not likely to be widely encountered in practice, thereby making it difficult for graduates to communicate effectively with their nursing and health care team colleagues. Obviously, there is no one right answer to this debate. The key question to consider is whether or not the concepts that are central to a theory—nursing or otherwise—truly are congruent with the beliefs and values of the majority of faculty, because that is what a statement of philosophy must reflect.

The inductive approach can be most useful to faculty when developing or refining their philosophical statement; rather than selecting concepts from existing theories or policy statements or other literature, the faculty themselves generate concepts to include in the philosophy. Case Study 7.1 illustrates this process and serves as an example.

Another approach that might be used combines deduction—drawing on existing literature, standards, or policy documents—with induction, or generating ideas "from the ground up" by interviewing faculty. An individual faculty member—one who is viewed as a leader in the group, who is respected and trusted by her or his peers, who has good writing skills, and who is knowledgeable about curriculum development—may be asked to talk to faculty about their beliefs about human beings, society and environment, and so on and use that input to draft a statement of philosophy that incorporates what faculty expressed. This draft could then be circulated to all faculty for comment, editing, and revision. The original writer would then revise the statement based

CASE STUDY 7.1   Developing a Statement of Philosophy Using an Inductive Approach

All faculty in the School of Nursing were asked to list no more than five bullet items that express what they believe about each concept in the metaparadigm: human beings, society and environment, health, nurses and nursing, and education and teaching–learning. The responses in each category were then compiled and faculty—in small groups—then engaged in an analysis of the items listed for each.

These working groups also were asked to note the frequency with which specific ideas were mentioned, thereby identifying those points where there is great agreement and those where only one or a few faculty identified an idea. The fact that only a single faculty member or few faculty identified a particular belief or value, however, did not necessarily mean that it would be discarded because it is possible that other faculty simply did not think of that idea as they were creating their own lists or that other faculty did identify the idea but did not include it because they were limited to five bullet items.

The compilation from each working group was then shared with the entire faculty. At this point, all faculty were asked to review the compilations, a discussion about the meaning and significance of the statements in each category ensued, the three to five statements faculty believed were most critical to

include in the philosophy were selected, and dialogue followed about why those statements were selected, what they meant to individuals, and so on. A draft statement of philosophy—one that evolved from an inductive, bottom-up process—was then written by an individual or small group and circulated to faculty for comment, further discussion, final revisions, and approval.

As you read the case study, keep these questions in mind:

1. What are the advantages of asking faculty, initially, to list no more than five things they believe about the metaparadigm concepts?
2. How could the discussion of the working group's compilation regarding the meaning and significance of the statements in each category begin to clarify faculty beliefs that will serve as the basis for the development and implementation of the curriculum?
3. Once the final draft of the philosophy is completed through the process described, does it remain "carved in stone" throughout the subsequent curriculum development processes, or can it be revised/refined as new insights arise from ongoing discussions?

on feedback from colleagues and present the new statement to the group for discussion and dialogue. This back-and-forth process would continue until there is consensus about what to include in the statement.

In either of these scenarios, or when a philosophical statement already exists but is being reviewed for possible updating and revision, simple online, anonymous surveys or in-person response technology (e.g., "clickers") can be used to get a sense of faculty agreement or endorsement. With this approach, each sentence in the draft (or existing) philosophy is listed as a separate item and faculty are asked to indicate the extent to which they agree (e.g., Strongly Agree, Agree, Disagree, or Strongly Disagree) with it. Instead of using the entire sentence as the item to be responded to, it may be more helpful to use phrases or major concepts within each sentence as the item. Regardless of the degree of detail in each item, the anonymous responses can then be

compiled, the results shared with the entire faculty, and discussions held to explore the meaning of the data obtained.

Finally, the entire process—whether it involves starting from an existing philosophy or creating a new one—can be prompted or stimulated by the thinking of those outside the school of nursing. For example, faculty may be assigned to review major contemporary documents or reports—for example, the Carnegie study (Benner et al., 2010), the *Future of Nursing* report (National Academies of Sciences, Engineering, and Medicine, 2021), accreditation standards, or published articles about employers' assessment of what new graduates can and cannot do. In reviewing those reports, faculty might identify values that are expressed or implied; beliefs about patients and nurses; or societal expectations related to health, health care, and the role of the nurse. Those values and beliefs could then be compiled and faculty asked to reflect on the extent to which they are aligned with the beliefs of the faculty. Through an iterative process such as one of those described previously, the group could then craft its own statement of philosophy, one that has been informed by the larger context in which the educational programs exist.

Regardless of the process used, it is critical that all faculty be involved and that adequate time and safe environments be provided for faculty to disagree, struggle, contemplate, rethink, debate, and "do philosophy." Ending the process prematurely is not likely to be wise. It also is important to remember that this is an iterative process that will continue, to some extent, throughout all of the subsequent steps of curriculum development. For example, the statement of philosophy may have been endorsed and approved-in-concept by faculty, but as various groups work on developing course syllabi, they may generate questions about "what we really meant" by something in the philosophy. Should this occur, it would be worthwhile to revisit the philosophical statement and make revisions to it if such revisions will lead to greater clarity about its meaning.

The preceding discussion has focused exclusively on the role of faculty in the creation or revision of the school's philosophy. It is assumed that school administrators (e.g., dean, program chair) are faculty who also must be involved in this process. Additionally, consideration should be given to including students in dialogue about beliefs and values. In the end, however, the final document must reflect what faculty believe and are guided by regarding human beings, society and environment, health, nurses and nursing, and education and teaching–learning.

The final statement of philosophy should be clearly written, internally consistent, and easily understood and should give clear direction for all that follows. It should be long enough to clearly express the significant beliefs and values that guide faculty actions but not excessively detailed, as expressions of detail (rather than fundamental beliefs) often are more congruent with the work that must be done in formulating the conceptual framework, end-of-program outcomes, and curriculum design. Later chapters in this book explore those subsequent curriculum development steps in detail (see Fig. 7.1), so only

a few examples of how the philosophy gives direction to the development, implementation, and evaluation of the curriculum are offered here.

IMPLICATIONS OF THE PHILOSOPHICAL STATEMENT FOR THE CURRICULUM

If the statements included in the school of nursing's philosophy reflect what the faculty truly believe—and are not merely words on a page to "get the task done"—then those values should be evident in how the curriculum is designed, how it is implemented, and how it is evaluated. Examples of this influence are presented in Table 7.2 as "If–Then" statements. Case Study 7.2 addresses the implications of a philosophical statement for a nursing program's curriculum.

It is hoped that these examples, combined with the detail provided in subsequent chapters, reinforce the importance of the philosophy. Faculty aim to establish positive relationships with students, clinical partners, alumni, administrators, and each other; one way to achieve that goal is to be clear about the values we share and, more importantly, to "live" those values in everything we say and do.

CASE STUDY 7.2 Implications of a Philosophical Statement for a Nursing Program Curriculum

Faculty within a school of nursing have completed the revision of the philosophy statement for their nursing programs. The following beliefs and values were included in the newly revised statement:
- We believe that nurses are scholars, leaders in health care, and advocates of health care equity
- We believe that, as individuals, students have unique learning needs
- We believe the education environment should be designed to value and support teaching–learning innovations

1. Based upon these statements, what values are the faculty articulating for inclusion in the curriculum?
2. How might the adoption of these statements change faculty teaching practices?

TABLE 7.2   Examples of "If–Then" Statements Regarding Implications of a Philosophical Statement for the Development, Implementation, and Evaluation of a Curriculum

IF the philosophical statement says...	*THEN* one would expect to see...
We believe that human beings should have choices regarding what they do...	Free, unrestricted elective courses in the curriculum or choice among several courses to meet a degree requirement (e.g., English)
We believe that human beings engage in deliberate action to achieve goals...	Opportunities throughout the curriculum for students to write their own learning goals and collaborate with faculty or clinical staff to design unique learning experiences to achieve those goals
We believe that individuals reflect unique and diverse cultural, ethnic, experiential, and socioeconomic backgrounds...	Face-to-face or virtual experiences with a wide variety of patient populations and within communities having a range of resources and challenges
We believe that health can be promoted, maintained, or regained...	Equally distributed clinical learning experiences in wellness settings, with patients and families who are managing chronic illnesses, and in acute care settings
We believe that nurses are scholars who practice with scientific competence and intellectual maturity...	Courses and learning experiences that expose students to the concept of scholarship, what it means to be a scholar, and how one develops and maintains scientific competence
We believe that nurses must be prepared to provide leadership within their practice settings and for the profession as a whole...	Courses and learning experiences that help students appreciate the differences between leadership and management, study nursing leaders, and reflect on their own path toward becoming a leader
We believe that nurses collaborate with patients and other professionals as equal yet unique members of the health care team...	Face-to-face or virtual experiences where nursing students learn with students preparing for other professional roles, dialogue with or interview members of other health care professions, or undertake projects that call for interprofessional collaboration to meet the health needs of a patient population or community
We believe that the goal of teaching is to awaken the learner's natural curiosity...	Problem-based learning experiences where students must identify what it is they need to know to address a problem, seek out that information, judge its quality, ask questions about established practices, and so on
We believe that education involves nurturing students and pulling them forth to a new place...	A program evaluation plan that incorporates open forums with students about the extent to which they feel nurtured, supported, and challenged by faculty; dialogue with graduates about how their educational experience changed them as human beings; and surveys of students and alumni regarding the contributions they have made in their practice settings and to the profession

CHAPTER SUMMARY: KEY POINTS

- Articulating a philosophy that addresses faculty values regarding human beings, society and environment, health, nurses and nursing, and teaching/learning is essential to ensure that the curriculum is relevant, internally consistent, and effective in preparing students for new professional roles.
- "Doing philosophy" is hard work, but it is important and valuable work that has implications for faculty and our practice as teachers, as well as for our students.
- "Doing philosophy" may prompt us to attend more deliberately to affective domain learning

and identity formation as we design learning experiences.
- "Doing philosophy" may challenge us to ask new questions about our practice as teachers and seek answers to those questions through rigorous pedagogical research efforts.
- "Doing philosophy" directs us to seek out new teaching strategies and evaluation methods that better facilitate student learning.
- The philosophical foundations of the curriculum extend far beyond mere program designs and course syllabi.

REFLECTING ON THE EVIDENCE

1. How can a school's philosophy serve to distinguish it from other schools, all of whom are guided by Board of Nursing requirements, accreditation standards, or licensing expectations that are more alike than different? Similarly, how can the philosophy serve to prepare graduates to bring a unique perspective to the way they implement their nursing roles?
2. What are the most effective ways by which faculty can ensure that the program's statement of philosophy is not just a statement in a handbook but actually used to influence the students' learning experiences and future nursing practice?
3. What support, guidance, and preparation do faculty need as they "do philosophy" and engage in the work of articulating, discussing, and debating values and beliefs that may challenge usual practices, suggest different relationships between teachers and students, or point out inconsistencies between what we say and what we do as educators?
4. How does an institution's mission influence the development of the philosophy statement of a school of nursing?

REFERENCES

Astin, A. W. (1997). *What matters in college? Four critical years revisited*. Jossey-Bass.
Benner, P., Sutphen, M., Leonard, V., & Day, L. (2010). *Educating nurses: A call for radical transformation*. Jossey-Bass.
Bevis, E. O. (1989). *Curriculum building: A process* (3rd ed.). National League for Nursing.
Colley, S. L. (2012). Implementing as change to a learner-centered philosophy in a school of nursing: Faculty perspectives. *Nursing Education Perspectives*, 33(4), 229–233.
Dewey, J. (1944). *Democracy and education: An introduction to the philosophy of education*. The Free Press.
Diekelmann, N. (2002). "Too much content …" Epistemologies' grasp and nursing education. *Journal of Nursing Education, 41*(11), 469–470. https://doi.org/10.3928/0148-4834-20021101-04.
Diekelmann, N., & Smythe, E. (2004). Covering content and the additive curriculum: How can I use my time with students to best help them learn what they need to know? *Journal of Nursing Education, 43*(8), 341–344. https://doi.org/10.3928/01484834-20040801-06.
Emerson, R. W. (1921). In E. Emerson (Ed.), *The complete writings of Ralph Waldo Emerson*. Wm. H. Wise & Co.

Fawcett, J. (1984). The metaparadigm of nursing: Present status and future refinements. *Image. The Journal of Nursing Scholarship, 16*(3), 84–86.

France, A. (1920). The crime of Sylvestre Bonnard. *In The works of Anatole France in an English translation (L. Hearn, Trans.).* J. Lane Publishers.

Giddens, J. F., & Brady, D. P. (2007). Rescuing nursing education from content saturation: The case for a concept-based curriculum. *Journal of Nursing Education, 46*(2), 65–69.

Gordon, S. (1991). *Prisoners of men's dreams: Striking out for a new feminine future.* Little: Brown.

Greene, M. (1973). *Teacher as stranger: Educational philosophy in a modern age.* Wadsworth.

Hardin, P. K., & Richardson, A. J. (2012). Teaching the concept curricula: Theory and method. *Journal of Nursing Education, 51*(3), 155–159. https://doi.org/10.3928/01484834-20120127-01.

Mossop, L., Dennick, R., Hammond, R., & Robbe, I. (2013). Analysing the hidden curriculum: Use of a cultural web. *Medical Education, 47,* 134–143. https://doi.org/10.1111/medu.12072.

National Academies of Sciences, Engineering, and Medicine. (2021). The future of nursing 2020–2030: Charting a path to achieve health equity. The National Academies Press. https://doi.org/10.17226/25982.

Orem, D. E. (1971). *Nursing: Concepts of practice.* McGraw-Hill.

Ozolins, I., Hall, H., & Peterson, R. (2008). The student voice: Recognising the hidden and informal curriculum in medicine. *Medical Teacher, 30*(6), 606–611. https://doi.org/10.1080/01421590801949933.

Palmer, P. (2007). *The courage to teach: Exploring the inner landscape of a teacher's life.* Jossey-Bass.

Roy, C., Sr. (1980). The Roy adaptation model. In J. P. Riehl & C. Roy (Eds.), *Conceptual models for nursing practice* (pp. 179–188). Appleton Century Crofts.

Snyder, M. (2014). Emancipatory knowing: Empowering nursing students toward reflection and action. *Journal of Nursing Education, 53*(2), 65–69. https://doi.org/10.3928/01484834-20140107-01.

Tabak, N., Adi, L., & Eherenfeld, M. (2003). A philosophy underlying excellence in teaching. *Nursing Philosophy, 4*(3), 249–254.

Tanner, C. A. (2010). Transforming prelicensure nursing education: Preparing the new nurse to meet emerging health care needs. *Nursing Education Perspectives, 31*(6), 347–353.

Thistlethwaite, J. E., Forman, D., Matthews, L. R., Rogers, G. D., Steketee, C., & Yassine, T. (2014). Competencies and frameworks in interprofessional education: A comparative analysis. *Academic Medicine, 89*(6), 869–875. https://doi.org/10.1097/ACM.0000000000000249.

Valiga, T. M. (2017). Do schools of nursing truly value excellence in teaching? Actions speak louder than words. *(Guest Editorial). Journal of Nursing Education, 56*(9), 519–520. https://doi.org/10.3928/01484834-20170817-01.

Valiga, T. M. (2018). Curriculum models and development. In M. H. Oermann, J. C. De Gagne, & B. C. Phillips (Eds.), *Teaching in nursing and role of the educator: The complete guide To best practice in teaching, evaluation, and curriculum development* (2nd ed, pp. 321–330). Springer.

Watson, J. (2008). *Nursing: The philosophy and science of caring (Rev. ed.).* University Press of Colorado.

8

Curriculum Models for Undergraduate Programs[*]

Sarah M. Billings-Berg, DC, DNP, RN, CNE

Preparing nurses at the undergraduate level has never been more challenging and complex. The explosion of new approaches to health and health care has created academic opportunities and demands to continually assess curricular models. Furthermore, in this era of unprecedented societal, cultural, political, and educational change, opportunities exist for nursing faculty to develop undergraduate curriculum that are less bound to traditional and historical requirements, making it possible for faculty to more easily be innovative in addressing nursing and health care issues. Nursing faculty who develop and revise undergraduate curricula should consider a systematic approach to ensure alignment of content organization, learning outcomes, pedagogy, assessment strategy, and student learning experiences (Neville-Norton & Cantwell, 2019).

This chapter centers on undergraduate nursing curricula with discussion of the spectrum of approaches in undergraduate programs, including promotion of seamless academic progression at multiple levels. The chapter also discusses aspects of undergraduate curriculum models, including considerations relevant to planning and decision making, that are influencing each level of entry into practice. Faculty who are teaching in undergraduate programs must reflect on the factors that continue to shape nursing education models and design curricula to meet future needs.

PURPOSE OF UNDERGRADUATE CURRICULA IN NURSING

In general, undergraduate curricula provide the pathway for learners to become competent in entry-level practice knowledge, skills, and attitudes in a field of study and to prepare learners to become effective citizens in a complex society. The contributions of higher education graduates greatly enhance the productivity and fiscal solvency of the geographical areas in which they work and live—a benefit that extends far beyond the graduate's personal and professional growth. Universities and colleges have long recognized this, and the missions of many institutions of higher education reference the preparation of their graduates who contribute to a just society through valuing the arts and sciences, engaging in research that addresses societal needs, embracing diversity, and contributing to the global good.

Undergraduate nursing curricula contribute to these broader goals but are focused primarily on preparing students for entry into practice. In addition, some undergraduate curricula are designed as academic progression models for registered nurses (RNs) to achieve a bachelor of science in nursing (BSN) degree or licensed practical or vocational nurses (LPNs/LVNs) to pursue a degree leading to the opportunity for RN licensure. Other undergraduate programs are designed to attract students with an academic degree in another discipline who wish to pursue nursing as a second, or even third, career. This array of pathways is important in a profession such as nursing with multiple educational degrees and more than one

[*]The author acknowledges the work of Susan M. Hendricks, EdD, RN, CNE in the previous edition of the chapter.

licensure entry point. Learners are not one-size-fits-all and need options in addition to a traditional 4-year baccalaureate nursing degree. The development of new and creative approaches to nursing education, e.g., career ladder and accelerated programs, offers nontraditional learners more choices about how they earn their degree(s).

In the United States the supply of nurses has been increasing, and the proportion of nurses prepared at the baccalaureate level has also steadily increased. Additionally, undergraduate curricula leading to registered nurse licensure provide a strong foundation for students to pursue graduate education and prepare for careers as educators, leaders, administrators, informaticians, researchers, and advanced practice nursing roles.

Responding to Major Calls for Reform

Within the nursing profession, undergraduate curriculum must respond to the needs of society *and* be attuned to the needs of its students. Most recently, the COVID-19 pandemic has drawn focused attention to the nursing profession and has exacerbated the already existing nursing shortage. Government officials, national, state and private health care organizations, and the general public have a vested interest in and concern for the need to increase the number of nurses in practice, nationally and globally. The pandemic has increased pressures on higher education institutions to enroll more students in nursing and other health care-related programs and find ways to graduate students more quickly while maintaining high-quality outcomes. The urgency to implement multiple pathways in nursing education at all levels of practice has not been stronger. In recent years educators have implemented the recommendations espoused by landmark reports such as the initial Institute of Medicine's (IOM, 2011) *Future of Nursing Report* and the 2021 follow-up, *The Future of Nursing 2020–2030: Charting a Path to Achieve Health Equity* (National Academy of Medicine, 2021). Reports such as these galvanized nurse educators to create a number of degree progression initiatives and engage in programmatic and curriculum reform.

Calls for additional content in curriculum have continued, including calls for preparing prelicensure students for enhanced roles in primary care practice (Dolansky et al., 2022), inclusion of veteran-centric care (Rose et al., 2020), and attention to LGBTQ+ health care needs (McNiel & Elertson, 2018; Sherman et al., 2021). Additionally, emphasis on complex community and public health, social determinants of health and health disparities, global disease spread, and disaster preparedness have surfaced as contemporary content requisites. Faculty planning undergraduate curricula must discern priorities regarding what students need to learn to practice safely and effectively to deliver care to patients, families, and communities across a spectrum of care situations, in community and acute care settings. Faculty must design learning experiences that consider learner needs and stakeholder expectations. Furthermore, as the care environment advances to include multiple clinical settings and modalities, such as telehealth, precision medicine, and technology-enhanced patient applications, faculty must update curricular delivery and outcomes to include technology-driven competencies.

Responding to External Stakeholder Expectations

The effect of stakeholder expectations on prelicensure nursing education cannot be overstated. For example, significant national and international reports often create calls to action and demands curricular revision. State boards of nursing, nursing accrediting agencies, professional organizations, and the US Department of Education also have tremendous influence on both the design and delivery of undergraduate education. State boards of nursing are variable in how prescriptive they are relative to nursing curriculum, but they do influence content taught, clinical requirements (both in types of setting and hours completed), faculty/student clinical teaching ratios, and, in some cases, pedagogy. Faculty engaged in curriculum revision should identify these requirements early in the planning process. National nursing accreditation standards also influence the criteria to be met in curricular design and implementation. Curricular alignment with professionally recognized standards, such as the Quality and Safety Education for Nurses (QSEN, 2022) *Competencies*, the National

League for Nursing (NLN, 2010) *Outcomes and Competencies*, and the American Association of Colleges of Nursing (AACN, 2021) *The Essentials: Core Competencies for Professional Nursing Education*, is paramount in rigorous curricula.

In addition to professional accreditation standards, parameters set by state or federal legislation or colleges/universities can also impact curriculum design. Credit limits, clinical contact hours, general education requirements, and other rules about the organization of the curriculum must be understood before curriculum design or change begins. Faculty should consider additional factors when making curricular decisions, including the institution's mission, learners' needs, philosophical beliefs about teaching, learning and evaluation, and the needs of the health care agencies and communities served by the school's graduates. See Chapter 27 for additional information about program evaluation and Chapter 28 for a further discussion of the accreditation process.

The process of curriculum design is a complex and creative activity. Principles of curriculum organization and leveling and use of a theoretical framework or another organizing approach to guide curriculum design should be carefully considered (Neville-Norton & Cantwell, 2019); these are discussed in full in Chapters 6 and 7.

Because of the significant commonalities and standards of curricula in nursing, curricula across multiple schools often share many similar features. This does ensure that new graduates have been exposed to knowledge and competencies that are universally accepted to be essential to practice, but having a large body of knowledge that faculty perceive to be essential can also be daunting to organize and deliver. Curricula in nursing must be constructed to entice, retain, and graduate a diverse population of new nurses who are able to progress to higher educational levels with few impediments. Curricula must also be efficient and free of redundancies. Today's learners are financially conscious and seek out pathways that best fit their lifestyle and timeline and incur the least amount of debt possible while still leading to achievement of their professional goals.

TYPES OF UNDERGRADUATE NURSING PROGRAMS

Undergraduate nursing education offers multiple pathways to individuals who desire to pursue a nursing career. This wide array of certificates and degrees grew from historical movements and societal need at different points in time and continues to provide multiple entry points into the profession. Curricula that are designed to promote academic progression and stackable credentials are increasingly available in an effort to facilitate nursing workforce growth, increase diversity in nursing, and promote the pursuit of advanced nursing degrees. This section provides an overview of the different types of undergraduate nursing programs and discusses characteristics of each. Table 8.1 summarizes the various aspects of each type of undergraduate program.

Practical and Vocational Nursing Programs

Practical nursing (PN) programs, also known as vocational nursing (VN) programs in some regions of the United States, provide an opportunity for many individuals to first enter the nursing workforce. The primary purpose of the PN program is to prepare graduates as caregivers to provide basic nursing skills such as administering medications. However, state nurse practice acts, which define the LPN/LVN scope of practice, vary, sometimes widely, from state to state. Now, more than ever, it is vital to the nursing workforce and health care consumers that LPN/LVNs are working to the full extent of their licensure. Licensed practical nurses work under the direction of a registered nurse, advanced practice provider, or physician. Faculty developing and revising practical nursing curricula must be attuned to the scope of practice in the state that the program is offered and provide learning opportunities reflecting that level of practice. Practical nursing programs are typically 10 months to one year in length. The PN/VN program curriculum includes a limited foundation in the arts and sciences and is primarily focused on the care provider role. PN/VN programs are often situated in technical colleges, community colleges, vocational schools, private stand-alone centers, and more recently career and technical centers that

TABLE 8.1   Characteristics of Four Types of Undergraduate Nursing Programs

Type of Nursing Program	Purpose	Degree Received/ Degree Granting Institution	Role of Graduate	Curriculum Plan	Employment Setting
Practical/ Vocational Nursing	Prepare students to provide direct patient care under supervision of RN or MD	Diploma/cer- tificate from state-approved technical or vocational school	Provide direct care to individual patients and in some instances administer medications	12–18 months; curriculum focused on foundational technical and communication skills	Hospitals, clinics, physicians' offices, long-term care, home care
Registered Nursing: Diploma Program	Prepare graduates to provide care to individ-uals, work in teams, and manage groups of patients in structured settings	Diploma affiliated with clinical agencies or free-standing degree-granting institutions	Care pro-vider, team member in structured settings	Curriculum typically includes gen-eral education courses taken at affiliating col-lege/university; includes nurs-ing courses in adult, pediatric, maternity, psy-chiatric nursing and leadership. Average pro-gram length is 3 years	Employed in structured set-tings, primarily in acute care settings, physi-cian offices
Registered Nursing: Associate Degree Program	Prepare graduates to provide care to individ-uals, work in teams, and manage groups of patients in structured settings	Associate of arts/sciences degree from technical or community college	Care pro-vider, team member in structured setting	60 credits in 2 years; 30 credits from general edu-cation courses and 30 credits from nursing courses	Employed in structured set-tings, primarily in acute care settings, physi-cian offices
Registered Nursing: Baccalaureate Degree	Prepare a professional nurse to promote, maintain, and restore health of individuals, groups, and community	Bachelor of Science in Nursing degree from a college or university	Care provider, leader, and manager; global citizen, interprofes-sional team member	8 semesters; 120 credits, 60 credits general education courses, 60 credits nursing	Employed in structured and unstruc-tured settings, including acute care, long-term care, commu-nity, home care, case management

previously only offered high school-level learning opportunities. The increased availability of LPN/LVN programs promises to increase diversity in nursing and provide opportunity for entry into practice for previously isolated students who faced socioeconomic and/or geographic or other types of access barriers.

LPN/LVNs are typically employed in structured environments such as hospitals, clinics, outpatient surgery centers, and long-term and home care settings. The demand for nurses at the LPN/LVN level is growing significantly, mainly because of the expanded need for nursing care for the aging "baby boomer" population in long-term and home care settings. Acute care settings are also redefining how they utilize LPN/LVNs in their staffing mix. An emerging trend in many inpatient care settings is a team nursing approach that places an LPN/LVN at the core of the team with RN oversight. This approach promotes LPN/LVNs working at the full scope of their practice and reduces the demands on the RN, making them more available to focus on higher-level patient care concerns.

The importance of the growing role for the LPN/LVN in the nation's health care system and the importance of developing curricula that adequately prepare LPN/LVNs for this role was previously addressed in the NLN's (2014b) *Vision for Recognition of the Role of Licensed Practical/Vocational Nurses in Advancing the Nation's Health.* One challenge facing nurse educators developing curricula for PN/VN programs is the relative lack of established national PN/VN curricular standards with identified outcomes and competencies for the preparation of the PN/VN. One such resource for nurse educators is the *NLN Practical/Vocational Nursing Curricular Framework* (2014a), which has been developed for PN/VN curricula based on the NLN's *Outcomes and Competencies* model (2010). As of 2020, the NCSBN reported that there were more than 996,154 active LPN/LVN in the United States (National Council of State Boards of Nursing [NCSBN], 2020).

Individuals who are first licensed as LPN/LVN frequently return to school to pursue licensure as RNs, thus increasing their levels of responsibility and accountability within the health care environment. Providing avenues of academic progression

TABLE 8.2 **Ivy Tech Community College Practical Nursing Program**		
Prerequisite Courses: Anatomy & Physiology I, Student Success Elective, English Composition, Introduction to Psychology		
Year 1	**8-Week Term**	**Courses**
	1	• Fundamentals of Nursing • Nursing Lab • Anatomy & Physiology II
	2	• Medical Surgical Nursing I • Medical Surgical Nursing I Lab • Anatomy & Physiology II
	3	• Pharmacology for Nursing • Medical Surgical Nursing II • Medical Surgical Nursing II Clinical
	4	• Maternal-Child Nursing • Maternal-Child Nursing Clinical
	5	• Geriatric/Complex Medical Surgical Nursing III for the Practical Nurse • Geriatric/Complex Medical Surgical Nursing III for the Practical Nurse Clinical

Courtesy Ivy Tech Community College, Indiana.

for LPN/LVNs that acknowledge and grant credit for their previous learning and experience continues to be an important component of nursing education academic progression models. Table 8.2 provides one example of a practical nursing program curriculum plan provided by Ivy Technical Community College.

Diploma Programs (RN)

Diploma programs for preparing registered nurses represent the first curriculum model developed for training nurses in the late 19th and early to mid-20th centuries. Initially affiliated with hospitals, there are few remaining diploma programs today, with the Accreditation Commission for Education in Nursing (ACEN, 2021) listing 29 accredited diploma programs in 2022, down from 33 listed in 2018. The states with the highest concentration of diploma programs are New Jersey and Pennsylvania, with 5 and 15, respectively. Most of today's diploma schools of nursing are affiliated with health care systems or medical centers, but a small number are programs within institutions of higher education.

Diploma programs prepare nurses who provide direct patient care in a variety of health care settings. The programs are designed to be completed in 2 to 3 years with an emphasis on clinical practice. General education courses in the biological and social sciences are typically provided through affiliation with a local college or university or are prerequisites for program entry. These college course credits can commonly be applied toward a baccalaureate degree in nursing if the student chooses to continue their education and they are earned at an accredited institution.

Associate Degree Programs

Associate degree in nursing (ADN) programs, which most commonly award the associate of science in nursing (ASN) degree, were first envisioned in 1952 by Mildred Montag in response to a critical nursing shortage. As originally conceived by Montag, the intent of the associate degree programs was to prepare in 2 academic years a technical nurse who would provide direct patient care in acute care settings. Associate degree programs are very popular, and associate degree-prepared nurses are significantly contributing to meeting workforce needs in many health care settings. An ASN degree is often used as a stepping stone for nurses looking for RN-level entry to practice but do not wish to commit to a 4-year traditional program. As acute care agencies push for greater numbers of baccalaureate-prepared nurses, mainly in response to the IOM's call in the *Future of Nursing* (2011), the trend is clear that many associate degree–prepared nurses are returning to school to pursue baccalaureate or graduate nursing degrees, often supported by their employers. Employers are hard-pressed to limit nursing staff hiring to those with baccalaureate nursing degrees and so commonly require associate degree-prepared employees to attain a BSN within a certain amount of time of hire. This approach allows the employee to benefit from tuition reimbursement offered by

their employer and the employer gains a BSN-prepared nurse.

Associate degree programs are often situated in technical and community colleges and have served local community needs for a registered nursing workforce for years. With the complexity of the professional nursing role increasing along with the expectations for practice in rapidly changing health care environments, many associate degree nursing programs have responded by partnering with baccalaureate institutions to facilitate the academic progression of students from the associate degree to the bachelor's degree. Some states have granted legislative authority for community colleges to expand their mission to offer bachelor's degrees in nursing and to facilitate academic progression of their associate degree graduates. Many institutions are embracing the 2 + 2 model and have implemented an in-house RN to BSN program to complement their associate degree program.

One challenge inherent in associate degree nursing education is the difficulty of incorporating a large body of complex information and skills into a degree offered in two years. Some programs have responded in the past by increasing the credits in the program beyond the typical number of 60 credits (with 50% or more of the credits in nursing courses) in a 2-year degree, a solution that may extend the program length but not to the extent of the student receiving a bachelor's degree. As more attention is placed on the costs of higher education and the amount of student loan debt incurred by students, the number of credits required in all associate degree programs (regardless of discipline) is often highly scrutinized, with some state legislation mandating that associate degree programs be limited to 60 academic credit hours. It is important for faculty who design and revise curriculum plans for ASN/ADN programs to carefully consider the number of credits they are requiring in their programs and consider ways to ensure that the curriculum remains free of excess credit hours.

The curriculum of associate degree programs commonly consists of nursing courses that include content related to the practice of adult medical–surgical, pediatric, maternal-child, and mental health nursing care, focused most intently on what is needed to succeed in the first RN role, consistent with the NCSBN Licensure Examination test plan (NCSBN, 2019). Some programs also include additional topics including management, community health, gerontology, and research. Because the NCSBN has responded to changes in the practice environment and is implementing the Next Generation NCLEX, most nursing programs leading to licensure as an RN have widened their focus to teach principles and concepts related to the management of care, such as prioritization, delegation, and managing a team of patients, but more importantly, the concept of sound clinical judgment in relation to these facets of nursing. The emphasis on critical thinking and pertinent clinical judgment in patient care situations has prompted associate degree faculty to revise curricula and reframe what and how content is presented to learners, with strong consideration of the relatively accelerated curricular timeline in associate degree delivery and keeping the program credit total at or around 60.

Students completing the ADN are prepared to enter practice in structured health care settings.

In response to future workforce needs and employment patterns, faculty teaching in associate degree programs instill in their students a sense of lifelong learning and the expectation of advancing their initial education to the baccalaureate or higher level. Facilitating the academic progression of associate degree-prepared nurses through innovative curriculum models is essential. As previously discussed, employer support for ADN and prepared nurses is a key element in facilitating academic progression. Table 8.3 provides one example of an associate degree nursing program curriculum plan from Sandhills Community College.

Baccalaureate Degree Programs

The purpose of the baccalaureate program is to prepare a professional nurse with a broad background in arts and sciences and civic and global engagement to promote, restore, and maintain the health of patients, families, groups, communities, and populations. Baccalaureate degree (BSN, BS, and BA) programs are traditionally offered by 4-year colleges and universities, with approximately 120 credit hours, of which 50% or more of

TABLE 8.3 Sandhills Community College Associate Degree Program

Academic Year	Fall Term	Spring Term
Year 1	• Anatomy & Physiology I • Writing & Inquiry • Intro to Health Concepts • General Psychology	• Anatomy & Physiology II • Writing/Research in Disc OR • Professional Research & Reporting • Health-Illness Concepts • Health Care Concepts
Summer Term	• Holistic Health Concepts • Development Psych	
Year 2	• Microbiology • Family Health Concepts • Health System Concepts • Introduction to Sociology	• Complex Health Concepts • Humanities/Fine Arts Elective

Courtesy Sandhills Community College.

the credits are allocated to nursing coursework. The graduate of a baccalaureate nursing program is prepared to deliver care in clinical agencies, homes, community, and public health settings. In addition to content related to specific nursing areas, baccalaureate curricula also include concepts related to nursing leadership and management, community and population health, nursing theory and research, health policy and advocacy, health care ethics, group and team dynamics, evidence-based practice, quality and safety, informatics, global health, and contemporary professional issues.

The baccalaureate curriculum offers a strong foundation of liberal arts and sciences in addition to nursing courses. The program may be designed to require students to take prerequisite courses in the sciences, arts, and humanities in their first academic year before admission to the nursing major, or students may be directly admitted to the nursing program and take these courses concurrently with nursing courses. Depending on the mission of the college or university, baccalaureate programs may also have an emphasis on civic and global engagement, service, and social justice. Faculty are expected to build on concepts or learning outcomes discussed in general education courses and integrate these concepts throughout the nursing program.

It is imperative for the faculty to construct curricula that are flexible enough in adapting to changing practice expectations of baccalaureate-prepared nurses, especially as efforts continue to focus on enhancing the proportion of nurses prepared with a bachelor's degree (IOM, 2011; National Academy of Medicine, 2021). This growing evidence supports the need for more baccalaureate-prepared nurses in the workforce given the data showing increases in patient safety and patient care outcomes as a result of the practice of baccalaureate-prepared nurses. There is a continued need for nursing research to also look at patient safety and patient care outcomes data in BSN-prepared nurses who advanced via academic progression models versus second career and accelerated program preparation versus traditional 4-year preparation. Table 8.4 provides one example of a traditional 4-year baccalaureate degree nursing program curriculum plan provided by the University of North Carolina Wilmington.

Second Degree Entry Into Practice: Accelerated Baccalaureate Degree Programs

Coupled with increased workforce demands as a result of the aging population in the United States, and the exacerbated demands for nurses during a multiyear global pandemic, individuals holding a bachelor's degree in a field other than nursing may seek alternative career opportunities that may be more fulfilling or hold stronger job prospects. Nursing is often an excellent career option to consider. Many schools offering the baccalaureate nursing degree have designed a program track for students seeking a second degree. This BSN degree option is achieved in a short time in a fast-moving, densely packed curriculum that is focused on providing nursing knowledge and

TABLE 8.4	University of North Carolina Wilmington Pre-Licensure BSN Program	
Academic Year	**Fall Term**	**Spring Term**
Year 1	• Principles of Biology: Cells • Math Requirement • General Psychology • University Studies • University Studies	• General Chemistry • SOC 105 OR ECN 125 OR ECN 221 • Lifespan Human Development • University Studies • University Studies
Year 2	• Microbiology • Human Anatomy & Physiology I • PAR 101, 115, 205, 211 OR 215 • University Studies • University Studies	• Intro to Health Assessment • Clinical I: Foundations in Professional Nursing Practice • STT 210 OR STT215 OR QMM 280 OR PSY 225 • Human Anatomy & Physiology II
Year 3	• Pathophysiology/Pharmacology I • Clinical Application of Therapeutic Nutrition • Clinical II: Adult Health I • Research in Nursing • University Studies	• Clinical III: Mental Health Nursing • Clinical IV: Maternal-Infant Nursing • Gerontology Nursing • Pathophysiology/Pharmacology II • University Studies
Year 4	• Issues, Trends, & Health Policy • Clinical V: Pediatric Nursing • Clinical VI: Community Health Nursing • University Studies	• Clinical VII: Adult Health II • Leadership & Management • Clinical VIII: Capstone

Courtesy University of North Carolina Wilmington.

is sometimes referred to as an accelerated degree program. These second-degree nursing programs facilitate acquisition of a bachelor's degree and create pathways for graduates to continue their education to obtain a master's or doctoral nursing degree. Students entering the profession through this route are often nontraditional students and many have experienced a professional work life and bring a variety of skill sets to the learning environment. Table 8.5 provides one example of an accelerated baccalaureate degree nursing program curriculum plan provided by Norwich University.

DESIGNING UNDERGRADUATE CURRICULA TO SUPPORT ACADEMIC PROGRESSION

Because the profession of nursing has many different degrees that lead to practice at the PN/VN and RN levels, effective planning for academic progression is critical in supporting workforce growth. Academic progression models in nursing education exist to reduce duplication of course work and facilitate transition across the academic continuum. Vermont Technical College offers a prime example of the career-ladder approach to nursing education in the 1 + 1 + 2 model provided in Table 8.6. Progression through the practical nursing program, associate degree program, and RN to BSN program allows students to join the nursing workforce after year 1 as an LPN (after taking the NCLEX-PN) and continue into the second-year associate degree program. Once graduates complete year 2, they are eligible to take the NCLEX-RN and begin their registered nursing career while also continuing in the RN to BSN program. This pathway is highly desirable for nontraditional learners who want to pursue nursing as a career but are not keen on enrollment in a more traditional 4-year baccalaureate degree program. This example encompasses both LPN to RN progression and RN to BSN progression, both of which are discussed in the following sections.

TABLE 8.5 **Norwich University Accelerated BSN Program**			
Prerequisite Courses: Human Anatomy & Physiology I & II, Microbiology, General Chemistry I & II, Organic OR Biochemistry, Statistics, Developmental Psychology, Sociology Elective, 21 Additional Elective Credits			
Academic Year	**Summer Term**	**Fall Term**	**Spring Term**
Year 1	• Focus on Nursing • Nutrition & Health Promotion • Health Assessment Across the Lifespan • Simulation for Nursing • Pathopharmacology for Nurses	• Research for Evidence-Based Practice • Technology & Informatics in Healthcare • Care of the Adult 1 • Care of the Adult 1 Practicum	• Client, Psychological/Mental Health Problems • Client, Psychological/Mental Health Problems Practicum • Nursing Leadership • Care of Women-Childbearing Family • Care of Women-Childbearing Family Practicum • Care of Children/Child Rearing • Care of Children/Child Rearing Practicum
Year 2	• Care of the Adult II • Care of the Adult II Practicum • Care at End of Life • Management Course • Sociology Course	• Coordinator of Care • Coordinator of Care Practicum • Promoting Health in Communities • Promoting Health in Communities Practicum • Nursing Capstone	N/A

Courtesy Norwich University.

TABLE 8.6	Vermont Technical College's Academic Progression Model: 1 + 1 + 2 Career Ladder		
Academic Year	**Fall Term**	**Winter/Spring Term**	**Spring 2 (PN Program)**
Year 1: Practical Nursing Certificate	• Principles & Practices of Nursing I • Principles & Practices of Nursing I Lab/Clinical • Nurse/Client Relationship Anatomy & Physiology I • Introduction to Nutrition	• Principles & Practices of Nursing II • Principles & Practices of Nursing II Clinical Anatomy & Physiology II • Human Growth & Development	• Principles & Practices of Nursing III • Principles & Practices of Nursing III Clinical
Year 2: Associate Degree	• Principles & Practices of Nursing IV • Principles & Practices of Nursing IV Clinical • LPN to RN Trends & Transitions • Introduction to Psychology • English Composition • Microbiology	• Principles & Practices of Nursing V • Principles & Practices of Nursing V Clinical • Technical Communication • Math for Health Professions • Arts/Humanities Elective	
Year 3: RN to BSN	• Statistics • RN to BSN Transitions • Nursing Informatics • Pathophysiology & Assessment • Palliative Care OR • Transitions of Health Care Reform	• Healthcare Systems • Abnormal Psychology • Sociology Elective • Teaching & Learning OR • Health Promotion Across the Lifespan	
Year 4: RN to BSN	• Bioethics • Research & Evidence-Based Practice • Nursing Leadership & Management	• East & West Holistic Healing • Global Health • Community Health	

Courtesy Vermont State University.

Academic Progression Models for Associate Degree and Diploma Prepared Registered Nurses to the BSN

Courses in RN to BSN programs typically include additional courses in liberal education to meet general education requirements and to provide graduates with exposure to a broad educational background. Nursing courses in RN to BSN programs usually encompass areas of focus that are minimally addressed or not included in associate degree or diploma programs. Most RN to BSN programs include coursework in community and public health, nursing leadership or management, research and evidence-based practice, informatics, and global health, in addition to exposure to topics of concern to professional nurses, such as professional communication, health care ethics, and health policy. Many RN to BSN programs also include capstone learning experiences, facilitating the achievement of a culmination of learning outcomes. Participation in clinical nursing courses is an expected aspect of

this academic progression model, often occurring through the use of precepted coursework.

Designing curricula that facilitate academic progression in a "seamless" manner has become a significant national movement in the nursing profession (Angel, 2020). Due to the now-exacerbated nursing shortage, it is not likely that the profession will eliminate any entry point into licensed practice in the coming years. Further, because nursing has multiple educational levels of entry and the call for nurses to advance their education to meet society needs, academic progression is one of the most important initiatives in undergraduate curriculum today.

In 2015 leaders from 25 states were convened by the Robert Wood Johnson Foundation (RWJF, 2015) and the Tri-Council for Nursing to advance the academic progression in nursing (APIN) movement. The RWJF's (2015) support of the APIN program led to the creation of nine state-level coalitions to support seamless academic progression model development and implementation. Although the

APIN project concluded in 2019, nursing's focus on academic progression continues to grow.

Taking APIN's lead, many states and institutions have implemented innovative academic progression plans developed to increase numbers of baccalaureate- and advanced degree-prepared nurses to meet market demands for nursing leaders, educators, and advanced practice nurses. However, there is still a significant need to increase capacity of RN to BSN programs and encourage academic progression (Gorski & Polansky, 2019).

Meyer (2017) noted that the IOM's *Future of Nursing* report recommendation to increase the number of baccalaureate-prepared nurses did not lead to the end of associate degree programs but instead spurred collaboration and articulation agreements between degree programs. Program designs vary and depend on the philosophy of the nursing faculty and the expectations of the parent institution. The most common include the RN to BSN program and the RN to MSN program, which may bypass or grant the BSN during the period in which the MSN is being earned. These collaborative curricular models are increasingly common, and the advantages to students include a clear path toward the BSN, reduction of unnecessary barriers to progression, early introduction to the idea of academic progression and lifelong learning as a professional expectation, and often a community of peers who are engaged in similar progression. For schools of nursing, such models help ensure a strong pipeline of nurses advancing in education, using resources across multiple types of institutions effectively, and forming creative partnerships with academic, employer, and government stakeholders. Importantly, academic progression plans help overcome the efficiency lost in moving from one degree program to another in a profession with multiple entry points into practice.

Academic Progression Models for Licensed Practical/Vocational Nurses

Students make the choice to begin nursing careers as LPNs or LVNs for a variety of reasons. For example, students may seek a short time to program completion, early entry into the workforce, a faster increase in earning potential, and program access and affordability. The most common

academic progression models for LPN/LVNs are LPN/LVN to ASN and LPN/LVN to BSN. These progression models offer a reentry point on the pathway to registered nursing practice. The relatively short program duration, lower debt potential, and increased accessibility tend to draw a greater proportion of ethnically, racially, and economically diverse students, individuals from disadvantaged personal and academic backgrounds, nontraditional adult learners, and students who may have learned English as a second or additional language. In nursing, a profession that has not achieved diversity goals in many areas, this entry point into registered nursing is a mechanism that could help the profession become more diverse (Jones et al., 2018). Successful programs provide robust student supportive services to enhance reading comprehension, to develop writing skills, and to overcome financial obstacles in a student-centered environment.

It is expected that nurse educators will continue to design academic progression options that facilitate educational transition for individuals licensed as PN/VNs. Given the complexity among academic progression program options, faculty and leaders who are able to design and implement these flexible undergraduate curriculum models are needed. With academic progression models, faculty must make decisions about how to recognize and credit previous learning experiences. This may be accomplished through articulation agreements, advanced placement opportunities, credit transfers, and validation of previous learning through testing and portfolios.

As the nursing profession seeks to increase the number of nurses prepared with baccalaureate and higher degrees, academic progression models will continue to provide a quality, cost-effective means of supporting career mobility and accomplishing this goal. Faculty must use creativity and out-of-the-box thinking to consider innovative clinical models of instruction which reinforce the classroom learning experience (Case Study 8.1). Curricula should consist of structured and unstructured learning experiences that build on prior knowledge and abilities of the learner. These nursing curricula must be constructed to maximize the use of the latest learning technology, including

CASE STUDY 8.1 Expanding a Community College Practical Nursing Program

A faculty member is teaching at a small community college with a practical nursing program that grants a certificate in practical nursing. The practical nursing (PN) program is 1 year in length and typically enrolls 25 students each fall and has 20–22 graduates each summer. Students are mostly nontraditional and there is no residential option on campus. The PN program is delivered at one campus that is centrally located in the state. There is a larger state university located about 30 minutes away that has a 4-year baccalaureate degree program and mostly enrolls traditional residential college students. They graduate 40–45 BSN graduates each year.

The state legislators have recently shown an interest in the nursing workforce shortage and are inquiring about what resources the community college and larger state university would need to graduate more nurses each year. The PN program's nursing director has asked the faculty member and another colleague to lead the development of a plan for moving forward with expansion of the practical nursing program.

1. What additional information would the faculty want to know about the community college PN program when considering expansion?
2. What data, feedback, and input should the faculty consider collecting to inform their proposed development plan?
3. What potential opportunities with the state university might the faculty consider? Should the state university be included in the planning process?
4. What potential barriers might there be to the program's expansion?

impact nursing practice and, ultimately, patient outcomes. For example, the recently updated *The Essentials: Core Competencies for Professional Nursing Education* (AACN, 2021) focuses on competency-based education for prelicensure registered nursing baccalaureate and master's degree programs, as well as advanced-level nursing. The revised core competencies focus on the requisite knowledge, skills, and attitudes necessary for contemporary nursing practice.

Additionally, *The Future of Nursing 2020–2030: Charting a Path to Health Equity* (National Academy of Medicine, 2021) *emphasizes the need for* flexible and diverse nursing education pathways to create more opportunities for nurses to obtain a BSN or higher degree. Concurrent enrollment design is an innovative approach that allows nursing students to be working toward two different degree levels at the same time, enabling nurses to fast-track earning a BSN, sometimes within the same concurrent timeframe as earning an associate's degree. Designing concurrent ADN and BSN curricula that are aligned and complementary is key to promoting student success in this alternative pathway. Concurrent enrollment programs may be attractive to students who are looking for a more efficient, nontraditional option (Gentry & Graves, 2022). Curriculum design in concurrent enrollment programs is an area that would benefit from more nursing education research.

As faculty update, revise, and develop curricula for undergraduate learning, consideration of organizing phenomena is important to keep in mind. Chapter 6 discusses the curricular design models of concept-based curricula, competency-based education, and block curricula in more detail.

Academic-Practice Collaborations, Partnerships, and Consortia

In today's complex social system nursing practice and education cannot afford to operate in silos. Nursing education programs that engage in partnerships with health care agencies, other schools, state and local government, and community centers situate their practice in a position of strength. Such partnerships can strengthen the relevance of the curriculum, align resources to achieve a common goal, and often lead to solutions to problems

human patient simulation, that supports innovative teaching pedagogies and transformative learning environments.

CURRICULAR DESIGNS FOR UNDERGRADUATE NURSING CURRICULA

One of the ongoing challenges faced by faculty designing undergraduate curricula is staying abreast of the many different calls for curriculum reform from professional organizations, institutes, and research findings that have the potential to shared by all stakeholders. Key leaders recognize that nursing educators and administrators alike may have missed opportunities for collaboration and full partnership, thoroughly breaking down silos between practice and academia.

Even in health systems that are not characterized as academic health systems, partnerships between health care agencies and schools of nursing may prove effective in addressing local health problems while providing excellent clinical education opportunities. One example of such a partnership is a dual appointment or dual services agreement entered into by the academic institution and the clinical partner. In this model the clinical partner agrees to appoint a qualified staff member as the clinical instructor for a designated group of students. The instructor remains an employee of the partner facility, and the institution gains a knowledgeable and competent clinical instructor for their students without going through extensive recruitment efforts. Implementing this type of model requires consideration of multiple elements, including scheduling, staffing, clearly delineating job duties and the instructor role, finances, and program support.

Employer-sponsored cohorts are another example of an academic-practice partnership. This type of cohort can take on many shapes and sizes, but the key expectations are that an employer supplies robust support for their employees or future employees to matriculate through a local nursing program. The employer may provide education and lab space or work with the academic institution to identify such spaces, provide instructional resources via a dual appointment, support students financially through tuition reimbursement or wraparound costs to the student, and prioritize diverse clinical experience opportunities. As an example, Vermont Technical College has developed employer-sponsored cohort models with several local health care facilities, including Central Vermont Medical Center and Dartmouth Hitchcock.

CURRICULAR MODELS SUPPORTING TRANSITION TO PRACTICE

The undergraduate curriculum also must prepare learners who are ready to function in a dynamic and increasingly complex health care environment upon graduation. Many undergraduate curricula are designed to culminate in clinical practice, capstone, or immersion experiences that allow students to experience the full responsibilities of the nurse's role before graduation under the guidance of an experienced nurse in practice. These clinical experiences begin the transition process of moving from student to practicing nurse. Increasingly, however, the nursing profession is recognizing that new graduates benefit from a supported environment that continues throughout the first year of practice.

Facilitating transition into practice is not a new concern. Since the 1970s, faculty and new graduates alike have recognized that the transition to practice is a challenge for most new nurses (Hampton et al., 2021). Today's new nurses begin to practice in a health care environment that is complex and fragmented. Many novice nurses experience difficulties adjusting to the full realization of the expected responsibilities of the RN's role, struggling to adapt to the demands of the workplace. As a result of these concerns, increasing attention has been placed on developing strategies to facilitate new graduates' transition to practice. One such strategy is the introduction of curricular programs in health care agencies to support transition to practice. These transition programs are referred to as residency programs.

Nurse Residency and Transition to Practice Programs

The IOM (2011) *Future of Nursing* report recommended the creation of nurse residency programs (NRPs) to facilitate RNs' transition to practice. In 2018 the American Academy of Nursing (AAN) issued a call for health care employers to be required to provide a nurse residency program for all new nursing graduates (Goode et al., 2018). Warren et al. (2018) report that the cost of the residency program is offset by the benefit of not hiring and orienting a new employee when nurses are retained beyond the first year of employment. With today's even more complex health care environment, partnerships have evolved into a key element of successful residency programs. Davis et al. (2021) discuss the successes of state- and regional-level collaboratives in implementing a standardized NRP in several states. It is incumbent upon residency program leaders and coordinators to recognize opportunities for collaboration, which will likely improve new nurse retention and strengthen academic-practice partnerships.

The average length of a residency program is 12 months. Residency programs are typically the product of collaborative partnerships between education and practice institutions and differ from a clinical agency orientation program, which focuses more on agency policies and procedures. The curriculum for such programs can be variable depending on the health care institution and the position of the nurse residents. NRPs currently exist in a variety of health care settings. While mostly major medical centers and large health care systems have developed NRPs, smaller community-based hospitals, home health providers, and even long-term care facilities are also developing NRPs for their newly graduated nurses.

Most NRP programs include general topics such as patient safety, evidence-based practice, clinical judgment, teamwork, disaster preparedness, and population health paired with an opportunity for clinical practice with a preceptor in an area of the residents' choice. There are some commercially provided NRP curriculum models on the market that health care institutions can purchase in which to participate (Goode et al., 2018). Some programs offer academic credit or continuing education contact hours. The NCSBN developed the Transition to Practice Program, which includes a five-course series focusing on communication and teamwork, patient- and family-centered care, EBP, quality improvement, and informatics (NCSBN, 2022) NRPs can integrate the NCSBN's series into their curriculum by having residents concurrently complete the modules. Well-structured NRPs have clearly defined outcomes and competencies encompassing the concepts listed above.

With a widening gap in nursing expertise developing in clinical practice and the need to improve the retention of new nurses, it can be expected that the planning, implementation, and evaluation of residency programs will continue to be a priority for the nursing profession. Faculty can anticipate being engaged in collaborations with their health care partners to create and implement such programs

(Case Study 8.2). Residency leaders and coordinators should additionally consider state and regional collaborative efforts to grow the number of NPRs that are evidence based with clearly structured curricula and competencies. There is also a push for well-established, evidence-based NRPs to become

---

CASE STUDY 8.2   Starting a Nurse Residency Program

A faculty member at a semiurban private institution in the northeastern United States teaches in a traditional 4-year BSN program that typically enrolls 50 new students each fall. The program is largely face to face and the students are a 50/50 mix of traditional campus residents and nontraditional local commuters. Approximately 65% of the program's graduates remain in the greater metropolitan area after program completion. This BSN program performs the majority of their clinical experiences at the area's major medical center.

While in the clinical setting, the chief nursing officer (CNO) at the medical center approached the faculty member about starting a nurse residency program (NRP) for the program's graduates who are hired by the medical center. The CNO is hoping that by developing a NRP for the program and increasing the collaboration between the medical center and the institution, it will increase the medical center's recruitment and retention of baccalaureate-prepared nurses. The faculty member shares the project idea with the program's chief academic nursing administrator, who is also excited about the idea and approves release time for the faculty member to work on a formal collaborative proposal for the NRP.

1. What initial data should the faculty propose collecting when planning the NRP proposal?
2. When considering curricular content, what potential structure and components would be important for the faculty to include in the proposal?
3. What advantages does the NRP collaboration potentially create for the academic nursing program and the medical center? Are there any possible disadvantages that should be considered?
4. How can the nursing program and the medical center use a pathway model to recruit students into the BSN program?
5. How does the community benefit from such a partnership?

nationally accredited. As of 2022, the Commission on Collegiate Nursing Education (CCNE, n.d.) listed 39 NRPs as accredited on their website.

DEVELOPING AND REVISING UNDERGRADUATE CURRICULUM

Faculty are responsible for the development and revision of the curriculum. Faculty involved in updating or developing curricula should have a firm understanding of content but also accreditation and professional standards such as QSEN Competencies (2022), NLN *Competencies for Graduates of Nursing Programs* (2010), and *The Essentials: Core Competencies for Professional Nursing Education* (AACN, 2021). Chapter 6 discusses the faculty's participation in the change process related to curriculum development and revision in detail.

In addition to being cognizant of professional organization recommendations and accreditation requirement updates, faculty should strive to remain up to date on curricular trends in the nursing education literature. Regularly reviewing at least one nursing education peer-reviewed journal informs faculty of creative and innovative approaches to nursing education and curricular revision. Attendance at a national nursing education conference each academic year also supports faculty awareness of new approaches to undergraduate teaching and learning strategies. The volume of ideas can be both overwhelming and inspiring, but it is important for faculty to carefully consider what changes are appropriate for their program(s). A careful analysis of the proposed curriculum changes should be conducted by faculty and include feedback from administration, students, and external stakeholders such as clinical partners. Accelerated curricula and concurrent programming, career ladder progression models, and credit for previous degrees and experience, as well as competency-based curricula, are some current trends to explore.

EMERGING ISSUES IN UNDERGRADUATE NURSING CURRICULUM

Emerging issues in health care, nursing, and higher education will continue to have a significant influence on how undergraduate nursing curricula are designed and implemented. One of the greatest challenges facing faculty lies in defining how the roles of nurses will need to transform to meet evolving and changing health care needs and translate these changes into relevant curricula. For example, in response to the COVID-19 pandemic faculty must enhance a number of concepts across multiple levels of nursing education, including infection prevention, vaccination, telehealth, mental health, and public and global health considerations. Responding to a health care environment that focuses more on ambulatory and community-based health care has not traditionally been a primary focus in undergraduate nursing education, but this will need to change. Students will require learning experiences that facilitate an understanding of health promotion, illness prevention, and management of chronic illness. As the age of the population in the United States increases, the need for more nurses who are skilled and interested in gerontological nursing will continue to rise, and planning curriculum that addresses care of older adults will be key (Gray-Miceli & Morse, 2019).

Another curricular area that requires major change and innovation is the clinical teaching models currently in use in undergraduate education. Although some new clinical models have emerged in recent years, far too many programs continue to rely on clinical teaching models that are decades old. Faculty need to consider how best to design clinical learning experiences that will facilitate the development of clinical reasoning skills in learners and ultimately affect patient outcomes (Halstead, 2018).

Ensuring a successful transition into entry-level nursing practice and retaining new nurses in the profession is a major challenge, one that will require the collaborative efforts of education and practice. Such efforts will include maintaining congruence between nursing curricula and contemporary nursing practice, further developing and evaluating the outcomes of initiatives such as nurse residency programs that will help new graduates with the transition into nursing practice, and establishing mechanisms to retain and advance the education of experienced nurses in the workforce. There also will continue to be an emphasis placed on interprofessional education and the development of learning experiences that expose learners to collaborative practice concepts.

Contemporary articulation models that are flexible in design, supported by broad course and credit transferability, and packaged to maximize the use of students' time will continue to be designed. Nursing faculty will need to explore innovative curricular models that yield effective means by which to design and implement consortia to effectively utilize scarce faculty resources across programs. Academic progression models that are student centered and creative to support a career-ladder approach to nursing education are a key strategy in increasing the nursing workforce and facilitating entry to practice at multiple levels.

Faculty will also be required to go beyond a focus on the use of instructional technology in the classroom and provide expanded learning experiences

for students that focus on the use of technology in the clinical setting. Telehealth, electronic health records, and clinical judgment that is supported by the use of technology are major health information technology-driven patient care initiatives in which nurses will be required to demonstrate competence (Halstead, 2018). Students must have the opportunity for learning experiences in these areas in their undergraduate programs.

In the world of higher education the nursing profession has long been the source of much educational innovation. The issues identified here are critical to the future of nursing education, but by no means are they an exhaustive listing of the issues that nursing faculty must consider as they design future nursing programs and curricula. The innovation and creativity that nursing faculty have demonstrated in the past will continue to identify them as leaders in professional and higher education into the future.

CHAPTER SUMMARY: KEY POINTS

- Academic progression models provide multiple pathways for students to pursue in undergraduate nursing education.
- Potential students need to review the types of nursing programs available and strongly consider which pathway provides the best career path for them.
- Faculty need to be aware of the various nursing entry levels and certificate/degree options, as well as scope of practice considerations for each role as they design program curricula.
- Practical/vocational nursing programs provide an initial entry point into a nursing career for many individuals and have the potential to increase diversity in the nursing workforce.
- Undergraduate academic progression pathways must be creative, flexible, and seamless

to make the most of previous education/credits and be attractive to potential students.
- Academic-practice partnerships and consortia are increasingly important in supporting innovative programming and clinical experience opportunities.
- Nurse residency programs and transition to practice models are essential to increase new nurse acclimation to the work environment, clinical judgment, and retention.
- Maintaining contemporary undergraduate nursing education programs require faculty to remain alert to emerging nursing education considerations, including enhancing global and population health content, increasing focus on nursing care of older adults, and creative clinical learning experiences.

REFLECTING ON THE EVIDENCE

1. What emerging trends and issues in curriculum development do you envision needing to address in the next 2 years? Five years?
2. Review the curriculum development process for an undergraduate program. What potential

barriers and facilitators to curriculum development and revision can you identify in the process?
3. An undergraduate program plans to integrate content about communication skills for patient

safety into the curriculum. Using an existing curriculum, consider how you will approach integrating these skills into the curriculum.

4. Review the nurse practice acts for practical/vocational nurses and registered nurses from two or three different US state boards of nursing. Compare and contrast the curriculum and educational requirements for nursing programs in those states that you find, and reflect on the ways in which these regulations affect the development of a curriculum plan.

REFERENCES

Accreditation Commission for Education in Nursing. (2021). *Accredited programs*. http://www.acenursing.org/

Angel, L. (2020). Best practices and lessons learned in academic progression in nursing: A scoping review. *Journal of Professional Nursing*, 36(6), 628–634. https://doi.org/10.1016/j.profnurs.2020.08.017

American Association of Colleges of Nursing (AACN). (2021). *The essentials: Core competencies for professional nursing education*. https://www.aacnnursing.org/Portals/42/AcademicNursing/pdf/Essentials-2021.pdf

Commission on Collegiate Nursing Education (CCNE). (n.d.). *CCNE-accredited entry-to-practice nurse residency programs*. https://www.aacnnursing.org/CCNE-Accreditation/CCNE-Accredited-Programs

Davis, K., Warren, J., Nusbaum, S., Rhoades, J., Liss, D., Ricords, A., & Cadmus, E. (2021). Expanding nurse residency programs through regional and statewide collaborative partnerships. *Nurse Leader*, 19(5), 521–524. https://doi.org/10.1016/j.mnl2021.01.006

Dolansky, M., Nikstenas, C., Badders, A., Brannack, L., & Burant, P. (2022). Assessment of primary care content in a nursing curriculum. *Nurse Educator*, 47(1), E7–E11. https://doi.org/10.1097/NNE.0000000000001086

Gentry, S. S., & Graves, B. A. (2022). Experiences of graduates from concurrent enrollment programs in nursing. *Teaching and Learning in Nursing*, 17, 27–30. https://doi.org/10.1016/j.teln.2021.06.014

Goode, C. J., Glassman, K. S., Ponte, P. R., Krugman, M., & Peterman, T. (2018). Requiring a nurse residency for newly licensed registered nurses. *Nursing Outlook*, 66(3), 329–332.

Gorski, M. S., & Polansky, P. (2019). Accelerating progress in seamless academic progression. *Nursing Outlook*, 67, 154–160. https://doi.org/10.1016/j.outlook.2018.11.008

Gray-Miceli, D., & Morse, C. (2019). Curricular innovations for teaching undergraduate nursing students care of older adults. *Nurse Educator*, 44(3), E7–E10. https://doi.org/10.1097/NNE.0000000000000583

Halstead, J. A. (2018). The future role of the nurse educator. In J. Halstead (Ed.), *NLN core competencies for nurse educators: A decade of influence*. Wolters Kluwer.

Hampton, K. B., Smeltzer, S. C., & Ross, J. G. (2021). The transition from nursing student to practicing nurse: An integrative review of transition to practice programs. *Nurse Education in Practice*, 52. https://doi.org/10.1016/j.nepr.2021.103031

Institute of Medicine, (2011). *The future of nursing: Leading change, advancing health*. The National Academies Press.

Jones, C. B., Toles, M., Knafl, G. J., & Beeber, A. S. (2018). An untapped resource in the nursing workforce: Licensed practical nurses who transition to become registered nurses. *Nursing Outlook*, 66, 46–55. https://doi.org/10.1016/j.outlook.2017.07.007

McNiel, P. L., & Elertson, K. M. (2018). Advocacy and awareness: Integrating LGBTQ health education into the prelicensure curriculum. *Journal of Nursing Education*, 57(5), 312–314. https://doi.org/10.3928/01484834-20180420-12

Meyer, D. (2017). Academic progression in nursing, reviewing the past 5 years. *Teaching & Learning in Nursing*, 12(2), 176–177. https://doi.org/10.1016/j.teln.2017.01.002.

National Academy of Medicine, (2021). *The future of nursing 2020–2030: Charting a path to health equity*. The National Academies Press.

National Council of State Boards of Nursing. (2019). *2019 NCLEX-RN test plan*. https://www.ncsbn.org/testplans.htm

National Council of State Boards of Nursing. (2020). *National nursing database: A profile of nursing licensure in the U.S.* https://www.ncsbn.org/national-nursing-database.htm

National Council of State Boards of Nursing. (2022). *Transition to practice program*. https://www.ncsbn.org/transition-to-practice.htm

National League for Nursing (NLN). (2010). *Outcomes and competencies for graduates of practical/vocational, diploma, associate degree, baccalaureate, master's, practice doctorate, and research doctorate programs in nursing*. Author.

National League for Nursing. (2014a). *NLN practical/ vocational nursing curriculum framework guiding principles.* https://www.nln.org/docs/default-source/ uploadedfiles/default-document-library/ nln-practical-nursing-framework-guidelines-final. pdf?sfvrsn=6cd9df0d_0

National League for Nursing. (2014b). *Vision for recognition of the role of licensed practical/vocational nurses in advancing the nation's health.* Author.

Neville-Norton, M., & Cantwell, S. (2019). Curriculum mapping in nursing education: A case study for collaborative curriculum design and program quality assurance. *Teaching and Learning in Nursing, 14*(2019), 88–93. https://doi.org/10.1016/ jteln.2018.12.001

Quality and Safety Education for Nurses (QSEN). (2022). *QSEN competencies.* https://qsen.org

Robert Wood Johnson Foundation. (2015). *Thinking together in new ways: Advancing academic progression in nursing.* https://campaignforaction.org/ our-network/grantee-and-award-programs/ academic-progression-in-nursing/

Rose, A. Y., Roach, A. D., Lloyd-Penza, M., Miller, C., Cooper, M., & Messecar, D. (2020). Veteran-centric content integration into a baccalaureate nursing curriculum. *Journal of Nursing Education, 59*(7), 400–404. https://doi.org/10.3928/01484834-20200617-09

Sherman, A. D. F., Cimino, A. N., Clark, K. D., Smith, K., Klepper, M., & Bower, K. M. (2021). LGBTQ+ health education for nurses: An innovative approach to improving nursing curricula. *Nurse Education Today, 97.* https://doi.org/10.1016/j.nedt.2020.104698

Warren, J. I., Perkins, S., & Greene, M. A. (2018). Advancing new nurse graduate education through implementation of statewide, standardized nurse residency programs. *Journal of Nursing Regulation, 8*(4), 14–21. https://doi.org/10.1016/ S2155-8256(17)30177-1

9

Curriculum Models for Graduate Programs*

Sandy L. Carollo, PhD, MSN, ARNP

Graduate nursing education is sitting at the crossroads of transformation. The changing higher education climate, variable learning styles of students, and public expectation for practice-ready advanced practice nurses require a closer examination and adaptation of pedagogies relevant to a new class of learners who will challenge traditional teaching models. Driven by a rapidly changing health care system, diverse learners, faculty shortages, and advancing technologies, a time for change has come. Attention to the areas of academic-practice partnerships, holistic applications, faculty development, and competency-based education would be well advised. This chapter describes the progression of graduate nursing education in the United States, as well as emerging curriculum models and trends in teaching and learning in master's and doctoral nursing programs.

HISTORICAL DEVELOPMENT OF GRADUATE NURSING EDUCATION

Formal graduate nursing education can be traced as far back as the 1930s when the specialty of nursing administration was recognized as an area of graduate study for nurses. In the 1950s, and supported by funding from the Kellogg Foundation, 13 universities launched graduate nursing programs to prepare students for the nurse administrator role.

---

*The author acknowledges the work of Karen Grigsby, PhD, RN, in the previous edition.

In 1963 a federally commissioned study was undertaken in which nursing faculty were identified as possessing minimal educational preparation for teaching. The subsequent report, *Toward Quality in Nursing: Needs and Goals* (US Department of Health, 1963), identified the need for additional funding for nursing programs, ultimately supporting the 1964 Nurse Training Act that promoted advancement in graduate nursing programs.

In the 1960s, fueled by challenges with access to care in underserved communities, a new role for nursing was established, the role of nurse practitioner (NP). This role allowed nurses with specialized education to offer care commonly reserved for physicians. Dr. Loretta Ford, is recognized as the cofounder (with Dr. Henry Silver) of the first NP program. While serving as a public health nurse in the 1960s in Denver, Colorado, Ford and her physician colleague, Silver, identified a gap in health care access for rural families. Together they developed a model that provided advanced practice training for community-based nurses. This program moved to the national arena in the early 1970s and served as the foundation for advanced practice nursing worldwide.

In the 1970s Nurse Practitioner education took place primarily at the graduate level. During this time there was expansion of graduate nursing programs, many of which offered a focus on clinical specialties. Specialty roles included clinical specialist, NP, researcher, and nurse administrator. The 1980s saw an increased interest in clinical specialty and decreased enrollment in the nurse administrator track. The 1990s and early 2000s were focused on developing new advanced practice programs.

In 2008 the consensus model for APRN regulation emerged, and in 2011 the Institute of Medicine (IOM) released a report, *The Future of Nursing: Leading Change, Advancing Health*, which focused on improving the nation's health by strengthening the nursing workforce. Recommendations included increasing the number of doctorally prepared nurses, curricula revision with an emphasis on competency-based outcomes, emphasis on student diversity, and employer incentives. This document became the blueprint that propelled changes in nursing education and the nursing workforce over the next decade.

MASTER'S PROGRAMS IN NURSING

Table 9.1 lists types of graduate nursing degrees and examples of focus areas of study. Nursing master's degree programs offer multiple pathways to achieve advanced practice roles from leadership to clinical specialty, education, policy, and more (AACN, 2022d). Some of the available tracks for master's degree programs include entry-level master's programs for students with an existing bachelor's or graduate nonnursing degree; RN to MSN programs for RNs prepared at the associate degree level, which incorporate baccalaureate level nursing content early in the program; BSN to MSN programs which build on BSN competencies and are typically focused on specialty areas; and dual master's programs for students with interest in two complementary study areas including MSN/MBA,

MSN/MPH, and MSN/MHA (AACN, 2022d). Practice roles tied to these tracks include Clinical Nurse Leader, Clinical Nurse Specialist, Nurse Administrator, Nurse Educator, Public Health Nurse, Nurse Informaticist, Nurse Practitioner, Certified Registered Nurse Anesthetist, and Certified Nurse Midwife (AACN, 2022d).

Master's programs have evolved over the years, with waxing and waning of role relevance, while there has been movement in the profession toward doctoral preparation for advanced practice roles. Currently, while many MSN programs continue to exist, there remain questions about the benefit of continuing to provide the MSN degree option.

In the early 1950s there were very few nursing master's degree programs and wide variability in covering master's graduate competencies. The Southern Council on Collegiate Education (SCCEN) was formed in the southern states and Western Interstate Commission for Higher Education (WICHE) was formed in the western states to address overcoming challenges facing curriculum in the master's degree programs. Each organization planned new programs and revised curricula related to clinical content and competencies at the master's level. By 1962 enrollment in masters programs had doubled. During the 1970s, role development included the areas of CNS, educator, administrator, and researcher (Ervin, 2018). As the popularity of the CNS role increased, fewer nurses selected the role of researcher, educator, or

TABLE 9.1	**Types of Graduate Nursing Degrees and Examples of Focus Areas of Study**	
	Education	**Program Focus**
Clinical Practice	*MSN–Master of Science in Nursing*	*Clinical Focus* • Clinical Nurse Leader (CNL)
APRN- Advanced Practice Registered Nurse	*MSN* *DNP–Doctor of Nursing Practice*	*Clinical Focus* • Nurse Practitioner (NP) • Clinical Nurse Specialist (CNS) • Certified Registered Nurse Anesthetist (CRNA) • Certified Nurse Midwife (CNM)
Non-Clinical Specialties	*MSN* *DNP* *PhD* *EdD*	*Nonclinical Focus* • Nurse Administrator • Nurse Informaticist • Nurse Educator • Nurse Researcher

administrator. As this trend grew, programs preparing educators and administrators at the master's level were either eliminated or relegated to supporting courses for programs focused on preparing the CNS (Egenes, 2018).

The NP role emerged during the 1970s, initially as certificate programs, and later moved to a master's degree in the early 1980s. A new addition to the master's level, NP programs included developing skill in political activism to influence legislative changes needed to allow NPs to practice to the full scope of their preparation. Efforts to influence legislators to make changes in state laws so that NPs can practice to their full scope continues today (Egenes, 2018). In the latter half of the 1980s the practice trend toward specialty care prompted shifts in curricular content for NP programs with a greater emphasis on clinical areas. (Ervin, 2018). Today, there are questions being raised by the profession about the continued need for master's programs as the focus shifts to doctoral preparation for nurse practitioners, administrators, researchers, and educators. Some programs are phasing out their master's programs to encourage nurses to move directly into doctoral preparation, while other programs continue to offer master's programs in addition to doctoral programs (Scheckel, 2018). Some in the profession are concerned that eliminating master's programs could create a shortage of advanced practice nurses prepared to deliver direct patient care in the clinical setting. The debate and dialogue about the future of master's degree nursing programs will continue into the foreseeable future.

The Clinical Nurse Leader: The Advanced Generalist

In response to a fragmented and misaligned health care system, the clinical nurse leader (CNL) role emerged in 2003 (AACN, 2022c). AACN assumed the leadership of moving this role forward in 2004 including development of scope of practice and credentialing requirements (AACN, 2022c). The role was established with a master's level education requirement, and as a generalist prepared to practice in all health care settings to improve patient outcomes and to coordinate and promote evidence-based practice. The intended emphasis for this role was for clinicians to work collaboratively within a team incorporating a focus to engage in outcomes-based practice using quality improvement strategies. The CNL is prepared to deliver support aimed at microsystems and care at the point of contact with the patient. The Veterans Administration was an early adopter of this role with the intent to positively influence care of veterans and concentration on team-based, safe, quality, and cost-effective care to patients (USDVA, 2016). As of September 2021, 8,749 nurses have been certified as CNLs since 2006, with the greatest number of graduates practicing in California and within acute care inpatient facilities (AACN, 2021b). While the number of certified CNLs has increased, the number of new graduates and the number of CNL programs has decreased (AACN, 2021b).

The CNL role has not been without controversy. As the CNL role was first introduced, some questioned the need for this role because CNSs also are prepared to deliver care to populations. However, the differentiation between the two roles has become clearer as the CNL role has become better understood. The CNS is recognized as an advanced practice nurse who is an expert clinician in a particular specialty or subspecialty of nursing practice. The CNL works at the microsystem level to manage and coordinate client care, whereas the CNS designs, implements, and evaluates patient-specific and population-based programs of care. Ultimately, the CNL works in partnership with the CNS, and both contribute to the delivery of safe, efficient, effective, quality care.

Advanced Practice Registered Nurse Role

The American Association of Colleges of Nursing (AACN, 2022b) categorizes APRNs as nurse practitioners (NPs), clinical nurse specialists (CNSs), certified registered nurse anesthetists (CRNAs), and certified nurse midwives (CNMs). Each of these roles focuses on a specific population or setting to deliver care to individuals, families, or communities.

While all four roles are considered specialty driven, the NP, CRNA, and CNM are involved in direct patient care, while the CNS additionally offers macro-level impact (Mohr & Coke, 2018).

Programs offered at schools/colleges of nursing vary depending on faculty credentials and population need within the area where the program is offered. Nursing programs may elect to not prepare APRNs at the MSN level, choosing to prepare APRNs only at the doctoral level. As the DNP degree has developed, some programs have elected to eliminate the MSN program option and educate APRNs only at the DNP level. Other programs continue to offer APRN education at both the MSN and DNP levels.

As stated previously, APRN preparation at the MSN level is in flux currently as programs address population needs within the area they serve and school/college resources. The Council on Accreditation (COA) for CRNAs has endorsed doctoral education requirements by 2025. Further, all accredited CRNA programs are required to offer doctoral education by January 1, 2022 (COA, 2020). CNMs, who provide primary health care services for women and newborns, acknowledge the value of doctoral education; however, the American College for Nurse Midwives (ACNM) continues to require a master's degree for entry into midwifery practice (ACNM, 2019). The National Association of Clinical Nurse Specialists does support the DNP for future entry to practice, with 2030 being the date by which CNS must obtain the degree to retain their ability to practice (NACNS, 2015).

Other Foci for MSN Programs

In addition to the APRN roles of CNS, NP, CNM, and CRNA, and the role of CNL, other foci are available. Nurses who desire to teach in nursing programs or who want to serve in leadership roles in either clinical or academic organizations may enroll in MSN programs to prepare for specialized roles. There are MSN programs with curricula specifically designed to prepare nurses as educators or administrators. Nurses who are enrolled in APRN programs and aspire to become educators or administrators can also choose to add graduate course work in education and/or administration to their plan of study. Education coursework is especially helpful for nurses who want to combine a practice role as an APRN with an educator role.

There are other roles that require graduate nursing education, for example, public health nurse and nurse informaticist, who are prepared to integrate technology into nursing care so that communication is enhanced across disciplines, costs of care are reduced, efficiencies are increased, and quality of care is improved. Additionally, nurses who wish to focus on genetics or forensics also need graduate nursing education to prepare them within this specialty area (AACN, 2022a). Any of these roles require not only an advanced graduate nursing degree but certification within the specialty.

DOCTORAL PROGRAMS IN NURSING

Doctoral education for nurses has existed since the 1920s. Originally, doctoral programs prepared nurses for administrative and teaching roles. Because nursing had not established doctoral programs at this time, nurses were required to seek access through other programs, including the disciplines of education, sociology, and psychology. The first doctoral program available to nurses was offered in 1924 at Teachers College, Columbia University, where graduates earned an EdD degree (Scheckel, 2018). This limited access to non-nursing-specific programs continued through the 1960s.

Although master's programs were growing in number in the 1970s, nurse leaders were advancing the idea that nursing needed its own theory base to be recognized as a discipline and a profession that could stand alone rather than borrow theory from other disciplines. Doctoral programs in nursing were initially created to stimulate the development of nursing theory and research and prepare nurses to teach; development of these programs surged in the later part of the 20th century (Scheckel, 2018). These programs resulted in a PhD with a focus on nursing science and research.

The clinical doctorate in nursing emerged as recognition developed that more emphasis was needed for clinical application. The first nursing clinical doctoral program designed to focus on clinical practice opened at Boston University, which offered the DNSc, a clinical doctorate for nursing. In 1979 Case Western University launched the ND, nursing doctorate, which prepared individuals for basic licensure plus application of advanced knowledge in clinical practice areas. Both the ND and DNSc served as precursors to the current doctor of nursing practice (DNP) degree. Amid confusion regarding the focus of the early nursing doctoral degrees, and as the expansion of DNP programs has been realized, the PhD and DNP have emerged as the current titles in use today with a focus on research for the PhD and practice for the DNP. There are also efforts supporting a dual PhD–DNP, which would enhance ties between the two doctoral degrees to bridge research translation (Graves et al., 2021).

The Doctor of Nursing Practice Degree

The DNP is a practice-focused terminal degree to prepare graduates to provide leadership in the development and implementation of clinical knowledge in specialized areas of advanced practice (AACN, 2020b). In 2004, after 4 years of task force review, the AACN endorsed doctoral-level preparation expectations for entry to practice for advanced nursing practice (AACN, 2020b).

Factors influencing this move include a rapidly changing and complex health care environment, emphasis on patient care quality, safety and cost, and response to a 2005 National Academy of Sciences address (in *Advancing the Nation's Health Needs: NIH Research Training Programs*) to establish a clinically based doctorate to prepare nurses as practitioners and as clinical faculty (AACN, 2020b).

In 2006, AACN endorsed *The Essentials of Doctoral Education for Advanced Nursing Practice*, which outlines competencies and curricular components. Additional documents have been provided by AACN to provide support for institutions developing a DNP and/or transitioning from an MSN to a DNP. In 2008, the Commission on Collegiate Nursing Education (CCNE) started accrediting DNP programs. In 2014, a national study titled The DNP by 2015: A Study of the Institutional, Political, and Professional Issues that Facilitate or Impede Establishing a Post-Baccalaureate Doctor of Nursing Practice Program found widespread support for the value of the DNP within nursing education (AACN, 2020b).

The original 2015 target deadline set by AACN for transition to DNP for entry to advanced practice has not been met. In response to this, in April 2018, NONPF committed to moving all NP education to the doctoral level (DNP) by 2025 (NONPF, 2018). As of 2020, all 50 states and the District of Columbia offer DNP programs. As of 2019, nationwide, 357 programs were enrolling students and 106 schools were planning new DNP programs (AACN, 2020b).

The DNP degree is considered a terminal degree in nursing practice. Although not intended to prepare nurses for positions as educators, the DNP degree does provide a terminal degree credential that many institutions accept as qualification for a faculty position and thus can be instrumental in addressing the profession's shortage of nursing faculty. If DNP graduates are dually prepared as nurse educators and advanced practice nurses, they would be well positioned to educate all levels of students and to close the practice–education gap (Tyczkowski & Reilly, 2017).

The development of DNP programs proliferated early in the 21st century, and some nurse leaders began voicing concerns that the introduction of the DNP degree would lead fewer nurses to enter PhD programs, master's preparation for NPs would be eliminated, and APRNs would no longer be focused on providing care to people, especially individuals and families living in areas with limited access to health care providers. At this time, the number of PhD programs remains relatively stable with minimal growth, while DNP programs have continued to grow in number (AACN, 2020b). The profession continues to debate the continuing value of the MSN degree for the preparation of APRNs. The controversy surrounding the issue of DNP degrees as the entry into advanced nursing practice has economic, societal, and health care delivery implications. The DNP degree is regarded as the highest level of advanced nursing practice that focuses on translating new knowledge into practice and developing evidence-based practice.

With the AACN's mandate for the DNP degree to be the entry into advanced practice, questions are raised as to how to prepare a nurse for advanced practice while at the same time developing skills in leadership and systems change. Some leaders argue that engaging young nurses to advance to the DNP degree immediately after completing their BSN degree limits the contributions they can make to the profession, whereas others see an economic benefit for the student and a means of improving health care delivery. To address this concern, programs are developing integrated curricula that incorporate the AACN Essentials and NONPF competencies (NONPF, 2017). To date, the discussion continues while programs determine how best to address these recommendations.

The PhD in Nursing Degree

The PhD in nursing degree is designed to prepare nurse scientists who are committed to the generation of new knowledge and can steward the discipline and educate the next generation of nurse scholars. PhD programs focus on developing researchers who have a strong scientific understanding within the discipline of nursing and related disciplines. Additional areas of focus include research design, data analysis, dissemination of findings, and collaboration (AACN, 2022e).

Some PhD programs in nursing also provide a focus of study in nursing education. These programs mentor students by involving them in a community designed to stimulate students' thinking about their own research agenda and by providing opportunities to prepare grants and manuscripts and initiate a program of research.

Programs of study include both postbachelor's to PhD and postmaster's to PhD formats and can be accomplished in 3 to 5 years of full-time study or 5 to 8 years of part-time study. Program delivery varies from traditional on-campus coursework to fully online programs to a hybrid approach that uses a blending of both on-campus and remote coursework to deliver the program.

As DNP programs have seen increased enrollment and number of programs (AACN, 2020d), PhD programs have seen enrollment flattened to trending down. Reportedly, research-focused programs increased from 78 in 1999 to 145 in 2019 (Penn Nursing, 2020). Despite this increase in programs, the enrollment has declined over the last 5 years. In response to this issue the University of Pennsylvania invited 41 representatives from education, government, and professional and philanthropic sectors to dialogue about the future of PhD education. Synthesis of the discussions is serving as a catalyst for next steps for the PhD (Penn Nursing, 2020). One area that is gaining traction is the interest in dual PhD–DNP degrees (Loescher et al., 2021).

The Doctor of Education Degree

Early in the 20th century, nurses who wanted to teach chose to attend doctoral programs in schools of education. Schools of education offered PhD and Doctor of Education (EdD) programs ("the practice doctorate" in education). As nursing doctoral programs developed, nurses had more choices about the type of doctoral program they could attend and some chose PhD or DNSc (DNS) programs in schools of nursing, while others chose to obtain their degree from schools of education to focus their studies on preparing to teach in programs of nursing. Nurses who want a focus on education for their doctoral program can still select an EdD program today. Because of the emphasis on preparing nurse educators at the doctoral level, several schools of nursing are now offering an EdD in nursing.

A national study completed by King et al. (2020) indicated that the greater part of respondents believe that the need for nurse educators with a terminal degree is greater than the number available. Further, the doctoral degree options of the PhD, which focuses on research, and the DNP, which focuses on practice, align poorly with career aspirations focused on nursing education. Even the EdD does not offer the depth of discipline-specific content requisite for this role. For this reason, a new degree, the doctorate in nursing education (DNE), has been proposed (Oermann & Spalia King, 2019). This degree would cover best practices in teaching-learning, curriculum design and development including clinical practice, and curricula evaluation. The EdD and DNE may collaborate with the school of education on a given campus, which can offer foundational courses and major areas of concentration in education.

CURRICULUM MODELS FOR GRADUATE PROGRAMS

Curriculum models for graduate nursing education have become varied, with a number of program models designed to facilitate academic progression to graduate-level preparation. The quality of graduate nursing education programs is maintained in part through the admission of well-qualified students. This section describes various graduate curriculum models and student qualifications.

Student Qualifications

Despite a national nursing shortage, qualified applications are being turned away in large numbers, including nurses seeking entry into graduate programs. AACN reported in 2019 that more than 8,000 eligible applicants were not accepted to master's programs and more than 3,000 were not accepted into doctoral programs (AACN, 2020a,c).

A variety of factors influence a student's admission to graduate study. Overall, students are evaluated for their potential for success in academic progression within their chosen program.

Realizing that one element is not enough to predict success, and in an effort to create a diverse student body, a number of programs have initiated a holistic admissions process. This allows for a comprehensive review of multiple criteria. Admission criteria vary from school to school and program to program, and Table 9.2 offers a number of potential requirements, prerequisites, and expectations before enrollment. See Case Study 9.1 for further discussion related to student admission criteria.

In addition to general graduate school requirements, graduate nursing programs typically require additional criteria. As noted, this varies depending on the program of study. For example, a writing sample may be a requirement in a PhD program, whereas a requirement of 2 years of clinical practice in a CCU and a CCRN may be an expectation for someone entering a CRNA program. While many graduate programs require a BSN, there are RN to MS and RN to DNP programs available for applicants without a bachelor's degree and these are considered bridge programs. There are also direct-entry MSN programs for applicants who hold a bachelor's degree in a discipline other than nursing. Admission criteria include strong work and academic histories with minimum 3.0 GPA, completion of all prerequisites, and often a GRE. Letters of reference are generally requested and should include both

TABLE 9.2 Examples of Graduate Program Admission Criteria

Requirements
- BSN or MSN from accredited institution
- GPA 3.0 or higher
- Letters of reference (academic and professional)
- Statement of professional goals
- Current, unencumbered RN license and work experience (1–2 years depending on specialty)
- Preadmission testing including GRE or MAT
- Professional resume
- Writing sample (publication or graded paper)
- Preadmission interview

Academic Prerequisites
- Statistics/research
- Basic health assessment course in undergraduate program
- Chemistry
- Biology
- Anatomy & Physiology

Additional Expectations at Enrollment
- Immunizations, boosters, and titers
- Health history and physical exam
- Liability insurance
- Background check
- CPR/ACLS (depending upon specialty)
- Drug test

professional and academic endorsement. For anyone who has been out of school for more than 5 years, references should include a supervisor or manager who can speak to relevant experience. A detailed resume will provide work experience, licensure, and certification credentials, which may be additional requirements for some programs. A statement of professional goals or an essay may be requested and is an opportunity for applicants to articulate strengths, future plans, and research interests. Standardized preentry exams such as the Graduate Record Exam (GRE) or Miller Analogies Test (MAT) continue in some programs, while others are eliminating them completely, and some offer waivers for students with higher GPAs or prior degrees. Finally, in research-focused doctoral programs it is important for the research interests of the student to be consistent with the research interests of the faculty they will be working with.

CASE STUDY 9.1 **Admission Criteria for Advanced Practice Nursing Programs**

A public university offering a DNP with specialty tracks for FNP and PMHNP held admissions review in January each year for entry in September. The admissions criteria included a minimum GPA requirement, completion of BSN degree, official transcripts, unencumbered nursing license, CV, letters of recommendation, written goal statement, and response to written interview questions. Not listed as a requirement, but an area of faculty debate, was the requirement of 1 year of full-time practice as a BSN-prepared nurse. Several faculty felt strongly that advanced practice students must have experience in practice to have the background necessary to be successful in the program. Other faculty articulated that a 1-year practice requirement would place unreasonable barriers on student academic progression and that concurrent practice with enrollment in the program should be supported. The institution made no changes to the applicant requirements at the time but later added an additional expectation for applicants that 1-year full-time practice is preferred.

1. What would be disadvantages of admitting a licensed RN without practice experience to an APRN program? What would be the advantages to this approach?
2. What strategies can faculty implement if admitting RN students to APRN programs without clinical experience to support student success?
3. If considering 1-year full-time clinical practice as a requirement for admission to an APRN program, should the type of clinical practice be a consideration?

Program Designs for Master's Education

Graduate nursing programs are often selected by working students who are dedicated to advancing their education but who may have challenges with other commitments including work and family. As adult learners, they recognize that more education equates to more opportunity, whether that is with practice focus on direct patient care, teaching, research, administration, or other.

Graduates of master's level nursing programs are prepared to engage in a number of advanced roles including direct care and nonclinical roles. Master's education builds on foundational knowledge covered in undergraduate bachelor's nursing programs. For students attending bridge programs where the student is not required to have a BSN, the foundational content is covered in the early terms of the master's program. Graduates of master's degree programs are also prepared to enter a research or practice-focused doctoral program.

Since 1986 AACN has provided direction for nurse educators in baccalaureate and higher degree nursing program, including the publication of professional standards to guide curriculum development. Historically this has been offered through a degree-related format. *The Essentials of Masters Education in Nursing* was published in 2011 and has been replaced by the 2021 document titled *The Essentials: Core Competencies for Professional Nursing Education*. This document offers a framework for academic preparation of nurses at multiple levels including entry-level and advanced-level nursing education.

The Essentials: Core Competencies for Professional Nursing Education provides a plan for seamless academic progression and includes transition to competency-based education. The 10 competency domains and 8 foundational concepts threaded within the domains (Table 9.3) provide the framework for this new model. Within each domain there are two levels: one for entry level and another for advanced level and specialty care (AACN, 2021). While the newest version of The Essentials has been approved, it will be several years until full implementation. Professional standards for graduate curriculum based on specialty can be found through other organizations including the National Organization of Nurse Practitioner Faculties (NONPF) NP competencies, National League for Nursing (NLN) core competencies for nurse educators, and the American Organization for Nursing Leadership (AONL) nurse leader competencies.

Master's programs vary in length and focus, as well as credit hours required for graduation, which may range from 30 to 45 credits. This variance is related to multiple factors including program design, credits required, clinical hour requirements, and current education level of applicant. Most students with a BSN can complete a master's

TABLE 9.3 2021 AACN Nursing Education Core Competencies and Domain Concepts

Core Competencies	Domains
1 Knowledge for nursing practice	Clinical judgment
2 Person-centered care	Communication
3 Population health	Compassionate care
4 Scholarship for nursing discipline	Determinants of health
5 Quality and safety	Diversity, equity, and inclusion
6 Interprofessional partnerships	Ethics
7 Systems-based practice	Evidence-based practice
8 Informatics and health care technologies	Health policy
9 Professionalism	
10 Personal, professional, and leadership development	

(From American Association of Colleges of Nursing. The *Essentials: Core Competencies for Professional Nursing Education*.)

degree in 1.5 to 2 years of full-time study. Students attending part-time will take longer to complete their program.

MSN programs may offer their courses or the entire degree program fully or partially online, thus increasing scheduling flexibility. Additionally, the online format makes the program accessible to underserved areas of the country and allows students to remain in their communities during the program and upon graduation.

Although many master's programs require an earned baccalaureate in nursing for admission, increasing numbers of academic progression models facilitate individuals obtaining a nursing master's degree via an accelerated pathway. Individuals with an associate degree in nursing, an undergraduate degree in another discipline, or a graduate degree in another discipline can enter a nursing master's program and graduate with an MSN degree.

Postmaster's certificates (PMCs) are program options that allow students with a previous master's degree in nursing to obtain credentials in another specialty. These alternate-entry master's programs are designed to reflect achievement of the baccalaureate and master's outcomes and to prepare the student to take the RN licensing examination (if they enter the program without a nursing degree) and the appropriate certification examination. The design of curriculum models varies depending on the college or university where they are offered, but the underlying intent is to prepare individuals with basic and advanced nursing knowledge and skills so that they can enter the workforce easily.

Program Designs for Doctoral Education

Doctoral curricula tend to be unique to each institution. Because the PhD and the DNP degrees have different purposes and goals, their program design is significantly different.

DNP Program Design

The DNP degree is a terminal degree that is practice focused. DNP programs are designed to prepare graduates to provide leadership in the development and application of clinical knowledge in specialized areas of advanced practice (AACN, 2022b). Graduates of this program type focus on practice that is innovative and evidence based, applying research findings to practice rather than generating the evidence for practice. Curricula for DNP programs can vary significantly, from programs that initially prepare graduates for practice as an advanced practice nurse to programs that focus more on leadership in systems-level indirect care roles, such as administration.

DNP programs reside in colleges and schools of nursing, and they are under the direction of the college or school of nursing. Therefore DNP programs are accredited by either the Accreditation Commission for Education in Nursing (ACEN), the National League for Nursing Commission for Nursing Education Accreditation (NLN CNEA), or the Commission on Collegiate Nursing Education (CCNE).

DNP programs have several points of entry (e.g., postassociate degree, postbaccalaureate degree, postmaster's degree, and nonnursing degree). Individuals entering DNP programs without a baccalaureate or master's nursing degree may need to complete general education courses and nursing bridge courses before beginning DNP course work. Bridge courses are designed to allow the student to obtain knowledge and skills that were not present in their previous degree programs. Typically, a student's transcript is reviewed and a specific plan of study is designed for the individual to ensure they are prepared for DNP work. Graduates from DNP programs are expected to provide the leadership for implementing evidence-based practice and, with the appropriate preparation to assume a teaching role, they could also serve as clinical faculty to teach in nursing programs. DNP programs require an additional 35 to 40 credit hours over the master's level, and the length of time to complete the DNP degree depends on the previous academic experiences a student brings to the program. A postmaster's DNP may be completed with 2 years of full-time study, whereas a BSN to DNP program may require 4 or 5 years of full-time study.

The AACN established *The Essentials of Doctoral Education for Advanced Nursing Practice* in 2006 and they have been used by faculty to guide curriculum development. These essentials include scientific underpinnings for practice, organizational and systems leadership for quality improvement and systems thinking, clinical scholarship and analytical methods for evidence-based practice, information systems and technology and patient-care technology for the improvement and transformation of health care, health care policy for advocacy in health care, interprofessional collaboration for improving patient and population health outcomes, clinical prevention and population health for improving the nation's health, and advanced practice (AACN, 2017d). As noted under the master's program design section, in 2021 AACN approved *The Essentials: Core Competencies for Professional Nursing Education*, in which DNP competencies are covered. In April 2022 the National Task Force (NTF) document 2022, Standards for Quality Nurse Practitioner Education, was endorsed by multiple National Nursing Organizations including the American Association of Colleges of Nursing (AACN), the American Association of Nurse Practitioners (AANP), the American Nurses Credentialing Center (ANCC), the Commission on Collegiate Nursing Education (CCNE), the National Certification Corporation (NCC), the National Organization of Nurse Practitioner Faculty (NONPF), and the National League for Nursing Commission for Nursing Education Accreditation (NLN CNEA).

PhD Program Design

Doctoral programs in nursing that award the PhD are research focused with a program outcome of preparing graduates to engage in knowledge generation and dissemination. As researchers and scholars, a PhD-prepared nurse is trained to examine and address complex health and health care questions. Curricula in nursing PhD programs typically consist of coursework related to nursing philosophy and theory construction; statistics and research methodology; state of the science nursing knowledge; social, political, and ethical issues; and teaching and mentoring (AACN, 2022e).

The majority of PhD nursing programs require a master's degree in nursing for entry; however, with a focus on increasing the number of doctorally prepared nurses (AACN, 2020), many programs are offering the option of completing master's level work as part of the requirements for the PhD degree. This design approach is seen with the BSN to PhD programs. Another option for students who hold a bachelor's or graduate degree in another discipline is the AE–PhD program design. The first year of the program includes an intensive line up of foundational nursing courses and experiences designed to prepare the student to meet RN licensure requirements. Students who enter the PhD program with a master's degree will usually engage in full-time study for approximately 3 years and complete a dissertation. Students who enter a PhD program with a baccalaureate nursing degree usually study full-time for 5 years and complete a dissertation. These timelines are extended for many students, as they choose to pursue part-time study, if allowed by the program. Students who enter BSN to PhD programs need support from faculty to make the transition directly from baccalaureate course work to doctoral course work. Schools handle this transition using a variety of strategies. Some schools assign an advisor for the doctoral course work and an advisor for the clinical area in which the student is pursuing advanced knowledge. Other schools integrate these students into classes with more experienced RNs and mentor students into understanding the practice world as they learn how to generate research from a theoretical perspective.

While PhD programs reside in colleges/schools of nursing, they are under the direction of the college or university's graduate school. Therefore nursing PhD programs are not accredited by nursing accrediting bodies. Instead, these programs are subject to periodic external and internal academic review procedures following criteria established by the institution within which they reside.

Upon completion of coursework and before writing the dissertation, students typically must complete a qualifying examination to demonstrate their ability to conduct research that is grounded in science and to be eligible to enter into the final stage of the program. The process used for the qualifying examination varies depending on the institution, but it is common to have a written or oral component—frequently both. For many students, this is a major milestone and may serve as the first step in the dissertation process with the designation of PhD candidacy following completion.

Graduates of PhD programs are required to conduct independent research and prepare a document communicating the process and results of the research. This document historically has been a dissertation. Currently, faculty in many PhD programs are reconsidering the value of a lengthy dissertation and are allowing options for presenting the results of the student's research. These may include writing one or more manuscripts to submit for publication or even digital products that could include motion, sound, and graphics (Graves et al., 2018).

Academic Progression Models for Graduate Education

The *Future of Nursing* reports (2011 and 2021) recommended higher levels of education through seamless academic progression. To meet this recommendation, an examination of learner demographics may be in order. In 2018 AMN Health care made available the report *Survey of Millennial Nurses: A Dynamic Influence on the Profession*, which outlines future academic and profession goals of practicing nurses by generation. In this report responses are clustered by age: Millennials (age 19–36), Generation X (age 37–53), and Baby Boomers (age 54–71). Table 9.4 outlines the responses (AMN Healthcare, 2018).

Academic progression is a process used to facilitate individuals obtaining higher degrees in a timely manner without duplicating or repeating previous course work. For example, common examples of academic progression models in colleges of nursing are those that facilitate RNs without a BSN degree to achieve a graduate nursing degree. Such programs allow nurses to more rapidly assume an advanced practice role. Academic progression models can help facilitate RNs who are usually working full-time while attending school part-time to obtain a graduate degree. Part-time graduate program offerings allow the nurse to remain in the workforce while attending school. Academic progression models can also help facilitate underrepresented minority students achieving a graduate degree, thus preparing a pipeline of underrepresented student populations qualified to assume faculty roles in schools of nursing. An example of an academic progression program that advances underrepresented ethnic minority students to a doctoral degree is a bridge program in which different institutions partner to provide direct access. This may include an articulation agreement between institutions.

TABLE 9.4 Future Academic and Professional Goals by Generation			
	Millennials	**Generation X**	**Baby Boomers**
Seek leadership role	36%	27%	10%
Pursue academic progression	71%	56%	20%
Pursue APRN role	49%	35%	12%

Articulation Agreements

Another example of an academic model that promotes entry into a graduate program for nurses without a BSN degree is the use of articulation agreements between schools offering MSN programs and community colleges that offer associate degree programs. Sometimes referred to as "bridge" or "transition" programs, the curriculum of the nursing baccalaureate and master's programs are analyzed to identify what content is needed by nurses holding the associate degree to ensure that all BSN and MSN outcomes are met. Using this model means that nurses can enter the workforce as an advanced practice nurse more quickly than if they took the more traditional approach of the RN to BSN program and then applied for entry into a graduate program to obtain a master's nursing degree.

In 2012, the Robert Wood Johnson Foundation (RWJF) awarded 4-year grants to nine states to facilitate the development of academic progression models. These grants provided the financial support to establish academic progression in nursing initiatives to address the IOM recommendation to increase the number of nurses with a doctoral degree by 2020 (RWJF, 2013). Although the RWJF funding ended in 2017, the academic models created through this initiative continue to serve as examples for other schools/colleges. These academic progression models are creating innovative educational pathways for all nursing degrees to facilitate a more rapid transition to advanced practice (Gerardi, 2017). Curriculum designs for these programs ensure that essentials for the BSN, MSN, and/or DNP are met regardless of whether the earlier degrees are conferred. This trend is likely to continue in the future and will increasingly be achieved through the formation of collaborative efforts and partnerships.

Graduate/Postgraduate Certificate Programs

Graduate certificate programs, also referred to as postgraduate certificate programs, are available to advanced practice nurses who already have a master's degree or a DNP degree and want to add another specialty focus to their current practice as an APRN. For example, a nurse prepared as a family NP may return to school to obtain a postgraduate certificate in psych-mental health. This additional education will allow the nurse to sit for certification as a psych-mental health NP and then to provide services within the scope of practice for both specialties. This approach is especially useful for nurses who practice in rural and community settings such as clinics or emergency rooms.

Postgraduate certificates are available in other specialties besides advanced practice areas. For example, nurses may return to school to obtain postgraduate certificate in nursing education, leadership, health care informatics, palliative care, or health care ethics, just to cite a few possibilities, thus enhancing their career options.

Professional standards exist to help guide faculty in the curricular design of postgraduate certificate programs for NP programs. Faculty who develop curricula for a postgraduate certificate program for NPs prepared in a different specialty use the criteria provided in the *Standards for Quality Nurse Practitioner Education* (NTF, 2022) to evaluate the knowledge and skills needed for the advanced practice nurse to obtain a postgraduate certificate in another NP specialty. Typically, this is done using a gap-analysis process, which compares the applicant's previous education and work experiences with expected outcomes of another specialty. This process supports the rigor of a program offering while providing the applicant with credit for work already completed.

Academic Progression for Doctoral Programs: BSN to PhD and BSN to DNP

A number of academic progression models are being developed to specifically facilitate acquisition of a doctoral degree earlier in a nurse's career. Typically, in the nursing profession, individuals return to school to seek a doctorate after years in practice. Although this work experience is beneficial to the individual and to nursing, nurses can be more effective at advancing the profession by achieving doctoral degrees earlier in their careers. Thus BSN to PhD and BSN to DNP program models have developed, and nurses who are relatively new to the profession are being encouraged to enter these programs earlier in their careers. Some programs also offer DNP to PhD certificates or degrees for students who wish to combine their practice skills with a research focus.

One of the challenges facing nurses who want to apply to a nursing doctoral program is how to select the best program for them. Should they obtain a PhD, which would prepare them as a nurse scientist, or should they obtain a DNP, which would prepare them to translate knowledge into practice? It is important that they consider their career goals and aspirations when selecting doctoral programs. Faculty can help applicants understand their options, and whether a PhD program or DNP program is best for that person.

REGULATION OF THE APRN ROLE

As graduate programs preparing advanced practice nurses expanded enrollment and produced corresponding growth in the APRN workforce, it became apparent that uniformity in preparing and credentialing APRNs was needed. Drawing on collaboration from professional nursing organizations, regulatory agencies, and accrediting bodies, the APRN *Consensus Model for APRN Regulation: Licensure, Accreditation, Certification & Education* was developed. The purpose of this model is to describe regulatory requirements in four areas: licensure, accreditation, certification, and education (LACE). Several important outcomes related to APRN education have resulted from these collaborative efforst.

National Organization of Nurse Practitioner Faculties

The National Organization of Nurse Practitioner Faculties (NONPF) is an organization formed by NP faculty to promote quality NP education, influence policy to advance NP education, foster diversity, promote scholarship of NP educators, and strengthen resources to sustain NONPF. Along with the National Council of State Boards of Nursing (NCSBN) and other professional organizations, NONPF has been instrumental in leading the development of the APRN Consensus Model. In 2009 NONPF conducted a study, funded by NCSBN, focused on clarification of NP titles, clinical hours, and credentialing. The outcomes of this study identified inconsistency in how higher education institutions market programs, offerings for specialty and subspecialty tracks, and titling of

the same. Adoption of the consensus model would move institutions toward an approach that is standardized (NONPF, 2021). In 2009 NONPF offered clarity on the NP role and in 2011 a position statement on the distinction of acute and primary care NP roles with amendment in 2013. The consensus model provided the framework for these writings, as well as reference for implementation of the model (NONPF, 2021).

NONPF developed the first core competencies for NPs in 1990, with subsequent revisions including the current competencies applying to all entry to practice NPs regardless of a master's or doctoral degree, in 2017. Since 1995, NONPF has worked closely with NTF to provide resources for faculty and program evaluation guidelines for NP programs. As with the core competencies, there have been revisions over the years. The 6th edition, titled *2022 Standards for Quality Nurse Practitioner Education*, was approved in April of 2022 (https://www.aacnnursing.org/Portals/42/CCNE/PDF/NTFS-NP-Final.pdf).

The APRN Consensus Model

LACE are the essential components to preparing and transitioning an APRN to practice. Individual state licensing boards hold the final decision regarding who is licensed as an APRN, as well as role recognition, scope of practice, and criteria for entry to practice, including certification options. Variability in regulatory requirements has created obstacles for APRNs to move from state to state and has placed limitations on patient access to APRN care. In 2008, with a focus on uniform APRN regulation and a goal of allowing APRNs to practice to the full extent of their education, a consensus model was developed. This model, developed thorough the collaboration of 40 nursing organizations, provides a framework for regulation, ensures patient safety, and serves to improve access to APRN care. If adopted, it allows APRN license portability and mobility between states. The model uses a 28-point scoring system to determine state progress toward adopting model requirements. This scoring system allows one point for adopting each of the seven components for each role (Box 9.1). The target to fully implement this model by 2015 has not been met (NCSBN, 2022a,b). As of January 2022, 26

BOX 9.1 Components of APRN Consensus Model

Title	APRN–Advanced Practice Registered Nurse
Roles	CNP–Certified Nurse Practitioner CNS–Clinical Nurse Specialist CRNA–Certified Registered Nurse Anesthetist CNM–Certified Nurse Midwife
License	RN and Advanced Practice Licensure
Education	Graduate education
Certification	Successful completion of national certification examination
Independent Practice	Full independence to practice without MD oversight
Full prescriptive authority	Full prescriptive authority without MD oversight or collaborative agreement

states, Guam and the Northern Mariana Islands had received 28 points making them 100% eligible for implementation, yet only North Dakota and Delaware were considered compact states (https://www.ncsbn.org/APRN_Consensus_Grid_January2022-1.14.22.pdf).

Institute of Medicine/National Academy of Medicine Reports

The Institute of Medicine was established in 1970, and in 2015 became the National Academy of Medicine, one of three academies under the National Academies of Sciences, Engineering, and Medicine (National Academies) umbrella (NAM, 2021). The mission of the National Academies has been and continues to be to promote health by advancing science and technology (NAM, 2021). Several landmark reports examining the state of health care in the United States have offered recommendations for changes in the health care system and education of professionals working in these systems, including advanced practice nurses. They were published by the Institute of Medicine (IOM), beginning in the late 1990s. These reports have stimulated many changes within graduate nursing programs to meet the needs of society.

Crossing the Quality Chasm (IOM, 2001) identified the need for restructuring the health care system to promote safe, effective, timely, efficient, and equitable health care. In 2003 the IOM recommended that all health professionals be educated to deliver evidence-based, patient-centered care and that all professionals work in interdisciplinary teams using quality improvement strategies and informatics. In 2011, with the support of the Robert Wood Johnson Foundation, the IOM published *The Future of Nursing: Leading the Change, Advancing Health*. In this document, recommendations were made to strengthen health care and health care delivery including areas focused on health care professional education (IOM, 2011). Specifically important to graduate education are the recommendations for full practice authority, seamless academic progression, full partnership with other members of the health care team, and doubling the number of doctorally prepared nurses by 2020 (IOM, 2011). In 2021 the National Academies released the report titled *The Future of Nursing Report, 2020–2030: Charting a Path to Achieve Health Equity* (National Academies of Sciences, Engineering and Medicine, 2021). This report builds on the 2011 publication and reinforces nursing's role in impacting noticeable change on health, health care, and health care delivery. Specifically called out is the area of health equity which ties the importance of APRN practice authority and the consensus model to improve access and quality of care (NCSBN, 2021). The report calls for education to examine curricula for opportunities to strengthen the future clinician's ability to navigate difficult and complicated cases that are impacted by health disparities related to social, economic, and environmental issues.

CURRICULUM DEVELOPMENT FOR GRADUATE PROGRAMS

Graduate-level programs build on the mission and philosophy of the school of nursing in which the program resides. Faculty teaching in graduate programs are responsible and accountable for designing, implementing, and evaluating the curriculum (AACN, 2018).

As graduate programs are developed, faculty must determine which professional standards are appropriate for incorporation into the curriculum as established for a particular specialty. For example, the AACN developed *The Essentials of Master's Education* (AACN, 2011) and *The Essentials of Doctoral Education for Advanced Practice* (AACN, 2006), which faculty have used when developing graduate programs. The most newly adopted document, *The Essentials: Core Competencies for Professional Nursing Education* (AACN, 2021a), provides the most current standards for advanced practice nursing and will be gradually phased in by graduate nursing programs over the next few years. The NLN has established scope of practice and competency statements for nurse educators: academic nurse educators, academic clinical nurse educators, and novice academic nurse educators (NLN, 2020).

These competencies for nurse educators are used to guide graduate curriculum development for nurse educator programs.

NONPF (2017) has established core competencies for NP curricula and the National Task Force on Quality Nurse Practitioner Education (NTF, 2016; 2022) established criteria for the evaluation of NP programs. Programs that prepare APRNs are required to provide a stipulated number of clinical hours in the students' program and to maintain student-faculty clinical ratios that follow the national guidelines (NTF, 2016; 2021). A minimum of 500 clinical hours of supervised direct patient care has traditionally served as the minimum expectation for NPs. The 2021 NTF criteria revisions called for 1,000 hours, which had been a source of concern for some schools and organizations within the profession. For example, the NLN provided a response to the NTF criteria citing lack of evidence to support the recommendation and "unintended consequences" to include impact on goals to increase diversity and additional cost to both students and institutions that will be required to secure additional clinical faculty, sites, and preceptors, all during a shortage of available faculty (NLN, 2021). The *2022 NTF Standards for Quality Nurse Practitioner Education*, endorsed by multiple national organizations in April 2022, stipulates that a minimum of 750 direct patient care clinical hours be required.

National certification is available for all NP specialties in addition to CNLs, nurse educators, nurse administrators, and nurse informaticists. It is an expectation, by most programs, that graduates will complete national certification whether required for employment or not. National certification is required for all APRNs, and it is an expectation that the curriculum of graduate programs preparing APRNs will design the curriculum in such a way that their graduates will be eligible to take the certification examination for their specialty area.

Curriculum Design for Graduate Programs

Rapid changes in health care demand that traditional curriculum designs for graduate nursing education, which have historically been content based, be transformed to meet evolving changes in the health care environment. Various curriculum designs are emerging in response to this need.

Competency-Based Curriculum Design

A key curriculum design that needs to be considered in the development of graduate programs is the competency-based curriculum. This is an expectation in the newest *The Essentials: Core Competencies for Professional Nursing Education* document (AACN, 2021a). A competency-based curriculum focuses on the knowledge, skills, and attitudes that encompass professional nursing practice and begins with agreement from stakeholders on the expected outcomes and associated competencies, and it ends with implementation and evaluation of the outcomes. Because this design is cyclical, there is no true ending to the process. As the health care environment changes and places new demands on health care practitioners, outcomes and competencies are updated as programs are required to adapt to ensure that new competencies are taught and evaluated.

Collaborative Curriculum Designs

Collaborative curricular designs can be adapted to improve efficiency within schools of nursing that offer multiple specialties at the master's or doctoral level. This is especially critical given the shortage of nurse faculty that exists today. Collaborative curricula are designed to meet the common needs of learners across specialties. The faculty of each graduate specialty examines their curriculum plans, identifies common outcomes and competencies, and then designs a graduate curriculum that shares content, as appropriate, across specialties. This can increase the efficiency within a school that prepares NPs for several specialties. This type of design calls for core courses such as pharmacology and health assessment to be taught across the specialty programs and then population-focused courses to be taught within the specialty. This design mandates that faculty critically examine the overlaps in content and determine methods of teaching that promote collaboration among nursing faculty while streamlining content that is population specific.

Another example of a collaborative curriculum design, and likely the forerunner of the dual doctoral degree trend, is the collaboration of PhD and DNP students working together on their final program projects, such as dissertation and capstone projects (Eaton et al., 2017). This type of collaboration necessitates faculty within the same school/college to understand the differences in the two types of doctoral program outcomes while also educating students on how to work together after graduation so that knowledge and evidence are synthesized and practice outcomes are improved.

The Nursing Education Xchange (https://winnexus.org) is another example of a collaborative model that has been established as a national consortium to offer courses for PhD and DNP programs. Schools of nursing participate in the consortium by contributing online courses and faculty to teach them and by making these courses available to students in participating schools. As a result of the consortium, a greater variety of courses are available than any one school might be able to offer its students (Eaton et al., 2017).

TEACHING IN GRADUATE PROGRAMS

The quality of graduate nursing education programs is maintained through the appointment and selection of well-qualified faculty. According to AACN, in 2019, faculty vacancies in the United States were almost 8%, with over 50% as full-time positions and more than 90% either preferring or requiring doctoral preparation (AACN,

2020a,c). Adding to this information that less than 3% of nurses hold PhD or DNP degrees, it is no wonder that the nursing profession has a faculty shortage.

Many graduate programs include curriculum focused on clinical and administrative emphasis rather than teaching, and this has likely contributed, among other issues, to the shortage of doctorally prepared faculty (Harris, 2019). Faculty who teach in graduate programs must hold at minimum a master's degree, and for those teaching in an APRN specialty area, clinical expertise with certification, and current practice is an expectation. In addition to clinical expertise, faculty teaching in a DNP program should have the requisite experience to teach the courses for which they are responsible. Depending on the curriculum, this can include such topics as health policy, epidemiology, complexity science, leadership in complex systems, and health care technology.

Given the nature of the curriculum in DNP programs, it is likely that the faculty will be interdisciplinary in nature. Faculty who teach in PhD programs are expected to have an active research program to mentor PhD students in their development as nurse scientists, and in research-intensive institutions there may be funding expectations. There must be a critical mass of faculty in a school of nursing who are active researchers to support a PhD program. Faculty must be both excellent teachers and scholars to effectively guide and advise students in their development as researchers. As members of the scientific community, faculty disseminate their research findings through publications in peer-reviewed journals and presentations at scientific conferences. PhD students learn by participating with their faculty in their research and dissemination of the findings (Joseph et al., 2021).

Assessing Graduate Student Readiness for Progression and Graduation

Teaching in graduate programs is both challenging and rewarding. Many issues appear that require faculty to have skillful conversations about what is best for the program and to ensure that students have the knowledge and skills necessary for the career they are planning.

One such example is faculty responsibilities related to the qualifying examination. It is common for students enrolled in a PhD program to take a qualifying examination. This exam is designed to test the student's knowledge of a field and the critical and analytical skills needed for success as a researcher and scholar. Although the requirements for both the qualifying examination and dissertation vary with institutions, it is a common expectation that faculty will serve as mentors, advisors, and chairs for students. Typically a faculty member is assigned the role of major advisor to a PhD student and has the responsibility to guide the student in course selection and formation of a minor concentration and, in general, serve as a resource as the student progresses through the curriculum. Major faculty advisors may chair the qualifying examination committee, bearing primary responsibility for developing the examination according to the school's policies. The major faculty advisor may also chair the dissertation committee and guide the student in the selection of other dissertation committee members.

In some schools it is the student's responsibility to select a dissertation chair and committee members. Regardless of the selection process, it is the responsibility of the qualifying examination and dissertation committee members to ensure that the student has met the expected competencies and outcomes of the PhD program and is ready to graduate. It is important that the graduate faculty have collectively determined the expected outcomes of the program so that evaluating student outcomes can be accomplished with some measure of objectivity.

Progression and graduation requirements for students enrolled in DNP programs tend to vary based on the expected program outcomes. Some programs follow a format similar to the PhD programs and require a student to take a comprehensive examination before progressing to a scholarly inquiry project. The comprehensive examination process may include a written examination, a self-reflection synthesis demonstrating integration and synthesis of all coursework and practice activities, and an oral examination. Other DNP programs do not require a comprehensive examination. However, all DNP programs require the student to complete a scholarly inquiry project that is designed to improve health care delivery or form health policy. Some schools recognize the scholarly inquiry project as a comprehensive examination that ensures competence of DNP students. The DNP final project must meet specific guidelines. The submission of an integrative or systematic review, portfolio, or group/team project does not meet the expectations of scholarly work at this level. Box 9.2 offers a list of requirements for the final DNP project as outlined by the AACN Essentials (2021).

For students advancing to clinical practice, DNP residencies and fellowships have been identified as beneficial, but there is debate about where these are best placed, pre- or postgraduation. If placed pregraduation, the cost is covered by the student; if postgraduation, the cost is often absorbed by the employer (McCauley et al., 2020).

Preparing Faculty to Teach at the Graduate Level

Preparing faculty to teach at the graduate level is a challenge faced by all schools of nursing. There are a number of factors that play into recruitment and retention of qualified faculty to teach in graduate programs including workload, mentor support, and ability to maintain clinical practice. Additional barriers include the areas of financial obligations for academic preparation and noncompetitive faculty salaries (Harris, 2019). With the current shortage of nursing faculty, it is imperative that nurses who want to teach are prepared for the role.

BOX 9.2 Inclusion Items for DNP Final Project

- Identify an area of interest with clinical importance and practice value
- Include areas of planning, implementation, evaluation, sustainability, and implications for future study
- Identify change that impacts outcomes
- Include requisite systems focus
- Illustrate implementation
- Identify a sustainability plan
- Demonstrate an evaluation process
- Provide groundwork for future inquiry

Successful teaching at the doctoral level, in particular, requires a unique skill set. In addition to a solid foundation in nursing science, research, and scholarship, strong writing and oral skills, and a firm grasp on societal, policy, and ethical issues affecting their area of scholarly expertise, faculty need to be able to impart that knowledge and mentor students in the beginning development of their own program of research or clinical practice expertise. Developing such a relationship with students requires a commitment of time and energy to help students conceptualize their research or clinical projects and implement them successfully. It is also important for faculty to be skilled in teamwork and negotiation to help them participate in dissertation and project committees in a manner that is supportive to students and creates an environment for objective evaluation of student outcomes. Faculty who are new to teaching at the graduate level, especially in doctoral education, will require mentoring of their own to help them adjust to the role.

Not all individuals hired into a faculty role have pedagogical course work as part of their graduate program to help them prepare for the educator role. To be effective educators, faculty must be prepared in the science of pedagogy for both classroom and clinical teaching. Some schools deal with this issue by requiring that new faculty take courses to prepare them with the knowledge and skills necessary to teach using a variety of strategies that promote active engagement of students. Effective clinical supervision is another area for faculty skills development. Finally, faculty new to the teaching role in APRN programs must learn how to work effectively with preceptors and understand the responsibilities of the student, preceptor, and faculty in the precepting relationship. If faculty do not take formal course work in nursing education, it is important to establish faculty development programs that provide new faculty with the skills and knowledge needed for success in the teaching role at the graduate level. Mentoring by experienced educators is essential to promote the success of faculty moving into teaching at this level.

Graduate faculty must balance the roles of teaching, practice, scholarship, and service to advance their own careers in academia. Experienced doctoral faculty are required to mentor younger doctoral faculty on how to be successful in all of these areas. Aging faculty may positively contribute as coaches and through their many years of experience, leadership, and teaching. Interprofessional teaching opportunities offer additional avenues for support as new faculty transition into their roles. Faculty teaching in PhD programs must be scholars who can not only mentor and coach younger research scholars in teaching PhD students but additionally support new faculty in conducting and disseminating their own research through grant development and implementation, publication in peer-reviewed journals, and presentations at scientific meetings. Faculty teaching in DNP programs must be scholars who can mentor and coach younger DNP-prepared faculty to teach, practice, and develop and implement scholarly projects and disseminate their scholarly projects through publication in peer-reviewed journals and presentations at appropriate meetings. Developing teaching skills and practice skills in faculty who enter academia after completing a BSN to DNP or BSN to PhD program must be considered when developing a program to assist faculty to be successful in academia. Faculty development needs to ensure success in the teaching role vary depending on the individual requiring individualized plans to help each person be successful.

FUTURE TRENDS IN GRADUATE EDUCATION

Nursing education, and especially graduate nursing education, takes place within a broader social context. It is essential that institutions offering graduate nursing programs stay abreast of opportunities that will contribute to generating graduates ready for a complex practice environment.

Graduate students have demonstrated an increased interest in online and asynchronous learning, which tends to offer more flexibility for working and nurses living in rural environments. Harlan et al. (2021) indicated that the top five preferred teaching strategies for online coursework include PowerPoints with voiceover, case studies, demonstrations, guest speakers, and simulations.

While PowerPoint lecture is losing favor in most learning environments, the rationale posed for this strategy is to target audience access by impacting more than one sense (visual and hearing). Other strategies identified as effective teaching options for graduate students include journal reading, debates, and discussion boards. Additional teaching trends that have been supportive for graduate programs include a greater emphasis on gaming use in flipped classrooms.

Numerous trends that affect the future of graduate education continue to emerge in health care and higher education, and faculty make changes to program curricula based on these changes. The area of telehealth, while not new, gained significant attention during the COVID-19 emergence when access to health care was limited. According to Koonin et al. (2020), telehealth use increased by 154% between 2019 and 2020. Implications to practice include access to care, reduced disease exposure for care providers and patients, and best use of resources including personal protective equipment (PPE) and patient use of facilities. This is one practice area, with positive implications, where changes are likely to be retained and where graduate nursing student preparation will be needed. Another area that is emphasized in the *Future of Nursing 2020–2030* document is the opportunity to address inequities and sociocultural inequality in health care. This will include curricula content emphasizing antibias training, cultural competency, community outreach, public health, and access to affordable care in diverse urban and rural settings.

Another area drawing attention in the same document is the importance of developing and maintaining strategic partnerships. *AACN's Vision for Academic Nursing* (2019) recommends expansion of formal academic practice partnerships. See Case Study 9.2 for further discussion of the value of partnerships. Schools are encouraged to develop strategies to promote opportunities to develop and strengthen relationships. Box 9.3 offers elements to consider when developing these partnerships.

BOX 9.3 Components of a Strong Strategic Partnership

- Clear and measurable goals with timelines
- Outline mutual expectations
- Mutual planning and collaborative efforts
- Open communication
- Formative and summative evaluations
- Balance of power

CASE STUDY 9.2 The Value of Partnerships

One rural public institution with a long history of offering nursing programs including PhD and MSN degree programs decided to move forward with adding a postmaster's DNP in the early 2000s. By mid-2000, the institution was facing severe state budget cuts and difficulty recruiting doctorally prepared faculty. With strong community support, including some well-established strategic partnerships, and faculty interest in supporting this initiative, planning continued. Long-standing faculty who were not doctorally prepared were recruited to complete the program, as an internal mechanism for establishing a pool of doctorally prepared DNP faculty. The institution has for many years offered distance learning and hybrid courses for the Masters and PhD program, and this format was utilized for the DNP as well. The institution has statewide partnerships including many in rural areas where nurses may not have had access to higher education without the distance learning option. Thus the hybrid format was attractive to many students residing in rural communities. For the partners, this offered an opportunity to gain well-trained and educated advanced practice nurses who could fill patient access issues. Additionally, for the institution, this approach reduced clinical placement challenges, as relationships were established and mutual planning had occurred.

1. One of the barriers associated with clinical placement in rural settings is a lack of confidence and experience in practitioners serving as preceptors for NP students. What resources and trainings would be helpful in supporting new clinical preceptors, especially those in rural settings?
2. Mutual and shared goals are essential to the success of clinical partnerships. What areas of focus should be addressed in establishing and maintaining collaborative relationships?

CHAPTER SUMMARY: KEY POINTS

- Challenges to current teaching models for graduate nursing students include the changing higher education climate, variable learning styles of students, and public expectation for practice-ready advanced practice nurses.
- Formal graduate nursing education has been available since the 1930s, progressing to include advanced practice specialty categories for nurse practitioners, clinical nurse specialists, certified nurse anesthetists, and certified nurse midwives.
- Other graduate nursing specialty areas include public health nursing, nurse informaticist, and focus in the areas of leadership, education, genetics, and forensics.
- The DNP is a practice-focused terminal degree focused on specialty areas of advanced practice. Starting in early 2000, it has continued to grow in popularity with the degree option available in all states.
- The PhD is designed to prepare nurse scientists as researchers. PhD students are recommended to select a program where the student research interest aligns with that of the faculty.
- A new degree, the doctorate in nursing education (DNE), has been proposed to focus specifically on nursing education focus rather than an additional content area for existing DNP and PhD programs.
- Appointment of well-qualified faculty to teach in graduate nursing programs continues to be a concern. Contributing factors include workload, administrative support, noncompetitive salaries, and clinical practice hour requirements.
- Graduate curricula are moving from a content-based format to a competency- or outcomes-based format.
- Nurse educators are provided direction through professional standards for graduate curriculum, including those offered for core competencies and those for specialty areas.
- Graduate program accreditation is offered through the Accreditation Commission for Education in Nursing (ACEN), the National League for Nursing Commission for Nursing Education (NLN CNEA), and the Commission on Collegiate Nursing Education (CCNE).
- The APRN Consensus Model is aimed at providing uniformity in licensure, accreditation, certification, and education between states and ensuring mobility to practice between states. As of January 2022, only 26 states, Guam and Northern Mariana Islands have reached a point of readiness to adopt the model.

REFLECTING ON THE EVIDENCE

1. Think about your current graduate program affiliations. Do you have strong community support and strategic partnerships? What factors have influenced the success of these partnerships? How could they be strengthened?
2. What are the areas of your graduate nursing program where you notice adjustments are needed to prepare students to promote health equity, reduce health disparities, and improve population health?
3. Think about your current graduate program admission requirements. Are they supportive of academic progression, or do they pose barriers?
4. Do you think that one year of full-time practice should be a requirement to enter an advanced practice program? Why or why not?
5. A dual PhD–DNP degree has gained support. How do you envision this credential being utilized in the workforce?
6. There is a lack of clarity regarding where nursing education belongs in nursing programs, and there is discussion about the benefits of a doctorate in nursing education (DNE) degree that would serve as a terminal practice degree for nursing education. What do you think about this proposed degree? Do you think it would positively or negatively impact the DNP and PhD?

REFERENCES

American Association of Colleges of Nursing (AACN). (2006). *The essentials of doctoral education for advanced practice.* https://www.aacnnursing.org/DNP/DNP-Essentials

American Association of Colleges of Nursing (AACN). (2011). *The essentials of master's education in nursing.* https://www.aacnnursing.org/Portals/42/Publications/MastersEssentials11.pdf.

American Association of Colleges of Nursing (AACN). (2018). *Standards, procedures, & guidelines.* https://www.aacnnursing.org/CCNE-Accreditation/Accreditation-Resources/Standards-Procedures-Guidelines

American Association of Colleges of Nursing (AACN). (2020a). *Fact sheet: Nursing faculty shortage.* https://www.aacnnursing.org/portals/42/news/fact-sheets/faculty-shortage-factsheet.pdf

American Association of Colleges of Nursing (AACN). (2020b). *DNP fact sheet.* https://www.aacnnursing.org/News-Information/Fact-Sheets/DNP-Fact-Sheet

American Association of Colleges of Nursing (AACN). (2020c). *Special survey on vacant faculty positions for academic year 2018–2019.* https://www.aacnnursing.org/Portals/42/News/Surveys-Data/Vacancy18.pdf

American Association of Colleges of Nursing (AACN). (2020d). *DNP trends in enrollment and graduation.* https://www.aacnnursing.org/Portals/42/Downloads/Board/DNP-Data-Sheet.pdf

American Association of Colleges of Nursing (AACN). (2021a). *The essentials: Core competencies for professional nursing education.* https://www.aacnnursing.org/AACN-Essentials

American Association of Colleges of Nursing (AACN). (2021b). *Commission on nurse certification.* https://www.aacnnursing.org/portals/42/CNL/CNLStats.pdf

American Association of Colleges of Nursing (AACN). (2022a). *APRN education.* https://www.aacnnursing.org/Teaching-Resources/APRN

American Association of Colleges of Nursing (AACN). (2022b). *Doctor of nursing practice (DNP) tool kit.* Retrieved from https://www.aacnnursing.org/DNP/Tool-Kit

American Association of Colleges of Nursing (AACN). (2022c). *Clinical nurse leader: About the CNL.* https://www.aacnnursing.org/CNL/About

American Association of Colleges of Nursing (AACN). (2022d). *Master's education.* https://www.aacnnursing.org/Nursing-Education-Programs/Masters-Education

American Association of Colleges of Nursing (AACN). (2022e). *PhD education.* https://www.aacnnursing.org/Nursing-Education-Programs/PhD-Education

American College of Nurse Midwives (ACNM). (2019). *Position statement.* http://www.midwife.org/acnm/files/acnmlibrarydata/uploadfilename/000000000079/PS%20Midwifery%20Education%20and%20Doctoral%20Preparation%2020190927.pdf

AMN Healthcare. (2018). *Survey of millennial nurses.* https://www.amnhealthcare.com/amn-insights/nursing/surveys/survey-of-millennial-nurses-2018/

Council on Accreditation. (2020). *Position statements.* https://www.coacrna.org/about-coa/position-statements/

Eaton, L., Gordon, D., & Doorenbos, A. (2017). Innovation in learning: PhD and DNP student collaborations. *Journal of Nursing Education, 56*(9), 556–559.

Egenes, K. (2018). History of nursing. In G. Roux & J. Halstead (Eds.), *Issues and trends in nursing: Practice, policy, and leadership* (pp. 3–27). Jones & Bartlett.

Ervin, S. (2018). History of nursing education in the United States. In S. Keating & S. Deboor (Eds.), *Keating's curriculum development and evaluation in nursing education* (pp. 5–28). https://doi.org/10.1891/9780826186867

Gerardi, T. (2017). The academic progression in nursing initiative: The final year outcomes. *Journal of Nursing Administration, 47*(2), 74–78.

Graves, J. M., Postma, J., Katz, J. R., Kehoe, L., Swalling, E., & Barbosa-Leiker, C. (2018). A national survey examining manuscript dissertation formats among nursing PhD programs in the United States. *Journal of Nursing Scholarship, 50*, 314–323. https://doi.org/10.1111/jnu.12374.

Graves, L. Y., Tamez, P., Wallen, G. R., & Saligan, L. N. (2021). Defining the role of individuals prepared as a doctor of nurse practice in symptoms science research. *Nursing Outlook, 69*(4), 542–549. https://doi.org/10.1016/j.outlook.2021.01.013. Epub 2021 Mar 6. PMID: 33750612; PMCID: PMC8410634.

Harlan, M., Roszenweig, M., & Hoffman, R. (2021). Preferred teaching/learning strategies for graduate nursing students in wen-enhanced courses. *Dimensions of Critical Care Nursing: DCCN, 40*(3), 149–155.

Harris, J. (2019). Challenges of nursing faculty retention. *The Midwest Quarterly, 60*(3), 251–270.

Institute of Medicine (IOM), (2001). *Crossing the quality chasm: A new health system for the 21st century.* National Academies Press.

Institute of Medicine (IOM), (2011). *The future of nursing: Leading change, advancing health.* National Academies Press.

Joseph, P., McCauley, L., & Richmond, T. (2021). PhD programs and the advancement of nursing science. *Journal of Professional Nursing, 37*(1), 195–200.

King, T. S., Melnyk, B. M., O'Brien, T., Bowles, W., Schubert, C., Fletcher, L., & Anderson, C. M. (2020). Doctoral degree preferences for nurse educators: Findings from a national study. *Nurse Educator, 45*(3), 144–149.

Koonin, L. M., Hoots, B., Tsang, C. A., et al. (2020). Trends in the use of Telehealth during the emergence of the COVID-19 pandemic—United States, January–March 2020. *Morbidity and Mortality Weekly Report, 69*, 595–1599. http://doi.org/10.15585/mmwr.mm6943a3 external icon.

Loescher, L., Love, R., & Bdger, T. (2021). Breaking new ground? The dual (PhD-DNP) doctoral degree in nursing. *Journal of Professional Nursing, 37*(2), 429–434.

McCauley, L. A., Broome, M. E., Frazier, L., Hayes, R., Kurth, A., Musil, C. M., Norman, L. D., Rideout, K. H., & Villarruel, A. M. (2020). Doctor of nursing practice (DNP) degree in the United States: Reflecting, readjusting, and getting back on track. *Nursing Outlook, 68*(4), 494–503. https://doi.org/10.1016/j.outlook.2020.03.008.

Mohr, L. D., & Coke, L. A. (2018). Distinguishing the clinical nurse specialist from other graduate nursing roles. *Clin Nurse Spec, 32*(3), 139–151.

National Academies of Sciences, Engineering and Medicine. (2021). *The future of nursing 2020–2030: Charting a path to achieve health equity.* https://www.nationalacademies.org/our-work/the-future-of-nursing-2020-2030#:~:text=Nurses%20play%20a%20key%20role%20in%20the%20health%20system.&text=The%20National%20Academy%20of%20Medicine,family%2Dfocused%20care%20into%202030

National Academy of Medicine (NAM). (2021). *About the national academy of medicine.* https://nam.edu/about-the-nam/

National Council of State Board of Nursing (NCSBN). (2021). *Policy briefing-the future of nursing report 2020–2030: Charting a path to achieve health equity.* https://www.ncsbn.org/15924.htm

National Council of State Board of Nursing. (2022a). *APRN consensus grid January 2022.* https://www.ncsbn.org/APRN_Consensus_Grid_January2022-1.14.22.pdf

National Council of State Board of Nursing. (2022b). *APRN campaign for consensus: Moving toward uniformity in state laws.* https://www.ncsbn.org/campaign-for-consensus.htm

National League for Nursing (NLN) (2020). *Nurse educator core competencies.* http://www.nln.org/professional-development-programs/competencies-for-nursing-education/nurse-educator-core-competency

National League for Nursing (NLN) (2021). *NLN response to the criteria for the evaluation of nurse practitioner programs* (6th ed.). http://www.nln.org/newsroom/news-releases/news-release/2021/09/03/nln-response-to-the-criteria-for-evaluation-of-nurse-practitioner-programs-(6th-ed)

National Organization of Nurse Practitioner Faculty (NONPF). (2017). *Nurse practitioner core competencies.* http://c.ymcdn.com/sites/www.nonpf.org/resource/resmgr/competencies/npcorecompetenciesfinal2012.pdf

National Organization of Nurse Practitioner Faculty (NONPF). (2018). *The doctor of nursing practice degree: Entry to nurse practitioner practice by 2025.* https://cdn.ymaws.com/www.nonpf.org/resource/resmgr/dnp/v3_05.2018_NONPF_DNP_Stateme.pdf

National Organization of Nurse Practitioner Faculty (NONPF). (2021). *Consensus model for APRN regulation.* https://www.nonpf.org/page/26?&hhsearchterms=%22consensus+and+model%22

National Task Force on Quality Nurse Practitioner Education (NTF). (2016). *Criteria for evaluation of nurse practitioner programs.* https://www.nonpf.org/page/15.

National Task Force on Quality Nurse Practitioner Education (NTF). (2022). *Standards for quality nurse practitioner education* (6th ed.). https://www.aacnnursing.org/Portals/42/CCNE/PDF/NTFS-NP-Final.pdf

National Task Force (NTF). *APRN roundtable (2021). The updated national task force criteria for evaluation of nurse practitioner programs.* https://www.ncsbn.org/2021_APRN-Roundtable-MBBigley.pdf

Oermann, M., & Spalia King, T. (Hosts). (2019, December 11). *Doctor of Nursing Education: Proposed new degree in nursing* [Audio podcast episode]. In nurse educator podcast-nurse educator tips for teaching. Nurse Educator. https://nurseeducatorpodcast.libsyn.com/doctor-of-nursing-education-proposed-new-degree-in-nursing

Penn Nursing News Archives. (2020). *Re-envisioning the nursing PhD degree.* https://www.nursing.upenn.edu/details/news.php?id=1865

Robert Wood Johnson Foundation (RWJF). (2013). *The case for academic progression: Why nurses should advance their education and the strategies that make this feasible.* http://www.rwjf.org/content/dam/farm/reports/issue_briefs/2013/rwjf407597

Scheckel, M. (2018). Nursing education: Past, present, and future. In G. Roux & J. Halstead (Eds.), *Issues and trends in nursing: Practice, policy, and leadership* (pp. 31–61). Jones & Bartlett.

Tyczkowski, B., & Reilly, J. (2017). DNP-prepared nurse leaders: Part of the solution to the growing faculty shortage. *The Journal of Nursing Administration, 47*(7/8), 359–360.

United States Department of Health, Education, and Welfare. (1963). *Toward quality in nursing: Needs and goals.* https://play.google.com/books/reader?id=ZCFtAAAAMAAJ&pg=GBS.PP2&hl=en

United States Department of Veterans Affairs (2016). *Office of nursing services (ONS): Clinical nurse leader (CNL).* https://www.va.gov/NURSING/practice/cnl.asp

10

Designing Courses and Learning Experiences

Martha Scheckel, PhD, RN

The purpose of the curriculum is to create a learning environment that presents students with a cohesive body of knowledge, attitudes, and skills necessary for professional nursing practice. The curriculum is implemented by and for faculty and students through learner-centered courses and learning experiences. This chapter focuses on designing courses and learning experiences for effective implementation of the teaching–learning process, whereby students become educated for self-development and various nursing roles in society. Designing courses and learning experiences cannot be accomplished through a casual, hit-or-miss approach; instead, they must be thoughtfully and cohesively developed to provide students with the opportunities necessary to achieve the intended curriculum outcomes.

LEARNER-CENTERED COURSES

There is an increased emphasis on learning and learner-centered instruction, shifting the focus in education from teacher-centered instruction. In teacher-centered instruction teachers direct the delivery of content, often through lectures. Teaching-centered instruction has an insufficient effect on helping students learn (Patel-Junanker, 2018). Freire (2006) most notably names teacher-centered instruction "banking" education, whereby students become receptacles for information. Historically, schools of nursing have adopted banking models of education. This adoption has been largely driven by nurse educators' concerns that students need content to be prepared for nursing practice. Students do need discipline-specific

knowledge to provide safe and effective nursing care. However, an overreliance on providing content through teacher-centered instruction can impede students from integrating theory and practice, which requires active rather than passive engagement in learning (Benner et al., 2010; Neilsen, 2016; Sterner et al., 2019).

There are many ways of providing learner-centered courses in nursing education. Huston et al. (2018) suggest that students can be better prepared than they currently are for nursing practice through disruptive learner-centered innovations. According to Hutson, such innovations require teachers to move away from the podium and PowerPoints and "design and orchestrate experiences that are interactive and engaging" (p. 30) through strategies such as:

1. Asking intriguing and challenging questions
2. Assigning students to complete concept-mapping
3. Asking students to complete journaling activities
4. Using flipped classroom techniques

COURSE DESIGN PROCESS

Course design follows a sequential process, starting with course outcomes that are aligned with broader program outcomes and ending with specific lesson plans. Although a sequential process is described here, the process is, in fact, iterative and integrative as the course design unfolds. Courses may be designed by a faculty team or an individual with subject matter expertise. Instructional designers, a resource often available at teaching resource centers at many universities, are an asset to the course development process.

Predesign

Course design begins with an understanding of the learning background and experience of the students who will enroll in the course and identifying how the course fits within the overall academic program outcomes, competencies, and curriculum framework. During the predesign stage, faculty also should review any prerequisite, concurrent, or other courses if the course being developed is a part of a sequence. If the course has been taught previously, student course evaluations can provide additional insight for course revision and development.

Before writing course outcomes, faculty will find it essential to do an environmental scan and review recommendations from national health care organizations; influential reports with recommendations for nursing education; and recommendations from professional nursing organizations about essential competencies, concepts, and content related to the course. State regulatory and national accrediting agencies may also have prescriptive statements about course content and credit hour allocation.

Course Outcomes and Competencies

Course outcomes and competencies are derived from end-of-program (terminal) and program-leveled (year or semester) outcomes and indicate what students should know, be able to do, and value at the end of the course. Although faculty use terms in different ways, the term *learning outcome* (as opposed to the term *objective*) is less restrictive and more appropriate in a learner-centered environment. Regardless of the term used, these "behavioral indicators" activate the curriculum, direct the choice of learning materials, guide the development of learning activities, and communicate to students what they are expected to learn and how they will be evaluated. Course learning outcomes and competencies therefore must be written at appropriate levels to be relevant to clinical practice, easily understood by students, and guide evaluation of student attainment of the learning outcomes.

Moving From Course Content to Concepts

Once learning outcomes are written, faculty can make decisions about which concepts and content to include in the course. Typically, faculty develop and teach courses related to their expertise with the content and may be inclined to include all that is known about the subject. However, they also must design the course to fit within the curriculum and the level of practice for which the student is being prepared, emphasizing salient concepts.

To shift the focus of the course from content to concepts and prevent overburdening the course with content, faculty can design the curriculum by determining the concepts that are most linked to patient care or the phenomenon under study, using a concept-analysis approach that is organized yet intuitive to students (Giddens, 2021). Faculty create a concept-based curriculum by carefully selecting and categorizing concepts and integrating them across the curriculum. Ignatavicius (2019) describes a 12-step approach to concept-based curriculum development that begins with review and revision of the nursing program's mission and philosophy; includes development of student learning outcomes, concepts, and exemplars; and ends with selecting clinical experiences and activities that are conceptually based. According to Ignatavicius, this approach requires faculty to develop learning opportunities that include selected exemplars, which promotes deep conceptual learning. The assumption is that, in a concept-based curriculum, students make conceptual linkages in a manner that develops conceptual thinking as they progress through the curriculum (Giddens et al., 2019).

Organizing Concepts and Content Into Learning Modules

Once core concepts and concept-related content are established, the next step is to organize related material into learning modules. Learning modules can be organized in a variety of ways: using a logical sequence from beginning to end (e.g., across the lifespan or by topic), following a sequential process (e.g., the management process), sorting by complexity (from simple to complex or from concrete to abstract), using a body systems approach, or, in the instance of case-based or problem-based learning, inquiring about a particular problem. Regardless of how the concepts and content are organized, the structure should be evident to students, be consistent throughout the course, and be designed to facilitate achievement of student learning outcomes. See Box 10.1 for an example of an organizing module for a healthcare ethics, policy, and advocacy undergraduate course. Additionally, Case Study 10.1 includes an example of how to create learning modules for clinical courses.

Designing Lesson Plans

Once the learning modules are organized, faculty design lesson plans within each of the modules, which include the following general guidelines (see an example of a lesson plan in Box 10.2):

1. Purpose: Clearly and succinctly outline what students will learn, including relevance.
2. Program and Course Outcomes and Competencies: Identify program, level, and course outcomes and competencies *most* related to the lesson.
   - This identification allows students to understand the module's foci and allows faculty to determine how course lesson plans address program, level, and course outcomes and course competencies, as well as potential gaps in concept and content coverage.
3. Lesson Outcomes: Delineate what students will be able to demonstrate at the end of the lesson.
   - When writing lesson outcomes, faculty should consider what students will need to learn for "real-world" nursing practice.
4. Assignments: Describe assignments so that students understand expectations for learning experiences.
   - List all assignments in course syllabi, specifying assignment instructions and elaborating on assignments in class sessions or online forums.
   - Develop assignments to be consistent with course, program, and lesson outcomes.
   - Create assignments that include active learning strategies (see Chapter 16).
5. Evaluation strategies: Students need to be informed how faculty will measure learning and what strategies or rubrics they will use to do so.
   - It is important to link the evaluation strategies to achievement of the lesson outcomes to ensure consistency and coherency of course delivery.

BOX 10.1   Example of a Learning Module in a Healthcare Ethics, Policy, and Advocacy Course

Learning Module 1: Overview of Healthcare Ethics, Policy, and Advocacy
- History of ethics, policy, and advocacy
- Models and theories related to ethics, policy, and advocacy
- Change agency in ethics, policy, and advocacy
- Application of the principles and practices of ethics, policy, and advocacy

---

CASE STUDY 10.1   Creating Learning Modules for Clinical Courses

A group of undergraduate nursing faculty received a grant to incorporate integrative nursing principles and practices into the curriculum. To begin, they explored the literature on integrative nursing practice. To enhance their work, they also identified individuals with expertise in various healing practices and conducted deep listening sessions with them to learn about their work. They invited these content experts to coauthor the modules with faculty. During the course design process, the faculty and content experts created created modules that included: module name and purpose, program and course outcomes, and competencies related to expected student learning outcomes. Relevant readings and interactive assignments were identified. To assess student learning, formative evaluation strategies were developed, which required students to reflect upon their learning and describe how they would apply what they learned to their nursing practice.

1. Considering content-laden curricula in nursing programs, how do these modules perpetuate or mitigate content saturation?
2. Does this case study reflect a learning experience that is a disruptive learner-centered innovation?
3. How does the learning experience developed for this course illuminate the affective learning domain?

(Case study courtesy of the St. Thomas School of Nursing, St. Paul, Minnesota.)

BOX 10.2   Lesson Plan: Undergraduate Healthcare Ethics, Policy, and Advocacy Course

Module 1:

Purpose:
- Learn the historical overarching principles of ethics, policy, and advocacy as a foundation for being an agent of change in nursing practice and health care.

Selected Program Outcomes Related to the Lesson:
- Promotes the common good through ethical, moral, and socially just nursing care for people and populations through health promotion, disease prevention, and emancipatory praxis.
- Demonstrates advocacy, professionalism, and leadership skills, including leading self to lead others, self-care, lifelong learning, and clinical excellence.

Selected Course Outcome Related to the Lesson:
- Explain principles and practices of ethics, policy, and advocacy in nursing practice and health care.

Outcomes Related to This Lesson:
- Describe the history of ethics, policy, and advocacy in nursing practice and health care.
- Describe historical exemplars of nurses acting as change agents through application of ethical principles, political competence, and advocacy.

Assignments:
- Read assigned chapters in textbook

- Interview a Registered Nurse, asking the following: Describe a nurse or health care provider who influenced your ability to address and resolve an ethical dilemma; create a policy; or advocate for a patient, family, community, or group. Write a one-page deidentified summary of the story or situation, including a one-sentence summary describing how this influence was similar to or different from the historical exemplars discussed in class. Be prepared to share the story or situation and sentence in class in small groups. Each small group will report to the class what they learned about ethics, policy, and advocacy in relation to being a change agent in nursing or health care.

Evaluation Strategies:
- Interview rubric
- Group discussion rubric
- Examination #1
- Be prepared to identify:
  - historical examples of nursing's impact as change agents.
  - strategies for mentorship to develop political competence.
  - examples of the ethics of influencing policy.
  - ways to overcome barriers to advocacy.

Lesson plan example adapted from the St. Thomas School of Nursing, St. Paul, Minnesota.

University of St. Thomas Susan S. Morrison School of Nursing, St. Paul, Minnesota.

Time commitment must be considered when determining lesson plan design, with the time allotted proportional to the significance of the concepts and content, the students' ability to learn the material, and the length of the course.

DESIGNING LEARNING EXPERIENCES

Successful implementation of course designs requires careful construction of student-centered learning experiences within courses. Well-designed learning experiences provide students with the opportunity to develop higher-order thinking and clinical decision-making skills and help them synthesize content and concepts (Leighton et al., 2021). Examples of learning experiences include participating in simulations, using case studies, completing writing assignments such as journaling, analyzing narratives of patients' experiences, developing concept maps, engaging in discussions or debates, and using computer-mediated activities and resources such as computer-assisted instruction and the internet (see Chapter 16 for additional examples).

Learning experiences can be designed for use by individual students, pairs of students, or groups of students. The learning experiences can be required assignments or optional, supplemental, or remedial activities and can take place in class or online or in the clinical setting or be assigned as part of class preparation. The learning experiences should be reflected in the syllabus and be related to the achievement of the identified program outcomes and related student learning outcomes. Faculty should also ensure that they are designing learning experiences that facilitate student progression across the curriculum, enabling students to grow professionally and acquire the expected skills and competencies.

The learning experiences within lesson plans should be congruent with program, level, course, and student learning outcomes and competencies and provide information about how students will be evaluated. For example, the lesson plan in Box 10.2 states the purpose of the lesson. The purpose is linked to related program and course outcomes. Identifying student learning outcomes for each lesson plan helps students specifically understand *what* they will be able to do upon completion of the learning experience. The learning experiences or assignments reflect *how* students will acquire the expected competencies and achieve the identified student learning outcomes. The evaluation strategies describe to students how their learning will be measured and feedback about their performance provided to them.

In addition, it is important that faculty plan and organize class time so that students enjoy and benefit from a variety of learning experiences. Variety helps prevent faculty and students from becoming bored and makes it more likely that faculty can accommodate different learning style preferences. Regardless of the learning experiences, faculty should consider the three major principles when designing learning experiences:
1. Use of structured or unstructured learning experiences
2. Use of active, passive, or both passive and active learning strategies
3. Use of the learning domains (cognitive, affective, and psychomotor)

These principles are outlined in more detail in the following sections.

Structured and Unstructured Learning Experiences

When designing learning experiences, it is important to consider when to use structured or unstructured experiences. Structured learning experiences are often faculty directed and include learning strategies that guide learners through activities to meet course outcomes. Unstructured learning experiences, originating from Bruner's discovery learning (Bruner, 1977) and, more recently, *inquiry-based* learning (Lehtinen & Viiri, 2017), are designed to allow students to acquire knowledge and skill with much less specific direction from faculty while also meeting course outcomes.

Structured Learning Experiences

A structured learning experience consists of a clear, concise description of the purposes, outcomes, and competencies related to the experience and the content and processes to be used while engaged in the experience. Specific directions are provided to learners, outlining a logical sequence that indicates the steps to be followed, the time for the experience, and the method to be used to report its completion.

A well-structured learning experience allows students to function with independence and creativity while working to achieve expected learning outcomes. For example, when assigning students a reading assignment, providing specific suggestions related to the desired outcomes assists students to focus on the essential concepts. Faculty may choose from several methods for students to share outcomes related to their learning experiences. For instance, students may be asked to do the following:
1. Complete an answer sheet that will be evaluated by peers and/or faculty.
2. Write and submit a summary report addressing the concept, content, or process.
3. Present a report to the class.
4. Discuss the experience with their peers, individually or in groups.
5. Lead a discussion among their peers of the major points, issues, or problems that arose during their learning experience.

These examples can be used separately or in combination with each other. Faculty may also choose to allow the student to select the preferred method of sharing.

Unstructured Learning Experiences

Unstructured learning experiences can be an effective way to promote active learning and student engagement. Discovery learning is believed to do the following:

1. Promote a disposition toward inquiry.
2. Promote independent thinking and enhanced problem solving.
3. Stimulate student motivation and interest.
4. Improve knowledge retention.
5. Facilitate transfer of learning by stimulating the student to seek and find relationships between information and the situation at hand.

In an unstructured learning experience students may be given an assignment in which they apply their knowledge, skills, and experiences either to a specific faculty-designated situation or to a situation of their choice that fits a general profile described by faculty. The situation may be an actual event in the practice setting or an event that is depicted through simulation, case study, or a form of media. For example, a learning outcome in a community health nursing course may be for students to become familiar with the kinds of activities and interactions that occur during a community meeting. Students would be directed to attend a community-based meeting of their choosing as a participant–observer. The meeting could be a support group for a particular health problem, a meeting of constituents with their legislator, a town board meeting, or a neighborhood association meeting. Students could be given the option of describing their experience verbally in class or at a clinical conference or by writing about it in a journal. A major limitation associated with discovery learning is the need for students to adapt to self-directed learning that is student centered rather than teacher centered (Morris, 2019).

Selecting Learning Materials and Resources

Faculty have responsibility for choosing course learning materials as part of the course design process. When choosing learning materials, faculty should consider how the materials will support students' learning needs and the achievement of expected learning outcomes. The selected learning materials should also be aligned with the course design and the program's teaching and learning philosophy. Ensuring easy access to materials and instructions on their use, providing rationale for selected readings, and explaining how the materials relate to course concepts and evaluation methods are ways to effectively use learning materials to support students' learning needs.

In addition, faculty need to consider the best use of prepackaged resources offered by textbook companies and other publishers. Such materials require a thorough review and critique by faculty before deciding to adopt them for use. Creating a rubric with criteria to evaluate such resources can help faculty conduct a good assessment of the utility of the materials for use in the course. This approach helps to ensure that prepackaged resources are intentionally chosen to contribute to the course's learning goals and are linked to the overall curriculum. Asking students to purchase and use prepackaged materials without a critical examination of them may be costly and result in poor learning outcomes.

It is also important for faculty to consider use of e-books. E-books have become increasingly available. Compared with print copies, e-books offer a number of advantages, such as lower costs, availability, accessibility, portability, and searchability. However, Gloekler and Lucus (2021) indicate that there is a learning curve involved in proficient use of e-books and that some nursing students may prefer print books. Nonetheless, the growth of e-books and the diversity of student learning styles necessitates that faculty prepare for use of these electronic resources.

To promote judicious use of materials and resources, faculty can develop custom-designed course packs. Faculty may find that course packs with readings that include web-based resources, selected chapters from various textbooks, and journal articles that are pertinent to the course better facilitate learning. Faculty can create course packs for print production or use e-reserve systems at the library.

When selecting learning resources and materials, faculty should consider employing learner-centered approaches to select course materials. Martin (2018), for example, suggests providing students with personal voice and choice by providing them with opportunities to access resources and create knowledge at their own pace, place, and path, which moves beyond teacher-selected use of static textbooks. Perhaps this means giving students a menu of resources to use or asking them to participate in creating such a menu.

Passive and Active Learning

In designing courses and learning experiences it is important to take into consideration theories that explain the learning process. Many of these theories are behaviorally, cognitively, or socially based and include, but are not limited to, constructivism, brain-based learning, experiential learning, and adult learning. Other learning theories are situated in phenomenology and postmodernism, among other philosophical origins. Common to each of these theories is the idea that learning may be a passive or an active process. Students typically experience both types of learning throughout their educational career. See Chapter 14 for an in-depth discussion of learning theories.

Passive Learning

Passive learning occurs when students use their senses to take in information from a lecture, reading assignment, or some form of audiovisual media. Passive learning provides faculty with the opportunity to present a great deal of information within a short period, and they can select and prepare in advance lecture notes, handouts, and audiovisual media. Faculty, especially if they are novice educators or teaching new content, usually feel more comfortable with these teaching methods because they can present the information in a controlled environment.

Because many students have been socialized to passive learning, they often prefer this approach. Important concepts and content are identified for students in a concrete manner that helps them organize the material in a meaningful way. With passive learning, students tend to have lower anxiety levels and feel secure in their belief that listening to a lecture, reading the assignments and handouts, taking notes, and copying information from audiovisual media will provide them with all or most of the information they need to be successful in the course.

However, there are disadvantages to passive learning activities. Passive learning activities may leave faculty with little opportunity to understand how well students are learning the content. Unless designed otherwise, the time used for presentation of the content may leave little time for questions, clarification, or discussion. Students may not feel comfortable letting faculty know that they do not understand key points or relationships; furthermore, they may be reluctant to ask questions in class to clarify their misunderstandings. Students may be unable to articulate what it is they do not know or understand. Additionally, listening to a presentation, taking notes, and copying from printed media require little cognitive effort from students and no consistent use of higher-level cognitive skills. Even reading activities, although important, do not provide students with opportunities to apply the concepts about which they are reading. Although many students may prefer passive learning, over time, passive learning experiences tend to become tedious.

Active Learning

Active learning "involves students 'doing things' and reflecting on what they are doing" (Misseyanni et al., 2018, p. 1). There are numerous benefits of active learning such as increasing accountability for learning, fostering a sense of belonging in the classroom, and improving perceptions of the relevance of content (Auerbach et al., 2018).

"Flipped" classrooms and team-based learning are examples of active learning strategies. The use of active learning strategies is discussed further in Chapter 16.

There can be some disadvantages associated with active learning. Faculty need to be aware of content areas and concept relationships that usually pose difficulty for students to grasp. They also need to be responsive to intercultural learning needs of students that, if not managed using culturally responsive pedagogies, can discourage active learning (Markey et al., 2021). The shift to active learning paradigms may be stressful for faculty, particularly when trying these approaches with large groups of students. Faculty may also have concerns about receiving less favorable evaluations from students. It is important for faculty to receive support from administration and their peers if active learning strategies are to be successfully incorporated into teaching practice.

DOMAINS OF LEARNING AND LEARNING EXPERIENCES

Historically, faculty use Bloom's taxonomy (Anderson & Krathwohl, 2001; Bloom, 1956) to address the cognitive, psychomotor, and affective domains of learning and identify the level at which students need to demonstrate competencies that lead to achievement of expected learning outcomes. These domains mirror the knowledge, attitudes, and skills that nursing students need to practice safely and effectively. Figs. 10.1, 10.2, and 10.3 illustrate the categories of each domain. Each domain is hierarchical, with learning presented in ascending order of complexity. When designing learning experiences, faculty need to identify the domains best suited to the learning experiences. Faculty also need to write clear and measurable learning outcomes using action verbs to express the desired domain behavior. The use of action verbs helps faculty communicate to students' expectations for achievement of outcomes. What follows is a description of each domain with examples of action verbs and learning outcomes with the verbs and an example of learning experience within each domain.

Cognitive Domain

The emphasis in the cognitive domain of learning is on knowledge. From a nursing perspective, it is important to emphasize the highly complex aspects of this domain. Example action verbs are as follows:
- Remembering: Define, list, label, select, locate, match
- Understanding: Explain, describe, interpret, summarize, predict
- Applying: Solve, apply, use, calculate, relate, change
- Analyzing: Compare, classify, differentiate
- Evaluating: Reframe, critique, support, assess
- Creating: Design, compose, create, formulate, develop

The following examples of learning outcomes in a nursing leadership and management course demonstrate how the cognitive domain can be used to depict varying levels of complexity:
1. **Identify** leadership and management theories applicable in an acute care setting. (Remembering)
2. **Describe** conflict resolution strategies to promote teamwork in an acute care setting. (Understanding)
3. **Compare** the role of a nurse manager in an acute care setting with the role of a nurse manager in a long-term care facility. (Analyzing)

An example written for a community health nursing clinical learning experience illustrates a learning outcome in the cognitive domain with a corresponding learning experience.

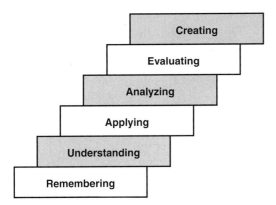

FIG. 10.1 Cognitive domain.

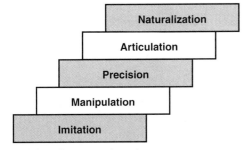

FIG. 10.2 Psychomotor domain.

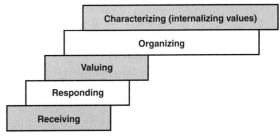

FIG. 10.3 Affective domain.

Learning outcome: Apply principles of population health to fall prevention in a community-based setting for older adults.

Learning experience: In preparation for a community-based clinical experience in a respite center for older adults, read at least two evidence-based articles about fall prevention scales designed to assess fall risk in older adults. Be prepared to discuss clinical settings where the fall prevention scales are most applicable for assessing fall risk among older adults. Following your clinical experience, briefly journal about how your experience in the respite center setting changed your view of the use of fall prevention scales in this setting and for this population. Be prepared to share your views in the post clinical conference and discuss any possible alterations needed in fall-risk assessments for this clinical setting.

This learning experience requires that students become knowledgeable about fall prevention scales for use in older adults before they have a clinical experience at the respite center. They will use this knowledge to formulate ways to conduct fall-risk assessments in community settings. The affective domain is an interdependent domain in this experience because it facilitates valuing what their knowledge of fall-risk assessment in a community setting can mean to preventing falls in the nonhospitalized older adult population.

Affective Domain

The affective domain of learning encompasses attitudes, beliefs, values, feelings, and emotions. The aspects of this domain are organized along a continuum of stages of internalization that reflect changes in personal growth, moving from an external to an internal locus of control (Krathwohl et al., 1964). Faculty often find this domain the most difficult to incorporate into learning and the most challenging to assess. Example action verbs are as follows:

- Receiving: Ask, choose, select, locate
- Responding: Discuss, perform, recite, read, help
- Valuing: Differentiate, form, justify, report, share
- Organizing: Alter, arrange, formulate, order, synthesize
- Characterizing: Propose, influence, revise, question, solve

The following examples of learning outcomes in a health assessment course demonstrate how the affective domain can be used to illustrate the acquisition of professional values and attitudes:

1. **Choose** appropriate professional communication skills when interviewing a client. (Receiving)
2. **Justify** the need for applying cultural competence skills when conducting health assessments. (Valuing)
3. **Revise** assessment approaches based on the uniqueness of the person in their environment. (Characterizing)

An example written for a community health nursing course illustrates a learning outcome in the affective domain with a corresponding learning experience.

Learning outcome: Arranges for patients and families to participate in decisions about self-care practices in the management of chronic illness.

Learning experience: Before class, read the assigned article about a patient newly diagnosed with diabetes. The patient describes the importance of learning to care for his diabetes from family members who also have diabetes. Focus on what the patient values most in learning from his family members about how to manage his self-care. In your small learning groups discuss how you might respond to the knowledge the patient has gained from his family and how to use this knowledge to design an individualized patient education plan for self-management of his diabetes.

Because this learning experience focuses on patient values and the students' responses to these values, it addresses the affective domain of learning. The cognitive domain is the interdependent domain because students need to be knowledgeable about diabetes management to design a patient education plan that discerns which aspects of the patient's knowledge gained from his family are therapeutic and which indicate further education is necessary.

Psychomotor Domain

The psychomotor domain of learning addresses the development of manual or physical competencies and is the domain that faculty use most often in developing nursing skills and competencies related to clinical practice. Students initially learn skills through imitation and manipulation and with repetition eventually internalize the skills. Internalization of skills may not occur until students gain experience as licensed nurses, where the repetition eventually requires little conscious thought. Example action verbs are as follows:

- Imitation: Repeat, imitate, follow, show
- Manipulation: Move, manipulate, assemble, display
- Precision: Be consistent, Be precise, demonstrate
- Articulation: Adapt, alter, change, connect, display
- Naturalization: Create, revise, vary, alter

The following examples of learning outcomes in a medical–surgical nursing course demonstrate how the psychomotor domain promotes skill competency development:

1. **Assemble** the supplies needed to safely and aseptically change intravenous tubing for a given patient following demonstration by a nurse preceptor. (Manipulation)
2. **Demonstrate** safe technique in the insertion of a Foley catheter on assigned patients. (Precision)
3. **Adapt** psychomotor skills to provide patient-centered care based on patient needs. (Articulation)

The following example of a simulated learning experience illustrates a learning outcome in the psychomotor domain with a corresponding learning experience.

Learning outcome: Demonstrate administration of an intravenous (IV) infusion.

Learning experience: Before demonstrating the administration of IV fluids in a simulated learning scenario, review the steps involved in IV fluid administration. During a simulated patient-care scenario, demonstrate administering a primary maintenance IV solution, including attaching the primary fluid tubing, inserting the IV tubing into the IV pump, setting the appropriate rate of fluid administration, and assessing the IV site. Be prepared to discuss possible complications of IV fluid administration.

Although this learning activity is designed to focus primarily on skill development in the psychomotor domain, the cognitive learning domain is an interdependent domain because students need to use knowledge about proper administration of IV fluids, complications of administration, and an understanding of an IV site assessment. The affective domain is also an interdependent domain because students need to value answering patient questions about an IV infusion.

EVALUATING COURSES AND LEARNING EXPERIENCES

Designing courses and learning experiences requires faculty to determine how they will evaluate student learning and calculate and assign grades. Where possible, it is desirable for students to be able to choose among several options with regard to how their work will be evaluated and graded. Students deserve to be informed about when they will be evaluated and the purpose of the evaluation.

Evaluation of teaching and learning is a continuous process. Two common types of evaluation are *formative* and *summative evaluation*. These types of evaluation are briefly described in this chapter and are further discussed in Chapter 23. Another type of evaluation, also described later in this chapter, is the prior learning assessment (PLA). This type of evaluation is often used as an approach to grant credit for prior learning to facilitate postsecondary degree completion.

Formative Evaluation

Formative evaluation is conducted while the teaching–learning process is unfolding. Faculty use formative evaluation to (1) appraise learning experiences while they are developing and using them; (2) assess student learning and ability to apply the content; and (3) identify any difficulties that occur during implementation of the learning experience.

Students use formative evaluation to (1) appraise the effectiveness of their learning strategies; (2) determine the extent to which they are grasping the knowledge, skills, and attitudes presented in the course; (3) identify the need for additional clarification of the material; and (4) recognize the need for further study.

Clearly differentiating between learning and evaluation and allocating specific time for each purpose is essential. Faculty need to communicate to students the purposes of formative evaluation and how the process is being used to support their learning.

Collecting systematic verbal and written feedback about their learning from students at regular intervals is an integral and essential component of the teaching–learning process and can easily and effectively occur during class time. These data enable faculty to monitor student progress and design appropriate strategies to improve student achievement. One means by which to engage in formative evaluation and monitor student progress is the use of classroom assessment techniques.

Classroom Assessment Techniques

Classroom assessment techniques (CATs) are informal evaluation tools and procedures used to assess student learning. They involve immediate, continuous interaction between the student and teacher to validate, clarify, and facilitate learning. CATs can be used to assess students' attitudes and knowledge about course concepts, study habits, or even reactions to teaching strategies used in particular courses. Angelo and Cross's (1993) classic work describing various CATs remains a relevant resource for faculty seeking ideas about how to successfully integrate CATs into their teaching practice. Angelo and Cross's three phases of developing and using CATs are planning, implementing, and responding.

Planning phase.   During the planning phase, the teacher selects a particular class or learning experience in which to implement the CAT. The teacher needs to clearly identify the goal of the CAT and the desired information to be gained and select a CAT that is the best fit for assessing the goal. To effectively use a CAT, the teacher should focus on assessing one specific goal. For example, the teacher may want to gather feedback regarding students' unanswered questions about the concepts being discussed or the most confusing aspect of the lesson being taught.

Implementation phase.   The CAT may be implemented before, during, or after a class or learning experience. The class content can be taught, with administration of the CAT following, or the CAT can be administered first to set the stage for the rest of the classroom discussion. The timing of the administration of the CAT depends on the goal of the classroom assessment and the particular content of the learning experience. After implementing the CAT, the teacher must examine and organize the results of the CAT into a meaningful framework that will help inform how the teacher can most effectively use the information obtained.

Responding phase.   The responding phase involves reporting the results of the CAT to the students and represents the final step in the administration of a CAT. The feedback is interpreted, organized, and presented in a manner that will enhance student learning. To maximize benefit to students' learning, the teacher should present results of the CAT to the students as soon as they are available. The less time it takes students to receive results, the greater the effect on student learning outcomes.

The last activity in the responding phase is reflection (Angelo & Cross, 1993). The teacher evaluates the use of the CAT. Did the CAT accomplish the goal established during the first phase? Did implementation of the CAT occur as planned? Did the outcome of the CAT enhance student learning? How did the students respond to the use of the CAT? What did the teacher think about the use of the CAT?

Answering these questions and others posed by the teacher completes the three phases of using a CAT. However, reflection on the experience usually stimulates further action. Use of another CAT, repeated use of the same CAT at a later date, redesign of a learning experience, and even course revision are some of the future actions that may result from the evaluation. See Box 10.3 for an example of a CAT.

Summative Evaluation

Summative evaluation is conducted by faculty to measure student outcome achievement and course and program effectiveness. Faculty use summative evaluation at specified points in time throughout students' course of study for the purpose of determining whether students have met expected

BOX 10.3 Classroom Assessment Technique: Minute Paper

Description: A quick and efficient way to collect data about student learning. The teacher asks students to write short responses to questions such as "What was the most important thing you learned in this class?" or "What important question remains unanswered?"

Purpose: Assesses to what extent students are learning and facilitates any needed adjustments in instruction.

Exemplar: A faculty who is teaching concepts related to family theories anticipates students will struggle to differentiate the various theories. In class students work together on case studies that require them to apply various family theories to a clinical family-care situation. At the end of the class session, the faculty asks students to share any remaining questions they have about the family theories in the course's web-based discussion forum. After reviewing the posted responses, the faculty identifies points of confusion that still exist and using this information develops additional learning materials, which are shared with students to further assist student learning.

Caution: Although the Minute Paper is a very effective classroom assessment technique (CAT), if this technique is overused or poorly used, students may not take the CAT seriously. Therefore it is important to prepare questions that will effectively obtain adequate information to assess student learning.

Note: A teacher implemented the Exemplar in a nursing classroom. The remaining aspects of this example are derived from Angelo and Cross (1993), pp. 148–153.

outcomes. For example, midterm examinations in a course or an end-of-program portfolio of learning are forms of summative evaluation. It is important for faculty to align summative forms of evaluation with program and course outcomes and the culmination of student learning outcomes. It is also important to construct and describe summative evaluation measures so that students understand the areas of learning that will be measured and evaluated.

There is great utility in linking program, course, and student learning outcomes to summative evaluation strategies. However, faculty efforts in using summative evaluation to measure learning do not stop there. Faculty can also use the results of summative evaluation methods to determine the effectiveness of learning experiences used during courses.

Nonetheless, research demonstrates that for summative evaluation to be reliable and valid, faculty must achieve competencies in conducting such evaluations (National League for Nursing, 2022). For example, Helminen et al. (2016) conducted a review of the literature about summative evaluation in clinical education and suggested that faculty must have orientation to the evaluation process to assure consistency in results. This orientation is imperative to ensure validation that students have achieved competencies in the provision of safe and quality nursing care. Faculty therefore must participate in faculty development to develop expertise in summative evaluation. Such competence can enhance the accuracy of summative evaluation methods and promote effective use of evaluation results.

Once faculty have developed summative evaluation strategies that are aligned with expected student learning outcomes and engaged in a process to ensure rigor of the methods they use, they need to use summative evaluation results to facilitate planning appropriate revisions to the learning experiences. See Case Study 10.2 for an example of how using evaluation data can lead to changes in teaching strategies.

Regardless of the summative evaluation strategies faculty use, it is imperative that they work together to examine evaluation results, use an evidence base to adjust learning experiences, and evaluate implementation of new summative evaluation strategies. These efforts can help ensure effective use of summative evaluation methods.

Prior Learning Assessment

A prior learning assessment (PLA) is "the process by which an individual's experiential learning is assessed and evaluated for purposes of granting college credit, certification, or advanced standing toward further education or training" (Klein-Collins & Hudson, 2018, p. 4). PLAs originated in 1974 through the American Council on Education's College Credit Recommendation Service to help adults obtain college credit for

CASE STUDY 10.2   Evaluating Student Learning Outcomes

Faculty in one school of nursing were concerned that pharmacology examination scores and National Council Licensure Examination preparation assessments were lower than desired. They noted that students experienced difficulty demonstrating expected competencies in medication administration in the clinical setting. Their evaluation of the examination scores and the students' clinical performance indicated a need for an evidence-based learning experience that integrated the skills, knowledge, and attitudes related to medication administration. Faculty reviewed the literature on strategies for teaching pharmacology and determined that objective structured clinical examination (OSCE) could be effective in improving students' pharmacology competencies. The faculty designed and implemented a pharmacology OSCE scenario focused on medication administration. Initial findings from this experience suggested an increase in pharmacology examination scores and improved clinical performance in medication management.

1. What learning domains would the use of an OSCE address in a simulated learning scenario?
2. How would you evaluate the student learning outcomes associated with the newly developed OSCE? Would you consider it to be an example of a formative evaluation of student performance or summative evaluation? What might be most appropriate in this given situation?
3. How would you develop a rubric to evaluate the student outcomes related to this learning experience?

BOX 10.4   Ten Standards for Assessing Learning

1. Credit or competencies are awarded only for evidence of learning, not for experience or time spent.
2. Assessment is integral to learning because it leads to and enables future learning.
3. Assessment is based on criteria for outcomes that are clearly articulated and shared among constituencies.
4. The determination of credit awards and competence levels is made by appropriate subject matter and credentialing experts.
5. Assessment advances the broader purpose of equity and access for diverse individuals and groups.
6. Institutions proactively provide guidance and support for learners' full engagement in the assessment process.
7. Assessment policies and procedures are the result of inclusive deliberation and are shared with all constituencies.
8. Fees charged for assessment are based on the services performed in the process rather than the credit awarded.
9. All practitioners involved in the assessment process pursue and receive adequate training and continuing professional development for the functions they perform.
10. Assessment programs are regularly monitored, evaluated, and revised to respond to institutional and learner needs.

From Council for Adult and Experiential Learning (n.d.). *Ten standards for assessing learning*. Retrieved from https://www.cael.org/ten-standards-for-assessing-learning

courses and examinations completed outside of traditional degree programs (American Council on Education, 2021).

The need for PLAs is important as it can facilitate college completion, particularly for students of color, those with low income, and immigrants (García & Leibrandt, 2020). Subsequently, the PLA has become an important method for assessing learning, with evidence that some methods such as portfolio assessment (documenting prior learning) and standardized examinations are associated with college persistence and completion rates (Klein-Collins & Hudson, 2018).

To ensure appropriate assessment of prior learning, the Council for Adult and Experiential Learning (n.d) provides *Ten Standards for Assessing Learning* that should be used in determining whether to grant credit for prior learning (Box 10.4).

DEVELOPING THE COURSE SYLLABUS

A course syllabus is required for all academic courses, including those taught on campus or through the use of technology (online, videoconference, etc.). The course components and learning experiences should be clearly and succinctly described in the course syllabus. A well-developed syllabus serves as a contract between faculty and students and as a student guide to achieving learning outcomes. It is expected that students will receive the syllabus on or before the first day of class so that they will have a clear understanding of course requirements before the class begins. The syllabus also explains how learning will be assessed, evaluated, and graded. Equally important, the syllabus sets the tone for the course by introducing the faculty and the faculty's philosophy, university, school, and course policies and norms for attendance and behavior to be demonstrated during the course; as such, it should be written with a learner-centered focus. In a classic article Harnish et al. (2011) stated that it is important to include characteristics that create warm or welcoming syllabi (see Table 10.1). Evidence suggests that creating such syllabi can, in fact, support students' mental health needs, increasing likelihood that they will seek help during times of stress (Gurung & Galardi, 2021). The syllabus for a learner-centered course also explains the roles of the faculty and students in the teaching–learning process and conveys the attitudes and behaviors that will promote active and effective learning.

A *full* course syllabus includes essential information about the course, course implementation, university and school policies, and norms for expected behaviors. The various components of a full course syllabus (see Box 10.5) are described in the following sections.

Faculty should be knowledgeable about which components of the syllabus they have the autonomy to change and which they do not. For example, the course title, description, allotted credit hours, prerequisites and corequisites, grading scales, and course objectives (outcomes) are all determined by the program or institution and cannot be modified without obtaining the appropriate program and institution-level approvals. Course assignments and evaluation strategies may often be changed by the faculty responsible for teaching the course. Faculty should familiarize themselves with the policies of their program before modifying any existing course syllabi.

An *abbreviated* form of the syllabus may be developed as required by the institution or program and contains basic information about course

TABLE 10.1	Six Characteristics of a Warm Syllabus
Characteristic	**Description**
Positive or friendly language	Helps students feel comfortable and welcome. Example: Office Hours—"I am readily available to provide individual assistance by appointment."
Rationale for assignments	Motivates students by clarifying how assignments relate to course objectives and their learning. Example: Assignment—"The worksheet questions for this course are designed to help you develop your clinical reasoning skills about nursing practice."
Self-disclosure	Provides students with awareness of a teacher's interpersonal style. Example: Learning Resources—"We all experience the need to have help with learning new knowledge at some point in our lives. This list of learning resources will support your learning in this course."
Enthusiasm	Increases students' active learning and a teacher's effectiveness. Example: Course Topical Outline—"Consider the positive impact of research and how evidence-based nursing practice has changed lives and contributed to health and well-being."
Compassion	Acknowledges unexpected events and life circumstances. Example: Attendance—"Attendance is expected. However, please contact me if you have an unforeseen event such as a death in the family or illness."
Humor	Increases students' active learning and a teacher's effectiveness. Example: Teaching Philosophy—"Please beware the use of cartoons is common in this course, and are designed to stimulate your attention to the course content."

Harnish, R. J., McElwee, R. O., Slattery, J. M., Frantz, S., Haney, M. R., Shore, C. M., & Penley, J. (2011, January). Creating a foundation for a warm classroom climate: Best practices in syllabus tone. *Observer, 24*.

BOX 10.5   Example of a Full Syllabus for an Undergraduate Nursing Course

Nursing 610: Healthcare Ethics, Policy, and Advocacy
Class Sessions: Face-to-face
Credit Hours: 3
Catalog Course Description
  Students will ascertain concepts and theories to practice safe and ethical care within an advocacy framework. Emphasis will be on ethical principles, health policy analysis, political competence, and principles and practices of advocacy in the context of the spheres of care (disease prevention/promotion of health and well-being, chronic disease care, restorative care, and hospice/palliative/supportive care), whole-person wellness, social determinants of health and health equity, health care advocacy and systems change, and interprofessional collaboration.

Course Outcomes
At the completion of this course, the student will be able to:
1. Investigate historical perspectives on ethics, policy, and advocacy in nursing practice and health care.
2. Critique ethical principles and theories, including relational ethics, in nursing practice and health care.
3. Demonstrate decision-making in situations of ethical or legal uncertainty and values conflict.
4. Critique health policies, using multiple vantage points.
5. Appraise policymaking and regulatory processes, using multiple vantage points.
6. Organize approaches to policy and regulation to influence policy-makers on issues of social determinants of health and health equity, health care advocacy, and systems change.
7. Select principles and practices of advocacy for the quality provision of nursing and health care.
8. Design leadership strategies to advocate for quality nursing practice and health care.

Prerequisites: *Nursing 550 Complex Nursing Care I*
Brief Topical Outline:
1. Ethical analyses processes and approaches
2. Ethical comportment in clinical and professional relationships
3. Treatment consent and refusal, coercion, end-of-life care, and privacy
4. Current or controversial issues and ethical dilemmas
5. Political philosophy
6. Policy and regulatory-making, formation, and implementation

7. Political analysis
8. Policy and politics in government, workforce, associations, and interest groups
9. Stages and components of advocacy
10. Advocacy toolkits
11. Barriers to advocacy
12. Developing agency

Course Faculty:
Names and ranks, contact information, office hours with provision for "arranged" office hours to accommodate student schedules

Faculty Philosophy of Teaching and Learning:
Faculty in this course believe in active learning and the development of healthcare ethics, policy and advocacy knowledge, and skills and attitudes inclusive of and beyond those you have acquired to date. They also believe in democratic learning, where students and teachers partner in meeting learning outcomes.

Teaching and Learning Strategies:
You will learn through assigned readings, online learning groups, case studies, presentations, and written assignments.

Course Materials, Resources, Required Texts:
All required and optional texts and other learning resources should be listed on syllabus.

Evaluation:
Learning experiences and corresponding assessments and grading:

Advocacy Reflection Paper	20%
Legislative Outreach Project	20%
Simulated Case Study	20%
Ethical Analysis Case Study	20%
Health Policy Brief	20%
Total	100%

Course Grading Scale:
The final course grade will be based on the following scale:

A = 94–100	C = 80–84
AB = 92–93	CD = 78–79
B = 87–91	D = 74–77
BC = 85–86	F = 73 and below

BOX 10.5   Example of a Full Syllabus for an Undergraduate Nursing Course—Cont'd

Assignments:
Extensions on assignments may be arranged by contacting the course instructor before the deadline. If an extension is not requested, a penalty for late assignments may be applied as outlined in the student handbook.

Formatting and Submission Guidelines:
APA format is required for all papers. Please refer to the *APA Manual* (7th edition). In addition, papers will be submitted via an antiplagiarism software package.

Attendance:
The course runs: MONDAY 8 a.m.–11 a.m. Attendance is required as outlined in the student handbook.

Accommodations for Students With Disabilities:
Students with disabilities should contact Disability Services to establish reasonable accommodations.

(Syllabi adapted from the St. Thomas School of Nursing, St. Paul, Minnesota.)

---

requirements such as course name, credit hours, description, and objectives (outcomes). Some schools publish the abbreviated syllabus on the website and offer full course information in electronic or print format at the beginning of the course.

Course Information

The following course information should be included in the syllabus: title, description, credit hours, prerequisites, corequisites, outcomes, teaching–learning strategies, learning experiences, topical outline, policies and procedures, assessment and evaluation strategies, and the grading plan and scale. In addition, faculty should list all course meeting dates. If the course meets in varied locations throughout the semester or through the use of technology, such as online at synchronous or asynchronous times, it is imperative to indicate this information at the outset. Because the syllabus is an implied contract between the student and faculty, all involved must plan to adhere to the syllabus as written and distributed. Any changes to the course syllabus after the syllabus has been shared with the students and the course is underway should be made only in rare instances and as needed to enable the students to meet the learning outcomes set forth in the syllabus.

Faculty Information

Faculty should include basic information such as name, rank, office hours, general availability, and contact information, with the preferred way of contacting faculty. Faculty should also note the hours of their availability inside and outside of scheduled class time. If providing phone or electronic contact information, it is appropriate for faculty to delineate when students are welcome to contact faculty and for what reasons. Faculty can also provide a short description of their philosophy of the teaching and learning process to help students understand how they view the roles and responsibilities of the teacher and learner.

Course Materials and Resources

In this section faculty can provide information about required and supplemental readings such as textbooks, journal readings, and other relevant course resources. A bibliography and listing of course-relevant websites may also be included.

Course Requirements

A section of the full syllabus should include course requirements, including information about class attendance and participation, assigned and optional learning experiences, clinical assignments, examinations, and written work. Faculty also should specify the consequences of not meeting course requirements and whether there are options for completing late or missed requirements, particularly in courses with clinical experiences.

Course Grading Policies

In the full syllabus faculty can provide detailed information about the course grading scale, assignments, and how they will be graded. The use of rubrics facilitates clarity about the criteria that will be used to grade assignments. Students should also be made aware of the percentage of the overall course grade each assignment represents. Faculty should provide due dates for assignments and tests, procedures for test makeup, information on the use of optional graded assignments, and procedures for late papers and projects, and they should inform students when results from tests and papers will be available.

Study and Technology Assistance

If the campus or school provides resources to assist students with study and writing skills, this information can be noted in the syllabus. Faculty can also make suggestions for how students can learn the course material and how students can form their own study groups. For courses with reliance on the use of technology to achieve the expected student learning outcomes, the syllabus should also include a section on technology requirements to successfully complete the course and how to access technology support. Students enrolled in online courses should also be instructed on how to obtain all institution and program student support services made available to students enrolled on campus.

Course, Program, and Institution Policies

Each nursing program and institution has its own set of policies with specified consequences related to codes of conduct, academic honesty, incivility, criminal acts, student privacy, and resources for students with disabilities or special needs. Information about required criminal background checks and substance testing should also be provided as pertinent to the program and course. Information regarding program and institutional policies can be provided in the syllabus with links to appropriate institution or school websites.

Course Norms

Course norms are guidelines for behavior in the classroom. Course norms can be written to describe expectations for individual and group participation and active learning within the class, when the use of computers and cell phones is acceptable, how to handle arriving late or leaving early, and how to prevent and manage other annoying or uncivil behavior (see Chapter 15). At the beginning of each course, faculty should spend time in dialogue with students, explaining and answering questions, soliciting input from the students, and modifying the syllabus as appropriate. Clark (2017) notes that

clarifying expectations at the outset of the course helps promote desired classroom behavior. Faculty can ask students to commit to the behaviors specified in the syllabus in writing; in online courses faculty can ask students to send an email or post in the discussion forum indicating their agreement with the document. Faculty can also engage in dialogue with students to gain insight into the students' own expectations about the behavior of their faculty and peers. The syllabus then becomes a learning contract that can be reviewed and referred to throughout the course. Case Study 10.3 addresses a strategy to norm classroom behavior.

CASE STUDY 10.3 Establishing Course Norms

Nursing faculty in an undergraduate nursing program expressed concerns to the director about poor student class attendance. They informed the director that they tried administering graded quizzes at the start of class to incentivize attendance. The director suggested that faculty use end-of-class reflections rather than beginning-of-class quizzes. The reflections required students to write a one-sentence response to one of the following questions of their choice and enter the response into the learning management system: What element of this class session was most meaningful to you? What element of this class session requires more clarity? What element of this class session do you want to know more about? Students were awarded five points for their responses. Faculty analyzed responses for patterns and themes, which often indicated additional learning needs. They came to each class session with a report for students of these needs and used learning strategies to reinforce additional learning needs. Students valued this response and attendance subsequently increased. The faculty were so pleased with this small change to classroom management that they included a description of it in syllabi to norm behavior at the start of each course.

1. Why did this small change in creating course norms have such a positive outcome?
2. How is this type of course norm a form of formative learning assessment?
3. How does documenting this approach as a course norm in the syllabus align with characteristics of warm syllabi?

EVALUATION OF COURSE DESIGN

Once the course and syllabus are sufficiently developed—and before their use with students—faculty can request internal and external review from peers and other curriculum experts. Teaching colleagues can review the syllabus for content accuracy, completeness, congruence with the curriculum, and compliance with program and institutional policies. For additional and external review, faculty can consult curriculum and course design experts at the campus teaching center, if available, or faculty content experts from other disciplines. Ultimately, the course syllabus represents the expected learning outcomes of the course and is the document that is submitted to the course review process as designated by the school of nursing and the college.

CONSTRAINTS TO COURSE DESIGN AND LEARNING EXPERIENCES

Constraints to designing courses and learning experiences may arise from faculty, students, time, and resources. Although it may not be possible to eliminate all constraints, by making a careful assessment of each source of constraint during the planning phases, faculty will be able to avoid many pitfalls. Faculty can gain an appreciation of the benefits and limitations of the course design and learning experience after implementing them, reflecting on how students responded, and assessing how the experience contributed to learning. Taking time to debrief after course delivery helps faculty decide whether to repeat, revise, or delete the activity. Table 10.2 presents a summary of the sources of constraint in selecting and implementing learning activities.

Faculty Constraints

Some constraints in designing courses and learning experiences arise from faculty. A faculty member's lack of teaching experience in an academic setting or in teaching students at the course level assigned may have an effect on course design. Faculty are more likely to design courses and select appropriate learning experiences when they have a reasonable understanding of the cognitive

TABLE 10.2 Sources of Constraint in Choosing and Implementing Learning Activities

Source	Constraint
Faculty	Faculty–student ratio
	Lack of experience
	Lack of knowledge of course content
	Lack of understanding of students' knowledge and skills
	Personal attributes
	Personality
	Vocal qualities
Students	Distractions
	Inability to use equipment and technology
	Lack of prerequisite knowledge and skills
	Resistance to active participation
	Stress and anxiety
	Student–faculty ratio too large
Time	Inadequate for activity
	Inadequate for debriefing
Resources	Copyright restrictions
	Inadequate clinical or classroom facilities
	Inadequate funds
	Unavailable audiovisual equipment
	Unavailable electronic technology

abilities, knowledge base, and life experiences of their intended learners. Overestimating or underestimating the abilities and experiences of students can undermine the intended value of the designed learning experience and affect the students' ability to engage in the course work.

Novice faculty—and even experienced faculty who are teaching a new course—may not possess an adequate command of the content and processes required by the course and learning experiences. As a result, they may not be comfortable responding to student questions, problems, or issues that may arise during the course. Students may raise questions and issues that faculty may not consider as being related to the course or bring forth perspectives not anticipated by the faculty. Consulting with faculty who have previously taught the course or who have had experience teaching the same level of students can provide valuable input to consider when designing the course and learning experiences. Because courses and learning experiences should be learner centered, faculty must be prepared to be flexible and deal with any ambiguity that may arise and take advantage of the opportunity to learn from students as they process the course experience. Feedback from students about the different ways they interpreted the course design and learning experiences can be used as points of discussion and thus expand the course and the learning experiences.

Demands on students outside the classroom can complicate and put constraints on faculty. Retaining standards and rigor while providing appropriate academic expectations for students with numerous job and family demands makes teaching a challenge and can have major implications for pedagogy. Learner-centered classrooms can mitigate challenges teachers face from students who experience demands outside the classroom.

Tomlinson (2021) suggests giving students more control over learning by changing the traditional power relationships between the teacher and students from one where the teacher is viewed solely as the expert to one where responsibility for learning becomes a partnership between students and teachers. The change in power relationships can occur through viewing teaching and learning within these five key areas: (1) curriculum is making meaning; (2) instruction is facilitating learning; (3) assessment is charting a course; (4) management is leading for success; and (5) environment is designed for flexibility. Tomlinson purports that using these key elements helps students mature in voice, agency, collaboration, and decision making because they share responsibility for learning with teachers. The power relationship in learner-centered classrooms promotes inclusiveness, responds to students' needs, and accounts for diversity. However, Tomlinson emphasizes that changing power relationships does not mean abrogating legitimate responsibility for which a teacher is required by law, education, and experience to ensure students' academic progress.

Faculty may have personal attributes that interfere with their ability to establish a climate that engages student interest in learning. Having a soft or poor-quality voice, talking too fast or too slow, or speaking in a monotone may make it difficult for students to pay attention to and follow verbal presentations. Faculty with reserved or shy personalities or those with a matter-of-fact orientation may be perceived by students as distant, aloof, or uncaring. Personal habits that faculty may be unaware of may also be distracting for students and interfere with their ability to fully focus on the learning experience. Although students may be reluctant to share some of their perceptions about faculty's personal attributes, inviting a colleague to attend a class can provide helpful input that can be used to improve classroom performance.

Student Constraints

Student constraints may be a result of the number of students enrolled in a course. Large numbers of students in a course may affect the faculty's ability to get to know students personally, address various learning styles, and ensure students have a comparable learning experience. The student/faculty ratio may make a particular course or learning experience labor and time intensive.

Students may lack some of the prerequisite knowledge and skills required for a course or learning experience, knowledge and skills that faculty reasonably anticipated the students would possess. There are usually some students, regardless of the clarity of the activity and the directions, who do not grasp the course content or the goal of a learning experience. Distractions such as uncomfortable classroom temperature and mechanical noise in the classroom environment may also interfere with learning activities. Students working in groups may also create enough noise to interfere with the learning of students who prefer a quiet environment to concentrate.

Resistance to participation in learning experiences is another constraining force. Students socialized to a passive learning model may be resistant to engaging in learning experiences that require active participation. Students may perceive learning experiences as a form of busywork that has little or no meaning for them and not accept them as meaningful experiences.

Students may not have the skill or experience in using the resources, equipment, or electronic technology required for a learning experience.

Faculty should carefully assess the possible student constraints to learning each time they teach the course. Student constraints are variable and likely to be different each time the course is taught with a new group of learners.

Time Constraints

Time is an all too common constraint in teaching. Faculty must carefully weigh the trade-off between faculty-centered and learner-centered learning experiences when determining how to use class time most effectively. For all courses and learning experiences, faculty must prioritize and then select the outcomes or competencies and the related content and processes. Faculty must also assess the complexity of the course and learning experiences to ensure that they can be accomplished given the ability of the students and the allotted time.

For courses and learning experiences to be meaningful and worthwhile, adequate time needs to be allowed for both students and faculty to actively plan and participate in the course and its learning experiences. Time should also be allowed for debriefing after the completion of the learning experiences within courses. Although the need to debrief depends on the nature of the learning, debriefing is an important part of learning, and it has several benefits for both students and faculty. It extends the learning process as students share what they did with their peers, it enables faculty to gain a more comprehensive perspective of the kinds of thinking processes students use, and it provides an opportunity for students to identify issues that came up during the learning experience. Faculty can use this information as the basis for further discussion of issues and problems relevant to the student's immediate learning situation. Information gleaned from students about their difficulties with the directions, elements, or focus of the experience itself is useful to faculty when deciding whether to retain, revise, or discard the experience.

Resource Constraints

Resources may be another source of constraint. The resources used to support courses and learning experiences include clinical facilities, learning resource centers, physical examination rooms, classrooms, instructional supplies and equipment, print materials, audiovisual equipment, computer-assisted instructional programs, and a variety of information technologies. The use of a particular learning experience or type of experience, for example, may not be possible because of a lack of the appropriate resources needed to implement the experience.

Information technology, email, and other electronic messaging and conferencing systems are useful tools that can be used as a vehicle for designing courses and learning experiences. Although faculty may inform students in advance of the course that skill and experience in using technology are required, students may report that they are too busy to allocate the time to acquire the necessary training on their own time. In addition to time, money may also be a barrier. Faculty who teach courses that incorporate the use of technology need to consider how students will be oriented to the technology so that their learning experiences are not negatively affected.

CHAPTER SUMMARY: KEY POINTS

- Learner-centered approaches to course design prevent and promote learner engagement.
- Course design involves a series of sequential steps that are iterative, starting from the course predesign phase and concluding with the development of lesson plans and evaluation strategies.
- Course design requires faculty to make decisions about when to use structured and unstructured learning experiences and should include predominantly active rather than passive learning strategies.
- Faculty must use cognitive, psychomotor, and affective learning domains to create measurable student learning outcomes, which include action verbs most suitable for the desired level of learning.

- Formative and summative evaluation methods are an essential part of course design, and faculty should plan to use both to assess learning needs and evaluate the extent to which learning has occurred.
- Course syllabi are a contract between teachers and students and must be thoughtfully

designed with attention to incorporating a warm and inviting tone.
- It is important for faculty to continuously assess faculty and student constraints that impede effective course design and learning experiences and act to mitigate these constraints.

REFLECTING ON THE EVIDENCE

1. Review an existing course for its congruence with disruptive learner-centered innovation (Huston et al., 2018). How can the course be modified to reflect these innovations?
2. Analyze a course syllabus for linkages between the course description, program and course objectives, competencies, concepts, learning experiences, evaluation methods, and learning resources. Are the course elements interconnected?
3. Analyze the course objectives for inclusion of the cognitive, affective, and psychomotor domains.

Is there a balance among the domains? If not, what is the rationale for an imbalance?
4. Compare and contrast formative and summative evaluation. Cite an example of when it is appropriate to use each type of evaluation in the teaching/learning process.
5. Reflect on faculty and student constraints to course design and learning experiences. What are antecedents of constraints where proactive actions can be used to mitigate constraints?

REFERENCES

American Council on Education. (2021). *About learning evaluations.* https://www.acenet.edu/Programs-Services/Pages/Credit-Transcripts/About-Learning-Evaluation.aspx

Anderson, L. W., & Krathwohl, D. R. (2001). *A taxonomy for learning, teaching, and assessing: A revision of Bloom's taxonomy of educational objectives.* Longman.

Angelo, T. A., & Cross, K. A. (1993). *Classroom assessment techniques: A handbook for college teachers.* Jossey-Bass.

Auerbach, A. J., Higgins, M., Brickman, P., & Andrews, T. C. (2018). Teacher knowledge for active-learning instruction: Expert–novice comparison reveals differences. *CBE-Life Sciences Education, 17*(1), 1–14. https://doi.org/10.1187/cbe.17-07-0149

Benner, P., Sutphen, M., Leonard, V., & Day, L. (2010). *Educating nurses: A call for radical transformation.* Jossey-Bass.

Bloom, B. S. (Ed.), (1956). *Taxonomy of educational objectives. Handbook 1: Cognitive domain.* Longman.

Bruner, J. (1977). *The process of education.* Harvard University Press.

Clark, C. (2017). *Creating & sustaining civility in nursing education* (2nd ed.). Sigma Theta Tau International.

Council for Adult and Experiential Learning. (n.d.). Ten standards for assessing learning. https://www.cael.org/ten-standards-for-assessing-learning

Freire, P. (2006). *Pedagogy of the oppressed: 30th anniversary edition.* Continuum International Publishing Group.

García, C. & Leibrandt, S. (2020). *Recognition of prior learning in the 21st century: The current state of higher learning policies.* https://www.clasp.org/sites/default/files/publications/2020/11/The-Current-State-of-PLA-Policies.pdf

Giddens, J. F. (2021). *Concepts for nursing practice* (3rd ed.). Elsevier.

Giddens, J. F., Caputi, L., & Rodgers, B. (2019). *Mastering concept-based teaching: A guide for nurse educators* (2nd ed.). Elsevier.

Gloekler, L., & Lucas, D. (2021). Nursing students' preferences in test taking, e-books, and learning styles: A longitudinal study. *International Journal of Nursing Education, 13*(1), 152–159. https://doi.org/10.37506/ijone.v13i1.13333

Gurung, A. R., & Galardi, N. R. (2021). Syllabus tone, more than mental health statements, influence intensions to seek help. *Teaching of Psychology,* 1–6. https://doi.org/10.1177/0098628321994632

Harnish, R. J., McElwee, R. O., Slattery, J. M., Frantz, M. R., Haney, C. M., Shore, C. M., & Penley, J. (2011). Creating a foundation for a warm classroom climate: Best practices in syllabus tone. *Observer,* 24.

http://www.psychologicalscience.org/index.php/publications/observer/2011/january-11/creating-the-foundation-for-a-warm-classroom-climate.html

Helminen, K., Coco, K., Johnson, M., Turunen, H., & Tossavainen, K. (2016). Summative assessment of clinical practice of student nurses: A review of the literature. *International Journal of Nursing Studies, 53,* 308–319. https://doi.org/10.1016/j.ijnurstu.2015.09.014

Huston, C. L., Phillips, B., Jeffries, P., Todero, C., Rich, J., Knecht, P., Sommer, S., Lewis, M.P. (2018).The academic-practice gap: Strategies for an enduring problem. *Nursing Forum, 53,* 27–34.

Klein-Collins, R., & Hudson, S. (2018). *Do methods matter? PLA, portfolio assessment, and the road to completion and persistence: A study of prior learning assessment and adult students' academic outcomes at four LearningCounts partner colleges.* https://files.eric.ed.gov/fulltext/ED593472.pdf

Krathwohl, D., Bloom, B., & Masia, B. (1964). *Taxonomy of educational objectives. Handbook II: Affective domain.* Longman.

Lehtinen, A., & Viiri, J. (2017). Guidance provided by teacher and simulation for inquiry-based learning: A case study. *Journal of Science Education and Technology, 26*(2), 193–206. https://doi.org/10.1007/s10956-016-9672-y

Leighton, K., Kardong-Edgren, S., McNelis, A. M., Foisy-Doll, C., & Sullo, E. (2021). Traditional clinical outcomes in prelicensure nursing education: An empty systematic review. *Journal of Nursing Education, 60*(3), 136–142. https://doi.org/10.3928/01484834-20210222-03

Markey, K., O'Brien, B., Kouta, C., Okantey, C., & O'Donnell, C. (2021). Embracing classroom cultural diversity: Innovations for nurturing inclusive intercultural learning and culturally responsive teaching. *Teaching and Learning in Nursing, 16*(3), 258–262. https://doi.org/10.1016/j.teln.2021.01.008

Martin, K. (2018). *Learner centered innovation: Spark curiosity, ignite passion, unleash genius.* IMPress.

Misseyanni, A., Lytrasp, M. D., Papadopoulou, P., & Marouli, C. (Eds.), (2018). *Active learning strategies in higher education: Teaching for leadership, creativity and innovation.* Emerald Publishing.

Morris, T. H. (2019). Adaptivity through self-directed learning to meet the challenges of our ever-changing world. *Adulty Learning, 30*(2), 56–66. https://doi.org/10.1177/1045159518814486

National League for Nursing. (2022). *NLN core competencies for academic nurse educators.* https://www.nln.org/education/nursing-education-competencies/core-competencies-for-academic-nurse-educators

Neilsen, A. (2016). Concept-based learning in clinical experiences: Bringing theory to clinical education for deep learning. *Journal of Nursing Education, 55*(7), 365–371. https://doi.org/10.3928/01484834-20160615-02

Patel-Junanker, D. (2018). Learner-centered pedagogy: Teaching and learning in the 21st century In G. Kayingo & V. M. Hass (Eds.), *The health professions educator: A practical guide for new and established faculty* (pp. 3–11). Springer Publishing Company, LLC.

Sterner, A., Hagiwara, M. S., Ramstrand, N., & Palmér, L. (2019). Factors developing nursing students and novice nurses' ability to provide care in acute situations. *Nursing Education in Practice, 35,* 135–140. https://doi.org/10.1016/j.nepr.2019.02.005

Tomlinson, C. A. (2021). *So each may soar: The principles and practices of learner-centered classrooms.* ASCD.

11

Interprofessional Education and Collaborative Practice

Elizabeth Speakman, EdD, RN, FNAP, ANEF, FAAN

INTRODUCTION

The literature is replete describing the role of nurses in team-based care delivery as a result of global events. Many accounts are within the context of historical, societal, political, and economic events. For example, occupational therapists and nurses worked collaboratively with patients to regain optimal functioning during the polio epidemic and nurses, physicians, and pharmacists worked with GIs during World War II who contracted illnesses on foreign soil to find treatment modalities. The recent global pandemic can be categorized as another historical event, although slightly different because the pandemic has had a significant impact on nurses personally. Nurses worked in unprecedented conditions, with fear of personal death, loneliness, and isolation from family and friends, having to act as a surrogate family member for individuals dying without loved ones. Additionally, the barriers to health care access, along with restricted mobility, and/or fear of infection have created unprecedented challenges in many countries because of the recent pandemic (WHO, 2021). Today little is known about the long-term effect of a nurse's moral distress related to care for patients during COVID-19 health care crisis (Lake et al., 2021). We do know that during these dire conditions, nurses and in fact all members of the health care team have had to collaborate and rely on each other more.

While nurses played an irreplaceable role during the recent pandemic, they also experienced psychological changes related to ambiguity, fear, and moral distress (Zhang et al., 2020). "It has been 100 years since a global event has had an impact on nursing education in the United States and around the world equal to that of the COVID-19 pandemic. Both World War I and the influenza pandemic of 1918 to 1920 led to transformations in nursing education, including standardization of training and professionalization of the field. The COVID-19 pandemic has already led to innovations that are likely to shape the future of nursing education" (National Academies of Sciences, Engineering, and Medicine, 2021, p. 231). The COVID-19 pandemic highlighted the need for team-based care and accentuated the value and need for collaborative approaches to care.

When health emergencies arise, hospital management often needs to develop proactive contingency plans and long-term planning and preparedness (Zaghini et al., 2021). For many institutions, the use of team-based care approaches was part of the COVID-19 response contingency plan. Did our rapid response to the pandemic consider resilience, staff burnout, and/or the long-term impact it will have on care delivery? In fact, very early data suggests that the rate of burnout is significant and needs to be addressed. This data also suggests that working collaboratively helped with not only care delivery but also morale. COVID-19 is driving remarkable and unprecedented transformations within care delivery and the health care industry. Michaelic & Lamb 2020 suggest that working in interprofessional teams can help with resiliency and dilution of traditional hierarchical care models and helps individuals manage their stress. Furthermore, Tannenbaum et al. (2021) note that the use of interprofessional teams using effective teamwork and coordination is best positioned to overcome the unprecedented challenges of the COVID-19 pandemic. Team app-roaches to care delivery are not a new phenomenon; in fact the renewed interest prepandemic was rooted in recognizing that care delivered by an interprofessional team was more likely to result in better patient outcomes.

As previously described, health care providers, including nurses, have been experiencing moral distress and burnout as a result of the pandemic care challenges. Bowles et al. (2019) further described the role of the nurse on health care teams as critical to optimizing patient safety and workforce satisfaction, which is linked to improved patient outcomes, patient experience, health care quality, and cost per capita. Nurses are and have always been integral members of the health care team.

This chapter addresses the influence of interprofessional education (IPE) and collaborative practice (CP) on health care delivery and more specially its effect on nursing curriculum. The definition of IPE and CP as defined by the World Health Organization (WHO) in 2010 has not changed. For the purposes of this chapter, IPE will continue to be defined as occurring "when students from two or more professions learn about, from and with each other to enable effective collaboration and improve health" and CP as when "multiple health workers from different professional backgrounds work together with patients, families, care providers and communities to deliver the highest quality of care" (p. 7). Finally, this chapter describes approaches in which nursing faculty can provide IPE experiences in the classroom, simulation, and CP experiences in live clinical, community learning environments and through telehealth learning experiences. It is important to note that the goal of IPE and CP in the learning environment is to prepare clinicians to engage in team-based care—interprofessional collaborative practice (IPCP), in the health care environment.

A HISTORICAL PERSPECTIVE ON INTERPROFESSIONAL COLLABORATION

Conversations from those on the front line of care are now suggesting that they are holding the value of teamwork and teamwork in higher esteem (Michaelic & Lamb, 2020). But this narrative has not always been the sentiment. In the past five decades IPE had primarily focused on classroom curriculum and prepared students to be "collaboration ready" after graduation (Brandt et al., 2018). Ironically, documents like *Educating for the Health Team*, a report of the 1972 Institute of Medicine (IOM) conference that explored health care practitioners engaging in teamwork and, more than two decades later, the Health Professions Commission report, which concurred with the need to require interdisciplinary competence in all health professionals (O'Neil, 1998), were not actualized. Further, the IOM (1999; 2001; & 2003) published white papers that recommended that educators and practice develop interdisciplinary team approaches to care, warning that the effect would be great if silos remained the status quo among health care professionals. The subsequent WHO report of 2010 supported and described the benefits of coordinated education and experiential learning and workforces that use IPE and CP models (Flood et al., 2021).

But despite these publications, early health care education and practice continued to only dabble in IPE, and in fact, many early IPE learning experiences included the use of solo professions role playing other members of the health care team. What has been learned from the past about the reality of IPE and CP education is that students who graduated from well-intended, accredited institutions were not prepared to practice team-based care because they were taught in an "old" health care system that did not offer opportunities to practice teamwork skills or shared decision making (Speakman, 2017; Brandt et al., 2018). It was not until several later reports, the 2011 Interprofessional Education Collaborative Expert Panel (IPEC) competencies (updated in 2016), and health profession education accreditation associations requiring IPE and CP learning outcomes that educators and clinicians could begin to conceptualize and then actualize how IPE and CP could be achieved. This marks the resurgence of the IPE and CP movement. Fig. 11.1 illustrates the updated 2016 core competencies and subcompetencies that can be integrated throughout the prelicensure learning continuum and the professional practice settings (IPEC, 2016, pp. 9–10).

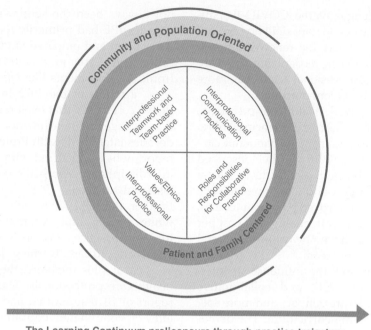

The Learning Continuum prelicensure through practice trajectory

FIG. 11.1 Interprofessional collaboration competency domain. (From Interprofessional Education Collaborative. [2016]. *Core competencies for interprofessional collaborative practice: 2016 update.* Interprofessional Education Collaborative.)

NATIONAL STANDARDS FOR INTERPROFESSIONAL EDUCATION AND COLLABORATIVE PRACTICE

Arenson (2017) described the IPEC core competencies as the logistical elements of team-based care. The IPEC competencies were specific and achievable outcomes. The publication of the IPEC competencies provided structure and process for health professions education and led to an increase of IPE and CP in health care education. Additionally, the competencies now emphasize the role of the patient as a member of the health care team (Flood et al., 2021). Box 11.1 illustrates the latest IPEC model (2016) and lists the four core competencies: values and ethics, roles and responsibilities, interprofessional communication, and team and teamwork. It is intended that the core competencies serve as a framework that can be integrated into the curricula of health professions programs. The core competencies are crucial to success in health care team settings, and nurses can best use these skills to lead

or engage other members of the health care team (Speakman, 2017; Speakman et al., 2016).

While health care education moved quickly to adopt and incorporate these competencies, the clinical arena has lagged. It was theorized that it is easier for health care educators to find the similarities in curriculum to embed students in interprofessional learning opportunities, but in the clinical environment health care professionals practice differently under their own scope of practice. Clinical education models also differ. Nursing clinical education is often unit based as nursing students are assigned to a clinical unit with a clinical instructor and are not imbedded into the health care team as other health professions students may be as they are assigned to follow their preceptor throughout the organization. Brandt et al. (2018) raised the question of how to prepare students to practice in new models of care when they are practicing in traditional models. They continue to posit the need to "inoculate" existing students to embrace interprofessional values and behavior.

BOX 11.1   IPEC Core Competencies for Interprofessional Collaborative Practice

Values and Ethics	Roles and Responsibilities	Interprofessional Communication	Team and Teamwork
Work with individuals of other professions to maintain a climate of mutual respect and shared values.	Use the knowledge of one's own role and those of other professions to appropriately assess and address the health care needs of the patients and to promote and advance the health of populations.	Communicate with patients, families, communities, and professionals in health and other fields in a responsive and responsible manner that supports a team approach to the promotion and maintenance of health and the prevention and treatment of disease.	Apply relationship-building values and the principles of team dynamics to perform effectively in different team roles to plan, deliver, and evaluate patient-/population-centered care and population health programs and policies that are safe, timely, efficient, effective, and equitable.

Interprofessional Education Collaborative Expert Panel (IPEC). (2016). *Core competencies for interprofessional collaborative practice: Update.* Retrieved from. https://www.ipecollaborative.org/resources.html

Even with IPE and CP becoming an essential value to health care education and practicing, the ability to sustain IPE programming can be a challenge (NCICLE, 2021). Faculty are responsible to design and implement learning experiences to facilitate acquisition of the knowledge, skills, and attitudes represented in the competencies. Recently published IPE and CP literature supported developing more robust learning experiences to foster student development and ability to perform in high-functioning teams in the clinical environment. Ketcherside et al. (2017) and Speakman (2017) specifically remarked that nursing students should be provided with IPE and CP opportunities to demonstrate acquisition of interprofessional behaviors and competencies. A subsequent study conducted by Coleman et al. (2017) found that students' ability to work in teams influenced students' perceptions of their team skills and patients' perception of care improved.

It is important to note that the IPEC core competencies are a framework and can be used to assess and evaluate students' acquisition of the core competencies. However, widespread integration of IPE and CP in health professions curricula remains challenged by perceived and actual barriers at the institutional, program, faculty, and student levels. While the value of team-based learning continues to thrive, a continued concern about infrastructure required to develop, implement, evaluate, and sustain effective

IPE and CP in health professions programs exists. Institutional strategic plans need to include references to the benefits of interprofessional learning and collaborative care opportunities (NCICLE, 2021). Now with the increasing use of telehealth and the availability of connectivity as an important part of advancing interprofessional practice, there is an increasing need for accreditation bodies to develop and implement competencies related to the use of telehealth technology (DuBose-Morris et al., 2021). The following sections elaborate on the IPEC core competencies of values and ethics, roles and responsibilities, interprofessional communication, and team and teamwork. Interprofessional practice that places the patient as a central member of the team leads to improved patient outcomes. This team-based approach represents the creation of a synergy of high-quality patient care and a core measure of how to provide safe and efficient patient care (Wei et al., 2020).

Values and Ethics

"Work with individuals of other professions to maintain a climate of mutual respect and shared values. IPEC (2016, p. 11)."

Interprofessional values and related ethics are an important new part of crafting a professional identity, one that is both professional and interprofessional in nature. Professional values and ethical behavior have always been tenets of nursing practice and are major concepts integrated throughout nursing curricula. This is a common thread for all health profession programs, and this mutual competency lends itself quite nicely as the basis of joint interprofessional learning experiences. However, it is important to note that teaching interprofessional student teams requires strategies that acknowledge diverse learning styles and perspectives and maintains a sensitivity to the various professions' identities (Willgerodt & Zierler, 2017). Values and ethics fall within the area of sensitivity to professional identities. Furthermore, Schot et al. (2020) recommend the use of clear common rules and adequate organizational arrangements to help interprofessional teams to get to know one another.

Team-based learning, values clarification, case studies, reflective thought, interprofessional grand rounds with debriefing opportunities, and simulations are examples of teaching and learning strategies that can be effective in facilitating interprofessional student learning. IPE and CP community-based learning experiences and virtual experiences also offer students many opportunities to examine their personal ethos and develop a team value framework. Unlike the inpatient clinical environment, the community setting is less physically and emotionally prescriptive. How one chooses to live and care for themselves or another, and how well the community can meet the needs of an individual, can challenge a student's belief system and ethos. Providing students with team-based CP experiences in diverse community settings promotes the student teams' ability to develop a collective moral compass and respect for each other. This is also true of virtual learning experiences where students learning and working together in interprofessional teams create "a climate of mutual respect and shared values" (IPEC, 2016, p. 10).

Roles and Responsibilities

"Use the knowledge of one's own role and those of other professions to appropriately assess and address the health care needs of patients and to promote and advance the health of populations (IPEC, 2016, p. 12)."

Learning to be interprofessional requires an understanding of how professional roles and responsibilities complement each other in patient-centered and community/population-oriented care. To fully engage in IPE and CP, it is important for team members to understand each other's roles and responsibilities; it is also essential for each member of the team to be able to clearly articulate to each other their own roles and responsibilities in patient care (IPEC, 2016). Nurses, by the nature of their profession, are accustomed to working with other health care professionals. However, there is no assurance that a nurse understands the role and responsibilities of the other health care providers or that those other health care providers necessarily understand the nurse's role. Such understandings need to be intentionally cultivated in environments characterized by mutual respect and trust.

Developing a reciprocal understanding of the roles and responsibilities of the many members of the health care team should begin in the educational setting. Hence students must be prepared to learn "how to use the knowledge of one's own role and those of other professions to appropriately assess and address the health care needs of patients and to promote and advance the health of populations" (IPEC, 2016, p. 10). The transformation from a uniprofessional care team to an interprofessional team requires a shift in culture, a change in a hierarchical mindset that embraces the uniqueness of each professional role while simultaneously cultivating a collaborative team (Khalili & Price, 2021). Faculty can work collaboratively to create opportunities to engage nursing students with other members of the health care team. For example, team debriefings after rounding in the clinical setting, interprofessional case study presentations in the classroom, either in a face-to-face or virtual platform, and simulated learning activities are just a few strategies that can bring student teams of health care providers together to discuss patient-care scenarios and consciously require them to articulate how their role and responsibilities complement other team members' contributions, forming a collective goal for the patient's care.

The patient or individual has a different role in the community from the one they have in the inpatient care setting. Community-based IPE and

CP learning experiences offer an additional perspective—the role of the community and its stakeholders in the health care delivery system. Some examples of community learning opportunities include having student teams complete home assessments and windshield surveys and/or hosting health fairs and health promotion activities in community sites. Community health IPE and CP experiences are an effective way to develop authentic learning experiences for students (Grace & Coutts, 2017).

Interprofessional Communication

"Communicate with patients, families, communities, and professionals in health and other fields in a responsive and responsible manner that supports a team approach to the promotion and maintenance of health and the prevention and treatment of disease IPEC (2016, p. 13)."

Communication competencies help professionals prepare for collaborative practice. Communicating a readiness to work together initiates an effective interprofessional collaboration. The process of interprofessional communication is complex and prone to misunderstanding (Coolen et al., 2020). Although nursing education prepares students at all levels to strive to be effective communicators, the implementation of interprofessional communication means that all health professionals have equal responsibility to demonstrate leadership and raise concerns with each other within the IPCP team. Each team member also has equal value in managing and delivering safe and effective patient care. According to IPEC (2016), "Learning to give and receive timely, sensitive, and instructive feedback with confidence helps health professionals improve their teamwork and team-based care" (p. 13). However, feeling empowered and safe enough within the team to speak and possibly challenge another health professional who either has seniority or is perceived to hold positional authority can be a challenge. Whether a real or perceived hierarchy exists, a nurse may feel intimidated about speaking up or even more hesitant to make recommendations.

"Communicating with patients, families, communities and professionals in health and other fields in a responsive responsible manner that supports a team approach to the promotion and maintenance of health and the prevention and treatment of disease" (IPEC, 2016, p. 10) is an important skill to master. Nurse educators must find communication practice opportunities such as the SBAR (situation, background, assessment, and recommendation) technique to help students develop confidence in speaking up within the IPCP team. The use of simulations can be an effective strategy in facilitating students becoming more confident in their SBAR communication skills and using clear affirmative communication techniques in practice will have a major effect on safe and effective patient care delivery. The SBAR tool can be used in a variety of clinical settings as an effective means of communicating critical patient information (Coolen et al., 2020). Implementing SBAR training sessions with students from multiple professions has the potential to teach nurses how to frame any conversation and feel free to offer recommendations. More information can be found at http://www.ihi.org/resources/Pages/Tools/sbartoolkit.aspx.

Another opportunity for building communication competencies is the use of a TeamSTEPPS program that uses standardized communication techniques to promote patient safety practices. Implementing a standard approach, health care profession can respond more effectively and quickly, which can transform the health care culture that promotes patient safety (Agency for Healthcare Research and Quality, n.d.). Simulation is an ideal modality to teach TeamSTEPPS, using the safe space scenarios to learn how to treat patients successfully and safely (Duffy et al., 2017). Furthermore, the use of digital and telecommunication implemented during the COVID-19 pandemic further underlines the need for developing and implementing effective communication interprofessional learning activities (Jones et al., 2020).

Team and Teamwork

"Apply relationship-building values and the principles of team dynamics to perform effectively in different team roles to plan, deliver, and evaluate patient/population centered care and population health programs and policies that are safe, timely, efficient, effective, and equitable IPEC (2016, p. 14)."

Working in teams involves sharing one's expertise and relinquishing some professional autonomy to work closely with others. Shared accountability, shared problem-solving, and shared decision-making are characteristics of collaborative teamwork and working effectively in teams.

The gestalt of learning the tenants of IPE and CP is to be prepared to practice IPCP effective teamwork. Nurses must be comfortable with assuming a leadership role on the team and with being effective team members. As previously discussed, nurses routinely work in teams, but are these teams always effective at working together to produce quality care outcomes? Interprofessional teams can only be effective if team members understand each other's roles and everyone is comfortable speaking up and engaging in an open discussion. For many nurses, especially novice nurses, assuming a leadership role on the team can be intimidating. Learning to be an effective team member and patient advocate requires practice that must include building equitable relationships. Understanding the mechanisms underlying interprofessional collaboration can enhance collaborative practice care (Wei et al., 2020).

Nursing students can learn to engage in teamwork in a variety of ways. For example, experiencing team-based learning in either face-to-face or virtual classrooms with peers or group project assignments with students from other disciplines, including those outside the health professions, can help the student develop the group dynamic skills necessary to be an effective team leader and member. Interprofessional simulation activities, experiential learning experiences in clinical settings with other health care providers, and community-based interprofessional service-learning projects with a variety of community members are just a few examples of how faculty can intentionally foster the development of teamwork skills in the curriculum. The literature on IPCP states that teamwork has the potential to positively affect patient outcomes. High-functioning care teams work together, collaborating in collective problem-solving and decision-making processes. Interestingly, Michaelic and Lamb (2020) describe the unprecedented changes in frontline care because the COVID-19 pandemic has changed providers' perceptions of

teamwork, leaning now toward team-ness, solidarity and collectivity, and hierarchy. Conversely Sukhera et al. (2021) warn that tension in interprofessional teams that impacts trust and collaboration may be the result of larger social, physical, organizational, and historical influences. Using the four IPEC core competencies as a framework for IPE and/or CP learning experiences provides students with the ability to work more efficiently in IPCP teams with the aim of improving population health (IPEC, 2016). Providing team training in academia can develop more cohesive relationships with common goals empowering every team member to practice at the top of their license.

EFFECT OF INTERPROFESSIONAL EDUCATION AND COLLABORATIVE PRACTICE ON PATIENT OUTCOMES

Promoting IPE and CP early and often in the learning environment yields the greatest possibility for establishing and promoting relationships that can be strengthened over time in IPCP clinical environments. The demand for IPCP is related to improving patient-care outcomes. IHI originally developed the Triple Aim framework with a goal of optimizing the performance of the US health care delivery system (Berwick et al., 2008; IHI, 2007). The Triple Aim framework had three goals: to improve the patient's experience of care, to improve population health, and reduce per-capita costs of health care, as represented in Fig. 11.2 (IHI, 2007). The Triple Aim framework reenforced the importance

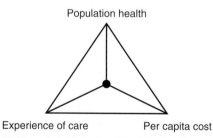

FIG. 11.2 The Institute for Healthcare Improvement Triple Aim Framework. (The Triple Aim framework was developed by the Institute for Healthcare Improvement in Cambridge, Massachusetts [http://www.ihi.org]. Reprinted with permission.)

of interprofessional health care would eventually lead to improved health outcomes, better care, better health, better value, and better work experience (Bouchaud et al. 2017, Khalili & Price, 2021).

Additional goals have now been added to the original Triple Aim framework. The Quadruple Aim framework adds the element of attaining joy in work, acknowledging that even the best performing health care delivery systems experience provider burnout. Burnout has a direct correlation to poor patient experiences since staff who find joy in their work are more likely to engage in higher level of patient care and engagement (http://www.ihi.org/communities/blogs/the-triple-aim-or-the-quadruple-aim-four-points-to-help-set-your-strategy). The significance of job satisfaction and joy in nursing cannot be overlooked. It is indisputable that being a nurse is challenging. Patient care and health care delivery systems are complex, and nurses need to enter the workforce prepared to work in teams, feel empowered to speak up, and know their opinion and input is valuable. Placing students in team experiences yields the best chance of preparing students to work and speak up earlier in their careers rather than later. The IOM recommended that nurses should be full partners on the health care team, contributing their unique perspective and expertise and having opportunities for interprofessional collaboration and leadership development (IOM, 2011, 2015). For nurses to achieve these skills and beliefs in practice, they should be learned when they are students.

But simply being part of a team does not always achieve all the criteria in the Quadruple Aim framework, especially "joy in working." To reach this level of satisfaction, teams must have a productive, trusting relationship that boosts mutual respect and common goals and in which one can feel appreciated and understand another's opinion has merit (Perlo et al., 2017). The COVID-19 pandemic underscores the need for health care educators to continue to develop innovative ways to have students engage in interprofessional education (Jones et al., 2020). This is especially needed today as we prepare students to become front-line providers. Tannebaum et al. note that teamwork has become more central and challenging during the pandemic to care delivery but posit that crises

can stimulate individuals' willingness to cooperate and tackle a shared predicament (2021). While the triple aim remains the standard of how care delivery should be done, the addition of the fourth aim acknowledges that the first three aims must be accomplished by creating a joyful work environment. The inability to add the fourth aim will lead to failure and unsustainable quality patient care (Nundy et al., 2022).

Another disparity highlighted in part by the COVID-19 pandemic is health care inequity. The recent report, *The Future of Nursing 2020–2030: Charting a Path to Achieve Health Equity*, examines the role of nursing in reducing health inequities while attending to cost, utilizing technology, and maintaining patient and family-focused care delivery. Concomitantly, it has been suggested that a fifth goal (aim) be added to the IHI Triple Aim Framework, creating the "Quintuple Aim" that would focus on quality evidence-based care to encourage health equity (Nundy et al., 2022). Nurses have always been mindful of the social determinants of health and health equity. Using collaborative care models that examine the entirety of the health care experience is a crucial factor in moving toward actualizing this goal.

DEVELOPING AN ORGANIZING CURRICULUM FRAMEWORK FOR INTERPROFESSIONAL EDUCATION AND COLLABORATIVE PRACTICE

Creating an organizing framework for the curriculum of any educational program provides faculty with a way of organizing knowledge and skills and is critical to achieving the desired educational outcomes. Although not designed specifically for IPE, the Kirkpatrick model (Kirkpatrick & Kirkpatrick, 2010) is one framework that is frequently used in IPE to evaluate student learning. The Kirkpatrick Model guides the training process using real data to evaluate and understand how training impacts organizations (Smith, 2020). The IPE community has acknowledged the value of the Kirkpatrick model, which is implemented both nationally and internationally. The Kirkpatrick model has been described as a simple but fairly accurate way to measure adult learning or training (LaDuke, 2017). Finally, it can also be used as the basis of an evaluation plan for IPE/CP programming by examining student mastery of the Kirkpatrick levels.

First developed in 1954, the Kirkpatrick model has four components to evaluate educational program effectiveness. Level 1, the reaction level, evaluates how a participant reacts to the training and education programs. Level 2, the learning level, evaluates how much the participant has learned from the actual training. Level 3, the behavior level, evaluates how the participants apply what they learned to their work setting. Level 4, the results level, evaluates the formative outcomes of the training and education programs. The Kirkpatrick model was modified with the addition of a new dimension called return on expectations (ROE). ROE is the practitioner's approach to determining the organizational value of the training and the degree to which the organization's expectations have been satisfied (Kirkpatrick & Kirkpatrick, 2010).

To achieve the desired ROE and effect on patient outcomes, interprofessional learning opportunities should be integrated into the curricula of health professions programs and offered on a continuous basis, using a variety of teaching strategies. When collaborative practice teams can demonstrate effective behaviors, improved health care metrics such as better health of patients or populations and subsequent reduced cost can be achieved (Arenson, 2017). Box 11.2 outlines some examples of how the Kirkpatrick model can be used in the evaluation of interprofessional learning activities.

Preparing the Institution and Faculty for Implementation of Interprofessional Education and Collaborative Practice

Incorporating IPE activities and CP initiatives into the curriculum can require changing institutional culture. Many IPE champions report that they receive pushback from other faculty and clinicians because it is perceived that the system they are currently using appears to meet their needs in implementing the curriculum. When discussing and planning IPE and CP activities, it is important for faculty to understand that incorporating IPE and CP learning experiences is not just a curriculum add-on. In fact, IPE and CP learning experiences can be incorporated into many patient-care situations in a variety of settings. One means by which to highlight the benefits of IPE is reminding faculty and administrators of the importance of students learning to provide care in teams so they can more effectively provide team-based care as practitioners. One of the outcomes of the COVID-19 pandemic is a growing understanding of the importance of health providers to engage in increased levels of collaboration, shared responsibilities, upskilling, and greater fluid boundaries (Langlois et al., 2020). The pandemic highlighted the importance of team approaches to care delivery and underscored the value and importance of integrating interprofessional education and collaborative practice initiatives in health care education.

Box 11.3 is a guide to planning IPE and CP learning initiatives. Some faculty may already have experience with IPE and CP and can serve as faculty champions for those who have less

---

BOX 11.2   Application of the Kirkpatrick Model in Interprofessional Education

Reaction	Learning	Behavior	Results
What did the student think and feel about experiencing interprofessional collaboration? How did the student react to the learning activity? Was the response favorable?	How well did the student learn the intended content? Did the student acknowledge an increase in knowledge of interprofessional collaboration?	To what extent was the student able to effectively apply teamwork and communication techniques?	In the health care environment, what were the outcomes resulting from students' learning and practicing in interprofessional collaborative teams?

BOX 11.3 **Guide to Planning Interprofessional Education and Collaborative Practice Initiatives**

- Decide who should participate in planning the experience, ensure representation from each discipline, and find a mutually convenient time to meet.
- Identify key information needed from each discipline to facilitate planning.
- Determine learner level that will be involved in the learning experience, striving for congruency among the various student populations.
- Describe and discuss various program curricula and influence of program accreditation standards.
- Consider placement of clinical learning experiences within the curricula. Use IPEC competencies as a framework for the design of learning activities
- Create a consensus on desired project outcomes using the Core Competencies for Interprofessional Collaboration as a guide.
- Avoid trying to align the entire curriculum of multiple programs. Focus interprofessional efforts where the curricula intersect in some manner (schedule, clinical rotations, common concepts, etc.). Outline the program, deciding who, what, when, where, and how.
- Develop program elements including goals, concepts to be covered, and how the program will be evaluated
- Identify a common time to host the program and a location that ensures easy access by all students.
- Identify needed administrative support and resources to implement the program. Examine and select reliable and valid evaluation tools to measure program outcomes (https://nexusipe.org/measurement-instruments).
- Consider using a systematic plan to facilitate program implementation and evaluation using the core competencies for interprofessional practice.

experience. There must be a concerted effort to orient faculty on the components of IPE and CP. The following activities can help prepare nursing faculty to engage in IPE:

- Seek advice and resources from national IPE champions and use up-to-date IPE and CP resources. The *Journal of Interprofessional Care* and the *Journal of Interprofessional Research and Education* along with the National Center for Interprofessional Practice and Education [NEXUS] (https://nexusipe.org) have a plethora of resources that faculty can use to plan, implement, and evaluate IPE and CP programs. In addition, the National League for Nursing (2017) published the *Guide to Effective Interprofessional Education Experiences in Nursing Education*, which includes an IPE readiness assessment and detailed exemplars of IPE and CP learning activities and *Interprofessional Education Collaborative Practice: Creating a Blueprint for Nurse Educators [NLN Press]*.
- Complete the IPE readiness assessment found in the *Guide to Effective Interprofessional Education Experiences in Nursing Education* to help identify what efforts need to be taken before starting an IPE and/or CP program. Understanding the needs before embarking on an IPE and/or CP

project can diminish or eliminate barriers and pitfalls when implementing programming.
- Identify a rationale for participating in IPE. The IOM (2011) report *Future of Nursing: Leading Change, Advancing Health*, the IOM (2015) progress report on the impact of the *Future of Nursing*, and *The Future of Nursing 2020–2030 Charting a Path to Achieve Health Equity* report can be used to frame faculty discussions and provide context to the importance of integrating IPE and CP into nursing programs.
- Review your programs' accreditation standards and the standards of other health professions' disciplines that may be participating in the IPE and/or CP proposed program. Understanding how IPE and/or CP initiatives can support meeting accreditation standards is often helpful when identifying rationale for implementation of IPE and CP programming. Identifying the overlapping accreditation standards of other health professions programs can be used to frame a discussion of common interprofessional goals for all programs.
- Identify faculty champions for leading the integration of IPE into the curriculum and assign mentors to help less experienced faculty. If mentors are not available within your institution, seek out other

institutions that have already incorporated IPE and/or CP into their curriculum. Searching the literature may also help you identify IPE champions who may be willing to speak to you or the group and serve as faculty mentors.

- Seek collaborating partners from interdisciplinary colleagues within your own institution and other local and regional colleges, universities, and health care agencies. Although it is important to explore various types of IPE and CP initiatives that will work in a specific learning environment, it is also important to learn with and from others. Forming local or regional consortiums and partnerships, reviewing the literature for examples of successful IPE programs, and sharing outcomes from such collaborative efforts can be helpful activities. Provide time for faculty to debrief after implementing an IPE initiative to evaluate the experience, acknowledge the lessons learned, and explore new ways to advance IPE in the curriculum.
- Consider developing online interprofessional learning activities. While interprofessional socialization is different in the online format, providing additional resources, facilitating intentional interactions, and developing social networks among learners can foster interprofessional learning and provide students with a broader interprofessional community (Khalili & Orchard, 2020; Langlois et al., 2020).

INTEGRATING INTERPROFESSIONAL EDUCATION AND COLLABORATIVE PRACTICE INITIATIVES INTO THE CURRICULUM

Providing nursing students with interprofessional education learning opportunities enhances their ability to engage in collaborative practice (Labraguea et al., 2018). Designing IPE and CP initiatives for implementation into the curriculum can be a daunting task because it requires collaboration and coordination with other professions. However, the accreditation standards of most health professions programs include expectations related to providing students with IPE (Langlois et al., 2020), so seeking opportunities for

> **CASE STUDY 11.1 Integrating IPE into the Curriculum**
>
> A nurse faculty is approached by a physical therapy faculty with a request to develop an IPE project. When the nurse faculty mentions this opportunity casually in a faculty meeting, the faculty member is told by some colleagues that "there is simply no room in the curriculum to add another thing" and discussion of the topic is dropped. The faculty wants to continue to pursue the IPE opportunity but is uncertain of how to proceed.
>
> 1. What would be the best approach for the nurse faculty in continuing to pursue this IPE opportunity with their faculty colleagues?
> 2. What evidence could the nurse faculty use to support the case for implementing IPE learning activities?
> 3. What other methods could the nurse faculty have used to announce to their colleagues the request for a collaborative IPE initiative with the physical therapy program?

collaborating with other health professions faculty hold benefits for all program (see Case Study 11.1).

As plans for introducing IPE into the curriculum are developed, it is important to focus initially on obtaining the support of senior leaders in the institution, as this can have a significant effect on how much buy-in will be received from others (Speakman et al., 2016). Part of the proposal to senior leadership should include references to the health professions' accreditation standards to demonstrate the importance of incorporating IPE into the curricula. Once institutional support has been secured and an IPE readiness assessment conducted within the programs, it is important to bring any interested parties to a development meeting. Securing the support of administrators, staff, faculty, and students eases the ability to implement organizational culture change and IPE curriculum reform (Speakman et al., 2016). This preliminary step is an essential means to reducing the risk of failure to progress because of barriers and challenges not dealt with at the time of programming inception.

The greatest challenge to implementing IPE is usually finding a common time for the learning experiences and resolving competing schedules. Pardue et al. (2017) suggest using a framework that faculty can use to design, implement, and evaluate IPE. It is also important to consider the appropriate level of students from multiple programs to participate in any given learning activity. Depending on the desired learner outcomes, the faculty may decide to partner students of comparable educational levels. For example, students in their first year of clinical experience, such as first-year nursing students, may be partnered with first- or second-year medical, pharmacy, or physical or occupational therapy graduate students. However, there may also be value to partnering less experienced students with students who are further along in their educational program to foster learning among peers. Subsequently it may be appropriate to partner second-year nursing students with third- or fourth-year medical, pharmacy, or physical or occupational therapy, or physician assistant students, as all students are engaged in clinical experiences. The goal is to have students from different professions engaging and dialoguing with one another, building those important interpersonal relationships.

Sometimes nursing programs are the only health professions program offered by the institution. If the institution does not have other health-related degree programs, faculty can reach out to other academic disciplines. Humanities, environmental or bench sciences, computers and technology, and justice and law are a few examples of disciplines that require teamwork and can be collaborative partners in addressing health care issues. Seeking out these academic partners gives students an opportunity to learn the effective collaboration and communication skills they need as practicing nurses to address complex health care situations requiring the expertise of varied disciplines.

See Box 11.4 for an exemplar of an IPE and/ or CP initiative that can be used in either academic health centers and/or small colleges or

---

BOX 11.4   Activity Exemplar Title: Emergency Training

Type of Activity: Simulation
Purpose of Activity: The purpose of this activity is to provide students with an opportunity to practice patient-centered and team-based care in a simulated emergency environment.

Learning Objectives
- Discuss the importance of emergency preparedness
- Identify the roles of different health professionals and laypeople in dealing with an emergency
- Recognize opportunities to use emergency preparedness skills in emergency situations
- Apply emergency preparedness skills to deliver high-quality patient care

Target audience and maximum number of participants: various student professions, both health related and non–health related; maximum student number determined by room size and the simulation capacity.

Preparation for the Activity: Training Presentation: This activity involves an element of surprise as the students are brought to the activity under the pretense of training or a meeting, unaware that they are about to do an emergency simulation. The first step is to determine the skill or knowledge you want the students to put into practice during the activity.

Specific examples include general emergency management training, teamwork skills, such as conflict management, or a protocol for wound care or heart failure.

Develop a training presentation on the topic. Emergency Environment: Then, determine the emergency environment. The idea is for the students to have to immediately put the skill or protocol into practice after the didactic presentation during an emergency simulation. The environment can be as complex or simple as you desire. An example of a complex environment is an explosion at a public event or shopping mall with many injured patients and limited medical supplies on hand. A simpler example is a patient in an exam room experiencing cardiac arrest.

If your institution doesn't have access to resources to create an emergency environment, consider doing role play without a simulated environment after the training presentation.

Simulation Materials: Determine if you want to use manikins or live actors to play the simulated patients. Based on the emergency scenario you select, gather the supplies needed. Supplies could include theatrical elements, such as artificial blood, a fog machine, or debris, and medical supplies such as a stethoscope, sling, ice pack, inhaler, and medication.

Simulated Patient
Scenarios: Develop patient scenarios for the emergency environment requiring students to evaluate each patient's condition and how to treat him/her. The patient scenarios should be customized to the

Continued

BOX 11.4   Activity Exemplar Title: Emergency Training—cont'd

different professions represented among the participants and to the number of participants. Also, if your institution does not have access to students of multiple health-related professions, this activity is an opportunity to partner with non-health-related professions for general disaster preparedness skills. Example patient conditions include a twisted ankle, a fractured forearm, hypoglycemia in a diabetic, and asthma attack in a known asthmatic. Incorporate elements that beg for the skill or protocol to be used to ensure students are focusing on it, in addition to handling any other simulation factors.

Training Presentation: A facilitator presents the training to the students. Simultaneously, the simulation environment is being set up in a different room that is hidden from the students' view to maintain the element of surprise. Toward the end of the presentation, an actor enters the room to alert the students of the simulated emergency and set the scene. The actor could play the role of a firefighter who enters and says, "We need your help! You are now in a shopping mall and there has been an explosion and there are injured people in the room next door who need medical attention! For your safety, you will not be able to leave the room. Also, there are no medical supplies beyond what is present in the room. Please follow me and disperse yourselves among the injured."

Simulation: The students then file into the simulation room, which has been furnished to look like a disaster (use of fog machine, ceiling debris on the ground). There are simulated patients on gurneys with various injuries or ailments around the room and medical supplies in the room are visible.

Once the simulations are underway, a simulated paramedic announces that one ambulance has arrived and that the students need to determine which patients are in the most acute condition. At this point, the students should begin the shared decision-making process and begin communicating across the room about each patient's condition. A patient is taken away in an ambulance once the group has reached consensus. The simulations finish once all patients are treated.

Debriefing: A facilitator then calls for the simulation to end and all students should stop treating patients. Students should remain at their patient stations and debrief initial reactions to the simulation experience with their facilitator. If the simulated patients are live actors, they can also contribute to the conversation by discussing their satisfaction with or observations

about the team dynamics and problem-solving abilities of the students who treated them.

Sample Discussion Questions for Students
- How did you address issues around communication and safety during the scenario?
- How did your team work together?
- Did you feel mutual support?
- Was there a team leader?
- What communication or teamwork skills did you use to communicate with one another?
- To the team leaders?
- Can you walk us through the thought process around the medical management of your patient?
- What might you do differently next time?
- What are two to three main takeaways from this scenario?

Timeline of Activity
- 60-Minute training presentation—by facilitators
- 30-Minute emergency simulation—by simulated patients and facilitators
- 5-Minute small group debriefing—by facilitators
- 20-Minute large group debrief—by facilitators

Pre-Work for Students: Variable based on the training presentation, could include readings or reviewing a PowerPoint presentation for the didactic portion of the program.

Coordination Needs: Before Event
- Recruit faculty members to be facilitators and simulation specialists to help construct the emergency.
- Determine event date and reserve two rooms for the training and the simulation.
- Develop training presentation, emergency environment, and simulated patient scenarios.
- Gather materials needed for the simulation; faculty and simulation support staff at your institution may be able to assist.
- Advertise the event to students and gather a list of students planning to attend.
- Order any food or other supplies for event (as needed).
- Email students an event reminder with date, time, and location close to event date. In your communication with students before the event, leave out information about the emergency simulation to maintain the element of surprise.
- Print any handouts for students and attendance sheet to track student participation (as needed).

From National League for Nursing. (2017). *Guide to effective interprofessional education experiences in nursing education.* https://www.nln.org/docs/default-source/uploadedfiles/default-document-library/ipe-toolkit-krk-012716.pdf universities. As previously noted, the NLN *Guide to Effective Interprofessional Education Experiences in Nursing Education* (nln.org) and Speakman (2017) *Interprofessional Education and Collaborative Practice: Creating a Blueprint for Nurse Educators*, can provide additional exemplars for implementation in program curriculum.

IPE and CP Learning Partnerships

Creating and crafting IPE and CP initiatives in colleges, universities, and/or academic health centers can be challenging. The complexity of the organizations, the challenges of competing schedules and not finding other IPE/CP champions can be daunting. There also may not be a preexisting culture of collaboration within the institution. The key to addressing these issues is to create partnerships with other institutions and programs with similar needs and goals. Designing and planning teamwork and communication opportunities does not require the environment of an academic health center that has other health profession programs. Institutions can engage in IPE and CP initiatives in several ways. For example, nursing faculty can meet with faculty from another program and identify common IPE and CP competencies that address each program's outcomes and develop a collaborative learning activity to facilitate meeting those outcomes.

Since most people are familiar with using teleconferencing to support class meetings, an IPE program can be implemented virtually. Using virtual programming creates many possibilities that are limited by face-to-face interaction. Scheduling conflicts can be minimized since no travel is required and it expands opportunities for students at a distance to participate in the learning experiences. It is important to develop interprofessional virtual experiences to prepare student for telehealth and virtual collaboration. Cowperthwait et al. (2020) described a virtual freeze-frame learning activity that can be adapted to a web-based platform as a promising opportunity for an interprofessional learning experience. Furthermore, DuBose-Morris et al. (2021) support this notion and recommend that health professions education prepares the next generation of interprofessional telehealth care providers with the competencies necessary to practice with the use of technology. As health care educators begin to incorporate more telehealth and virtual interprofessional learning opportunities, a clear set of telehealth competencies like the IPEC core competencies needs to be developed and measured. Developing formal telehealth competencies will help prepare future health care providers to competently meet population health and public health care needs (DuBose-Morris et al. 2021).

All health professionals recognize the need for teams of providers to work collaboratively toward collective health care goals and improved patient outcomes. Nursing, medicine, and many other health professions have noted their commitment to collaborative IPE and CP care (Jones & Phillips, 2016). Providing nursing students with diverse opportunities can only enhance their ability to work in teams by understanding the variety of roles represented in health care.

Additional strategies for developing IPE learning experiences include seeking out opportunities to engage in collaborative research and grant submissions as well as collaborating on scholarship endeavors such as publications and presentations. Such strategies can be used to support the faculty research agenda. Finally, developing a true collaborative culture within the institution can be accomplished by offering a designated IPE course that addresses the national core competencies and enrolls students from multiple disciplines.

Organizing Interprofessional Education and Collaborative Practice Experience

The individual competencies organized under each of the four core competency domains can be thought of as behavioral learning objectives and can be linked to learning activities and assessments of interprofessional effectiveness (IPEC, 2016). To reiterate, the foundation of IPE and CP and ultimately IPCP is teamwork and communication. Therefore nursing students should be given ample opportunities to interact and engage in teamwork learning experiences with a variety of health care professionals or paraprofessionals to practice collaborative, team-based, patient-centered care. Placing students in a variety of interprofessional CP experiences will facilitate students' ability to achieve the four IPEC core competencies (see Case Study 11.2).

CASE STUDY 11.2 **Placing Students in Interprofessional Collaborative Practice Experiences**

A clinical instructor notices that physician providers conduct bedside rounds on the unit at around the same time each day, and many of the students are assigned to the patients for whom the physician group is providing care. The clinical instructor decides to suggest that the nursing students be included in the bedside rounds of their patients.

1. Is it appropriate for the clinical instructor to ask that the nursing students be part of the rounding on their assigned patients?
2. What strategies would best assist the students to communicate with the other members of the team?
3. What topics should the instructor include in a CP post conference debriefing?

Ensuring that each faculty and program can have input into what works for his or her respective college or school has the greatest potential in overcoming any logistical challenges. To develop IPE and CP learning experiences requires nursing faculty to persist in participating in collaborative curriculum planning efforts with other health professions faculty (Speakman, 2017, p. 3). Changing the culture of noncollaboration can be a challenge, but the addition of IPE in accreditation standards and guidelines of most health education professions has been helpful and will continue to move organizations toward a culture of collaboration. The following sections contain examples of how faculty can create interprofessional learning opportunities for nursing students.

Natural Interprofessional Relationships

Natural interprofessional relationships refers to the pairing of nursing students with one or more students from medicine, pharmacy, occupational and physical therapy, physician assistants, diet and nutrition, and social work health care education programs. For the most part, these students are in program plans of study that include didactic and experiential clinical experiences with patients with chronic and episodic health care needs and therefore are most likely to naturally engage with nursing students on the clinical unit. For these partners, interprofessional teamwork can be demonstrated in the classroom and in clinical and simulated learning environments and can be done in community sites. Some ideas include the following:

- Develop an interprofessional case study with partners from other disciplines. Have students work in teams to discuss how each profession might manage the care of the patient, creating an interprofessional plan of care.
- Invite an interprofessional team of experts to interact with students, either face to face or online, and explain their role in the delivery of patient care. Although such a learning experience can be designed and offered to a single student discipline, providing such an experience to students representing multiple disciplines is more powerful.
- Implement a simulated case study regarding a clinical incident or disaster preparedness with an interprofessional team of students. Providing opportunities to practice teamwork, communication skills, and clinical decision making in a simulated environment is a low-risk learning experience and will help students build confidence in implementing these skills in the clinical environment.
- Engage nursing students with other members of the health care team in a rounding experience on the clinical unit. If possible, have the students complete a patient assessment together and jointly present findings during a debriefing experience after the rounding activity.
- Work with students from multiple disciplines to host a health or science fair in the community. Students can conduct a community assessment together and work in teams to plan and deliver health promotion activities to both adults and children living in the community. Students can then debrief on how each of their professions approaches community engagement and what they learned from working with individuals from other programs.
- Develop virtual clinical learning experiences. Use telelearning modalities where students can engage in virtual joint patient assessment and

care planning. This allows students to remain "in situ" at their respective clinical placements while collaborating with other members of the health care team.

Designed Interprofessional Relationships

Designed interprofessional relationships refers to pairing nursing students with one or more of the groups of students enrolled in education, theater, law, psychology, biological and chemical science, radiological science, music, art, or business programs. For these partners, interprofessional activities that foster teamwork might be limited to the classroom setting with the potential simulation, clinical, or service-learning experience. Some ideas include the following:

- Develop a case study with partners from other disciplines. Have students form interprofessional teams to discuss management of the scenario described in the case study. Students should discuss their respective professional roles and responsibilities. As a team, define how their professions intersect in managing the scenario.
- Invite students from multiple professions to attend a common classroom experience to form teams to work on team-building skills using such block-building exercises as Zoom wordless book (https://www.zoombook.com), Paper Chain building, and Lego. During debriefing, have the students describe the techniques they employed during the group process.
- Develop a simulation case study with partners from other disciplines on disaster preparedness, having students practice teamwork and communication skills in interprofessional teams.
- Design a community service-learning or joint clinical opportunity. Have students collaborate on an interprofessional care plan or project activity. Confer a joint postconference and discuss the tenets of teamwork and communication.
- Work with a local senior center, school, or after-school program. Have the students develop and provide an age-appropriate teaching program. Debrief with the students on how each member approached the topic and the effectiveness of teamwork and the use of communication skills.

- Engage with students from theater programs or local theater companies to serve as medical actors using case study or simulation interprofessional activities (https://www.theatre.udel.edu/getting-involved/healthcare-theatre).

Student Considerations With Interprofessional Education and Collaborative Practice

Students are not immune to the challenges of organizational culture change. For some students, engaging in IPE and/or CP is a change from what they previously experienced and for others, it might be contrary to their beliefs and understanding of the role of the nurse in health care. It is important to create an orientation program for students and include the rationale and expectations for IPE and CP learning experiences. Frankel et al. (2017) note that groups who have a shared understanding will experience a higher degree of teamwork and a greater communication experience.

Incorporating the concepts of IPE and CP into the curriculum should not be considered an add-on; it is a teaching strategy. Teaching strategies for IPE are much like general teaching strategies and those principles outlined in Chapter 16. Among the curricula of health professions programs, there are common foundational concepts to be applied to the delivery of patient care. Similarly, each health profession has accreditation standards that include IPE and CP learning experiences. Beginning with this common core of knowledge and the accreditation metrics provides the intersection to build interprofessional learning experiences for students.

FUTURE CONSIDERATIONS FOR IPE AND CP: THE ADDITION OF TECHNOLOGY

"The retention crisis can be addressed by developing innovative strategies to suit the unique needs of nurses today and beyond the pandemic" (Gaffney, 2022, p. 25). The recent pandemic has shown health care clinicians and educators the need to be prepared for untoward events. Early pandemic "silver lining" theories assert that the increased use of team-based approaches had a positive impact on patient care. In addition, the use of virtual platforms has allowed a shift from traditional learning to online modalities, and traditional patient care to telemedicine modalities. This was also true of IPE and CP learning experiences. LeBlanc (2020) suggests that educators need to rethink and shift their face-to-face IPE learning to online platforms. Similarly, Kahili (2020) describes the value of case studies, virtual simulation, and webinars with frontline workers.

Langlois et al. (2020) stated that "Collaboration at all levels is a crucial ingredient for an effective health service response during major health emergencies. Interprofessional education (IPE) is a key vehicle to foster collaborative practice, and investment in IPE, particularly during health crises is arguably more important than ever" (p. 587). Therefore this chapter suggests incorporating advanced technology like simulation and telecommunication when creating and implementing IPE and CP initiatives. Labraque et al. (2018) state that simulation activities that prepare students for interprofessional practice are crucial to prepare future collaborative practitioners. The increased use of telemedicine has also shown to be a viable option to meet patients' health care needs. In fact, early adopters are encouraged by the increased acceptance of this modality. But the issues that existed prior to the pandemic continue today; not enough clinicians have had formal education requiring them to engage in "on the job training," and even more health care educators lack the knowledge on how to train students in telemedicine. For the most part, telehealth technology training is vendor driven and focuses on the technical aspects and not on etiquette needed by health care providers (Gustin et al., 2020). It is important the health care systems and providers, who rapidly employed telemedicine during the pandemic, do not underestimate the need to develop key principles to mitigate the potential unintended consequences of virtual care delivery (Perry et al., 2021).

CHAPTER SUMMARY: KEY POINTS

- The team approach to care can provide consistent, safe, quality, patient-centered care.
- Students who engage in interprofessional learning experiences and have ample opportunities to practice effective communication skills in team-based approaches will have the greatest potential to affect patient-centered care through their practice upon graduation.
- IPE and CP learning experiences that are incorporated into an institution's educational goals and offer educators and practitioners the physical space and protected time to develop and implement collaborative learning opportunities and physical space for these collaborative experiences will have the greatest potential for success (NCICLE, 2021).
- The literature is replete with demonstrating the value and impact of team-based approaches to care delivery on patient outcomes.
- Nurses need to invest in their future to promote purposefulness and direction (Graber et al., 2021). Nurse educators need to develop IPE and CP learning opportunities to prepare students to practice in a collaborative health care delivery system.
- The pandemic highlighted the need for collaboration among many members of the health care team and as a result the health care system experienced a growth in team-based care. Langlois et al. (2020) suggest that the pandemic offers health care clinicians and educators a unique opportunity to make sure they retain what has been served well by IPE and CP.
- The current pandemic offers a unique opportunity for educators, practitioners, researchers, and consumers of interprofessional education and collaborative practice. While the pandemic may not last long, the impact of COVID-19 is going to change our personal, professional, and academic lives for years to come. Intentional critical reflection on approaches and envisioning what is to be learned will be crucial to enabling future advancements in the field of IPE and collaborative practice (Langolis et al., 2020, p. 590).

▮ REFLECTING ON THE EVIDENCE

1. What evidence supports the need to engage nursing students in interprofessional teams when delivering patient care?
2. What is the impact on IPCP when students learn to be effective team leaders and members?
3. What strategies can you use in your academic environment to create IPE and CP learning opportunities? Whom can you identify as potential academic and clinical partners in establishing such learning opportunities?
4. When designing an IPE or a CP program for your curriculum, what challenges would you anticipate needing to address to successfully implement the program? What factors exist within the environment that can be helpful in supporting program implementation? What resources do you need?
5. What elements would you include in a plan designed to evaluate the effectiveness of your IPE and CP program? What is the value of creating a systematic evaluation plan for IPE or CP activities? How current are the IPE and CP learning activities being developed and implemented at your institution?
6. What accreditation standards exist that require students to engage in IPE and CP learning activities?
7. What has been the impact of the COVID-19 pandemic on implementing IPE and CP at your institution? Is there an opportunity to use IPE and CP learning opportunities virtually?

REFERENCES

Agency for Healthcare Research and Quality. (n.d.). *TeamSTEPPS*. https://www.ahrq.gov/teamstepps/index.html

Arenson, C. (2017). Core Competencies and the Kirkpatrick model: a framework for interprofessional education and collaborative practice. In E. Speakman (Ed.), *Interprofessional education and collaborative practice: creating a blueprint for nurse educators*. National League for Nursing.

Berwick, D. M., Nolan, T. W., & Whittington, J. (2008). The triple aim: Care, health, and cost. *Health Affairs, 27*(3), 759–769. https://doi.org/10.1377/hlthaff.27.3.759.

Bouchaud, M. T., Sicks, S., & Mills, C. (2017). Mobilization and organizing interprofessional education and collaborative practice: Examining the challenges and opportunities. In E. Speakman (Ed.), *Interprofessional education and collaborative practice: Creating a blueprint for nurse educators*. National League for Nursing.

Bowles, J. R., Batcheller, J., Adams, J. M., Zimmermann, D., & Pappas, S. (2019, April/June). Nursing's leadership role in advancing professional practice/work environments as part of the quadruple aim. *Nursing Administration Quarterly, 43*(2), 157–163. https://doi.org/10.1097/NAQ.0000000000000342.

Brandt, B. F., Kitto, S., & Cervero, R. M. (2018). Untying the interprofessional Gordian Knot: The national collaborative for improving the clinical learning environment. *Academic Medicine, 93*(10), 1437–1440. https://doi.org/10.1097/ACM.0000000000002313.

Coleman, M. T., McLean, A., Williams, L., & Hasan, K. (2017). Improvement in interprofessional student learning and patient outcomes. *Journal of Interprofessional Care, 8*, 28–33. https://doi.org/10.1016/j.xjep.2017.05.003.

Coolen, E., Engbers, R., Draaisma, J., Heinen, M., & Fluit, C. (2020). The use of SBAR as a structured communication tool in the pediatric non-acute care setting: Bridge or barrier for interprofessional collaboration. *Journal of Interprofessional Care* https://doi.org/10.1080/13561820.2020.1816936.

Cowperthwait, A., Graber, J., Carlsen, A., Cowperthwait, M., & Mekulski, H. (2020). Innovations in virtual education for clinical and simulation learning. *Journal of Professional Nursing, 37*, 1011–1017.

DuBose-Morris, R., McSwain, S. D., McElligott, J. T., King, K. L., Ziniel, S., & Harvey, J. (2021). Building telehealth teams of the future through interprofessional curriculum development: A five year mixed methodology study. *Journal of Interprofessional Care* https://doi.org/10.1080/13561820.2021.2005556.

Duffy, J. J., Forstater, A. T., & Pettit, A. M. (2017). Interprofessional education and simulation: Building a culture of communication and teamwork for patient safety. In E. Speakman (Ed.), *Interprofessional education and collaborative practice: Creating a blueprint for nurse educators*. National League for Nursing.

Flood, B., Smythe, L., Hocking, C., & Jones, M. (2021). Interprofessional practice: The path toward openness. *Journal of Interprofessional Care* https://doi.org/10.1080/13561820.2021.1981264.

Frankel, A., Haraden, C., Federico, F., & Lenoci-Edwards, J. (2017). *A Framework for Safe, Reliable, and Effective Care*. White Paper. Institute for Healthcare Improvement and Safe & Reliable Healthcare.

Gaffney, T. (2022). Retaining nurses to mitigate shortage. *American Nurse*, 17(1), 14–16. 25.

Graber, J., Saylor, J., Jackson, A., & Hayes, E. (2021). A living legacy for nurses. *Nursing Management*, 52(9), 43–48.

Grace, S., & Coutts, R. (2017). An interprofessional health assessment program in rural Amateur sport. *Journal of Interprofessional Care*, 31(1), 115–117. https://doi.org/10.1080/13561820.2016.1244176.

Gustin, T. S., Kott, K., & Rutledge, C. (2020). A guide for preparing interprofessional teams for successful encounters. *Nurse Educator*, 45(2), 88–92. https://doi.org/10.1097/NNE.00000000000006.

Institute for Healthcare Improvement (IHI). (2007). *The IHI triple aim initiative*. http://www.ihi.org/Engage/Initiatives/TripleAim/Pages/default.aspx

Institute for Healthcare Improvement (IHI). (2010) *SBAR technique for communication: A situational briefing model*. http://www.ihi.org/resources/Pages/Tools/sbartoolkit.aspx

Institute of Medicine. (1972). *Educating a health care team: Report of the conference*. National Academies Press.

Institute of Medicine. (1999). *To err is human: Building a safer health system*. National Academic Press.

Institute of Medicine. (2001). *Crossing the quality chasm: A new health system for the 21st century*. National Academies Press.

Institute of Medicine. (2003). *Health professions education: A bridge to quality*. National Academies Press.

Institute of Medicine. (2011). *The future of nursing: Leading change, advancing health*. National Academies Press.

Institute of Medicine. (2015). *Assessing progress on the IOM report the future of nursing*. http://nationalacademies.org/hmd/reports/2015/assessing-progress-on-the-iom-report-the-future-of-nursing.aspx

Interprofessional Education Collaborative Expert Panel (IPEC). (2016). *Core competencies for interprofessional collaborative practice*. https://www.ipecollaborative.org/resources.html

Jones, B., & Philips, F. (2016). Social work and interprofessional education in health care: A call for continued leadership. *Journal of Social Work Education*, 52(1), 18–29. https://doi.org/10.1080/10437797.2016.1112629.

Jones, T. A., Vidal, G., & Taylor, C. (2020). Interprofessional education during the COVID-19 pandemic: Finding the good in a bad situation. *Journal of Interprofessional Care*, 34(5), 633–646. https://doi.org/10.1080/13561820.2020.1801614.

Ketcherside, M., Rhodes, D., Powelson, S., Cox, C., & Parker, J. (2017). Translating interprofessional theory to interprofessional practice. *Journal of Professional Nursing*, 33(5), 370–377. https://doi.org/10.1016/j.profnurs.2017.03.002.

Khalili, H., & Orchard, C. (2020). The effects of an IPS-based IPE program on interprofessional socialization and dual identity development. *Journal of Interprofessional Care*, 1–11. https://doi.org/10.1080/13561820.2019.1709427.

Khalili, H., & Price, S. L. (2021). From uniprofessionality to interprofessionality: Dual vs dueling identities in healthcare. *Journal of Interprofessional Care* https://doi.org/10.1080/13561820.2021.1928029.

Kirkpatrick, J. D., & Kirkpatrick, W. K. (2010). ROE's rising star: Why return on expectation is getting so much attention. *T&D: Magazine for the Association of Talent Development*. Retrieved from https://www.kirkpatrickpartners.com/Resources/ROEs-Rising-Star

Labrague, L. J., McEnroe-Petitte, D. M., Fronda, D. C., & Obeidata, A. A. (2018, August). Interprofessional simulation in undergraduate nursing program: An integrative review. *Nurse Education Today*, 46–55. https://doi.org/10.1016/j.nedt.2018.05.001.

LaDuke, P. (2017). How to evaluate training: Using the Kirkpatrick Model. *Professional Safety*, 62(8), 20–21.

Lake, E. T., Narva, A. M., Holland, S., Smith, J. G., Cramer, E., Rosenbaum, K., French, R., Clark, R., & Rogowski, J. A. (2021). Hospital nurses' moral distress and mental health during COVID-19. *Journal of advanced nursing*. Advance online publication https://doi.org/10.1111/jan.15013.

Langlois, S., Xyrichis, A., Daulton, B. J., Gilbert, J., Lackie, K., Lising, D., MacMillan, K., Najjar, G., Pfeifle, A. L., & Khalili, H. (2020). The COVID-19 crisis silver lining: Interprofessional education to guide future innovation. *Journal of Interprofessional Care*, 34(5), 587–592. https://doi.org/10.1080/1356 1820.2020.1800606.

LeBlanc, P. (2020). *COVID-19 has thrust universities into online learning—how should they adapt? Education Plus Development. Brookings*. https://www.brook-ings.edu/blog/education-plus-development/.

Michaelic, B., & Lamb, G. (2020). COVID-19 and team-based healthcare: The essentiality of theory-driven research. *Journal of Interprofessional Care*, 34(5), 593–599. https://doi.org/10.1080/13561820.2020.1801613.

National Academies of Sciences, Engineering, and Medicine. (2021). *The future of nursing 2020–2030: Charting a path to achieve health equity*. The National Academies Press. https://doi.org/10.17226/25982.

National *Center for Interprofessional Practice and Education*. https://nexusipe.org/

National Collaborative for Improving the Clinical Learning Environment. (2021). *NCICLE pathways to excellence: Expectations for an optimal clinical learning environment to achieve safe and high-quality patient care, 2021*. https://doi.org/10.33385/NCICLE.0003

National League for Nursing. (2017). *Guide to effective interprofessional education experiences in nursing education*. https://www.nln.org/docs/default-source/uploadedfiles/default-document-library/ipe-tool-kit-krk-012716.pdf

Nundy, S., Cooper, L. A., & Mate, K. S. (2022, January). The Quintuple aim for health care improvement: A new imperative to advance health equity. *JAMA* https://doi.org/10.1001/jama.2021.25181.

O'Neil, E. H. (1998). *Recreating health: Professional practice for a new century*. Pew Health Professions Committee.

Pardue, K. T., Konrad, S. C., Morton, J., & Mason, T. A. (2017). Community-based interprofessional education: Partnerships promoting health and well-being. In E. Speakman (Ed.), *Interprofessional education and collaborative practice: Creating a blueprint for nurse educators*. National League for Nursing.

Perlo, J., Balik, B., Swensen, S., Kabcenell, A., Landsman, J., & Feeley, D. (2017). *IHI framework for improving joy in work*. IHI White Paper. Institute for Healthcare Improvement. www.ihi.org.

Perry, A. F., Federico, F., & Huebner, J. (2021). *Telemedicine: Ensuring safe, equitable, person-centered virtual care*. IHI White Paper. Institute for Healthcare Improvement. www.ihi.org.

Schot, E., Tummers, L., & Noordegraaf, M. (2020). Working on working together. A systematic review on how healthcare professionals contribute to inter-professional collaboration. *Journal of Interprofessional Care*, 34(3), 332–342. https://doi.org/10.1080/1356 1820.2019.1636007.

Smith, D. (2020, March 11). A complete guide to the Kirkpatrick Model of training evaluation. https://www.bizlibrary.com/blog/training-programs/kirkpatrick-model-training-evaluation/

Speakman, E. (2017). *Interprofessional education and collaborative practice: Creating a blueprint for nursing education*. National League for Nursing.

Speakman, E., Tagliareni, M. E., Sherburne, A., & Sicks, S. (2016). *A guide to effective interprofessional education experiences in nursing education toolkit*. http://www.nln.org/docs/default-source/default-document-library/interprofessional-education-and-collaborative-practice-tool kit1.pdf

Sukhera, J., Bertram, K., Hendrikx, S., Chisolm, M., Perzhinsky, J., Kennedy, E., Lingard, L., & Goldszmidt, M. (2021). Exploring implicit influences on interprofessional collaboration: a scoping review. *Journal of Interprofessional Care*. https://doi.org/10.1080/13561820.2021.1979946.

Tannenbaum, S. I., Traylor, A. M., Thomas, E. J., & Salas, E. (2021). Managing teamwork in the face of pandemic: Evidence-based tips. *BMJ Quality & Safety*, 30, 59–63. https://doi.org/10.1136/bmjqs-2020-011447.

Wei, H., Webb Corbett, R., Ray, J., & Wei, T. L. (2020). A culture of caring: The essence of healthcare inter-professional collaboration. *Journal of Interprofessional Care*, 34(3), 324–331. https://doi.org/10.1080/1356 1820.2019.1641476.

Willgerodt, M. A., & Zierler, B. K. (2017). Faculty development in interprofessional education and collaborative practice. In E. Speakman (Ed.), *Interprofessional Education and Collaborative Practice: Creating a Blueprint for Nurse Educators*. National League for Nursing.

World Health Organization (2010). *Framework for action on interprofessional education & collaborative practice*.

World Health Organization (2021). *WHO's 7 policy recommendations on building resilient health systems*.

World Health Organization. http://www.who.int/hrh/nursing_midwifery/en/

Zhang, Y., Wei, L., Li, H., Pan, Y., Wang, J., Li, Q., Wu, Q., & Wei, H. (2020). The psychological change process of frontline nurses caring for patients with COVID-19 during its outbreak. *Issues in Mental Health Nursing*, 41(6), 525–530. https//doi.org/10.1 080/01612840.2020.1752865.

Zaghini, F., Fiorini, J., Livigni, L., Carrabs, G., & Sili, A. (2021, September/October). A mixed methods study of an organization's approach to the COVID-19 health care crisis. *Nursing Outlook*, 69(5), 793–804. https//doi.org/10.1016/j. outlook.2021.05.008.

12

Fostering Social Responsibility Through Service-Learning*

Caitlin Krouse, DNP, FNP-BC, RN

The health care system is becoming ever more complex, which creates a challenge for nurse educators who are responsible for preparing the next generation of nurses with the many skills needed to care for diverse populations. Nurses are called not only to provide high-quality, safe care for patients, families, and communities but also to implement this care with cultural competence, social responsibility, and a deep understanding of personal bias and social determinants of health (SDOH). *The Future of Nursing 2020–2030: Charting a Path to Achieve Health Equity* (National Academy of Medicine [NAM], 2021) has specifically called for a strengthened nursing curriculum to ensure graduates are prepared to promote health equity in a changing America.

As such, nurses' jobs do not start and stop with direct patient care. Nurses are expected to be ever-more present in leadership, advocacy, and policy roles. The Code of Ethics (American Nurses Association, 2015) states that nurses, in all roles and settings, must advocate for patients, protect human rights, work to reduce health disparities, and integrate social justice into their practice. These are strong words with a very clear message. However, to live out this message, nursing students must be given the tools in their education to put the directive into action.

Fortunately, the use of a service-learning pedagogy in nursing education is a known way to enhance students' knowledge and implementation

of these important lessons into practice. When implemented successfully, service-learning can have significant benefits for students, colleges/universities, patients, and communities.

THE NEED FOR SERVICE-LEARNING IN NURSING EDUCATION

The past decade has fostered an increased understanding of the significance SDOH have on patient outcomes. The COVID-19 pandemic, for example, highlighted the health disparities across the United States and global world. The critical need for health equity is increasingly evident in literature. As nurses respond, nursing education is being scrutinized to ensure broad competencies are achieved in graduates so that they are prepared to address the ever-changing needs of patients, the complex health care system, and beyond.

The American Association of Colleges of Nursing (AACN, 2021) published *The Essentials: Core Competencies for Professional Nursing* to capture core nursing competencies. This document emphasizes the need to optimize equitable care to vulnerable populations. It states, "Nursing education needs to ensure an understanding of the intersection of bias, structural racism, and social determinants with healthcare inequities and promote a call to action" (AACN, 2021, p.4). The "promote a call to action" aspect is crucial for educational learnings to evoke real change in nursing practice.

However, while nursing competencies are more fully inclusive of the broad skills required by today's nurse, educational programs have fallen

*The author acknowledges the contributions of Carla Mueller, PhD, RN in previous editions of this chapter.

short in fully integrating and achieving these skills over the years (NAM, 2021). Improved instruction is needed on topics such as cultural humility, implicit bias, and trauma-informed care; these topics must be threaded throughout the entire nursing curriculum rather than briefly covered in stand-alone courses and must be paired with community-based experiential opportunities (NAM, 2021).

It is essential to expand the nursing classroom beyond the physical walls of a university, the virtual walls of an online course, and the traditional nursing clinical experience. Simply covering content in an academic setting alone does not provide students with the sufficient knowledge, skills, and attitudes to advance health equity; applying this content to experiential community learning is critical for mastering competencies (NAM 2021; National League for Nursing [NLN] 2019; Sharma et al., 2018). Service-learning opportunities allow students to work with interprofessional groups, community/governmental organizations, and diverse populations to evaluate health and health care from a broader system level.

The Future of Nursing: Campaign for Action (2019), NLN (2019), and NAM (2021) have all recently promoted innovative community experiences in nursing education. NLN (2019) directed faculty to "create partnerships with community agencies to provide experiences that intentionally expose students to address the impact of [SDOH] on patients, families and communities." Community-based education allows students to engage with community partners to prepare them for the essential work of participating in and leading partnerships that address SDOH (NAM, 2021). Having experiences outside the traditional health care system to see the impact that other sectors, like government agencies and nonprofit organizations, have on the health and wellness of individuals and communities is transformative.

OVERVIEW OF SERVICE-LEARNING

Service-learning is an education pedagogy that utilizes meaningful community service experiences and critical reflection to transform academic learning and encourage civic participation. Through service-learning, students are asked to apply academic skills and knowledge to "real world" community needs, issues, or problems; students can develop leadership skills, cultural competence, and a sense of civic responsibility congruent within the tenets of social justice and social change.

Service-learning is not merely volunteerism, nor is it a substitute for a field experience or practicum that is a normal part of a course. Instead, the focus of the service-learning is on meeting both the needs of the community and the nursing curriculum. Sigmon (1994) described it best in stating that the relationship between service and learning must be equal; the emphasis is not placed on the service (SERVICE-learning) nor the learning (service-LEARNING), but the balance of the two. Both the recipient and the student equally benefit from the experience.

Furco (1996) also captured the service-learning continuum by placing it at the center of other hands-on learning experiences. On the service side of the spectrum, volunteerism and community service primarily benefit the recipient. On the learning end, the beneficiary of field education and internships is the student. Service-learning lies perfectly in the center.

Often the terms *service-learning* and *experiential learning* are used interchangeably, but they are distinct entities. Experiential learning includes hands-on work and has the mastery of work-related skills as its major goal. Traditional nursing clinical experiences are an example of experiential learning; their focus is on the student's learning. In contrast, service-learning involves work that meets actual community needs, has a goal to foster a sense of civic responsibility, and includes structured time for student learning and reflection. Key differences between service-learning and experiential learning are summarized in Table 12.1.

While service-learning is a great tool to address gaps in nursing education, nurse educators do not understand it well in comparison to traditional clinical experience (Dombrowsky et al., 2019). Both service-learning and clinical education can help achieve competencies in cultural competence, skill development, teamwork, leadership, and application of theory to practice, yet service-learning does outperform in providing a broader perspective of health care and fostering students' creativity,

TABLE 12.1   Differences Between Traditional Learning and Service-Learning

	Traditional Learning	Service-Learning
Location	Classroom	Classroom, community
Teacher	Professor	Professor, preceptor or facilitator, patients
Learning	Activities	Collaboration with the community partner
	Writing	Writing
	Examinations	Examinations
	Passive	Active
	Authoritarian	Shared responsibility
	Structured	Reflective
	Compartmentalized	Expansive, integrative
	Cognitive	Cognitive and affective
	Short-term	Short-term and long-term
Reasoning	Deductive	Inductive
Evaluation	Professor	Professor, preceptor or facilitator, community partner, self-assessment by students

independence, and self-confidence (Dombrowsky et al., 2019). Additionally, a systematic review of 51 articles found that academic service-learning nursing partnerships sustain educational standards and processes, improve academic outcomes, strengthen capacity for collaborative practice and interprofessional education, prepare nurses of the future, enhance community services and outcomes, and allow for innovative academic nursing partnerships (Markaki et al., 2021).

Many colleges and universities now recognize the importance of service-learning for their students and community. Each school may engage in it differently because of their unique institutional missions and traditions. Some universities embrace service-learning as a philosophy or part of their spiritual mission, while others see it as their commitment to civic responsibility or as a way to foster community partnerships. Regardless of the reason for utilization of service-learning within the academic setting, the benefits are numerous.

BENEFITS OF SERVICE-LEARNING

Service-learning in the curriculum provides opportunities for students to attain personal,

professional, and curriculum goals. It contributes to the overall educational experience of the college or university and thus provides benefits to the institution, as well. Finally, and importantly, service-learning benefits the community in which it occurs and the individuals it serves.

Benefits to Students

Research has found that students who participate in service-learning work harder, are more engaged in their courses, and are more likely to gain skills in communication, leadership, and collaboration than those who do not participate in service-learning (Jacoby, 2015). For nursing students, service-learning experiences have been found to enrich the learning experience, increase confidence in problem-solving, use knowledge and skills, optimize potential to full-scope practice, teach civic responsibility, and enhance life-long learning (Markaki et al., 2021). The social effect of service-learning includes the increased orientation to volunteerism, increased political and global awareness, development of cultural competence, and improved ethical decision making (Richard et al., 2016).

Service-learning facilitates academic inquiry by connecting theory and practice, enhancing disciplinary understanding and understanding of complex material, bringing greater relevance to course material, and helping students generalize their learning to new situations on a continuum of focus from individuals to families and communities within a broader context of care (Taylor et al., 2017). Service-learning experiences also develop critical thinking, communication, collaboration, leadership, and professional skills.

Embedding research into the service-learning experience provides a unique opportunity to engage students in learning outcomes, especially for courses that do not already have a clinical component or other authentic learning experience (Horning et al., 2020). Horning et al. (2020) built a service-learning experience for BSN students that aligned with the AACN Essentials. Students applied knowledge of sciences to evidence-based care and were able to understand how research informs evidence-based practice. It also provided an opportunity for students to enhance communication skills and practice therapeutic relationships with patients and families (Horning et al., 2020).

Although the majority of service-learning occurs in undergraduate programs, graduate programs in nursing are increasingly exploring community engagement to further develop students' leadership skills, sense of responsibility, understanding of health care issues, and cultural competence in addition to enhancement of their critical thinking skills and learning of academic content (Bryant et al., 2017). Graduate students engaged in service-learning improved in knowledge and understanding of health care issues, research ethics and methods, advocacy regarding health policy and social justice, and cultural competence (Bryant et al., 2017).

Benefits to Faculty

Identifying benefits to faculty is key to obtaining buy-in because of the time commitment involved. Even though faculty may not be on site with students directly supervising the service activities, significant faculty time commitment is required to plan the assignment, obtain community partners, read student journals, and facilitate reflection sessions. Faculty who link service-learning activities in their courses with their research and service interests have increased commitment to continuing its use.

Some universities have adopted the Boyer model of scholarship, which enlarged the scholarship perspective to include teaching, service, and practice, in addition to research. By enlarging the scholarship perspective, Boyer (1990) believed that there would be a stronger connection between universities and the communities they served (see Chapter 1). This scholarship model facilitates integration of service learning into the faculty member's academic role and promotion and tenure requirements. To maximize the impact of involvement in service-learning on their tenure and promotion portfolio, faculty should promote scholarship and transformation of knowledge by measuring effectiveness of service-learning in courses they teach, documenting outcomes, and discussing results publicly. Increasing visibility of integration of service-learning into their courses and students' service-learning work by leading discussions at their university, presenting at professional conferences, and publishing in scholarly journals enhances credibility as an expert teacher. Submission for competitive grants to support continued scholarship related to service-learning would also strengthen the promotion and tenure portfolio.

Benefits to the Institution

Service-learning also has institutional benefits, as students who participate in service-learning report a greater satisfaction with their college experience and are more likely to graduate (Jacoby, 2015). Other benefits include invigoration of the campus educational culture, development of a strong sense of campus community, increased institutional visibility, enhanced appeal to potential donors, and retention of students. It invigorates the campus culture by increasing students' engagement in their own learning, revitalizing faculty, and allowing faculty to mesh service projects with research interests.

The interdisciplinary nature of service-learning helps the campus regain a strong ethos of community, keeps students and faculty more engaged in the life of the college, and contributes to student retention. When service-learning experiences are timed early in the program, the student retention rate can be increased because students develop self-efficacy and an understanding of the field of study. Increased institutional visibility contributes to increased student recruitment by providing a visible link between the community and the institution and by providing a perception of access to higher education to community members who have not believed higher education to be within their reach. Service-learning enhances the institution's appeal to potential donors by providing a direct link between the college and the community, and it appeals to donors interested in community service educational reform (Pellietier, 1995).

For nursing education, service-learning has been found to decrease faculty and preceptor turnover rates, save costs for onboarding and training new nurses, strengthen the ability for collaborative and interprofessional practices, and improve innovative academic nursing partnerships (Markaki et al., 2021). Educational institutions across the country are looking to recruit and retain their nursing faculty, along with strengthening community partnerships; service-learning accomplishes these important goals.

Benefits to the Community

The community benefits when colleges and universities include service-learning and other civic engagement outcomes in their academic programs. For example, research has found that students who participate in service-learning are more connected to their communities and are more likely to choose a service career. These students also have a deeper understanding of complex social, racial, and cultural issues, and they display reduced stereotypical thinking. Finally, graduates who participated in service-learning are more likely to become involved in public policy and political work to evoke change (Jacoby, 2015).

Broadly, as has been previously discussed, there is a critical need to ensure nurses have been equipped with the knowledge, skills, and attitudes necessary to care for diverse populations, with the ultimate goal being that nurses can lead solutions to address health disparities which cause poor patient outcomes and increased health care

costs. These same issues contribute to a cycle of poverty that can torment a community, including a sicker and more disabled working-age population. Therefore, preparing nurses to address social determinants and provide culturally competent care through service-learning experiences can benefit communities across our globe. Exposure to vulnerable populations through these experiences can also drive graduates to work with vulnerable patients and communities.

At the core of service-learning is balance between service and learning, in which both the student and community benefit. A unique demonstration of this can be found in the research by Tillman et al. (2020). They used a multiinstitutional event to offer free health and dental services to poor and underserved patients utilizing students from interprofessional disciplines, including nursing. Their findings captured a significant change in students' perspectives of those living in poverty, including an increased belief that disease burden impacts finances and ability to work and that poor people are unhealthy due to added stressors and lack of access to care (Tillman et al., 2020). Consistent with other research that also suggests service-learning can have a positive impact on students' attitudes, students demonstrated an improved likelihood of empathy and advocacy for those living in poverty (Tillman et al., 2020). The community at large and the students themselves mutually benefit from these improved perspectives and decreased biases and stereotypes.

There are more direct community benefits, as well. After all, service-learning is providing an actual service to the community. When implemented correctly, service-learning identifies a community need and, through collaborative work with partners and stakeholders, a project is designed to meet this need. For example, Horning et al. (2020) found that the service-learning project greatly benefited the families that participated, as they had individualized attention from students that allowed for tailored education specific to the families' needs that would not have otherwise been possible. Additionally, Phlypo et al. (2018) found that utilizing a service-learning project in undergraduate dental education improved the oral health in residents with intellectual disabilities and had a positive impact on the local community.

SERVICE-LEARNING AS AN EDUCATIONAL MODEL

Kolb's (1984) theory of experiential learning has been widely used as a theoretical basis for designing and analyzing service-learning programs. Reflective observation about the experience is essential to the learning process. It links the concrete experience to abstract conceptualizations of that experience. Learning is increased when students are actively engaged in gaining knowledge through experiential problem solving and decision making. Use of reflection is built on the work of Kolb (1984) and Dewey (1916, 1933, 1938). In service-learning, reflection is both a cognitive process and a structured learning activity. Effective reflection fosters moral development and enhances moral decision making.

Delve et al. (1990) developed a service-learning model based on theories of moral decision making and values clarification. Their model includes five phases of development: exploration, clarification, realization, activation, and internalization. It illustrates that service-learning is developmental, providing students with an opportunity to move from charity to justice as they become more empathetic. Without that empathy and caring, the student will not come to recognize the members of the patient population as valued individuals in the larger society and as sources for new learning (Delve et al., 1990).

The pedagogy of service-learning has powerful flexibility. It can be based on subject matter or on learning process; it can connect theory and practice; it integrates several different approaches to knowledge and uses of knowledge; it encourages learning how to learn; and it can focus on a wide range of issues, problems, and interests (Taylor et al., 2017). It also lends itself to problem-based learning and case study methodologies.

BEST PRACTICES IN THE IMPLEMENTATION OF SERVICE-LEARNING IN THE CURRICULUM

As faculty consider integrating service-learning into the curriculum, they must first identify a need within a community that requires the collaboration of community partners to problem solve. Community agencies are true partners in design, implementation, and evaluation of the experience. The cocreated experience promotes social responsibility and its dedication to social change. It provides students with a learning opportunity in the "real world" that they would otherwise be unlikely to experience, pushing them to utilize and enhance their knowledge and skills in new ways.

While service-learning may be a separate course within the college curriculum, it is often integrated into one or more existing courses. When this occurs, it is essential that a "once and done" service-learning experience is not simply added as an additional course requirement. Faculty members must intentionally and strategically thread the concepts of service-learning throughout the entire course(s). See Box 12.1 for best practices in integrating service-learning into the curriculum.

Support Structures

Faculty support is important to cultivating success. Support begins with campus and school administrators who value service-learning and will commit resources to its implementation in the curriculum. Although universities have embraced service-learning, they have been slow to implement support systems needed for effective implementation. Faculty can organize a faculty service-learning committee or advisory board to provide needed support. This group could be an invaluable advocate of service learning as a teaching tool (Gallagher et al., n.d.). The committee can establish faculty handbooks and guidelines for service-learning courses, sponsor lunch-and-learn sessions on service-learning for particular departments or the entire college, develop webinars, ensure that faculty receive continuing education units for attending service-learning workshops, and organize faculty development opportunities regarding service-learning pedagogy. This committee also encourages the development of interdisciplinary professional relationships and provides an avenue for sharing ideas, successes, and failures.

The goal of planning is to work for sustainability of service-learning throughout the curriculum. Funding can be obtained from the community,

BOX 12.1 Best Practice for Integrating Service-Learning Into the Curriculum

- Add service-learning to the syllabus as a teaching strategy.
- Give credit for learning in relation to the course, not for service alone.
- Create rubrics, exams, papers, and reflection assignments as evaluation metrics.
- Tie service-learning outcomes to course objective and curricular outcomes.
- Ensure the service-learning activity is experiential and not observational.
- Place emphasis on guided reflection before, during, and after the service-learning experience. Dissemination and debriefing can be integral components.
- Assess and evaluate the service-learning with faculty, students, and community partners; incorporate feedback to improve the experience.
- Service-learning must enhance learning by allowing application of the theoretical principles taught in the classroom setting.
- Service-learning must allow students to use their knowledge and skills to address human and community needs.
- Service-learning must develop a sense of caring, cultural awareness, social responsibility, health advocacy, and civic engagement.
- Service-learning must promote collaboration and teamwork.
- Service-learning must have reciprocity so that students, faculty, and community partners are empowered and act both as teachers and learners.
- Service-learning should increase exposure to diversity and vulnerable populations to enhance students' cultural competency.

from grant funding available locally and nationally, and often from the college or university itself. Although service-learning is not expensive, it does require time for planning and course development and the personnel to make the arrangements. A number of colleges and universities have a service-learning office or coordinator. Staff from this office provide assistance in structuring the program, identifying community partners, and placing students according to mutual needs.

Integrating service-learning experiences into the curriculum requires careful planning. The experience must be developed and resources acquired before the course is offered. Identifying enthusiastic faculty champions and faculty development is key to success.

Challenges

Some of the challenges to implementing service-learning result from ordinary budgetary constraints in higher education. Multiple departments and programs compete for limited resources. Those beginning a service-learning initiative may need to search for external funding sources and rely on the goodwill of faculty members willing to spend extra time learning about service learning and then incorporating it into their courses without extra compensation.

Institutions that lack a dedicated service-learning office may struggle with organization and effective evaluation strategies. When funding issues prevent the establishment of a service-learning office, a service-learning council composed of faculty members from each department on campus can provide direction for faculty development, coordinate student learning activities with community agencies, evaluate service-learning experiences, and facilitate the sharing of information.

Convincing faculty members to adopt service-learning as an effective pedagogical device can also be a challenge. This resistance is understandable because of the time and effort involved in incorporating it into courses. Faculty members involved in service-learning often serve as the best change agents as they extol the benefits of service-learning, including increased student engagement in the learning process and increased sense of collegiality because of their intradisciplinary and interdisciplinary activities.

Challenges encountered by faculty include time constraints, students' commitments to work and family, and faculties' and community partners' heavy workloads. Community partners may struggle with orienting new students each semester and with the lack of students during summer break. There are also challenges when service-learning experiences last more than one semester or students taking multiple courses with service-learning components are to remain at the same community agency to increase continuity.

Planning Development for Faculty New to Service-Learning

Planning for a change to service-learning begins with faculty development that may be available from the academic institution, conferences and workshops, and independent study. These resources will help faculty obtain essential information about how to design and implement service-learning. For example, Johns Hopkins University Schools of Public Health, Nursing, and Medicine is now offering the Service-Learning Academy to train faculty in this important pedagogy and advanced service-learning teaching methodologies.

Development should include an exploration of the meaning of service and its place in the educational arena. It is important that faculty understand that service-learning does not compromise academic rigor; instead, it enriches and extends learning (Gallagher et al., n.d.). Faculty should be educated on the differences between shallow and deep experience and the importance of collaboration with the community agency. Training should also emphasize that the practical considerations involved in planning include establishing good relationships with community agencies, identifying the types of experiences suitable for the course content, finding agency representative supervisors, structuring the types of activities, identifying the time commitment involved for students, and collaborating with the agency in scheduling the activities.

Preparation links the service-learning activities to specific learning outcomes and prepares students to perform the activities. Reinforcement should be given that the service needs to be challenging, engaging, and meaningful to the students, and it must focus on meeting an actual community need that students can perceive as important and relevant to their own development.

Preparation also includes finding agencies for student placement. Students involved typically work in voluntary not-for-profit community or public tax-supported service agencies and organizations that provide services that meet people's actual needs. Agencies and programs are selected on the basis of their congruence with the academic program or course and student goals and objectives. Faculty must also assess the agency's capacity for students and determine that the students' abilities are a match for the agency's needs.

Although careful planning prevents many problems, faculty members should be prepared for the unexpected and some loss of control. Occasionally the needs of community agencies change (e.g., because of funding cuts or receiving a grant), there may be conflicts between agencies' needs for services and students' schedules, or there may be dissatisfaction. Sources of dissatisfaction may include students' perception of inequality of time investment between groups, failure of the reality of the situation to match expectations, and problems in communication. Regular communication with community partners and students will help catch problems in their initial stages. Faculty members may need to intervene to prevent the escalation of problems and to renegotiate expectations.

Faculty development provides an explanation of a new pedagogy for many and establishes a common definition and a sound knowledge base. Faculty will need to rethink their role as sole transmitter of knowledge as they move to a facilitation and guidance role. This role change may be uncomfortable and awkward at first. Consultants can be an invaluable aid in this early development process, and many campuses have offices of service learning that can provide or assist with faculty development.

It is also helpful for faculty to make contact with faculty in other colleges to identify what others have been doing and how they felt during the initial process. The internet can be a means of making contact with other faculty involved in service learning. The internet can also be a source of information about starting service-learning programs, sample course descriptions, syllabi, electronic mailing lists, faculty involved in service-learning, funding resources, and best practices. Some of the most widely recognized internet resources are:
1. Campus Compact: https://compact.org
2. Corporation for National and Community Service: https://www.nationalservice.gov

3. Learn and Serve, National Service-Learning Clearinghouse: http://www.servicelearning.org

Developing Placement Sites

During the development process, faculty should be provided assistance in developing placement sites. Anstee et al. (2008) presented a process model for incorporating service learning into an academic class. The six stages of their model were "(a) establishing community collaboration, (b) partnering in the classroom, (c) student training, (d) delivering the service, (e) returning to the classroom, and (f) reporting to the stakeholders" (p. 599). Selecting a placement site and establishing collaboration within the community are important early steps.

It is important to match the type of community organization and service with the institutional mission of the college when service-learning experiences are being planned. Before making plans regarding service placements, faculty should conduct a community needs assessment and develop a resource inventory, either informally through personal and telephone contact or formally through surveys or needs assessments. Community agency staff are invaluable in determining where students are needed the most and what the greatest need is. Allowing community partners to control the identification of the service helps ensure that projects meet agency needs. Involvement of agency staff in the planning process also helps educate community agencies about service-learning. Community advisory boards often help ensure continual contact between agencies, students, faculty, and staff and ascertain evolving community needs.

Student safety is also an issue, and the agency and school have a responsibility to choose sites that are appropriate for the students' safety needs. Development of an informed consent form and exploration as to whether the organization carries liability insurance for volunteers enhances clarity of responsibility and minimizes student risks. Gallagher et al. (n.d.) provide sample forms to assist faculty who are new to service-learning.

Once placement sites have been determined and projects are finalized, preceptors must be identified. Faculty also need to set dates for student orientation and initial meetings.

Communication With Students and Preparation for Service-Learning

Once service-learning experiences have been planned, students must be engaged. Faculty can use groups such as the student nurses' association, student government, the student life office, and campus publicity mechanisms (e.g., newspaper, radio station, online learning system bulletin boards) to inform students about service-learning. Often courses or service-learning components of courses are open to students from a variety of disciplines, and faculty should distribute the course announcements widely. Service-learning's best promoters are its own students, who attract other students by word of mouth.

Once student placements and focus of the service have been selected, preparation must extend to the classroom setting. Conceiving of service-learning as simply a matter of mutually beneficial service ignores the important concept of readiness for the encounter. Radest (1993) introduced the idea of *solidarity:* "the name of my relationship to the stranger who remains unknown—only a person in an abstract sense—but who is, like me, a human being. Solidarity is then a preparation for the future and at the same time a grounding in the present" (p. 183). Sheffield (2005) noted that "Radest's concept of solidarity develops into a disposition toward democratic interaction and service" (p. 49) and that academic preparation for the encounter is essential. Preparation develops a sense of understanding in students that gives increased meaning to the service and a realization that the strangers are much like them, further developing the sense of solidarity.

Preparation should include exploration of social issues and an introduction to the service environment and the people who will be encountered. It can take the form of reading materials from the agency, reading text-based materials, exploring material available on the internet, or viewing films and should be accompanied by discussions to prepare students for the service experience. Preparatory classroom activities should have an overall goal of enhancing understanding and helping the stranger become familiar. Preparation also brings participants a greater understanding of diversity, the ability to embrace and celebrate differences, and a realization of their ethical responsibility to connect with others in the community. This understanding is the learning component essential to service-learning; without it, service would simply be volunteerism.

Written project descriptions, contact information, and a schedule of initial meetings should be available for students on the first day of class for students to select from. Organization before the start of the semester ensures that students get started on projects promptly and are likely to complete projects within the semester time limit.

Students must be prepared for the service-learning experience with appropriate content knowledge and skills, understanding of learning objectives, timeline for the experience, project guidelines, and information about the community organization. It may be helpful for the faculty member to have a faculty mentor experienced in service-learning attend class to help field student questions and concerns.

Planning Learning Activities

Service-learning can be used as an experientially based pedagogy to bring excitement and vitality to the classroom, to assist community members in need while at the same time learning from them, and to provide students with information and experiences through which they can engage in critical reflection about society's needs and one's responsibility to the community. During faculty development, faculty currently involved in service-learning can provide examples of how they have implemented this pedagogy. They can then facilitate faculty identification of additional opportunities that may be discovered from a number of sources. Faculty may identify appropriate situations for service-learning from their own service activities in a wide variety of community agencies. Opportunities may also be suggested by friends, colleagues, agency personnel, or students, or they may be found in the professional or secular literature. When faculty have identified potential service-learning experiences that seem to be appropriate for the course, discussions and negotiations are held with the agency staff.

Legal issues also need to be considered when planning service activities. Any time a student performs service off campus in conjunction with coursework, liability issues can arise. Faculty should seek legal counsel from the college or university regarding activities with potential liability, just as legal counsel is sought when contracts with clinical agencies are established. Institutional review board approval should be sought if students are collecting data as a part of their service-learning projects.

Student activities are planned so that they relate to the course objectives and content (Gallagher et al., n.d.). Community agencies offer many opportunities for students to collaborate with the agency to fulfill unmet needs. Some service experiences will involve assessment, others work in ongoing programs, and still others work on development and implementation of new programs or services. During the final phase of the service experience, students who have developed new programs should work with agency partners to establish plans for sustainability. Students should compile materials to facilitate this continuation. Although the community agency should be an active partner throughout the activity, a summary meeting with the stakeholders should be held to close the service experience.

EXAMPLES OF IMPLEMENTING SERVICE-LEARNING IN THE NURSING CURRICULUM

The nursing literature provides a wealth of examples for ways to integrate service-learning into the curriculum. Types of agencies and programs that could be used for nursing students engaged in service-learning include working with underserved and vulnerable populations with different forms of impairment or disability, preventive health and health care facilities (both freestanding and mobile), social welfare agencies, child and adult day care programs, Head Start, Meals on Wheels, senior centers, youth services, a center serving teenage parents, a mission for homeless parents or individuals reentering the community after incarceration, civic leagues, drug education programs, and groups or committees related to health disparities or health policy.

The COVID-19 pandemic accelerated many partnerships among community stakeholders. For example, Johns Hopkins University School of Nursing partnered with the Baltimore Neighborhood Network at the beginning of the pandemic to create a phone-based support service for older adults as a way to combat social isolation (Gresh et al., 2020). All aspects of quality service-learning were adhered to; a community need was met while also achieving student learning outcomes and implementing critical reflection.

Many universities utilize college breaks as the perfect time to implement service projects as a part of a service-learning course. For example, Saint Mary's College and the University of Notre Dame offer service-learning courses that run the length of a semester, with a service trip offered during spring or summer break. They have domestic and international opportunities in their Summer Service-Learning Program and their International Summer Service-Learning Program that includes grant funding to ensure all students have the chance to attend without financial concern (University of Notre Dame, 2015).

In health majors, the opportunities are endless (see Case Study 12.1). Undergraduate students can provide health, social, and developmental screenings; create health-related handouts for parents; read safety storybooks to children; and assist with classroom activities. Graduate family nurse practitioner students can work in freestanding or mobile health clinics focusing on impoverished or underserved populations, provide sports physicals for students, and provide primary health care and education at a clinic located at a homeless shelter. Graduate midwifery students have developed enhanced curriculum for midwives in Haiti, policies and training for their communities such as pregnancy self-care, well baby care, or limiting the use of restraints on pregnant and laboring women or youth in prisons. Doctoral students could provide health policy or research assistance for professional or nonprofit organizations.

Designing service-learning to reinforce interprofessional education and team-based care is an excellent teaching strategy. For example, nursing students could offer blood pressure screenings and education about hypertension while partnering with dietetic students who could teach people to prepare a low-cost meal following the dietary approaches to stop hypertension (DASH) diet. These students can work together in preparation for the event and reconvene for reflection after the event. Interprofessional education opportunities increase high-quality patient care and give students a deeper appreciation for the various scope of practices within distinct professions (see Case Study 12.2).

Service-learning approaches are often integrated into global health experiences to provide students an opportunity to understand diverse cultures, develop a sense of global citizenship, and acquire an appreciation for global health concepts (see Chapter 13). Service-learning experiences can

---

CASE STUDY 12.1 Considerations for Integrating Service-Learning Into a Course

A faculty new to teaching wants to incorporate service-learning into the course. The faculty had a meaningful service-learning experience as a student and can contribute expertise to developing a service-learning component for a 16-week, 6-credit didactic and clinical junior-level course in a baccalaureate program. The course focuses on care for vulnerable populations and social determinants of health.

1. What should these faculty consider when working with colleagues to integrate a service-learning experience into this course?

CASE STUDY 12.2 Considerations for Developing a Multidisciplinary Service-Learning Plan

A homeless shelter has asked the faculty at a university health science center to help them develop plans for managing communicable diseases such as COVID-19 at their shelter. The university has a mission of civic engagement and has charged the schools of nursing, medicine, and public health to work with the shelter and develop a plan. The plan will include students from each of the schools who will participate in the service-learning project.

1. What should the faculty from the school of nursing consider in working with this group?

also help students develop cultural humility and an understanding of cultural differences within a community (see Chapter 17).

Adapting Service-Learning for Distance Education

Service-learning has traditionally been structured as a part of an on-campus nursing program. However, as more and more programs move in whole or in part to distance education, consideration must be given to service-learning experiences for this student population.

Service-learning for distance learning students can occur in a number of ways. First, the student in a distance-delivered course can identify a community partner in their local community for a service experience and take advantage of online and videoconferencing learning technologies. An asynchronous forum can be used for discussions with opportunities for reflection. Descriptions of agencies and service projects used by on-campus students can be posted online to help distance education students find comparable experiences within their own community. Faculty members worked collaboratively with students to finalize arrangements with those agencies.

Second, students enrolled in an online program could travel to an international site for a service-learning experience together with other students enrolled in the course (whether online or on-campus).

Third, the service could become e-service-learning. This would overcome the traditional time and geographical boundaries and allow students to conduct indirect service to the community. E-service-learning provides opportunities for engagement, skill building, and practical experience that might otherwise be limited or lacking in an online course; e-service-learning requires both the student and the community partner to have access to technology (chat rooms, email, videoconferencing, Skype, wikis, or discussion boards), but it removes the traditional geographical boundaries. Best practices for e-service-learning include providing training on any technology that will need to be used, creating clear written communication of expectations between students and community partners, scheduling meeting times to enhance communication, and maintaining faculty engagement throughout the service-learning experience. With use of these guidelines, service-learning opportunities can be expanded to distance education students. See Chapter 21 for more information on distance learning.

Incorporating Reflection

Reflection is a critical and essential aspect of service-learning that further differentiates it from volunteerism, community service activities, and nursing students' clinical experiences. Reflection must be an active, persistent, thoughtful, and intentional consideration of the service activity that includes the student's behavior, practice, and achievement. Within the reflective process, students must respond to basic questions such as "What am I doing?", "Why am I doing it?", and "What am I learning?" They also should critically examine their actions, feelings, and thoughts. During this examination and while responding to the questions posed, students contemplate, think, reason, and speculate about their service experiences.

Reflection is a learning tool that serves to maximize students' highly individualized learning experiences by linking the service experiences with the learning objectives established for the course and curriculum. Reflection combines cognitive and affective activities in a way that bridges the gap between the service experience and the course.

Reflection also provides opportunities for students to improve their self-assessment skills and have insights that help build on their strengths. Because reflection and self-assessment are skills that require development, many students new to service-learning find faculty facilitation and journaling helpful with the reflective process.

One common approach to stimulate reflection is to have students keep a journal or engage in directed writing that faculty read and respond to frequently throughout the course. Journals allow students to record thoughts, observations, feelings, activities, questions, and problems encountered and solved during the service-learning experience. If students are working on a service-learning project as a team, a team journal can be used to promote interaction between team members on project-related issues and to introduce students to different perspectives on the project. The team concludes its work with a collective reflection on the service-learning. Students often have difficulty initially with separation of event observation and reflection and integration of course concepts.

To assist the process, students can use a multicolumn journal with observations, course concepts, and reflection in separate columns. Using common prompts can be quite helpful, as well, such as the reflective model developed by Rolfe et al. (2011), the What, So What, Now What? "What?" asks students what the problem is and what their role is in the situation. "So what?" prompts students to think about why this project matters to their learning and their communities. "Now what?" is a broader question encouraging students to think of future needs and responses.

It is recommended to grade journals as satisfactory/unsatisfactory instead of using points or letter grades to decrease students' fear of expressing their ideas and their perception of being judged. Use of a journal grading rubric helps students to more clearly understand journal expectations and provide consistency in faculty grading. The rubric can include assessment for linking prior knowledge/feelings/values with new knowledge/feelings/values, examples of transformation in perspectives and behaviors, and committing to future actions that improve practice.

Service-learning provides opportunities for students to work with a multicultural, underserved sector of society that has a variety of needs and challenges and are deemed disadvantaged in some way—be it through social class, age, race, ethnicity, sexual orientation, ability, or any combination of these. Generally, those providing service have more advantages than those they are serving, so concerns about racism and other biases, injustice, power, and oppression should figure prominently in postservice discussions. Effective reflection regarding multicultural service-learning can provide a transformative experience that reinforces caring and social responsibility and has the potential to create long-term social change.

Reflection is most effective when it is continuous, connected, contextual, and challenging. Continuous reflection involves reflection before, during, and after the service-learning experience.

Connecting service-learning with classroom learning assists students to develop a conceptual framework for their service project and to apply concepts and theories learned in class to the experience. Faculty responsibilities include designing reflection activities, coaching students during reflection, monitoring students' reflections, and providing feedback. Faculty may need training to effectively mentor students in reflective thinking, and this should be included in initial development opportunities. Faculty who want ideas on reflection activities can find a wealth of information available on the internet.

Reflection must be appropriate for the context and setting of the experience. Some service-learning experiences lend themselves to formal methods of reflection, such as written papers with a writing prompt with a specific focus, whereas others are best suited to informal discussions where students can share exemplars, what they have learned, and the connections they have made. Smit and Tremethick (2017) reported that their study showed that students who participated in an online discussion had a higher level of reflective thinking and discussed a wider variety of topics than students who completed a written reflection. Other informal methods include poems, songs, videos, and artwork.

Whether formal or informal methods are used, reflection should challenge students to think in new ways, question their assumptions, and formulate new understandings and new ways of problem solving.

Including service partners in the reflective dialogue enhances communication and increases the depth and breadth of learning. Without an emphasis on dialogue between individuals and community partners, reflection becomes one sided, focusing on the isolated views and perceptions of the individual student without coming to an understanding of each person's perspective.

Portfolios can be developed to organize materials related to the service-learning project and document reflection, accomplishments, and learning outcomes. Other reflective activities include small-group discussions and presentations that relate the service experience to classroom concepts, introduce students to different perspectives, and challenge them to think critically about the service experience. It is helpful for faculty to pose a few questions to guide the discussion, but students should also be allowed to freely discuss and reflect on ideas and issues. In such discussions, students often disclose expectations and myths about the service experience. Themes that may emerge during reflections include social analysis of community needs, health disparities, and the importance of civic responsibility. A journal or final reflective paper based on the writing done during the semester can provide a comprehensive description of students' learning.

Bringle and Hatcher's (1996) guidelines help clarify the nature of effective reflection activities in a service-learning course. Effective reflection activities:

1. Link the service-learning experiences to the learning objectives
2. Are designed, structured, and guided by faculty
3. Are planned so that they occur across the span of service-learning experience
4. Permit faculty feedback and assessment of progress and learning
5. Foster the clarification and exploration of values

Debriefing

After the experience, debriefing is essential to reinforce classroom theory, allow students to share differing experiences, and reinforce the sense of solidarity that was developed. Debriefing adds to the intentional nature of the service experience and facilitates a dialogue between students who may have been placed in different locations throughout the community. Debriefing can be combined with an evaluation of the service experience. Community partners can also be engaged in the debriefing experience and share their views of outcomes of the experience and what effect the service-learning had on the agency in which the students served.

Evaluation

After the completion of service-learning, the community partner, faculty, and students should evaluate the usefulness of the service project in meeting their needs, the strengths and areas for improvement of the service project, and student performance. Faculty should evaluate student outcomes and the contribution of the experience to overall curriculum goals. Evaluation of students' achievement is based on the students' learning and not merely on their experience or participation in the service activities. Faculty, the agency supervisor, and students' self-assessment provide the evaluation data.

Many faculty administer preservice and postservice surveys that measure students' attitudes toward community service and civic responsibility and toward their coursework. Such instruments not only help faculty evaluate their students and assess the usefulness of service-learning but also help students see how much they have learned and how their attitudes may have changed because of their service-learning experience. In addition to the short-term course evaluation, a systematic long-term follow-up of students helps determine any additional learning that may have occurred after the course is completed.

CHAPTER SUMMARY: KEY POINTS

- Service-learning can prepare nurses for work with diverse populations through increased awareness and knowledge of social determinants of health, cultural competence and humility, social responsibility, and implicit bias. It also supports the growth of professional nurses who are prepared to serve in leadership, advocacy, and policy roles.
- Universities, communities, and students all benefit from service-learning. Universities can expect increased student retention and graduation rates. Strategic partnerships among universities and organizations can identify and fill community needs. Students who participate in service-learning are often inspired to continue to work for social justice as engaged citizens in their communities.
- Service-learning is not just a one time addition to a course or academic program service activity. It must be thoughtfully woven into the curriculum of one or more courses with opportunities for student reflection.

REFLECTING ON THE EVIDENCE

1. How does service-learning help nursing students develop social responsibility?
2. In what ways is service-learning similar to and different from a nursing clinical practicum experience?
3. A sequence of three courses in a curriculum focus on the social determinants of health. How could a service-learning experience be integrated into these courses?
4. How can tenure-track faculty best integrate service-learning into the scholarship of teaching area of their portfolio?
   a. What aspects of integrating service-learning into a course best illustrates scholarship of teaching? What supporting evidence can they add to their portfolio?
   b. Where can faculty disseminate the results of their scholarly work related to service-learning?

REFERENCES

American Association of Colleges of Nursing. (2021). *The essentials: Core competencies for professional nursing education.* https://www.aacnnursing.org/Portals/42/AcademicNursing/pdf/Essentials-2021.pdf

American Nurses Association. (2015). *Code of ethics for nurses.* American Nurses Publishing.

Anstee, J. L. K., Harris, S. G., Pruitt, K. D., & Sugar, J. A. (2008). Service learning projects in an undergraduate gerontology course: A 6-stage model and application. *Educational Gerontology, 34*(7), 595–609.

Boyer, E. L. (1990). *Scholarship reconsidered: Priorities of the professoriate.* The Carnegie Foundation for the Advancement of Teaching.

Bringle, R. G., & Hatcher, J. A. (1996). Implementing service learning in higher education. *Journal of Higher Education, 67*(2), 221–239.

Bryant, K., Matthews, E., & DeClark, L. (2017). Integration of service-learning into a doctoral level qualitative research methodology course. *Nurse Educator, 42*(6), 288–302.

Delve, C. I., Mintz, S. D., & Stewart, G. M. (1990). Promoting values development through community service: A design. *New Directions for Student Services, 50*(2), 7–29.

Dewey, J. (1916). *Democracy and education.* Macmillan.

Dewey, J. (1933). *How we think.* Heath.

Dewey, J. (1938). *Experience and education.* Macmillan.

Dombrowsky, T., Gustafson, K., & Cauble, D. (2019). Service-learning and clinical nursing education: A Delphi inquiry. *Journal of Nursing Education, 58*(7), 381–391.

Furco, A. (1996). Service-learning: A balanced approach to experiential education. *Expanding Boundaries: Serving and Learning, 1,* 2–6. The Crop for National Service.

Future of Nursing: Campaign for Action. (2019). http://futureofnursing.org.

Gallagher, L., Planowski, E., & Tarbell, K. (n.d.). Elevate the experience. Faculty guide to service-learning: Information and resources for creating and implementing service-learning courses. University of Colorado Denver: Experiential Learning Center. http://www.ucdenver.edu/life/services/ExperientialLearning/foremployers/Documents/UC%20Denver%20Faculty%20S-L%20Guide.pdf.

Gresh, A., LaFave, S., Thamilselvan, J., Batchelder, A., Mermer, J., Jacques, K., Greensfelder, A., Buckley, M., Cohen, Z., Coy, A., & Warren, N. (2020). Service learning in public health nursing education: How COVID-19 accelerated community-academic partnership. *Public Health Nursing, 38,* 248–257.

Horning, M. L., Ostrow, L., Beierwaltes, P., Beaudette, J., Schmitz, K., & Fulkerson, J. A. (2020). Service learning within community-engaged research: Facilitating nursing student learning outcomes. *Journal of Professional Nursing, 36*(6), 510–513.

Jacoby, B. (2015). *Service-learning essentials: Questions, answers and lessons learned.* Jossey-Bass.

Kolb, D. A. (1984). *Experiential learning: Experience as the source of learning and development.* Prentice Hall.

Markaki, A., Prajankett, O., Shorten, A., Shirley, M. R., & Harper, D. C. (2021). Academic service-learning nursing partnerships in the Americas: A scoping review. *BMC Nursing, 20,* 179.

National Academy of Medicine. (2021). *The future of nursing 2020–2030: Charting a path to achieve health equity.* https://nam.edu/publications/the-future-of-nursing-2020-2030/

National League for Nursing. (2019). *A vision for integration of the social determinants of health into nursing education curricula.* http://www.nln.org/docs/

default-source/default-document-library/ social-determinants-of-health.pdf?sfvrsn=2

Pellietier, S. (1995). The quiet power of service learning: Report from the National Institute on Learning and Service. *The Independent, 95*(4), 7–10.

Phlypo, I., De Tobel, J., Marks, L., De Visschere, L., & Koole, S. (2018). Integrating community service learning in undergraduate dental education: A controlled trial in a residential facility for people with intellectual disabilities. *Special Care in Dentistry, 38*(4), 201–207.

Radest, H. (1993). *Community service: Encounter with strangers*. Praeger.

Richard, D., Keene, C., Hatcher, J. A., & Pease, H. (2016). Pathways to adult civic engagement: Benefits of reflection and dialogue across difference in higher education service-learning programs. *Michigan Journal of Community Service Learning, 23*(2), 60–71.

Rolfe, G., Freshwater, D., & Jasper, M. (2011). *Critical reflection in nursing and the helping professions: A user's guide*. Palgrave Macmillan.

Sharma, M., Pinto, A. D., & Kumagai, A. K. (2018). Teaching the social determinants of health: A path to equity or a road to nowhere? *Academic Medicine, 93*(1), 25–30.

Sheffield, E. C. (2005). Service in service-learning education: The need for philosophical understanding. *The High School Journal, 89*(1), 46–53.

Sigmon, R. L. (1994). *Serving to learn, learning to Serve: Linking service with learning*. Council for Independent Colleges Report.

Smit, E. M., & Tremethick, M. J. (2017). Value of online group reflection after international service-learning experiences: I never thought of that. *Nurse Educator, 42*(60), 286–289.

Taylor, W., Pruitt, R., & Fasolino, T. (2017). Innovative use of service-learning to enhance baccalaureate nursing education. *Journal of Nursing Education, 56*(9), 560–563.

Tillman, P., Thomas, M., & Buelow, J. R. (2020). Impact of service learning on student attitudes toward the poor and underserved. *Nurse Educator, 45*(6), 316–320.

University of Notre Dame. (2015). *Center for Social Concerns*. https://socialconcerns.nd.edu/

13

Global Health and Curricular Experiences

Mary E. Riner, PhD, RN, CNE, FAAN

This chapter addresses global health education from multiple curricular perspectives to support nurse educators in developing students' knowledge, skills, and attitudes for providing care in an increasingly globalized world community. By integrating global perspectives into nursing education, students will be better prepared to address cultural issues important to providing care to diverse populations, whether it is for newly arrived persons in their local community or in an international community. The chapter introduces the concept of global health, offers strategies to assist nurse educators in preparing themselves for including global health learning experiences in their teaching, and provides information about how to advance global health through curricular and education abroad experiences.

GLOBAL HEALTH

Global health encompasses the multiple strands of education, research, and practice that prioritize improving health and achieving health equity for all people in the global community. Global health is concerned with the health issues that transcend national boundaries and governments and calls for globally coordinated actions that can determine the health of people. International health, on the other hand, indicates a relationship between two or more countries focused on one or more health issues of mutual concern.

The benefit of including global health learning experiences in nursing education is to develop a nursing workforce prepared to provide high-quality care that is culturally appropriate for each person in a health care organization or community setting. In a seminal *Health Affairs* article Betancourt et al. (2005) call for focused cultural competence education as a potential strategy for addressing health inequities, in which nurses play a key role. Cultural competence in health care describes the ability of systems to provide care to patients with diverse values, beliefs, and behaviors, including tailoring delivery to meet patients' social, cultural, and linguistic needs. Cultural humility involves self-reflection about one's own beliefs and cultural identity in order to learn about and better understand another's culture. Developing cultural humility and providing culturally competent care may mean the student cares for individuals of different cultures from theirs, either in the student's home country or in another country where the student may visit or live. Students also need to develop interprofessional competence in being team members with health professionals who may come from another country and have migrated, either voluntarily or because of hostile conditions that created unsafe environments for them and their families. Nurses, as members of their local community, need to be informed and engaged citizens to ensure a civil and peaceful environment that honors all residents of the community.

In light of evolving human and nature interactions, as people continue to respond to changing climate conditions, it is expected that exposure to new viruses will constantly challenge the global health community. The recent pandemic involving a new coronavirus has highlighted nurses' central roles in prevention, control, and care of populations impacted by emerging diseases.

Nurses will be involved in interprofessional and international teams that must be skilled in epidemiological methods of tracking emerging infections, engaged in research to develop and bring to readiness medications and vaccines to respond to outbreaks, and prepared to protect themselves and their patients while providing care and finally to evaluate the effectiveness of the health care systems' efforts.

Global Health Competencies and Goals of International and Federal Agencies

It is beneficial to understand the resources available to guide the development of students' global health knowledge, skills, and attitudes. WHO has developed overarching competencies for all health care workers that address core personal conduct, management, and leadership. Professions developed by the Consortium of Universities in Global Health (CUGH) include those specific to nursing and include more generic competencies for interprofessional use. In addition, the Association of Schools and Programs of Public Health developed a competency model for use with local and global populations. These competency categories are useful for developing individual courses, certificates, or global health undergraduate and graduate programs (Box 13.1).

Torres-Alzate (2019), after conducting a review of the literature, proposes a framework for nursing global health competencies. The framework is grounded in the dimension of nursing core values and principles, which include social justice and equity, holistic care, advocacy, health as human right, sustainability, and collaboration. This conceptual framework can be adapted by educators across multiple health issues and settings.

Healthy People 2030 (https://health.gov/healthypeople) sets data-driven national objectives to improve health and well-being of the American people. Healthy People 2030 identifies leading causes of poor health and objectives that educators and agencies can use to focus their efforts. They are interprofessional in nature and call for collaborative action from multiple sectors of society to work together for a healthier citizenry. For example, the recommended adult vaccination schedule now includes an objective that people over 19 years of

---

> **BOX 13.1   Global Health Competencies for Health Professions Programs**
>
> The Consortium of Universities in Global Health (CUGH) initially developed nursing competencies to guide curriculum development.
>
> The major areas of nursing-specific competencies include:
> - Understanding the global burden of disease
> - Health implications of migration, travel, and displacement
> - Social and environmental determinants of health
> - Globalization of health and health care
> - Health care in low-resource settings; and health as a human right and development resource (Wilson et al., 2012).
>
> Competencies specific to public health that have been developed also include:
> - Capacity strengthening
> - Collaborating and partnering
> - Ethical reasoning and professional practice
> - Health equity and social justice
> - Program management
> - Sociocultural and political awareness
> - Strategic analysis
>
> (Association of Schools and Programs of Public Health, n.d.).

---

age be vaccinated. Future professionals as well as those in practice can use Healthy People 2030 to learn about current recommendations for advising people and developing agency policy. The plan is updated every 10 years through an extensive input process and includes measurable objectives.

In the global context Sustainable Development Goals (SDGs) are part of the World Health Organization's work to improve health around the world (United Nations Development Programme, n.d.). They address multisectoral goals that support population health and include economic stability, education access and quality, health care access and quality, neighborhood and built environment, and social and community context. Countries are encouraged to tailor the global SDGs to their context.

As the United Nations' health arm, the WHO is the primary agency concerned with global health. One of the areas of responsibility is to provide guidance and respond to pandemics. WHO, through its network of educators and practitioners, issued the COVID-19 Strategic Preparedness and Response Plan (SPRP) aimed at guiding the coordinated actions needed at national, regional, and global levels to overcome the ongoing challenges in response to COVID-19, address inequities, and plot a course out of the pandemic (World Health Organization, n.d.).

Global Perspective in Higher Education

The benefits of global learning further the purpose of a liberal arts education. Using a consensus process, the American Association of Colleges and Universities (AACU) asked faculty from across the United States to develop a rubric of indicators for global learning. These indicators include global self-awareness, perspective taking, cultural diversity, personal and social responsibility, understanding global systems, and applying knowledge to contemporary global contexts (AACU, n.d.). These indicators can be tailored for use in developing learning experiences within a class period, a threaded case that extends across multiple classes, a course, or to integrate global learning into an entire curriculum. They are also useful in general education course requirements that are part of a nursing program.

Many universities and health care agencies have developed mission statements that include developing global competence as an aspect of the curriculum or service (Box 13.2). To further the intent of a mission statement with a global perspective, a university may develop principles or learning goals to guide curricular development across the institution. One university included a specific undergraduate principle of learning focused on diversity and how students could demonstrate it (Box 13.3). Additionally, the AACU has developed areas of global learning to be used for developing a program or course rubric to assess learning (Box 13.4).

Global Health Perspectives in Schools of Nursing

Many schools of nursing have established centers for global health that focus on and promote international initiatives. These often include hosting visiting scholars, managing student exchanges and study abroad programs, developing and sustaining partnerships with schools in other countries, and

> **BOX 13.2   University Mission Statement With Global Focus**
>
> Provide a liberal arts education that develops learners' capacity to think freely, critically, and humanely and to conduct themselves with honor, integrity, and civility. Graduates will be prepared for life-long learning, personal achievement, responsible leadership, service to others, and engaged citizenship in a global and diverse society.
> (Washington and Lee University, n.d.).

> **BOX 13.3   Undergraduate Principles of Learning Related to Diversity**
>
> Definition: the ability of learners to recognize their own cultural traditions and to understand and appreciate the diversity of the human experience
> Learners are expected to demonstrate this by:
> - Understanding society and culture
> - Comparing and contrasting the range of diversity and university in human history, societies, and ways of life
> - Analyzing and understanding the interconnectedness of global and local communities
> - Operating with civility in a complex world
> (Gregory, 2015).

facilitating collaborative research partnerships. As knowledge and skill in global health become increasingly important, particularly in light of pandemics, schools are finding it important to incorporate learning objectives that prepare students to locate and use national and international best practices. Nursing schools are finding it crucial to develop strategic goals that focus resources for advancing global health and promoting global engagement for their faculty and students. Increasingly, these initiatives involve collaborative efforts with other professions and disciplines to promote interprofessional education and practice.

Role of Professional Nursing Associations in Advancing Global Health

Professional nursing associations have been involved in advancing global nursing education and practice (Table 13.1). Some have developed accrediting standards related to global health

BOX 13.4   Rubric to Assess Student's Attainment of Global Learning Goals

- Effectively addresses significant issues in the natural and human world based on articulating one's identity in a global context.
- Evaluates and applies diverse perspectives to complex subjects within natural and human systems in the face of multiple and even conflicting positions.
- Adapts and applies a deep understanding of multiple worldviews, experiences, and power structures while initiating meaningful interaction with other cultures to address significant global problems (cultural, disciplinary, and ethical).
- Takes informed and responsible action to address ethical, social, and environmental challenges in global systems and evaluates the local and broader consequences of individual and collective interventions.
- Uses deep knowledge of the historical and contemporary role and differential effects of human organizations and actions on global systems to develop and advocate for informed, appropriate action to solve complex problems in the human and natural worlds.
- Applies knowledge and skills to implement sophisticated, appropriate, and workable solutions to address complex global problems using interdisciplinary perspectives independently or with others.

Adapted with permission from "VALUE: Valid Assessment of Learning in Undergraduate Education." Copyright 2019 by the Association of American Colleges and Universities. http://www.aacu.org/value

TABLE 13.1   Organizations Involved in Global Nursing Leadership

Organization	Weblink
American Association of Colleges of Nursing	http://www.aacn.nche.edu/
Commission on Graduates of Foreign Nursing Schools International, Inc.	http://www.cgfns.org/
Global Alliance for Leadership in Nursing Education and Scholarship	http://ganes.info/Home.php
International Council of Nurses	http://www.icn.ch/
National League for Nursing	http://www.nln.org/
Sigma Theta Tau International	http://www.nursingsociety.org/
World Health Organization	http://www.who.int/en/

in nursing education that builds a strong and diverse nursing workforce to advance the health of our nation and the global community" (NLN, 2017, p. 2). The *Vision* statement recognizes the nurse as a global citizen with a commitment to culturally responsive health care, both nationally and internationally.

In 2014 the Sigma Theta Tau Nursing International (STTI) Honor Sorority established the Global Advisory Panel on the Future of Nursing & Midwifery (GAPFON) to identify global health care issues, specifically related to a voice and vision for nursing (STTI, 2018). This work was in response to the United Nations' announcement of the 2030 Agenda for Sustainable Development, which provides targets for advancing the well-being of people and countries globally (STTI, 2018). GAPFON sought to align economic, social, and environmental pathways for the advancement of global health and to identify how nursing and midwifery could take the lead in such endeavors. The results of the regional dialogue sessions identified the need for global leadership presence as the core issue, crossing policy, practice, and education arenas.

for schools of nursing. Other organizations have developed position papers and toolkits in support of global health or focus on preparing nurses educated outside of the United States for licensure in the United States.

Nursing accrediting agencies have broad standards for advancing global health. For example, *The Essentials: Core Competencies for Professional Education* (American Association of Colleges of Nursing [AACN], 2021) addresses global health in baccalaureate and masters programs with a program outcome to compare and contrast local, regional, national, and global benchmarks to identify health patterns across populations.

A Vision for Strengthening Nursing Education for Global Health Engagement, developed by the National League for Nursing, promotes "excellence

The Global Alliance for Leadership in Nursing Education and Science (GANES, n.d.) comprises national associations involved in accrediting schools of nursing. They regularly meet to discuss issues of accreditation for further understanding of national environments and how they inform accreditation standards.

The Commission on Graduates of Foreign Nursing Schools International, Inc. (CGFNS) serves the global health care community by providing a comprehensive suite of credential assessment products to meet specific needs. The commission's (CGFNS, n.d.) main area of work focuses on assessing preparation of nurses educated outside the United States for seeking a state nursing license in the United States.

The International Council of Nurses (ICN) is a federation of more than 130 national nurses associations. Through member countries, ICN focuses on advancing quality nursing care, effective health policies, nursing knowledge, and promoting the respect of the profession. The ICN hosts a biennial congress that brings together leaders from all the member national nurses associations to consider areas of advancement in nursing. In addition, ICN offers policy and leadership training events to prepare nurses for leading country-level initiatives.

ADVANCING GLOBAL HEALTH THROUGH INTERNATIONALIZING THE NURSING CURRICULUM

Internationalizing the curriculum refers to varied approaches and components, including education abroad programs, foreign language courses, interdisciplinary or area programs, and the provision of programs or courses that focus on requirements of professional practice and citizenship (Leask, 2015; Robertson, 2014). A successfully internationalized curriculum emphasizes a wide range of teaching and learning strategies designed to develop graduates who demonstrate international perspectives as professionals and as citizens (Oxford Brooke University, n.d.). This requires rethinking curriculum so that graduates in all academic programs are equipped to live and work successfully in both local and global communities.

Program Level Changes

Faculty have considerable authority and accountability in the design and content of nursing curriculum. The curriculum adopted will play a key role in shaping learners' personal and professional values, attitudes, and behaviors. It is not only the subject matter of the curriculum but also the pedagogical strategies used that serve to develop the learner's global perspective.

Many definitions describe the intent of designing curricular experiences to promote development of global perspectives. One of the more succinct is from the National Association of Foreign Student Advisers (NAFSA), an association of professionals in international higher education. NAFSA (n.d.) describes internationalizing the curriculum as the Internationalization is the conscious effort to integrate and infuse international, intercultural, and global dimensions into the philosophy of postsecondary education. The core issue for nursing is to focus on a curriculum that includes global and cultural aspects in a range of courses across a program.

An internationalized curriculum needs to be more than individual faculty deciding to include learning experiences. Ideally, international components are threaded into program outcomes and course objectives across the curriculum. An example of how a BSN program can thread a global perspective of women's health issues across courses is shown in Table 13.2. Although this example demonstrates a focus on one population, it is clear that by tailoring broad program outcomes to a specific population, faculty efforts allow for deeper learning about one population. In a graduate program students may focus a scholarship project on a specific ethnic population represented in the local community to further their knowledge of unmet health care needs and issues of access to services. Many communities have more than one refugee/migrant population, and faculty will need to teach skills that cross multiple ethnicities. Using the idea of concept-based learning, learners can learn skills for one population that are transferable to additional populations.

Teaching in an internationalized curriculum requires educators to develop current knowledge of key health conditions affecting communities

TABLE 13.2   International Perspective of Women's Health Threaded Across a BSN Curriculum

Course	Learning Objective	Types of Learning Resources
Health Promotion	Identify incidence of overweight/obesity nationally and internationally	Show world maps of the changing incidence
Discipline of Nursing	Understand nursing discipline within the global context	International Council of Nurses Statement of the Practice of Nursing
Maternal Health	Describe incidence of maternal mortality within the United States and globally	United Nations Family Planning
Child Health	Childhood immunization rates by country	World Health Organization
Mental Health	Describe the incidence and treatment of maternal depression globally	Journal research
Adult Health	Compare and contrast the leading causes of death among women of reproductive age by country	World Health Organization data
Leadership and Management	Identify issues for managing OB-GYN services for immigrant/refugee populations in the local community	Clinical nurse managers in local health facilities

around the globe and in specific countries that may be exemplars in the curriculum. This involves educators accessing resources to develop specific knowledge about health conditions of global interest and disciplinary knowledge about nursing and health care in other countries

Locally Based Global Learning Experiences

When the goal is to internationalize the nursing curriculum, there is a need to address local opportunities available to most, if not all, students.

This can be carried out in a variety of ways while addressing specific course objectives and broader program outcomes. Developing partnerships with local refugee serving agencies can provide a way to present issues in class or during practicum experiences from the refugee and agency advocacy staff perspectives. Following an evolving global health event, like the COVID-19 pandemic, can be incorporated into a epidemiology segment or course. Many learners take foreign language courses and complete certificates and minors. This serves to prepare them to provide culturally appropriate care for different language groups in their community. Didactic courses can include unfolding case studies about leadership skills needed to effectively care for refugee populations.

Communities often comprise more than one ethnicity and may represent countries around the world. For nurses to provide high-quality care, they must have the capacity to understand, appreciate, and communicate with individuals whose background is different from the nurse's. Whether the nurse educator is providing clinical learning experiences in an acute, subacute, or community-based setting, there are a wealth of opportunities for learners to engage with international patients and populations. Although exposure to international communities may happen as part of any clinical, the educator who is intentional about developing learners' abilities to provide high-quality, culturally sensitive care for people from other countries will likely be more successful in achieving curricular goals. As a beginning step, faculty may need to extend their knowledge of the international populations represented in the local community. Ways the educator can do this include:

- Inquiring of facility managers about the ethnicity and country background of the patient population
- Using Data USA (https://datausa.io/) to learn about the demographic profile in the local community, specifically ethnicities represented

- Meeting with community and health care leaders about the international communities they serve
- Meeting with the school/university community liaison
- Reading broadly about the nationalities represented
- Talking with members of the international community about life in the United States and their health
- Developing some language capacity to talk with people in their native language
- Continuing professional education

Learning goals and experiences will be different depending on the type of course the educator is teaching. For didactic courses, the learning activities may involve readings, online investigations, videos, guest speakers, role play, and presentations.

Another strategy is to focus on a single health concern with the goal of promoting learners' knowledge of the issue from a global perspective. For example, maternal mortality is considered a key indicator of how well a community is able to support its residents. By exploring maternal mortality patterns in countries with varying income levels, learners can begin to understand the linkage of poverty with health. On the other hand, by showing maps of countries of the world depicting longevity and country income, students can learn that high-income countries may not have the highest longevity. This can be followed by readings and discussions about the social determinants of health and how they influence health and well-being.

For a learning goal involving issues of acculturation of a local refugee community, the instructor might use a multipronged approach. This can include experiences that allow students to learn the history of how the ethnic group came to settle in the local community and about the refugee camp where the individuals stayed before coming to the United States, the conditions in their home country that caused them to leave, and the experiences from the refugees through in-person presentations or videos.

It is important for educators to assess the outcomes of their teaching efforts in promoting learner competence in caring for international populations. The instructor can identify specific outcomes targeted for the course, the learning experiences the students will engage in, and evidence that supports learner achievement of the outcomes. Box 13.5 provides an example based on inclusion of the program goal of students developing deep knowledge about the health needs of a local Burmese refugee population. For example, an educator whose intent is for learners to demonstrate cultural sensitivity in providing holistic nursing care to Burmese individuals, families, communities, and populations may discuss decision-making patterns among traditional Burmese families. Evidence of learning could involve discussing a learner's clinical experience in postconference

---

BOX 13.5 Program Outcomes Integrated into a Leadership Course

- Finds and uses a variety of sources of evidence as a basis for clinical reasoning and decision making in providing care to a patient, family, or community.
- Demonstrates cultural sensitivity in providing holistic nursing care to individuals, families, communities, and populations.
- Is a knowledgeable care coordinator who facilitates patients' access to resources across the continuum of health care environments that meet their evolving health care needs.
- Demonstrates understanding and consideration for how patients may be affected by local health care policy, financing mechanisms, and regulatory issues.
- Engages in ethical and legal professional behavior that is culturally sensitive to the Burmese patient.
- Promotes improved outcomes for patients by using effective communication skills with patients and families, and interprofessional team members.
- Provides professional care for the patient across diverse health care environments.
- Demonstrates accountability for leading and managing resources within an organization to promote quality care and safety for patients.
- Embraces and employs innovations in information management and technology in the delivery of quality care to patients.

Adapted from Riner, M. (2017). *BSN Program Outcomes.* Indiana University School of Nursing.

about how a decision for further treatment of a young woman was jointly made with her husband and extended family.

A range of resources from university study abroad programs and agencies that support and promote study abroad experiences are available to guide the educator in developing an internationally focused learning experience, including developing cultural competence. For either undergraduate or graduate programs, the experience may be a short one occurring during one class session that is embedded in a semester-long course; for example, a healthy populations course when discussing specific health problems such as heart disease. Or it may be in a semester-long global health course. For graduate programs, the issues will be more complex clinically and organizationally and require deeper understanding of cultural mores, community and health care resources available to an immigrant or refugee, and knowledge of facilities mission and resources for serving specific language groups. See Case Study 13.1 to begin developing a locally-based global learning module.

CASE STUDY 13.1 Developing a Locally Based Global Learning Module

The School of Nursing faculty are developing a new undergraduate curriculum. Currently faculty are focused on how best to integrate a wide range of cultural competence experiences across the curriculum. The previous curriculum included a separate culture course. However, the new design does not allow for a stand-alone course. A faculty and three colleagues have been asked to present a strategy focused on immigrant and refugee health and health care services. The group has decided to recommend a threaded case-study module that will include multiple courses and be based on an extended family from a large refugee population living in the local community.

1. What strategies will be helpful to the group to develop their own knowledge of this local refugee population?
2. How will the group learn about health care agencies serving the population and what their nurse leaders identify as important for new nurses to know?
3. What recommendations can the group make to tailor the unfolding case study module objectives for integration across multiple courses?

INTERNATIONAL CLINICAL EXPERIENCES

Education abroad programs involve students engaging in educational opportunities in a country other than their own. Traditionally, these programs involved study for a semester or academic year but recently students can participate in these programs during a summer semester, intersessions, or during a break in the semester. In a study of schools of nursing in the United States about their use of international clinical experiences in their programs, McNelis et al. (2019) found that 27% of schools included these experiences. The experiences were most often embedded in a community health nursing course.

Students benefit in many ways from participating in a study abroad program. In terms of global citizenship this may include personal enrichment, enhanced self-concept clarity, enlargement of the learner's worldview, development of personal confidence in navigating an unfamiliar environment, development of new relationships, and development of intercultural communication skills (Adam et al., 2018; Dwyer & Peters, n.d.). Benefits extend to future career development and may include experiencing a different health care system, increasing awareness and interest in global issues, and heightening awareness of global health security and equity as a component of US foresight policy (Wilson et al., 2012).

Purpose and Program Development

The design of study abroad programs can influence the type of outcomes achieved (Engle & Engle, 2003). It is important to develop a clear rationale for the type of learning experience, the location, and the specific learning goals that will guide the program design. Study abroad programs generally have cultural competence goals embedded in the global learning goals.

Engle and Engle (2003) identify components of program design to be considered, including length of learner stay; language competence; context of academic work within learner group or provided at host nation higher education institution; types of learner housing in terms of home stay, dorms, or commercial; provision for guided/structured cultural interaction and experiential learning;

and guided reflection on cultural experience. The level of the program can be advanced by longer stays that progress from a few days, weeks, or a month to a summer, semester, or academic year. Nursing schools have generally found it difficult to offer programs longer than a few weeks because of curricular design and learner progression practices.

Within the health disciplines, education abroad programs often center around learning about another country's health care system in terms of national health insurance, design of delivery, discipline-specific roles, and education. This can be done as a course with a group of learners or an internship or residency. It can include only nursing learners or learners from other health-related disciplines. Another important component is to design experiences for learners about the country's history, politics, culture, and economic systems for deeper learning (McDermott-Levy et al., 2018).

The trend in health service-learning programs has been changing as a result of thoughtful consideration of the effect of unprepared learners and unlicensed faculty providing care in another country. New standards are being promoted that recommend learners not to engage in providing care for which they are not qualified and without institutional faculty supervision (Lasker et al., 2018). The Unite for Sight organization has developed Global Health University, which provides online education programs for a wide range of learners planning to go abroad for service or mission trips. The approach taken provides valuable information that first seeks to do no harm (Unite for Sight, n.d.).

Academic Framework

The program goal should leverage the unique opportunities available within the community and health care organizations abroad. Program leaders need to provide clear information, with substantive detail, about the full range of intended purpose and design including pre-departure, onsite, and returned home aspects. Since learners generally participate in study abroad experiences at times of identity and value development as emerging adults (Harper, 2018), they will come with a variety of motivations, as well as personal biases. Personal interviews

with applicants is a way to begin understanding what they anticipate, how they will prepare, personal issues that may need to be addressed, and support they have for undertaking the experience. This interview serves as a basis for further developing the learner/mentor relationship.

The program needs to be guided by academic policies of the home institution and host instructions. Learners and faculty need to be aware of these policies, the support available to ensure they are carried out, and their personal responsibilities for complying with them.

According to Goode (2008), faculty fill a variety of roles, including dean of students, logistical coordinator, intercultural guide, and academician (Box 13.6). Four types of cultural mentoring behaviors that faculty can anticipate include: expectation setting, explaining the host culture, exploring self in culture, and facilitating connections (Niehaus et al., 2018). The educator needs to be prepared to supervise research, if that will be a component of the program. Policies and procedures of the home institution and host institution for conducting research need to be followed.

Institutional Support

Institutional support should ensure that the program is adequately funded and staffed. The funding must be sufficient for safe and high-quality learning experiences that include cocurricular experiences that enhance academic learning. The educator needs to be qualified and fairly compensated so that they have adequate time to develop, deliver, and evaluate the program. Funding sources for both students and faculty may be available from the school or university office of international studies or from grant funding. Faculty may need to make a site visit before offering the course to learners. This allows the opportunity to meet people, visit various learning and community sites, and develop a general sense of the location. Funding for this part of program development must also be allocated in advance.

If clinical experiences are included in the program, faculty must arrange for supervision of nursing students by licensed nurses in the local community. Attention needs to be given to the demands placed on host health care and

BOX 13.6   Roles of Faculty Leading Study Abroad Programs

- The dean of students role is something faculty often have not been involved with and requires taking on a mindset of counselor and a casual demeanor that invites students to share difficulties as they arise.
- For the logistical dimension, it is very helpful to have support either within the office or through a contracted onsite organization to assist with scheduling, housing, and transportation. In addition, it is helpful to have a clear understanding of how the program will be financed, including student fees, coverage of faculty salary and expenses, and covered costs for in-country host agencies.
- The intercultural dimension of operating the program involves the faculty developing location-specific knowledge and relationships with key individuals involved in supporting the program.
- The academic dimension involves the specific learning objectives, design of the learning experiences, assessment of learning, and academic mentoring.

Faculty Director Dimension	Responsibilities
Dean of students	Student social life, student group dynamics, student mental health, student physical health, student safety, and student conduct, including alcohol use
Logistical	Attaining university program approval, marketing and recruitment, scheduling, administration, staff management, and budgeting
Intercultural	Familiarity with the education abroad program sites ahead of time and intellectual insights about the culture of the sites to share with students
Academic	Course development, teaching, grading, and academic mentoring

Adapted from Goode, M. L. (2008). The role of faculty study abroad directors: A case study. *Frontiers: The Interdisciplinary Journal of Study Abroad, 15*, 149–172.

educational personnel, agencies, and local communities that are involved in arranging the visit. Participating in the education abroad program may take needed time and energy away from other pressing demands of their roles. It may be appropriate to compensate host agencies for their effort. See Case Study 13.2 for beginning to develop a study abroad program plan.

Partnership Development

Many institutions and schools of nursing have established strategic partnerships abroad and invested effort over many years to ensure sustainability of the relationship. When the institution has an international strategic partnership, the school of nursing can benefit from collaborating with interdisciplinary colleagues from their home campus and infrastructure that may be in place in the host institution and community. Partnerships indicate a mutuality of benefit, and nurse educators participating in a partnership need to be mindful of equity issues that allow the host country partner to benefit. There may be times when the educator is involved in gaining entry into the community and establishing a partnership. This needs to be attended to with cultural sensitivity and respect. Engaging in effective partnership and sustainment principles and practices will facilitate a high-quality educational experience (Hayward & Li, 2018; Riner & Broome, 2014).

Developing Student Learning Outcomes

The student learning outcomes or educational objectives serve as the guideposts for designing and assessing the program. They should articulate with the course, program, and institutional goals. Process and outcome assessment should be conducted regularly to measure learning and learner development (West, 2015). Process assessment is valuable during the program, as it gives the instructor feedback on how well the planned activities are being received by the learners and the local community. If adjustments are needed, they can be made as feasible during the onsite portion of the course. Outcome assessment allows for decisions about the quality of learning achieved, resource use, and fit within the range of education abroad experiences offered by the institution.

CASE STUDY 13.2 Developing a Study Abroad Plan

The university board of trustees has recently published a new 10-year plan that includes increasing the number of students who participate in study abroad courses. Over the 10-year period, the goal is for each school to increase the number of students participating in these programs by 10% each year. The dean of the school of nursing has asked the undergraduate program coordinator to support the development of a faculty-led study abroad program. In addition to providing an international learning experience for students, the dean hopes the program will serve to deepen faculty, staff, and student understanding of a large refugee population in the local community. Since this is a new endeavor, what elements should the undergraduate program coordinator include in a plan for how to accomplish this work? The undergraduate program coordinator has met with but is not actively engaged with staff of the Office of Study Abroad in the Center for International Affairs at the university. The undergraduate coordinator has attended sessions at a national nurse educator conference on study abroad and considers contacting the speakers for more information.

1. In developing the plan the undergraduate program coordinator is considering whether this should be an observational or clinical service experience. What are best practices for nursing students providing clinical service during study abroad programs?
2. What resources might the university have to help the undergraduate program coordinator prepare a proposal for the program?
3. What kind of support will the school need to provide to faculty who agree to lead study abroad programs?

Assessment of learner outcomes is important to consider while designing the program. Nurse educator research in this area is evolving and has primarily relied on small single-class samples, often with instructor-developed tools. Increasingly, institutions are taking an inclusive approach to assessing learner outcomes and are asking learners from all approved programs to complete a common tool. This allows evaluation of the total education abroad effort and can identify programs where learners assess their learning as greater. One such tool is the Global Perspective Inventory (Braskamp et al., 2008), which has established reliability. Two tools developed for assessing cultural competence with established reliability and in use over time are Camphina-Bacote's *Inventory for Assessing the Process of Cultural Competence Among Healthcare Professionals—Revised* (1998) and the *Cultural Competence Self-Assessment Questionnaire* (Mason, 1995).

Selecting Students and Student Code of Conduct

Information about a program needs to be transparent and include purpose, eligibility, selection process, and financial costs, including for the travel component and academic credit. Academic advisors and the faculty program director can be helpful in assisting learners to think about where in their program of study an education-abroad experience might best fit. The availability of scholarships can increase learner participation, and all sources of possible funding can be given to learners with application due dates.

Preparation of Students and Predeparture Planning

Sessions in advance of departure are useful in preparing students for academic and social/cultural experiences. These sessions generally include personal safety and health issues, including securing overseas travel health insurance. Learners also need information about getting their passport, visa, and immunizations. The faculty may elect to have students book flights together or have them arrange their own flights with information on where to meet in country, such as at the airport, a hotel, or a university.

Preparing students for the local culture and health care experience can occur in a variety of ways. Some of these include speakers from the country, students who previously participated in the program, videos, language practice, assignments that require research and presentation in class or posting to an online course site, and reviewing key cultural norms and expressions of cultural sensitivity. Learning about a country's major health concerns and how the health care system operates provides foundation information for onsite experiences. Exploring the nursing education and licensure systems can inform students of similarities and differences with the United States (Baker et al., 2021).

Learners need to know the appropriate dress for various activities they will engage in, such as a visit to health care agencies that may require a laboratory coat, a community agency in casual professional dress, or an orphanage where jeans are acceptable. This prepares the learner for demonstrating cultural humility.

Security issues may include registering with the Smart Traveler Enrollment Program (STEP) on the website of the US Department of State (https://step.state.gov/step). Parents and others may need information on how to contact the academic institution in case of emergency if they are not able to get in touch with the learner. Likewise, the academic institution needs to have information on how to contact a learner's parent/guardian if needed.

Onsite Arrival

Upon arrival, learners benefit from an orientation to living arrangements and the local neighborhood. Time to acclimate to the environment may be needed. A review of the details of scheduled activities orients participants so that they can be prepared for departures, length of time away from lodging, types of dress, what they will be doing and with whom, and when they will be returning each day.

It is important to have clear standards of conduct and how violations will be dealt with so that faculty and students are clear about the consequences and resulting violations. This needs to occur before departure and onsite as well.

Onsite Learning Strategies

Learning strategies used during the onsite program activate the purpose of the study abroad experience. A wide range of strategies are used to meet the program's learning goals. Some of these are observation, visits to health care agencies, interviews with residents and community leaders, participation in providing care, and pairing with local students and providers, to name a few.

Frequent debriefing sessions after the experience can be useful in helping learners reflect on information learned from presenters, tours, and walking within the community; sharing emotional reactions; and linking readings to experiences.

Journaling about their experiences encourages student reflection on activities, their response to them, and what they are learning. This can lead to transformation in their self-perception, deeper insights into their experiences, and ways to understand challenging situations. When reflection assignments are linked to course materials, learners can demonstrate the achievement of course learning objectives. Reflection assignments can be designed for different purposes. Reflection prompts that are designed for intercultural learning may include the student's:

1. Experience of cultural difference
2. Adjustment during the international experiences
3. Collaboration with people from a different culture
4. Experience communicating or speaking the local language
5. Specific skills, knowledge, or abilities they used or the new ones they have gained through this international experience.

A model used in service-learning programs locally and globally is the DEAL Model for Critical Reflection (Ash & Clayton, 2009). This model engages students in clearly describing the experiences to help clarify what happened. This is followed by an examination of the experience during which the students describe how they responded to the situation and how course materials and goals are linked to the experience. The final part is for the student to describe what they learned, why it matters, and how they will use the new learning in the future. Box 13.7 provides phrases for use in prompting student reflections.

Additionally, social media has become a popular way for learners to communicate in real time about their experiences through blogs, Facebook, Instagram, and Twitter. Social media can engage those in the home community, such as friends, family, student peers, and the larger academic community. It is important, however, for educators to communicate and expect students to engage in ethical photography practices while abroad. Reputable organizations provide ethical and culturally sensitive questions and guidelines for individuals to consider as they think about what kinds of photos to take to document their experience (Unite for Sight, n.d.).

BOX 13.7 Study Abroad Reflection Prompts for Clinical Experiences

1. Describe your clinical learning experience. Look at it objectively and in some detail to address what occurred using the questions *who, what, when, where, and how.*
2. Examine the experience from the perspective of what happened in relation to your clinical objectives; what academic materials were relevant such as models, concepts, or principles; and what skills were used or could have been used.
3. Articulate learning (individually; in writing): *I learned that ... I learned this when ... This learning matters because ... In light of this I will ...*

Data from Ash, S. L., & Clayton, P. H. (2009). Generating, deepening, and documenting learning: The power of critical reflection in applied learning. *Journal of Applied Learning in Higher Education, 1,* 25–48.

Postexperience Debriefing

Bringing the class back together a few weeks after returning home can help with reentry shock that often occurs, especially when students from the United States have visited a health care agency in a low-resource community. Students can share responses they receive from sharing their experience with friends, family, and sponsors who may have made financial contributions to their trip. This is often a time for sharing photos and reviewing program highlights. It can be combined with submitting final course assignments, such as a paper. At this time, students can complete course evaluations, surveys from the university, or other tools evaluating the program.

INTERNATIONAL STUDENTS ENROLLED IN COURSES/PROGRAMS IN US SCHOOLS OF NURSING

International Students and Fellows

Since the mid-1950s, the United States has been a destination of choice for international students and has experienced an increasing number of students seeking academic degrees and short-term experience like postdoctoral studies and research fellowships. Reasons given have been the quality of education, a welcoming culture, and the prospect of employment in the United States after graduation. In recent years the number of international students has declined. Among the key factors for this decline were the rising cost of US higher education, high numbers of student visa delays and denials, a difficult political environment for immigrants under the Trump administration, and expanded opportunities to study in other countries. The COVID-19 pandemic further aggravated these dynamics. Closures and limited access to US embassies and consulates, travel restrictions, and personal safety considerations have complicated visa issuance and travel plans of international students. While the current national and global environment is evolving, there continues to be a demand for US education among international students (Migration Policy Institute, 2021).

Planning for Arrival

The process of applying to a school of nursing generally occurs in connection with applying for admission to the academic institution and requesting the necessary visa documents. Preparing to receive an international student involves working with institutions' international office as they have official responsibilities in relation to federal education requirements. Preparation also includes ensuring arrangements are made for housing; tours and acculturation orientations to the school, campus, and community resources; and ensuring they know how to access educational resources like learning centers, the library, writing center, and student counseling services. It is important to be clear about expectations for the educational experience and standards of academic conduct. Providing one or more peer students can help them with the transition, particularly cultural aspects of the university as well as the local community (Kim et al., 2017). In short, retention of international students is a joint responsibility of faculty, academic advisors, English-language program staff, and student affairs professionals on campus (Mamiseishvili, 2012).

Preparing Course Faculty for Supporting International Student Learning

Faculty new to teaching international students will want to develop a mindset that welcomes them not only to the class but to the program, university, and community. Giving attention to acculturation issues will help the student adapt to US educational norms and practices. The roles and methods employed by many US nursing faculty may be unfamiliar to international students, who are accustomed to teachers adopting an authoritarian role and who primarily lecture and hold formal office hours. For nursing faculty who adopt a more informal approach, this may need to be explained in terms of US egalitarian values. The integration of active learning strategies within the classroom may be unfamiliar and require additional coaching. Pairing the international student with a home student can also be helpful in the social adjustment that may be causing stress. The Berkeley Center for Teaching and Learning (2017) provides suggestions that educators can use to support international students.

Students from another country may have different experiences regarding acceptable behavior or academic conduct. This can include permissible receiving and giving of help from and to fellow students, citing material from another source, and taking examinations. It is useful to make expectations clear, provide rehearsal opportunities, and make clear what assistance will be provided during examinations, such as having a dictionary available to look up an unfamiliar word.

In the United States critical thinking is highly valued, but in many countries this is not emphasized, as it may seem confrontational and challenging to the teacher's expertise (Tan, 2017). Students may need help understanding the value and developing the skills needed to be successful with new teaching/learning modalities. Pedagogy like the flipped classroom, problem-based learning, and simulation may also require additional explanation for international students.

There are a variety of ways students can meet the established course goals. Considering how they may need to be adapted to make the experience relevant for the international student and usable when they return home will make the learning experience more valuable to the international student. In addition, this can engage home students in learning more about nursing in their peers' country. While maintaining evaluation expectations, strategies may need to be modified as well. International students may need more time to complete an examination, may request prereads of written assignments, and can be encouraged to work with a coach for presentations.

CHAPTER SUMMARY: KEY POINTS

- Educators need to be prepared to address global health within the curriculum that promotes students learning about and being prepared to provide culturally appropriate care in local and global settings.
- Global health competencies, guidelines, and toolkits can guide course and program development.
- National and international professional nursing organizations provide consensus guidelines to develop best practices and standards for global nursing and nurse educator preparation.
- Internationalizing the curriculum involves a wide range of learning opportunities that engage the learner in understanding and preparing to function in their discipline across national borders.
- Nurse educators can employ course-specific strategies to promote cultural competence for refugee and immigrant populations in local communities.
- Using institutional resources regarding international learning goals, standards, and accepted practices assists nurse educators in receiving approval for study abroad programs and proposals.
- Employing an academic framework guides the development of study abroad programs that are academically rigorous and support overall program outcomes.
- Strategic international partnerships require sustained commitment, demonstrated humility, and equity that allows all partners to benefit from the program.
- Study abroad courses require selection of students, predeparture orientation, onsite experiences and debriefing, and post experience reflection.

- Effectively serving international students in the nurse educator's home institution requires administrative support, comprehensive planning for successful integration into academic life, and support for the personal well-being of students.

REFLECTING ON THE EVIDENCE

1. To start adding a global component to your didactic course, use Healthy People 2030 to identify a key national health condition and review the student learning outcomes. Can the outcome be tailored to include understanding the prevalence of the condition in other countries? Where might you find information about the condition outside the United States?
2. In a clinical course during which your students engage with newly arrived refugees, there is a course goal for students to demonstrate culturally tailored care. How might you help students learn to access information about current health, cultural, and political conditions in the patients' country and incorporate it into their care plan?
3. You and a colleague are planning to take a group of nursing students abroad. What are key clinical, service-learning, and host country issues to address and how will you go about developing your proposal to present to administrators of your school?

REFERENCES

Adam, H., Obodaru, O., Lu, J. G., Maddux, W. W., & Galinsky, A. D. (2018). The shortest path to oneself leads around the world: Living abroad increases self-concept clarity. *Organizational Behavior and Human Decision Processes*, 145, 16–29.

American Association of Colleges of Nursing (AACN). (2021). *The essentials: Core competencies for professional nursing education*. https://www.aacnnursing.org/Essentials

American Association of Colleges and Universities (AACU). (n.d.). *Global learning VALUE rubric*. https://www.aacu.org/value/rubrics/global-learning

Ash, S. L., & Clayton, P. H. (2009). Generating, deepening, and documenting learning: The power of critical reflection in applied learning. *Journal of Applied Learning in Higher Education*, 1, 25–48.

Baker, C., Cary, A. H., & da Conceicao Bento, M. (2021). Global standards for professional nursing education: The time is now. *Journal of Professional Nursing*, 37(1), 86–92.

Berkeley Center for Teaching and Learning. (2017). *Creating conditions for (international) "student success*. https://teaching.berkeley.edu/creating-conditions-international-student-success.

Betancourt, J., Green, A., Carrillo, J., & Park, E. (2005). Cultural competence and health care disparities: Key perspectives and trends. *Health Affairs*, 24(2), 499–505.

Braskamp, L.A., Braskamp, D.C., Merrill, K.C., & Engberg, M. (2008). *Global Perspective Inventory (GPI): Its purpose, construction, potential uses, and psychometric characteristics*. https://www.researchgate.net/publication/239931705_Global_Perspectives_Inventory_GPI_Its_Purpose_Construction_Potential_Uses_and_Psychometric_Characteristics

Commission on Graduates of Foreign Nursing Schools International, Inc. (n.d.) *Mission statement and goals*. Retrieved from http://www.cgfns.org/

Dwyer, M.M., & Peters, C.K. (n.d.). *The benefits of study abroad*. https://www.iesabroad.org/study-abroad/news/benefits-study-abroad#sthash.2Zw7gln1.dpbs

Engle, L., & Engle, J. (2003). Study abroad levels: Toward a classification of program types. *Frontiers: The Interdisciplinary Journal of Study Abroad*, 9(1), 1–20.

Global Alliance for Leadership in Nursing Education and Science. (n.d.) *Resources*. http://ganes.info/

Goode, M. L. (2008). The role of faculty study abroad directors: A case study. *Frontiers: The Interdisciplinary Journal of Study Abroad*, 15, 149–172.

Gregory, J. (2015, July). *PULs*. https://ctl.iupui.edu/Resources/Preparing-to-Teach/PULs

Harper, N. J. (2018). Locating self in place during a study abroad experience: Emerging adults, global awareness, and the Andes. *Journal of Experiential Education*, 41(3), 295–311.

Hayward, L., & Li, Li. (2017). Sustaining and improving an international service-learning partnership: Evaluation of an evidence-based service delivery model. *Physiotherapy Theory and Practice*. https://doi.org/10.1080/09593985.2017.1318425.

Healthy People, https://health.gov/healthypeople

Kim, Y. K., Collins, C. S., Rennick, L. A., & Edens, D. (2017). College experiences and outcomes among international undergraduate students at research universities in the United States: A comparison to their domestic peers. *Journal of International Students, 7*(2), 395–420.

Lasker, J., Aldrink, M., Balasubramaniam, R., Caldron, P., & Compton, B. (2018). Guidelines for responsible short-term global health activities: developing common principles. *Globalization and Health, 14.* https://doi.org/10.1186/s12992-018-0330-4.

Leask, B. (2015). A conceptual framework for internationalisation of the curriculum. *Internationalizing the Curriculum, 26–40.*

Mamiseishvili, K. (2012). International student persistence in US postsecondary institutions. *Higher Education, 64*(1), 1–17.

Mason, J.L. (1995). *Cultural competence self-assessment questionnaire: A manual for users.* http://www.racialequitytools.org/resourcefiles/mason.pdf

McDermott-Levy, R., Leffers, J., & Mayaka, J. (2018). Ethical principles and guidelines of global health nursing practice. *Nursing outlook, 66*(5), 473–481.

McNelis, A., de Leon, K., Whitlow, M., & Fitszpatrick, J. (2019). Current state of international clinical experiences in US prelicensure nursing programs. *Nursing Education Perspectives, 40*(5), 291–294.

Migration Policy Instiute. (2021). http://www.migrationpolicy.org

National Association of Foreign Student Advisers. (n.d.). *Internationalizing the curriculum.* https://www.nafsa.org/about/about-international-education/internationalization

National League for Nursing. (2017). *A vision for expanding US nursing education for global health engagement.* https://www.nln.org/detail-pages/news/2017/05/16/NLN-Vision-for-Strengthening-Nursing-Education-for-Global-Health-Engagement

Niehaus, E., Reading, J., Nelson, M. J., Wegener, A., & Arthur, A. (2018). Faculty engagement in cultural mentoring as instructors of short-term study abroad courses. *Frontiers, 30*(2), 77–91.

Oxford Brooke University. (n.d.). *Internationalising the curriculum resource kit.* http://www.brookes.ac.uk/services/cci/resourcekit.html

Riner, M., & Broome, M. (2014). Sustainability of international partnerships. In M. J. Upvall & J. Leffers (Eds.), *Global health nursing: Building and sustaining partnerships.* Springer Publishing Company.

Robertson, J. (2014). *Internationalizing the curriculum at home: Creating global citizens locally.* Valencia College. http://events.valenciacollege.edu/event/internationalizing_the_curriculum_at_home_creating_global_citizens_locally_4872#.Wkp581WnE_M.

Sigma Theta Tau International. (2018). *Global advisory panel on the future of nursing & midwifery: Bridging the gaps for health.* https://www.sigmanursing.org/connect-engage/our-global-impact/gapfon

Tan, C. (2017). Teaching critical thinking: Cultural challenges and strategies in Singapore. *British Educational Research Journal, 43*(5), 988–1002.

Torres-Alzate, H. (2019). Nursing global health competencies framework. *Nursing Education Perspectives, 40*(5), 295–299.

Unite for Sight. (n.d.). *Global Health University.* http://www.uniteforsight.org/global-health-university/

United Nations Development Program. (n.d.). *United Nations sustainable development goals.* https://www.undp.org/sustainable-development-goals

Washington and Lee University. (n.d.). *Mission statement.* https://www.wlu.edu/about-wandl/non-incautus-futuri/mission-statement

West, C. (2015). Assessing learning outcomes for education abroad. *International Educator, 24*(6), 36.

Wilson, L., Harper, D. C., Tami-Maury, I., Zarate, R., Salas, S., Farley, J., Warren, N., Mendes, I., & Ventura, C. (2012). Global health competencies for nurses in the Americas. *Journal of Professional Nursing, 28*(4), 213–222. https://doi.org/10.1016/j.profnurs.2011.11.021.

World Health Organization. (n.d.). *How is WHO responding to COVID-19?* https://www.who.int/emergencies/diseases/novel-coronavirus-2019/who-response-in-countries

14

Theoretical Approaches to Teaching and Learning in Nursing*

Diane M. Billings, EdD, RN, ANEF, FAAN

Teaching and learning in nursing are grounded in theoretical approaches that faculty can use to understand how students learn and choose strategies to facilitate learning. Theoretical approaches draw on theories from a variety of disciplines like education, sociology, psychology, philosophy, and information science, as well as from nursing science and evidence-based practices to guide the teaching-learning process. Theories provide a perspective on the complex nature of the students' learning needs, the interaction of students with their faculty, the learning environment, and the subject matter. Learning theories focus on processes used to bring about changes in either the way in which students perform or the way in which they understand or organize elements in their environment and provide the structure that guides the selection of teaching strategies and student-centered learning activities.

Faculty can use learning theories across all levels of academic programs, in all domains of learning, in all types of clinical settings, and in distance learning environments. The use of a particular theoretical approach is determined by the faculty's beliefs about learning and provides the assumptions that underlie the approaches used in their teaching. Being cognizant of how to use various learning theories is a prerequisite to effective teaching. When choosing which theories to use, faculty must consider those that support the school philosophy, align with the curriculum design, meet student learning needs, and complement their

*The author acknowledges the work of Lori Canedela, EdD, FNP in previous editions of the chapter.

own teaching. Because learning tasks in nursing are complex and diverse, faculty may use one or more theories in their practice depending on the students' learning needs, the nature of the content, and its application to clinical practice.

While theoretical approaches are also used to inform curriculum design, describe students' learning styles, guide specific strategies like simulations, and provide frameworks for evaluation, these are discussed in the relevant chapter. This chapter includes those theoretical approaches pertinent to teaching and learning. For each learning theory, there is a description of the main premise, a discussion of its implication for teaching and learning in nursing, and suggestions for using the theory in practice.

BEHAVIORAL LEARNING THEORIES

The main premise of behaviorism is that all behavior is learned and can be observed and then shaped and rewarded to achieve appropriate and desired ends. Behaviorism focuses on helping students change their behavior in a way that can be observed as they acquire the skills, knowledge, and attitudes necessary for becoming a nurse. Changes in behavior occur through a series of learning cues when practice and positive reinforcement are used to achieve learning (Ertmer & Newby, 1993; Skinner, 1953). Reinforcement is an essential condition for learning because reinforced responses are remembered. This was demonstrated in a study conducted on 159 students by Gebauer et al. (2012), who found that students who opted for pregrading via feedback on a written assessment performed better on the final written paper.

286   UNIT III   Teaching and Learning

Implications for Teaching-Learning (See Box 14.1)

Principles of behaviorism are used in classrooms, clinical settings, simulation centers, and learning resource centers. The organization of instruction is directed by behavioral objectives (now called learning outcomes) that can be specified, and behavior can be observed, improved, and evaluated. Behaviorist principles are appropriate for structured situations in which the learning outcomes can be clearly established in a step-by-step sequence such as using the steps of the nursing process, clinical judgment or reasoning models, and in which the desired behavior can be defined, learned, and observed.

Behaviorism tends to be faculty centered because it is the role of the faculty to write behavioral objectives (currently written as learning outcomes) that identify the behavior to be attained and then design learning experiences that will elicit the desired behavior as students participate in learning activities like simulations, skills demonstrations and practice, case studies, questioning, prompts, role play, and clinical experiences (see Chapters 16, 18, and 19). It is also the role of the faculty to offer positive reinforcement through ongoing feedback. Faculty's focus is on what the student is doing correctly while making suggestions for improving incorrect behavior. Student attainment of learning goals is monitored by looking for behavior patterns demonstrated over a period.

Students use the behavioral objectives (or learning outcomes) as a guide for what is to be learned. Students work to achieve and demonstrate the desired behavior and plan the time needed to practice as much as necessary to attain the desired behavior. Student motivation for achievement is obtained from the tangible rewards that reinforce the desired behavior.

COGNITIVE LEARNING THEORIES

Cognitive learning theories focus on the internal learner environment and the mental structures of thinking rather than the observed behavior. Drawing on work by Bruner (1964) and Gagne (1985), this theoretical approach emphasizes information processing rather than the behavior that results from thinking, as was emphasized by the behaviorists. Prior learning, information processing, storage retrieval, and activation affect how and what is learned (Fressola & Patterson, 2017). The learner is actively engaged in making meaning between what has been known to what is new. Different aspects of memory (sensory, working and long-term) all function to process information, but it is the long-term memory that is best able to retain it for long periods of time. In this theory, memory is viewed as a complex organized system in which information is processed through three components of the memory system: sensory register, short-term memory, and long-term memory. The goal of learning is to practice information for retention in short-term memory so that the information will move to long-term memory for later recall.

Cognitive theory emphasizes mental processes and knowledge structures that can be inferred from behavioral indices. It is concerned with mental processes and activities that mediate the relationship between stimulus and response. In cognitive systems of learning, behavior is not automatically strengthened by reinforcers; the reinforcers provide affective and instructional information. The focus is on mental processes that

---

BOX 14.1   Behavioral Learning Theory: Implications for Teaching-Learning

Premise	Role of Faculty	Role of Student
Behavior is learned by being shaped by feedback to obtain desired results	• Faculty is coach and provides feedback • Write behaviorally focused learning outcomes • Choose learning experience • Use teaching prompts to elicit behavior • Give positive and informational feedback to observed behavior (written work; skills practice; clinical experiences) • Assess changes in behavior indicating attainment of learning outcome	• Study content and practice skills to attain learning outcomes • Use deliberate practice strategies • Receive feedback to guide improved skills, knowledge, attitudes

include perception, thinking, knowledge representation, and memory, with emphasis on understanding and acquisition of knowledge, not merely on acquiring a new behavior or learning how to perform a task.

Information processing is an important aspect of cognitive learning. In this theory memory is viewed as a complex organized system in which information is processed through three components of the memory system: sensory register, short-term memory, and long-term memory. The goal of learning is to practice information for retention in short-term memory so that the information will move to long-term memory for later recall and use.

Cognitive theories define learning as an active, cumulative, constructive process that is goal oriented and dependent on the student's mental activities. Learning is an internal event in which modification of the existing internal representations of knowledge occurs. Learning is processing information; it is experiential and formed by a person's experience of the consequences.

Two related cognitive theories with relevance to nursing are cognitive load theory and cognitive continuation theory. *Cognitive load theory* considers the amount of effort required to learn. As the amount and complexity increase, cognitive abilities to learn can be overwhelmed (Schumacher et al., 2013). Hammond's *Cognitive Continuation Theory*, discussed by Cadar et al. (2005), uses continuums to make sense of how judgments and decisions are derived. The continuums are composed of cognition and task properties. Tasks requiring low-level cognition can be done rapidly and more intuitively. More structured, complex tasks require slower, more deliberate, analytical cognitive processing time. The middle area of the continuum is called the area of quasirationality and is where many judgments and decisions are made. It does require some intuition and analysis.

Implications for Teaching-Learning (See Box 14.2)

In a cognitivist approach to learning students have active rather than passive roles in the instruction and a new responsibility for learning. Faculty assign learning experiences that will provide students an opportunity to learn how to think by using teaching strategies like simulation with debriefing, reflection papers in which students synthesize information from what they have learned and experienced to application to patient care, and case students in which student apply information learned to realistic clinical scenarios. Students discover meaning by taking in information, processing it, and storing it in memory to subsequently apply it to patient care.

CONSTRUCTIVIST LEARNING THEORIES

Constructivism as a learning theory is based on the work of Piaget (1970a, 1970b, 1973), Vygotsky (1986/1962), and Bandura (1977). Constructivism holds that learning is development (Fosnot, 1996) and that assimilation, accommodation, and

BOX 14.2 **Cognitive Learning Theory: Implications for Teaching-Learning**		
Premise	**Role of Faculty**	**Role of Student**
Focus on changes in mental structures of thinking and learning as opposed to observed behavior; information is processed through sensory input, working memory, and long-term memory	• Faculty is facilitator, guide; helps students develop thinking skills • Choose learning activities that require students to paraphrase (verbally or in writing) what they have learned • Use case studies to help students apply learning to patient care • Use reflection strategies to help students consolidate learning in long-term memory • Use debriefing strategies • Use student presentations, posters, papers that require application of learning	• Develop metacognitive skills to reflect on what they are learning • Use learning strategies of paraphrasing, summarizing • Use learning strategies of self-testing and practice testing to ensure understanding of content they are learning and how to apply it to clinical practice

construction of knowledge are the basic operating processes in learning. Constructivists believe that learners build knowledge to make sense of their experiences and that those learners are active in seeking meaning. Students form, elaborate, and test their mental structures until they get one that is satisfactory. In the constructivist paradigm knowledge representation is open to change as new knowledge structures are added to the existing foundational structure and connections.

Constructivism is also helpful in understanding how interactive social situations foster learning. Social constructivist views involve both individual cognition and social interactions in the learning process.

From this perspective, also known as *social interactivist*, construction of knowledge is enhanced because of interactions with others (Hean et al., 2009). Packer and Goicechea (2000) described this as learning via communities of practice. According to the authors, learning is constructed in those social types of settings.

Implications for Teaching-Learning (See Box 14.3)

Using constructivist approaches to learning suggest faculty should focus on learner participation which includes learning from others. Faculty create a safe and comfortable learning environment that encourages students to engage with one another in expression of creative ideas and novel thought (Powell & Kalina, 2009).

Hunter and Krantz (2010) used a constructivist learning approach in a graduate nursing course on cultural diversity and competence using student group assignments including discussion and reflection activities. Assignments were structured to require reconciling differences and developing awareness of others' views. In both face-to-face and online student groups (n = 76) significant changes were noted from pre- to posttest scores on the Campinha-Bacote IAPCC-R scale.

Siemens (2005) has discussed constructivism as connectedness, using principles of chaos, complexity, network, and self-organization theories to understand today's learners. Learning is internal but is also connected to the complex information coming from organizations and networks. It is vital for learning to be current, be up to date, and be able to quickly assess the accuracy, quality, and relevance of information.

SOCIAL LEARNING THEORY

In social learning theory, as proposed by Bandura (1977), learning involves active information processing. The basic premise of social learning theory is that people can learn through observation (such as role modeling) and that individual mental state (such as value perceived) affects all learning. Students learn by observing others as models of behavior. A key component of this theory is that students who believe they can perform well have high self-efficacy and will be able to take on

BOX 14.3	**Constructivist Learning Theory: Implications for Teaching-Learning**	
Premise	**Role of Faculty**	**Role of Student**
Learning occurs in interaction with others (faculty, classmates, health care professionals, patients)	• Faculty is facilitator of learning environment • Structure learning activities to involve students with others. • Encourage collaboration in learning and in evaluation (test-taking) • Use team-based learning • Engage students in peer tutoring • Use role playing, debate and simulation • Teach students teamwork and how to collaborate; if learning produces an outcome to be graded, determine how to evaluate both individual and group contributions	• Students work together in pairs or groups • Students learn to take responsibility for their contribution to the group • Give peer feedback • Use civil communication skills to interact with others and to call out inappropriate group behavior

complex tasks with confidence. The goal of learning is to develop self-efficacy. The environment, cognition, and behavior all interact through a series of processes that consist of attention (such as complexity and value), retention (remembering, coding, mental images), reproduction (trying it and observing how it went), and motivation (compelling reason) to affect learning and performance. Learning is best able to occur when accompanied by social interaction.

Implications for Teaching-Learning (See Box 14.4)

Social learning theory with its emphasis on self-efficacy is used in nursing education to guide teaching-learning strategies such as role play, simulation, and clinical learning experiences to develop students' self-efficacy. Bandura's theory is also used as a framework for nursing education research (Lasater et al., 2015).

SOCIOCULTURAL LEARNING

Sociocultural learning theory (SCT) is attributed to Lev Vygotsky. Although acknowledging a biological base to the human development potential and recognizing cognitive learning theory such as that suggested by Piaget, Vygotsky (1986/1962)

believes that learning involves (1) cognitive self-instruction, (2) assisted learning, and (3) the zone of proximal development (ZPD). The main tenet of SCT is that learning is interactive and occurs in a social context. Students interact with an expert (faculty, clinician) to assume increasing responsibility for mastering the knowledge, skill, or attitude. Assisted learning requires that a senior learner (clinician, preceptor, faculty) provide the learner with the necessary support to allow the learner to eventually solve the problem. The senior learner gradually withdraws instruction and coaching as the student gains independence. Support includes clues, affirmation, reducing the problem to steps, role modeling, and giving examples. Real learning occurs in the ZPD, the point at which the learner cannot solve the problem alone but has the potential to succeed and can do so with assistance. The teacher or facilitator must understand what the learner has mastered and what comes next.

Implications for Teaching-Learning (See Box 14.5)

Sociocultural learning theory can be used in the classroom, online, and in the clinical or laboratory setting. The faculty work with the student in the ZPD and provide "scaffolding" or necessary support while the student is learning and then withdraw the support as the student demonstrates mastery. To facilitate further learning, faculty recognize learners' zones of proximal development and provide assistance through encouragement, affirmation, role modeling, and the breakdown of steps. They support students and motivate them to learn through the use of innovative teaching strategies, such as discourse around socially learned traditions (Erdogan, 2016; Phillips & Vinton, 2010). Sanders and Sugg (2005) discussed the actions of faculty as assisted performance that includes feedback and cognitive structuring. The focus is on student development through participation with others. Faculty must be comfortable in letting learning emerge and trust the student when "scaffolding" is withdrawn.

Faculty can encourage student identification of the sociocultural nature of their previous learning through personal reflection, storytelling, and comparisons between textbook or clinical examples

BOX 14.4	Social Learning Theory: Implications for Teaching and Learning	
Premise	**Role of Faculty**	**Role of Student**
Learning occurs in social contexts; students are influenced by interactions with others and the environment	• Create opportunities for students to interact with each other, faculty, health professionals • Use strategies like collaborative learning; team-based learning; think-pair, share; group projects • Encourage peer review and peer mentoring	• Assume responsibility for own role within group • Be open to and respectful of perspectives of others • Learn and use team skills

BOX 14.5   Sociocultural Learning: Implications for Teaching-Learning

Premise	Role of Faculty	Role of Student
Sociocultural learning, according to Vygotsky, involves learning in the zone of proximal development (ZPD) in which the faculty provides support (a scaffold) while the student is in early stages of learning and as the student develops knowledge, skills, abilities gradually withdraws the support (scaffold)	• Faculty provide support (a scaffold) by coaching, role modeling, providing feedback, guides decision making and withdraws the support as the student develops confidence and provides safe nursing care	• Students are responsible for identifying need for support and how to request it

and their own experience. Encouraging students to communicate in their own voice in both written and oral presentations can serve to both illuminate and enrich individual and peer learning. Scaffolding techniques to be constructed or gradually diminished based on student needs include modeling, feedback, instruction, questioning, and cognitive structuring.

Group interactions in activities such as examination of issues from an actual clinical day promote sociocultural learning. Debriefings following simulation activities provide rich opportunities for feedback and learning. Authentic case studies can be used to foster questioning, dialogue, and even debate among student groups. This may be enhanced if cases are given that are complex and contain less than all of the information needed. Peer and McClendon (2002) noted that teachers need to focus on connection-making activities, such as peer and reciprocal questioning techniques and cooperative learning. Sociocultural learning aimed at constructing new knowledge can also be used in interprofessional education (Hean et al., 2009; Sthapornnanon et al., 2009).

Students are responsible for their learning by communicating and collaborating with others. This includes reflection, sharing, and questioning as ways to learn from others. Students participate in the design and evaluation of learning. Students may discover the meaning by presenting analogies, using and describing prior knowledge and experiences, and having dialogues with faculty and peers about real-life situations that require application of the content. With faculty and peer support and scaffolding, students can acquire an increased self-awareness about what is known and become aware of how the new knowledge fits into their existing knowledge structure. Student reflection on the meaning of the content and the learning experiences is a process they can use to enhance and extend their learning.

SITUATED (AUTHENTIC) LEARNING, SITUATED COGNITION

The premise of situated learning is that teaching and learning occurs in real-world situations that will provide opportunities for students to develop skills important to practice, including providing safe patient care, collaborating with team members, making safe clinical decisions, and communicating effectively. Situated learning occurs in the context of the actual nursing practice setting. The goal is to bring the "real" world into the academic setting so that students are better prepared to navigate the complex and often ill-defined environments in which they will ultimately be employed. There is a blending of instruction within actual communities. Students confront issues and solve problems in the context of where they are occurring (Edmonds-Cady & Sosulski, 2012). Rule (2006) notes that these situations are typically open ended and require investigation through multiple sources, collaboration with others, and individual and group reflection. An important aspect of situated learning is situated cognition or thinking embedded in the context in which it occurs. Benner et al. (2010) note that situated learning is the hallmark of nursing education and, in their call for transformation of nursing education, recommend a shift from teaching decontextualized knowledge to teaching for a sense of salience and situated cognition through a closer integration of classroom and clinical experiences.

Implications for Nursing Teaching-Learning (See Box 14.6)

When using situated learning as a foundation for learning, faculty can design learning experiences like case studies, unfolding case studies, role play, and simulation that provide the context for patient care. Learning in clinical settings is essential to immerse students in situations they will experience in actual nursing practice.

The role of the student is to focus on learning for application in clinical practice. There is less emphasis on memorization, with increased learning and practice for synthesizing information for safe and quality patient care.

BRAIN-SCIENCE-BASED LEARNING

Previously, the brain was thought to develop only before birth and childhood. However, it is now known that the brain continues to develop and adapt throughout life as a result of learning. These changes can be observed by neuroscientists who study the architecture of the brain through various direct imaging techniques and mapping how each individual neuron operates. Scientists use imaging to study how learning, aging, and disease affect the brain and are studying how biochemical activity influences learning through neurotransmitters that can affect memory and retention of learning. Dopamine and acetylcholine, for example, are linked to motivation and increased attention, while cortisol, increased in times of stress, can impair learning.

Neuroscience also finds that brains learn differently at different ages. Working memory capacity may be similar for simple tasks, but younger learners maintain more working memory when tasks become more complex. Inhibitory control (blocking distracting interferences), affect cognitive processing speed, and long-term memory. Auerbach et al. (2011) conducted a national study and determined that the population of young people, ages 23 through 26, use technologies to play complex, fast-paced, highly visual video games and engage in all types of social media. The rapid and ongoing use of such technologies affects the neuroplasticity of the brain, specifically chemical processing and development of some neural networks. These learners are used to multitasking and moving attention quickly from one thing to another.

Cognitive neuroscience blends brain science and psychiatry to understand the relationship of the brain to emotions and behavior. Findings from cognitive neuroscience indicate that relationships, experience, and context play an important role in learning. Complex and interconnected functions in the brain work to process incoming information from memory or outside senses and route for immediate action, elimination, or further processing and storage.

BOX 14.6	Situated Learning: Implications for Teaching-Learning	
Premise	**Role of Faculty**	**Role of Student**
Learning is situated in an actual or simulated clinical context in which students can apply knowledge, skills and abilities and develop a professional identity	• Faculty design real-world contexts in which students can use knowledge, skills, abilities learned in the classroom in a clinical context • Connect classroom learning to clinical learning experiences • Use simulations of complex clinical problems • Assign virtual/digital experiences to prepare students for real-world situations • Use role play to provide context and practice • Use preconference, prebriefing to prepare students for clinical practice • Use postconference and reflection activities to help students link knowledge to clinical experience	• Students actively engage to prepare for clinical practice and give safe patient care rather than learning for recall • Reflect on patient care given during the clinical experience as well as after the experience to solidify clinical knowledge, skills, and abilities

Brain-science-based learning or brain-based learning focuses on the optimal conditions for the brain to learn (Connell, 2009). The way the brain learns is affected by multiple factors, including time of day, nutrition, and stress (Jensen, 2008). Twelve principles of brain learning have been advanced by Caine and Caine (1991). Three of these include the idea that the learning brain continues to develop patterns and reconstruct itself, emotions are essential to pattern development, and learning can be enhanced through nonthreatening challenges.

Emotional thought is also related to cognitive function and involves multiple areas of the brain and several processes of decision making, memory, and learning. Thoughts trigger emotions and can be influenced by external information or body sensations (Immordino-Yang & Damasio, 2007). Emotions in learning have been used to further understand connections such as cognitive patterning motivation and actual engagement and effort (Immordino-Yang & Damasio, 2007).

Implications for Teaching and Learning (See Box 14.7)

Using findings from neuroscience and cognitive neuroscience, faculty can maximize student learning by understanding that (1) learning is influenced by brain development; brains of younger adults are different from those of students who have had more experience; and (2) learning is influenced by biochemical processes that can increase or decrease motivation and attention, enhancing the conditions under which the brain learns best like being relaxed, participating in learning activities that are authentic and complex, and processing experiences to develop meaning (Gozuyesil & Dikici, 2014). Faculty can teach students to be aware their emotions can affect motivation and learning. Having positive feelings (emotions) and motivation to learn will increase a student's capacity to take in and process information. Lee et al. (2022) redesigned three courses in a baccalaureate program during a time of national stress using principles from brain science like using case studies prior to class to increase student preparation, using videos and recorded lectures to create "brain links," and quizzing to reinforce learning. They found that students' grades improved when

BOX 14.7 Brain-Science-Based and Deep Learning: Implications for Teaching-Learning

Premise	Role of Faculty	Role of Student
Brains develop and learn in different ways at different ages; young adults have different ways of processing information than older adults Learning is influenced by neurochemicals precipitated by stress, nutrition, time of day	• Construct learning outcomes and activities in the higher levels of all domains of learning • Guide students to apply what they are learning to a clinical context • Teach students to manage stress • Establish a productive learning environment • Provide opportunities for practice and retrieval • Use interleaving strategies to help students embed learning	• Learn to manage stress • Practice retrieving information to assess learning for application (retrieval-based learning) • Practice connecting new information to previously learned information • Relate learning to application of content to clinical practice

compared with students in the previous offerings of the courses.

Learning is also fostered through activities that require knowledge construction and connection to previous learning. Examples include authentic case studies that adapt based on new content and initial responses; simulations; group projects; in-depth, multifaceted exploration of a patient; and reflection on how and why decisions are made.

Metanalytical research conducted by Gozuyesil and Dikici (2014) examined 31 studies and the effect of academic achievement using brain-based learning. The results indicated higher academic achievement in those who had been exposed to brain-based learning. Gulpinar et al. (2015) discussed the optimal brain/mind learning environment as one of relaxed alertness where students feel safe and have minimal threats and orchestrated alertness and where faculty have designed experiences to help students concentrate on new information while using memory and active processing throughout to solve problems and situations.

Gozuyesil and Dikici (2014) found that students in a course using brain-based learning strategies demonstrated greater academic achievement than traditional teaching methods. Students' learning was maximized when students were in a state of relaxed alertness, immersed in authentic and complex experiences, and actively processing experiences to develop meaning.

Having students from different age groups and in various stages of brain development can present challenges for faculty. For example, when working with young adults, faculty must engage their short attention span, need for immediate feedback, and diverse stimulation. Taking advantage of their proficiency in using various technologies, faculty can use technologies like steaming videos or group exercises in which information on the internet must be obtained and applied. Revell and McCurry (2010) noted the need to adopt the use of technologies, such as response systems (clickers or phone apps) in the classroom, to promote critical thinking, communication skills, and engagement.

DEEP LEARNING

Deep learning occurs when students focus their learning to understand information for meaning and application and have a reason and motivation to understand a particular subject. Deep learning is contrasted with surface learning, in which students memorize information for short-term application, such as passing an exam. Strategic learning is a combination of deep and surface learning, where students are both goal oriented and also doing only what is necessary to acquire the information. (Whittmann-Price & Godshall, 2009). According to DeLotell et al. (2010), there can and should be deep meaningful connection between students and the course content.

Implications for Teaching and Learning (See Box 14.7)

Deep learning can be fostered in classroom or clinical settings that offer the time and space for interactive discourse. Faculty can create opportunities for students to learn facts and concepts for application in clinical settings. Case studies, unfolding

case studies, simulation, and clinical learning experiences facilitate deep learning. Concept mapping also promotes deep learning (Hay, 2007) as well as teaching questions to prompt thinking. Students need to regularly assess their learning and be actively engaged in the learning process with peers and teachers. Students benefit through a more conceptual understanding that fosters meaning and relevance (Clare, 2007). Takase and Yoshida (2021) found from a systematic review of literature about undergraduates' approach to learning and their academic achievement that there was a positive relationship between nursing students' use of deep learning strategies and their academic achievement and a negative relationship between the use of the surface approach to learning and achievement.

Students have responsibility for developing deep learning skills. These can include completing preclass assignments such as reading, completing a case study, and then participating in class with the intention of learning course material for application to clinical practice (Case Study 14.1). Students can use retrieval strategies such as using practice tests (see Chapter 16) to activate long-term memory.

CASE STUDY 14.1   Deep Learning

Faculty in a pathophysiology course have noticed that students are not able to apply what they have learned in the classroom to clinical practice. Item analysis test results indicates the students have difficulty with questions that require application of content to scenario-based questions. When faculty ask the students about their study habits, they admit to studying the facts in the textbook several days before the test. The faculty want to help students learn information for application to practice.

1. What theoretical approaches to learning can the faculty use to improve student learning?
2. What teaching-learning strategies will foster deep learning.

ADULT LEARNING THEORY

According to Adult Learning Theory (ADL), adults learn in ways that are different from children. Knowles advanced the theory in the 1980s and has updated it through the years (Knowles et al., 2015).

The term *andragogy* is used to refer to the education of adults, in contrast to *pedagogy*, the term used for the education of children. Knowles described adult learners as persons who do best when asked to use their experience and apply new knowledge to solve real-life problems. Adult learners' motivation to learn is more pragmatic and problem centered than that of younger learners. Adults are more likely to learn if they view the information as personally relevant and important. The basic assumptions about adult learners are that they are increasingly self-directed and have experiences that serve as a rich resource for their own and others' learning. Their readiness to learn develops from life tasks and problems, and their orientation to learning is task centered or problem centered.

Four characteristics of adult learners are that (1) they lead lives with different roles and responsibilities; (2) they tend to learn by participating and negotiating; (3) as they progress through life, their focus and the meaning they assign to aspects of life are continually being refined; and (4) they may have some anxiety related to their learning (Fressola & Patterson, 2017). The following additional characteristics of adult learners have been described by Jackson and Caffarella (1994):

1. Adults have more and different types of life experiences that are organized differently from those of children.
2. Adults have preferred differences in personal learning style.
3. Adults are more likely to prefer being actively involved in the learning process.
4. Adults desire to be connected to and supportive of each other in the learning process.
5. Adults have individual responsibilities and life situations that provide a social context that affects their learning.

The learning behaviors of adults are shaped by past experiences; their maturity and life experiences provide them with insights and the ability to see relationships. Adults are not content centered; adults are self-directed and motivation to learn is internal (Goddu, 2012). They are problem centered and need and want to learn useful information that can be readily adapted. Adults need a climate that enables them to assume responsibility for their learning.

The basic assumptions about adult learners are that they are increasingly self-directed and have experiences that serve as a rich resource for their own and others' learning. Their readiness to learn develops from life tasks and problems, and their orientation to learning is task centered or problem centered.

Implications for Teaching and Learning (See Box 14.8)

Because adults may have anxiety and even fear academic failure, faculty must create a relaxed, psychologically safe environment while developing a climate of trust and mutual respect that will facilitate student empowerment. Faculty facilitate, guide, or coach adult learners. Although faculty assume responsibility for being the content expert, a collaborative relationship and use of the democratic process are essential with adult learners. Faculty can design meaningful learning

BOX 14.8   Adult Learning Theory: Implications for Teaching-Learning

Premise	Role of Faculty	Role of Student
Adult learners are self-directed and shaped by past experiences	• Accept students' experience and expertise they bring to the learning situation; build on past experiences • Avoid embarrassing students; students fear failure and ridicule • Empower students to assume responsibility for their learning and to be successful • When practical, provide choice in learning experiences to meet student's motivation and learning needs • Choose relevant learning experiences	• Determine own learning needs within context of the course or experience • Monitor own progress toward goals

activities so that learning transfer becomes a reality. Learning activities should stimulate and encourage reflection on past and current experiences and be sequenced according to the learners' needs. Faculty attend to adult learners' needs and concerns as legitimate and important components of the learning process; this helps ensure that their learning experiences are maximized.

Course materials and learning experiences should be sequenced according to learner readiness.

Learning activities should include independent study and projects that focus on inquiry and experiential techniques. Field-based experiences such as internships and practicum assignments provide experiential learning. Reflective journals, critical incidents, and portfolios are other types of activities that allow adult learners to introduce their past and current experiences into the content of the learning events. These activities also help learners make sense of their life experiences, providing added incentive to learn. Evaluation is shared with the students and peers; students should have some options for selecting the methods of evaluation.

The use of adult learning principles actively involves students and stimulates the use of a wider variety of resources as students work collaboratively with others to achieve their personal learning objectives. Students must be able, with support from faculty and peers, to determine their own learning needs and work collaboratively in negotiating their learning experiences. Self-directedness and the ability to pace learning and monitor progress toward completion of goals are essential attributes of adult learners.

THEORY OF INTELLECTUAL AND MORAL DEVELOPMENT

The theory of intellectual and moral development features an understanding of how college students come to understand knowledge and the ways in which they develop the cognitive processes of thinking and reasoning. William Perry (1970) proposed that college students pass through a predictable, developmental sequence of positions from simple to complex thinking. Learners move from viewing truth in absolute terms of right-and-wrong, dualist thinking to a more elaborate

set of viewpoints. At any point in time, however, further development may be halted or suspended. Growth is usually not linear and usually occurs in fluctuating surges. Students develop the ability to abstract and weigh information to problem-solve in specific situations. In the end, students understand that making a commitment is necessary to become oriented to a world of relativism and develop a personal identity in a pluralistic world.

Implications for Teaching and Learning (See Box 14.9)

Findings from studies in which Perry's model was used in nursing have particular relevance because of the responsibility faculty have for preparing graduates with highly developed moral and

---

BOX 14.9 Theory of Moral and Intellectual Development: Implications for Teaching-Learning

Premise	Role of Faculty	Role of Student
Students progress through developmental stages as they develop thinking and reasoning skills; from simple to complex thinking; from concrete to abstract; from absolutes like right vs. wrong	• Establish supportive relationships with students that encourage development of broad thinking skills • Create a learning environment where students are safe in expressing their views and listening to the views of others • Seek opportunities for students to develop a professional identity, ethical and moral behavior appropriate to the profession	• Reflect on own values and their beliefs about right and wrong • Identify their own thinking patterns (concrete vs. conceptual; right vs. wrong) and how they affect their learning • Develop openness to perspectives of others • Use respectful communication skills

intellectual skills and the ability to deal with uncertainty when they provide care in an increasingly complex society and health care system. Valiga (1988) summarized several variables identified through research with Perry's model that relate to moral and intellectual development. Variables that pertain to the student include age, sex, socioeconomic status, verbal fluency, student's hometown population, educational motivation, and learning style preference. Variables related to the development and implementation of the curriculum and courses include the subject matter discipline of the curriculum, the amount of structure and flexibility, the degree of challenge and support given, the types of course assignments, the nature of student–peer interactions, the openness of student–faculty relationships, and the degree of fit between the students' positions in the Perry model and the learning environment.

Valiga (1988) found in her study that at the beginning and at the end of the academic year, most of the students were at the dualistic stage. Although some showed no change, a few gained almost two positions, moving them into the relativism stage.

Faculty using Perry's model are attentive to developing not only intellectual capacity but also the ethical and moral capacity of the students. Faculty develop an open, honest, and supportive partnership with students while facilitating intellectual growth. Valiga (1988) recommended that faculty design curricula that require students to have organized experiences with other students who have alternative ways of thinking, reasoning, and viewing the world. These experiences should be introduced during freshman year. Requiring courses in different disciplines that provide gradual degrees of complexity should be part of the curricular design. Interprofessional courses can provide situated learning that blends complexity and uncertainty with the collaboration necessary for successful clinical practice (Sargeant, 2009).

When using Perry's theory, students must be willing to be socialized to the college experience and risk entering into new experiences with others whose backgrounds and views are different from their own. Having an open and receptive attitude and a disposition to become comfortable in revealing aspects of the self is important. Students' being aware of the importance of their active participation in new and challenging experiences that will stretch their cognitive abilities is beneficial for their development. Students can also expect that progression through school will bring increased intellectual demands, challenging faculty expectations, and some disruptions in their sense of certainty about their world.

Students who developmentally focus on certainty or absolute answers may be stressed to develop answers to contextual situations that exist in nursing practice. These students may adopt a negative attitude about the amount of time and effort required to meet the program and course objectives. Thus the context of their learning becomes a negative experience in and of itself.

HUMANISM

Humanism, sometimes referred to as the *human potential movement*, became an important force during the 1970s as a strong reaction to the excessive use of behaviorism and focus on skills development. Humanistic psychologists (Combs, Glasser, Kohlberg, Learn, Leininger, Maslow, and Rogers) were concerned with motivating students for growth toward becoming self-actualized. Individual behavior is described according to the person rather than the observer. Humanistic education has been defined as an educational practice in which the teaching-learning process emphasizes the value, worth, dignity, and integrity of all individuals.

The humanistic approach supports and promotes the dignity of the individual, values students' feelings, and promotes the development of a humanistic perspective toward others. Learning is defined as a process of developing one's own potential with the goal of becoming a self-actualized person.

Implications for Teaching-Learning

Educators adopting a humanistic approach use learning experiences that emphasize the affective aspects of development, promoting the students' sense of responsibility, cooperation, and mutual respect. Honesty and caring are considered equally important as the learning goals that focus on the cognitive and psychomotor domains. Humanistic education involves a climate in which there is recognition and valuing of individual freedom and worth. It may be used in academic courses, continuing education courses, staff development programs, and personal development seminars and courses.

Faculty create a learning environment that fosters and promotes self-development by establishing an informal and relaxed climate. This can be accomplished by taking a few minutes at the beginning of the first few classes to use "icebreaker" strategies that invite students to mingle and become acquainted with each other and the teacher. One way to help students learn the behaviors consistent with the humanistic movement is through modeling. Faculty can model the desired behaviors and attitudes that are integral components of humanistic education: being a caring, empathetic person and demonstrating genuineness while being consistently respectful of self and others. Faculty's recognition of themselves as a colearner in educational transactions encourages more egalitarian student–teacher relationships. Faculty help students recognize and develop their own unique potential by facilitating their growth process. This may be facilitated by praising students' positive behaviors, asking students to draw on and share their own experiences, asking questions that enable students to contribute to discussions, and elaborating on students' responses and questions.

Students are responsible for their own learning; determine their own needs, goals, and objectives; and conduct self-evaluations. Students become actively engaged in the learning process, assume responsibility, are open to discussion, and are able to use reflection and introspection. In addition, students adopt the respectful and caring behaviors modeled by faculty.

HUMAN CARING

The human caring theory developed by nurse theorist Watson (Sitzman & Watson, 2018; Watson, 2011) integrates within a human science orientation concepts and principles drawn from the humanistic-existentialist perspective and feminist philosophy, as well as from phenomenology. The primary concepts of the theory are:

- Practice of loving-kindness and equanimity
- Authentic presence: enabling deep belief of others (patient, colleague, family, etc.)
- Cultivation of one's own spiritual practice toward wholeness of mind/body/spirit—beyond ego
- "Being" the caring-healing environment
- Allowing miracles (openness to the unexpected and inexplicable life events)

The main premise of this theory is caring for self and others based on a moral, ethical, and philosophical foundation of love and values. It assumes all persons are caring (Eggenberger et al., 2012). Essential to the theory is the use of 10 carative factors, which are vital in caring for one another. The 10 factors are promoting transpersonal teaching–learning; assisting with gratification of human needs; systematically using a scientific (creative) problem-solving caring process; exhibiting humanistic-altruistic values; promoting and accepting expressions of positive and negative feelings; instilling and enabling faith and hope; allowing for existential-phenomenological spiritual dimensions; cultivating sensitivity to one's self and other; providing a supportive, protective, corrective mental, social, and spiritual environment; and cultivating sensitivity to one's self and others (Watson, 1989, 2011). These factors move thinking from the more curative realm to one in which caring of self and others in the moment is a treatment unto itself.

Implications for Teaching-Learning

Watson's theory of caring and the practices of caring have been used as a model for teaching in the classroom and clinical practice and as a curriculum framework. The goal of the caring curriculum is to create an educational experience in nursing that is more in accord with true education and consistent with the professional nursing philosophy and values that are an integral part of contemporary nursing practice, research, and education. Caring is active and reflective. Strategies such as reflection are ways to develop further insight (Levy-Malmberg & Hilli, 2014).

Content and student learning experiences must be based on the science of human caring and grounded in and derived from the actual reality of lived experience as ascertained from phenomenology rather than merely the content that nurse educators have traditionally taught or the content as they believe it should be. Although theory traditionally has been taught to inform practice, in the new models, theory and practice are viewed as informing each other. A restructured focus of learning is based in clinical practice and uses content as the substance to actively involve students in scholarly endeavors.

Human caring has been used as a framework for nursing leadership (Britt Pipe, 2008) and as a framework for nursing curricula. Incorporation of caring concepts in the curriculum can lay a solid foundation for how future practice is perceived and realized.

Faculty implementing a caring curriculum work to discover ways to eliminate adversarial relationships with students; faculty also strive to maintain open, honest, caring, and supportive relationships. It is within this context that faculty create a climate and structure that promotes the desired learning environment. Faculty develop and model the spirit of inquiry that helps students to develop maturity in their learning and cognitive abilities. The content selected is basic to what is needed in accord with the program's philosophy and desired graduate outcomes. Faculty focus their efforts on helping students see beyond the information presented to discern the underlying assumptions.

To provide students with an in-depth educative learning experience, faculty function in different roles and become experts in learning and in the subject matter (Case Study 14.2). Frequent use of instructional strategies that facilitate active learning, such as the use of questioning and dialogue, is important. Faculty-initiated dialogues with students focus on developing the attributes of intellectual curiosity, caring, caring roles, ethical ideals, and assertiveness. Dialogues occur within the context of a spirit of inquiry and should stimulate and enhance faculty and student learning as meanings of the content are explored.

Students assume responsibility for active learning and seek support and guidance from faculty. It is important that students shift their conception of faculty as authority figures to that of colleagues in the

---

CASE STUDY 14.2   Using Theoretical Approaches to Guide Selection of Teaching-Learning Strategies in a Course

Faculty in a school of nursing with baccalaureate and master's degree programs are revising the curriculum in both programs to align with the mission statement of the institution and the faculty's philosophical beliefs about caring, service, and health. The faculty are redesigning their courses to consider theoretical approaches to choosing teaching-learning strategies that align with the redesigned curriculum.

1. What factors should the faculty consider as they develop their courses?
2. What teaching-learning strategies will be appropriate for the revised mission statement and philosophical beliefs?

---

learning enterprise because students are expected to function as active participants in the decision-making structure. Changes in the faculty's relationship with students promote an energized climate in which faculty become allies with students. Students' active engagement in the teaching-learning process allows more opportunities for faculty to observe increases in students' self-esteem, self-confidence, and competence. Students experience an increase in their internal motivation and sense of responsibility.

NARRATIVE PEDAGOGY

Narrative pedagogy is a commitment to practical discourse in which knowledge is gained through the experiences of teachers, students, and clinicians. The framework has been developed by nurse theorists Diekelmann (2001) and Ironside (2003). As an interpretive pedagogy grounded in phenomenology, narrative pedagogy focuses on exploring, deconstructing, and critiquing experiences and embraces multiple epistemologies, ways of knowing, and practices of thinking (Diekelmann, 2001). Narrative pedagogy is the collective interpretation of common experience that encourages shared learning. It is not intended to replace other types of teaching but has true application as a complementary pedagogy in nursing courses (Walsh, 2011).

A 12-year study produced nine themes from interview texts obtained from teachers, students, and clinicians (Diekelmann, 2001). The experience of learning and teaching is articulated in the common and shared experiences of what is really important in nursing education as the concernful practices of schooling, learning, and teaching. outlined by Diekelmann (2001).

Ironside (2003) conducted a qualitative study of nursing faculty and students to find out what teaching (or learning) in a narrative pedagogy classroom was like. Two themes were discovered. One was thinking as questioning to discover what else there is and what other ways there are to think of the topic versus finding the "best" answer. The other theme is related to the capacity for preserving uncertainty and fallibility. Developing thinking like this in nursing students is beneficial, considering the massive amount of incoming information, diverging views, and chaos that defines clinical practice in the 21st century. In another qualitative study Ironside (2006) found that using narrative pedagogy encourages dialogue and interpretation in a community of learning. The focus was on finding meaning in nursing practice and exploring alternate views.

Implications for Teaching-Learning

Narrative pedagogy is the dialogue and debate among and between teachers, students, and clinicians that questions both what is concealed and what is revealed. Faculty construct activities for content and skills acquisition by encouraging meaning making in students relative to stories about experience. This can be done through the narratives of others—for example, viewing and discussing a movie, presentation, or book (McAllister et al., 2009). Gazarian (2010) describes how students can use digital media to tell their stories. This strategy makes use of the visual and musical aspects of computers. Through listening and responding to stories and personal perceptions, knowledge is developed in context. Sheckel and Ironside (2006) conducted a phenomenological study on how student thinking is affected by use of narrative pedagogy. A subtheme of cultivating interpretive thinking emerged, exemplified by students' discussion of what it meant to be able to make their own clinical assignments. Questions and discussion around stories enact narrative pedagogy as a means for shifting thinking from what is known to what is important and needs to be known.

The concernful practices offer a climate of productive dialogue among and between clinicians, teachers, and students. Faculty must develop an understanding and skill in using the nine themes of concernful practices to expose the hidden understandings and provoke new possibilities in nursing education. Faculty must also understand the nature of the interpretive pedagogies in contrast to and along with conventional pedagogy. Faculty will likely engage in personal and professional introspection because the nine concernful practices will illuminate both positive and negative attributes. Students share the responsibility for discourse and deconstruction with clinicians and faculty.

Narrative pedagogy fits well with aspects of constructivism, cognitive learning, and social learning concepts. It can be helpful as one alternative to lecture as students learn and create meaning through story sharing (Beard & Morote, 2010).

UNDERSTANDING HOW NURSES DEVELOP CLINICAL PRACTICE SKILLS: NOVICE TO EXPERT

The development of nursing knowledge, skills, and abilities does not end at graduation, and developing expertise requires continuous orientation and education for current practice as a nurse progresses throughout their career. Benner (1984), a nurse educator, used the Dreyfus model of skill acquisition, to explain the differences in proficiencies of nurses at various levels. The Benner model describes these levels as novice (more concrete level of knowledge; needs close supervision), advanced beginner (developing more working knowledge of practice, more use of judgment; needs overall supervision), competent (increasing working knowledge of practice, mostly able to use own judgment), proficient (growing depth of understanding of practice and of nursing, responsible for self and some others), and expert (authoritative knowledge of practice and discipline, responsible for self and others, creates new interpretations beyond standards). Thus, while student nurses may graduate as novices or advanced beginners, they will pass through five stages as they fully develop their expertise as nurses.

Implications for Teaching-Learning

Although the novice-to-expert model was developed with practicing nurses in mind, it is relevant to nursing students who progress in levels of knowledge and experience throughout their nursing program. Faculty must first understand what level of students they are working with, such as those in the first semester versus the final semester of the program as well as what learning and experiences they have previously had. Faculty, and preceptors, must also understand that they may be approaching student learning from the perspective of the "expert" while the student is a "novice" and requires support. Throughout the learning process, faculty can use strategies that prompt student self-reflection on what is known, what needs to be learned, and how it can be learned. Continual assessment of student performance in didactic and clinical settings is necessary to adjust teaching. The novice to expert model is also useful when designing capstone experiences and elective courses in academic programs as well as the development of internship, orientation, and residency programs to foster transition to practice in clinical agencies.

CHAPTER SUMMARY: KEY POINTS

- Theoretical approaches to teaching and learning are the foundation for understanding how students learn and what teaching strategies faculty can use to facilitate student learning.
- Theoretical approaches to teaching and learning can be used in all academic programs, with all types of students, in all domains of learning, and in a variety of classroom and clinical settings.
- Each theoretical approach has varying degrees of usefulness depending on the faculty's philosophy about teaching; the nature of the curriculum; the setting in which the teaching is to occur; student characteristics; and the purpose, nature, and content of the course. Within these contextual variables, faculty need to weigh the advantages and disadvantages of each theoretical approach and select those that are most appropriate for their courses and students.
- Using a theoretical approach to learning ensures that faculty will serve as designers, facilitators, coaches, guides, and mentors and students will construct, create, use, and apply knowledge, skills, and abilities to provide safe patient care. There is constant interaction as faculty create the environment and contextual learning experiences and the student assumes control over learning through active engagement.

REFLECTING ON THE EVIDENCE

1. What do you believe about how students learn? Which theoretical approach (approaches) discussed in this chapter aligns (align) with your beliefs about teaching and learning?
2. Review a course syllabus. What theoretical approaches to teaching and learning are used in the course? Are they clearly stated for students? Do the theoretical approaches guide the use of teaching-learning strategies? Do the theoretical approaches align with the rest of the curriculum?
3. Should faculty use one or more learning theories in their course? What factors would guide this decision? What are the advantages and disadvantages of using just one theoretical approach vs. several? If using more than one theoretical approach, how do the various approaches complement each other? Conflict with each other?
4. Using a study that focuses on teaching-learning in nursing, identify the theoretical perspective in the study. How did that perspective guide the study? What were the implications for teaching and learning?
5. For your teaching portfolio or dossier, write a statement about your beliefs about using theoretical approaches in your teaching. Describe the educational context, the students, and the content of your course while answering the question, how do the theoretical approach(es) align with the context of your course?

REFERENCES

Auerbach, D. I., Buerhaus, P. I., & Staiger, D. O. (2011). Registered nurse supply grows faster than projected amid surge in new entrants ages 23–26. *Health Affairs, 30*, 2286–2292.

Bandura, A. (1977). *Social learning theory.* Prentice Hall.

Beard, K., & Morote, E. S. (2010). Using podcasts with narrative pedagogy: Are learning objectives met? *Nursing Education Perspectives, 31*(3), 186–187.

Benner, P. (1984). *From novice to expert.* Addison-Wesley.

Benner, P., Sutphen, M., Leonard, V., & Day, L. (2010). *Educating nurses: A call for radical transformation* (Vol. 15). John Wiley & Sons.

Britt Pipe, T, (2008). Illuminating the inner leadership journey by engaging mindfulness as guided by caring theory. *Nursing Administration Quarterly, 32*(2), 117–125.

Bruner, J. (1964). The course of cognitive growth. *American Psychologist, 29*, 1–15.

Caine, R.N., & Caine, G. (1991). Making connections: Teaching and the human brain. http://www.eric.ed.gov/PDFS/ED335141.pdf.

Cadar, R., Campbell, S., & Watson, D. (2005). Cognitive continuum theory in nursing decision making. *Journal of Advanced Nursing, 49*(4), 397–405.

Clare, B. (2007). Promoting deep learning: A teaching learning and assessment endeavour. *Social Work Education, 26*(5), 433–446.

Connell, J. D. (2009). The global aspects of brain-based learning. *Educational Horizons, 88*, 28–39.

Diekelmann, N. (2001). Narrative pedagogy: Heideggerian hermeneutical analysis of lived experiences of students, teachers, and clinicians. *Advances in Nursing Science, 23*(3), 53–71.

DeLotell, P. J., Millam, L. A., & Reinhardt, M. M. (2010). The use of deep learning strategies in online business courses to impact student retention. *American Journal of Business Education, 3*(12), 49–55.

Edmonds-Cady, C., & Sosulski, M. R. (2012). Applications of situated learning to foster communities of practice. *Journal of Social Work Education, 48*, 45–64.

Eggenberger, T. L., Keller, K. B., Chase, S. K., & Payne, L. (2012). A quantitative approach to evaluating caring in nursing education. *Nursing Education Perspectives, 33*(6), 406–409.

Erdogan, N. (2016). Sociocultural perspective of science in online learning environments. *International Journal of Education in Mathematics, Science and Technology, 4*(3), 1–12.

Ertmer, P. A., & Newby, T. J. (1993). "Behaviorism, Cognitivism, Constructivism: Comparing critical features from an instructional design perspective.

Performance Improvement Quarterly, 64(4). https://doi.org/10.1111/j.1937-8327.1993.tb00605.x.

Fosnot, C. T. (1996). *Constructivism: Theory, perspectives and practice.* Teachers College Press.

Fressola, M. C., & Patterson, G. E. (2017). *Transition from clinician to educator.* Jones & Bartlett Learning.

Gagne, R. M. (1985). *The conditions of learning and theory of instruction* (4th ed.). Holt, Rinehart, and Winston.

Gazarian, P. K. (2010). Digital stories: Incorporating narrative pedagogy. *Journal of Nursing Education, 49*(5), 287–290.

Gebauer, J., Janicki, T., & Yayacicegi, U. (2012). Multiple submissions and their impact on the "path of learning." *Information Systems Education Journal, 10*(2), 40–46.

Goddu, K. (2012). *Meeting the challenge: Teaching strategies for adult learners. Kappa Delta Phi, 48*(4), 169–173.

Gozuyesil, E., & Dikici, A. (2014). The effect of brain-based learning on academic achievement: A meta-analytical study. *Educational Sciences Theory & Practice, 14*(2), 642–648.

Gulpinar, M., Isoguli-Alkac, U., & Yegan, B. (2015). Integrated and contextual basic science instruction in preclinical education: Problem-based learning experience enhanced with brain/mind learning principles. *Educational Sciences Theory & Practice, 15*(5), 1215–1228.

Hay, D. B. (2007). Using concept maps to measure deep, surface, and non-learning outcomes. *Studies in Higher Education, 32*(1), 39–57.

Hean, S., Craddock, D., & O'Halloran, C. (2009). Learning theories and interprofessional education: A user's guide. *Learning in Health and Social Work, 8*(4), 250–262.

Hunter, J. L., & Krantz, S. (2010). Constructivism in cultural competence education. *Journal of Nursing Education, 49*(4), 207–214.

Immordino-Yang, M. H., & Damasio, A. (2007). We feel, therefore we learn: The relevance of affective and social neuroscience to education. *Mind, Brain, and Education, 1*(1), 3–10.

Ironside, P. (2003). New pedagogies for teaching thinking: The lived experiences of students and teachers enacting narrative pedagogy. *Journal of Nursing Education, 42*(11), 509–516.

Ironside, P. M. (2006). Using narrative pedagogy: Learning and practising interpretive thinking. *Journal of Advanced Nursing, 55*(4), 478–486.

Jackson, L., & Caffarella, R. S. (1994). Experiential learning: A new approach. Jossey-Bass.

Jensen, E. (2008). *Brain-based learning: The new paradigm of teaching* (2nd ed.). Corwin Press.

Knowles, M. S., Holton, E. F., & Swanson, (2015). *The adult learner: The definitive classic in adult education and human resource development* (8th ed.). Taylor & Francis Group.

Lasater, K., Mood, L., Buchwach, D., & Dieckelmann, N. F. (2015). Reducing incivility in the workplace: Results of a three-part educational intervention. *The Journal of Continuing Education in Nursing, 1*(46), 15–26.

Lee, A. S., Owings, C. R., Johnson, J. M., & Carruth, M. (2022). Brain science-based innovative collaborative teaching to facilitate nursing education. *Journal of Nursing Education, 61*(3), 62–166.

Levy-Malmberg, R., & Hilli, Y. (2014). The enhancement of clinical competence through caring science. *Scandinavian Journal of Caring Sciences, 28*, 861–866.

Packer, M. J., & Goicechea, J. (2000). Sociocultural and constructivist theories of learning ontology, not just epistemology. *Educational Psychologist, 35*(4), 227–241.

Peer, K. S., & McClendon, R. C. (2002). Sociocultural learning theory in practice: Implications for athletic training educators. *Journal of Athletic Training, 37*(4), S136–S140.

Perry, W. G. (1970). *Forms of intellectual and ethical development in the college years: A scheme.* Rinehart & Winston.

Phillips, J. M., & Vinton, S. A. (2010). Why clinical nurse educators adopt innovative teaching strategies: A pilot study. *Nursing Education Research, 31*(4), 226–229.

Piaget, J. (1970a). Piaget's theory. In P. H. Musen (Ed.), *Carmichael's manual of psychology* (pp. 703–752). Wiley.

Piaget, J. (1970b). *Structuralism.* Basic Books.

Piaget, J. (1973). *To understand is to invent: The future of education.* Grossman.

Powell, K. C., & Kalina, C. J. (2009). Cognitive and social Constructivism: Developing tools for an effective classroom. *Education, 130*(2), 241–250.

Revell, S. M. H., & McCurry, M. K. (2010). Effective pedagogies for teaching math to nursing students: A literature review. *Nurse Education Today, 33*(11), 1352–1356.

Rule, A. C. (2006). Editorial: The components of authentic learning. *Journal of Authentic Learning, 3*(1), 1–10.

Sanders, D., & Sugg, D. (2005). Strategies to scaffold student learning: Applying Vygotsky's zone of proximal development. *Nurse Educator, 30*, 203–207.

Sargeant, J. (2009). Theories to aid understanding and implementation of interprofessional education. *Journal of Continuing Education in the Health Professions, 29*(3), 178–184.

Schumacher, D. J., Englander, R., & Carraccio, C. (2013). Developing the master learner: Applying learning theory to the learner, the teacher, and the learning environment. *Academic Medicine, 88*(11), 1635–1645.

Sheckel, M. M., & Ironside, P. M. (2006). Cultivating interpretive thinking through enacting narrative pedagogy. *Nursing Outlook, 54*(3), 159–165.

Siemens, G. (2005). Connectivism: A learning theory for the digital age. *International Journal of Instructional Learning and Technology, 2*(1), 3–10. http://www.elearnspace.org/Articles/connectivism.htm.

Sitzman, K., & Watson, J. (2018). *Caring science, mindful practice: Implementing Watson's human caring theory* (2nd ed.). Springer Publishing.

Skinner, B. (1953). *Science and human behavior.* Free Press.

Sthapornnanon, N., Sakulbumrungsil, R., Theeraroungchaisri, A., & Watcharadamrongkun, S. (2009). Social constructivist learning environment in an online professional practice course. *American Journal of Pharmaceutical Education, 73*(1), 10.

Takase, M., & Yoshida, I. (2021). The relationships between the types of learning approaches used by undergraduate nursing students and their academic achievement: A systematic review and meta-analysis. *Journal of Professional Nursing, 37*(5), 836–845.

Valiga, T. M. (1988). Curriculum outcomes and cognitive development: New perspectives for nursing education. In E. Bevis (Ed.), *Curriculum revolution: Mandate for change* (pp. 177–200). National League for Nursing.

Vygotsky, L. (1986/1962). *Thought and language.* MIT Press.

Walsh, M. (2011). Narrative Pedagogy and simulation: Future direction for nursing education. *Nurse Education in Practice, 11*, 216–219.

Watson, J. (1989). Transformative thinking and a caring curriculum. In E. O. Bevis & J. Watson (Eds.), *Toward a caring curriculum: A new pedagogy for nursing* (pp. 51–60). National League for Nursing.

Watson, J. (2011). *Human caring science: A theory of nursing.* Jones and Bartlett Learning LLC.

Whittman-Price, R. A., & Godshall, M. (2009). Strategies to promote deep learning in clinical nursing courses. *Nurse Educator, 34*(5), 214–216.

15

Managing Student Incivility and Misconduct in the Learning Environment

Susan Luparell, PhD, RN, CNE, ANEF and Jeanne R. Conner, DNP, APRN, FNP

Student learning is greatly impacted by the quality of the learning environment that surrounds them in classroom and clinical settings. Learning is best fostered in environments in which students feel supported and free to express diverse viewpoints. Civil behavior demonstrates respect for others and engenders mutual trust and open communication.

On today's campuses of higher education, experiences with student incivility have become more common among faculty of various disciplines, and there may even be an increasing incidence of incivility among nursing students (Patel & Chrisman, 2020). Beyond the impact on the learning environment, poor behavior among health care team members can result in negative patient outcomes (Hicks & Stavropoulou, 2020). Thus it is incumbent upon nurse educators to ultimately help students understand and appreciate the impact of their behavior on patient care. Faculty have a responsibility to create a learning environment that promotes civility and fosters student learning.

How can faculty ensure that the learning environment supports a quality teaching and learning experience for all? This chapter explores issues related to incivility in classroom and clinical settings. Instructional strategies are discussed to assist faculty in achieving a robust and engaging learning environment while also helping students develop appropriate professional comportment.

Specifically, this chapter explores methods to nurture and support learning and describes effective responses for situations in which student behavior could disrupt the learning environment wherever it may be, with an emphasis on (1) understanding a continuum of student misconduct, (2) preventive strategies, (3) proactive response strategies, and (4) effective use of campus resources.

The learning outcomes of this chapter include gaining an understanding of incivility in the learning environment and an understanding of specific steps faculty can take to minimize disruptions in the learning environment. The content of this chapter is based on case law, statutory law, research, and many years of collective experience working with college students and college student misconduct. As a cautionary note, it is strongly recommended that faculty consult with the administrators responsible for student conduct at their institution, their immediate supervisor, campus police, and campus legal counsel regarding issues specific to their institution.

INCIVILITY IN THE HIGHER EDUCATION ENVIRONMENT

Most experienced faculty will tell you that they derive pleasure from working with students much of the time. However, on occasion, interactions between students and faculty may be uncomfortable, slightly challenging, or even distressing. Despite the "ivory tower" moniker, the academy, as a microcosm of society, is not immune to the problems of society. Incivilities of various types and among various individuals can and do occur in higher education. However, this is an aspect of the teaching role that tends to surprise novice faculty and befuddles even experienced faculty.

Both faculty and students report having experienced incivility in nursing education (Aul, 2017;

Clark et al., 2020; Courtney-Pratt et al., 2017; Rose et al., 2020; Sauer et al., 2017). Since the first national study exploring this topic in nursing education found that all faculty respondents had experienced students being late, inattentive, or absent from class, and more than 90% reported student cheating as a problem (Lashley & de Meneses, 2001), additional work has confirmed that student incivility remains a problem (Eka & Chambers, 2019), is perceived by many faculty to be worsening over time (Luparell & Frisbee, 2019a), and may even be more prevalent in nursing than in other disciplines (Wagner et al., 2019). Faculty occasionally experience more serious episodes of misconduct, including verbal or physical abuse, albeit less frequently (Ziefle, 2017). Additionally, incivility in the online learning environment is becoming increasingly common (De Gagne et al., 2016; Kim et al., 2020; Perfetto, 2019). Stress in both faculty and students has been identified as contributing significantly to uncivil behavior in nursing education, which was further exacerbated by the COVID-19 pandemic (Aloufi et al., 2021; Clark et al., 2020; Rawlins, 2017; Urban et al., 2021).

Although the majority of this chapter addresses how student misbehavior can be managed, it is important that faculty have an appreciation for the overall context in which misconduct and incivility occur. Student misconduct and incivility rarely occur in a vacuum, and poor student behavior and incivility may be influenced by a broad spectrum of variables, including stress levels, lack of trust in the educational process, personal experience, and a culture of incivility within the overall environment. Thus, the thoughtful educator should consider multiple variables when considering how to best prevent and manage conduct problems in the classroom environment.

In both the general workplace and in nursing education, experts suggest that incivility is reciprocal in nature (Courtney-Pratt et al., 2017; Patel & Chrisman, 2020). If student misbehavior is viewed as a form of communication, it necessitates that we view it in a broader context that includes student interactions with faculty and the learning environment. There is evidence to suggest that faculty play a pivotal role in establishing classroom behavioral norms and also may contribute to the problem in a

---

> **BOX 15.1** **Uncivil Faculty Behaviors**
>
> - Unresponsive to student needs
> - Targeting students, attempting to weed out
> - Setting students up to fail
> - Encouraging students to leave program
> - Unprofessional behavior
> - Defensive behavior
> - Verbal abuse: berating, belittling, yelling, name calling
> - Threatening failure
> - Favoritism, unfair treatment
> - Rigid expectations for perfection
> - Scare tactics
> - Violations of due process
> - Arrogance
> - Making unannounced course changes

---

variety of ways. In another landmark study, Boice (1996) concluded that faculty are the most crucial initiators of incivility in the classroom. Poor teaching and learner assessment skills may lead to student frustration and misbehavior (Nodeh et al., 2020). Additionally, lack of instructor willingness to address classroom incivility sends a message that such behavior is acceptable (Andersen et al., 2019). Furthermore, students sometimes experience incivility at the hands of faculty and clinical agency staff (Aul, 2017; Courtney-Pratt et al., 2017; Tecza et al., 2018). Example behaviors that students may identify as uncivil on the part of faculty and staff can be found in Box 15.1.

STUDENT BEHAVIOR AND PROFESSIONAL IDENTITY FORMATION IN NURSING

Professional identity in nursing has been defined as "a sense of oneself, and in relationship with others, that is influenced by characteristics, norms, and values of the nursing discipline, resulting in an individual thinking, acting, and feeling like a nurse" (Godfrey & Young, 2020, p. 363). Four domains of professional identity have been identified and include knowledge, values and ethics, nurse as leader, and professional comportment, which is defined as "a nurse's professional behavior, demonstrated through presence, words, and actions" (Brewington & Godfrey, 2020, p. 201).

When viewed through the lens of professional identity formation, faculty should embrace the opportunity to address inappropriate behavior as a necessary responsibility to facilitate students' professional development. For example, faculty should understand that the priority goal of nursing education is not merely to transfer knowledge and skills to students but rather to help students come to fully identify as nurses (who subsequently have a specific set of knowledge and skills). This is an important distinction. Otherwise, novice faculty may be tempted to address poor behavior from the disciplinary point of view, emphasizing how breaching of established rules and expectations affects and frustrates others. This is not a student-centered approach and typically does not compel students toward professional development and sustained behavioral change. If faculty are able to help students appreciate how poor behavior impacts their own professional identity formation, students may be more internally motivated to change. Additionally, an emphasis on professional identity formation expands the criteria by which student performance might be evaluated. For example, it permits assessment beyond traditional knowledge and skills acquisition.

A CONTINUUM OF MISCONDUCT

In considering student conduct, one approach does not fit all. It is important to examine each incident in terms of the behaviors observed and reported. It is also vital to use a framework from which to evaluate student behavior. With few exceptions, institutions of higher education develop policies or documents to support and inform expectations of civil behavior and conduct. These are described in many ways, such as a student code of conduct, an honor code, student rights and responsibilities, or some other variation. These policies provide the filter through which one takes a set of observed and reported behaviors and considers the extent to which a specific situation may or may not violate a code of conduct. It is the responsibility of faculty to familiarize themselves with their program's policies.

A Continuum of Student Behaviors

Annoying acts	Administrative violations	Criminal conduct

FIG. 15.1 A continuum of student behaviors.

It has been posited that uncivil behaviors fall on a continuum from relatively benign to more egregious (Clark, 2017b). Though benign behaviors occur more commonly (Wagner et al., 2019), they can still exert significant negative consequences on the environmental culture (Patel & Chrisman, 2020; Rose et al., 2020). For purposes of analyzing student behaviors in the academic setting, all behaviors fall within one or more of the following three categories: (1) annoying acts, (2) administrative violations, and (3) criminal conduct (Fig. 15.1). It is possible that a single behavior, such as stealing a test, can be both an administrative violation and criminal conduct. It is also possible that a behavior repeated over time, such as interrupting a lecture, can be considered both an annoying act and an administrative violation. Occasionally a lecture disruption might be annoying, but the behavior moves from annoying to a violation of campus policy if the disruptions persist after the student has been counseled that the behavior exceeds reasonable limits. Regardless of where the behavior may lie on the continuum, it is critically important to create a teaching approach wherein faculty are in a position to observe student behaviors objectively. The focus should be on actions and not on emotion, rumor, or innuendo. Furthermore, it is important that faculty remain cognizant of student behaviors and their potential effect on learning to consider at the earliest opportunity the extent to which student actions fall within this framework. Awareness is the first step in managing the learning environment. Box 15.2 lists examples of student misconduct that fall within the categories of annoying acts, administrative violations, and criminal conduct.

Annoying Acts

Annoying acts are behaviors that may not be desired but do not violate an administrative code of conduct. Annoying acts are usually included in the institution's policy informing the student

BOX 15.2   Examples of Student Misconduct in the Classroom

Annoying Acts

- Sleeping in class
- Talking in class
- Discourteous or inappropriate comments
- Being uncooperative or disengaged
- Arriving late to class or leaving early
- Poor hygiene
- Distracting eating or drinking
- Texting or using social media during class

Administrative Violations

- Dishonesty; false accusations or information; forgery; alteration or misuse of any university document, record, or identification
- Disorderly conduct
- Actions that disrupt the academic process
- Failure to comply with directions of authorized university officials
- Cheating, plagiarism, fabrication

Criminal Conduct—Also Can Be Considered Administrative Violations

- Threats of violence against self or others
- Actions that endanger oneself or others in the university community
- Physical or verbal abuse
- Possession of firearms
- Conduct that is lewd, indecent, or obscene
- Intimidation, harassment, stalking
- Alcohol or drug possession or sale
- Theft

CASE STUDY 15.1   Addressing Annoying Acts

A first-semester student appears emotionally needy and does not seem to have any friends in class. Lately, the student has started interrupting others during in-class discussion. The other students don't listen and have asked not to be in a laboratory group with the student.

When the student's behavior begins to disrupt the faculty's ability to lecture in class and the students' ability to learn, the faculty decides to meet with the student at the end of one class session. During the meeting, the faculty lets the student know that they are valued as a student, but recently, it has been noticed that the student has begun interrupting students during class discussion. The faculty asks the student about their studies and how they feel the class is progressing. The student mentions that they are having a tough time making friends in the program and at times feels very alone and isolated. The faculty lets the student know that their comments are valuable but that they also need to allow other students to be heard. The faculty points out that listening is a part of learning and that they would like the student to wait and allow fellow students time to make their points in class. The faculty also lets the student know that making friends is important and studying in groups is helpful to learning. The faculty suggests that the student talk with a counselor at the campus counseling center to gain some ideas on how to develop these friendships on campus. As a follow-up to the meeting, the faculty sets a time to meet in 3 weeks to talk about the student's class work and overall progress in the program.

1. What are some learning activities that would allow students to intentionally practice and develop effective interpersonal communication skills?
2. How can faculty communicate and establish consensus in the classroom regarding the professional behaviors expected as a member of the learning group?

of behaviors that are or are not expected of the student. Student conduct policies can address poor interpersonal communication skills, such as monopolizing class discussion, and discourteous, abrasive, aggressive, or hard-to-get-along-with behaviors. Annoying acts may also include poor time- or life-management skills, entering class late or leaving class early, or repeated excuses for poor performance. Case Study 15.1 addresses annoying acts in the classroom.

Individual faculty perception plays a role in identifying annoying acts, and what exactly constitutes improper behavior, such as use of cell phones and texting during class, may not be viewed the same by both faculty and students alike and

perceptions may be influenced by cultural differences or personal biases. Nonetheless, faculty are in a position to interpret behaviors relative to usual classroom norms and the professional norms of a discipline and thus make informed judgments about behaviors that fall outside of those norms.

From a student developmental perspective, addressing annoying behaviors in the learning environment offers a tremendous opportunity to assist the student toward professional comportment. It is important for the educator to be mindful of the manner used to communicate with a student regarding annoying behaviors. In confronting students regarding annoying behaviors, faculty are keeping small problems small and possibly avoiding an escalation of behaviors along the continuum. The risk-management level is low, but over time these types of behaviors can escalate. Although these behaviors are at the more benign end of the continuum, it is best to document any observed behaviors and interactions with students regarding their conduct.

The key to faculty appropriately responding to annoying behaviors is to stay grounded in the learning experience. When talking with students about annoying behaviors, faculty should remain focused on the importance of the learning environment and on the goal of meeting or exceeding the course learning objectives. Faculty are not simply asking the student to be polite or thoughtful; they are exploring with the student how their behavior is not serving them or the rest of the learning community. Often students are startled to learn that their behavior may be negatively influencing others' perceptions of them. Based on these authors' experience, it is most likely that once faculty have met with a student who displays annoying behavior, brought these behaviors to the attention of the student, and suggested new behaviors, no further misconduct will occur. In fact, coaching sessions can often lay the foundation for a productive teaching–learning–mentoring relationship.

From a professional standpoint, it is important to note that, left unchecked, these annoying acts may later manifest themselves in the professional workplace (Luparell & Frisbee, 2019b). Clearly and consistently holding students accountable for their actions has an immediate effect on the individual as a learner and a future effect on the individual in his or her professional life. Though it is tempting to consider them rather inconsequential, annoyance behaviors—and any follow-up with students in response to them—should be documented. Repeated infractions and ongoing patterns of improper behavior can provide valuable insight into a student's

willingness to incorporate constructive feedback in his or her professional development.

Administrative Violations

Administrative violations are behaviors that violate an administrative code of conduct. Administrative violations include a variety of behaviors that significantly disrupt the learning process, such as acts of intimidation or harassment. These behaviors may be motivated by a desire to gain an academic advantage through scholastic misconduct, such as cheating, plagiarism, or fabricating results. Because codes or policies of student conduct are unique to each institution, it is strongly recommended that faculty acquaint themselves with their institution's code to know when a student may have violated policy. Chapter 3 further discusses the ethical issues related to academic dishonesty. Case Study 15.2 addresses administrative violations.

From a developmental perspective, there may be an opportunity to assist the student, but this will depend on the incident and the student's disposition and attitude toward change. For instance, an incident involving an alcohol-impaired student coming to an on-campus class that has zero tolerance for such behavior would limit faculty's ability to work with the student in a coaching capacity. On the other hand, in the case of plagiarism or cheating resulting from poor time management, though consequences to the behavior may still be levied, there also may be an occasion to provide guidance and resources to the student to develop time management skills. If faculty have reason to believe that a student has violated the campus student code, the best approach is to document the faculty's observations, when reasonably possible, talk with the student, and engage the student to fully understand the situation. If after talking with the student it continues to appear that a violation has occurred, then documentation of the student's behavior should be referred to the appropriate administrative officer as prescribed by campus policy.

It is important to communicate with the student regarding any allegations of misconduct. When confronting students regarding possible violations, the sooner faculty confront the student, the better. It might be advisable for faculty to contact their department chair for assistance in talking with the

CASE STUDY 15.2 Addressing Administrative Violations

A student has started to dominate classroom conversations. The student often becomes angry and visibly agitated, using incendiary language when interacting with other students. The student constantly challenges the material the faculty presents. The faculty decides to talk with the student, describing their behaviors in class, and how the faculty would like the student to participate in class discussion in the future, emphasizing the importance of working cooperatively with the other students in the class. The student begins to argue with the faculty and refuses to consider the request to reflect on their own conduct. The student blames other students who have "disrespected" them. During the next class, the student's behavior escalates and is disruptive to the point that the faculty is not able to cover the material planned for that day. The faculty decides to forward a referral to the department chair for review and advice as to next steps.

The department chair receives the documentation and informs the faculty that two other faculty have sent similar reports about the student over the past year. The department chair contacts the dean of students' office and forwards all three referrals for review and action. The student's lack of cooperation makes it difficult to approach them developmentally, and their response pushes the situation to a level that violates administrative policies. The risks to manage are increasing as well, which makes it important to involve other campus offices.

The department chair, associate dean, and faculty member meet with the student. A behavioral contract is drawn up between the department chair and the student. The student agrees to adhere to the standards set in the faculty's class. The student's conduct is referred to the dean of students for administrative review as a violation of the student code of conduct.

1. What are some strategies you can employ that incorporates knowledge of your institution's student conduct code into course orientation?
2. How would you respond if one of your students approached you early in the semester, stating they did not feel safe in class when a particular student was in the room?

student. When faculty confront the student immediately, they avoid an escalation of behaviors along the continuum. The risk-management level is moderate, but over time these types of behaviors can escalate and increase the administrative severity and the possibility of the behavior violating local, state, or federal law. These behaviors should be documented, as should interactions with students regarding their conduct. Faculty should expect that the incident will be referred to the appropriate administrative office for disciplinary review.

Criminal Conduct

Criminal conduct can be characterized as behaviors that violate local, state, or federal criminal law. Criminal conduct includes a variety of behaviors that significantly disrupt the learning process, such as threats or acts of violence, stalking, intimidation, harassment, possession of firearms, drugs, alcohol, or theft. Because local and state laws can vary and the application of the law to college populations can vary as well, it is strongly recommended that faculty acquaint themselves with the practices at their institution. It is also recommended that faculty discuss these legal issues with their dean and colleagues so that they become familiar with the historical context and institutional practice. Case Study 15.3 addresses the criminal conduct of students on campus.

Title IX of the Education Amendments of 1972 prohibits discrimination based on sex, including filming and the continuum of sexual violence. Historically, Title IX has been enforced inconsistently on campuses across the nation, with the issue often clouded because of drug or alcohol use by those involved. Guidance in the application of Title IX states that sexual violence "refers to physical sexual acts perpetrated against a person's will or where a person is incapable of giving consent" (United States Department of Education, 2020, para. 1). Although recently, there have been discussions about the exact manner in which accusations against students should be handled; in general, the statute calls for definitive steps to be taken by school administrators to end sexual harassment and violence (Ellman-Golan, 2017). To promote a safe learning environment and comply with Title

---

CASE STUDY 15.3 Addressing Criminal Behaviors

A student is a senior in the last year of the nursing program. The student has struggled academically throughout the program and has difficulty working with others in the clinical setting.

About 3 weeks into the semester, another student reports to the faculty that the student is very angry with a fellow student in class and has vandalized the student's car to "get even." The faculty contacts the dean, who contacts the campus police and the dean of students' office.

The campus police investigate the allegations and criminal charges are brought against the student by the police. The dean of students initiates administrative disciplinary proceedings, and the student is placed on disciplinary probation until she completes her degree. The student is moved to another class and is told to have no contact with the student whose car was vandalized. A condition of the student's probation is to attend counseling.

1. Besides following institutional policy, what is the rationale for contacting the dean with this report rather than reporting directly to campus police?
2. How should the faculty manage the conversation if other students have questions about this incident involving two of their fellow students on campus?

IX, faculty should act on and report all suspected incidents of sex discrimination or violence in a timely manner, regardless of whether the victim chooses to report the incident to law enforcement.

Acts that are determined to be criminal limit the extent to which a student can be assisted and should be quickly relegated to campus and local law enforcement personnel for investigation and disposition. For instance, an incident involving one student threatening to injure a fellow student limits faculty's ability to work with the student in a coaching capacity. If faculty have reason to believe that a student has acted criminally, the best approach is to document their observations and immediately report the observations to the appropriate campus law enforcement personnel.

When criminal conduct is suspected, it is important for faculty to inform their immediate supervisor (e.g., department chair) of the incident and contact campus law enforcement. Not only are these valuable resources to guide management of the situation, but federal law such as the *Clery Act* requires that certain crimes be cataloged by higher education institutions and reported to the public (U.S. Department of Education, 2016). Each situation will dictate the faculty's role regarding any further engagement with the student regarding her or his behavior. In many cases, the student's faculty may know the student well and could become a vital resource as to the most constructive approach to take with the student to minimize any threat of violence or disruption to the student and to the greater learning community. The risk-management level is high, and all exchanges with the student should be carefully coordinated with campus law enforcement and the campus office responsible for student conduct to limit an escalation of criminal conduct.

The campus administration may further hold the student accountable for an administrative violation of the student code of conduct after an investigation of the alleged behavior. It is important to understand that a university or college cannot and should not insulate the student from being held accountable for criminal actions. These behaviors should be well documented. Faculty should expect that the incident will be referred to the appropriate administrative unit for disciplinary review. Pursuing a single incident through multiple levels of the university and pursuing both criminal and administrative action is not considered double jeopardy; rather, it is a result of multiple jurisdictions properly responding to a single behavior.

PREVENTING INAPPROPRIATE BEHAVIOR

With an emphasis on preventing inappropriate behavior altogether, this section describes a series of actions that faculty can implement when managing a learning environment. These strategies can be applied to learning in a conventional classroom, in off-campus settings, and in online learning environments. It is also recommended that faculty within a department discuss these strategies and adopt common practices when practical. Students will notice common practices from class to class, which may help reinforce these strategies.

Establishing Behavioral Expectations From Day One

An important first step in managing the learning environment is taking early action to prevent problematic behavior (Clark, 2017a; Kamolo & Njung'e, 2021; Tharani et al., 2017). This can be done in a variety of ways, including being attentive to creating a climate of civility from day one of class. Novice faculty tend to assume that college students intrinsically understand professional behavioral expectations of them. This may be a false assumption. It is imperative that appropriate behavior be explicitly described, both in the syllabus and on the first day of class.

In the course syllabus, faculty should express their goals and expectations for the learning environment. The program or institution may also have specific expectations or policies that faculty are required to insert into syllabi. The syllabus is a performance agreement between faculty and students. As such, it is an opportunity to express the ground rules and guidelines for engagement. This is the time that faculty should outline student behaviors that matter most to them as educators, including expectations for interpersonal interactions.

It is also important to emphasize and verbally discuss the behavioral expectations with the entire class on the first day, as doing so elevates their importance in the minds of students and also provides an opportunity for clarification. Open discussion of behavioral expectations also helps foster student trust and confidence in the instructor, since they quickly see that the faculty has put intentional thought into establishing a positive classroom culture and is being transparent about it. For those who may be unsure how to transition to a discussion about behavior expectations, some sample scripts are provided in Box 15.3.

Unfortunately, many students may perceive feedback on poor behavior to be punitive based on previous educational experiences. Students' transition into a professional role affords faculty the opportunity to reset their perceptions about the importance of behavior to their success as nurses. Faculty should keep the discussion positive, indicate the behaviors they wish to see demonstrated by students, and explain the relationship

> ### BOX 15.3   Suggested Scripts for Initiating Conversations about Class Behavior
>
> After welcoming the students on day one and discussing the course in general, work the following language into the conversation at an appropriate point:
>
> - "It's really important to me that everyone feels welcomed and respected at all times in this course. So, let me share what I'd like to see us all commit to in terms of class behavior so that everyone can flourish here." (And then communicate expectations.)
> - "I'm really committed to creating a classroom experience where every person can flourish and find success. You may not have ever considered that we have the opportunity to collectively create the environment we want. So as our first class activity, let's together decide how we'd like to treat each other." (And then lead in an exercise to have students cocreate classroom expectations.)
> - "I'm really committed to helping you each become safe and competent nurses, and this may be a personal goal of yours as well. Did you know that the way the health care team treats each other is directly linked to patient safety? Because it is, it's important that we all constantly develop our interpersonal skills. Therefore, as one of the first important lessons in this class, I want to talk about the way I expect us to treat each other and why it is important."

of professional behavior to patient care outcomes. Faculty should also connect these behaviors to the achievement of the learning outcomes established for the course, particularly outcomes related to safe patient care. Some faculty (e.g., Clark, 2017b) advocate for the co-creation of classroom behavioral norms with the students themselves. With guidance from faculty, students can have a voice in what they expect from one another and how they will hold one another accountable to maximize learning for all.

For example, if students arriving to class on time and remaining through the entire class period is an important component of the learning environment, then express this expectation in the syllabus and indicate the rationale for this expectation. It is also recommended that faculty provide students with a way to manage these expectations. If a student knows that they will not be able to arrive at a class on time, what should the student do? Should the student not attend at all? Should the student call faculty in advance of the class and discuss the need to arrive late? Is there a place (e.g., the back row of the class) that has been designated as an area where students who arrive late or must leave early should sit so that they do not disrupt the learning of others?

Clearly discussing and also stating expectations in writing to students from the first day together helps students understand the behaviors faculty expect from the outset. This approach also provides faculty with a guide in case a student acts in a manner that has been previously determined unacceptable. As instructors, faculty are in a position to set standards that students must meet. These standards may be both academic and behavioral. The key is that they are clearly expressed and

---

BOX 15.4 Examples of Text for the Syllabus

Teaching–Learning Philosophy

My expectation is that you are a self-motivated learner. By the end of the semester, you will have invested your time, energy, and resources to complete this course and I want you to be successful. My responsibility as your instructor is to provide a context and environment that supports your learning through mindful, intentional curriculum that guides your investigations and learning. I expect you to be an involved, active member of this learning community who will contribute with thorough preparation, active discussion participation, and timely participation in course activities. I further expect that you will treat everyone, including the instructor, with respect and civility. Learning in this course takes place through lectures, readings, written analysis, reflective discussions, critical reflection, and written assignments.

Class Expectations

This course will be most successful when all participants commit to developing a learning community in which the beliefs of all may be discussed in an open, civil, and understanding environment. Everyone will be expected to consider multiple perspectives, engage in critical reflection, and take intellectual risks built on one's confidence in the course content. Class activities will focus on critical analysis of (1) course readings, (2) case study scenarios, (3) group work, and (4) research findings. Your personal experiences are important but require critical reflection and analysis. Hence the ability to interact with the material in a personal and self-reflective manner is essential.

Professional Expectations

Becoming a professional is not simply a matter of possessing a degree. Becoming a professional is agreeing to a set of standards of behavior now, as a student, that models the behavior that will be expected of you once you complete your professional program.
1. Be on time. Arrive 10 minutes before your expected time and be prepared to begin class or laboratory.

Leave with plenty of time in case you encounter delays.
2. Be present every day. Your instructor has created specific lesson plans with the expectation that you will be present every class day. On what should be a rare occasion, it is imperative that if you are unable to keep your commitment, you contact your instructor as soon as possible. Ask the instructor about the best way to communicate with them. Write down his or her email or phone number and have it with you at all times.
3. Be professional. Maintain a professional attitude and be positive! You never get a second chance to make a first impression.
4. Know what is expected of you every day. Read your syllabus. Note all course obligations on your calendar and check your calendar daily.
5. Leave your cell phone off and out of sight. Focus on being present in the class and with your work.
6. Collegiality. Now, as a student, and in the future, as a professional, you will interact with and work extensively with your peers and colleagues. Work to be a positive influence and a productive colleague to your peers. Demonstrate value and appreciation for all others by treating them respectfully.
7. Ethics. As a student, learn and reflect on the ethical expectations of the profession and begin reflecting on your current daily decisions within an ethical context. Realize that the decisions and choices you make every day build on your ability to make decisions and actions on behalf of others you will be responsible for in the future.
8. Collaboration. As a professional, you will collaborate with patients, family members, and other professional colleagues in providing care. As a student today, you will be expected to collaborate in a positive, civil, and mutually beneficial way that will build your skills and understanding of working with groups of people to achieve a common goal.

consistently expected of all students. Three sets of sample language are offered for your consideration in Box 15.4. The examples are suggestions and should be customized to support the established culture and values of your particular program and university or college.

Expectations for behavior should also be clearly established in online classes. Although information can be shared in text format, for a more impactful approach, faculty can consider posting a video of themselves talking about their goals for student success and the behavioral expectations they have for themselves and students. Using one of the many apps available now, faculty can also have students cocreate the class expectations.

Reviewing the Institutional Code of Conduct

With expectations clearly outlined in the syllabus, the first class meeting of the semester is a time to give added meaning to the importance of the course behavioral expectations by emphasizing them in class. In addition to sharing faculty expectations particular to the course, it is also appropriate to inform students about any policies that the institution has established to guide student conduct. It is recommended that faculty briefly address the sections of the institutional student conduct policy that have meaning for the specific learning objectives of the course. This is the time for faculty to describe their expectations and interpretations of the code. It is also appropriate for faculty to provide positive examples of the behavior they wish to see exhibited by the students and engage the students in a discussion about these expectations. One exercise is to ask the students to describe annoying or disruptive behaviors they have seen from their fellow classmates in other classes and to talk about how important it is that each person agree to not act in a manner that disrupts learning in the classroom.

Being Transparent

Another way in which faculty can minimize problematic behavior is to be as transparent as possible with students regarding development of assignments and rationale for decision making and grading (Andersen et al., 2019). Students may respond disruptively when they disagree with grading decisions, when they receive an unsatisfactory clinical grade, or when they receive a failing grade for a course, particularly if the student perceives that the grading decisions are unfair (Rawlins, 2017). Perceptions that an instructor acts in an arbitrary manner, especially where grades are concerned, may result in a student misbehaving out of frustration. Therefore, open communication about how the course has been developed and how decisions have been made serve to decrease student perceptions that an instructor's actions are arbitrary or even malicious.

Establishing a Trusting and Caring Environment

As a measure to prevent incivility, faculty should develop immediacy skills that help foster a sense of closeness between faculty and students and are perceived by students to demonstrate caring (Teach the Earth, n.d.). For example, instructors who exhibit behaviors such as smiling, making eye contact, appropriate vocal inflections, and active listening tend to experience fewer forms of discourteous or disruptive behavior by students (Weger, 2018). Additionally, a trusting relationship between student and faculty is essential to creating an environment in which students can mature professionally (Ackerman-Barger et al., 2021; Tharani et al., 2017). Strategies for fostering a sense of immediacy may be found in Box 15.5.

Additionally, faculty frequently need to deliver critical feedback that is constructive in nature. It is false to assume that students understand the well-meaning and professional motives behind providing such feedback; they are often unprepared to receive feedback that is not wholly positive. Consequently, it is beneficial to elucidate the purpose of constructive feedback in students' professional development. A sample script for initiating this discussion can be found in Box 15.6. Once the underlying basis of trust has been established, a more conducive environment is created for the give-and-take of constructive feedback.

Educational Interventions to Promote Civility

Nursing faculty can help students mitigate and manage incivility on their own to improve the culture of nursing education. Educational interventions including cognitive rehearsal therapy (CRT), role play, debriefing, online modules, and journal clubs have resulted in positive outcomes (Clark & Dunham, 2020; Courtney-Pratt et al., 2017; Kamolo & Njung'e, 2021; Rose et al., 2020; Sanner-Stiehr, 2018). Some mindfulness interventions to improve stress management and mood among nursing students demonstrated promising results, though the quality of the studies included was variable (Aloufi et al., 2021). Merkel et al. (2020) reported positive student response to a quality improvement project created by a faculty and student team to promote a culture of civility. Acknowledging that increased stress contributes to incivility, education for self-care and stress management is vital for success as a nursing student and later as a practicing nurse (Bartlett et al., 2016).

RESPONDING TO INAPPROPRIATE BEHAVIOR

When faculty have reason to believe that a student may be acting inappropriately, there are six steps to use when responding to allegations of misconduct (Box 15.7):

1. *Gather and document information.* The information should objectively describe the student's actions and note the date, time, and others who were present.
2. *Engage the student about behaviors observed.* At the earliest time possible, meet with the student privately to discuss the behaviors that have been observed. This meeting will inform the student of faculty concerns, allow the student to express his or her perspective on the situation, and provide an opportunity for the student to understand how the behavior affects others and is disrupting the learning outcomes of the course. The script provided earlier in the chapter may be helpful here.

BOX 15.5 Strategies to Foster Immediacy

- Learn and call students by name. In large classes, have students make and place "name plates" on their desk so that you can call them by name.
- Enthusiastically welcome students to each class session.
- Make eye contact with students in and between classes.
- Arrive to class early to engage students or answer last-minute questions. Stay a few minutes after class to do the same.
- Make appropriate small talk with students before class and at breaks. For example, ask students how their weekend was or if they watched the big game.
- Say 'thank you' to students when they ask questions, share ideas, or respond to questions in class, even if they are off base.
- Smile and nod affirmatively when speaking with students.
- Avoid crossing arms or other negative nonverbal communication.
- Be encouraging. Add high-fives or fist bumps to students who consent to it.

BOX 15.6 The Role of Trust in Giving Constructive Feedback

"Providing you with feedback on your performance and progress is a crucial component of this course. Although that feedback often will be positive and address your strengths, at times, I may need to share constructive feedback that focuses on areas that are not as well developed. I am willing to trust that you want this feedback to meet your educational goals. I ask that you trust that my sole motivation for giving you this feedback is to help you be successful in your development."

BOX 15.7 Steps for Addressing Inappropriate Behavior

1. Gather and document information.
2. Engage the student about behaviors observed.
3. Focus on the behavior.
4. Outline required new behaviors.
5. Outline consequences of compliance and noncompliance.
6. Refer unresolved or risky cases to other campus resources.

3. *Focus on the behavior.* Faculty should always focus on what the student did and not be swayed by ancillary aspects, such as the extent to which one knows or likes the student or the student's academic record. For instance, high-achieving students are just as likely to plagiarize as average students. It is important to be consistent in what is expected from students.

4. *Outline required new behaviors.* The purpose of meeting with the student is to first explore with the student concerns about her or his behavior. If after talking with the student the concerns remain valid, then the second goal of the meeting is to discuss with the student how the behavior should change in the future. Working with the student to change any annoying acts provides the greatest opportunity for a collaborative discussion between the student and the faculty. Any administrative violations of the code of conduct should be documented and forwarded to the appropriate administrative office and, depending on campus policy, may be followed up administratively in addition to actions the faculty has discussed with the student. All criminal conduct should be immediately forwarded to the appropriate campus office and may limit faculty's ability to outline new behaviors.

5. *Outline consequences of compliance and noncompliance.* Faculty interactions with the student should conclude with the hope that the student will decide to make different choices and will choose to comply with the standards that faculty and the campus have established. However, it is also important to be clear with the student that, should he or she fail to comply and continue to disrupt the learning environment, there will be additional follow-up that may include further sanctions.

6. *Refer unresolved or risky cases to other campus resources.* If at any time faculty are working with a student and it comes to their attention that the student's misconduct is not being resolved as planned, or if there is evidence that the incident may escalate in terms of level of disruption or safety to either the faculty or other students, the situation should automatically be referred to other campus resources.

Provide Effective Behavioral Feedback

Students often are unaware of how their behaviors are perceived. In a trusting environment in which the student's professional development is a priority, faculty have a responsibility to provide concrete and specific feedback regarding behaviors that may impede a student's progress. A template for crafting such a discussion has been shared elsewhere (Luparell, 2007) and may be found in Box 15.8. It is important to note that the script provides

---

BOX 15.8   Sample Script for Giving Feedback Related to Problematic Behavior

Hi _____,

Thank you for coming in to see me. Remember the first day of class when we talked about the role of trust in giving feedback? I have some feedback to share with you now that may be a bit difficult to hear. Please remember that I'm sharing it with you so you can successfully meet your goal of becoming a competent nurse. When you do _____, it leaves me with the impression that _____.

   If I have that impression, it's likely that others may have it as well. If you are okay with people drawing this conclusion about you, then keep on doing what you are doing. If you are not comfortable with people potentially drawing this conclusion, you may want to consider a change.

The following is an example of the script put to use with a student who does not put good effort into completing postclinical paperwork:

Hi Mary,

Thank you for coming in to see me. Remember the first day of class when we talked about the role of trust in giving feedback? I have some feedback to share with you now that may be a bit difficult to hear. Please remember that I'm sharing it with you so you can successfully meet your goal of becoming a competent nurse. When you turn in your clinical packet so insufficiently completed, it leaves me with the impression either that you really don't understand what is going on with your patient or that you are a bit of a slacker. If I have that impression, it's likely that others may have it as well in response to this quality of work. If you are okay with people drawing the conclusion that you really don't understand what you are doing or that you are a slacker, then keep on doing what you are doing. If you are not comfortable with people potentially drawing these conclusions, you may want to consider a change.

students with the choice to continue the behavior or not, based on whether they are concerned with the outcomes of their behavior. Students almost always choose to discontinue the annoying behavior. However, if the behavior continues, you will need to address it more assertively by requesting unequivocally that it stop.

Know Whom to Contact for Consultation

Sooner or later, faculty will need to seek consultation regarding a student's behavior. There are important legal underpinnings that must guide faculty when addressing student misbehavior. See Chapter 3 for a more detailed discussion of the legal implications associated with disciplinary action for student misbehavior. In particular, students retain their constitutional rights of free speech and due process, and these rights must be considered when addressing student misconduct. However, most novice nurse educators are not well acquainted with the legal aspects of education. For this reason, it is important to seek assistance from knowledgeable individuals at the outset.

Every college or university has designated individuals who respond to issues regarding student behavior. There are no consistent titles or standardized credentials, and every institution, through its history, context, mission, vision, values, and goals, has constructed individualized approaches to how student behavior is managed. It is best if faculty reacquaint themselves annually with the key people on campus who should be consulted regarding student behavior concerns.

Consultants can include staff from such offices as the dean of students, counseling, advising, student health services, student ombudsman, student advocate, faculty professional development, student affairs, student life, human resources, or the campus police. Faculty are encouraged to inquire of their faculty colleagues and administrators as to which offices and staff have provided helpful counsel in the past, depending on the student's situation. Faculty should also know who is responsible for administering the institutional student code of conduct. It is helpful to have established a working relationship with these individuals in advance of contacting them with a particular student concern. The key point is that, as instructors, faculty

are supported in responding to student conduct in the classroom and have the institutional support of other professionals with specialized expertise in handling student issues.

Know When to Call for Consultation

Just as important as knowing whom to call for consultation is knowing when to call for consultation and when to refer an unresolved matter to others. Quite often, faculty dwell on an unresolved matter with a student much longer than necessary, which is distracting to the teaching and learning experience for the entire class. Let us assume that during the first class, a faculty member has outlined the behaviors that are expected from students to facilitate learning. Let us further assume that discussion of behavioral expectations also included identification of the student conduct code, with statements detailing how the code provides institutional support for the faculty's expectations. If the faculty member has outlined student behavior expectations in the syllabus, met with the student, and made the student aware that his or her behavior is not meeting the standard that has been set for the class, and the student either refuses or is unable to change the behavior to meet the expected standard, then the faculty member should immediately consult with others, such as the department chair, to identify other ways to work with the student or to request a referral to another office on campus. As mentioned earlier, the timing of a referral also depends on the unique circumstances and the continuum of behaviors observed. If at any time faculty feel their safety or the safety of others is at risk, then campus law enforcement should immediately be contacted. If, on the other hand, faculty are responding to an annoying act, then they may wish to meet with the student on repeated occasions to address a variety of issues that are adversely affecting the student's academic success.

Documentation and Communication

It is important for faculty to keep notes of student behaviors that have been observed. Faculty may observe behaviors that are not desired but that do not violate the established classroom standard or the campus student code. One reason to note these "below the radar" behaviors is that they can escalate to a level that would ultimately violate the classroom standard or the campus student code. At that point, it would be helpful when faculty meet with a student to be able to note the specific patterns of behaviors observed. Students are often surprised that faculty have taken note of problematic behaviors and want to talk with them about their conduct.

Keeping personal notes may also be helpful if faculty need to refer an incident to others. The information important to document includes time, day, and place where the behavior was observed. It is also important to use descriptive and not evaluative statements. To say that the student was "rude" is not helpful, but to document that "the student has arrived late to four of the last six classes, which disrupted the class lecture when the student attempted to locate a seat in class" is helpful, because it is specific and allows the faculty to talk with the student in a way that focuses on student behaviors and not on how the faculty may feel about those behaviors.

There is often a misunderstanding among faculty and staff throughout colleges and universities regarding documentation and communication of students' behaviors and students' privacy rights. These misunderstandings center on an interpretation of federal legislation called the Family Educational Rights and Privacy Act (FERPA). Pursuant to FERPA (U.S. Department of Education, 2020a), faculty and staff may and, in fact, should share information about a student when a "legitimate educational interest" exists. Matters of classroom management, student conduct or misconduct, and behaviors of concern fall within a legitimate educational interest. The Department of Education acknowledges there is a balance between students' rights to privacy and the university's responsibility to ensure stability and public safety. As such, the institution may disclose a student's educational records without the student's prior written consent under the FERPA exception for disclosure to school officials with legitimate educational interests. Therefore you should communicate with your department chair when you become aware of possible student behavioral concerns. It is good practice to keep the department chair updated as to any documentation, meetings, or other actions regarding student behavior issues.

Discipline as an Educational Experience

Faculty may want to simply eject a student from a class because the faculty is offended or annoyed or feels that the student has acted in a disrespectful manner, but it is vitally important for faculty to frame their interactions with the student within an educational framework. Setting standards of conduct within a learning environment is part of the educational and professional preparatory experience. Students learn that there are standards of conduct and consequences for not meeting these standards, which contribute to their preparation for their postdegree work. Developing the discipline and focus to arrive to class on time will contribute to students' ability to effectively complete work-related duties and help increase their understanding of the importance of collegiality, connectedness, and teamwork as a means of achieving a quality working environment. The integrity required to ethically complete laboratory work by submitting only the results that they have personally calculated and not use the work of other students is the same integrity that will be required of graduates when they are in the workforce completing work-related reports.

CAMPUS RESOURCES

As stated previously, it is recommended that faculty become familiar with the services, programs, and personnel who staff their institution's campus support resources before they actually need their assistance. Campus resources can include counseling services, student health services, police, department chair, dean of students, and services for students with disabilities. Depending on the history and context of the institution, there may be other support services, including campus ministries and specialized centers for specific populations of students, such as women; people of color; veterans; indigenous students; or lesbian, gay, bisexual, transgender, queer, or questioning (LGBTQ+) students. Regarding behaviors of concern that rise to the level of safety for individuals or groups, universities have increasingly established formal committees that convene to conduct a broad review of a student's behavior to coordinate a comprehensive and organized response. Coordination of a team of professionals who can work together to assess threats and identify problems is preferred to individual faculty working alone. It is best to have multiple offices come together on a case-by-case basis and form a team to assess the situation and achieve the desired results. One easy way to develop relationships with these support services is to invite personnel from one or two of these offices to present introductory information about their offices to faculty within the nursing program and to explore how and when students should be referred as a part of the program's faculty professional development activities.

INCIVILITY IN THE ONLINE ENVIRONMENT

Misconduct and incivility issues associated with remote or online education may manifest in various ways (Campbell et al., 2020). In both synchronous and asynchronous environments instructors may witness rude, offensive, or insensitive comments or obvious trolling and active embarrassment of others. Distracting or inappropriate onscreen activity or blatant hijacking of a live videoconference are also known to occur. Inappropriate behavior may be less obvious to faculty working to manage asynchronous discussions or providing a class by videoconference to dozens or more students attending by individual video feeds.

The principles for preventing and managing student incivility in the online setting are the same as for in-person classes. Behavioral expectations must be clearly spelled out at the start of the class, including proper "netiquette" (Donathan et al., 2017). To establish a more personal, caring environment, faculty can improve social presence and instructor–student interaction using a variety of means, including the use of short videos or podcasts prepared by the instructor so that students may see and hear the instructor explain the expectations and why they matter. Timely responses to student questions and class contributions with individualized feedback and encouragement

foster a sense of trust and community (Campbell et al., 2020; Donathan et al., 2017). Online instructors are encouraged to address incivility in the learning environment promptly and to hold offenders accountable (De Gagne et al., 2019; Perfetto, 2019). Though it is tempting to manage online misconduct using electronic communication, a videoconference or phone call minimizes the likelihood that the message is misconstrued.

ADDITIONAL IMPLICATIONS FOR FACULTY PRACTICE

Novice faculty are frequently unprepared for the diverse challenges that arise in classroom management. It is important to recognize early that faculty are likely to experience some degree of student misconduct in their teaching career. *Thus it is wise for faculty to consider in advance how to respond in specific situations.* Working with students effectively and managing the classroom learning environment in a manner that meets or exceeds the learning objectives of the course requires instructors to consider how they will manage the learning environments for which they have accepted responsibility. Faculty may find it helpful to consider their emotional assets, as discussed in Goleman's (2005) work on emotional intelligence. His work is a helpful guide for developing the faculty's role as a learning facilitator and developing strategies for engaging students in interventions regarding their conduct.

It is tempting to ignore inappropriate behavior or avoid having difficult conversations with students. However, there are foundational tenets in nursing that serve as a compelling rationale for action. For example, most nursing education programs have established objectives or standards related to professional behavior. Additionally, the *Code of Ethics for Nurses* (American Nurses Association, 2015) states that the "nurse creates an ethical environment and culture of civility and kindness, treating colleagues, coworkers, employees, students, and others with dignity and respect…" (p. 20), and also that "disregard for the effects of one's actions on others, bullying, harassment, intimidation, manipulation, threats, or violence are always morally unacceptable behaviors" (p. 20). Likewise the Code notes that educators are responsible for ensuring that our "graduates possess the knowledge, skills, and moral dispositions that are essential to nursing" (p. 28). When students consistently behave inappropriately, there is an argument to be made that they do not meet the ethical standards of the profession.

Unwillingness or inability to address poor behavior may have more far-reaching implications than have previously been acknowledged. Horizontal violence and disruptive behavior are unfortunate phenomena in health care and have been linked to negative patient outcomes (Hicks & Stavropoulou, 2020; Olson & Stokes, 2016; The Joint Commission, 2021). Evidence exists that poorly behaving students may subsequently behave poorly as practicing nurses. For example, physicians who have been disciplined for unprofessional behavior were more likely to have displayed problem behavior as students (Fargen et al., 2016). Specific to nursing, Luparell and Frisbee (2019b) conducted a large national study to explore nursing faculty knowledge of poorly behaving or uncivil students who went on to demonstrate uncivil or unprofessional behavior as practicing nurses. Over one-third of the faculty respondents (n = 688 of 1869) reported knowing of a former badly behaving student who went on to demonstrate bad behavior in practice.

To effectively manage the learning environment, faculty need to appropriately and effectively manage their own emotions. Nursing faculty experience negative emotions when subjected to student incivility, including feelings of decreased self-esteem, a loss in their confidence as teachers, resentment related to the time involved in documenting student misconduct incidents, and a loss of motivation to teach (Andersen et al., 2019; Kamolo & Njung'e, 2021). It is paramount that faculty be cognizant of their own feelings about students and their personal responses to student misbehavior. Feelings such as fear, anxiety, anger, and sadness can cause faculty to avoid engaging students, which not only impairs ability to manage the environment but also limits faculty ability to facilitate student development. These feelings can also skew faculty observations of student behavior. If a faculty member believes that a student is acting inappropriately but remains reluctant to engage the student in a discussion about these behaviors, the faculty's feelings may be an underlying issue that needs to be addressed as well. Many schools offer faculty development opportunities to assist faculty to learn strategies for effective student conferences.

As faculty engage with their students in learning experiences, a key to effective management is maintaining sensitivity to others' feelings and concerns and the ability to consider others' perspectives. Awareness of possible generational and cultural differences in understanding of and response to behavioral expectations and consequences may assist faculty in engaging with students in a positive manner. Additionally, perceptions of what constitutes uncivil behavior may vary among students and faculty (Kamolo & Njung'e, 2021; Patel & Chrisman, 2020). These differences in perceptions between faculty and students further illustrate the importance of faculty being explicit about the behaviors that are expected of students at the very initiation of the learning experience.

Rights and responsibilities of both students and faculty in the academic environment are guided by constitutional law, state law, and institutional policy. Private and public colleges and universities have been treated differently by the courts in that private institutions are seen more as private corporate entities and public institutions are considered to be agents of the government (Kaplin & Lee, 2014). Regardless of the type of institution, see Box 15.9 for an example of the rights and responsibilities that are generally held as good practice when working with students in a learning setting.

If an institution or program does not have clearly established expectations for the behaviors of both students and faculty, these policies should be developed (Clark, 2017a, 2017b). In addition to faculty development activities, student development activities should be provided by the institution to assist students in coping with the multiple stressors many are facing in their lives and to help students identify appropriate and inappropriate behaviors.

Lastly, when contemplating the consequences of student incivility directed at faculty, program leaders should contemplate the general well-being of the faculty workforce. Student incivility has been linked to decreased faculty job satisfaction, intent to leave, and faculty turnover (Andersen et al., 2019; Eun-Jun & Hyunwook, 2020).

BOX 15.9 Conduct Guidelines and Grievance Procedures for Students

Students Have the Right to
- Expect confidentiality of personal information (with exception of directory information)
- Appeal any university status (e.g., scholastic suspension, financial aid suspension, conducts sanction)
- File a grievance against appropriate university employees or processes
- Voice dissent of university decisions and processes
- Have support to pursue changes to university policy

Faculty Have the Responsibility to
- Provide students with timely information regarding important aspects of the course, including students' obligations and responsibilities concerning both academic and personal conduct
- Be prompt and well prepared for class meetings and be timely and fair in grading assignments and exams
- Refrain from considering personal information such as race, religion, age, and political beliefs in matters of academic evaluation

- Be available to students and post liberal office hours at hours convenient to students

Students Have the Responsibility to
- Be prompt, well prepared, and regular in attending classes
- Submit honest representations of one's own work and in a timely fashion
- Act in a respectful manner toward other students and instructors in a way that does not detract from the learning experience
- Respect the personal and property rights of others
- Meet the course and behavior standards as defined by the instructor
- Seek assistance from the instructor and other appropriate student resources as needed
- Enjoy and participate in university programs

Adapted from the *Montana State University Conduct Guidelines and Grievance Procedures for Students*. http://www.montana.edu/policy/student_conduct/ and http://www.montana.edu/deanofstudents/studentrights.html

---

CHAPTER SUMMARY: KEY POINTS

- Professional comportment has been established as a key domain of professional identity in nursing, and faculty are instrumental in helping students to develop their professional identities.
- Inappropriate student behavior may typically be classified as an annoying act, an administrative violation, or criminal conduct.
- Faculty have a responsibility to establish student behavioral expectations and address inappropriate student behavior in order to foster professional comportment.

- Faculty should take proactive measures to establish behavioral expectations, such as listing expectations in the syllabus, discussing expectations in class, and explaining why behavior is important to safe patient care.
- Inappropriate behavior should be addressed promptly, drawing on relevant policies and in collaboration with appropriate personnel, and with the goal being to foster student growth and development.

REFLECTING ON THE EVIDENCE

1. A student snaps irritably at you when you smile and greet them upon entering the classroom. Seeing your surprised facial expression, they tell you they are tired, stressed, and upset as they just saw the poor grade they earned on yesterday's exam. The student reports taking extra shifts at work and requests an opportunity for extra credit to improve their grade. How might you best address this behavior to achieve change while preserving the student–teacher relationship?

2. A student requests an appointment to discuss an interaction they had during a college laboratory experience in which a fellow student made sexually suggestive comments to them. How would you go about handling this situation? How, if at all, would you handle it differently if a faculty member was the one making the remarks?

3. How do students learn what it means to be a professional nurse? What steps do you see yourself taking in future classes to better establish your expectations for student behavior?

4. What are some teaching strategies that would target the affective domain related to professional comportment? That is, how could you help students develop an internal desire to behave professionally at all times?

5. Review your institution's code of student conduct and the behavioral health resources available to your students. What additional resources exist at your institution to guide you in managing problematic student behavior? Who are the appropriate personnel who could assist you?

REFERENCES

Ackerman-Barger, K., Dickinson, J. K., & Martin, L. D. (2021). Promoting a culture of civility in nursing learning environments. *Nurse Educator*, *46*(4), 234–238. https://doi.org/10.1097/NNE.0000000000000929.

Aloufi, M. A., Jarden, R. J., Gerdtz, M. F., & Kapp, S. (2021). Reducing stress, anxiety and depression in undergraduate nursing students: Systematic review. *Nurse Education Today*, *102*(2021), 104877. https://doi.org/10.1016/j.nedt.2021.104877.

American Nurses Association, (2015). *Code of ethics for nurses with interpretive statements*. American Nurses Publishing.

Andersen, P., McAllister, M., Kardong-Edgren, S., Westmoreland Miller, C., & Churchouse, C. (2019). Incivility behaviours exhibited by nursing students: Clinical educators' perspectives of challenging teaching and assessment events in clinical practice. *Contemporary Nurse*, *55*(4–5), 303–316. https://doi.org/10.1080/10376178.2019.1634480.

Aul, K. (2017). Who's uncivil to who? Perceptions of incivility in pre-licensure nursing programs. *Nurse Education in Practice*, *27*, 36–44. https://doi.org/10.1016/j.nepr.2017.08.016.

Bartlett, M. L., Taylor, H., & Nelson, J. D. (2016). Comparison of mental health characteristics and stress between baccalaureate nursing students and non-nursing students. *Journal of Nursing Education*, *55*(2), 87–90.

Boice, B. (1996). Classroom incivilities. *Research in Higher Education*, *37*(4), 453–486.

Brewington, J., & Godfrey, N. (2020). The professional identity in nursing initiative. *Nursing Education Perspectives*, *41*(3), 201–201. https://doi.org/10.1097/01.NEP.0000000000000667.

Campbell, L. O., Jones, J. T., & Lambie, G. W. (2020). Online academic incivility among adult learners [Article]. *Adult Learning*, *31*(3), 109–119. https://doi.org/10.1177/1045159520916489.

Clark, C. M. (2017a). An evidence-based approach to integrate civility, professionalism, and ethical practice into nursing curricula. *Nurse Educator*, *42*(3), 120–126. https://doi.org/10.1097/NNE.0000000000000331.

Clark, C. (2017b). *Creating and sustaining civility in nursing education* (2nd ed.). Sigma Theta Tau International.

Clark, C. M., & Dunham, M. (2020). Civility mentor: A virtual learning experience. *Nurse Educator*, *45*(40), 189–192. https://doi.org/10.1097/NNE.0000000000000757.

Clark, C. M., Landis, T. T., & Barbosa-Leiker, C. (2020). National study on faculty and administrators' perceptions of civility and incivility in nursing education. *Nurse Educator*, *46*(5), 276–283. https://doi.org/10.1097/NNE.0000000000000948.

Courtney-Pratt, H., Pich, J., Levett-Jones, T., & Moxey, A. (2017). "I was yelled at, intimidated and treated unfairly": Nursing students' experiences of being bullied in clinical and academic settings. *Journal of Clinical Nursing*, *27*(5–6), e903–e912. https://doi.org/10.1111/jocn.13983.

De Gagne, J. C., Choi, M., Ledbetter, L., Kang, H. S., & Clark, C. M. (2016). An integrative review of cybercivility in health professions education. *Nurse Educator*, *41*(5). https://doi.org/10.1097/nne.0000000000000264.

De Gagne, J. C., Hall, K., Conklin, J. L., Yamane, S. S., Roth, N. W., Chang, J., & Suk Kim, S. (2019). Uncovering cyberincivility among nurses and nursing students on Twitter: A data mining study. *International Journal of Nursing Studies*, *89*(2019), 24–31. https://doi.org/10.1016/j.ijnurstu.2018.09.009.

Donathan, L. N., Hanks, M., & Dotson, A. T. (2017). Minimizing incivility in the online classroom. *Radiologic Technology*, *89*(1), 88–91.

Eka, N. G. A., & Chambers, D. (2019). Incivility in nursing education: A systematic literature review. *Nurse Education in Practice*, *39*, 45–54. https://doi.org/10.1016/j.nepr.2019.06.004.

Ellman-Golan, E. (2017). Saving Title IX: Designing more equitable and efficient investigation procedures. *Michigan Law Review, 116*(1), 155–186.

Eun-Jun, P., & Hyunwook, K. (2020). Nurse educators' experiences with student incivility: A meta-synthesis of qualitative studies. *Journal of Educational Evaluation for Health Professions, 17*, 1–15. https://doi.org/10.3352/jeehp.2020.17.23.

Fargen, K. M., Drolet, B. C., & Philibert, I. (2016). Unprofessional behaviors among tomorrow's physicians: Review of the literature with a focus on risk factors, temporal trends, and future directions. *Academic Medicine, 91*(6), 858–864. https://doi.org/10.1097/acm.0000000000001133.

Godfrey, N., & Young, E. (2020). Professional identity. In J. F. Giddens (Ed.), *Concepts of nursing practice* (3rd ed.). Elsevier Publishing.

Goleman, D. (2005). *Emotional intelligence.* Bantam Books.

Hicks, S., & Stavropoulou, C. (2020). The effect of health care professional disruptive behavior on patient care. *Journal of Patient Safety, Publish Ahead of Print* https://doi.org/10.1097/PTS.0000000000000805.

Joint Commission. (2021). *Quick safety 24: Bullying has no place in healthcare.* https://www.jointcommission.org/resources/news-and-multimedia/newsletters/newsletters/quick-safety/quick-safety-issue-24-bullying-has-no-place-in-health-care/bullying-has-no-place-in-health-care/

Kamolo, E. K., & Njung'e, W. W. (2021). Interventions for addressing incivility among undergraduate nursing students: A mixed study review. *International Journal of Caring Sciences, 14*(1), 476–486.

Kaplin, W. A., & Lee, B. A. (2014). *The law of higher education* (5th ed.). Jossey-Bass.

Kim, S. S., Lee, J. J., & De Gagne, J. C. (2020). Exploration of cybercivility in nursing education using cross-country comparisons. *International journal of environmental research and public health, 17*(19). https://doi.org/10.3390/ijerph17197209.

Lashley, F. R., & de Meneses, M. (2001). Student civility in nursing programs: A national survey. *Journal of Professional Nursing, 17*(2), 81–86.

Luparell, S. (2007). Dealing with challenging student situations: Lessons learned. In M. H. Oermann & K. T. Heinrich (Eds.), *Challenges and new directions in nursing education: 5. Annual review of nursing education* (pp. 101–110). Springer.

Luparell, S., & Frisbee, K. (2019a). *Faculty attitudes and beliefs about nursing student incivility: A national survey.* [Unpublished manuscript]. College of Nursing, Montana State University.

Luparell, S., & Frisbee, K. (2019b). Do uncivil nursing students become uncivil nurses? A national survey of faculty. *Nursing Education Perspectives, 40*(6), 322–327. https://doi.org/10.1097/01.NEP.0000000000000491.

Merkel, R., Olsen, J., Pehler, S., Sperstad, R., Sisto, H., Brunsell, K., & Mades, H. (2020). An innovative civility intervention created by a faculty and student action research team. *Journal of Nursing Education, 59*(4), 214–217. https://doi.org/10.3928/01484834-20200323-07.

Nodeh, Z. H., Tayebi, Z., Aghabarary, M., & Tayebi, R. (2020). Nursing students' experience of faculty incivility: A qualitative exploratory study. *Nursing Practice Today, 7*(2), 121–130.

Olson, L. L., & Stokes, F. (2016). The ANA Code of Ethics for nurses with interpretive statements: Resource for nursing regulation. *Journal of Nursing Regulation, 7*(2), 9–18.

Patel, S. E., & Chrisman, M. (2020). Incivility through the continuum of nursing: A concept analysis. *Nursing Forum, 55*(2), 267–274. https://doi.org/10.1111/nuf.12425.

Perfetto, L. M. (2019). Preparing the nurse of the future: Emergent themes in online RN-BSN education. *Nursing Education Perspectives, 40*(1), 18–24. https://doi.org/10.1097/01.NEP.0000000000000378.

Rawlins, L. (2017). Faculty and student incivility in undergraduate nursing education: An integrative review. *Journal of Nursing Education, 51*(12), 709–716. https://doi.org/10.3928/01484834-20171120-02.

Rose, K., Jenkins, S., Mallory, C., Astroth, K., Woith, W., & Jarvill, M. (2020). An integrative review examining student-to-student incivility and effective strategies to address incivility in nursing education. *Nurse Educator, 45*(3), 165–168. https://doi.org/10.1097/NNE.0000000000000719.

Sanner-Stiehr, E. (2018). Responding to disruptive behaviors in nursing: A longitudinal, quasi-experimental investigation of training for nursing students. *Nurse Education Today, 68*(2018), 105–111.

Sauer, P. A., Hannon, A. E., & Beyer, K. B. (2017). Peer incivility among prelicensure nursing students: A call to action for nursing faculty. *Nurse Educator, 42*(6), 281–285. https://doi.org/10.1097/NNE.0000000000000375.

Teach the Earth. (n.d.). *Immediacy in the classroom: Research and practical implications.* https://serc.carleton.edu/NAGTWorkshops/affective/immediacy.html

Tecza, B. M., Boots, B. K., Mains, B. C., Dryer, L. D., Oertle, D. L., Pontius, C. J., Cantu, C. L., Olney, A., McElroy, S., & Teasley, S. (2018). Incivility toward nursing students in clinical rotations: Measuring the incidence and testing interventions. *JONA: The Journal of Nursing Administration, 48*(11), 585–590. https://doi.org/10.1097/NNA.0000000000000684.

Tharani, A., Husain, Y., & Warwick, I. (2017). Learning environment and emotional well-being: A qualitative study of undergraduate nursing students. *Nurse Education Today, 59*(2017), 82–87. https://doi.org/10.1016/j.nedt.2017.09.008.

United States Department of Education. (2020, January 16). *Sex-based harassment.* https://www2.ed.gov/about/offices/list/ocr/frontpage/pro-students/issues/sex-issue01.html

Urban, R. W., Smith, J. G., Wilson, S. T., & Cipher, D. J. (2021). Relationships among stress, resilience, and incivility in undergraduate nursing students and faculty during the COVID-19 pandemic: Policy implications for nurse leaders. *Journal of Professional Nursing, 37*(6), 1063–1070.

U.S. Department of Education, Office of Postsecondary Education. (2016). *The Handbook for Campus Safety and Security Reporting, 2016 Edition.* https://www2.ed.gov/admins/lead/safety/handbookfsa.pdf

U.S. Department of Education. (2020a). *FERPA* Model notification for postsecondary officials. https://studentprivacy.ed.gov/resources/ferpa-model-notification-postsecondary-officials

Wagner, B., Holland, C., Mainous, R., Matcham, W., Li, G., & Luiken, J. (2019). Differences in perceptions of incivility among disciplines in higher education. *Nurse Educator, 44*(5), 265–269. https://doi.org/10.1097/NNE.0000000000000611.

Weger, H. (2018). Instructor active empathic listening and classroom incivility. *International Journal of Listening, 32*(1), 49–64. https://doi.org/10.1080/10904018.2017.1289091.

Ziefle, K. (2017). Incivility in nursing education: Generational differences. *Teaching and Learning in Nursing, 13*(1). https://doi.org/10.1016/j.teln.2017.09.004.

16

Evidence-Based Teaching Strategies to Promote Learning*

Ann M. Stalter, PhD, RN, MEd

Employing evidence-based teaching strategies that promote nursing student engagement and active learning is an essential element of the faculty role (Halstead, 2019). There is substantial evidence indicating that engaged students are more likely to meet expected learning outcomes (National Survey of Student Engagement, 2016, 2017, 2018, 2019, 2020) and to apply learned concepts in practice settings (Kinzie, 2017). Additional evidence of the benefit of using teaching strategies that engage students has emerged as faculty met the challenge of teaching in reconfigured and often virtual classrooms (Harris & Bacon, 2019; Jowsey et al., 2020; Rao, 2019). This challenge has called upon faculty to adapt trusted teaching strategies and try new ones. This chapter draws on that evidence which has increased in depth and rigor in recent years and begins by describing the teaching-learning process and explaining the role of faculty in choosing *teaching* strategies that will engage students in their own learning and the role of the students in using *learning* strategies that will ensure transfer of knowledge to clinical practice. The chapter concludes with a description, advantages and disadvantages, and supporting evidence for using a variety of teaching strategies.

TEACHING-LEARNING PROCESS

Teaching and learning are reciprocal processes in which faculty choose strategies that will help

*The author acknowledges the work of Janet M. Phillips, PhD, RN, ANEF in the previous editions of this chapter.

students meet program, course, and lesson learning outcomes and students assume responsibility for using learning strategies that best promote their own learning. The faculty's role is to choose strategies embedded in theory and supported by evidence that will promote student engagement and translate it into safe and high-quality nursing practice. The role of the student is to complete preclass assignments, participate in the learning process and postclass reflection, and link learning from the classroom to patient care in the clinical setting.

Teaching Strategies

Faculty are influenced by a number of variables when determining which strategy to use that will best meet student learning outcomes. Faculty must make decisions that are guided by learning theory and align strategies with the students' previous courses and learning experiences. Further, faculty must consider the domain of learning and the appropriate level of the domain, as well as provide a variety of strategies that engage the student in the learning process. Faculty must also consider strategies that are compatible with their own teaching experience, expertise, and the resources available for implementing their teaching plans. Finally, faculty, particularly newly employed faculty, must develop the confidence to try new teaching approaches, challenge students, and overcome barriers that impede learning. As Soroush et al. (2021) found, experienced instructors, because they have higher self-confidence in their teaching abilities, are more efficient in helping students achieve course objectives. Ultimately, the intent of using evidence-based teaching strategies is to prepare students for providing safe, quality, patient-centered care. Principles for choosing teaching strategies are described below.

Meet Program, Course, Lesson Learning Outcomes, and Clinical Competencies

The choice of a teaching strategy in nursing courses is to enable students to attain learning outcomes at the program, course, and lesson levels and to acquire clinical competencies. Every decision about using teaching strategies must link back to learning outcomes and forward to evaluation strategies.

Integrate Curricular Threads of the Institution

The nursing curriculum is embedded in the institution in which in resides and that provides the foundation for student learning throughout the academic program. When choosing teaching strategies, faculty must also need to consider those that facilitate the program outcomes of the institution. Many colleges and universities have identified high-impact practices (HIP) that are associated with college success. The Association of American Colleges and Universities (2021) describe the following as HIPs: First-year seminars and experiences; a core curriculum; learning communities; writing intensive courses; collaborative assignments and projects; opportunities for students to participate in research with faculty; e-portfolios; internship or field experiences; study abroad; and culminating senior experiences such as a capstone project.

High-impact practices support engaged learning, increase retention, and provide evidence of offering students a quality education as defined by various aspects of the Higher Learning Commission Criteria for Accreditation (2022). The general rule of thumb among undergraduate programs is for all college students to experience at least one HIP during their first year and another HIP again during senior year (Kuh & Kinzie, 2018). Commonly coupled HIPs are first-year seminars and experiences with a culminating senior experience. Within nursing programs, these coupled HIPs may involve first-year orientation bootcamps that focus on successful study skills (Hughes et al., 2020) and a final capstone course where students

are precepted by a registered nurse in a clinical setting (Robertson & Disch, 2021).

Provide Students an Opportunity to Learn and Apply Content

According to Bloom's revised taxonomy (Anderson & Krathwohl, 2016), learning in the three domains of learning occurs at various levels. Faculty must consider the level of the domain that the strategy addresses. For example, a strategy that provides information such as that can occur during a lecture or assigning textbook readings will engage students at the lower levels of the domain, while a strategy such as a case study will require the students to apply information to a real-world situation.

The flipped classroom strategy, in which students acquire basic knowledge before coming to class and apply it during the class (Evans et al., 2019), takes advantage of this principle by setting the expectation that students will learn the content prior to coming to class where the faculty has designed an in-class activity that will challenge the student to apply what they have learned.

Connect Learning to Clinical Practice

The goal of teaching in the classroom is to prepare students to acquire the knowledge, skills, and abilities to provide safe patient care. Strategies such as clinical case studies, simulations, and role play are well suited to helping students link what they learn to how they plan care for patients.

Encourage Diversity of Ideas and Promote Civil Communication

Selecting teaching strategies focuses not only on helping students learn content but also can provide a forum in which students can learn how to work in teams and to share ideas respectfully. For example, collaborative work groups, team-based learning (TBL), and think-pair-share strategies encourage students to engage in dialogue in which students can offer different perspectives. Faculty can configure groups to ensure diversity by assigning groups using random numbers or drawing a group number from a box.

Appeal to Varied Learning Styles

Students learn in different ways (see Chapter 2). To address students' learning style preferences, where possible, faculty can provide options for learning or participating in learning activities. Faculty can take advantage of the increased availability of multimedia and technical capabilities by recording lectures and offering assignments that allow student choice while, at the same time, accommodating special learning needs.

Develop a Professional Identity

An important learning outcome for all academic programs in nursing is for the students to be able to develop the ethical, moral, thinking, and judgment abilities that are the essence of the profession. Faculty can incorporate strategies in their course that contribute to the development of each student's ability to acquire these attributes. Strategies such as role play, debate, reflection papers, and journal writing can contribute to shaping a student's professional identity.

Learning Strategies

Students have a responsibility to be actively engaged in their own learning and spend the time required to learn course content in a way that they can retrieve it to provide safe and high-quality patient care. The strategies below can be included in student study skills and success programs that introduce the importance of developing effective approaches to learning.

Retrieval Practice

Retrieval practice is the act of recalling from memory recently learned information (Agarwal et al., 2021; Hattie, 2018). The purpose of retrieval is to strengthen memory (Froehlich & Rogers, 2022). Memory strengthening exercises are demonstrated through self-quizzing, where students ask themselves questions that prompt recall of information (Brown et al., 2014) that can be applied to patient care and making clinical judgments (van Peppen et al., 2021). Nursing students at all levels of education can ask themselves: (1) What content have I just reviewed? (2) What new vocabulary, terminology, and/or concepts have I discovered? (3) What

are the key points for me to understand? (4) How do these key points build upon what I understand about the topic? (5) How will I use this information to plan care for patients? (6) How will this help me make safe clinical decisions and judgments?

Spaced Practice

Spaced practice is the act of reviewing information more than one time but allowing for processing time between the next practice session (Brown et al., 2014). The strategy is contrasted with massed learning or cramming in a single study session (Corwin Visible Learning, 2021; Ohio State University Veterinary Program, n.d.). In spaced practice, self-quizzing is performed within 15 minutes to 4 hours of time proximity to the first encounter of new information. Self-quizzing occurs again several days later and should continue until retrieval of responses is consistently accurate. As new material is introduced, the learner should ask how any new information relates to what has been previously learned (Latimier et al., 2021). Quizlet (2022). A free website for creating flashcards, has a built-in feature for helping students with spaced practice. It has been identified as a successful strategy among Saudi Arabian nursing students taking anatomy and physiology (Cabalsa et al., 2022), among Taiwanese nursing students taking a pathology course (Huang et al., 2021), and among American nursing students completing presimulation clinical activities (Dodson & Ferdig, 2021). Spaced practice has also been used among graduate students taking statistics (Immekus, 2019) and among actively practicing nurses to improve knowledge of atrial fibrillation and anticoagulation (Ferguson et al., 2019).

Interleaving

Interleaving is the act of mixing related topics during the learning process. Interleaving is contrasted with blocked learning, where before moving on to the next topic, each topic is learned in its entirety (Brown et al., 2014). For example, during a study period, a student might need to review four concepts. Interleaving requires that the student dedicates time to concept 1, then some time to concepts 2, 3, and 4. After a short break, the student rotates back through the concepts, in a rearranged order, using different retrieval strategies. By reorganizing the concepts, students are pushed to retrieve information from both working and long-term memories, leading them to make new connections between all the concepts (Brunmair & Richter, 2019; Chen et al., 2021). Thus interleaving improves the brain's ability to differentiate and discriminate between concepts while strengthening memory associations (Chen et al., 2021). Interleaving has been effective in helping nursing students learn mathematical computations in medication administration processes (Zwart et al., 2021) and to employ safe pharmacological nursing actions (Phillips & Ford, 2021). Interleaving has also been found to improve nurse practitioner students' abilities for accurate differential diagnosing (Graber et al., 2018).

Elaboration

Elaboration is the act of enriching learning content with detail during the learning process. The technique helps students make meaningful connections between their lives and what they've previously learned and grasp new concepts (Brown et al., 2014; Hattie, 2018; Ong et al., 2022). Examples of elaboration pertaining to nursing focus on across the lifespan recipients of care, health and illness, and/or professionalism (Giddens, 2019) and expand the ideas of culture and spirituality to include health behaviors. Concepts specific to health and illness broaden thinking from pathophysiologic or biologic responses to the students personally having a hand in the fostering of healing responses. Concepts specific to professionalism support standards of care such as ethics, quality, and safety relevant to developing policies and systems of care that support human flourishing. Elaboration concentrates on understanding differences and similarities between related ideas, which requires advanced reasoning and critical analysis (Brown et al., 2014).

The strategy can involve two methods: Elaborative interrogation or self-explanation. *Elaborative interrogation* uses the Socratic method of repeatedly asking "why" so that answers are deeply processed. *Self-explanation* is when students generate explanations in a way that new information is integrated with existing knowledge, thereby creating new neural pathways (Bartsch & Oberauer, 2021). Regardless of which type of elaboration students employ, when using elaboration, nursing students can think about the concepts in terms of how they apply to clinical practice. A key safety message faculty should provide when using elaborative interrogation is that once a nursing student can no longer answer the question "why" a nursing action is being taken, the action should not be performed without collaborating with the instructor, preceptor, or an experienced nurse. Makhene (2019) emphasized the need for nurses, especially nurse practitioners, to use Socratic inquiry to facilitate critical thinking. Kuzma et al. (2019) showed how this can be accomplished with advanced practice nursing students during standardized patient debriefing experiences to improve cultural humility.

Reflection

Reflection is a metacognitive activity that helps students examine what they know, what they think they know, and what they do not understand (Brown et al., 2014; Guo, 2022). Reflection affords learners the opportunity to step away from actively learning long enough to contemplate what they have learned and how they can improve future performance to fill knowledge gaps. It is not a recess from studying, so it should involve a journaling exercise, or another creative reflection assignment aimed at thoughtful student-centered and meaningful learning (Box 16.1). Reflection helps to develop critical thinking skills and confidence and to set new learning goals. According to Scheel et al.'s (2021) scoping review, reflection is broadly used as an effective way to assist nursing students in developing competent skills and judgment for working in clinical settings. Pleshkan and Boykins (2022) substantiated that reflection is a key cognitive activity for transitioning a registered nurse into the nurse practitioner role.

Generation

Generation is the act of predicting an answer to a question before the answer is given (Brod, 2021). It is attempting to solve a problem before the solution is offered (Brown et al., 2014). Students exhibit

	BOX 16.1	Reflection Assignments

	Assignment	Rationale
1	Setting goals	Creates a growth-focused attitude by establishing and reinforcing student-oriented outcomes that are specific, measurable, attainable, realistic, and time framed.
2	Clinical journals with faculty-developed prompts/questions containing verbs that advance learning to higher-order thinking (remembering to creating)	Journaling and questioning can prompt deep insights by asking students to respond to questions that elicit deeper thinking and application of information to patient care. • To remember what was learned, ask: What did you accomplish from the clinical experience? (remembering level) • To understand what was learned, ask: What was important about what you did during your clinical experience? (understanding level) • To apply what was learned, ask: Where or how can you use this clinical experience again? (applying level) • To analyze what was learned, ask: What were your patterns of behavior or nursing actions during this clinical experience? (analyzing level) • To evaluate what was learned, ask: What was one thing that you learned from this clinical experience, how well did you perform, and/or what could you do differently next time to have a better clinical outcome? (evaluation level) • To extend into the future what was learned, ask: How can I use this knowledge in other clinical settings or in my practice to improve health outcomes across individuals, families, groups, communities, or systems? (creating level)
3	Reflective drawing	Students draw a one-page image or images to represent a concept or experience pertinent to learning objectives and/or mastery of them
4	Vlogging	Using a reflection prompt such as those listed in Assignment 2 above, students prepare a video where they can share their thoughts, feelings, drawings, or the like in a creative, on-camera experience
6	Scrapbooking	Growth across time is shared in a scrapbook format
7	Cubing	A die cube is created with the questions prepared in Assignment 2. Students sit in groups, taking turns tossing the die and answering the questions

generation when trying to answer end-of-chapter questions before they read the chapter. Math students exhibit generation by working to answer homework problems before class lectures. This example is translated to nursing as faculty prepare students for safe medication administration by having them solve dosage calculation and drip rate problems ongoingly prior to taking exams or going to clinical (Gregory et al., 2022; Thelen, 2022).

On the other hand, Hoogerheide et al. (2019) found that generating multiple-choice test questions resulted in lower test performance than restudying of textual material. This is mentioned because it is common practice for faculty to have nursing students generate mock test questions and answers as an exam preparation activity. The

evidence suggests this type of teaching strategy may not be effective because students may lack the skills for properly designing test questions that test single concepts such as those without double negatives or that use absolutes such as *never* or *always*. Nursing students also need test items that expand beyond factual knowledge such as critically analyzing and applying clinical judgments. Overall, generation reinforces how retrieval and spaced practices combined with interleaving are essential for making connections because generation teaches the brain to anticipate connection-making.

Burt (2021) established foundational information regarding evidenced-based teaching strategies to increase nurse practitioner student diagnostic accuracy. Specifically, nurse practitioner students were asked to solve written case studies while explaining out loud how they predicted patient needs and diagnoses. Explanations using biological rationale correlated with accurate diagnostic scores, $r(35) = 0.49$ ($p < 0.002$) (Burt et al., 2021). These statistically significant findings suggest that faculty should prompt nurse practitioner students to self-explain clinical features consistent with underlying biologic clinical manifestations.

Calibration

Calibration involves taking action to align judgments of what one knows and doesn't know with an objective opinion to avoid assuming that mastery has occurred and being surprised by failure when formally tested. More precisely, calibration is being able to accurately assess what students do and do not know. Accurately gauging effective learning is difficult because of *illusions of knowing*, which is the belief that understanding has been mastered when learning has not at all occurred (Gutierrez de Blume, 2022). Zawadzka and Hanczakowski (2020) describe several illusions of knowing that interrupt learning. These include false memories, hindsight bias, the feeling of knowing, fluency illusions, memory conformity, false consensus effect, and Dunning-Kruger Effect (Box 16.2). To offset these illusions, Gutierrez de Blume (2022) recommended that faculty provide opportunities for group studying, attending office hours, and participating in practice test sessions, as these can be very helpful in accurately calibrating knowledge.

Griffith et al.'s (2021) scoping review cites calibration as a strategy that nurse practitioner students use to avoid errors and make unbiased diagnostic decisions. They inferred that the ultimate means of avoiding error was to employ team-based decisions using specific strategies such as seeking second opinions and using clinical practice guidelines, algorithms, and/or mnemonic devices to stimulate the retrieval of learned information.

BOX 16.2   Illusions of Knowing That Interrupt Learning

	Illusions of Knowing	Definitions
1	False memories	A phenomenon where people recall memories that did not occur or that happened differently than they actually did.
2	Hindsight bias	A phenomenon where people perceive past events as having been more predictable than they actually were, and mostly comes across as overconfidence with predicting answers and solving problems.
3	The feeling of knowing	When a learner predicts his or her own knowledge prior to answering a question or solving a problem. It is the proverbial *psyching oneself out*. As an interrupter of knowing, the learner imposes that he/she does not know and therefore inaccurately exhibits knowing anything about the topic presented.
4	Fluency illusions	A phenomenon where people believe false information is correct after there has been repeated exposure.
5	Memory conformity	A phenomenon where others' memories when shared with a learner influence an individual's memory to agree with others' memories regardless of truth.
6	False consensus effect	A phenomenon where people assume their choices, behaviors, personal qualities, characteristics, and beliefs are pervasive across society and/or the general population.
7	Dunning-Kruger effect	A phenomenon where people with low abilities overestimate their ability to achieve or where people with high abilities underestimate their abilities to achieve.

Data from Zawadzka, K., & Hanczakowski, M. (2020). Knowing more or thinking that you know more? Context-dependent illusions of knowing. In A. M. Cleary and B. L. Schwartz (Eds.), Memory Quirks: The Study of Odd Phenomena in Memory (pp. 175–189). Routledge.

Mnemonic Devices

Mnemonic devices use key words, rhyming words, or acronyms to link new learning with prior knowledge (Brown et al., 2014; Hattie, 2018). Mnemonic devices use visual and/or acoustic cues to creatively engage learners (Maheshwari & Kaur, 2019) and create cognitive structures that facilitate retrieval of learned information (Brown et al., 2014). Mnemonic devices used in nursing offer opportunities to learn complex terms such as cranial nerves (On old Olympus' Towering Tops, a Finn and German viewed some hops); symptoms and diseases such as causes of and assessment for dementia (**D**rugs, **E**yes/ears, **M**etabolic/endocrine disorders, **E**motional issues, **N**eurological disorder/nutrition, **T**umors/trauma, **I**nfection, and **A**lcoholism); nursing actions such as resting, icing, compressing, and elevating a wound (RICE); and giving report using the Situation-Background-Assessment-Recommendation (SBAR) approach (World's Database of Medical Mnemonics, 2022). Hurst et al. (2022) found that mnemonics helped licensed health care professionals learn and recall cholinergic toxidromes during an advanced hazmat life support class. The recall was sustained up to 4 years later ($p < 0.001$).

Equitable Learning

Equitable learning is the deliberate act of manipulating the classroom environment so that learning outcomes are achieved by all students regardless of backgrounds or identities (Agarwal et al., 2021; Epstein et al., 2020). The goal of equitable learning is to help students develop a strong sense of self and to advance a culture of acceptance so that bias and systemic racism are minimized and mitigated (Hanover Research, 2017). Oruche et al. (2022) employed equitable learning to prepare nurse practitioner students to recognize socially determined health inequities and global health issues.

TEACHING STRATEGIES

Bloom's revised taxonomy (Anderson & Krathwohl, 2016) can be used to categorize teaching strategies at various levels of the domains of learning. The knowledge dimension (or the kind of knowledge to be learned) is composed of four knowledge types: (1) factual, (2) conceptual, (3) procedural, and (4) metacognitive. *Factual knowledge* refers to the basic content students must know to be familiar with a discipline or to solve problems in it. *Conceptual knowledge* refers to the relationships between the basic fundamentals within a larger configuration that enable them to function together. *Procedural knowledge* refers to skills, techniques, and methods needed for specific disciplines. *Metacognitive knowledge* is the awareness of one's own cognition in addition to cognition in general. Table 16.1 has examples of knowledge dimensions, definitions, and exemplar teaching strategies.

Learning objectives and outcomes for the knowledge types can be created using the six cognitive process dimensions of Bloom's revised taxonomy: (1) remember, (2) understand, (3) apply, (4) analyze, (5) evaluate, and (6) create (see Chapter 10). Examples of select teaching strategies for student engagement are listed alphabetically in the four knowledge types (Anderson & Krathwohl, 2016) in the following sections and may be used across classrooms, skills and simulation labs, and clinical and online environments. Specific teaching strategies for simulations may be found in Chapter 19, technology-supported learning activities in the connected classroom may be found in Chapter 20, and teaching at a distance in Chapter 21.

Factual Knowledge

Nursing students must learn both the basic factual knowledge at levels of remembering and understanding, but also at the higher levels of being able to analyze and create. Faculty can use a combination of strategies such as lectures, peer learning, seminars and group discussions (small or large), and/or TBL to help students acquire foundational facts. Other teaching strategies can also be used, such as textbook reading assignments and/or games that require recall of facts.

Lecture

Lecture involves a faculty (or student) providing factual information in an oral presentation, typically accompanied by PowerPoint slides to focus students' attention or provide an outline for organizing the content. Lectures can also be recorded

TABLE 16.1   Exemplar Teaching Strategies by Knowledge Dimensions of Revised Bloom's Taxonomy

Knowledge Dimensions	Definition	Exemplar Teaching Strategy
Factual	Basic content students must know to be familiar with a discipline or to solve problems in it	Lectures, peer learning, seminar, small and large group discussions, and team-based learning
Conceptual	Relationships between the basic fundamentals within a larger configuration enabling them to work together	Argumentation, debate, structured controversy, cooperative learning and group assignments, mind mapping and concept mapping, role play
Procedural	Skills, techniques, and methods needed for specific disciplines	Demonstration, games, imagery and mindfulness, poster, self-learning modules, writing
Metacognitive	The awareness of one's own thinking	Case study, interprofessional education, portfolio and e-portfolio, problem-based learning, questioning and Socratic questioning, reflection and journal writing

Data from Anderson, L. W. & Krathwohl, D. R. (Eds.) (2016). A taxonomy for learning, teaching, and assessing: A revision of Bloom's taxonomy of educational objectives. Longman.

using presentation software for students to use prior to class as preparation for application activities that may be used in class or after class as a review. Garrison et al. (2021) emphasized that short, prerecorded lectures (15 minutes or less) of chunked information prevent cognitive overload and allow learners to efficiently process new information. Pike et al. (2022) used this approach to improve oral health in a primary care pediatric nurse practitioner program.

Teaching tips. When using lecture as the primary teaching strategy, faculty should consider integrating other activities that require higher-order thinking such as application and creation to accompany the lecture. Worksheets and prompts designed to target misconceptions are effective in helping students to make cerebral connections (McConnell et al., 2017). Using a case study that draws on content presented in the lecture or using practice test questions to prompt retrieval of information are also ways to increase student engagement and application of factual knowledge.

Consider scaffolding as a means of integrating lectures. For example, follow this sequence: (1) pretest learner knowledge, (2) use short audio lectures to introduce new concepts (e.g., stages of labor), (3) employ varied practice strategies to reinforce knowledge (e.g., flashcards, practice test questions, case studies), (4) assess knowledge (e.g., give a quiz), (5) provide in-class activities to promote discovery about the concept (e.g., case study about a laboring mother), (6) provide simulation or lab activities to practice applying the concept to practice (e.g., high fidelity manikin gives birth), (7) reinforce understanding after a real-world clinical experience (e.g., post conference discussion or clinical reflection journal), and (8) evaluate knowledge through posttests (quantitative internal source of evidence) and include clinical agency feedback (qualitative internal source of evidence).

Tennyson et al. (2022) integrated scaffolding with technology to establish microlearning strategies and connectedness among student cohorts. Nurse practitioner students increased understanding of lecture material using videos, blogs, smartphones, virtual reality, gaming, and social media.

Advantages and disadvantages. When choosing lecture as a teaching strategy, faculty must consider the course learning outcomes and the advantages and disadvantages of this strategy. Unless developed by students, lectures tend to be teacher centric and rely on the ability of the faculty to make the presentation engaging. While being an efficient way to ensure students are familiar with foundational content, lectures tend to encourage student's ability to memorize the information rather than learn it to apply it to patient care. Scaffold sequencing can advance student learning from memory to performance.

Evidence. See Bristol et al. (2019); Gallegos and Nakashima (2018); Garrison et al. (2021); McConnell et al. (2017); Pike et al. (2022); Silva et al. (2022); Sanaie et al. (2019); and Tennyson et al. (2022).

Peer Learning

Peer learning draws on sociocultural theory (Chapter 14) that provides evidence that students learn from others including their classmates. Learning from peers occurs when students share information, collaborate to solve problems, or engage in dialogue that offers a variety of perspectives. In class, faculty can structure situations in which students work in groups and use strategies such as Jigsawing, collaborative writing and testing, and solving case studies. Peer learning can also be used to pair students from different levels in the curriculum or degree program in which beginning students learn from more experienced students and the experienced students have an opportunity to solidify their own learning and develop mentoring and teaching skills. Students also use peer learning when they form study groups outside of the classroom.

Another aspect of peer learning is through positive and corrective feedback. Faculty assign peers to take turns teaching and evaluating one another, which gives students the opportunity to participate in competency or performance evaluation. Liang et al. (2021) compared self, peer, and supervisor assessments to evaluate nurse practitioner professional competence. They (Liang et al., 2021) found competence scores by supervisors were significantly lower than self or peer assessments (F = 10.07, p < 0.001), implying that adding a peer perspective to professional competency assessment may help identify or fill knowledge gaps that potentially impact quality and safety of patient care. This is consistent with peer review being one of the most common preferred teaching strategies for graduate nursing students (Harlan et al., 2021).

Teaching tips. A clear connection must be made between the objectives and the strategy, or students will think working with their classmates is not a good use of their time. Create a possible list of topics or allow students to choose what they are interested in to promote active student learning. Creating relevance to the learning objectives will help focus student learning. Informal meetings between faculty and students may help clarify and structure questions used to promote in-class discussion. If using a peer learning model that incorporates peer mentors across programs to enhance student learning experiences, pairing first-year students with third-year students supports student confidence and teamwork skills (Cust, 2018). If using peer assessment to determine competency, make sure to incorporate clear performance measures so that feedback is meaningful for the learner.

Advantages. Peer learning provides opportunities for students to explore concepts from multiple points of view. Faculty can structure peer learning experiences so that they also promote reflection, critical analysis, and application of knowledge in context. Peer learning can be used in a variety of situations, including student interest groups, peer review of student work, group tests, digital storytelling, and peer mentoring. From these, students can gain self-efficacy in learning and practice, empowering them with both a voice and mindset to make safe, ethical decisions.

Disadvantages. Peer learning requires faculty to focus continually on the relevance of peer assignments because students may feel as if they are not learning what they need to know from their peers. Faculty must provide mentoring students with adequate preparation to serve as peer support. Faculty may need to assist learners to focus or refocus on concepts being discussed throughout the course. Student evaluation may be challenging if not all students are participating equally. And quiet students may need encouragement, whereas assertive students may try to monopolize the group. Guidelines and performance criteria are necessary for the learning activities.

Evidence. See Cust (2018); Choi et al. (2021); Harlan et al. (2021); Liang et al. (2021); Markowski et al. (2021); Pålsson et al. (2021); and Putri and Sumartini (2021).

Seminar and Small or Large Group Discussions

A seminar is a meeting for an exchange of ideas in some topical area; it may also involve a guided discussion of concepts. Interprofessional assignments can enhance student engagement and active learning, but a clear connection of the seminar discussion to the course objectives is necessary, or students may perceive the seminar as an inefficient use of their time. Seminars ensure that students learn what they need to know and that they are supported in their academic and personal growth. This structure can be completed in the classroom or online, synchronously or asynchronously.

Small group discussions are used during class sessions to expand on reading assignments and/or lecture content. Students are placed into groups of no more than six students and given a challenge as an opportunity to solve a problem by exploring or investigating the newly presented information (Zou et al., 2019). Some examples of challenges for small group discussions are mystery diagnoses, crossword puzzles, escape rooms, and "conver-stations."

Mystery diagnoses are used to enhance critical reasoning (Iverson et al., 2018). They have been successfully used in teaching nurse practitioner students; however, use with undergraduate students has been applied to chemistry (Mahaffey, 2020), biology (Church, 2021), and pathophysiology (Ogilvie, 2019). In essence, students are given information about their patient who enters a clinic, emergency room, or another clinical setting. Information on primary health problems, medication history, lab values, and the like are given. Students work together to determine what is wrong with the patient and make a plan for nursing interventions.

Crossword puzzles are assigned to complement small group discussions as a means of enhancing concept retention at the remembering and factual levels of Bloom's taxonomy. Crossword puzzles can be assigned cumulative or noncumulative. As *noncumulative* assignments, small groups create crossword puzzles that contain weekly content for other student groups in the class to solve.

Cumulative assignments have small groups create crossword puzzles that contain information they learned previously in the class and for the class as a whole to solve. Crossword puzzles have been incorporated across all levels of nursing education, including master's and doctoral courses (Torres et al., 2022).

Escape rooms are also used to complement small group discussions. They are a popular and highly motivating teaching strategy that allows students to recall and apply knowledge gained in class (Gómez-Urquiza et al., 2019) and assist in developing skills in both communication and teamwork (Reed, 2020). Faculty create a fictitious imprisonment setting where students use hands-on or online interactions to solve puzzles and decipher clues to free themselves. The strategy has been successfully employed among a variety of students and courses (Veldkamp et al., 2020) including helping nurse practitioner students practice clinical decision-making skills (Casler, 2022).

Conver-stations is a teaching approach developed by Wessling (2019) that uses movement to stimulate student-led small group discussions. Faculty prepares enough questions for class groups of 4–5 students per table, which is referred to as a station. That is, a class of 30 would have 6 tables, so 6 total questions would need to be developed by faculty before the class session. The six questions build in complexity, where the first question is easier and the last one is more challenging. To begin, groups are assigned and the class is provided with the first question. Each student takes 1 minute to think about and write down a response to the question. Then, the groups at each table discuss their responses as the faculty member roams the room, reminding students to take notes about key ideas. The faculty determines when the conversation needs to shift, the conversation is paused, and the second question is offered to each table. After the second question is presented, the faculty member directs two students (rotators) from each table to move to a different table before groups discuss the newly presented question. This process is repeated until all rotators have cycled through each station. Once all rotators are back at the original station, the students spend a few minutes formulating a collaborative answer to the last question presented.

Each station group elects a representative to present their answer to the class.

Large group discussions are used to promote deeper learning engagement with recently presented content. They take quite a bit of faculty preparation and help students form professional opinions regarding the relevance of content to practice. Some examples of ways to implement large group discussions are *Talking Stick, A day in the life of a client with...,* and *Six Hats Plus One.* When these strategies are used, they require students to receive clear, succinct directions.

The *Talking Stick* strategy fosters discussion from reticent students while establishing boundaries with students who monopolize conversations. The strategy is also used in clinical practice during staff meetings (Welch & Parker, 2020), inferring its appropriateness to use with graduate students. While handing a talking stick to a student, faculty ask questions pertaining to a process and/or solution to a complex scenario. Each student takes turns holding the talking stick, which serves as a talking ticket. That is, the student holding the stick is the only one permitted to speak. When a student holds the stick, they are to discuss what they think or feel about the question. Faculty establishes the amount of time one can speak, but the student holding the stick passes it to any student of their choice. The stick cannot be given to any one person a second time until all students in the class have spoken. For large classes, faculty may need to pass the stick out in phases consistent with content delivery (i.e., concept 1 is presented then discussed, next concept 2 is presented then discussed, and so on).

A day in the life of a client with... is a strategy described by Herrman (2019) where student groups select or are assigned a disease, condition, or lifestyle. The students look up information on symptoms, vital statistics, social determinants of health, treatment plans, medication side effects, lab values, activities of daily living, and the like. They create a fictitious patient and describe a day in the life of the person. The group presents the information to the class as a whole, which can be accomplished by integrating a nursing care plan, health teaching/disease prevention intervention, or policy statement.

Vos (2018) activates this strategy using practical examples for nurse practitioners to apply to their practices. For example, they provides practical activities and exercises to help clients make meaning of and accept diseases, conditions, or lifestyles. This strategy would also be useful with students in any nursing program.

Six Hats Plus One is a teaching strategy developed by de Bono (1985) used to cultivate insights about decision-making. Since then, it has been used in nursing education to nurture ethical decision-making, professional identity, advocacy, and empathy in a practical and civil manner (Morsy & Darweesh, 2021; Tsimane & Downing, 2020). The strategy employs the use of seven differently colored hats (white, red, yellow, green, blue, black, and purple) to represent varying opinions/perspectives. Tsimane and Downing (2020) used de Bono's (1985) hats to explain a model to facilitate transformative learning with both graduate and undergraduate nursing students.

As a topic is discussed, hats are passed around the room until everyone has worn each color one time. For example, the person wearing the white hat represents facts; responses are objectives and composed of neutral opinion and statistics. The person wearing the red hat is emotional and passionate; responses are gut level, nonfiltered, biased views. The person wearing the yellow hat focuses on the logical positive and is optimistic; responses are hopeful and positive. The person wearing the green hat is creative and energetic; responses are growth oriented. The blue hat donner is the controller and planner, controlling all the other hat wearers; responses are leader oriented and limit setting in nature. The person wearing the black hat represents the logical negative and is pessimistic/cynical; responses are cautionary and judgmental. The person wearing the purple hat is invested in the outcome; responses pertain to program success, profits, and future-oriented returns on investment. To expedite the process, several same-color hats can be passed about (except for blue) to add lively and timely discussion.

Teaching tips. To have an effective discussion, faculty should select topics that will elicit a variety of responses and viewpoints. Faculty should ask open-ended questions and provide students with opportunities to critically think before expressing their thoughts and feelings. Clear guidelines are needed so that a vocal person (student or faculty) does not dominate the discussion. Student preparation time may be reduced by having students rotate as discussion facilitators, so the individual student is responsible for in-depth preparation of only a few topics. The teacher may be a part of the group, sometimes acting as a participant, a consultant, or the leader. Thus, it is important for faculty to serve as a role model and use effective facilitation and feedback skills. To promote participation and interactivity, faculty should employ technology-enhanced learning such as synchronized laptops and/or interactive multimedia presentations. Reflective writing assignments can be used to assess the effectiveness of seminar topics and/or discussions.

Advantages. Discussion allows for active student engagement with content. Discussion can facilitate comprehension and practical application of concepts. It allows teachers to act as role models for concept clarification and expert problem solving. Student's verbal presentation skills improve in discussion, as do thinking skills. Limited development time is required for faculty, but planning is still necessary to ensure effectiveness. In general, discussion does not typically require additional supplies such as handouts or audiovisuals, and students can learn group problem-solving techniques. However, select strategies such as the *Talking Stick* and *Six Hats Plus One* can require additional preparation and supplies.

Disadvantages. The structure requires that students possess adequate knowledge for active discussion and comprehension. This may require a great amount of student preparation time or may allow a student to "slip through" without sufficient knowledge or thinking skills. Students may require instruction on how to participate in seminars. Students must have the confidence and ability to express themselves while grappling with new experiences and difficult concepts.

Evidence. See Casler (2022); Church (2021); de Bono (1985); Gómez-Urquiza et al. (2019); Herrman (2019); Iverson et al. (2018); Mahaffey (2020); Morgan (2019); Morsy and Darweesh (2021); Ogilvie (2019); Reed (2020); Torres et al. (2022); Tsimane and Downing (2020); Veldkamp et al. (2020); Vos (2018); Welch and Parker (2020); Wessling (2019); and Zou et al. (2019).

Team-Based Learning

In team-based learning (TBL), faculty create teams of students to enhance student engagement and the quality of learning outcomes. Students may work in teams online or in class. Interprofessional teams enhance active learning and student engagement. TBL groups must be well formed and properly managed. Students are responsible for the quality of their individual and group effort and must be given frequent, timely feedback. Team assignments should be designed to promote both learning and team development. Students work together and earn group and individual grades. TBL is regarded as having the highest level of evidence for learning among health care professionals resulting in better academic and clinical outcomes, as it has been well studied across undergraduate, graduate, and professional groups (Joshi et al., 2022; Michaelson et al., 2008). TBL offers students opportunities to increase interpersonal skills such as active listening, caring/empathy, leadership, motivation, responsibility, and teamwork.

TBL follows a precise six-step process including (1) preassigned readings; (2) an Individual Readiness Assurance Test designed to measure what students learned from their preclass readings; (3) a group assignment with a multiple choice question, and a Team Readiness Assurance Test completed on a specific scratch-off form which provides immediate feedback for correct answers and that contains a correct answer designated by a star; (4) the ability for students to appeal incorrectly answered questions; (5) a faculty mini-lecture presented to clarify content that is misunderstood; and (6) transference of knowledge to fieldwork activities, requiring students to apply newly learned content (Michaelson et al., 2008).

Teaching tips. Keep group sizes at five to seven participants. Students stay in the same team for the duration of the course. Students are expected to prepare before the start of class and join their team at the beginning of class time. Set clear expectations for grading, with a rubric for either individual or group grades. Prepare the lessons before the course begins, such as creating preassigned reading lists and readiness tests including scratch-off forms, engaging mini-lectures, and coordinating fieldwork experiences.

Advantages. A TBL strategy can be used in large classes to give students the actual experience of working in a team to understand and apply content. As the group becomes accountable for earning grades, their learning increases student involvement with course content. Overall advantages include the generation of more ideas, diversity of opinions, and networking opportunities. In addition, conflict resolution skills can be enhanced, and collaborative decisions build ownership of solutions. Ultimately, implementation of TBL can yield effective learning and increase interpersonal skills, especially among interprofessional groups.

Disadvantages. TBL requires shifts of roles of faculty and student. It involves faculty time to learn the technique, and students need orientation to a different way of learning. Student scheduling issues may complicate group assignments. Other disadvantages of TBL are that student stress may increase if group conflict occurs, segregation of individuals can occur, reaching agreement can be difficult, decision-making takes more time, and it is easier for some individuals to avoid doing work while allowing other more extroverted and competitive individuals to take on leadership of the group outcome. Time and resources may be limited for effective faculty planning.

Evidence. See Alberti et al. (2021); Choi et al. (2021); Considine et al. (2021); Ironside and McNelis (2009); Joshi et al. (2022); Michaelson et al. (2008); and Nasim et al. (2022).

Conceptual Knowledge

Conceptual knowledge uses "interrelationships among the basic elements within a larger structure that enable them to function together" (Anderson & Krathwohl, 2001, p. 29). The main forms of conceptual knowledge teaching are argumentation, debate, structured controversy, and dilemmas; cooperative learning, collaborative learning, and jigsawing; mind mapping and concept mapping; and role play. In a concept analysis by Fletcher et al. (2019), conceptual

knowledge was described as a process that results in enhanced synthesis and analysis of complex ideas, improved problem solving, and translation of theory to practice.

Argumentation, Debate, Structured Controversy, and Dilemmas

There are a variety of strategies such as arguments, debates, controversies, case studies, and dilemmas that require students to not only be familiar with content and underlying concepts but also to use evidence to engage in dialogue to support a particular position. These strategies develop critical thinking and clinical judgment skills, along with developing oral presentation skills. One effective strategy to foster ethical decision-making in debates is Mock Trials.

Mock Trials is a strategy that helps students address legal/ethical conflicts pervasive in health care. The strategy takes quite a bit of preparatory effort because prior to class, faculty develop a courtroom vignette, legal documents that contain evidence, and the roles of the victim, nurse on trial, witnesses, and legal teams such as the jury, judge, prosecuting, and defense attorneys. The trial must be aligned with the course topics and student learning outcomes. Some topic examples underscore issues related to negligence, incompetency, medication administration errors, assisted suicide, confidentiality breach, treatment refusal, inadequate staffing, peer substance abuse, peer incompetence, coming to work sick, and work assignments that contradict personal religious beliefs. Students are assigned various roles with the ultimate goal of demonstrating fundamental knowledge and skill competencies associated with the topic (Cariñanos-Ayala et al., 2021; Herrman, 2019).

Teaching tips. When using debates and structured controversies, faculty must ensure that the topic that is the focus of the activity has several viewpoints that can be supported by evidence. Debate teams usually consist of five students: two students debate in favor of the topic, two debate in opposition to the topic, and the fifth acts as the judge. Structured debates typically include three phases: (1) a predebate phase where students seek evidence to defend their position; (2) a staging phase where students provide opening comments, present affirmative and negative viewpoints, and rebuttal; and (3) a postdebate activity where students summarize lessons learned and offer constructive criticism for future endeavors (Cariñanos-Ayala et al., 2021). Encouraging students to argue in opposition to their personal beliefs may increase student learning. Structured debate may be completed online or in the classroom. Interprofessional teams will enhance student engagement and active learning.

Advantages. Argumentation techniques help students develop analytical skills and the ability to recognize complexities in many health care issues. They broaden student views of controversial topics, and these techniques develop communication skills, increase students' ability to work in groups, and stimulate critical thinking through the development of analysis, synthesis, and evaluation. Thus, debate strategies foster students to achieve high-order knowledge and skills in Bloom's Taxonomy (Cariñanos-Ayala et al., 2021).

Disadvantages. Argumentation techniques require a significant level of knowledge about the subject on behalf of those participating in the debate and the audience. Students may need a tutorial on how to debate. Argumentation requires increased student preparation time. The confrontational aspect of debate can create anxiety and conflict for students without adequate confrontation skills, public speaking skills, or a strong sense of professional identity. The time cost is high when students are to work in groups.

Evidence. See Al-Jubouri (2021); Cariñanos-Ayala et al. (2021); and Fletcher et al. (2019).

Collaborative Learning, Cooperative Learning, and Jigsawing

Collaborative and cooperative learning are often used as interchangeable terms and evidence suggests that both collaborative and cooperative learning help to promote critical thinking (Zhang & Chen, 2021). Collaborative learning is student centered, whereas cooperative learning is teacher centered. In collaborative learning students organize and divide a faculty-directed assignment and the success of the group is dependent on the effort of individual members.

There are a variety of strategies that faculty can use to promote collaborative and cooperative learning.

Some examples of strategies of collaborative learning are: Stump your partner, fishbowl debate, and one-minute papers.

Stump your Partner (Cornell University, 2022) is used at the end of or at a midpoint of a lecture. Students are given a few minutes to create a challenging question regarding recently presented content. Each student in the class poses the question to a student sitting next to them. The student writing the question also provides the answer.

Fishbowl debate is a purposeful strategy for developing ideas that need description, explanation, evidence, perspective, and ethical/legal awareness. Fishbowl debate is accomplished by asking students to sit in groups of three. Students are assigned roles as the supporter, the opposer, or the equalizer. The equalizer decides which of the debaters is most convincing and why (Bodrožić-Brnić & Thiessen, 2022).

One-minute papers give student groups the opportunity to get a sense of what they have learned as a result of the classroom experience. Students are simply given 60 seconds at the end of a class to write down three things they have learned, to define concepts, and/or to inform the faculty member how useful the group exercise was for them (Lee & Saunders, 2020). One-minute papers can help faculty identify knowledge gaps and determine if teaching strategies used have been effective (Stevens, 2019). To be clear, one-minute papers are designated as an individual assignment but are turned in as a group bundle if they are to be graded.

Cooperative learning occurs when students with varied abilities are arranged into preassigned groups and rewarded in proportion to the group's success rather than individual success (Johnson & Johnson, 2018). Some examples of strategies of cooperative learning are three-step interviews, think-pair-share, graffiti wall, and jigsawing. Supplementary cooperative learning strategies and directions for employing them are available for faculty use (The Curators of the University of Missouri, 2021).

Three-step interviews is a strategy to help students communicate with each other and their patients and learn new roles. In groups of three, student pairs take turns interviewing each other until all three students have been an interviewer or have been interviewed. Then, student groups report what they learned to another triad. This strategy is effective in helping English as second language students become socialized in new cultures (Kamaliah, 2018).

Think-pair-share is implemented by faculty posing a question or topic to students to think about individually. Individual students then turn to a partner and share their thoughts or responses. Pair responses are then shared in a small group, large group, or the entire class. It has been used successfully to teach asthma medications among undergraduate nursing students (McClure & Brame, 2020).

Graffiti wall is a strategy for assessing prior knowledge. Students write comments or draw pictures to reflect their thoughts on a topic. The words or images should depict their experiences and emotions pertaining to the topic. Students can use arrows or geometric shapes to connect ideas. The class is asked to summarize and draw conclusions about what is seen on the wall (Robertson et al., 2020). Faculty take this information and build upon it across learning dimensions.

Jigsawing is another strategy to promote cooperative learning. The jigsawing technique organizes classroom activities in a way that drives students to become reliant on each other to be successful. Students are preassigned into home groups where they must complete a piece of an assignment or solve small problems, of which they will be required to present their solutions/answers to the class. When all groups are finished, the solutions are collated and synthesized to a greater lesson or conclusion. When the larger class processes the conclusion, greater understandings are formed (Goolsarran et al., 2020; McConnell et al., 2017). Cornell University's (2022) cooperative learning strategies offer explicit recommendations for implementing jigsawing. Home groups or teams should be formed using three to five students. Next, each home group member takes on a faculty-assigned role within the group. Members from each team with like roles form expert groups of 3–10 members. The faculty then provides time for expert team members to work together to become experts on the topic they are assigned. Expert team members then return home to share what they have learned. The information the experts come back with is needed for the home team to complete a cooperative task or to solve a larger problem (Case Study 16.1).

Ng et al. (2020) have prepared an open-access interactive workshop using the jigsaw method to enhance graduate student's (medical students, resident physicians, nurse practitioner students) knowledge in managing geriatric women's health topics such as menopause, osteoporosis, urinary incontinence, and abnormal uterine bleeding. The interactive workshop contains a plethora of teaching/learning materials including reading materials, student worksheets, facilitator guides, and pre-/posttests.

Teaching tips. When using collaborative or cooperative learning strategies, faculty must develop a clear teaching plan that includes how the groups will be structured, how many students will be in the group, what the role(s) of the student will be, if the results of the group work will be evaluated, and if the group will conduct peer review of each member giving feedback on the amount and quality of their participation.

Faculty should identify real-world situations that can be addressed by collaboration. Depending on the nature of the group project, a group of three to five diverse students is ideal. Group roles such as "leader," "recorder," "reflector," and "reporter" can be assigned by the faculty or students. Configuring the groups can be done in several ways. The simplest is to have students count off by the number to be in each group; this will ensure a random configuration of the group. When a specific viewpoint or expertise is needed in the group, faculty can ask all the students with the desired characteristics to line up by each characteristic and then randomly assign one person from that group to the collaborative group.

The teaching plan should allow sufficient time for students to assemble in their group, assign

CASE STUDY 16.1   Using Jigsawing to Help Students Learn Leadership Concepts

A core course in a graduate nursing program focuses on topics such as leadership and role transformation in an acute care setting. Students from all majors are required to enroll in this course. The faculty decides to use Jigsawing to integrate leadership and role transformation concepts relevant to all students and have created simulated "Mock Hospital." Students are divided into "home groups" of 5 to 10 students. The home group creates fictitious units, patient populations, missions, visions, and strategic plans. Each home team member takes on leadership roles like Chief Nursing Officer, Chief Financial Officer, Legal Counsel, Chief of Staff, Clinical Pharmacist, Chair of the Ethics Board, Patient Ombudsman, Union Representative, or Quality Improvement Coordinator. The course lead faculty serves as a narrator who presents units with unique challenges such as critical staffing needs, grievances, sentinel events, a fire, natural disaster, bankruptcy, active shooter scenarios, lawsuits, staff strikes, preparing for a Joint Commission and Magnet status survey, and other similar scenarios. Each unit works to solve the challenge using leadership management concepts such as strategic planning, budgeting, root cause analysis, or Plan-Do-Study-Act cycles.

Each "like" role meets to discuss how they as nurse experts should guide the home group. After the experts return home, the home group students cooperate to resolve their challenge and present a short report to the entire class as to what they learned about leading and managing in a complex health care system.

1. What are the advantages of using a collaborative learning strategy such as Jigsawing to engage students in real-world situations?
2. What is the role of the faculty to help students put the pieces of the jigsaw puzzle together?
3. How should faculty configure collaborative groups?
4. What is the best size for a collaborative group?
5. Should the work of the students be assessed? Evaluated? Graded?
6. What are the disadvantages of using Jigsawing?
7. What teaching tips might help foster a cooperative learning environment?
8. What evidence supports this teaching strategy?
9. How could this case study be revised to be offered in online classrooms, synchronously versus asynchronously?

roles, and determine their approach to working on the task at hand. The plan should also include time in the end for each group to report the results and then for the entire class to debrief the experience and ensure that the key points that contribute to attaining the learning outcome have been discussed by the entire class.

Advantages. Cooperative learning and similar activities promote active and reflective learning and encourage teamwork. Cooperative learning reduces learner anxiety and increases learner self-confidence because specified role designations reduce learner confusion. Cooperative learner activities that join academic and clinical experiences can increase assessment and technical skill (Zhang & Chen, 2021). Thus, cooperative learning activities provide opportunities for students to become accountable for their own and others' actions, so designated roles enhance the group's dynamics' skills which in turn foster learning success. One-minute papers provide students with a sense of having a voice in their educational experience. Jigsawing has received mixed but mostly positive reviews from

students (McConnell et al., 2017). Jigsawing helps build comprehension; encourages cooperative learning among students; and improves listening, communication, and problem-solving skills. Also, cooperative learning can help students accomplish large learning assignments and projects more efficiently.

Disadvantages. Students may resist frequent use of group assignments. There is a possibility that not all students will participate equally. Student scheduling issues may complicate preparation of group assignments, and student stress may increase if group conflict occurs. The main factor for determining effectiveness is the level of cooperation among group members and the ability to attain the intended learning outcome.

Evidence. See Bodrožić-Brnić and Thiessen (2022); Cornell University (2022); Goolsarran et al. (2020); Johnson and Johnson (2018); Kamaliah (2018); Lee and Sanders (2020); McConnell et al. (2017); McClure and Brame (2020); Ng et al. (2020); Robertson et al. (2020); Saeedi et al. (2021); Silva et al. (2022); Stevens (2019); Curators of the University of Missouri (2021); and Zhang and Chen (2021).

Mind Mapping and Concept Mapping

Mapping strategies involve the learning of complex phenomena by diagramming concepts and subconcepts. Mind mapping places one main concept at the center of a page and poses related concepts surrounding it, forming a radial structure. *Mind maps* are used for generating and exploring ideas, brainstorming, and organizing information. *Concept maps* are visual–structural diagrams that help students organize diverse elements of a larger topic and form a tree-like structure. Concept maps are used for organizing information, analyzing complex issues, creating solutions, and taking action.

Both mapping exercises are good for group assignments, especially interprofessional groups with divergent conceptual knowledge. The faculty must identify the goal of the lesson before assigning mind mapping versus concept mapping exercises. Assignments without purposeful goals result in students preparing graphical representations of a concept, or system, in the form of charts, clouds, Venn diagrams, timelines, or infographics without consideration of how the concepts are interrelated. For example, a concept map assigned to help learners understand how various diuretics work is more meaningful to novice nurses if they first depict the concepts of renal functioning such as glomerular filtration, the sodium-potassium pump, and the loop of Henley. Thus, mind mapping and concept mapping assignments must be meaningful for influencing clinical judgment for safe nursing practice.

Mind mapping strategies have been used with graduate nursing students to facilitate the understanding of digital health technologies, critical thinking, and the comprehension of how technologies support both practice and patient care. Digital health technologies were defined as electronic health records, telehealth services, robotics, and mobile health through smartphones, wearables, apps, and other monitoring devices (Seckman & Van de Castle, 2021). Sullivan recommended having family nurse practitioner students work in small groups of three or four to develop "topic" maps on diagnoses found in primary care (2022, p. 42). Sullivan differentiated between topic and concept maps by stipulating that maps use bullet points to highlight the most pertinent information central to the diagnosis.

Teaching tips. Mapping strategies can be used to enhance conceptual knowledge and retention of learning outcomes. This teaching method is frequently used in clinical settings but is also effective in the classroom and online. Students can organize patient data before entering an actual patient encounter and then add to the map correlating new and existing data to better understand the clinical presentation of the patient. Grouping specific class content can also provide students with examples of mind mapping. Concept map software may be helpful when using this technique. Concept mapping can be an effective strategy for students with many learning styles.

Advantages. Mapping strategies encourage better understanding and recall of complex phenomena and are especially effective in stimulating long-term recall of like concepts. They require active involvement by the students in designing the maps to show relationships of concepts and develop conceptual thinking processes. They help students recognize similarities and differences among concepts, help clarify relationships between concepts, help link new information with information previously learned, and help students organize information and relate theories to practice. They enhance problem-solving skills and enhance knowledge retention compared to traditional assignments such as reading, lecture, writing assignments, or discussion. The method appeals to the visual learner. Software is available for mapping assignments.

Disadvantages. Mapping strategies require faculty to spend quite a bit of time at the beginning of the assignment to explain how to construct the map. Many students are "concrete thinkers" and may have difficulty understanding the higher-order relationships that mapping strategies are used to help students develop. Another disadvantage of using mapping strategies is that they may not appeal to auditory learners and they can be visually overwhelming if the assigned concept is large with layers of complexity. Both faculty and students may need to learn how to use mapping before this method can be used effectively.

Evidence. See Alfayoumi (2019); Garwood et al. (2018); Kaddoura et al. (2016); Seckman and Van de Castle (2021); and Wu & Wu (2020).

Role Play

Role play is a dramatic approach in which individuals assume the roles of others or pretend to be someone else such as a patient, family member, or member of the health care team. Role play may be scripted, unscripted, spontaneous, or semistructured interactions that are observed by others for analysis and interpretation of learning outcomes. It is an innovative and effective strategy that activates learning. This strategy can be used in class, online, or laboratory settings. Role play is also used among medical, anesthesia, and nurse practitioner students to determine critical thinking, clinical judgment, and competency. Typically role playing occurs as a patient-simulated scenario or via an Objective Structured Clinical Examination (OSCE). OSCEs are considered innovative evaluations that use systematic methods to objectively assess student performance. In the literature, OSCEs are differentiated from role playing and simulations in that OSCEs can involve real or simulated patients and/or actual clinical specimens.

Teaching tips. Faculty need to plan thoroughly for role play, but they also need to be prepared to monitor and modify student actions and reactions if necessary. Situations that involve conflicting emotions provide good scenarios for role playing. Examples can include death and dying, medical errors, acute mental health crisis, and dementia or elderly care. Typical organization of the role play involves briefing, setting the stage, and explaining the objectives, which is usually the shortest stage; running and acting out the role play, which may take from 5 to 20 minutes; and debriefing, discussion, analysis, and evaluation of the role-playing experience, which may last 30 to 40 minutes or more.

Debriefing is the most important stage of the role play, so students can clarify actions and alternative decisions can be explained, observation skills can be enhanced, and other interpersonal reactions can be anticipated. Video or audio recording of the role play may aid in the debriefing stage. The technique works best with small groups of students so that those who are not involved in the role play can become active observers. Students should be encouraged to respond naturally to the role play and avoid insincere acting. Having non-role playing students serve as observers is one method of offering peer feedback. Peer feedback should offer constructive criticism and be directed to the behaviors exhibited in the role play and not to specific students.

Advantages. Role play increases observational skills, improves decision-making skills, and increases comprehension of complex human behaviors. It provides immediate feedback about the interpersonal and problem-solving skills used in the role play and provides a nonthreatening environment in which to try out unfamiliar communication and decision-making techniques. Role play is also an effective way to develop affective learning such as ethical decision making and honesty when the role play is designed for an interaction between two or more individuals who must on the spot do the right thing.

Disadvantages. Students may be reluctant to participate if they do not feel as if it reflects real-life situations and is seen as simply play acting, or pretending. There is a high time cost for faculty to develop scenarios. Faculty who like to be in charge of the learning environment may be frustrated by this method. Stereotypical behavior can be reinforced, and role play can be a costly use of class time if it is not planned appropriately.

Evidence. See Dabbagh et al. (2020); Dorri et al. (2020); Nemec et al. (2021); and Sartain et al. (2021).

Procedural Knowledge

Procedural knowledge involves how to do something, methods of inquiry, and criteria for using skills, algorithms, techniques, and methods that are discipline specific. Teaching strategies relating to procedural knowledge are demonstration, games, imagery and mindfulness, posters, self-learning modules, simulation, and writing.

Demonstration. As a teaching strategy, demonstration is a method of communicating step-by-step processes using visual aids such as slide presentations, flip charts, posters, and/or models. Demonstration occurs when faculty perform an essential activity for the class in a systematic way. Safety and rationale for each step should be stressed during the performance. Whenever possible, faculty should involve students to assist with demonstrations.

As a learning strategy, demonstration requires that students show learning outcomes as projects, presentations, or learning objects, revealing to what degree they have met the learning objectives. Typically, learning demonstration is both a learning experience for the student and a means of evaluating academic progress by the educator. Whether used as a teaching or learning strategy, demonstration should be used for complex mental or psychomotor skill acquisition. It is appropriate for online, in-class, laboratory, and clinical assignments, as well as for interprofessional learning. Demonstration has been used with nurse practitioner students (Harlan et al., 2021) and with academic-service partnerships (Karikari-Martin et al., 2021). Nurse practitioner students ranked demonstration as the third out of 26 preferred teaching/learning strategies for web-enhanced course delivery.

Teaching tips. As a teaching strategy, faculty need to make sure objects used for demonstration are visible to all students, that clear, concise language is used so that students understand what is being demonstrated, and that students have the opportunity to ask questions and that answers are provided. After teacher demonstration occurs, students should return to the demonstration, showing the steps of the process clearly, from start to finish. Teachers should ask students to go through the process a second time, showing the rationale and allowing time for questions and provide for immediate, individual, supervised practice sessions. Video recordings may be used for student review before and after the demonstration. Demonstrations may be planned, implemented, reviewed, and revised through online videos.

Advantages. Visibly showing a multistep process often aids in retention. Complex skills become more understandable as a result of the demonstration, and demonstration allows an expert to model the skill. Tailored performance feedback enhances retention and procedural knowledge is enhanced for future problem-solving and metacognitive knowledge.

Disadvantages. Faculty demonstrations can go awry if models or aids do not work properly. There is a substantial time cost for practicing demonstrations, a high faculty workload involved in supervision of student practice times, and a high cost of supplies and equipment which may limit the amount of practice time available to students.

Students have differing levels of demonstration and skill-acquisition abilities. Students who quickly master skills may become uninterested while the others are practicing. Mastering psychomotor skills is usually very stressful for many students and requires faculty versed in formative and positive feedback, so realistic practice sessions benefit the entire class.

Evidence. See Harlan et al. (2021); Herrman (2019); and Karikari-Martin et al. (2021).

Games

An educational game is a learning activity with rules involving chance showcasing the players' knowledge or skill in attempting to reach a specific learning outcome. This strategy may be completed online or in class and is suited for interprofessional "icebreaker" assignments. Games can be used to increase student participation, foster social and emotional learning, and motivate risk taking. Gaming software is available for online use. Currently, evidence generated by gaming research is prominent in both education and nursing literature (see evidence below). For example, virtual games have been found to improve focus and spatial-temporal attention (Gallardo et al., 2018). Serious games promote teamwork and collaboration, especially among interprofessional groups (Fusco et al., 2022). Augmented reality facilitates high levels of student engagement (Menon et al., 2021). Competitive gaming has been used effectively to increase an understanding of advanced pathophysiology concepts among nurse practitioner students (Weiss, 2018). *Promote Your Favorite Organ* is a game created by advanced practice nursing students for peers to engage in challenging pathophysiological concepts and the management of disease processes. The impact the game had on grades was a 23% higher grade average and decreased course drop rates (Weiss, 2018).

Teaching tips. Use a gaming method for reinforcement of knowledge rather than introduction of new knowledge. Games must be well planned and aligned with learning outcomes. Also, establishing an open learning environment is crucial to learning with gaming. Faculty must appreciate that learning is student-to-student in this method. Debriefing after the game is critical, so students clearly connect the game with the important concepts. If faculty do not value gaming as a teaching strategy, they may unconsciously sabotage the game.

Advantages. Gaming increases student engagement and cognitive and affective learning, improves retention, is fun and exciting, increases learner involvement, motivates the learner, and can help connect practice experiences to theory. Students can learn from each other through the experience of the game; it is good for adult learners who take more responsibility for their own learning. Learners can receive immediate feedback in a learning situation and can also see the immediate application of theory to practice. Learning from gaming lasts longer compared with learning from traditional lecture.

Disadvantages. Gaming may be threatening to some learners, who may feel exposed if they are unsure of the answer. It may be time consuming and may be costly to purchase or develop. It may be difficult to evaluate the level of learning achieved through gaming if several players are involved. It may require a greater amount of space. It should have introductory and summary sessions and faculty must set guidelines so that the game remains educational.

Evidence. See Cerezo et al. (2022); Fusco et al. (2022); Gallardo et al. (2018); McEnroe-Petitte and Farris (2020); Menon et al. (2021); Pront et al. (2018); Sarker et al. (2021); Weiss (2018); and Xu et al. (2021).

Imagery and Mindfulness

Imagery and mindfulness include mental picturing, diagramming, or rehearsal before the actual use of the information in practice. The best use is in combination with other strategies (e.g., with physical practice in psychomotor skill acquisition). *Imagery* helps students recall information and improves comprehension. *Mindfulness* is a redirection activity that trains the brain to be in the present moment as opposed to focusing on the past or the future. Both imagery and mindfulness can be used to reduce stress and foster engagement within the classroom setting. Faculty must be able to guide imagery or mindfulness in a way that individuals and groups can respond. Mindfulness has been successfully implemented among family nurse practitioner students in first-semester clinical courses, resulting in statistically significant stress reduction ($p < 0.05$) (Conelius & Iannino-Renz, 2021).

Teaching tips. Create a scenario that mimics a real-life situation such as a walk on the beach. Use the scenario to demonstrate effective use of imagery. Relaxation techniques provide a good example of how to use imagery techniques. A supportive classroom environment is needed for the effective use of this strategy. This technique may be helpful for stress reduction for students and its application to nursing practice. Ideal times to implement imagery or mindfulness are a few minutes before an exam or just before performing a skill competency. Faculty should emphasize how students can apply this approach to practice such as to decrease fear with an anxious patient prior to an invasive procedure (Case Study 16.2).

Advantage. Imagery and mindfulness activates self-regulation in the brain and allows for effective decision making (Leyland et al., 2019). The techniques also provide superior learning of psychomotor skills when imagery is combined with physical practice. It may lead to the development of therapeutic and holistic nursing skills in practice.

Disadvantages. Individuals have varying levels of innate imagery skills, so some students may need to be taught how to conduct imagery. It does not provide a substitute for physical practice of a skill. Using imagery and physical practice of the skill will require more student study time than if only physical practice is used. Stress and performance fears may interfere with the productive use of imagery. It may require faculty development to implement imagery strategy.

CASE STUDY 16.2 Guided Imagery, "Walk on the Beach"

Faculty in a fundamental course have noticed that students are very anxious prior to each test. The teaching team plans to empower students to manage their anxiety for future tests. They decide to use a guided imagery strategy, "Walk on the Beach." The guided imagery experience lasts approximately 5 minutes. To begin the experience, the faculty uses a soft accepting and caring voice and, as the students enter the classroom, asks the students to be seated and turn off their electronic devices. The faculty passes out beach-scented lotions. Next, the faculty turns down the lights, turns on an overhead projector displaying a beach, plays an audio recording of wave sounds, and directs the students to close their eyes. Students sit comfortably and breathe, inhaling through their noses and holding their breath for four counts and exhaling out of their mouths for four counts. Students focus on their heart rate, noticing that their heart rate decreases while clearing their minds. Eventually, the faculty directs the students to envision a sunny day where they wade in the ocean and feel refreshed. When they open their eyes, they are instructed to stay mindful and safe as they take the test.

1. What other courses or content might benefit from guided imagery?
2. Under what circumstances might a guided imagery strategy not be useful?
3. What kinds of learner reactions should faculty expect from using a guided imagery strategy? Why?

Evidence. See Chen et al. (2021); Conelius and Iannino-Renz (2021); Leyland et al. (2019); and Windle et al. (2021).

Poster

A poster is a visual representation of learning outcomes. This project may be completed online, is well suited for peer or interprofessional learning, and provides opportunities for dissemination of knowledge. Posters can be used to set the stage for participating in professional conference poster presentations. Posters can be used in classroom, online, or clinical settings, including intra and interprofessional groups. Frequently, posters are assigned to graduate nursing students to improve scholarly writing, enhance oral presentations, and disseminate evidence-based practice projects and/or research activity (Arends & Callies, 2022; Vogt et al., 2021)

Teaching tips. When using posters, faculty should explain the difference between professional poster presentations and posters that are used to depict learning outcomes. Regardless of the type of poster that is assigned, students will need specific instructions about how to design it. Clear guidelines and criteria for the expected poster contents will need to be developed and presented to students. Evaluation criteria and techniques should be provided in the form of a rubric. Poster quality may be enhanced when artistic concepts are incorporated into the poster design. Software is available for creating visually pleasing posters. Space on posters can be made available by use of QR codes, allowing poster viewers to increase engagement and understanding (King, 2020). Another popular way to integrate posters into learning is the use of poster galleries. Students create eye-catching and informative posters and present them in gallery format; students move among a series of posters or other types of prompts and provide responses at each station. Finally, professional posters presented at conferences offer graduate students the opportunity to be socialized into the discipline and to communicate their research findings (evidence) with interested peers.

Advantages. Students can convey complex ideas through posters, and making posters can facilitate student creativity. Assessment of students' knowledge can be showcased through the use of posters. Students can receive feedback from peers and faculty. Students get a sense of achievement from producing posters. Posters provide the student with a sense of aligning academic experiences with clinical practice. The skills developed in the production of a poster may be valuable for students after graduation. Posters can be used to showcase student work publicly in professional conferences or student poster displays. Evaluation of posters by faculty or peers can be completed quickly using guidelines or grading rubrics. When poster galleries are paired with quizzing and/or lecture tutorials, students enjoy learning (McConnell et al., 2017).

Disadvantages. Faculty time is required to develop a poster assignment and evaluation techniques. The assignment can be frustrating to students who are not visual learners and some students may become more interested in the creative aspect of the poster than in the dissemination of knowledge.

Evidence. See Arends and Callies (2022); Hasanica et al. (2020); King (2020); McConnell et al. (2017); Rowe (2017).

Writing

Writing encourages learning through documentation of ideas in, for example, scholarly papers, informal journals, poems, and letters. Interprofessional scholarly writing may increase student engagement and active learning for dissemination of knowledge. Recent literature links writing with the development of critical thinking (Jefferies et al., 2018) and clinical judgment among nursing students (Smith, 2021). This is best accomplished through formative feedback, which strengthens scholarly writing activities, especially among graduate nursing students (Tornwall & McDaniel, 2022). The integration of the Association of American Colleges and Universities (2021) *The Essentials: Core Competencies for Professional Nursing Education*, Domain 9: Scholarship for Nursing Discipline affords students of all levels the opportunity to demonstrate the reporting of clinical inquiry, evidence gathering and appraisal, and translation of findings to practice processes (p. 37). However, some clinical experiences are difficult to describe. *The 55-word poem* is a strategy used to foster transformative growth, especially when students feel vulnerable and unprepared for the realities of human suffering.

Teaching tips. Teaching students how to write may increase the quality of student papers. Faculty should select writing assignments based on course learning outcomes. For example, an assignment to write a letter to a congressman supporting a car seat law might align with a health policy course where outcomes address participating in advocating for policies that protect vulnerable populations

across institutional, local, state, and federal levels. Faculty should structure the writing assignment with final grading in mind. Assess the paper in its entirety rather than concentrating on grammar and style issues. Incorporating peer review of drafts may stimulate thinking and critiquing skills and improve the quality of student papers (scholarship). Specific grading criteria decrease the amount of subjective grading. Time spent on grading can be decreased with a grading rubric. Increasing complexity in writing experiences across the curriculum increases the effect on stimulating higher-order thinking. Providing flexibility in topic selection for written assignments recognizes individual student learning needs and empowers students.

Many forms of writing can be used, such as journals, formal papers, creative writing assignments (e.g., poems or book reports), summaries of class content, letters to legislators and nurse administrators, and research critiques. Planned writing activities such as the 55-word poem create a classroom condition for deep learning and transformation of bias attitudes (Cusanno et al., 2022). Mentoring, reflection, and time to learn the different skills are suggested. Partnerships with students, faculty, and librarians may increase information literacy and online searching skills needed for writing academic papers. Writing manuscripts for publication involves more advanced academic writing skills; additionally, more specific instruction may be necessary.

Advantages. Writing stimulates higher-order thinking through active involvement with the literature, learning to judge the quality of the literature, organizing interpretation of the literature into logical sequences, and learning to make judgments based on what was learned. Students can discover their own beliefs and values when writing. Nurses write in many formats, and writing projects in an educational setting allow for learning different mediums and styles. Knowledge gained from the writing assignments can give confidence and helps empower students with their own ideas. This is ideal when intense emotions stifle how best to process lessons pertaining to the human condition (Soneru, 2021). Writing assignments such as the 55-word poem can help students find words to frame thoughts and feelings. Writing improves communication skills. In addition, there is a strong relationship between critical thinking skills in nursing practice and academic writing skills.

Disadvantages. Grading writing assignments can be subjective. Many students may feel unprepared to complete writing assignments, which may lead to students' increased frustration and stress. Students must understand the importance of learning through writing, or writing assignments will be viewed as superfluous work. There may be a high time cost for students to complete the writing assignments depending on how the assignment is structured. Writing assignments such as the 55-minute poem may not be enough to facilitate learning and to guide psyche. The faculty member needs to be prepared to refer students who have been traumatized by clinical events to other professionals such as clergy or mental health counselors. As with all writing assignments, there is typically a high time cost for teachers to grade. Faculty development may be needed before choosing this type of teaching strategy.

Evidence. See Association of American Colleges & Universities (2021); Carter and Townsend (2022); Cusanno et al. (2022); Jefferies et al. (2018); Smith (2021); Soneru (2021); Tornwall and McDaniel (2022); and White and Lansom (2017).

Metacognitive Knowledge

Metacognitive knowledge is knowledge of cognition in general, and the awareness and knowledge of one's own cognition. In other words, it is thinking about thinking and about what one knows. Strategies that invoke metacognition are ones that spark curiosity and challenge. Several formats can be used: case study, portfolio and e-portfolio, problem-based learning, questioning and Socratic questioning, reflection journal writing, and simulation.

Case study. *Case studies* represent an in-depth analysis of a real-life situation at a point in time as a way to illustrate class content. Case studies describe a person, event, or situation where students must apply clinical judgment that prevents disease, maintains health, or improves

a health condition (Heale & Twycross, 2018). Case studies apply didactic content and theory to real life, simulated life, or both. *Unfolding case studies* occur over several points in time, often from diagnosis of a health problem or admission to a health care facility through treatment and discharge. Originally developed by Glendon and Ulrich (1997), unfolding case studies have become a cornerstone in teaching quality and safety competencies that improve student learning outcomes (Sherwood & Barnsteiner, 2021). Unfolding case studies offer progressively revealed real-life clinical situations that offer students opportunities to build on previous knowledge and to connect theory to practice. Unfolding case studies enhance thinking processes and build connections to facilitate deep learning. These strategies are well suited for interprofessional or peer-group learning and may be completed online or in class. Unfolding case studies are also effective when used as in-class *Pop-Up Patient Activities* to prepare nurse practitioner students for telehealth experiences, virtual consultations, topic/concept maps, and certification exam reviews (Sullivan, 2022).

Teaching tips. A well-designed case that illustrates the most important learning outcomes is critical to the success of learning with this method. Unfolding case studies are those that progress or "unfold" over time. Before assigning a case study, analyze the case with the intent of determining the potential ways in which students could analyze the case, but be prepared for student questions and comments that previously have not been considered (e.g., be able to say, "I don't know" or "I haven't considered that before," if necessary). A safe, open, nonthreatening learning environment is crucial for active student participation. Cases should involve using the best available evidence to substantiate nursing actions. Faculty should develop criteria for the student to cite resources by using discipline-specific formatting and should address providing scientific rationale to support the student-recommended nursing interventions. At the conclusion of the assignment, provide a summary of the most important points and sources for more in-depth study. Assist in students' comprehension of critical concepts with the use of tools such as concept maps, chalkboards, flip charts, posters, or slide presentations.

Advantages. Case studies promote engaged learning beyond understanding and recall. Unfolding case studies allow students to use forethought to predict what might happen next when presented with a similar case in an actual clinical setting. Students like to guess what might happen next. Associating the practical with the theoretical helps many students recall important information. Case studies afford students the opportunity to solve problems in a safe setting without the fear or possibility of harming a patient.

Disadvantages. Case studies are most useful when they involve complex situations that require students to solve problems. They are effective when cases are simple and involve basic knowledge such as factual information. Developing cases is a time-consuming skill and using published case studies should be considered. Published case studies may carry financial costs. Case studies require the use of good questioning skills by the faculty. Poor student preparation may result in less learning. Case studies may frustrate students who desire content to be presented through more direct strategies such as lecture.

Evidence. See Glendon and Ulrich (1997); Sherwood and Barnsteiner (2021); and Sullivan (2022).

Portfolio and E-Portfolio

A *portfolio* is a dossier or collection of student work showcasing learning, achievement, and personal and professional development. Documentation of student skills from prior courses or life experiences can be used for assessing learning outcomes for a course or program or for professional development. This may be completed electronically and referred to as an e-portfolio. *E-portfolios* integrate information technology with electronic files. A scoping review identified that nursing student portfolios are helpful in mentoring student education (Mollahadi et al., 2018). Another review found that e-portfolios strengthened students' self-reflection, tracked student progress with skill acquisition, and increased teacher-student interaction (Sabet et al., 2022). A scoping review identified that e-portfolios scaffolded learning among multiple disciplines including across associate, baccalaureate, and graduate levels of nursing (Janssens et al., 2022).

Teaching tips. Students should be oriented on how to develop the portfolio or e-portfolio. Specifically, faculty should explain how to construct a portfolio. A content outline should provide the framework for the portfolio but not limit student creativity. The guidelines for portfolio construction and evaluation must be clear. Periodic assessment of portfolios should take place. Novice educators may want to seek consultation and assistance from experts before implementing portfolio requirements.

Advantages. Portfolios typically provide high student motivation because they control learning. Motivated students typically learn more. Portfolios help educators understand individual student goals and aspirations. They encourage student reflection on learning. Independent, self-confident, and self-directed students will excel with this method.

Disadvantages. Portfolios must be combined with reflective strategies to encourage student ownership of learning. They require alternative ways of thinking about the learning process by both educators and students. Students with low self-confidence will need much faculty assistance. The time involvement may be high for students in development of portfolios and for faculty in evaluation of portfolios. Unless students clearly see the objective of a portfolio, the work involved may be viewed as busy work. As with any assignment, portfolios must be meaningful. For example, e-portfolios offer Gen Z students the perception that they will receive instant, individual feedback in their electronic space as they prefer to receive feedback about what they have learned as opposed to tracking standardized test results (Demir & Sönmez, 2021).

Evidence. See Demir and Sönmez (2021); Janssens et al. (2022); Mollahadi et al. (2018); and Sabet et al. (2022).

Problem-Based Learning

Problem-Based Learning (PBL) is a strategy used to enhance students' abilities to critically evaluate and apply cumulated knowledge to solve actual clinical problems. PBL can be used to engage students at all levels of the curriculum as long as the problem to be solved is appropriate to the course learning outcomes and the level of the student's knowledge. PBL, when used in Master's and Doctoral programs, tends to be used throughout the entire program. Similar to case studies, faculty identify typical "problems" that the student would encounter in nursing practice and structure the problem to engage the students in appropriate solutions. As students work through the problem, they must follow three steps: (1) assess and analyze the problem, (2) collect evidence-based information that will contribute to solving the problem, and (3) summarize the findings, reflecting on both the problem's solution and the group's process used to solve it. PBL is usually adopted as an approach applied to the entire curriculum instead of concentrating on individual disciplines or nursing specialties.

This strategy can be completed online or in the classroom, and it can be used for interprofessional or peer learning. In a randomized controlled trial where nursing students using PBL were compared to a control group that did not use PBL, mean scores of patient safety-related knowledge, attitudes, and perceptions were statistically significant between the two groups after the PBL education ($p = 0.001$), where the PBL group patient safety-related knowledge, attitudes, and perceptions were significantly increased (Jamshidi et al., 2021). Statistically significant evidence supporting PBL in nursing education has become a consistent trend across international populations. According to a metaanalysis on PBL effectiveness, the strategy has positive effects on student satisfaction among medical and nurse practitioner students (Amir et al., 2022; Ibrahim et al., 2018).

Teaching tips. Develop realistic, comprehensive clinical problems that will prompt and advance intended learning outcomes. The case problem presented is typically accomplished through several scenes containing complex but realistic information that requires the students to process the available information into categories. Faculty workload can increase significantly, particularly during the development stages. PBL requires close collaboration between various disciplines if the case or curriculum is interdisciplinary. Orient students to the PBL approach and allow sufficient time for students to research the problem and discuss answers. Groups of 6–9 students are most effective for PBL. Faculty should make certain that students follow all steps in the PBL process to ensure learning occurs.

Advantages. PBL fosters active and cooperative learning. Students use skills of inquiry and metacognitive thinking along with peer teaching and peer evaluation. The problem can be developed in paper-and-pencil or electronic formats. Students often work in teams or groups. PBL can be used in interdisciplinary learning environments to develop roles and competencies of each discipline.

Disadvantages. PBL involves faculty time in developing the problem situation. Extensive time is needed for faculty to learn to use PBL. Students require orientation to the role of the learner in a PBL setting and must work through potential discrepancies in expectations and goals for learning. Student learning seems to be connected to the effectiveness of the case and the functioning of the group. It is difficult to use as a teaching technique when the class size is large.

Evidence. See Allert et al. (2022); Amir et al. (2022); Ibrahim et al. (2018); Jamshidi et al. (2021); and Park and Park (2022).

Questioning, Socratic Questioning, and Teaching Prompts

Questioning is an expression of inquiry—an interrogative sentence, phrase, or gesture—that invites or calls for a reply that goes beyond giving a factual answer. *Socratic questioning* involves probing questioning to analyze an individual's knowledge and thinking. *Teaching prompts* are questions that focus the students' attention on the knowledge and skills they are about to use for giving patient care. They are subtle cues or directions the faculty can give as a student is about to make a clinical judgment or perform a procedure. The purpose of questions, Socratic questions, and prompts is to help students uncover what they know and what they do not know in order to help them make connections among concepts. This strategy can be used in online courses or in classroom, clinical, or lab settings. When using interprofessional education methods, be sure that all students know the "language" of the participating professions and to refrain from using profession-specific jargon or slang. When using these strategies, it is helpful for faculty to remind the student that these questions are a part of a teaching situation, as questions can appear to be an evaluation of the students' knowledge or preparation to give care. Ultimately, questioning is used to stimulate critical thinking (Makhene, 2019; Yip, 2021) such as with advanced practice nursing students during standardized patient debriefing experiences (Kuzma et al., 2019).

Teaching tips. Questioning and prompts are effective strategies in both the classroom and clinical setting. They are also helpful in teaching a process such as the nursing process, delegation process, or clinical judgment process. When using this strategy, faculty should prepare a list of questions or prompts that can be used in relevant situations. Students may need to be informed that during questioning they will be pushed to a level of not knowing content and that they may experience stress from the questioning. When posing questions, faculty should be patient and allow about 10 to 20 seconds for students to respond, and then be prepared to use additional prompts if the student's response does not reflect the depth of thinking expected. Questions that use verbs consistent with Bloom's dimensions of learning will foster insight and higher-order thinking and judgment skills. Faculty must also consider if using questions and prompts in the classroom or clinical setting is appropriate when others are present.

Advantages. Using questions and prompts can promote higher-order learning and metacognition. Asking the questions gives faculty and the student insight into thinking processes and to intervene if the student's thinking is not based in evidence, there are errors in assumptions, or it would put patient safety in jeopardy.

Disadvantages. Questioning presumes a comprehensive knowledge of content. Preclass preparation by student and faculty must be thorough. Students cannot rely on a simple recitation of facts. They must

appreciate the inquiry process and be receptive to the learning process.

Evidence. See Kuzma et al. (2019); Makhene (2019); Seibert (2022); and Yip (2021).

Reflection and Journal Writing

Through this strategy, students detail personal experiences and connect them to learning outcomes. The most frequent use of reflection is through journal writing which serves to connect classroom theories and curriculum objectives to actual practice situations. The purpose of reflection and journal writing is to encourage students to contemplate clinical experiences and critically consider what happened, what was learned, and how to improve upon practice in the future. Oral and written reflections are equally as effective in helping students gain insight. This strategy may be completed online and is suited for group, peer, or interprofessional learning assignments and across all levels of education including graduate students (Guo, 2022).

Teaching tips. Set clear expectations for journal writing so that students know what is expected. Using different approaches to journal writing (e.g., writing learning objectives, summary of the experience, a diary, and focused argument) may increase student interest in the assignment. Thoughtful feedback (not necessarily lengthy feedback) from the teacher is important to student learning. Group discussions about the journals and what students are saying may increase learning for all students. Using specific thought-provoking questions in the journal enhances metacognitive thinking. Students may need to be taught how to conduct reflective exercises. Reflective journals are most often not graded with a letter grade. If so, grading rubrics will set clear expectations and provide guidelines for grading uniformly.

Advantages. Reflection promotes learning from experiences and helps students learn how to transfer facts from one setting to another. It encourages students to consider clinical experiences relative to didactic course content. Student-centered learning is especially valuable to adult learners. Reflection is helpful in demonstrating how to become a lifelong learner. It stimulates metacognitive thinking and provides a feedback loop between faculty and the student so that teaching emphasis can be adapted to enhance student learning. It can be used for all levels of nursing education.

Disadvantages. Educators may want to revert to the expert role rather than concentrating on the students' experiences; student-directed learning may frustrate some teachers and may stimulate unresolved conflict within some students. Faculty need to direct student learning through questioning and discussion that may cover topics for which they are not prepared. Students may see it as only a required exercise and not take the time to make appropriate use of the learning opportunity. There is a high time cost for faculty to construct reflection guidelines, read student reflections, and help individual students process their reflections; there is a high time cost for students to complete reflections.

Evidence. See Bjerkvik and Hilli (2019); Greenleaf Brown et al. (2022); Guo (2022); and Smith (2021).

CHAPTER SUMMARY: KEY POINTS

- In the teaching-learning process, faculty have responsibility for choosing appropriate strategies and learning activities, while the student has responsibilities to prepare, engage in, and use study skills that ensure their ability to provide safe patient care.
- Effective teaching emphasizes the importance of both faculty preparation for and student involvement in classroom experiences.
- Evidence for effective teaching has grown exponentially over the past decade, especially within nursing education.
- Evidence for effective teaching strategies across undergraduate and graduate students, as well as practicing nurses, is designated to offer faculty insight for effective selection and use.
- Bloom's revised knowledge dimensions (factual, conceptual, procedural, and metacognitive) guide nurse educators in selecting the best strategy for preparing graduates at all levels to safely practice in today's health care system.
- The major advantages of various teaching strategies is heightened faculty awareness of predicted successes and expected learning mastery.
- Taking into account the known disadvantages of specific teaching strategies can help faculty offset unintended or unsuccessful outcomes.

REFLECTING ON THE EVIDENCE

1. Foundational work about teaching and learning has often been derived from work in other disciplines such as education, psychology, and sociology. How might nurse educators build upon these studies?
2. How can nurse educators use research and evidence-based practice processes to transform nursing education while improving student learning outcomes?
3. Of the teaching strategies presented, which ones intrigue you the most as far as developing engaging classroom experiences for factual knowledge, conceptual knowledge, procedural knowledge, and metacognition? Which fit with your teaching "style"? Your level of confidence? Your students' needs?
4. How would you align teaching and learning strategies with the cognitive domains?
5. How would you integrate some of the learning/study strategies into a course or into the program curriculum?
6. What teaching strategies might you use to enable students to attain learning outcomes at the program, course, and lesson levels and to attain programmatic clinical competencies?
7. What additional evidence is needed for a strategy that you are considering using with a group of students?

REFERENCES

Agarwal, P. K., Nunes, L. D., & Blunt, J. R. (2021). Retrieval practice consistently benefits student learning: A systematic review of applied research in schools and classrooms. *Educational Psychology Review, 33*(4), 1409–1453.

Alberti, S., Motta, P., Ferri, P., & Bonetti, L. (2021). The effectiveness of team-based learning in nursing education: A systematic review. *Nurse Education Today, 97*, 104721.

Alfayoumi, I. (2019). The impact of combined concept-based learning and concept mapping pedagogies on nursing students' clinical reasoning abilities. *Nurse Education Today, 72*, 40–46. https://doi.org/10.1016/j.nedt.2018.10.009.

Al-Jubouri, M. B. (2021). Debate as a teaching strategy in nursing. *The Journal of Continuing Education in Nursing, 52*(6), 263–265.

Allert, C., Dellkvist, H., Hjelm, M., & Andersson, E. K. (2022). Nursing students' experiences of applying problem-based learning to train the core competence teamwork and collaboration: An interview study. *Nursing Open, 9*(1), 569–577.

Anderson, L. W., & Krathwohl, D. R. (2001). *A taxonomy for learning, teaching, and assessing: A revision of Bloom's taxonomy of educational objectives.* Longman.

Anderson, L. W., & Krathwohl, D. R. (Eds.). (2016). *A taxonomy for learning, teaching, and assessing: A revision of Bloom's taxonomy of educational objectives.* Longman.

Amir, S., Mehboob, U., Sethi, A., & Jamil, B. (2022). Problem-based learning: An overview of its process and impact on learning. *Pakistan. Journal of Physiology, 18*(1), 68–69.

Arends, R., & Callies, D. (2022). Dissemination enhancement in Doctor of Nursing Practice students. *Journal of Professional Nursing, 40*, 34–37.

Association of American Colleges & Universities (2021). High impact educational practices: What they are, who has access to them, and why they matte. *14*(3), 28–29. https://www.aacu.org/node/4084

Bartsch, L. M., & Oberauer, K. (2021). The effects of elaboration on working memory and long-term memory across age. *Journal of Memory and Language, 118*, 104215.

Bjerkvik, L. K., & Hilli, Y. (2019). Reflective writing in undergraduate clinical nursing education: A literature review. *Nurse Education in Practice, 35*, 32–41.

Bodrožić-Brnić, K., & Thiessen, T. (Eds.). (2022). Digitalization as a challenge for mindful leadership: *Mindful leadership in practice* (pp. 147–158). Springer.

Bristol, T., Hagler, D., McMillian-Bohler, J., Wermers, R., Hatch, D., & Oermann, M. H. (2019). Nurse educators' use of lecture and active learning. *Teaching and Learning in Nursing, 14*(2), 94–96.

Brod, G. (2021). Predicting as a learning strategy. *Psychonomic Bulletin & Review, 28*, 1839–1847. https://doi.org/10.3758/s13423-021-01904-1

Brown, P., Roediger, H., McDaniel, M., & Stick, M. I. (2014). *The science of successful learning.* The Belknap Press of Harvard University Press.

Brunmair, M., & Richter, T. (2019). Similarity matters: A meta-analysis of interleaved learning and its moderators. *Psychological Bulletin, 145*(11), 1029.

Burt, L. (2021). *Self-explanation use in nurse practitioner student diagnostic reasoning* [Doctoral dissertation, University of Illinois at Chicago]. Proquest.

Burt, L., Finnegan, L., Schwartz, A., Corte, C., Quinn, L., Clark, L., & Corbridge, S. (2021). Diagnostic reasoning: Relationships among expertise, accuracy, and ways that nurse practitioner students self-explain. *Diagnosis (Berlin, Germany), 9*(1), 50–58. https://doi.org/10.1515/dx-2020-0137.

Cabalsa, M., Samuel, V., Llaguno, M. B., & Mary Beth, M. R. (2022). Digital gamification: An innovative pedagogy for anatomy and physiology course among digital natives-nursing students. *Assiut Scientific Nursing Journal, 10*(28), 10–20.

Cariñanos-Ayala, S., Arrue, M., Zarandona, J., & Labaka, A. (2021). The use of structured debate as a teaching strategy among undergraduate nursing students: A systematic review. *Nurse Education Today, 98*, 104766. https://doi.org/10.1016/j.nedt.2021.104766.

Carter, H., & Townsend, D. R. (2022). A rationale for integrating writing into secondary content area classrooms: Perspectives from teachers who experience the benefits of integrating writing frequently. *Journal of Writing Research, 13*(3), 329–365.

Casler, K. (2022). Escape passive learning: 10 steps to Building an Escape Room. *The Journal for Nurse Practitioners, 18*(5), 569–574.

Cerezo, E., Aguelo, A., Coma-Roselló, T., Gallardo, J., & Garrido, M. A. (2022). Working attention, planning and social skills through pervasive games in interactive spaces. *IEEE Transactions on Learning Technologies, 15*(1), 119–136. https://doi.org/10.1109/TLT.2022.3155993.

Chen, O., Paas, F., & Sweller, J. (2021). Spacing and interleaving effects require distinct theoretical bases: A systematic review testing the cognitive load and discriminative-contrast hypotheses. *Educational Psychology Review, 33*(4), 1499–1522.

Chen, X., Zhang, B., Jin, S. X., Quan, Y. X., Zhang, X. W., & Cui, X. S. (2021). The effects of mindfulness-based interventions on nursing students: A meta-analysis. *Nurse Education Today, 98*, 104718.

Choi, J. A., Kim, O., Park, S., Lim, H., & Kim, J. H. (2021). The effectiveness of peer learning in undergraduate nursing students: A meta-analysis. *Clinical Simulation in. Nursing, 50*, 92–101.

Choi, S., Slaubaugh, M., & Tian, X. (2021). Integrating learning interpersonal skills through team-based learning (TBL) in a management course. *Journal of Education for Business, 96*(8), 498–509.

Church, F. C. (2021). Active learning: Basic science workshops, clinical science cases, and medical role-playing in an undergraduate biology course. *Education Sciences, 11*(8), 370.

Conelius, J., & Iannino-Renz, R. (2021). Incorporating a mindfulness program in a graduate family nurse practitioner program. *Journal of Holistic Nursing, 39*(4), 369–372.

Considine, J., Berry, D., Allen, J., Hewitt, N., Oldland, E., Sprogis, S. K., & Currey, J. (2021). Team-based learning in nursing education: A scoping review. *Journal of Clinical Nursing, 30*(7–8), 903–917.

Cornell University. (2022). *Examples of collaborative learning or group work activities*. Resource Library. https://teaching.cornell.edu/resource/examples-collaborative-learning-or-group-work-activities

Corwin Visible Learning Meta. (2021). *Spaced vs. mass practice*. https://www.visiblelearningmetax.com/influences/view/spaced_vs._mass_practice

Curators of the University of Missouri. (2021). *Cooperative learning strategies*. https://sites.google.com/a/emints.org/cooperative-learning-strategies/page2?authuser=0

Cusanno, B. R., Davidson, L. G., & Ketheeswaran, N. (2022). Fostering vulnerability, making brave spaces, and transforming worlds in 55 words: Writing 55-word stories for healthcare teaching, research, and practice. *Imagining new normals. Brave space-making through storytelling*, 319–348. https://www.researchgate.net/publication/358078995_Fostering_vulnerability_making_brave_spaces_and_transforming_worlds_in_55_words_Writing_55-word_stories_for_healthcare_teaching_research_and_practice/citation/download.

Cust, F. (2018). Increasing confidence of first-year student nurses with peer mentoring. *Nursing Times [online], 114*(10), 51–53. https://eprints.staffs.ac.uk/5520/.

de Bono, E. (1985). *Six thinking hats*. Penguin Books.

Dabbagh, A., Abtahi, D., Aghamohammadi, H., Ahmadizadeh, S. N., & Ardehali, S. H. (2020). Relationship between "simulated patient scenarios and role-playing" method and OSCE performance in senior anesthesiology residents: A correlation assessment study. *Anesthesiology and Pain Medicine, 10*(5), e106640. https://doi.org/10.5812/aapm.106640

Demir, B., & Sönmez, G. (2021). Generation Z students' expectations from English language instruction. *Journal of Language and Linguistic. Studies, 17*(1), 683–701.

Dodson, T. M., & Ferdig, R. E. (2021). Understanding nursing student choice in completion of presimulation activities. *Clinical Simulation in. Nursing, 59*, 52–60.

Dorri, S., Ashghali Farahani, M., Maserat, E., & Haghani, H. (2020). Comparison of role play and conventional training methods on long-term learning of nursing students. *Development Strategies in Medical Education, 7*(1), 61–77.

Epstein, I., Stephens, L., Severino, S. M., Khanlou, N., Mack, T., Barker, D., & Dadashi, N. (2020). "Ask me what I need": A call for shifting responsibility upwards and creating inclusive learning environments in clinical placement. *Nurse Education Today, 92*, 104505.

Evans, L., Bosch, M. L. V., Harrington, S., Schoofs, N., & Coviak, C. (2019). Flipping the classroom in health care higher education: A systematic review. *Nurse Educator, 44*(2), 74–78.

Ferguson, C., Hickman, L. D., Phillips, J., Newton, P. J., Inglis, S. C., Lam, L., & Bajorek, B. V. (2019). An mHealth intervention to improve nurses' atrial fibrillation and anticoagulation knowledge and practice: The EVICOAG study. *European Journal of Cardiovascular Nursing, 18*(1), 7–15.

Fletcher, K. A., Hicks, V. L., Johnson, R. H., Laverentz, D. M., Phillips, C. J., Pierce, L. N., Wilhoite, D. L., & Gay, J. E. (2019). A concept analysis of conceptual learning: A guide for educators. *Journal of Nursing Education, 58*(1), 7–15.

Fusco, N. M., Foltz-Ramos, K., & Ohtake, P. J. (2022). An interprofessional escape room experience to improve knowledge and collaboration among health professions students. *American Journal of Pharmaceutical Education, 86*(9), ajpe8823. https://doi.org/10.5688/ajpe8823.

Gallardo, J., López, C., Aguelo, A., Cebrián, B., Coma, T., & Cerezo, E. (2019). Development of a pervasive game for ADHD children. In A. Brooks, E. Brooks, & C. Sylla (Eds.), *Interactivity, Game Creation, Design, Learning, and Innovation*. Lecture Notes of the Institute for Computer Sciences, Social Informatics and Telecommunications Engineering (Vol. 265). Springer. https://doi.org/10.1007/978-3-030-06134-0_56.

Gallegos, C., & Nakashima, H. (2018). Mobile devices: A distraction, or a useful tool to engage nursing students? *Journal of Nursing Education*, 57(3), 170–173.

Garrison, C. M., Ritter, F. E., Bauchwitz, B. R., Niehaus, J., & Weyhrauch, P. W. (2021). A computer-based tutor to teach nursing trauma care that works as an adjunct to high-fidelity simulation. *CIN: Computers, Informatics, Nursing*, 39(2), 63–68.

Garwood, J. K., Ahmed, A. H., & McComb, S. A. (2018). The effect of concept maps on undergraduate nursing students' critical thinking. *Nursing Education Perspectives*, 39(4), 208–214.

Giddens, J. F. (2019). *Concepts for nursing practice E-Book*. Elsevier Health Sciences.

Glendon, K., & Ulrich, D. (1997). Unfolding cases: An experiential learning model. *Nurse Educator*, 22(4), 15–18.

Gómez-Urquiza, J. L., Gómez-Salgado, J., Albendín-García, L., Correa-Rodríguez, M., González-Jiménez, E., & Cañadas-De la Fuente, G. A. (2019). The impact on nursing students' opinions and motivation of using a "Nursing Escape Room" as a teaching game: A descriptive study. *Nurse Education Today*, 72, 73–76.

Goolsarran, N., Hamo, C. E., & Lu, W. H. (2020). Using the Jigsaw technique to teach patient safety. *Medical Education Online*, 25(1), 1710325.

Graber, M. L., Rencic, J., Rusz, D., Papa, F., Croskerry, P., Zierler, B., Harkless, G., Giuliano, M., Schoenbaum, S., Colford, C., Cahill, M., & Olson, A. P. J. (2018). Improving diagnosis by improving education: A policy brief on education in healthcare professions. *Diagnosis*, 5(3), 107–118.

Greenleaf Brown, L., Briscoe, G. S., & Grabowsky, A. (2022). The influence of journaling on nursing students: A systematic review. *Journal of Nursing Education*, 61(1), 29–35.

Gregory, L. R., Ramjan, L. M., Villarosa, A. R., Rojo, J., Raymond, D., & Salamonson, Y. (2022). Does self-efficacy for medication administration predict clinical skill performance in first-year nursing students? An inception-cohort study. *Teaching and Learning in Nursing*, 17(1), 77–83.

Griffith, P. B., Doherty, C., Smeltzer, S. C., & Mariani, B. (2021). Education initiatives in cognitive debiasing to improve diagnostic accuracy in student providers: A scoping review. *Journal of the American Association of Nurse Practitioners*, 33(11), 862–871.

Guo, L. (2022). How should reflection be supported in higher education? A meta-analysis of reflection interventions. *Reflective Practice*, 23(1), 118–146.

Gutierrez de Blume, A. P. (2022). Calibrating calibration: A meta-analysis of learning strategy instruction interventions to improve metacognitive monitoring accuracy. *Journal of Educational Psychology*, 114(4), 681–700.

Halstead, J. (2019). *NLN core competencies for nurse educators: A decade of influence*. National League for Nursing.

Hanover Research (2017, April). *Best practices in education equity*. https://www.wasa-oly.org/WASA/images/WASA/1.0%20Who%20We%20Are/1.4.1.6%20SIRS/Download_Files/LI%202017/May%2019%20-%20Best%20Practices%20in%20Educational%20Equity.pdf

Harlan, M. D., Rosenzweig, M. Q., & Hoffmann, R. L. (2021). Preferred teaching/learning strategies for graduate nursing students in web-enhanced courses. *Dimensions of Critical Care. Nursing*, 40(3), 149–155.

Harris, N., & Bacon, C. E. W. (2019). Developing cognitive skills through active learning: A systematic review of health care professions. *Athletic Training Education Journal*, 14(2), 135–148.

Hasanica, N., Ramic-Catak, A., Mujezinovic, A., Begagic, S., Galijasevic, K., & Oruc, M. (2020). The effectiveness of leaflets and posters as a health education method. *Materia Socio-Medica*, 32(2), 135.

Hattie, J.A. (2018). *Backup of Hattie's ranking list of 256 influences and effect sizes related to student achievement*. www.visiblelearningplus.com/content/250-influences-student-achievement

Heale, R., & Twycross, A. (2018). What is a case study? *Evidence-Based. Nursing*, 21(1), 7–8.

Herrman, J. W. (2019). *Creative teaching strategies for the nurse educator* (3rd ed.). FA Davis.

Higher Learning Commission (2022). *Criteria for accreditation*. https://www.hlcommission.org/Policies/criteria-and-core-components.html

Hoogerheide, V., Staal, J., Schaap, L., & van Gog, T. (2019). Effects of study intention and generating multiple choice questions on expository text retention. *Learning and Instruction*, 60, 191–198.

Huang, T. H., Liu, F., Chen, L. C., & Tsai, C. C. (2021). The acceptance and impact of Google Classroom integrating into a clinical pathology course for nursing students: A technology acceptance model approach. *PLoS One*, 16(3), e0247819.

Hughes, M., Kenmir, A., Innis, J., O'Connell, J., & Henry, K. (2020). Exploring the transitional experience of first-year undergraduate nursing students. *Journal of Nursing Education*, 59(5), 263–268.

Hurst, N. B., Grossart, E. A., Knapp, S., Stolz, U., Groke, S. F., Solem, C. R., & Walter, F. G. (2022). Do mnemonics help healthcare professionals learn and recall cholinergic toxidromes? *Clinical Toxicology*, 1–3.

Ibrahim, M. E., Al-Shahrani, A. M., Abdalla, M. E., Abubaker, I. M., & Mohamed, M. E. (2018). The effectiveness of problem-based learning in acquisition of knowledge, soft skills during basic and preclinical sciences: Medical students' points of view. *Acta Inform Medica*, 26(2), 119–124.

Immekus, J. C. (2019). Flipping statistics courses in graduate education: Integration of cognitive psychology and technology. *Journal of Statistics Education*, 27(2), 79–89.

Ironside, P., & McNelis, A. (2009). *Clinical education in prelicensure nursing programs: Results from an NLN national survey*. National League for Nursing.

Iverson, L., Connelly, S., & Potthoff, M. (2018). Teaching About zebras. *Journal of Nursing Education*, 57(2). 126–126.

Jamshidi, H., Parizad, N., & Hemmati Maslakpak, M. (2021). Problem-based learning; a new pathway towards improving patient safety-based communication skills in nursing students. *Journal of Preventative Epidemiology*, 6(2), e25.

Janssens, O., Haerens, L., Valcke, M., Beeckman, D., Pype, P., & Embo, M. (2022). The role of ePortfolios in supporting learning in eight healthcare disciplines: A scoping review. *Nurse Education in Practice*, 103418.

Jefferies, D., McNally, S., Roberts, K., Wallace, A., Stunden, A., D'Souza, S., & Glew, P. (2018). The importance of academic literacy for undergraduate nursing students and its relationship to future professional clinical practice: A systematic review. *Nurse Education Today*, 60, 84–91.

Johnson, D.W., & Johnson, R.T. (2018). Cooperative learning: The foundation for active learning. In S. Brito (Ed.), (2019). *Active learning—Beyond the future* (pp. 59–70). IntechOpen.

Joshi, T., Budhathoki, P., Adhikari, A., Poudel, A., Raut, S., & Shrestha, D. B. (2022). Team-based learning among health care professionals: A systematic review. *Cureus*, 14(1), e21252. https://doi.org/10.7759/cureus.21252

Jowsey, T., Foster, G., Cooper-Ioelu, P., & Jacobs, S. (2020). Blended learning via distance in pre-registration nursing education: A scoping review. *Nurse Education in Practice*, 44, 102775.

Kaddoura, M., VanDyke, O., Cheng, B., & Shea-Foisy, K. (2016). Impact of concept mapping on the development of clinical judgment skills in nursing students. *Teaching and Learning in Nursing*, 11, 101–107. https://doi.org/10.1016/j.teln.2016.02.001.

Kamaliah, N. (2018). Use of the three-step interview technique in teaching ESL speaking. *English Education Journal*, 9(1), 82–101.

Karikari-Martin, P., Zapata, D., Hesgrove, B., Murray, C. B., & Kauffman, K. (2021). Academic–service partnerships: Increasing the advanced nurse workforce. *Journal of Nursing Education*, 60(4), 190–195.

King, T. S. (2020). Using QR codes on professional posters to increase engagement and understanding. *Nurse Educator*, 45(4), 219.

Kinzie, J. (2017). The use of student engagement findings as a case of evidence-based practice. *New Directions for Higher Education*, 2017(178), 47–56. https://doi.org/10.1002/he.20233.

Kuh, G.D., & Kinzie, J. (2018). What really makes a "high-impact" practice high-impact? Inside Higher Education. https://www.insidehighered.com/views/2018/05/01/kuh-and-kinzie-respond-essay-questioning-high-impact-practices-opinion

Kuzma, E. K., Graziano, C., Shea, E., Schaller, F. V., Jr, Pardee, M., & Darling-Fisher, C. S. (2019). Improving lesbian, gay, bisexual, transgender, and queer/questioning health: Using a standardized patient experience to educate advanced practice nursing students. *Journal of the American Association of Nurse Practitioners*, 31(12), 714–722.

Latimier, A., Peyre, H., & Ramus, F. (2021). A meta-analytic review of the benefit of spacing out retrieval practice episodes on retention. *Educational Psychology Review*, 33(3), 959–987.

Lee, S.K., & Sanders, S.T. (2020). *Best practices in undergraduate nursing education: Concept-based curriculum*. Sigma Theta Tau Repository. https://sigma.nursingrepository.org/bitstream/handle/10755/21165/SKLee_Abstract.pdf?sequence=2

Leyland, A., Rowse, G., & Emerson, L. M. (2019). Experimental effects of mindfulness inductions on self-regulation: Systematic review and meta-analysis. *Emotion*, 19(1), 108.

Liang, H. Y., Tang, F. I., Wang, T. F., & Yu, S. (2021). Evaluation of nurse practitioners' professional competence and comparison of assessments using multiple methods: Self-assessment, peer assessment, and supervisor assessment. *Asian Nursing Research*, 15(1), 30–36.

Mahaffey, A. L. (2020). Mock urinalysis demonstration: Making connections among acid–base chemistry, redox reactions, and healthcare in an undergraduate nursing course. *Journal of Chemical Education*, 97(7), 1976–1983.

Maheshwari, S. K., & Kaur, P. (2019). Mnemonics and nursing. *International Journal of Nursing Science Practice and Research*, 5(2), 19–25.

Makhene, A. (2019). The use of the Socratic inquiry to facilitate critical thinking in nursing education. *Health SA Gesondheid*, 24. https://doi.org/10.4102/hsag.v24i0.1224.

Markowski, M., Bower, H., Essex, R., & Yearley, C. (2021). Peer learning and collaborative placement models in health care: A systematic review and qualitative synthesis of the literature. *Journal of Clinical Nursing*, 30(11–12), 1519–1541.

McClure, N., & Brame, C. (2020). Asthma medications: A think-pair-share-square activity for nursing students. *Nurse Educator*, 45(1), 16.

McConnell, D. A., et al. (2017). Instructional utility and learning efficacy of common active learning strategies. *Journal of Geoscience Education*, 65, 604–625.

McEnroe-Petitte, D., & Farris, C. (2020). Using gaming as an active teaching strategy in nursing education. *Teaching and Learning in Nursing*, 15(1), 61–65.

Menon, S. S., Wischgoll, T., Farra, S., & Holland, C. (2021). Using augmented reality to enhance nursing education. *Electronic Imaging*, 2021(1), 304.

Michaelson, L. K., Parmelee, D. X., McMahon, K. K., & Levine, R. E. (2008). *Team-based learning for health professions education: A guide to using small groups for improving learning*. Stylus.

Mollahadi, M., Khademolhoseini, S. M., Mokhtari-Nouri, J., & Khaghanizadeh, M. (2018). The portfolio as a tool for mentoring in nursing students: A scoping review. *Iranian Journal of Nursing and Midwifery Research*, 23(4), 241.

Morgan, R. (2019). Using seminars as a teaching method in undergraduate nurse education. *British Journal of Nursing*, 28(6), 374–376.

Morsy, A. A. I., & Darweesh, H. A. M. (2021). Effect of six hats thinking technique on development of critical thinking disposition and problem-solving skills of nursing students. *American Journal of Nursing*, 9(1), 8–14.

Nasim, A., Ghani, M., Kausar, S., & Khatoon, K. (2022). Effectiveness of problem-based learning in developing knowledge of undergraduate nursing students. *Annals of King Edward Medical University*, 28(1), 19–25.

National Survey of Student Engagement (NSSE). (2016). *NSSE annual results2016: Engagement insights: Survey findings on the quality of undergraduate education*. http://nsse.indiana.edu/html/annual_results.cfm

National Survey of Student Engagement (NSSE). (2017). *NSSE annual results2017: Engagement insights: Survey findings on the quality of undergraduate education*. https://scholarworks.iu.edu/dspace/handle/2022/23392

National Survey of Student Engagement (NSSE). (2018). *NSSE annual results2018: Engagement insights: Survey findings on the quality of undergraduate education*. https://scholarworks.iu.edu/dspace/handle/2022/23391

National Survey of Student Engagement (NSSE). (2019). *NSSE annual results2019: Engagement insights: Survey findings on the quality of undergraduate education*. https://scholarworks.iu.edu/dspace/handle/2022/25321

National Survey of Student Engagement (NSSE). (2020). *Overview*. https://nsse.indiana.edu/nsse/reports-data/nsse-overview.html

Nemec, R., Brower, E., & Allert, J. (2021). A guide to implementing role-play in the nursing classroom. *Nursing Education Perspectives*, 42(6), E163–E164.

Ng, P., Kranz, K., Abeles, R., Schwartz, D., & Lane, S. (2020). Using the Jigsaw teaching method to enhance internal medicine residents' knowledge and attitudes in managing geriatric women's health. *MedEdPORTAL*, 16, 11003. https://www.mededportal.org/doi/10.15766/mep_2374-8265.11003.

Ogilvie, J. M. (2019). The mysterious case of Patient X: A case study for neuroscience students. *Journal of Undergraduate Neuroscience Education*, 18(1), C1.

Ohio State University Veterinary Program, (n.d.). *10 learning strategies for rotations and courses*. https://otl.vet.ohio-state.edu/node/203

Ong, K. Y., Ng, C. W., Tan, N. C., & Tan, K. (2022). Differential effects of team-based learning on clinical reasoning. *The Clinical Teacher*, 19(1), 17–23.

Oruche, U. M., Moorman, M., deRose, B., Berlanga King, G., & Antisdel, J. A. (2022). Preparing nurse practitioner students to recognize health inequities and global health issues. *Indiana University Perdue University Indianapolis ScholarWorks Repository* https://scholarworks.iupui.edu/handle/1805/28422.

Pålsson, Y., Mårtensson, G., Swenne, C. L., Mogensen, E., & Engström, M. (2021). First-year nursing students' collaboration using peer learning during clinical practice education: An observational study. *Nurse Education in Practice*, 50, 102946.

Park, J. H., & Park, M. H. (2022). Effects of core fundamental nursing skills practical education based on problem-based learning. *The Korean Data & Information Science Society*, 33(2), 269–281.

Phillips, C. J., & Ford, K. (2021). The next gen pharmacology classroom: A quality improvement approach to transformation. *Teaching and Learning in Nursing, 16*(4), 379–383.

Pike, N. A., Kinsler, J. J., Peterson, J. K., Verzemnieks, I., Lauridsen, L., Love-Bibbero, L., & Ramos-Gomez, F. (2022). Improved oral health knowledge in a primary care pediatric nurse practitioner program. *Journal of the American Association of Nurse Practitioners, 34*(5), 755–762.

Pleshkan, V., & Boykins, A. D. (2022). Cognitive preceptorship: An emerging nurse practitioner role transition to practice model. *Journal of Professional Nursing, 39,* 194–205.

Pront, L., Müller, A., Koschade, A., & Hutton, A. (2018). Gaming in nursing education: A literature review. *Nursing Education Perspectives, 39*(1), 23–28.

Putri, S. T., & Sumartini, S. (2021). Integrating peer learning activities and problem-based learning in clinical nursing education. *SAGE Open Nursing, 7* 23779608211000262.

Quizlet (2022). *Home.* https://quizlet.com/

Rao, B. J. (2019). Innovative teaching pedagogy in nursing education. *International Journal of Nursing Education, 11*(4).

Reed, J. M. (2020). Gaming in nursing education: Recent trends and future paths. *Journal of Nursing Education, 59*(7), 375–381.

Robertson, B., & Disch, J. (2021). Improving quality and safety with transition-to-practice programs. In G. Sherwood, & J. Barnsteiner (Eds.). *Quality and Safety in Nursing: A Competency Approach to Improving Outcomes* (3rd ed., p. 560). Wiley-Blackwell.

Robertson, D. A., Padesky, L. B., & Brock, C. H. (2020). Cultivating student agency through teachers' professional learning. *Theory Into Practice, 59*(2), 192–201.

Rowe, N. (2017). Tracing the "grey literature" of poster presentations: A mapping review. Health *Information and Libraries. Journal, 31*(2), 106–124. https://doi.org/10.1111/hir.12177.

Sabet, R., Geckil, E., & Semra, K. (2022). Electronic-portfolio: A tool for nursing students' evaluation. *Genel Sağlık Bilimleri Dergisi, 4*(1), 62–67.

Saeedi, M., Ghafouri, R., Tehrani, F. J., & Abedini, Z. (2021). The effects of teaching methods on academic motivation in nursing students: A systematic review. *Journal of Education and Health Promotion, 10,* 271. https://doi.org/10.4103/jehp.jehp_1070_20

Sanaie, N., Vasli, P., Sedighi, L., & Sadeghi, B. (2019). Comparing the effect of lecture and Jigsaw teaching strategies on the nursing students' self-regulated

learning and academic motivation: A quasi-experimental study. *Nurse Education Today, 79,* 35–40.

Sarker, U., Kanuka, H., Norris, C., Raymond, C., Yonge, O., & Davidson, S. (2021). Gamification in nursing literature: An integrative review. *International Journal of Nursing Education Scholarship, 18*(1), 20200081. https://doi.org/10.1515/ijnes-2020-0081

Sartain, A. F., Welch, T. D., & Strickland, H. P. (2021). Utilizing nursing students for a complex role-play simulation. *Clinical Simulation in. Nursing, 60,* 74–77.

Scheel, L. S., Bydam, J., & Peters, M. D. (2021). Reflection as a learning strategy for the training of nurses in clinical practice setting: A scoping review. *JBI Evidence Synthesis, 19*(12), 3268–3300.

Seckman, C., & Van de Castle, B. (2021). Understanding digital health technologies using mind maps. *Journal of Nursing Scholarship, 53*(1), 7–15.

Seibert, S. A. (2022). Validated instructional resource to engage nursing students in critical thinking. *Teaching and Learning in. Nursing, 17*(3), 263–266.

Sherwood, G., & Barnsteiner, J. (Eds.). (2021). *Quality and safety in nursing: A competency approach to improving outcomes.* John Wiley & Sons.

Silva, H., Lopes, J., Dominguez, C., & Morais, E. (2022). Lecture, cooperative learning and concept mapping: Any differences on critical and creative thinking development? *International Journal of Instruction, 15*(1), 765–780.

Smith, T. (2021, April). Guided reflective writing as a teaching strategy to develop nursing student clinical judgment. *Nursing Forum, 56*(2), 241–248.

Soneru, C. (2021). Fostering resilience during COVID-19 epidemic through reflection and writing. *ASA Monitor, 85*(5), 13.

Soroush, A., Andaieshgar, B., Vahdat, A., & Khatony, A. (2021). The characteristics of an effective clinical instructor from the perspective of nursing students: A qualitative descriptive study in Iran. *BMC nursing, 20*(1), 1–9.

Stevens, T. E. (2019). Just one more thing: Getting the most out of one-minute papers. *Pennsylvania Libraries: Research & Practice, 7*(1), 38–45.

Sullivan, J. M. (2022). Flipping the classroom: An innovative approach to graduate nursing education. *Journal of Professional Nursing, 38,* 40–44.

Tennyson, C. D., Smallheer, B. A., & De Gagne, J. C. (2022). Microlearning strategies in nurse practitioner education. *Nurse Educator, 47*(1), 2–3.

Thelen, M. (2022). Medication competence: a concept analysis. *Nurse Education Today, 111,* 105292.

Torres, E. R., Williams, P. R., Kassahun-Yimer, W., & Gordy, X. Z. (2022). Crossword puzzles and knowledge retention. *Journal of Effective Teaching in Higher Education, 5*(1), 18–29.

Tsimane, T. A., & Downing, C. (2020). A model to facilitate transformative learning in nursing education. *International Journal of Nursing Sciences, 7*(3), 269–276.

Tornwall, J., & McDaniel, J. (2022). Key strategies in scholarly writing instruction for doctor of nursing practice students: A Q-methodology study. *Nurse Education Today, 108,* 105192.

van Peppen, L. M., Verkoeijen, P. P., Heijltjes, A., Janssen, E., & van Gog, T. (2021). Repeated retrieval practice to foster students' critical thinking skills. *Collabra: Psychology, 7*(1), 28881.

Veldkamp, A., van de Grint, L., Knippels, M. C. P., & van Joolingen, W. R. (2020). Escape education: A systematic review on escape rooms in education. *Educational Research Review, 31,* 100364.

Vos, J. (2018). *Meaning in life: An evidence-based handbook for practitioners.* Bloomsbury Publishing.

Welch, T. D., & Parker, K. (2020). Complex conversations: Tips, tools, and strategies. *Nursing Management, 51*(7), 11–13.

Weiss, J. A. (2018). Creative gaming: A new approach to engage students in pathophysiology. *The Journal for Nurse Practitioners, 14*(9), e177–e183.

Wessling, S. B. (2019). Conver-stations: A discussion strategy. *Teaching Channel.* https://www.teachingchannel.org/video/conver-stations-strategy.

White, B. J., & Lansom, K. S. (2017). The evolution of a writing program. *Journal of Nursing Education, 56*(7), 443–445. https://doi.org/10.3928/01484834-20170619-11.

Windle, S., Berger, S., & Kim, J. E. E. (2021). Teaching guided imagery and relaxation techniques in undergraduate nursing education. *Journal of Holistic. Nursing, 39*(2), 199–206.

World's Database of Medical Mnemonics, 2022. *About.* http://www.medicalmnemonics.com/cgi-bin/about.cfm

Wu, H. Z., & Wu, Q. T. (2020). Impact of mind mapping on the critical thinking ability of clinical nursing students and teaching application. *Journal of International Medical Research, 48*(3). 0300060519893225.

Xu, Y., Lau, Y., Cheng, L. J., & Lau, S. T. (2021). Learning experiences of game-based educational intervention in nursing students: A systematic mixed-studies review. *Nurse Education Today, 107,* 105139.

Yip, Y. C. (2021). Using Socratic inquiry to enhance critical thinking in nursing students. *Nursing2021, 51*(11), 13–16.

Zawadzka, K., & Hanczakowski, M. (2020). Knowing more or thinking that you know more? Context-dependent illusions of knowing. In A. M. Cleary & B. L. Schwartz (Eds.), Memory quirks: The study of odd phenomena in memory (pp. 175–189). Routledge.

Zhang, J., & Chen, B. (2021). The effect of cooperative learning on critical thinking of nursing students in clinical practicum: A quasi-experimental study. *Journal of Professional Nursing, 37*(1), 177–183.

Zou, P., Visayanathan, A., Whyte, C., Pak, A., Brathwaite, A. C., Zhu, Q., & Vanderlee, R. (2019). Successful vs. unsuccessful small group reflection: A narrative inquiry. *Journal of Nursing Education and Practice, 9*(5), 6. https://doi.org/10.5430/jnep.v9n5p6

Zwart, D. P., Goei, S. L., Noroozi, O., & Van Luit, J. E. (2021). The effects of computer-based virtual learning environments on nursing students' mathematical learning in medication processes. *Research and Practice in Technology Enhanced Learning, 16*(1), 1–21.

17

Multicultural Education in Nursing

Carolina G. Huerta, EdD, RN, FAAN

The United States has witnessed a time of historic change these past 5 years in terms of diversity, equity, and inclusion of minority groups and marginalized populations. The steady influx of thousands of immigrants crossing the Southern border and the relocation of many refugees that may eventually become legal US citizens will impact the economy, society, and most definitely, our educational systems. The deaths of George Floyd and Ahmaud Arbery are among several racially charged events that have led to the Black Lives Matter Movement and have also brought attention to the inequities that have existed for decades among racial and ethnic groups. As a consequence of the increased focus on racial inequities, it is now evident that there is a need for diversity in all aspects of our teaching, scholarship, and practice (Villarruel & Broome, 2020). The increased emphasis on diversity, equity, and inclusion has resulted in more racially and ethnically diverse student bodies that demand that nursing faculty demonstrate the ability to articulate and promote teaching practices that guide the success of students who are diverse (Zambrana et al., 2020). In order to produce diverse nurses, nursing education must first acknowledge that racist structures may be prevalent within nursing education and act to dismantle intrinsically embedded racism in schools of nursing (SON) (Thompson, 2021). Underrepresented minority nursing students face challenges that affect all aspects of their educational journey, including admission, progression, retention, and graduation. The profound changes in the nation's demographics are creating new realities for nursing faculty.

Data from the US Census Bureau demonstrate that racial and ethnic diversity has increased over the last 10 years. White non-Hispanic populations have decreased from 63.7% in 2010 to 57.8% in 2020. Hispanics now account for 18.7% of the total population, while Black or African American non-Hispanics account for 12.1% of the population. These statistics demonstrate that the US population is much more multiracial and more diverse than ever before (Jensen et al., 2021). According to the Pew Research Center, no other country has more immigrants than the United States. More than 40 million people in the United States were born in another country, accounting for 20% of the world's migrants. There is so much diversity in the United States that every country in the world is represented among US immigrants (Budiman, 2020). If these demographic trends continue, immigrants and their descendants are expected to account for 88% of the US population by 2065 (Budiman, 2020). With these population projections, academic institutions will undoubtedly be made up of groups of people who are disproportionally represented among the educationally underserved.

The profound changes in the nation's demographics are creating new realities for nursing faculty. There is a need to enhance diversity in the nursing workforce and a need to attract students from underrepresented groups in nursing. Nursing student statistics demonstrate that enrollment of minority nursing students increased from 77,265 to 184,050 from 2010 to 2019, that is, more than double the number of minority nursing students (National Advisory Council on Nurse Education and Practice, 2020). American Association of

Colleges of Nursing (AACN) (2020a) annual survey statistics indicate that there has been an increase in underrepresented minority students in recent years, with current data demonstrating that 37.9% of undergraduates and 37.1%, 33.8%, and 37.2% of all students in master's, research-focused doctoral programs, and doctor of nursing practice programs, respectively, are from racial and ethnic minorities.

Nursing faculty are the least diverse compared with other registered nursing positions. There are close to 27,000 nurse educators currently employed in the United States. The majority of nurse educators are White women (69.7%). Approximately 20% of all nurse educators are Black or African American or Hispanic or Latinx. Men comprise 12.1% of the total number of nurse educators and 14% of all nurse educators identify as LGBTQ+ (ZIPPIA, 2021). Those statistics indicate that the majority of culturally diverse and minority nursing students are being taught by nonminority nursing faculty, who may not know how to provide the support needed for their academic success. A lack of diversity among nursing faculty may send the message to students that the institution does not value diversity. This lack of diversity among nursing faculty may impact underrepresented minority students who are looking for role models to mentor them and provide community support (AACN, 2021a). Institutions of higher education have been asked by many nursing and philanthropic organizations to increase recruitment and strengthen graduation rates of underrepresented groups in nursing. Thus institutions of higher education must ensure that nurse educators are aware of the effect that a multicultural educational approach has on the success of minority and underrepresented nursing students.

A large body of social science research indicates that higher education is not immune from the inequities that occur in American society. Most of this research focuses on the experiences and outcomes of college and university students and indicates that Latinx, African American, and Native American students have lower rates of college enrollment and retention than White non-Hispanic students. In fact, research shows that college access and completion differ across racial and ethnic groups and that there are many systemic barriers to high-quality education for underrepresented minority students (American Council on Education, 2019). Nursing faculty must use new approaches for increasing the number of minority and ethnically diverse students by acknowledging that there are many factors that can influence their success and by designing culturally engaging environments and courses to meet the needs of all students that will ultimately result in students' academic success. Retention and graduation rates are major challenges for minority nursing students. These students face many barriers that may impede their academic achievement (Murray, 2021).

College enrollment totals have steadily declined by 1.67% yearly since 2010. It is estimated that there are 17.5 million undergraduates attending degree-granting institutions and 4.3 million enrolled in graduate school in American colleges. Approximately 19.5% of all student enrollments are Hispanic or Latinx, a 441.7 % increase since 1976. Female college enrollments have also increased by 34.7% since 1960 (Hanson, 2021). The percentage of college students who are Black has increased by 39.6% since 1976; however, Black student population has decreased by 10.1% since 2010. Ten percent (10%) of all students enrolled in colleges in the United States are Asian or Pacific Islanders and 0.07% are American Indian or Alaska Native, with no demonstrable increases since 1976. It is interesting to note that the White Caucasian non-Hispanic student demographic has also decreased by close to 35% since 1976, which is a significant amount. Although there has been an increase in minority enrollments, the fact is that close to 60% of all college and university students are White non-Hispanic (Hanson, 2021). These statistics are important to nursing schools as they attempt to recruit, enroll, and retain a student body reflective of the community in which the graduates will practice.

The nation's student population is becoming more diverse; however, the majority of full-time faculty positions in general continue to be filled by White men and White women. The demographics and culture of academia is distinctly White, heterosexual, and middle and upper-middle class.

According to the National Center for Education Statistics (NCES) (2021), 35% of all university faculty are female, thus reflecting some gender equity. In contrast, there have been few increases in faculty positions held by racially and ethnically diverse individuals. Only 25% of full-time faculty positions are held by people of color. In addition, among full-time tenured faculty at the rank of professor, only 19% were people of color (NCES, 2021). To describe this more clearly, 81% of the full-time college professorship are White non-Hispanic (DeWitty & Murray, 2020). White non-Hispanic faculty are more likely to be tenured compared with racial and ethnic female minorities. Achieving tenure gives faculty more privilege and more power in academic settings. Tenure gives academic freedom to professors to publish about thought-provoking issues. It also provides power to the tenured faculty through the stability of the position and allows for improved and open learning (Indeed, 2021). Because White non-Hispanic faculty are more likely to be tenured, they possess more power in higher education than other faculty of color. Women of color, in particular, continue to be underrepresented in academia. For example, in fall of 2018, women of color held only 11% of full-time faculty positions. Moreover, the percentage of women of color declined steadily with rising academic rank. Women of color composed 15% of instructors and lecturers, 15% of assistant professors, 17% of associate professors, and only 6% of full professors (NCES, 2020).

The lack of diversity in academia has implications for creating an inclusive learning environment, given that biases in academia still exist despite efforts for their elimination. The lack of diversity in nursing practice is also a source of concern. The Institute of Medicine's (IOM, 2020) *Future of Nursing 2020–2030: Charting a Path to Achieve Health Equity* clearly points out the need for increasing diversity in the health care workforce. The report focuses on system facilitators and barriers to achieving a diverse workforce, including gender, race, and ethnicity, across all levels of nursing education. Increasing the diversity in academic programs will increase diversity in the workforce and prepare students for addressing the social determinants of health and achieving health equity.

The purpose of this chapter is to provide guidance on creating a learning environment for nursing faculty, staff, and students that embraces nursing student inclusivity. This chapter begins with a discussion of key terminology and concepts that are foundational and relevant to nurse educators in understanding and providing an inclusive education to their multicultural nursing students. These concepts and key terms include: *diversity, equity,* and *inclusion.* Following the discussion of these essential concepts and terms, *multicultural* and *inclusive education* will be described, and faculty will learn how to create an inclusive environment for teaching and learning. The potential for *implicit bias* is included as possibly disrupting any attempt to deliver multicultural and inclusive educational environments. Implicit bias exists without an individual's conscious awareness and can affect a nursing faculty's understanding, decisions, and actions related to teaching diverse and marginalized students (Center for the Study of Social Policy [CSSP], 2019). The chapter also offers strategies for creating culturally responsive academic programs, curricula, and courses, with examples of instructional strategies and approaches essential to addressing diversity in the classroom and across the curriculum.

ESSENTIAL CONCEPTS AND TERMINOLOGY

Throughout this chapter, *diversity, equity, and inclusion* are described as central to the delivery of a nursing education that fosters learning for all students. The term *diversity* is very broad and refers to a variety of individuals, populations, and social characteristics. These characteristics include but are not limited to age, gender, race, ethnicity, sexual orientation, identity, family, geographic location, national origin, and religious beliefs. *Diversity* may also refer to language, physical, functional, and learning abilities and to socioeconomic status (AACN, 2021b). Some of the benefits of diversity in nursing education include producing professionals that can address health disparities and the social and structural determinants of health (AACN, 2021b, p. 5). *Equity* is the provision of different levels of support based on individual or group needs. The ultimate goal of equity is the achievement of fairness in outcomes. Understanding the need for equity requires recognizing that individuals/groups have unequal starting places (CSSP, 2019). *Inclusion*, on the other hand, refers to the environmental and organizational cultures where diverse faculty, students, and staff can thrive (AACN, 2021b). Integral to inclusion is being valued and welcomed equitably as decision-makers and collaborators (CSSP, 2019).

MULTICULTURAL EDUCATION

Multicultural education refers to teaching practices that promote educational equity among all students and improves their academic outcomes. Multicultural education strengthens the educator's awareness of the effect of culture on learning and promotes academic success for all students, including minority and underrepresented students. It utilizes a broad range of strategies to help students understand and appreciate the differences among themselves. Nursing faculty that use a multicultural educational approach can enhance learning and provide support for their diverse students. A multicultural approach to teaching incorporates values, beliefs, and perspectives of students from different cultural backgrounds. According to Banks (2013), all students—regardless of their defining characteristics such as gender, sexual orientation, social class, ethnicity, race, or cultural characteristics—are entitled to have an equal opportunity to learn. A multicultural education compels nursing faculty to see students as they are, instead of less than they are, and recognizes and builds on the strengths of the students (Mee, 2021). Multicultural education shares the same premise of addressing student learning outcomes and success as cultural competence does in addressing health disparities. Table 17.1 describes the differences between these two concepts.

Multicultural education has challenged educators and educational administrators to consider equality and inclusion for the benefit of all students. Banks (2013) outlined what he called the five dimensions of multicultural education. These dimensions include (1) content integration,

(2) knowledge construction, (3) equity pedagogy, (4) prejudice reduction, and (5) empowering school culture and social structure. Although not developmental, these five critical components of multicultural education emphasize planning and action steps in empowering cultural groups in the classroom setting. For example, content integration can be used by opening the classroom to dialogue, providing opportunities for students to learn diverse perspectives (e.g., non-Western), and supplying opportunities for reflection that can greatly enhance students' learning, which ultimately can support the provision of quality care. Prejudice reduction occurs when the teacher uses learning activities that help develop positive attitudes toward culturally diverse groups. Faculty who employ a multicultural approach in teaching diverse nursing students allow them to learn in a culturally relevant and responsive way. Faculty awareness of the importance of a multicultural education in the nursing classroom allows them to employ teaching strategies that will increase academic achievement, improve academic self-efficacy, increase cultural competence, and raise student political consciousness (Choi & Mao, 2021).

Faculty must first develop cultural knowledge, cultural sensitivity, and skills and become culturally competent themselves. Nursing faculty play a pivotal role in determining student success. They must be receptive to understanding their own biases and prejudices when teaching minority or underrepresented nursing students. Their assumptions about ways in which minority students learn and their intellectual capabilities can undermine students' academic success. Nurse educators should engage in introspection that will expose personal prejudices and stereotypes.

Cultural Knowledge

Cultural knowledge is the attainment of factual information about different cultural groups. Cultural knowledge goes beyond just knowing about a person's culture based on stereotypes. It involves an understanding of the person's central cultural characteristics, such as language, family structures, beliefs, values, and practices. Attainment of cultural knowledge requires that individuals possess a sense of *cultural humility*.

TABLE 17.1   Multicultural Teaching and Teaching for Cultural Competence

	Multicultural Teaching	Teaching for Cultural Competence
Focus	Creating curriculum and using instructional strategies and material to support diverse students (e.g., equity, justice)	Assisting students to learn about their own values, beliefs, and attitudes and those of individuals from other cultural backgrounds
Process	Developmental, a continuum	Developmental, a continuum
Knowledge assessment	Takes cultural background and attitudes, learning styles, biases, prejudices, and needs into account in planning for teaching and learning in diverse populations	Takes cultural background, attitudes, values, and beliefs into account to promote cultural understanding
Learning environment	Focuses on learning for diverse students, equity pedagogy Promotes respect for and among all students Ensures instructional materials are free of bias; facilitates use of extracurricular activities to assist student learning	Focus on varied aspects of culture in relation to patient care Promotes understanding and respect for all human variations Ensures inclusion of content about various cultures
Instruction	Allows student more responsibility and choices for learning Uses multiple ways of conveying information to facilitate student understanding	Promotes understanding Uses multiple strategies and approaches to facilitate knowledge acquisition
Teaching Strategies	Groups, instructional media, games, journals, ethnographies, guest speakers, panels, role play, textbooks, simulations, articles, discussion, reflection	Role play, games, vignettes, case studies and groups, media, popular books, visits to museums and other community settings, panels, interviews, storytelling, experiential immersion, exchange experiences, service-learning, ethnographies, workshops, educational programming, engagement
Assessing progress	Observe student engagement Curriculum and program review Course evaluation	Measurement of knowledge of cultural concepts (e.g., cultural awareness and cultural sensitivity, cultural competence), course evaluation, student evaluation of extent of perceived cultural competence
Evaluation	Student evaluation of course and instruction Faculty and student self-evaluation Peer evaluation of faculty; evidence of inclusive teaching External review of curriculum for multicultural education Student and alumni review of curriculum and instruction	Exams, writing, role playing discussions, simulation, abilities to provide appropriate cultural care

Cultural humility is defined as maintaining an interpersonal stance that is open to individuals and communities of varying cultures. It recognizes the importance of self-critique about differences in culture and an awareness of power imbalances between cultures (CSSP, 2019). Having cultural knowledge is important for faculty and students in the classroom and in clinical areas. Faculty can plan assignments for students to assess their own cultural knowledge. There are a variety of conceptual models and frameworks that faculty can use to assist students in acquiring cultural knowledge. For example, Giger and Davidhizar (2017) developed a transcultural assessment model that includes six cultural components: communication, time, space, social organization, environmental control, and biological variations. This model can be applied to any client or student of any culture. Such a model can help students learn about themselves and other individuals by using these components as a framework for assessment and for special assignments and points of reference in less formal conversations. Additional models have been identified in nursing that address the importance of cultural knowledge in caring for patients. Leininger (1970, 1993), in her Culture Care, Diversity, and Universality Theory, for example, was one of the first to synthesize caring and culture and described the importance of knowledge of cultural factors in the provision of competent care to patients. Additional models are Purnell's (2013) model for cultural competence that includes an organizing theory that purports that all cultures share similarities and that culture is a powerful force on interpretations and responses to health care (Purnell, 2019). Campinha-Bacote's (1999) model also focuses on cultural competence and delivery of health care services, which incorporates cultural knowledge, awareness, skill, desire, and encounters.

As knowledge is shared and as students seek to learn about specific cultural groups, faculty can ensure that students have knowledge of the concept of heterogeneity (e.g., variety, diversity, and differences in subgroups) as contrasted with the concept of homogeneity (sameness). An understanding of the differences must be manifested through the manner in which questions are phrased. The underlying point is to not make assumptions; in making cultural assessments, faculty should ask open-ended questions rather than direct questions. They should also recognize that cultural diversity and heterogeneity exist even among students who are thought to share the same culture.

CULTURAL UNDERSTANDING, CULTURAL KNOWING, CULTURAL SENSITIVITY, AND CULTURAL SKILLS

Cultural understanding is the recognition that there are multiple perspectives, multiple truths, multiple solutions, and multiple ways of understanding others. Developing intercultural readiness in nursing students is necessary. When faculty think of the importance of cultural understanding, it is usually in regard to caring for diverse patients (O'Brien et al., 2021). In reality, cultural understanding of nursing students is also essential to the success of the student in completing the nursing studies curriculum. Cultural understanding requires a willingness on the part of nursing faculty to see the student's worldview that reflects his or her values, norms, expressions, rites, and even taboos and myths. Faculty must shed any semblance of ethnocentrism or the notion that their own cultural beliefs and ways of life are superior to that of the student. Although it is rare to find a person who does not have a small degree of ethnocentrism, it is important for nursing faculty to perform a self-assessment to identify their ethnocentric patterns and behaviors. Both faculty and students must develop insights and learn that "one culture does not fit all." To assess students' cultural understanding, faculty should plan activities that have the potential for students to demonstrate an understanding of different cultures. In addition to clinical practice, students can actively engage in activities that highlight cultural understanding and cultural competence. A student who has an appropriate cultural understanding will recognize when values, beliefs, and practices of individuals are not compromised. *Cultural knowing* or personally knowing and recognizing the effect culture has on student learning is essential to producing positive student outcomes. Carper (1978) identified four fundamental ways or patterns of knowing. These patterns include empirical knowing, esthetic knowing, ethical knowing, and personal knowing or personal meaning that incorporates cultural knowing. Although empirical, esthetic, and ethical knowing patterns are important, personal knowing that includes cultural knowing is important to nursing education. The nurse faculty must consider the nursing student in his or her totality in the learning environment, a totality that includes the individual cultures of both the faculty and the student. To achieve cultural knowing, the nurse educator must first know themselves. Cultural knowing requires that the nurse faculty acknowledge the importance of culture to nursing education outcomes.

Cultural sensitivity develops as faculty and students come to appreciate, respect, and value cultural differences. Nurse faculty must be prepared to use best teaching practices to provide culturally sensitive and inclusive education. This type of education facilitates engaging and preparing culturally diverse students for the nursing workforce (Sommers & Bonnel, 2020). Because cultural sensitivity is not easily developed through classroom learning activities, an effective strategy is using clinical exchange experiences in a different part of the city or in different areas within the United States. Here, students have an opportunity to establish personal relationships with people who are from socioeconomic classes or cultural groups that are not the same as theirs. As a follow-up to these experiences, faculty can provide leading questions or points that will help students feel comfortable engaging in conversations. Cultural sensitivity is closely tied to the development of cultural competence. To develop cultural sensitivity, an individual must be open-minded, accepting with a nonjudgmental attitude, and have a positive self-concept

Cultural skill relates to effective performance when dealing with culturally diverse individuals. According to Campinha-Bacote (2002), cultural skill focuses on psychosocial, cultural, and physical assessments. Cultural skill is the ability to gather cultural data and use it effectively to achieve outcomes. For example, skill development in the area of communicating with others can be enhanced

through the use of interviews and visual media, the latter of which can be shown in segments and as time permits for discussion and evaluation of the effectiveness and ineffectiveness of the communication or interview techniques. Faculty can provide feedback and permit students to self-assess after select student activities that highlight culture. Evidence of skill development will be exhibited when beliefs, values, and practices are integrated into plans; when communication is effective; and when appropriate assessments and interventions are made. Cultural competence is by nature a skill evidenced through skill sets. See Box 17.1 for select student activities that highlight and increase cultural understanding, cultural knowing, cultural sensitivity, and cultural competence.

Cultural Competence

A goal of the nurse educator is to recruit, retain, and graduate diverse nursing students to meet the specific health care needs of the increasingly diverse patient population. Best teaching practices must be used to provide a culturally sensitive and inclusive nursing education and environment (Sommers & Bonnel, 2020). Because faculty are role models and cultural agents, they must possess necessary knowledge, skills, and attitudes to facilitate inclusive teaching and guide students to provide

---

BOX 17.1 Cultural Understanding and Cultural Competence Student Activities

- Book club discussions
- Cultural food buffet
- Case studies
- City tours
- Cultural self-assessment
- Cultural rounds
- Discussion groups
- Diversity portfolio
- Immersion experiences
- List and describe places lived
- Movie analysis
- Music potpourri
- Museum visits
- Photomontage of cultural scenes
- Role playing
- Values clarification exercises
- Vignettes

culturally competent care. It is equally important for faculty and students to have an awareness and understanding of their personal beliefs and how these may affect teaching and learning and patient care. See Table 17.2 for a tool to assess personal cultural competence.

Cultural competence has been defined as "the process in which the healthcare provider continuously strives to achieve the ability to effectively work within the cultural context of a client, individual, family, or community" (Campinha-Bacote, 2002, p. 54). Purnell and Paulanka (2008) defined

TABLE 17.2	Assessing Personal Cultural Competence
Ask specific questions relating to each of the attributes.	
Awareness	Am I aware of my personal biases, stereotypes, and prejudices toward cultures and/or people that are different from my own? To what extent am I aware?
	Am I aware that a limited English proficiency does not equate to ignorance or low intellectual capacity?
Knowledge	Do I have factual information on the similarities and differences between and among varying cultural groups, specifically regarding their health care practices, beliefs, and traditions?
Understanding	Do I understand that there are a variety of cultural factors that may contribute to why my students, peers, classmates, or patients may react the way they do? To what extent do I understand?
	Do I understand that there is a difference between race and ethnicity? If I don't understand, what can I do to change?
Sensitivity	Am I sensitive enough to convey to others that I appreciate, respect, and value their cultural differences? To what extent do I demonstrate sensitivity?
Cultural Interaction	Do I make deliberate efforts to make personal contact with individuals who are from a cultural group different from my own? Do I read books and articles, watch movies, or eat ethnic foods different from my own? Do I intellectually reflect on what I saw, read, heard, or ate? To what extent?
	Do I take advantage of exchange programs in my school such as study-abroad programs or mission trips that would take me to environments of people within my community that have a culture different from my own? Do I frequent cultural establishments in my community?
	Do I solicit information about individuals' cultural celebrations?
Cultural skill	Do I possess the skill sets to communicate effectively with my patients when I conduct a cultural assessment and a physical assessment that will provide evidence that I am appropriate, efficient, and safe? To what extent?
Cultural competence	Do I demonstrate competence to the extent that I could in my teaching about or in giving patient care? Identify the following outcomes that provide evidence of:
	• Facilitating or providing safe and satisfying care that respects the values, beliefs, and health practices of the patient
	• Integrating cultural beliefs, values, languages, and health practices of others in assessment plans and actual care
	• Examining the influence of culturally tied beliefs and practices on individual health care needs
	• Meeting cultural needs of individuals and their families
	• Incorporating cultural aspects of health and illness during assessments and communication, and in actual care
	• Applying national standards to facilitate the provision of appropriate care to individuals and families

cultural competence as developing an awareness of one's own existence, thoughts, and environments without letting it influence others from different backgrounds; demonstrating awareness and understanding of the patient's cultural background; respecting and accepting cultural differences and similarities; and providing congruent care by adapting it to the patient's cultural health care beliefs, values, and norms. Purnell (2013) identified the progression from cultural incompetence to cultural competence to include unconscious cultural incompetence, or not being aware that cultural knowledge is absent; conscious cultural incompetence, or being aware that knowledge is lacking; conscious cultural competence, involving a concerted effort to learn about cultures; and unconscious cultural competence, which includes automatically providing culturally competent care (p. 15). Campinha-Bacote et al. (1996) defined cultural competence as "a process, not an end point, in which the nurse continuously strives to achieve the ability to effectively work within the cultural context of an individual, family, or community from a diverse cultural and ethnic background" (pp. 1–2). This implies that one continuously strives to achieve; therefore it can be considered to be both developmental and a journey.

In addition, cultural competence has been described as existing on a continuum. Each provides a beginning point for faculty as they direct efforts to facilitate cultural competence understanding among students. Burchum (2002) identified eight attributes of cultural competence: cultural awareness, cultural knowledge, cultural understanding, cultural sensitivity, cultural interaction, cultural skill, cultural competence, and cultural proficiency. Likewise, Lister (1999) identified seven terms classified as a taxonomy: (1) *cultural awareness*, (2) *cultural knowledge*, (3) *cultural understanding*, (4) *cultural sensitivity*, (5) *cultural interaction*, (6) *cultural skill*, and (7) *cultural competence*.

Wells (2002) proposed a model of cultural competence that incorporates two phases: cognitive and affective. The cognitive phase involves acquiring knowledge, whereas the affective phase relates to changes in attitudes and behaviors. Both of these are considered developmental. In viewing the concept on a continuum, there is progression from lack of or limited knowledge to cultural knowledge and then awareness. Characteristics of the affective phase are the development of cultural sensitivity, cultural competence, and cultural proficiency. The components of cultural competence are similar in each of these models.

Preparing a culturally competent graduate is a goal of all nursing programs. To achieve this goal, instruction and activities should be directed toward the meanings, development of cultural confidence, attributes, assessment, instructional strategies, resources, and evaluation.

THE INCLUSIVE LEARNING ENVIRONMENT

Learning environments can be unequal power spaces, but when faculty adopt an inclusive learning environment, they foster a sense of belonging in students and increase their likelihood of academic success (Murray, 2021). Inclusive learning environments are places in which thoughtfulness, mutual respect, multiple perspectives, varied experiences, and academic excellence are valued and promoted. This is largely because of the fact that the faculty and students work together to create and sustain an environment in which everyone feels safe, supported, and encouraged to express their views and concerns. Inclusive learning environments occur intentionally and involve teaching strategies that take into consideration the needs of students from diverse backgrounds, learning styles, and intellectual abilities. Inclusive teaching strategies take thoughtful planning and intentionality. An inclusive teaching environment requires an awareness and sensitivity to the uniqueness of the class (Kachani et al., 2020). In the classroom, content is presented in a manner that reduces all students' experiences of marginalization and wherever possible helps students understand that individual experiences, values, and perspectives influence how they construct knowledge in any field or discipline.

To create an inclusive learning environment, everyone in the school is responsible for making students feel welcome and comfortable. In an inclusive environment, there must be mutual respect, a sense of trust, appreciation of diversity, equitable rewards and recognition, access to opportunity, and cultural competence. Managing dynamics that go beyond fitting in if one is different from the majority to messages of belonging and safety are crucial. The admission of diverse populations of students to SON directly affects factors such as the learning environment of the educational unit (campus wide and in the school of nursing), the social environment, and recruitment and retention. Therefore concerted efforts must be made to direct interventions that will have positive effects on all students. One important principle to follow in building inclusive teaching environments is to support a class climate that acknowledges the individuality of each student and fosters belonging for all students. Other important principles include selecting course content that recognizes diversity and is aware of barriers to inclusion and that maximizes self-awareness and commitment to inclusion (Columbia Center for Teaching and Learning, 2017).

Because most of the interaction among students and faculty occurs in the classroom and clinical agencies, faculty must be prepared to create a learning environment there that is sensitive to the dynamics of student interaction, to recognize and manage microaggressions and gender and linguistic biases, and to understand racial and ethnic differences in students' learning style. See Chapter 2 for a discussion on learning styles. Refer to Box 17.2 for strategies to create a welcoming and inclusive classroom.

Classroom Dynamics

Culturally competent education must be integrated into the nursing curriculum and be evident in the classroom. Minority nursing students face multiple barriers to successful program completion, including insufficient role models, bias, and lack of inclusion (Murray, 2021). One of the major barriers to learning for minority students is fear of participating in class and experiencing rejection

---

BOX 17.2 Strategies to Create a Culturally Inclusive Teaching and Learning Environment

- Make meaningful connections. Learn something about the students. Reach out to them and ask if they need help. Assign regular meeting times (standing appointments) for the students on a weekly basis. Inform the students that you are available to meet with them individually if they want.
- Include some information about your own cultural origin and any cross-cultural teaching and learning experiences you may have had over time. Sharing something about yourself helps students see a connection with you.
- Increase relevance of lectures and assignments. Connect assignments with student experiences. Ask students to respond to discussion boards online about their own experiences and have them connect these to the lecture and/or assignment.
- Ask students what pronouns they want used when referring to them. Some people do not use any pronouns and are called by their names.
- Many people use a combination of he, she, his, hers, and they. Using correct pronouns shows respect and helps in communication.
- Ask students what form of address they prefer. Take care to pronounce and to spell the name correctly. Use inclusive language that doesn't assume Western name forms. *Family* name, not *last* name;

given name, not *Christian* name. Students from more formal educational cultures, where status differences related to age or educational qualifications are important, might be uncomfortable addressing teaching staff by their given names. A compromise can be for students to use your title and given name (e.g., Professor Marie, Dr. Ivan).
- Be careful with the use of humor. The students may not understand your humor and believe that it is directed at them. Assign a mentor as a role model. Utilize ethnic role models if possible.
- Make nursing attractive. Use minority nurse images and culturally sensitive wording in written materials. Invite successful minority nurses in the community to present to the students so that they can see minority role models.
- Establish supportive networks of nurses and faculty from minority backgrounds as a support for minority students.
- Identify peer minority nursing students that can serve as mentors to incoming students.
- During silences, ask students to write down anonymously what they are feeling at the moment and why. Point to the similarities and differences between the responses to elicit discussion.

from their classmates. In the classroom, faculty must be aware of students' backgrounds and response patterns and how classroom norms and rules are forms of power. Faculty must also develop awareness of their own biases and responses to culturally diverse students. Faculty members who understand the barriers that minority students face and the effect of culture on their own teaching are better prepared pedagogically to address it in their students. Capitalizing on the opportunity from the beginning to create a welcoming environment will neutralize to a great degree the stress that comes with the feeling of not belonging. A caring pedagogy makes allowances for behaviors that are exhibited by students in the classroom even during moments of silence. It is especially important to stay learner driven and therefore student centered. This calls for an astute awareness of the adaptations that may be needed while simultaneously complementing participatory learning.

Microaggressions

The term microaggression was coined by Chester M. Pierce in 1978 after the Civil Rights era to bring attention to racist behavior that is subtle, stunning, often automatic, nonphysical insults directed toward minorities, especially people of color; lesbian, bisexual, gay, transgender, and queer (LBGTQ+) people; and women (Harwood et al., 2015). According to Ackerman-Barger et al. (2020), microaggressions foster exclusion and marginalize individuals. They serve as barriers to optimal learning for underrepresented and minority students in SON. Racial microaggressions are commonplace verbal or behavioral indignities that may be intentional or unintentional. These are usually subtle statements but they elicit negative emotions in the recipients and they may then feel conflicted (Ackerman-Barger et al., 2020). In addition to race, microaggressions are reported to be perpetuated on the basis of gender, sexual orientation, religious beliefs, and ability status. Refer to Table 17.3 for examples of microaggressions. The effect of continuing microaggressions to exclude racially diverse or minority students is real. At University of California, Davis, and Yale University, Ackerman-Barger et al. (2020) interviewed self-identified underrepresented medical and nursing students to get a better description of how racial microaggressions affected their learning. The data obtained showed consistent examples of microaggressions among all students, with

TABLE 17.3   Examples of Microaggressions

Culture and Learning	Statement or Behavior	Perceived Meaning of Statement
Ethnicity and race	When I look at you, I don't see color. There is only one race: the human race Being ignored in the classroom Where were you born? Where are you from? You seem to be more metropolitan than the other students here.	Denial of individual's racial and ethnic experiences. Denial of individual's ethnic and cultural being. Denial that racism or White privilege exists. Students from certain cultural groups are not valued. There is an implied assumption that a person of color is foreign born or not a US citizen. *The implication is that you seem more sophisticated than the students of color in the area.*
Gender	Anyone can succeed, man or woman, if he or she works hard. Getting an academic scholarship is easy for you because you are a double minority—a woman, and a woman of color.	No acknowledgment of unfair benefits because of gender Implied that achievements are not academically based.
Ability	You are so articulate. You are a credit to your race and community.	People of color may perceive this statement as negative and demeaning rather than positive and uplifting.

peers, faculty, and even structural elements of the curricula contributing to microaggressive behavior. Microaggression by teachers has been found to result in disengagement from educational advancement (Steketee et al., 2021). The implications of such studies indicate that educators need to think about any method of verbal exchange so as to eliminate statements that might be perceived as microaggressions.

When microaggressions occur, faculty or anyone present has the responsibility to manage the incident. The goal is to preserve the dignity of those involved:

- Be open to discussing, exploring, and clarifying what is felt and seen. In other words, "pay attention to the tension."
- Do a check-in. Watch body language and indications that students have checked out. This will do much to engender trust and positively seal a caring relationship.
- Be aware of stereotypes when a person discloses their racial or gender-related identities.
- Offer a simple "I'm sorry," which is all that may be called for in many instances.
- Reduce ambiguity and uncertainty, and make the invisible visible.
- Use the opportunity to educate all members of the community. Education holds one of the primary keys to combating and overcoming the harm that microaggressions deliver.
- Indicate at the outset that anyone present could unintentionally or intentionally commit these acts, especially through the language we use.

Managing the situation when one is involved as either the target or perpetrator requires particular acumen (Case Study 17.1). Sometimes the microaggression is used in the form of a compliment, such as "can you imagine that someone of your ethnicity is as smart as you are?" As the target of the microaggression, students may be left with the question, "did I really understand what he said?" Faculty and students can be open to exploring the possibility that one has acted in a biased fashion and controlling defensiveness. This involves suspending interpretation of behavior for those who challenge views and becoming aware of values, biases, and assumptions about human behavior.

CASE STUDY 17.1   Managing Microaggressions

A second-generation American student whose ethnicity is Hispanic is enrolled in an undergraduate nursing class. The faculty asks the student to remain in the classroom after all the students have completed an exam and left the classroom. As an MSN student in the education program who is being precepted by the faculty, you are present and actively listening to the faculty-student exchange. The faculty tells the student that they made the highest grade in the class and follows this with, "Congratulations. I was pleasantly surprised that you had no difficulty completing the exam and scored such a high grade. Are you from here? I imagine that you are probably from here because you are more articulate than some of the other students who were not born in this area."

1. Is what the faculty said considered microaggression? What is your responsibility in this case?
2. What would be your goal in addressing this incident?
3. How does microaggression affect the student's learning?

If faculty or students are working in a team when microaggressions occur, they should manage the process, not the content. This occurs by acknowledging the accuracy of statements when appropriate, helping individuals see the difference between intention and effect, encouraging individuals to explore how their feelings may be saying something about them, and enlisting the aid of others on the team by asking them what they see happening. When courage shows up, it is important for faculty to recognize, validate, and express appreciation for the individual's willingness to take a risk and to hold a courageous dialogue. By doing so, faculty model healthy relationship behaviors

GENDER AND LINGUISTIC BIAS

Everyone is capable of bias and therefore is not and cannot be all knowing and completely objective. It is possible to act in prejudicial or biased ways while sincerely believing that prejudice or biased thinking is personally rejected. People may be sincere in their rejection of biased or stereotypical thinking, yet their beliefs may be deeply engrained. Stereotypical thinking imposes certain characteristics on a group because of their race, ethnicity, nationality, sexual orientation, or even profession. While stereotypes may consist of all of the characteristics assigned to a group of persons, often they link various aspects of identity together and once absorbed may influence behavior without awareness or intent (Nittle, 2021). Thus for faculty, understanding their own biases and their students' beliefs and biases is a component of cultural due diligence and a prerequisite to establishing an inclusive learning environment.

In a class with diverse students, it is prudent and necessary for faculty to be attentive to responses by anyone in the class that may be perceived as dismissive or minimizing. Unconscious bias plays a part in the way faculty and students are perceived by others. Faculty and students can determine their biases by taking assessment tools, which can be a springboard for getting in touch with personal subconscious biases in a safe manner. The results can be transformative in terms of self-awareness. One source that helps develop self-awareness of personal biases is Harvard's Project Implicit. This site has online tests that are easily accessible at https://implicit.harvard.edu/implicit/iatdetails.html. Promoting equity in teaching also means that teachers are aware of subconscious biases and differential treatment. As psychologist Claude Steele's (2010) research indicates, even the fear that one will be judged according to extant stereotypes can depress academic performance. There are plenty of examples of bias and stereotyping in nursing education. Examples of bias include gender bias and reactions to students who are culturally and linguistically diverse. Examples of stereotyping students include expecting that Asian nursing students are superior intellectually to the other students or expecting the male students to do better on the medication math quizzes because males always outperform females in math.

Research on gender bias in classrooms and clinical environments has supported tendencies for faculty to interact with one gender more than another or to make assignments based on gender (Samuriwo et al., 2020). Specifically in classrooms with predominantly majority students, there is a tendency for teachers to interact with White male students more than they interact with women and men of color. With this awareness, teachers should make concerted efforts to provide equal treatment by engaging all students. This includes the quiet student who speaks up infrequently. Deliberate actions can be taken to accomplish this by devising a system for engaging students regardless of gender or ethnicity. One frequently used technique is placing index cards in an accessible manner where individuals can write their comments or questions anonymously or using the anonymous comment component of a learning management system survey tool. This provides insights into where students are struggling with concepts or have concerns that must be addressed.

With increasing numbers of male students in nursing programs, gender dynamics become important, and it is essential to deploy gender-neutral language unless specificity of gender affects the lesson being taught or the point being made. Gender-neutral language should also be reflected in examinations and any testing materials (see Chapter 24).

Nursing Education and LGBTQ+ Students

A discussion on gender bias must also include recognizing the need for improving LGBTQ+ cultural competence in nursing students. Gallup News (Jones, 2021) reports that 5.6% of U.S. adults identify as LGBTQ+. Those numbers have increased from 2017, when 4.1% of Americans identified as LGBTQ+. According to these statistics, approximately 0.6% of Americans are transgender, 3.1% identify as bisexual, 1.4% as gay, and 0.7% as lesbian. *Healthy People 2030* (HealthyPeople.Gov, 2020) has as one of its goals to improve the health, safety, and well-being of lesbian, gay, bisexual, and transgender people. This goal addresses the specific disparities and challenges faced by the LGBTQ+ community. According to King et al. (2021), there is a shortage of health care providers who are culturally competent in LGBTQ+ issues and this lack of cultural competence and discrimination still exists in nursing schools and perpetuates social norms that turn LGBTQ+ students away from nursing. King et al. (2021) found in their review of anatomy and physiology textbooks used by nursing students that the way LGBTQ+ people were portrayed violated ethical principles of nursing. Recommendations from this study included challenging nurse educators to consider the way that the LGBTQ+ community is portrayed and the impact that language, images, and classroom materials have on LGBTQ+ students and all students in general.

Cultural competence education that focuses on incorporating LGBTQ+ content in the nursing curriculum is effective in decreasing bias and prejudice and improving knowledge and attitudes among nursing students. Some strategies to incorporate this content in the curriculum may include group discussions, LGBTQ+-related clinical experiences, inviting panels of LGBTQ+ individuals to the classroom, analysis of LGBTQ+ literature and/or film reviews, and case studies. Simulation exercises and role playing may also increase knowledge of LGBTQ+-specific issues and reduce bias and prejudice. In addition to these strategies, nursing faculty must also take into consideration how students may want to be addressed. Pronouns communicate gender and gendered implications. Pronouns should be considered meaningful tools that communicate identities and experiences and can also communicate cultural, linguistic, and ethnic identities (Center for Sexual and Gender Diversity [CSGD], 2021). LGBTQ+ students face many challenges in higher education that may prevent them from being successful. Using the correct pronouns demonstrates a respectful and thoughtful classroom environment. According to CSDG (2021), there is no exhaustive list of pronouns to be used and most of them are commonly used. Many people choose one or a combination of the following pronouns: he, she, his, hers, they, theirs, them, and many more. Some people prefer not to use pronouns and want to be referred to by their name. Pronouns are very important when referring to transgender and nonbinary students. Improper use of pronouns may cause these students to experience intentional or unintentional misgendering on a daily basis.

Linguistic Bias

Faculty may also have a bias for students who are culturally and linguistically diverse. In fact,

nursing students with language differences are major challenges for faculty, thus causing students for whom English is not their first or only language to feel unsupported by the school and the faculty (Onovo, 2019). Nursing faculty that teach culturally and linguistically diverse students (CALD) face many challenges in teaching diverse student groups and may also feel unsupported and unprepared to do so. In a study conducted to ascertain the challenges faced by nursing faculty teaching CALD students, results indicated that faculty found language barriers and lack of support as the most challenging. Ultimately, these faculty found that they were unsupported and unprepared to teach and assess CALD students (Guler, 2022).

English-as-a-second-language (ESL) (or English-as-an-additional-language [EA]) students must be able to learn, write, take tests, and communicate with classmates and patients in two languages, first translating the concepts or communication into their own language and then back into English. For many ESL students, academic failure results from poor performance on multiple-choice examinations as a result of tests that contain linguistic errors. Mulready-Shick et al. (2020) found that linguistic modification of faculty-written test questions resulted in optimal readability and comprehension for students for whom English is a second language. If a student has an accent, challenges in communications may arise between the ESL student and other students or between the ESL student and faculty; class participation that requires verbal responses may be a challenge. In such situations, faculty may refer students to accent-reduction or modification programs. Keep in mind that accent modification is an elective service freely selected by the students who want to improve their accents. Freysteinson et al. (2017) reported favorable results for nursing and health care administration students who participated in a 12-week accent modification program. Findings indicated that the students perceived significantly higher self-esteem and overall competence in communicating after the accent-modification program.

Assumptions and beliefs undergird all interactions with others. For example, nonverbal behaviors such as frowns, furrowed brows, and intense concentration may not be deliberate behaviors;

instead, their use may be related to efforts to try to capture what is being voiced by the student, and faculty and students should seek to understand the meaning of the behavior rather than make assumptions about it. Unless clarified, these non-verbal behaviors may have an effect on students' future participation in discussions and classroom interactions. They may refrain from participation or not respond to or ask questions because of the panicky feelings they may experience at having to speak in class.

There are techniques that faculty can use to facilitate communication with ESL/EAL nursing students. Faculty can pay attention to techniques that are used for questioning, for example, asking "why" and "how" questions and encouraging and requesting students to respond, thus exploring "possibilities." An additional way to engage students in language use is to use a learning activity that requires them to write a question related to the assignment each week and ask them to read the question in class or small peer group. This activity has a high potential for opening dialogue, decreasing shyness, and enhancing community building with the class.

Furthermore, faculty must be willing to address students' affective issues that influence their feelings about English. There are many challenges encountered by students for whom English is not their first language. These challenges may include feeling that they are perceived differently, stress from assuming different cultural roles, lack of support services, and little to no orientation to the school (Merry et al., 2021). Nursing students for whom English is a second or additional language face many barriers related to a lack of faculty support, lack of any kind of mentorship, insufficient awareness of the different learning styles, racism and discrimination in the learning environment, and a lack of coping mechanisms (Onovo, 2019). In a study that explored the experiences and challenges of culturally diverse ESL nursing students, Onovo (2019) found that these students' learning experiences in the nursing program were overwhelming because the language barrier made it very difficult to understand the complex nursing concepts and the students felt that there was a lack of campus support and resources. Opportunities should be provided for informal conversations outside of the classroom. Choi (2016), in her description of a proactive nursing support program for ESL students, included the use of bimonthly group gatherings organized by faculty mentors. These gatherings not only provided a venue for social interaction but also explored a number of nursing education issues such as effective communication methods in clinical settings. Choi and Brochu (2022), in a study of EAL nursing students, found that the EAL students reported that an EAL nursing student support group helped in reducing barriers to success and provided them access to a variety of engagement and leadership opportunities. Having students attend group gatherings provides a forum for students to openly discuss issues and concerns in a supportive nonacademic environment. As a result, students have increased confidence in their abilities and may participate more frequently informally and increase participation in more formal classroom activities, including discussions.

Faculty must also be aware of students' use of voice registers. Joos (1967) found that it is socially acceptable to go down one register in the same conversation, but to drop two registers or more in the same conversation is to be socially offensive. Faculty must be sensitive to the subtleties in student vocalizations and the voice registers they use. For example, in some cultures, it may be appropriate to be what might be considered by the dominant culture as "soft spoken" or "loud." The vocal tone used can also be offensive and a barrier to effective communication. In their study on how vocal tone contributes to the identification of unspoken intentions, Hellbernd and Sammler (2016) found that a person's vocal tone can reveal intentions and thus affect interpersonal communication. Refer to Box 17.3, Tips on Managing Bias in the Classroom.

DEVELOPING INCLUSIVE EXCELLENCE IN ACADEMIC INSTITUTIONS, PROGRAMS, CURRICULA, AND COURSES

To meet the needs for diversity in nursing education and to prepare a workforce that is representative of the diversity of patients to be served,

---

BOX 17.3 Tips for Managing Bias in the classroom

- Do a cultural self-assessment to ascertain personal subconscious biases.
- Develop awareness of how you interact with minority, culturally diverse students.
- Use a system to engage students, such as index cards for anonymous comments/questions.
- Use gender-neutral terms when describing the nurse in class or in examinations.
- Address students by their preferred pronouns.
- Refer students to accent-reduction classes if needed.
- Find university learning assistance resources for students, such as a writing center.
- Be careful with your own nonverbal communication.
- Recognize student's nonverbal communication. For example, nods do not mean understanding or agreement; furrowed brows may mean deep concentration.
- Frame discussion questions in an open manner that allows multiple answers.
- Create a study guide for students.
- Provide an outline of your lecture that focuses on the main points.
- Allow students enough time to respond to questions; wait for 12–15 seconds for a reply.
- Recognize that voice register and vocal tone are important and at times not clear (speaking softly) or are offensive.

CASE STUDY 17.2 Creating a Culturally Inclusive Teaching and Learning Environment

A faculty has been assigned to teach Nursing Theory to graduate nursing students. This is the first graduate nursing course in which several exchange nursing students from Asia are enrolled. English is not their first language, though they have some proficiency in written English. On the first day of class, the faculty notices that the class is also quite diverse in terms of other races, ethnicities, and cultures. The faculty has extensive experience teaching nursing students but is a little apprehensive about teaching these very diverse students, including those who are identified as having English as an additional language (EAL). The faculty recognizes that for all of the graduate nursing students to be successful, the classroom environment must acknowledge the need for inclusivity and provide an inclusive approach to learning.

1. How can the faculty understand their own approach to creating an inclusive learning environment?
2. What principles could guide the faculty to achieve inclusive excellence in the classroom?
3. What strategies could the faculty use to create a culturally inclusive teaching and learning environment?
4. What legislation facilitates building a culture of inclusivity at the institutional level? What implications does that legislation have in providing a multicultural education to nursing students?
5. How can utilizing holistic admission criteria increase diversity in nursing student admissions? How does using holistic admission criteria differ from academic admission criteria?

---

administrators, staff, and faculty must build a culture of inclusivity at the institutional level and within the school of nursing and develop academic programs that embrace the strengths of all members of the academic community (Case Study 17.2). According to Appert et al. (2020), there are five principles that must be followed in academia in order to achieve inclusive excellence: establish and support a class climate that fosters belonging for all students; set explicit student expectations; select course content that recognizes diversity and acknowledges barriers to inclusion; design all course elements for accessibility; and reflect on one's beliefs about teaching to maximize self-awareness and commitment to inclusion. Additionally, a school must be able to recruit, retain, and graduate a diverse student body and support a culture of inclusivity in its programs, curricula, and courses.

Governmental and Legislative Issues

To ensure a culture of inclusivity for minority nursing students at the university level, the federal government has created policies and legislation that support accessibility and affordability for students of all backgrounds. Organizations like the American Nurses Association (ANA) and American Association of Colleges of Nursing (AACN) monitor federal policies closely and may even establish their own federal policy agenda. For example, AACN has established its 2021–2022 Federal Policy Agenda, which focuses on priority areas that include advancing higher education, the nursing workforce in addition to nursing research, and redefining models of care (AACN, 2021c). Within the higher education focus, AACN's agenda addresses the importance of diversity in education as a means to affect the classroom and professional environments. The focus is to remove barriers to higher education to provide accessibility for underrepresented racial and ethnic groups and those that are from an economically deprived background. Diversity in the workforce further ensures that patients will receive culturally appropriate and sensitive care. Increasing diversity to better match shifts in population will open career pathways and improve quality and population-centered care. Multicultural education in nursing requires that nursing faculty be aware of how legislation can affect nursing students and nursing education in general. Nursing faculty can, thus, monitor state and federal policies and become involved in advocacy for students and the nursing profession.

One example of legislation that has positively affected nursing students and nursing education is the Title VIII Nursing Workforce Reauthorization Act. This act provides the largest source of federal funding for nursing education. This funding is essential for universities and colleges that educate registered nurses who will be practicing in rural and medically underserved communities, expanding access to critically needed areas (AACN, 2020b). Title VIII also provides funding for the Loan Repayment Program, specifically targeting Substance Use Disorder.

Another example of legislation that has had a positive effect on nursing education is Title IX of the Education Amendments of 1972. Title IX was passed in 1972 and mandates equal treatment of all students, regardless of gender, if educated at an institution that receives federal financial aid. This legislation eliminates gender-based discrimination and ensures that all students have access to quality education (U.S. Department of Education, 2021). According to Kilpatrick (2018), Title IX changed education by allowing both sexes to enroll in the courses they want regardless of gender stereotypes, women to earn more degrees, and women to win at sports. Title IX also increased the number of women university professors and gives legal protection against discrimination to women who attend school while pregnant. This protection has also been extended against sexual assaults on campus. As a result of this legislation, Title IX requires that all institutions who receive federal funding designate a compliance coordinator who investigates infractions and implements guidance and regulations. Under Title IX, any person harmed by the university's failure to comply with the law may sue the school.

Institutional Values

Developing a culture of inclusivity begins at the institutional level and is made visible through explicit values for diversity and inclusivity; practices and procedures that support recruitment and retention of faculty, staff, and students from underrepresented populations; and policies that hold no tolerance for acts of discrimination. Whereas a diverse culture is open to a variety of perspectives, beliefs, cultures, religions, and sexual orientations, an inclusive culture brings this variety into the decision-making structures, academic programs, and classrooms; embraces it; and removes barriers to full engagement in the mission of the institution (Bleich et al., 2014). Bleich et al. (2014) identified six strategies that accelerate the development of an inclusive organization: (1) improve admission process; (2) reduce invisibility of underrepresented faculty, staff, and students; (3) create communities of support; (4) ensure that promotion and tenure structures are balanced; (5) eliminate exclusion; and (6) stand against tokenism. Additionally, colleges and universities and their SON must have statements about their commitment to diversity and inclusivity and specific campus conduct policies and procedures for discrimination related to age, gender, race, color, national origin, disability, and veteran status, among other factors.

Academic Programs

To establish inclusive learning environments at the school level, administrators and faculty can first assess their current environmental support for inclusion. Inclusive academic programs also have programs to support recruitment, admission, retention, and graduation of underrepresented students. In an effort to ensure that diversity and inclusion occurs for all students, colleges and universities have an office of diversity. Many SON are also addressing diversity, equity, justice, and inclusion by creating a position within the nursing school that addresses inclusive learning environments for students, faculty, and staff. The university office of diversity provides services and resources for minority and underrepresented faculty, staff, and students. Services are provided to persons with disabilities; LGBTQ+ persons; persons of disadvantaged economic status; and first-generation, nontraditional, or international students. This office also monitors compliance with the laws that govern colleges and universities in relation to diversity and inclusion and establishes benchmarks across the university or college to measure the progress made regarding diversity and inclusion. Both the university and the SON office of diversity are good resources for nursing students and nursing faculty. Nurse faculty may see that there is a need to refer a student to the SON or university diversity office if they are, for example, dealing with immigration status issues or are having difficulty enrolling at the university. Students who feel that they are experiencing bias, harassment, or discrimination should also be referred to the SON and/or the university office of diversity. Returning veterans might also find the diversity office helpful in providing resources, guidance, and assistance they may need to be successful. The university office of diversity is usually led by a chief diversity officer or a dean of diversity. Table 17.4 provides information on services that support an inclusive academic environment.

Recruitment

The changing US demographics and persistent health inequities highlight the need for the nursing profession to identify and implement best practices to recruit individuals from diverse racial and ethnic backgrounds and to ensure that these individuals graduate from nursing school. Thus nursing programs have a responsibility to recruit and retain men, LGBTQ+ people, first-generation college students, minorities, persons with disabilities, and those from disadvantaged backgrounds (DeWitty & Byrd, 2021; Relf, 2016). Successful recruitment requires that the SON cultivate relationships with

TABLE 17.4 **Services to Support an Inclusive Academic Program**	
Advertising materials	Should be recruitment and diversity friendly; brochures, leaflets, pamphlets, bulletins, and websites should reflect diversity by using minority nurse images. Advertisement materials are frequently examined as students and their family and faculty are searching for a school or seeking employment.
Campus and nursing programs	Should promote services that are needed by diverse populations. Academic and student services should be welcoming and reflect the potential population for the campus or school. Provide a variety of services, including mentors and peer tutors, time-management sessions, writing centers, inviting study areas, libraries, and equipment with representative population holdings. Enact gender-neutral and culturally appropriate language in policies. For recruitment and retention, provide faculty role models, diverse staff, and student populations (including men). Provide academic services inclusive of mentors and peer tutors.
Classroom	Should be designed for multipurpose use and diverse ways of learning; movable tables, chairs, and desks are useful for peer-to-peer interaction and small-group work.
Social environment	Plan events to bring students of diverse populations together for socialization and learning. Bring prominent and renowned speakers from a variety of ethnic groups and special program offerings.

prospective students and sources for prospective students such as school counselors, advisors at community colleges, and staff at potential feeder schools. Woods-Giscombe et al. (2020) found in a study on perceptions of minority baccalaureate nursing students that family and friends plus the media portrayal of nursing were major influences on the decision to pursue nursing as a career choice. The study found that there were many misperceptions about nursing and the nursing profession. Participants who did not have any personal exposure to nursing had a lack of knowledge of nursing and stereotypical images of nurses and the nursing profession. Recruitment of underrepresented minority students, thus, can begin as early as grade school at a time when students are making career choices. These programs involve sharing information about nursing as a career. Another strategy is for nursing programs to develop articulation agreements with high schools so that the students can transition to nursing programs once they graduate. These articulation agreements will establish partnerships or academic transition programs between high schools, BSN, and graduate programs that streamline the curricula to facilitate admission and progression to the next level of academic preparation (Bowles et al., 2020).

Financial support and scholarships dedicated to underrepresented minority students also aid in recruitment. In a study of second-degree minority or disadvantaged accelerated nursing students, DeWitty et al. (2016) found that competing priorities of finances and family responsibilities were the greatest challenges that these students experienced. The study also found that faculty support was the primary facilitator for program completion. Mentorship and academic and psychosocial support were found to be associated with increased enrollment and graduation for students participating in these programs.

Admission

Program admission criteria can also affect recruitment efforts. Admission requirements that depend solely on academic achievement may restrict minority student application and acceptance rates and limit the school's opportunities for having a more diverse student body. For example, Hampton et al. (2022), in a study of potential admission of Black students to RN programs in the South versus Northwest, and West, found that Southern programs relied very heavily on academic admission criteria, thus posing a potential admission barrier for Black students. The authors concluded that over 50% of all RN programs used academic metrics for admission and that even those that purported to use holistic admission criteria relied heavily on academic metrics as well. Across the country, nursing schools are rethinking the admission process and are implementing holistic admission criteria that focus on personal qualities, professional skills, and experiences in addition to evidence of academic achievements. The goal of the holistic admissions process is to admit diverse students who will excel academically and have those qualities needed for success in the work environment (Yung et al., 2021). Holistic admissions criteria may include appraisal of aptitude, characteristics, experiences, and academic metrics.

Retention

Once underrepresented minorities are admitted, nursing schools must also have programs in place to ensure student success. Barriers to success include lack of financial support, decreased family support, lack of English proficiency, lack of cultural competence, poor preparation for college, insufficient basic technology skills, nonresponsive academic advising, and lack of role models. Success programs seek to help students overcome these barriers. Success programs can include early identification of students at high risk for failure, mentoring, advising, study skills and test-taking skills programs, peer tutoring, use of social workers, writing centers, and empowerment sessions. Persistence and perseverance have been noted as powerful aspects of students' completion of a nursing program (Fagan & Coffey, 2019).

Preparation for Graduation and Transition to Practice

As students approach graduation, other strategies can be employed to prepare them for transition to practice. Licensing or certification examination preparation courses are helpful in preparing students to pass these examinations. Capstone courses, internships, and elective courses can prepare students for the realities of employment. Residency programs have proved successful in facilitating transition to practice and in the development of professional roles and acquisition of self-confidence (Wright & Scardaville, 2021). In addition to affecting transition and retention of graduates, residency programs have been found to provide greater employee satisfaction compared with those who did not participate in a residency program (Sampson et al., 2020). Courses within the curriculum focus on leadership, career, and professional development and prepare students to be lifelong learners and active members of professional nursing organizations.

The Curriculum

The curriculum should be designed using Universal Design principles (see Chapter 10). Diverse cultural content should be integrated throughout the curriculum. The multicultural model designed by Banks (2013) can be adapted to all levels of the curriculum. As Banks (2015) suggests, instructors must move beyond the initial level of integrating cultural artifacts such as names and holidays to an integrative level where students obtain more substantive information about cultural groups. Educators should make concerted efforts to exhibit attitudes of positive portrayal of diversity and indicate that diversity is valued. Exposing students to various cultural norms, health beliefs, and practices and a balanced assignment of reviewing articles and research written or conducted by faculty of color and members of the LGBTQ+ community or covering topics of concern to the marginalized are feasible first steps in diversifying the curriculum.

The expected curricular outcomes should be clearly identified and should guide didactic content, student assignments, and evaluation. In this way, students' progress toward cultural competence can be monitored and assessed as students move through the curriculum. The curriculum provides a framework for mapping and a set of criteria for evaluation. The results of the evaluation should exemplify the attainment of specific knowledge, skills, and attitudes.

Course Design

A thorough course analysis is a significant component of multicultural course transformation. The modification itself can present in various ways. Modifications to course design do not occur in isolation; that is, it is not ideal to only have the faculty who will teach the course be involved in the course design. Faculty who are involved in teaching in the particular program can be included in course design to ensure consistency among courses and building upon content from previous courses. A first step is to determine what the faculty wants the students to learn. The next step is to identify the expected outcomes and determine the course content. For example, after articulating that one goal for a course is to increase knowledge of bias and ethnocentrism as it relates to the study of various cultural groups, a faculty member may determine that the course's content includes various examples of cultural groups. However, the course may not facilitate opportunities for open and equitable exchanges of ideas and values. Therefore the transformative work may begin in the area of instruction for classroom and clinical practice.

Syllabus

Multicultural inclusion must be evident in the design of the course syllabus. The content is an essential element in the design of the syllabus. There are, however, other elements to consider, such as the tone conveyed, the opportunity for multiple perspectives, teaching activities appealing to diverse learners, and the extent to which the learning objectives aim at diversity. The syllabus should be welcoming and convey inclusiveness in tone and not be merely a list of rules and regulations important to the course. Because the syllabus is a contract with accompanying legal ramifications, faculty should ensure that the language used shows respect for differences and equity of opportunity. Most syllabi have references to disability services and sexual harassment and bullying policies, but often religious observance policies are missing. Having a religious observance policy in place and including it prominently in the syllabus sends a tangible cue of respect for all religious holidays, given that most college campuses follow the Christian calendar. The policy should indicate that it is the student's responsibility to inform the faculty member of religious holidays that conflict with any examinations, project due dates, or assignments so that other reasonable arrangements can be negotiated. Faculty who are serious about multicultural inclusion in their courses will make it clear that accommodations will be made if there are conflicts with religious holidays and observances. By assuming responsibility for notifying faculty of religious observances, students get practice for the work world, where such responsibilities will be theirs as well.

Course Materials and Instructional Resources

As educators choose instructional resources such as textbooks, virtual clinical experiences, or multimedia used as the foundation or to support teaching and learning, they should review all materials assigned to students and pay careful, close attention to implicit and explicit cues, wording, stereotypes, or generalizations. This also may mean that a variety of materials, articles, and media should be used to make up for deficits of limited information and examples in textbooks. Faculty should also examine teacher-made course materials for inclusion, exclusion, and bias. For example, course syllabi, handouts, worksheets, and evaluation instruments may inadvertently be written with culture or gender bias.

Additionally, special documentation such as books and web resources that include photos or illustrations may not include adequate racial, ethnic, or gender representation. To facilitate the availability of more unbiased instructional materials, faculty should seek peer evaluation and feedback from other faculty who teach in the program. Doing this provides faculty with suggestions on what content to include that supports a transformed curriculum.

Learning Activities

When students and faculty engage, four cultural encounters are involved: being a student, being a faculty member, learning in the academic institution or clinical practice setting, and being in a given country or region. If alliances are formed in a mutually respectful way, learning takes place in a bidirectional manner. Systems then can be developed to ensure that students have opportunities to engage in learning activities with peers from different racial and ethnic groups, peers with age or sexual orientation variations, and peers who are both male and female. In addition to student interaction, a diverse mix of experts from the community can be used for classroom activities as appropriate. These individuals, experts in their own right, are often willing to be involved in the education of students. Faculty should take advantage of the willingness of these individuals and use them to enhance inclusivity.

In the classroom, learning activities should be planned to facilitate knowledge acquisition and interaction and collaboration of diverse groups of students. Because all encounters are cultural encounters, each of these variations brings different experiences and perspectives. In other words, in the classroom faculty must move from lectures to activity and variety that promote an opportunity to interact with each other, seek understanding, and establish respect for diverse ways of learning, opinions, beliefs, and attitudes.

As cultural agents and role models, faculty can take actions that bridge gaps between students' cultures of origin and the campus culture. The implication here is to provide a variety of learning activities that appeal to varying styles of learning and for students to understand how their own learning style preferences affect their learning. There is evidence that cognitive and psychological traits affect learning styles, academic performance, and the engagement of students.

Using a variety of strategies and learning opportunities is particularly helpful to promote cultural understanding and competence. Faculty can assign students to write short papers describing themselves and then reflect on the descriptions. Encouraging students to accept invitations from individuals from a different ethnic or cultural group to special events such as weddings, graduations, parties, and rite-of-passage ceremonies can broaden perspectives.

Students and faculty should take advantage of programs both on campus and in the community. When faculty accompany students, they can encourage a shared, common experience whereby faculty can talk individually with students and explain what the student is seeing, learning, and possibly experiencing. Faculty can make a list of cultural events and establishments such as ethnic restaurants and special museums to share with students.

Promoting reflection among students increases self-awareness. Faculty can engage students by designing written assignments such as journaling logs or learning diaries. Requiring students to include a self-reflection section in their written clinical assignments after each clinical experience can also have value in promoting cultural competence and understanding. Personal letters written by and for the student have a dual purpose of addressing personal fears, feelings, assumptions, and expectations about a planned experience or about different racial and ethnic or age groups and later reflecting on the identified written content in preparation for writing a major paper. The connecting link between the initial letter and the reflection could be a service-learning experience. Students can read the letters after the experience and reflect on the initial letter in terms of similarities to and differences from their previous thoughts, feelings, and assumptions, thus providing an avenue for deeper reflection, meanings, and considerable learning. Refer to Box 17.2, Strategies to Create a Culturally Inclusive Teaching and Learning Environment.

Clinical Practice Courses

Emphasis should be placed on inclusive teaching and learning not only in classroom settings but also in clinical practice settings. As attention is given to making curricular and content changes, opportunities must also be provided for clinical practice so that knowledge is reinforced, skills are developed, and changes in attitudes occur. Although many studies identify barriers and facilitators to successful completion of nursing school by minority students, these barriers focus on academic factors in the classroom and usually fail to include the clinical education experiences of minority students. In a scoping study that focused on inclusivity and strategies to promote inclusivity in students enrolled in baccalaureate nursing programs, Metzger et al. (2020) found

that all minority students experienced some form of discrimination during their educational experiences. Nursing students experienced discrimination from faculty, peers, and clinicians in the clinical setting as well as in the classroom. This discrimination ranged from subtle to overt and in some instances involved policies that ignored the beliefs and or behaviors of minority groups and called for conformity to the dominant culture. In an integrative review of perceived barriers and facilitators to clinical education, Graham et al. (2016) found that minority students experience significant barriers in the clinical setting. These barriers include negative interactions between minority students and nursing clinical faculty, minority students and their peers, and minority students and nursing personnel. The review also found evidence of perceived and covert racism and discrimination in the clinical settings. Lack of attention to the educational clinical experiences of minority students is significant because clinical education has been found to be an important factor in the development of nursing skills and knowledge.

Many clinical experiences are structured for students to work with preceptors as their primary source of instruction and evaluation. Because of the power preceptors hold when working with students, there is a possibility that students may experience bias and racism in their precepted experiences. Johnson et al. (2021) recommend that faculty include preceptors in antiracism training sessions and review preceptor orientation programs to determine the need for including Diversity, Equity, and Inclusion strategies in these programs.

Communication is an important skill in clinical practice. To address the diversity of communication approaches, faculty can encourage students to actively observe different ways of communicating by summarizing news articles, watching television programs, and listening to the local news. When doing so, faculty should direct students to observe eye contact and mention that faculty and students with a Eurocentric background prefer eye-to-eye contact and often view others who do not look them in the eye as dishonest. Faculty can also use video clips with examples of communication interactions between health care team members and develop opportunities to practice different communication styles through the use of simulations and interprofessional simulations with the health care team members.

When selecting clinical placement sites, faculty should plan to use both inpatient and community-based facilities. Faculty should make concerted efforts to ensure that one in every five patients selected for student clinical learning experiences is from a different cultural group. Checklists or databases can be established for students and faculty to monitor and track the gender, age, racial and ethnic makeup, and socioeconomic status of patients assigned for care. When using these tracking systems, faculty should take the time to explain the systems being used and the rationale for their use with students.

By visiting urban areas or specific cultural districts, faculty can provide opportunities for students to view areas of the community that are different from their own and conduct an organizational climate audit as part of their assignment. For example, grocery stores, storefronts, houses of worship, health clinics, and businesses could be among the destinations. Often manufacturing plants and waste sites may be close to housing communities of the underserved. Students can be directed to books, movies, and stage plays that depict an image of life as experienced by varied cultures. To make these worthwhile experiences, faculty can assist students in developing focus points that can direct their observations, conversations, and discussions before and after the experience.

Immersion Experiences

Immersion experiences are another beneficial approach to integrating content, engaging students, and affording opportunities for reflection and the development of cultural competence. Faculty can use immersion experiences in several ways. One experience can be service-learning with agencies that serve culturally diverse populations or those that have a specific patient population. The benefits of immersion experiences are multifaceted. For example, Dyches et al. (2019) examined senior nursing students' experiences and learning during a cultural immersion service-learning trip to Haiti through the use of postexperience reflection. All student clinical experiences required that students complete a write-up on their daily interactions with patients. Issues related to how culture impacts care of patients along with examples were included in the write-up. The study found that students reported improved cultural understanding and self-perception. The results showed that students learned about social and cultural factors that impact nursing activities and health care. Conroy and Taggart (2016) also found that undergraduate and graduate nursing students who enrolled in a cultural immersion study abroad program indicated in their reflection assignments that they found the experience to be transformational in living and learning from the Chinese people. Another form of immersion is the use of ethnographies. *Ethnography* refers to a written presentation of qualitative descriptions of human social information based on fieldwork. It offers a close examination of social and cultural phenomena and allows for collection of data through an immersion experience in the natural setting. Ethnography allows students to acquire a deep understanding of cultural backgrounds and ethnocentricities among culturally different people. Ethnography is an excellent method for identifying phenomena that have cross-cultural implications.

Online Courses

Online learning is an established method for providing nursing education in the United States. Online courses can offer quality instruction to remote students, reach underserved populations, respond to the diverse learning styles through which, and paces at which, students learn, break down barriers of time and space, and give access to students with different languages and cultures. As a consequence of the COVID-19 pandemic, there has been an unprecedented shift to online and remote learning. This is true for all areas of higher education, and not just nursing. This shift has magnified inequities faced by underrepresented minorities and first-generation learners in higher education (Barber et al., 2021). Barber et al. (2021) conducted a study that focused on the delivery of completely online courses. This study surveyed enrolled students engaged in online learning to explore their experiences with COVID-19-related remote learning. The results showed that transitioning to remote learning was challenging for all students. However, results showed that underrepresented minority and first-generation college students were disproportionately impacted due to their competing familial responsibilities and economic insecurity. The study also found that there were many challenges for faculty who teach online.

Recognizing that instructional design cannot be culturally neutral is a first step in the process of developing culturally sensitive online course materials and resources. Teaching diverse students in an online environment requires understanding that the students' culture must be taken into consideration. Culture is discernible in online content and communication, most especially in online discussions and email communications. Clear norms and netiquette (network etiquette) must be established at the outset of the course to indicate key principles such as respect for diversity. The Columbia Center for Teaching and Learning (2017) has identified areas that are important for inclusive teaching and learning online and has included tips for including culturally responsive activities in online courses. Some of these tips are (1) reflecting on our own beliefs about teaching online to make sure that there is a commitment to inclusion; (2) acknowledging barriers to inclusion when selecting online course content and assignments; (3) engaging students by partnering with them in creating an environment that is supportive of their needs; (4) providing opportunities for students to interact with each other online (e.g., small group discussions); (5) being responsive to online students by having regular virtual office hours and periodically checking-in with the students, and (6) being flexible in terms of assignments and being mindful that not all students will have access to reliable internet software and hardware.

The roles of the student and the instructor in an online course may raise cultural issues. For instance, in some cultures it is considered inappropriate for students to question the instructor or the knowledge being conveyed in the course. The cocreation of knowledge and meaning in an online course, coupled with the instructor's role as an equal player in the process, may be uncomfortable for a student from this type of culture. Conversely, a student whose culture is more communal and in which group process is valued may feel uncomfortable in a course where independent learning is the primary mode of instruction.

Faculty can devise strategies to facilitate cultural engagement in online classrooms. For example, faculty can employ approaches to help students understand cultural differences such as discussing before the first days of class the cultural differences in online classroom dynamics in the United States in comparison with other cultures. Also, to enhance open communication in the online classroom using developmental approaches such as structured group exercises, permitting students to present written assignments verbally in small groups and progressing to the point at which the fear of participating in discussions is overcome have been reported as highly successful in achieving this aim. Online courses and experiences have the additional potential for linking classrooms for the purpose of establishing cultural exchanges through the use of virtual experiences. Additionally, faculty teaching online courses can facilitate students' awareness of their own beliefs and those of others by using peer-review learning strategies that provide more depth to individual learning. Online surveys and journals are two strategies for prompting these discussions.

Evaluation of Learning Outcomes

One of the most important responsibilities of the nurse educator is to ascertain whether students are achieving the course or program learning outcomes. Nursing education has come under public scrutiny to demonstrate accountability for the quality of the programs and ensure the competence of the practitioners who graduate from the nursing programs. With this increased focus on accountability and competence, assessment and testing practices are major responsibilities of the nurse faculty, who must ensure that all learning assessments are fair, appropriate, and equitable to all groups being assessed (Oermann & Gaberson, 2019). When evaluating underrepresented minority students, faculty must follow best practices in evaluation, such as having specific learning outcomes, providing opportunity for learning and practice, and providing clear guidelines for evaluation. For diverse nursing students, particularly those whose primary language is not English, testing and evaluation can become major challenges to their academic success. Much of the difficulty for these students centers around the inability to communicate in English, orally and in writing. As evaluation strategies, tests, written work, and clinical performance must be developed with the diversity and language abilities of the students in mind (see also Chapters 23, 24, and 25).

If an assessment is biased, the validity of the test and assessment scores for all students comes into question. Faculty must recognize that low test scores for a person with a disability may be because the student needed more time and not because of lack of knowledge, and approve accommodations as needed. Likewise, nurse faculty must recognize that minority students who are given linguistically biased assessments may have lower scores than their nonminority nursing student peers (Oermann & Gaberson, 2019). Teacher-made tests often are a source of unintentional multicultural bias. Faculty should follow American Psychological Association (2021) language guidelines for Equity, Diversity, and Inclusion and review current tests to remove any gender or cultural stereotyping; to avoid the use of American slang, idioms, or regional colloquialisms; and to use language that would be understood by all students.

One way to avoid these test errors is to have colleagues take the teacher-made test and provide a peer review (see Chapter 24); often colleagues can provide new insights because they have a fresh set of eyes and are more likely to find test construction errors and/or linguistic bias. Linguistic modification on exams may improve the students' test outcomes and increase the chances for student academic success. Linguistic modification is a process by which the language load of test items is reduced semantically and syntactically while the content and integrity of the items are maintained. For highly vulnerable students, every test becomes a test of language proficiency. To a greater degree than their native English-speaking peers, nonnative English speakers must process the language of tests and negotiate the cultural expectations embedded in them.

When faculty write tests, they must consider word frequency, word length, sentence length, and linguistic structures such as passive voice constructions, long noun phrases, long question phrases, prepositional phrases, conditional clauses, and constructions that are negative, abstract, or impersonal. In addition to linguistic bias, some test questions can also have cultural bias. Cultural bias refers to test items that contain references to a particular culture and that will be answered incorrectly by minority students. Linguistic bias occurs in poorly written questions that may require sentence completion, include items asking for priority actions without bolding or highlighting, or use clauses and unclear wording. All of these occurrences can have an adverse effect on a student's test scores, their self-worth, and ultimately their successful matriculation in a program.

Evaluating Student Work

When evaluating written work, faculty must consider the needs of students for whom English is not the first language and provide opportunities for students to receive feedback and review their work before grading. Doing so will require extra faculty effort, but the reward will be in seeing that the minority nursing student is succeeding. Grading rubrics should be used to clarify the elements of the written work that will be evaluated.

Clinical performance evaluation of nursing students is an important teaching responsibility of nursing faculty. Evaluation of students in the clinical arena depends on having clearly stated learning outcomes, opportunity to practice, and valid clinical assessment tools. Assessing clinical abilities in nursing students continues to be a major challenge. Evaluating students in the clinical arena is a basic nursing faculty responsibility, yet there is no consensus on the best ways to teach or evaluate clinical skills in nursing students (Marquez-Hernandez, 2019). When evaluating students from diverse cultures, faculty must take into consideration the challenges involved when any student is giving care to a patient who is from a different culture from their own (Case Study 17.2). In a qualitative study of faculty decision making in passing or failing a student in the clinical setting, DeBrew and Lewallen (2014) found that some of the faculty attempted to explain inappropriate student clinical behavior as being a result of cultural differences in communicating with clients. The authors concluded that deliberate, intentional, reflective practices will ensure that students are being evaluated appropriately. Faculty should develop a clear perspective on the benefits of clinical evaluation to faculty, students, and patients. Refer to Chapter 25 for more on clinical performance evaluation.

CHAPTER SUMMARY: KEY POINTS

- The United States has witnessed historic changes in the past 5 years. The increased focus on minority populations as a result of the Black Lives Matter Movement and the shift to online learning as a result of the COVID-19 pandemic have changed education in unprecedented ways.
- The increasing enrollments of diverse student populations in nursing programs provide opportunities for educators to be engaged in changes and to use current knowledge of multicultural education, equity pedagogy, and life experiences of diverse students to create a rich learning environment so that all students have an equal chance to achieve academically and professionally.
- The lack of faculty diversity in academia also has implications for creating an inclusive learning environment devoid of bias. Faculty must possess the knowledge, skills, and attitudes to facilitate inclusive teaching and guide students to become culturally competent.
- Best practices must be implemented to recruit, admit, and retain individuals from diverse racial and ethnic backgrounds, first-generation students, persons with disabilities, men, and LGBTQ+ people.
- Faculty must develop curriculum and course requirements that may include new modalities in presentation of content that explicitly state goals for cultural competence and cultural humility.

- Given that all encounters are cultural encounters and therefore teaching opportunities, faculty must develop inclusive learning environments in which all students are welcome, learn from each other, become empowered, manage differences, avoid bias, and learn to provide culturally competent care to their patients.
- Principles of inclusive excellence suggest faculty give consideration to course components including: managing the environment, content, instructional strategies, assessment of student knowledge, and classroom dynamics. This is particularly important as long as there are power inequities as in the workplace, the world, and academia.
- The use of teaching–learning strategies that incorporate concepts of equity, inclusiveness, and active engagement contribute to positive learning.
- Cultural competence may be used as an exemplar for applying some of the principles of multicultural education while at the same time facilitating an understanding of its value in quality care. By exemplifying cultural competence as a process or a journey, both academic leaders and students will realize that lifelong learning is inherent and a requirement for teaching, learning, and preparing graduates to work in a society that includes multiple diverse groups.

REFLECTING ON THE EVIDENCE

1. What are some purposes of multicultural education? What is incorporated in a multicultural teaching approach?
2. How do institutional values affect recruitment practices, curriculum, and diversity policies of the school of nursing?
3. How can faculty incorporate LGBTQ+ content into the curriculum? In the classroom?
4. What are some strategies that faculty can implement to make sure that exams are not linguistically biased?

REFERENCES

Ackerman-Barger, K., Boatright, D., Gonzalez-Colaso, R., Orosco, R., & Latimore, D. (2020). Seeking inclusion excellence: Understanding racial microaggressions as experienced by underrepresented medical and nursing. *Academic Medicine, 95*(5), 758–763.

American Association of Colleges of Nursing. (2020a). 2019–2020 *enrollment and graduations in baccalaureate and graduate programs in nursing.* https://www.aacnnursing.org/News-Information/Press-Releases/View/ArticleId/24802/2020-survey-data-student-enrollment

American Association of Colleges of Nursing. (2020b). *AACN applauds increased federal investments in nursing education and research.* https://www.aacnnursing.org/News-Information/Press-Releases/View/ArticleId/24546/Federal-Investments-FY20

American Association of Colleges of Nursing. (2021a). *Enhancing diversity in the workforce.* https://www.aacnnursing.org/news-information/fact-sheets/enhancing-diversity

American Association of Colleges of Nursing. (2021b). *Diversity, equity, and inclusion faculty toolbox.* https://www.aacnnursing.org/Portals/42/Diversity/Diversity-tool-kit

American Association of Colleges of Nursing. (2021c). 2021–2022 *Federal policy agenda.* http://www.aacnnursing.org

American Council on Education. (2019). *Race and ethnicity in higher education.* https://www.equityinhighered.org/

American Psychological Association. (2021). *Inclusive language guidelines.* https://www.apa.org/about/apa/equitydiversity-inclusion/language-guidelines.pdf

Appert, L., Bean, C. S., Irvin, A., Jungels, A., Klaf, S., & Phillipson, M. (2020). *Guide for inclusive teaching at Columbia.* Columbia Center for Teaching and Learning. https://mi.mcmaster.ca/app/uploads/2020/01/CTL-Inclusion-Guide-Web-082019.pdf.

Banks, J. A. (2013). Multicultural education: Characteristics and goals. In J. A. Banks & C. M. Banks (Eds.), *Multicultural education: Issues and perspectives.* John Wiley and Sons.

Banks, J.A. (2015). *Approaches to multiculturalism reform.* http://www.teachingforchange.org/wp-content/uploads/

Barber, P. H., Shapiro, C., Jacobs, M. S., Avilez, L., Brenner, K. I., Cabral, C., Cebreros, M., Cosentino, E., Cross, C., Gonzalez, M. L., Lumada, K. T., Menjivar, A. T., Narvaez, J., Olmeda, b, Phelan, R., Purdy, D., Salam, S., Serrano, L., Velasco, M. J., Marin, E. Z., & Levis-Fitzgerald, M. (2021).

Disparities in remote learning faced by first-generation and underrepresented minority students during COVID-19: Insight and opportunities from a remote research experience. *Journal of Microbiology and Biology Education, 22*(1). https://doi.org/10.1128/jmbe.v22i1.2457. 22.1.54.

Bleich, M. R., MacWilliams, B. R., & Schmidt, B. J. (2014). Advancing diversity through inclusive excellence in nursing education. *Journal of Professional Nursing, 31*(2), 89–94. https://doi.org/10.1016/j.profnurs.2014.09.003.

Bowles, W. S., Sharpnack, P., Drennen, C., Sexton, M., Bowler, C., Mitchell, K., & Mahowald, J. (2020). Beyond articulation agreements: Expanding the pipeline for baccalaureate nursing in Ohio. *Nursing Education perspectives, 41*(5), 274–279.

Budiman, A. (2020). *Key findings about U.S. immigrants.* Pew Research Center. https://www.pewresearch.org/?p290738.

Burchum, J. L. (2002). Cultural competence: An evolutionary perspective. *Nursing Forum, 37*(4), 5–15.

Campinha-Bacote, J. (1999). A model and instrument to address cultural competence in health care. *Journal of Nursing Education, 38*(5), 203–207.

Campinha-Bacote, J. (2002). *The process of cultural competency in the delivery of healthcare services: A culturally competent model of care.* Transcultural C.A.R.E. Associates.

Campinha-Bacote, J., Yahie, T., & Langenkamp, M. (1996). The challenge of cultural diversity for nurse educators. *Journal of Continuing Education in Nursing, 27*(2), 59–64.

Carper, B. A. (1978). Fundamental patterns of knowing in nursing. *Advances in Nursing Science, 1*(1), 13–23.

Center for Sexual and Gender Diversity. (2021). *Gender pronouns resource guide.* Duke University. https://studentaffairs.duke.edu/csgd.

Center for the Study of Social Policy. (2019). *Key equity terms & concepts: A glossary for shared understanding.* https://cssp.org/resources/key-equity-terms-concepts/

Choi, L. L. S. (2016). A support program for English as an additional language nursing students. *Journal of Transcultural Nursing, 27*(1), 81–85. https://doi.org/10.1177/1043659614554014.

Choi, L. L. S., & Brochu, N. (2022). English-as-an-additional-language nursing student support group: Student leadership and engagement. *Nursing Education Perspectives, 43*(1), 41–43. https://oce.ovid.com/article/00024776-202201000-00011/HTML.

Choi, S., & Mao, X. (2021). Teacher autonomy for improving teacher self-efficacy in multicultural classrooms: A cross-national study of professional development in multicultural classrooms. *International Journal of Educational Research, 105* https://doi.org/10.1016/j.ijer.2020.101711.

Columbia Center for Teaching and Learning (2017). *Guide for inclusive teaching at Columbia.* https://ctl.columbia.edu/resources-and-technology/resources/

Conroy, S. F., & Taggart, H. M. (2016). The impact of cultural immersion study abroad experience in traditional Chinese medicine. *Journal of Holistic Nursing, 34*(3), 229–235. https://doi.org/10.1177/0898010115602995.

DeBrew, J. K., & Lewallen, L. P. (2014). To pass or to fail? Understanding the factors considered by faculty in the clinical evaluation of nursing students. *Nurse Education Today, 34*(4), 631–636. https://doi.org/10.1016/j.nedt.2013.05.014.

DeWitty, V., & Byrd, D. A. (2021). Recruiting underrepresented students for nursing schools. *Creative Nursing, 27*(1), 40–45.

DeWitty, V. P., Huerta, C. G., & Downing, C. A. (2016). New careers in nursing: Optimizing diversity and student success for the future of nursing. *Journal of Professional Nursing, 32*(5S), S4–S13. https://doi.org/10.1016/j.profnurs.2016.03.011.

DeWitty, V., & Murray, T. (2020). Influence of climate and culture on minority faculty retention. *Journal of Nursing Education, 59*(9), 483–484.

Dyches, C., Haynes-Ferere, A., & Haynes, T. (2019). Fostering cultural competence in nursing students through international immersion experiences. *Journal of Christian Nursing, 36*(2), E-29–E-35. https://doi.org/10.1097/CNJ.0000000000000602.

Fagan, J. M., & Coffey, J. S. (2019). Despite challenges: Nursing student persistence. *Journal of Nursing Education, 58*(7), 427–430.

Freysteinson, W. M., Adams, J. D., Cesario, S., Belay, H., Clutter, P., Du, J., Duson, B., Goff, M., McWilliams, L. P., Nurse, R., & Allam, Z. (2017). An accent modification program. *Journal of Professional Nursing, 33*(4), 299–304. https://doi.org/10.1016/j.profnurs.2016.11.003.

Giger, J., & Davidhizar, R. (2017). *Transcultural nursing: Assessment and intervention* (7th ed.). Mosby.

Guler, N. (2022). Teaching culturally and linguistically diverse students: Exploring the challenges and perceptions of nursing faculty. *Nursing Education Perspectives, 43*(1), 11–13.

Graham, C. L., Phillips, S. M., Newman, S. D., & Atz, T. W. (2016). Baccalaureate minority nursing students perceived barriers and facilitators to clinical education practices: An integrative review. *Nursing Education Perspectives, 37*(3), 130–137.

Hampton, M. D., Dawkins, D., Rickman-Patric, S., O'Leary-Kelly, C., Onglengco, R., & Stobbe, B. (2022). Nursing program admission barriers in the United States: Considerations for increasing Black enrollment. *Nurse Educator, 47*(1), 19–25. https://doi.org/10.1097/NNE.0000000000001071.

Hanson, M. (2021). College enrollment & student demographic statistics. *Education Data Initiative* https://educationdata.org/college-enrollment-statistics.

Harwood, S. A., Choi, S., Orozco, M., Browne-Hunt, M., & Mendenhall, R. (2015). *Racial microaggressions at the University of Illinois at Urbana-Champaign: Voices of students of color in the classroom.* University of Illinois at Urbana-Champaign.

HealthyPeople.Gov (2020). *LGBT overview and objectives.* US Department of Health and Human Services. https://health.gov/healthypeople/objectives-and-data/browse-objectives/lgbt.

Hellbernd, N., & Sammler, D. (2016). Prosody conveys speaker's intentions: Acoustic cues for speech act perception. *Journal of Memory and Language, 88*, 70–86. https://doi.org/10.1016/j.jml.2016.01.001.

Indeed. (2021). *The role of tenure and why it is important. Career Development.* https://www.indeed.com/career-advice/career-development/the-role-of-tenure

Institute of Medicine. (2020). The future of nursing 2020–2030: Charting a path to achieve health equity. *National Academy of Sciences* https://nam.edu/publications/the-future-of-nursing-2020-2030/.

Jensen, E., Jones, N., Rabe, M., Pratt, B., Medina, L., Orozco, K., & Spell, L. (2021). *2020 U.S. Population more racially and ethnically diverse than measured in 2010.* United States Census Bureau. https://www.census.gov.

Johnson, R., Browning, K., & DeClerk, L. (2021). Strategies to reduce bias and racism in nursing precepted clinical experiences. *Journal of Nursing Education, 60*(12), 697–701.

Jones, J.M. (2021). *LGBT identification rises to 5.6% in latest US estimate.* https://news.gallup.com/poll/329708/lgbt-identification-rises-latest-estimate.aspx

Joos, M. (1967). The styles of the five clocks. In R. D. Abrahams & R. C. Troike (Eds.), *Language and culture diversity in American education.* Prentice-Hall.

Kachani, S., Ross, C., & Irvin, A. (2020, February 19). 5 principles as pathways to inclusive teaching. *Inside Higher Ed.* https://www.insidehighered.com/advice/2020/02/19/practical-steps-toward-more-inclusive-teaching-opinion

Kilpatrick, S. (2018). *Title IX: 5 ways it changed education for the better.* http://www.campusanswers.com/title-ix-positive-changes/

King, K. R., Fuselier, L., & Sirvisetty, H. (2021). LGBTQ+IA+ invisibility in nursing anatomy / physiology textbooks. *Journal of Professional Nursing* https://doi.org/10.1016/profnurs.2021.06.004.

Leininger, M. (1970). *Nursing and anthropology: Two worlds to blend.* Wiley.

Leininger, M. (1993). Culture care theory: The relevant theory to guide nurses functioning in a multi-cultural world. In M. Parks (Ed.), *Pattern of nursing theories in practice* (pp. 105–121). NLN Press.

Lister, P. (1999). A taxonomy for developing cultural competence. *Nurse Education Today, 19*(4), 313–318. https://doi.org/10.1054/nedt.1999.0642.

Marquez-Hernandez, V. V., Gutierrez-Puertas, L., Granados-Gamez, G., Rodriguez-Garcia, M. C., Gutierrez-Puertas, V., & Aguilera-Manrique, G. (2019). Development of a web-based tool to evaluate competencies of nursing students through the assessment of their clinical skills. *Nurse Education Today, 73,* 1–6. https://doi.org/10.1016/j.nedt.2018.11.010.

Mee, C. L. (2021). Insights from Dr. Kenya Beard on health inequities and multicultural education. *Teaching and Learning, 16*(3), A1–A2. https://doi.org/10.1016/j.teln.2021.03.005.

Merry, L., Visandjee, B., & Verville-Provencher, K. (2021). Challenges, coping responses, supportive interventions for international and migrant students in academic nursing programs in major host countries: A scoping review with a gender lens. *BMC Nursing, 20*(1), 1–37.

Metzger, M., Dowling, T., Guinn, J., & Wilson, D. T. (2020). Inclusivity in baccalaureate nursing education: A scoping study. *Journal of Professional Nursing, 36*(1), 5–14. https://doi.org/10.1016/j.profnurs.2019.06.002.

Mulready-Shick, J., Edward, J., & Sitthisongkram, S. (2020). Developing local evidence about faculty written exam questions: Asian ESL nursing student perceptions about linguistic modification. *Nursing Education Perspectives, 41*(2), 109–111.

Murray, T. (2021). Inclusivity: The margins or the mainstream? *Journal of Nursing Education, 60*(4). https://doi.org/10.3928/01484834-20210322-01.

National Advisory Council on Nurse Education and Practice. (2020). *Preparing nurse faculty and addressing the shortage of nurse faculty and clinical preceptors.* https://www.hrsa.gov/sites/default/files/hrsa/advisory-committees/nursing/reports/nacnep-17report-2021.pdf

National Center for Education Statistics. (2021). *Postsecondary education, chapter 2, the condition of education 2020.* https://nces.ed.gov/pubs2020/2020144.pdf

Nittle, N.K. (2021, February 7). *What is a stereotype?* https://www.thoughtco.com/what-is-the-meaning-of-stereotype-2834956

O'Brien, E. M., O'Donnell, C. O., Murphy, J., O'Brien, B. O., & Markey, K. (2021). Intercultural readiness of nursing students: An integrative review of evidence examining cultural competence educational interventions. *Nurse Education in Practice, 50.* https://doi.org/10.1016/j.nepr.2021.102966.

Oermann, M. H., & Gaberson, K. B. (2019). *Evaluation and testing in nursing education* (6th ed.). Springer Publishing Company.

Onovo, G. (2019). Fundamentals of nursing practice and the culturally diverse ESL nursing students: The students' perspectives for teaching and learning in nursing. *Teaching and Learning in Nursing, 14*(4), 238–245.

Purnell, L. (2013). *Transcultural health care: A culturally competent approach* (4th ed.). F.A. Davis Company.

Purnell, L. (2019). Update: The Purnell theory and model for culturally competent health care. *Journal of Transcultural Nursing, 30*(2), 98–105. https://doi.org/10.1177/1043659618817587.

Purnell, L., & Paulanka, B. (2008). *Transcultural health care: A culturally competent approach* (3rd ed.). F.A. Davis Company.

Relf, M. V. (2016). Advancing diversity in academic nursing. *Journal of Professional Nursing, 5*(5S), S42–S47. https://doi.org/10.1016/j.profnurs.2016.02.010.

Sampson, M., Melnyk-Mazurek, B., & Hoying, J. (2020). The MINDBODYSTRONG intervention for new nurse residents: 6-month effects on mental health outcomes, healthy lifestyle behaviors, and job satisfaction. *Worldviews on Evidence-Based Nursing, 17*(1), 16–23.

Samuriwo, R., Patel, Y., Webb, K., & Bullock, A. (2020). Medical students' perceptions of gender and learning in clinical practice: A qualitative study. *Medical Education, 54*(2), 150–161. https://onlinelibrary.wiley.com/doi/full/10.1111/medu.13959.

Sommers, C. L., & Bonnel, W. B. (2020). Nurse educators' perspectives on implementing culturally sensitive and inclusive nursing education. *Journal of Nursing Education, 59*(3). https://doi.org/10.3928/01484834-20200220-02.

Steele, C. M. (2010). *Whistling Vivaldi and other clues to how stereotypes affect us*. W. W. Norton and Company.

Steketee, A., Williams, M., Valencia, B., Printz, D., & Hooper, L. (2021). Racial and language microaggressions in the school ecology. *Perspectives on Psychological Science, 16*(5), 1075–1098. https://doi.org/10.1177/1745691621995740.

Thompson, R. A. (2021). Increasing racial/ethnic diversification of nursing faculty in higher ed is needed now. *Journal of Professional Nursing, 37*(4), A1–A3.

U.S. Department of Education. (2021). *Title IX and sex discrimination*. https://www2.ed.gov/about/offices/list/ocr/docs/tix_dis.html

Villarruel, A. M., & Broome, M. E. (2020). Beyond the naming: Institutional racism in nursing. *Nursing Outlook, 68*(4), 375–376. https://doi.org/10.1016/j.outlook.2020.06.009.

Wells, M. I. (2002). Beyond cultural competence: A model for individual development. *Journal of Community Health Nursing, 17*(4), 189–199. https://doi.org/10.1207/S15327655JCHN1704_1.

Woods-Giscombe, C. L., Johnson-Rowsey, P., Kneipp, S., Lackey, C., & Bravo, L. (2020). Student perspectives on recruiting underrepresented ethnic minority students to nursing: Enhancing outreach, engaging family, and correcting misconceptions. *Journal of professional Nursing, 36*(2), 43–49.

Wright, C., & Scardaville, D. (2021). A nursing residency program: A window into clinical judgement and clinical decision-making. *Nurse Education in Practice* https://doi.org/10.1016/j.nepr.2020.102931.

Yung, D., Latham, C., Fortes, K., & Schwartz, M. (2021). Using holistic admissions in pre-licensure programs to diversify the nursing workforce. *Journal of Professional Nursing, 37*(2), 359–365. https://doi.org/10.1016/j.profnurs.2020.04.006.

Zambrana, R.E., Allen, A., Higginbotham, E., Mitchell, J., Perez, D.J., & Villarruel, A. (2020). *Equity and inclusion, effective practices and responsive strategies: A guidebook for college and university leaders*. https://crge.umd.edu/2020/07/09/equity-and-inclusion-effective-practices-and-responsive-strategies-a-guidebook-for-college-and-university-leaders/

ZIPPIA. (2021). *Nurse educator demographics and statistics in the U.S.* https://www.zippia.com/nurse-educator-jobs/demographics/

18

Teaching in the Clinical Learning Environment

Paula Gubrud-Howe, EdD, RN, CHSE, ANEF, FAAN

Nursing education and particularly clinical education has responded with significant adaptations in response to the COVID-19 pandemic (NCSBN, 2022). Lack of access to traditional clinical practice has required educators to reexamine long-held assumptions regarding accepted practices in clinical education. The rapid pivot to virtual and online clinical experiences created an intense time of creativity and innovation. Most importantly, nursing programs developed new approaches, models, and practices focused on facilitating student integration of practice knowledge and competencies (Oermann, 2021). Nurse educators and practice partners are rethinking clinical education activity to include a variety of strategies, methods, and environments (Jones-Schenk, 2021).

In addition to an unprecedented shift in how clinical education is provided, practice has identified the need to assure new graduates are better prepared to make sound clinical judgments that promote safety and quality care across health care settings (Kavanagh & Szweda, 2017; Kavanaugh & Sharpnack, 2021). The National Council State Boards of Nursing (NCSBN) has responded to the call to improve clinical reasoning and judgment competency and has developed the NCSBN Clinical Judgment Model (NCSBN-CJM) with plans to revise the NCLEX to include more focus on questions designed to assure nurse candidates can demonstrate they are competent to provide sound clinical judgments (Dickison et al., 2019). The American Association of Colleges of Nursing (AACN) has also responded to the call for graduates who can make sound clinical judgments across nursing practice environments with a vision for academic nursing utilizing competency-based education based on ten essential competencies described as Domains (American Association of Colleges of Nursing, 2021; Giddens et al., 2022) and eight concepts that should be used to organize and assess baccalaureate and advanced practice nursing education. Clinical judgment is emphasized as a concept that should be integrated throughout all aspects of the curriculum including clinical education (Giddens et al., 2022).

Faculty must prepare graduates to practice in a health care system that emphasizes a culture of safety and quality, is patient centered, and includes community and population-based care. Graduates need to use technologically advanced skills for evidence-based practice and must attain competencies needed to practice as members and leaders of interprofessional health care teams. Clinical learning occurs in actual health care environments, virtual platforms, and in laboratory and simulation settings. Clinical learning environments provide opportunity for students to apply acquired knowledge and theory, use problem-solving skills to make sound clinical decisions, and acquire professional values necessary to work as competent and ethical nurses in a variety of established and evolving practice environments.

Clinical learning is a signature pedagogy (Benner et al., 2010) in the preparation of nursing students for today's health care environments and is a significant time and resource investment for students, faculty, and health care agencies. The rapid transition to virtual clinical experiences due to the COVID-19 pandemic combined (McKay et al., 2022, Oermann, 2021) with recent studies, demonstrate that reliance on a traditional model of clinical education is no longer feasible or necessary (Hill et al., 2020; McKay et al., 2022). Sole reliance on a clinical learning model featuring a faculty member designated to supervise and evaluate a small group of students who are each assigned to care for one or two patients in an acute care setting may not offer the intended opportunity to develop proficiency in nursing (Goers et al., 2022; Hill et al., 2020; McKay et al., 2022; McNelis et al., 2014). Nurse educators are implementing and evaluating learning activities in a variety of settings, using multiple modalities to assure students obtain the clinical competencies required in today's complex and multifaceted health care settings (Bowles et al., 2022; Donovan et al., 2022).

The purpose of this chapter is to describe the environments for clinical teaching and learning. The chapter also discusses traditional and new teaching methods, technology and models that facilitate application of knowledge, theory, and clinical reasoning in patient care situations. The chapter will address how the curriculum relates to clinical teaching and discuss the roles and responsibilities of clinical teachers.

CLINICAL LEARNING ENVIRONMENTS

The environment for practicum experiences may be any place where students interact with patients, their families, and populations for purposes such as acquiring needed cognitive skills that facilitate clinical reasoning and decision making, in addition to psychomotor and affective skills. The practicum environment, commonly referred to as the *clinical learning environment* (CLE), is an interactive network of forces within the clinical setting that influence students' clinical learning outcomes. The environment also provides opportunities for students to integrate theoretical nursing knowledge into nursing care, cultivate clinical reasoning and judgment skills, and develop a professional identity (Cant et al., 2021; Donovan et al., 2022).

The CLE introduces students to the expectations of the practice environment and the roles and responsibilities of health care professionals. To accomplish these outcomes, a variety of experiences are required in multiple settings. These settings may be special venues within schools of nursing or within acute care settings or communities. The clinical environment now includes virtual settings such as telehealth as a new modality for patient care and clinical learning (Donovan et al., 2022). Regardless of the setting, the clinical faculty must facilitate practice environments that are supportive for learning, provide learning activities that promulgate application of theory to practice, and promote development of a positive professional identity so that students will develop the knowledge, skills, and attributes needed to become competent and caring professionals (Cant et al., 2021). The following section describes these settings. Included among these are practice-learning centers such as learning labs, acute and transitional care, and virtual and community-based environments.

Understanding the Clinical Learning Environment

The CLE is vital to nursing education and includes settings where nursing care is provided or influences health policy. Common environments include hospitals, clinics, long-term care organizations, homecare agencies, and community-based health care organizations. Increased enrollment and limited access to traditional clinical learning sites have created the use and expansion of other clinical environments such as schools, workplace clinics, and neighborhood social service agencies such as homeless shelters and food banks. Advanced practice (AP) programs are experiencing significant challenges with finding clinical sites and preceptors that assure students meet the required number of hours focused on direct patient care. Telehealth in an emerging clinical environment as the pandemic increased use as a patient care environment (Eckhoff et al., 2022). Skill/clinical resource laboratories are an important aspect of the CLE and often include the opportunity for simulation-based experiences (SBE).

The CLE has been described as a place where students synthesize the knowledge gained in the classroom and make applications to practical situations. A number of forces affect attainment of expected learning outcomes, including the availability of staff for supervision and coaching and the degree of student-centeredness exhibited by the clinical teachers (Cant et al., 2021; Donovan et al., 2022. Additionally, opportunities available for students to pursue individual learning outcomes define the effectiveness of the clinical environment (Donovan et al., 2022). The extent to which the clinical environment values nurses' work and provides an adaptive culture that embraces innovation, creativity, and flexible work practices is another important aspect that sets the stage of effective learning (Cant et al., 2021; Hill et al., 2020).

These forces, coupled with the need to adjust to an environment that requires an integration of thinking skills and performance skills, may result in increased anxiety among students. Facilitating a supportive clinical environment involves comprehensive orientation of students to the environment, ensuring they are prepared to perform necessary skills, and encouraging the development of clinical reasoning (Donovan et al., 2022). Creating an environment that welcomes students, promotes learning, and facilitates praxis—the application of theory to practice—ensures learners become competent nurses (Sommer et al., 2021).

Clinical learning experiences in patient care environments have unique and complex challenges for the nurse educator to consider. Traditionally, undergraduate clinical rotations have consisted of short blocks of time spent on a unit caring for a patient or two, mostly performing nursing skills with little or no time dedicated to focus on integration of theory, application of critical thinking, and clinical reasoning. Often there was minimal focus on providing feedback or effective evaluation of the interventions performed. Additionally, the activity of the CLE can often focus on the operational aspects of the unit, resulting in an emphasis on completing tasks and maintaining unit schedules. Nursing staff are expected to meet productivity goals and are caring for patients who are extremely ill with multiple health care needs in complex and dynamic organizations. Nurses intuitively want to be good role models and nurture students but often do not have the time to do so. Faculty must balance the operational needs of the unit with the importance of ensuring that students receive feedback and focus on daily learning goals related to clinical reasoning, safety, socialization

into the profession, and clinical course outcomes. Graduate students tend to spend more concentrated time in fewer settings and work closely with a preceptor to master the competencies required for practice.

Clinical Learning Resource Centers

The Clinical Learning Resource Center (CLRC), also commonly called the skills lab, is a critical component of nursing program curriculum. Initial teaching and learning of psychomotor, cognitive, and affective skills in nursing education traditionally begin in a setting where students can practice and demonstrate mastery of the most common skills they are likely to use when caring for patients as new graduate nurses. The clinical learning center is used at several stages of students' learning to foster a nonthreatening and safe learning environment. These centers encourage guided experiences that allow students to practice and master a variety of psychomotor, affective, and cognitive skills. Skill/clinical resource lab is an essential component of AP nursing programs as well. AP students must master advanced skills depending on the specialty. Advanced skills such as suturing and central line placement are provided in the skills/clinical lab with ample time to develop mastery needed for providing safe patient care. Advanced physical assessment lab is a required component of AP nursing education.

The landmark study by Benner et al. (2010) identified a lack of clinical reasoning skills in nursing graduates and recommended transitioning designing skill development learning activities to incorporate contextualized learning. This means the psychomotor skills are contextualized, so the student practices the skill in the context of a case and includes more than memorizing the manual steps needed to complete a task. Embedding skills in a patient case and including documentation in the process provides the opportunity for students to learn the rationale and theory that influences providing safe and quality care. Additionally, designing learning in the skills lab should include asking the "what if" questions, so students learn to adapt the performance of skills to individual patient needs. For example, when teaching urinary catheterization, the teaching plan may ask how the student would adapt their approach to a patient who was confused and frightened or at a different age. Skills labs for AP students should be designed for the level of the learner to assure students contextualize the rationale for each skill-based intervention and provide patient communication when practicing.

Deliberate practice theory purports the learner needs repetitive practice to develop the level of mastery to ensure their skill proficiency is adequate to perform with actual patients in the clinical setting. Mastery learning uses deliberate practice theory and is associated with competency-based education. Mastery learning assumes all learners acquire essential knowledge, skill, and attitudes through deliberate practice and will demonstrate measurable performance behaviors to illustrate they are proficient in the well-defined desired learning outcome or competency (McGaghie, 2020). Performance feedback by someone who is a master of the skill is the defining characteristic of deliberate practice (Gonzalez & Kardong-Edgren, 2017; McGaghie, 2020). Mastery learning is typically not

time bound and relies on intentional learning on the part of the student. The time needed to demonstrate mastery is influenced by several variables: learner persistence, baseline aptitude, quality of instruction, ability, and desire to translate instruction into understanding and performance (McGaghie, 2020). Quality instruction related to clinical skill development involves several steps (McGaghie, 2020). An example of an instructional design created to facilitate mastery of clinical skills and the rationale for each step is outlined in Box 18.1.

Once the learner demonstrates mastery of the skill using a task trainer, faculty should contextualize the use of the skill in a simulated patient care situation. Deliberate practice theory recognizes the phenomenon of skill decay, which occurs when there is a long gap in time between initial mastery of the skill and actual use of the skill in patient care. Integration of deliberate practice requires periodic practice and review of skills with feedback to ensure skill mastery is maintained (Gonzalez & Kardong-Edgren, 2017; McGaghie, 2020).

BOX 18.1   Mastery Learning Approach to Teaching Psychomotor Skills

Instructional Activity	Rationale
Preparatory work—such as watching a live or recorded lecturette/discussion, reading a journal, or assigned chapter in a textbook, completing a quiz, reviewing standards of practice related to the skill.	This activity introduces or reintroduces the learner to the theoretical underpinnings related to the skill. For example, urinary catheterization requires the learner understand the facets of sterile technique. Potential complications related to the procedure can be considered. Standards of practice and institutional policy/procedure can be emphasized.
Real-life demonstration using a mid or high-fidelity manikin or a patient actor—the instructor/trainer demonstrates the skill in real time without providing teaching commentary—the instructor/trainer should interact with the simulated patient throughout the procedure. This step can occur in real time or through a digital recording.	This step allows the learner to observe what mastery of the skill looks like. For example, the demonstration of inserting a urinary catheter includes communicating with the patient during the procedure. Demonstrating mastery provides a mental frame for the learner, so they know what proficient performance looks like.
Instructor/trainer talk through—the trainer repeats the procedure while explaining each step and offers tips on how to perform the skill. The trainer/instructor may use a task trainer for this step allowing the learner to focus on the psychomotor aspect of the skill. This can be in real time or delivered through a digital recording. This step can be repeated multiple times using a recording.	This step breaks the procedural skill down into sequential steps. Provides opportunity for the learner to ask questions and clarify points. The trainer can repeat a particular step the learner wants to observe more closely.

BOX 18.1 **Mastery Learning Approach to Teaching Psychomotor Skills—cont'd**	
Instructional Activity	**Rationale**
Learner talk through—the trainee then directs the instructor/trainer on each step and psychomotor action as the instructor/trainer does the skill. A task trainer is typically used for this phase. The trainer provides cues and redirects the learner if the instructions conflict with standards of practice. This step is done in real time either in a clinical skills lab or using synchronous distance learning technology with camera capability.	Talking to the trainer/instructor through the lab reinforces the steps involved with performing the skill while reducing the cognitive load for the learner as they focus on the sequence and manual dexterity of the skill. A task trainer is used, so the student does not feel pressure to communicate and reassure the patient. Audio/visual recording of this step allows the student to review the cues and redirection while practicing.
Supervised Practice—earner does the skill with the instructor/trainer providing coaching cues and redirection when necessary—a task trainer is typically used in the phase. The learner practices until they feel confident in their ability to practice the skill independently. This step can be recorded so the learner can review and refine their own performance.	Formative feedback is an essential component of mastery learning because the learner gains knowledge, skill, and confidence as they move through their learning (McGaghie, 2020).
Learner practice—this step may not be required if the learner is able to demonstrate mastery of the psychomotor skill during supervised practice. The learner either independently practices the skill or collaborates with peers. This step occurs typically in the skill laboratory. An instructor/trainer is typically available to cue or redirect if the learner needs reassurance they are performing the skill correctly.	The time it takes for learners to develop confidence and demonstrate mastery will vary. Providing time, a place, and practice resources for learners to practice without the constraints of designated class time allows for a stress-free learning atmosphere.
Mastery demonstration—the learner performs the skill in a contextualized situation. The entire process of performing a skill in an authentic simulated environment is provided and the patient case history is presented. The skill is performed on a midfidelity, high fidelity, or patient actor. The learner receives the orders to perform the skill, interacts with the patient during the procedure, and documents according to standard practice. The learner is allowed to repeat this phase until proficiency is demonstrated. If the learner struggles, they may repeat the previous steps.	This phase of the process provides for contextualized learning, assures the learner is connecting the rationale for the skill/procedure while practicing the delivery of patient centered care in a learning centered environment.

Simulation-Based Experiences

The International Nursing Association for Clinical Simulation and Learning (INACSL) defines simulation-based experiences (SBEs) as "A broad array of structured activities that represent actual and potential situations in education, practice and research. These activities allow participants to develop or enhance knowledge, skills and/or attitudes and provide an opportunity to analyze and respond to realistic situations in a simulated environment" (INACSL Standards Committee, 2021).

The explosion of SBEs as a standard clinical learning activity is evident in the literature (Foisy-Doll & Leighton, 2018), and a robust multisite study validates the use of this modality in clinical education (Hayden et al., 2014). Each state's board of nursing regulates the use of SBE, determining the number of SBE clinical hours that can be used as a component of clinical education. Faculty need to access, know, and follow their state's regulatory requirements regarding SBE. AP programs use SBE but the time spent in simulation currently cannot be counted toward the number of required direct patient care hours required for certification (National Task Force [NTF], 2022).

INACSL has established, regularly updated, and published standards now called the Healthcare Simulation Standards of Best Practice addressing guidelines for the multiple aspects of SBE in health professions to include: professional development, prebriefing-preparation and briefing, simulation design, facilitation, debriefing process, operations, outcomes and objectives, professional integrity, sim-enhanced IPE, and evaluation of learning and performance (INACSL Standards Committee, 2021). Adherence to the INACSL standards ensures SBEs meet the intended clinical education outcomes and promote quality evidence-based learning in simulated clinical environments (see Chapter 19 for an in-depth presentation of SBE).

Virtual Clinical Learning Environments

The COVID-19 pandemic sparked a rapid transition from traditional clinical education to virtual experiences as many nursing programs prohibited students from practice in patient care settings (NCSBN, 2022). Consequently, the use of virtual simulation was used extensively and is increasingly accepted as a substitute for traditional patient care clinical experiences and site-based simulation (Shorey & Ng, 2021). Given the ongoing challenges of finding sufficient clinical experiences for students and the advancement of virtual technology, faculty are incorporating virtual clinical experiences made possible by online technologies that can create virtual clinical environments (Shorey & Ng, 2021). Virtual simulations use technology that virtually simulate hospitals 'units, clinics' communities, neighborhoods, and home environments. Virtual simulations create opportunities for clinical experiences that allow for practice focused on critical thinking, clinical reasoning, communication, and teamwork as a member of the interprofessional team (Fogg et al., 2020). Virtual patients are presented to individual or teams of students. Learners interact with a virtual environment and authentic clinical scenarios for the purpose of managing a patient problem. The computer-based technology supports clinical experiences that are flexible, reproducible, can be disseminated across a larger number of students, and permit access at times when traditional clinical environments are unavailable. Early research indicates virtual SBE can be meaningful and produce positive learning outcomes when the activities are well designed, sequenced appropriately, and the scenarios facilitate authentic interaction between the student and the patient (Fogg et al., 2020; Rim & Shin, 2021). Faculty should use the Healthcare Simulation Standards of Best Practice published by INACSL when designing virtual SBE to assure the learning experience meets best practices.

Virtual reality featuring haptic technology is emerging as a method to help student practice and develop fundamental psychomotor skills, such as Foley catheter insertion (Shorey & Ng., 2021). Students don virtual reality headgear and custom haptic technology to practice and master skill performance using game-based learning principles (Havola et al., 2020). This system of skill acquisition allows students to practice and maintain skill proficiency over time. Medicine and surgery have used haptic technology successfully for several years. As the technology continues to develop and becomes more affordable, it will likely become ubiquitous as a clinical education method to ensure students can perform skills safely before applying them in actual patient care situations (Coyne et al., 2021). See Chapter 19 for in depth discussion of simulation and technology.

Telehealth

Telehealth incorporates a broad range of technologies and methods for health care providers to deliver medical, health, and education interventions (Foster et al., 2021). Available technologies are expanding and utilization of the use of telehealth in patient care is expected to grow significantly to improve care for individuals and families who may experience challenges with access to health care resources and providers (Rambur et al., 2019). The COVID-19 pandemic has created even further demand in use of telehealth-delivered care. Authorities predict 30% of all patient visits will be provided virtually and health care consumers indicate they plan to continue to use telehealth post pandemic (Drees, 2020). Consequently, the role of nurses and especially AP nurses in telehealth is expected to increase significantly (Rutledge et al., 2021).

Emerging trends related to the increasing use of telehealth indicate entry-level and AP nursing education programs must integrate exposure to core competencies associated with telehealth care delivery and include practice experience as a component of clinical education (AACN, 2021; Eckhoff et al., 2022; Rambur et al., 2019; Rutledge et al., 2021). Rutledge et al. (2021) developed a comprehensive framework that can be used to design classroom and clinical learning experiences in telehealth. The Rutledge et al. (2021) framework is based on the 4P's of telehealth. The first phase clinical activity involves *Planning* for the implementation of a telehealth program. Rutledge et al. provide suggestions for clinical assignments for AP curriculum that addresses planning telehealth initiatives for health care systems. The second phase involves *Preparing* the provider for telehealth. In this phase, the provider is oriented to the equipment and software. The Preparing phase addresses telehealth etiquette and practice standards to use when providing care via telehealth. Both advance practice and prelicensure students should participate in this phase of clinical learning with telehealth. The third phase is *Providing* and incorporates three stages. In the first stage, the student studies the medical record which includes review of the patient history and reason for the visit. Once the learner has prepared for the telehealth encounter, contact using the technology is initiated with the patient. The second phase involves introductions of all parties involved in the encounter, establishing a shared understanding between the provider and patient of the reason for the visit, confirming expectations, and reconfirmation of consent. The student should also review how to handle technical difficulties with the patient should that occur. The next stage of the *Providing* phase involves conducting a history and physical assessment of the patient and focusing on the stated reason for the visit. This stage involves stating the problem or diagnosis and creating a plan of care. Documentation, making referrals as indicated, and scheduling follow-up visits should be included in this stage of the telehealth visit. The student

conducting the telehealth visit should be supervised and coached by a qualified preceptor or faculty throughout the encounter. The fourth phase of the 4P framework is *Performance* evaluation (Rutledge et al., 2021). Clinical educational activity in this phase includes developing an overall assessment plan for a telehealth program to include evaluating patient access, financial impact, the patient and provider experience, and effectiveness of the care provided. The fourth phase of the framework provides opportunity for learners to engage in health system evaluation processes (Rutledge et al., 2021) and can be used for a clinical learning activity with AP students and senior-level prelicensure focusing on leadership in the clinical setting.

Telehealth simulation is used increasingly in clinical education for undergraduate and AP students and includes interprofessional experiences designed to focus on collaboration between nursing and other disciplines (Eckhoff et al., 2022). Simulated telehealth has also been used to provide clinical learning experiences with motivational interviewing (Badowski et al., 2019). There are minimal studies reporting on the learning outcomes resulting from telehealth clinical experiences. As nurses take more accountability for managing chronic illness in community-based settings and leadership in initiating new and more effective care delivery systems (National Academies of Sciences, Engineering, and Medicine, 2021), the imperative for integrating telehealth standards of care and clinical learning experiences in both prelicensure and AP curriculum is needed to bridge the gap between education and practice (Foster et al., 2021).

Acute and Transitional Care Environments

Acute and transitional care environments provide clinical experiences for undergraduate and graduate students preparing for AP roles. Experiences in these environments enable undergraduate students to exemplify caring abilities and practice the use of cognitive, psychomotor, and communication skills as they interact with patients and their families. These environments have become increasingly complex. A sentinel multisite study found that the complexity relates to factors such as extensive use of technology (e.g., electronic health records), rapid patient and staff turnover, high patient acuity, and complex patient needs (McNelis et al., 2014). These sites are suitable for learning experiences that focus on providing care in complex clinical settings, and faculty must consider the level of the student, the focus of the experience, and the increased risk to patient safety when students have clinical assignments in these units. Acute care CLEs are recognized as appropriate for midlevel and senior students because of the acuity of patients and the complex environment. Faculty should match the level of the student to the setting so that beginning students will likely have better learning outcomes when early experiences emphasize stable and predictable workflow (Donovan et al., 2022).

Clinical Cases, Unfolding Case Studies, Scenarios, and Simulations

Simulated experiences that provide opportunities for students to integrate psychomotor, critical thinking, and clinical reasoning decision-making skills are equally valuable in assisting students to critically evaluate their own actions and reflect on their own abilities to apply theory to practice. The use of SBE is one example of using realistic scenarios to prepare students for clinical experiences, substitute for unavailable or unpredictable clinical experiences, or enhance clinical experiences in a safe environment. The use of SBE enhances the application of classroom theory to the practicum environment (Li et al., 2022). Students' learning with the SBE method can be enhanced, patient care can be optimized, and patient safety can be improved. Additional benefits may include enhanced learning in a risk-free environment, promotion of interactive learning, repeated practice of skills, and immediate faculty or tutor feedback (see Chapter 19 for additional discussion). Point of care cases, unfolding case studies, and scenarios are helpful in preparing students for clinical experiences, provide opportunity for students to encounter the trajectory of illness for patients across multiple settings (e.g., acute care, rehabilitation facility, and home), and allow for intentional design of clinical learning aimed at bridging the gap between classroom and practice (Li et al., 2022).

Community-Based Environments

As telehealth care delivery system and demands for value-based payment for health care evolve (Buerhaus & Yakusheva, 2022), nursing practice will transition from acute care hospital environments to home hospitals (Rauch & Malloy, 2020) and other outpatient and community settings. These changes have resulted in care provided through increased use of community agencies such as ambulatory, long-term, home health, and nurse-managed clinics; hospice; homeless shelters; social agencies (e.g., homes for battered women); physicians' offices; health maintenance organizations; and worksite venues and summer camps (National Academies of Sciences, Engineering, and Medicine, 2021).

The transition to community-based teaching requires the faculty to ensure that learning opportunities available in the clinical placement allow the student to achieve the learning objectives. The Future of Nursing 2020–2030 report (National Academies of Sciences, Engineering, and Medicine, 2021) established the importance of community and population-based clinical experience prepares students to address the Social Determinants of Health (SDOH). Academic-practice partnerships focused on care coordination and population health are a promising model to promote the role of nurses throughout the continuum of health care in effort to improve the health of communities and populations while decreasing costs (Nahm et al., 2022; Porter et al., 2020; Yoder & Pesch, 2020). Clinical supervision requires using technology such as being accessible by mobile phone and texting.

Establishing appropriate and sufficient learning experiences in the community may be difficult and challenging. These challenges often relate to economic constraints and the changes in nurse staffing patterns, with a resultant lack of time for professionals to facilitate skill development and serve as role models. These challenges may require faculty to be creative in their use and selection of resources within these environments and to consider establishing partnerships with the service agencies such a fire departments (Yoder & Pesch, 2020). Using community-based settings creates opportunity for critical thinking, understanding the health care system, and developing communication skills

(Zeydani et al., 2021). Faculty can provide other experiences using simulation or the clinical learning laboratory to assist students to develop proficiency in skills traditionally performed in the acute care setting.

Learner-Centered Clinical Education Environment

Every health care environment and specific unit within these environments has a culture. The culture of the immediate environment affects teaching and learning (Whitcomb et al., 2022). For example, the culture or patterns of actions and behaviors of the health care professionals can be observed in their attitudes, interactions, teamwork, and commitment to quality and safe patient care. Staffing levels, acuity of patients, anxiety of staff, and workload can influence these actions and behaviors. These aspects of the culture of the environment can in turn influence the time staff has to devote to students. The culture of the environment may also result in behaviors related to lateral violence. Lateral violence is often observed, witnessed, and verbalized by students. These verbalizations provide an opportunity for faculty to implement strategies and assist students with processing what they may be seeing, hearing, and feeling, and thus lessen the effects of these behaviors on students' learning. Faculty can hold debriefing sessions, listen to students' perceptions, and make concerted efforts to balance students' feelings and thoughts by using appropriate strategies to soften, yet not deny, the reality of the culture (Pusey-Reid & Blackman-Richards, 2022).

Clinical Environments for Advanced Practice Nursing

Clinical education environments for advance practice programs must be chosen to align with the Nurse Practitioner (NP) population specialty. The CLEs vary significantly depending on the foci of care (acute, primary, community) and must allow for opportunity to engage with the specialty population (i.e., adult, pediatric, psych mental health). Each specialty has distinct clinical requirements in terms of engagement with the patient population (Doherty et al., 2020) with the aim to develop AP clinical competency.

Some NP programs require students to identify their clinical sites and preceptors (Doherty et al., 2020). The National Task Force on Quality Nurse Practitioner Education calls for schools to assure all students have appropriate clinical site and preceptors (NTF, 2022). Additionally, the findings indicate schools must require faculty to increase oversite and supervision of clinical experiences (NTF, 2022). The minimum required number of direct patient care clinical hours is increasing from 500 to 750 (NTF, 2022), which will increase the demand for appropriate clinical sites and preceptors in a system that is strained by a lack of these required resources (Gigli & Gonzalez, 2022).

In summary, clinical environments for NP students are more focused on specific populations and must be chosen carefully to meet regulatory mandates. The role of program faculty is critical to assuring the clinical environment allows learners to meet course outcomes.

SELECTING HEALTH CARE ENVIRONMENTS FOR CLINICAL LEARNING

Regardless of the practice environment and level of program, faculty are responsible for selecting and providing oversite to assure CLEs within health care agencies and other organizations such as schools and social service agencies. Faculty must be aware of what policies and systems are in place within the program. Negotiating contracts that are congruent with the philosophies of the school of nursing and the agency should specify the rights and responsibilities of both. Determinations must be made about regulation and accreditation status, adequacy of staff, the patient population for needed experiences, expected course outcomes, and if the practice model is compatible with intended uses and curriculum needs. In addition, the adequacy and availability of physical resources (e.g., conference space) for students and faculty should be determined.

Finding a practice environment meeting all specified needs is becoming a challenge because of factors associated with the delivery of health care. For example, rapid patient turnover often means faculty must select available patients rather than those who best meet students' learning needs. This limitation in patient availability can create opportunities for faculty to be creative in the logistics in how learning experiences are selected and what teaching strategies are used. Regardless of the limitation, the role of the faculty is to assist students in making learning connections focused on application of content presented in the classroom to clinical practice. Dual clinical and classroom assignments for faculty may assist in making those necessary connections between clinical and classroom. "The very strength of pedagogical approaches in the clinical setting is itself a persuasive argument for intentional integration of knowledge, clinical reasoning, and skilled know-how and ethical comportment across the nursing curriculum" (Benner et al., 2010, p. 159). Thus, faculty have a significant role in helping students make the necessary connections between clinical and classroom experiences as they learn to think and act like a nurse (Donovan et al., 2022; Jesse, 2021) in spite of limitations for clinical learning in the health care environment.

Building Relationships Within Health Care Agency Environments

The ability of the clinical faculty to facilitate students' learning can be enhanced when an effective working relationship is established within the clinical agency. Effective relationships begin with effective communication, which must be practiced in an ongoing manner to maintain relationships and facilitate learning (Donovan et al., 2022). This requires having an understanding of the environment and the roles of the individuals within the environment, adapting teaching approaches to the situation, and establishing relationships aimed toward enhancing the educational experience. These elements do not exist in isolation but are patterned to dovetail with or complement other roles. Information should be shared continually, clearly, and consistently about goals, competencies, and expected outcomes; the level of students; practice expectations; the clinical schedule; and related information. Such information enables staff to assist with identification of appropriate experiences for students.

Inasmuch as clinical faculty have the primary responsibility for teaching and guiding students in the clinical environment, others often assist in the process. Therefore, the sharing of expectations with the staff is critical. Ensuring an orientation to the practicum environment and having students engage with staff early in the clinical experience promote positive student–staff interaction and provide opportunities for role clarification and the development of collegial relationships. A consistent demonstration of awareness of the mission and values of the agency through actions that are inherently respectful is crucial. Follow-up communication provides an avenue for those within the practice environment to keep abreast of changes.

Regardless of the location of the practice setting or the level of the program, faculty and nursing staff should provide an environment in which caring relationships are evident. The clinical practice environment should be a place where students feel they are accepted and their contributions are appreciated by individuals with whom they interact (Cant et al., 2021; Chicca & Shellenbarger, 2020a; Noone, 2022). The Future of Nursing 2020–2030 Report (National Academies of Science, Engineering and Medicine, 2021) declares nursing education programs must (1) challenge and eliminate practices that contribute to discrimination and racism and (2) embrace practices that support inclusive learning environments. The clinical teacher is responsible for assessing the inclusivity of the clinical environment assuring students are welcomed by the staff. A recent study found that underrepresented minority groups (UMG) learning in the clinical environment is optimal when faculty and staff are respectful, accepting, and encourage them (Metzger et al., 2020). The study also found that the success of UMG requires the clinical educator to intervene if discriminatory behavior occurs (see Case Study 18.1). The clinical educator may need to confront an individual engaging in inappropriate behavior and escalate the issue using the organizational structure (Chicca & Shellenbarger, 2020a; Pusey-Reid & Blackman-Richards, 2022). Role modeling inclusive behaviors such as warmth, support in obtaining access to learning experiences, direct communication, and willingness to engage in a learning-centered relationship, are considered essential aspects of

---

CASE STUDY 18.1 Managing Discrimination in the Clinical Environment

Students are in a labor and delivery unit in a small suburban community hospital. All students are meeting course objectives, completing weekly journals, and receiving positive verbal reports. During the midterm evaluation, a student begins to cry and tells the faculty they are assigned menial tasks such as folding laundry and stocking the supply room and have been excluded from attending several deliveries as staff explain certain patients will be uncomfortable with her in the room because of her brown skin color and accent.

1. How should the faculty handle the situation with the student?
2. How should the faculty handle the situation with the staff?

---

facilitating a positive CLE (Chicca & Shellenbarger, 2020a; Donovan et al., 2022).

Evaluating the Clinical Environment

Evaluating the clinical environment is an important activity included in the role of clinical educator. Many regulatory and accreditation standards include evaluation of the clinical environment as an aspect of required programmatic assessment. The Clinical Learning Environment, Supervision and Nurse Teacher scale (CLES+T) is commonly used worldwide to meet such requirements as reliability and validity of the instrument is well established (Cant et al., 2021). Nine questions included in the CLES+T address the student perceptions of the learning atmosphere in a particular ward or unit. The CLES+T has been used primarily in acute care settings and can be adapted for use in long-term care and other community-based settings (Cant et al., 2021). Johnson et al. (2021) suggest clinical sites should be assessed by the clinical faculty to assure the learning environment is free from bias and racism. They suggest assessing the clinical environment include targeted questions in a clinical environment assessment to include: "Did the instructor (or preceptor) create and maintain a learning environment free of racism" and "Did the student observe or experience racism in any interactions with faculty, (preceptors, or patients)?" (p. 700).

CLINICAL PRACTICUM EXPERIENCES ACROSS THE CURRICULUM

Understanding the Curriculum

The curriculum, composed of a series of well-organized and logical entities, guides the selection of learning experiences and clinical assignments, organizes teaching–learning activities, and informs the measurement of student performance. The curriculum organizational framework guides the planning of learning experiences in a logical, rational sequence with intent to align clinical learning activities with course outcomes. The curriculum is designed to build on prior knowledge and to reinforce the application of learning. Although this description of curriculum relates to process, this does not preclude faculty's use of creative and innovative methods in clinical environments. Creative methods have a high potential to motivate students and facilitate construction of knowledge to be applied in practice. Studies focused on perceptions of both clinical instructors and students indicate understanding the whole curriculum is a critical aspect of clinical instruction (Benner et al., 2010; Donovan et al., 2022; Hill et al., 2020). As students' progress and engage in varied practicum experiences, it is faculty's responsibility to interpret the curriculum and to describe the relationships between program outcomes, course competencies, and practicum experiences (Jesse, 2021).

Understanding the Student

Clinical experiences provide opportunities for students to practice the art and science of nursing, which enhances their ability to learn. To maximize these experiences, faculty must have full knowledge and understanding of each student (see also Chapter 2). The nursing student population is culturally diverse and includes members of varied age groups, many ethnic and racial groups, and an increasing number of men. This population is also likely to include persons with (or without) prior degrees from a variety of disciplines and those who possess many different health care experiences and technological skill levels. In addition, students differ in their learning styles, levels of knowledge, and preferences for learning experiences; therefore, faculty must make concerted efforts to balance the students' learning needs, interests, and abilities when selecting clinical experiences without losing sight of the curriculum and expected competencies and outcomes. Assessing the knowledge, culture, and skills of the learner can facilitate creating a positive, learner-centered experience for students (Chicca & Shellenbarger, 2020a). Completing a baseline assessment helps the faculty determine the students' beginning competencies related to knowledge, cognitive habits, critical thinking, clinical reasoning, decision making, and psychomotor and affective skills needed for learning in the CLE.

Selecting Clinical Practicum Experiences

Practicum experiences refer to all activities in which students engage in the practice of nursing. Such experiences are essential for knowledge application, skill development, and professional socialization. Practicum experiences are selected and planned to provide students with opportunities to work across settings and manage care for varied populations with emphasis on applying theory content from the classroom to the clinical experiences. Clinical experiences should include an emphasis on the nursing roles related to health promotion, disease prevention, managing patients with acute and chronic conditions, and palliative and end-of-life care. The Future of Nursing 2020–2030 report posits integrating the SDOH into all aspects of the curriculum including clinical education (National Academies of Sciences, Engineering, and Medicine, 2021). Selection of practicum learning experiences requires all faculty to be knowledgeable about teaching and learning in the clinical environment and have a sound understanding of the curriculum, the learners, and the learning environment. Clinical faculty should have in-depth understanding of course outcomes and know the competency evaluation process, criterium, and instruments used to assess student progression toward meeting clinical competency.

The practicum experiences should help students meet outcomes in a progressive, developmental manner. Experiences with patients from diverse populations and with different levels of wellness should be provided. Faculty should take advantage of opportunities to use their creative talents, clinical skills, and expertise to ensure that all students have opportunities to interface virtually or directly with a variety of patient populations.

As faculty begin to plan the clinical experience, it is essential to determine the learning goal for the day. The faculty then must seek and guide learning experiences that will allow the student to meet the daily clinical learning goals. For the beginning student, focused clinical experiences should be designed and facilitated to achieve specific competencies. Faculty should incorporate individual learning needs combined with course objectives and content to create focused, goal-oriented learning activities (Donovan et al., 2022). In a focused clinical learning activity, instead of providing all required care for one or two patients, students can focus on becoming proficient at a particular skill by practicing that skill for several patients. For example, students may interview several patients to work on communication skills, perform vital sign assessments on multiple patients to develop this skill set, or focus on learning standards of care in a specialty area. Organizing learning experiences allowing students to assign and delegate care or give and receive reports are other examples of focused clinical learning activities. The purpose of focused clinical learning is to design clinical learning experiences, focusing on repetitive practice related to a particular skill set. Focused experiences should integrate students' individual learning needs and focus on course outcomes (Donovan et al., 2022; Epp et al., 2022).

Other learning goals may emphasize facilitating students' ability to synthesize information, integrate didactic and clinical knowledge, develop clinical reasoning and judgment skills, and plan care for groups of patients (Benner et al., 2010; Gonzalez et al., 2021). Here, assignments that involve planning care for patients with complex needs and for multiple patients are appropriate. These *integrative* clinical experiences prepare students for transition to practice and typically occur toward the end of the program.

The selection of experiences should be consistent with the desired course and curriculum outcomes, which may be multiple and specific to the nursing program. For example, the expected outcomes for students in an undergraduate degree nursing program are different from those for students in a graduate degree program. Therefore, the learning experiences and clinical environment that are selected and the practice opportunities that are offered to students should be congruent with the program outcomes.

Interprofessional Clinical Education

Learning to collaborate with the many health care groups involved in patient care is increasingly becoming a fundamental competency expected of all health professionals. Through interprofessional clinical learning experiences, nursing students can learn to work collaboratively with a variety of health disciplines (Marion-Martins & Pinho, 2020). Therefore, students should be provided with opportunities to work as members of interprofessional teams and in practice environments where practice models are used for joint planning, implementation, and evaluation of outcomes of care. The goal of interprofessional education (IPE) is to foster development of teamwork competencies while enhancing contribution to each profession (Gonzales-Pascual et al., 2021; Williams et al., 2020).

Interprofessional simulations may assist students in health care disciplines such as nursing, medicine, pharmacy, and respiratory therapy to learn about the clinical management of a variety of patients. Several recent studies demonstrate interprofessional simulations improve knowledge, skills, and attitudes essential for collaboration in patient care (Sanko et al., 2020; Walker et al., 2019). Through shared learning, development of skills critical to collaborative communication and team functioning, and shared knowledge creation, interprofessional clinical education leads to trust and thoughtful decision making (Ganotice et al., 2022).

Nursing faculty are increasingly participating in teams and designing interprofessional clinical courses and learning experiences. Successful course development and implementation depend on faculty's commitment to the goal of interprofessional practice and a wide range of additional factors. For example, educators must demonstrate professional respect and role clarity. Educators must secure clinical facilities and develop schedules for clinical experiences that are compatible with the concurrent coursework and curriculum progression in each discipline. Other factors include identification of content and experiences

with similarities, differences, and overlaps, and clarification of autonomy and role interdependency. Success depends on the ability to identify philosophical similarities and differences in clinical practice and to establish clear communication through avenues such as frequent interdisciplinary clinical conferences.

An expected outcome of IPE is increased future collaboration among professionals (Ganotice et al., 2022; Marion-Martins & Pinho, 2020; von der Lanchken & Gunn, 2019). The assumption is that students who are taught together will learn to collaborate more effectively when they later assume professional roles in an integrated health care system. Rewards and benefits of interprofessional practice and education include clearer understanding of roles and better employment opportunities for graduates. The long-term outcome is improved access to care, quality care, and increased patient satisfaction and safety (see also Chapter 11).

Interprofessional clinical experiences are increasing as curriculum integrate the core competencies for interprofessional collaboration (Interprofessional Education Collaborative Expert Panel (IPEC), 2011). The core competencies were developed by six health care professional organizations in 2011 and updated in 2016 (Interprofessional Education Collaborative). Examples of IPE clinical experiences include rural health clinics (Walker et al., 2019), ambulatory care settings (Saunders et al., 2018); shadowing interprofessional team members in a clinical setting (von der Lancken & Gunn, 2019) and simulation scenarios designed specifically to promote the IPEC competencies (Marion-Martins & Pinho, 2020). The COVID-19 pandemic created obstacles to clinical education and may have created barriers to interprofessional clinical experiences. As the pandemic resolves, there will likely be an uptick in interprofessional learning activities.

Evaluating Experiences

Students are required to demonstrate multiple behaviors in cognitive, psychomotor, and affective domains. Consequently, clinical faculty must evaluate students in each of these areas. The evaluation must be both ongoing (formative evaluation) to assist students in learning and terminal (summative evaluation) to determine learning outcomes.

Constructive and timely feedback, which promotes achievement and growth, is an essential element of evaluation. For a discussion of clinical performance evaluation, refer to Chapter 25.

Scheduling Clinical Practicum Assignments

Although faculty schedule clinical practicum experiences to promote learning, there is ongoing dialogue about the best way to schedule experiences, with emphasis placed on the length of the experiences (hours per day, number of days per week, number of weeks per semester), the timing of the experiences in relation to didactic course assignments, and student needs. Faculty should consider course goals related to both theory and clinical courses and integration of theory content with clinical experiences when making scheduling decisions. Traditional approaches to undergraduate clinical education utilizing short blocks of rotations in various environments are being reconsidered due to a shortage of clinical sites and the increasing complexity of all patient care environments (Goers et al., 2022; McKenna et al., 2019). Clinical placements that allow students to spend longer periods of time or return to a unit reduce orientation and preceptor time (Goers et al., 2022).

When the learning goal is to integrate students into a clinical setting or when the students are working with a preceptor, students may work the same shift as the nurse with whom they are paired. Many acute care hospitals have an 8-hour shift option, whereas others have only 12-hour shifts. Giving students the opportunity to work the 12-hour shift affords the full scope of practice in any given nurse's day. Students are able to quickly see and experience the role of the nurse.

When scheduling clinical experiences, consideration of course outcomes and the quality of the clinical environment for learning should guide decisions for prelicensure and AP programs. Faculty must consider additional variables such as availability of patients, clinical facilities, course schedules, and student needs. Scheduling is frequently influenced by the desire to have concurrent classroom and clinical experiences so that knowledge can be transferred and applied immediately. Clinical scheduling can be further complicated by the need to coordinate schedules of students from more than one school of nursing. Ideal scheduling may not be a reality.

EFFECTIVE CLINICAL TEACHING

The roles and responsibilities required for clinical teaching are many and complex. In 2016 the National League for Nursing (NLN) developed a task group to explore the evidence about the roles and responsibilities of academic faculty performing the role of clinical nurse educator (NLN, 2022a). The NLN core competencies for clinical nurse educators are: (1) apply clinical expertise in the health care environment, (2) facilitate learning in the health care environment, (3) demonstrate effective interpersonal communication and collaborative interprofessional relationships, (4) apply clinical expertise in the health care environment, (5) facilitate learner development and socialization, and (6) implement effective clinical and assessment evaluation strategies (NLN, 2022a). These competencies were found to be an appropriate framework to support NP and undergraduate clinical educator competence (Sebach, 2022; Shellenbarger & Sebach, 2022)

Clinical teachers must understand the curriculum, use teaching skills to facilitate learning, interact with the staff in the clinical setting, and model expert nursing care. Effective clinical teaching uses multiple instructional techniques and teaching tactics to develop and adapt to the environment in which students have opportunities. The clinical instructor must facilitate relationships with staff and patients while implementing activities aimed at fostering mutual respect and support for students with each other while they are achieving identified learning outcomes. Faculty who teach in practicum environments are the crucial links to successful experiences for students and also work collaboratively with the nursing staff and administration to ensure patients involved with student learning receive safe and quality care.

Research about clinical teaching over time consistently indicates that effective clinical teachers are clinically competent, communicate clear expectations, are approachable, and can coach students through difficult patient situations (Donovan et al., 2022). Additionally, students indicate effective clinical teachers have knowledge of the clinical environment and curriculum, make clinical learning enjoyable through supportive actions, express empathy, and communicate passion for the profession (Subke et al., 2020). Making clinical learning enjoyable involves helping students connect theory to practice and applying clinical reasoning while using a patient-centered approach to addressing problems (Hill et al., 2020).

Being knowledgeable and being able to share practice wisdom with students in clinical settings is essential. Such knowledge includes an understanding of the theories and concepts related to the practice of nursing. Equally important is an ability to convey the knowledge in an understandable manner.

Nursing students experience stress and anxiety in clinical learning situations. Negative relationships with faculty can contribute to anxiety (Subke et al., 2020). The effective clinical teacher recognizes students' need for supportive and professional relationships and develops an interpersonal style that promotes a collegial learning environment. Behaviors such as showing appreciation for staff and treating students with respect, correcting mistakes without belittling, and being supportive and understanding of students' concerns are essential clinical teaching behaviors (Reising et al., 2018; Subke et al., 2020). A positive environment is significantly influenced by faculty who are available, set clear expectations, are approachable, and provide frequent formative feedback (Hill et al., 2020).

The literature points to the importance of building relationships between students and teachers early in the clinical course or rotation. Taking the time to identify each student's strengths, perceived challenges, and individual goals create positive expectations and prevent faculty from making assumptions and reacting to students' gaps in knowledge, misunderstandings, or poor performance. Unsubstantiated assumptions regarding student intent or motivation may be perceived by students as being disrespectful and can create unnecessary anxiety. Connecting with individual students early in the relationship assists faculty in determining the approach and strategies needed to meet students' learning needs (Subke et al., 2020).

Teacher confidence is another factor that enhances learning; teachers who lack confidence may create a climate that compromises approachability between themselves and the students they teach. A part of teacher confidence is establishing a foundation of nursing knowledge and developing the skills to convey that knowledge to students in an understandable frame (Reising et al., 2018). When clinical teachers use their nursing and teaching expertise to support learning, the teacher–student relationship is strengthened. Additional characteristics of effective teachers are listed in Box 18.2.

BOX 18.2 Characteristics of Effective Clinical Teachers

1. Create an environment that is conducive to learning that requires:
   - Knowledge of the practice area
   - Clinical competence
   - Knowledge of how to teach
   - A desire to teach
2. Be supportive of learners. Such support requires:
   - Knowledge of the learners
   - Knowledge of the practice area
   - Mutual respect
3. Possess teaching skills that maximize student learning. This requires an ability to:
   - Understand student learning needs
   - Learn about students as individuals, including their needs, personalities, and capabilities
4. Foster independence and accountability so that students learn how to learn.
5. Encourage exploration and questions without penalty.
6. Accept differences among students.
7. Relate how clinical experiences facilitate the development of clinical competence.
8. Possess effective communication and question skills.
9. Serve as a role model.
10. Enjoy nursing and teaching.
11. Be friendly, approachable, understanding, enthusiastic about teaching, and confident with teaching.
12. Be knowledgeable about the subject matter and be able to convey that knowledge to students in their practice areas.
13. Exhibit fairness in evaluation.
14. Provide frequent feedback.
15. Address bias and racism evident in the clinical environment.

Facilitating Development of Clinical Reasoning and Judgment

Safe and quality care requires nurses to make accurate clinical judgments amid uncertain situations (Tanner, 2006). Moreover, there are concerns that nursing education is not preparing new graduates to deliver safe, competent care in complex, rapidly changing patient care environments (Kavanaugh & Sharpnack, 2021; Kavanaugh & Szweda, 2017).

Skillful clinical reasoning requires the student to engage in reflection that considers multiple aspects of self, the patient, and the context of the situation at hand (Tanner, 2006). Effective clinical teaching requires educators to coach students as they learn clinical reasoning and judgment. In summary, clinical reasoning is a "complex process that uses cognition, metacognition, and discipline-specific knowledge to gather and analyze patient information, evaluate its significance, and weigh alternative actions" (Simmons, 2010, p. 1151).

Clinical judgment is the outcome of the clinical reasoning process and is defined as "an interpretation or conclusion about a patient's needs, concerns or health problems and/or the decision to take action (or not), and to use or modify standard approaches, or to improvise new ones as deemed appropriate by the patient's response" (Tanner, 2006, p. 204). Clinical reasoning occurs when an individual has the ability to reason about the details of a particular clinical situation and identify what is salient (Benner et al., 2010; Tanner, 2006). Effective and efficient clinical reasoning is derived from knowing the patient, grasping baseline data, and understanding the patient's response to the situation at hand (Tanner, 2006). Clinical reasoning requires knowledge, skills, and abilities grounded in evidence and facilitated through reflection in practice and on practice (Tanner, 2006). Prompting students to dialogue about their anticipatory thinking regarding a patient and situation provides the groundwork for deliberate clinical reasoning. Taking time to reflect about a circumstance after a difficult or challenging clinical situation is an essential clinical teaching strategy. Creating postclinical assignments and providing written feedback facilitates the habits of reflection that are important for developing expert practice.

Beginning students struggle with the ability to engage in clinical reasoning required to make sound judgments. The novice student does not have the ability to identify the subtle or relevant cues seen in a patient whose health condition is changing and for whom complications are beginning to occur. Faculty should coach students in identifying these subtle and relevant cues and start to collaborate with other health care professionals to provide the interventions needed to anticipate potential problems and consider the options for eliminating or treating complications (Gonzalez-Pascual et al., 2021).

Teaching behaviors that facilitate students' development in higher-order thinking skills include prompts to help students recognize the salient cues in a situation, prioritization, retrieval, and application of theoretical and factual knowledge from coursework. Most importantly, effective clinical instruction focuses on helping students think contextually with intent to understand the unique characteristics of the patient's situation at hand (Gonzalez-Pascual et al., 2021). Box 18.3 provides examples of strategies faculty can use to coach and facilitate clinical reasoning based on Tanner's updated clinical judgment model (Tanner et al., 2022).

Clinical teaching involves using motivational strategies to help students recognize the connections between classroom and theory while acknowledging their development toward attaining course and program competencies. Clinical faculty should discuss course goals and help student connect to the practicum arena, exhibiting enthusiasm about the profession, discerning student expectations, establishing feedback systems, and trying new and different teaching strategies. Using case studies, meaningful reflective activities, and other assignments such as concept maps helps students connect classroom content to prepare students for clinical and can bridge the gap between didactic courses and clinical learning experiences.

Effective clinical teaching involves the ability to optimize the environment to provide meaningful learning experiences focused on predetermined objectives. Facilitation of cooperative learning, active engagement, and the use of a variety of methods for learning leads to highly effective clinical learning (Gonzalez-Pascual et al., 2021).

BOX 18.3	**Facilitating Development of Clinical Reasoning**	

Tanner Model Aspect	Activity	Cues
Preencounter anticipatory thinking	Prebriefing—reflective dialogue or written guide	What do you think are this patient's primary problems? What prior experience do you have with similar patients? What do you know about these primary health problems? What do you want to know more about? How might the health problems this patient is experiencing be connected? What do you think is important to this patient? What cultural influences should be considered when caring for this patient? What are the standards of practice to consider when caring for this patient? Do you have any bias (positive or negative) regarding this patient or the situation to be aware of?
Noticing	One-on-one coaching Postclinical coaching Postclinical assignment	How did the patient's presentation align with your anticipatory thinking? Was there anything unexpected or surprising? What about this patient stands out as significant for further consideration?
Interpreting	One-on-one coaching Postclinical coaching Postclinical assignment	What do you think is going on with this patient? What is most important to address? What other possibilities have you considered? What data or information led you to identify this priority? What did you learn about the patient as a person that might influence your understanding of the priority problems? Did you rely on any hunches or emotions when considering this patient's problems? What cluster of signs and symptoms did you notice that led you to identify these problems? What standards of care are applicable to this patient's problem?
Responding	One-on-one coaching Postclinical coaching Postclinical assignment	What challenges did you experience when caring for this patient? How confident did you feel to manage this patient's care? What adaptations or changes from your initial plan did you make while caring for the patient? How did the patient respond to your care? How did other disciplines involved in this patient's care influence your interventions?
Reflection in practice	One-on-one coaching Postclinical coaching Postclinical assignment	What was the highlight of your time caring for the patient? Was there anything surprising that did not go as well as you expected? What would you do differently? Is there anything you need to learn more about, or skills you need to further develop to care for patients with similar situations? What strategies will you use to improve your care?

Questioning, Coaching, and Giving Feedback

Questioning students throughout the clinical day is an essential teaching skill to develop. Clinical environments are busy, and the responsibilities of the clinical faculty can create competing priorities. Consequently, it can be tempting to give information to students rather than ask questions. Giving information may seem like a timesaving strategy and is appropriate in circumstances involving a safety concern that must be addressed immediately. However, asking empowering questions (Davis & Wood, 2022; Gonzalez-Pascual et al., 2021; Hill et al., 2021) that elicit what a student knows allows the student to construct their own understanding and facilitates critical thinking and clinical reasoning. Questioning is an important strategy used to facilitate a transfer of knowledge from didactic to practicum (Cook, 2016; Gonzalez-Pascual et al., 2021).

Faculty should be cognizant that the type of questions can explore a range of salient topics during exchanges with students and should begin by asking questions that identify students' baseline level of knowledge and understanding. Cook (2016) describes several categories of empowering questions: clarifying questions, such as "can you tell me more about that?" or "tell me about the details that led to your assessment"; analytical questions, such as "what are the expected outcomes related to this decision?"; questions that address clinical reasoning in an ambiguous situation, such as "what did you notice that created a concern for this patient's progress?"; questions that challenge assumptions, such as "is there another possible explanation for this patient's condition?"; and questions that encourage students to develop solutions, such as "from what you know, what is the recommended course of action?"

Benner et al. (2010) recommend asking "what if" questions, so the student learns flexible and adaptive thinking. Examples of "what if" questions are: "how would the postoperative plan of care need to be altered if this patient were diabetic?" or "what if the oxygen saturation dropped to 85%, what would your first course of action be?" Faculty should also be mindful of the level of the learner and how questions are constructed. Faculty should avoid asking questions that provoke shame or embarrassment by consistently illustrating the student's deficits or gaps in knowledge. Educators can foster a positive climate for questioning by inviting questions and role modeling behaviors that value inquisitiveness and curiosity.

Coaching and providing feedback to students to help them develop clinical reasoning skillfulness involves a series of steps (Cook, 2016). Step one involves anchoring the student in their current level of knowledge and understanding by creating a dialogue that allows the learner to articulate what they know and do not know. Step two involves the teacher adding more pertinent knowledge and correcting misunderstanding and may involve demonstrating a skill. In step three, the learner applies the knowledge or performs the skill, and the teacher may need to provide prompts and cues to guide the student. Step four involves reinforcing the positive, identifying any needed improvements, and encouraging the student to reflect on applying what was learned in future situations.

Feedback, an essential element in teaching and learning, is described as information communicated to students for the purpose of improving their skillfulness (Cook, 2016). Feedback, when properly delivered, has a high potential for learning and achievement. In clinical practice, where assessments need to be made about the extent to which clinical competencies are met, clinical faculty have a variety of opportunities to offer feedback in response to performance behaviors relating to psychomotor and cognitive and affective actions. Regardless of the action, key considerations should be practiced. These considerations are *specificity, timing, consistency, continuity,* and *approach*. Approach is important because of its capacity to alleviate anxiety and enhance engagement (Thomas & Asselin, 2018).

Because of the variations in needs of students, each clinical experience provides opportunities for feedback. Creating a culture of reflection requires faculty to provide formative feedback as a standard practice as soon as possible after a skill or task is observed and should not be given only at documented, scheduled times for formative and summative evaluations. Faculty should be cognizant of those actions that require immediate interaction and those for which feedback can be delayed until a short time later—but not too much later. Methods must be identified to maintain data for providing timely feedback discerning both strengths and challenges with student performance. Faculty should create an efficient system for making brief written or electronic anecdotal or mental notes. The delivery of feedback can take multiple forms and depends on the situation. Face-to-face, time-sensitive, brief conferences (e.g., a few minutes) or electronic conversations or dialogue in a private area are examples of options.

Regardless of the method of delivery, guiding principles must be applied and the learning intent of feedback should be provided. Knowing how to give feedback regarding clinical performance and written clinical assignments is an important element of teaching. One method is to point out positive aspects of performance along with areas that require improvement. Some situations may provide an opportune time to role model. For example, if a student fails to integrate communication while performing a procedure, faculty can fill in the missing words. Such action may (or may not) alert the student to an "aha" learning moment: "I failed to communicate…." The faculty interjection could have a lasting outcome. See Chapter 26 for information about evaluating clinical learning and the delivery of feedback.

Debriefing and guided reflections are forms of feedback often used immediately after a clinical experience, nursing rounds, simulation, or presentation to determine the extent to which expectations were met and to identify any areas of concern. Structured debriefings typically involve three phases (Eppich & Cheng, 2015). In phase one, the faculty asks an open-ended question that allows the student to describe their feelings about the situation at hand. The faculty facilitate the debriefing so the learners transition the conversation from discussing feelings to describing facts to objectively review what happened, creating a shared mental model of the sequence of events and actions. In phase two, the participants analyze what happened and the actions that were taken. Accurate application of knowledge and appropriate actions that were taken are acknowledged and the rationales or thinking behind the actions are validated. Misunderstandings are uncovered and corrected through participatory dialogue. In phase three, the learners summarize what was learned and make a commitment to make improvements in performance through additional practice or study. Through the debriefing process, the discussion often evolves into identifying areas needing improvement. Although debriefing sessions generally take place in group settings (e.g., in clinical conferences), it is not uncommon for sessions to occur on a one-on-one basis. Faculty may take the lead by posing specific questions and listening to responses to guide further discussion.

PREPARING FACULTY FOR CLINICAL TEACHING

The preparation and development of faculty for clinical teaching require two distinct skill sets: competence in nursing and competence in teaching (Mann & De Gagne, 2017). Expert clinicians often have a desire to teach in the practicum area. Providing the faculty development needs of expert clinicians can be challenging. It can be very difficult to equip clinicians with teaching skills required to be an effective clinical teacher for those faculty who also maintain full-time clinical practices. Some have been preceptors, and further instruction, coaching, and guidance are required to fully attain the skills needed to make the transition to a new role as clinical teachers. These individuals should be encouraged and provided with information about where and how they can engage in activities that will facilitate their acquisition of the knowledge and skills required for the clinical teaching role. Consistent mentoring by experienced clinical faculty is an essential strategy for supporting the development of new clinical faculty (McPherson, 2019). The NLN Academic Clinical Nurse Educator Core Competencies serve as a guide for preparing and supporting new faculty (National League for Nursing, 2022b).

Orienting new faculty for clinical teaching is essential for assuming the role. Mandatory orientation with clear organizational structure based on intended outcomes promote new faculty satisfaction and reduce turnover (McPherson, 2019). Flexible scheduling should be considered as many clinical teachers also maintain a practice in patient care and work part-time as educators (McPherson, 2019). Online courses provide needed flexibility for meeting the challenge of educating clinical teachers who are making the transition from the role of expert clinician to that of clinical teacher. Essential topics to present include overview of the curriculum, legal-ethical guidelines, and agency framework. Strategies for facilitating learning in the clinical environment, coaching for clinical reasoning, how to deal with challenging students, formative and summative performance evaluation, and making patient assignments should be addressed in faculty development programs. Being an excellent clinical nurse does not mean that the nurse will be an excellent teacher and continued mentoring and support from experienced faculty will increase the likelihood of success.

In summary, effective clinical teachers are knowledgeable and know how to convey concepts to students in effective ways, are clinically competent, coach students to develop clinical reasoning and judgment, exhibit interpersonal skills that positively influence students' learning, and establish collegial relationships with staff in the clinical environment and other nursing program faculty. Clinical faculty need to be oriented, mentored, and provided with theoretical and experiential experiences to prepare them for the role. As nursing programs increase the reliance on nurses from clinical practice to assume clinical educator roles as a strategy to address the faculty shortage, research is likely to continue in this area (McPherson, 2019).

PREPARING STUDENTS FOR PATIENT CARE

Teaching for patient care should involve orderly and logical actions taken to accomplish educational goals. The actual selection and use of a particular strategy should be based on expected outcomes, principles of learning, and learner needs. This section focuses on several strategies commonly used in clinical teaching: patient care assignments, clinical conferences, teaching rounds, and written assignments.

Students may come to the health care environment not really understanding the standards in health care related to confidentiality. It is imperative that students know and understand the Health Insurance Portability and Accountability Act of 1996 (HIPAA) privacy and security regulations. It is the role of faculty to instruct students on the need to implement the HIPAA rules and regulations in all patient encounters. They are designed to protect the patient's right to privacy. Students should be informed of what they can and cannot do in relation to confidentiality, and these instructions must be enforced.

Patient Care Assignments

Patient care provides students with opportunities to integrate, synthesize, and use and further develop previously learned knowledge and skilled know-how. Some nursing clinical activities require students to prepare in advance for their clinical experience and may be preferred early in the curriculum. Students with minimal clinical exposure will benefit from studying the patient. Feeling prepared will influence the student's confidence and provide reassurance to the patient and staff overseeing patient care. Moreover, as discussed previously, the students' background knowledge will impact clinical reasoning making preparation an important aspect of teaching for clinical judgment (Tanner et al., 2022). Advance preparation commences with making clinical assignments, which may be the responsibility of the clinical teacher with input from nursing staff, the teacher and student together (especially useful for beginning students), the student alone, the student with guidance from the teacher, or the nursing and health care staff or preceptors. Allowing students some input in selecting clinical assignments encourages them to be self-directed and to choose experience integrating their personal learning needs. Refer to Box 18.4 for variables to consider when making patient assignments. Box 18.5 provides tips for making clinical assignments.

The selection of clinical assignments by students in collaboration with others has several benefits. It provides opportunities for students to select experiences that are based on personal learning needs, to experience a degree of control over their education, and to interact with practicing professionals during the process of selecting experiences. The extent to which students are permitted to self-select

BOX 18.4 Making Clinical Assignments

Variable	Considerations
Patient needs	Considering patient acuity is important to assure the student can participate in care and ensure the safety of the patient. Patients with complex and multiple health problems may not be an appropriate assignment for beginning students. Patients preparing for transition to home or community-based care may not align with learning needs when the learning objectives are focused on managing acute and complex health needs. Family needs should also be considered. Managing complex family dynamics may not be appropriate for beginning students.
Student needs and characteristics	The level of the student may warrant more guidance from the faculty. Faculty-led assignments are more appropriate for early clinical experiences. Student-led assignments are appropriate as the student progresses and becomes more self-directed. Late in the curriculum, the nurse preceptor and the student will likely make assignments using a collaborative learning centered approach.
Course objectives and content	Patient care assignments should be informed by the course objectives and content. Aligning classroom learning with clinical learning allows student to apply theory to practice and reinforces integration of experience to construct new knowledge.
Clinical environment	Knowing the current culture and climate of the learning environment is essential. When the environment is stressed due to complex patient load or understaffing, the clinical teacher may want to take a more active role in making patient assignments.

BOX 18.5 Tips for Making Assignments

New faculty often are at a loss in knowing where to begin. The following tips should assist new faculty to enhance their comfort level in implementing this task.
- Come to the unit with knowledge of specific student needs.
- Have an assignment sheet with a list of the students for the given day.
- Get input from those in charge and from the staff nurses.
- Talk to the nurse in charge and ask for brief suggestions about the patients on the unit. This simple act of communication is one way to build a trusting, supportive relationship with the staff on the unit, as they can be very helpful in guiding what patients will make for a good assignment.
- Make rounds and talk to all of the patients and family you plan to care for on the next day. Just a few minutes of chatting can assist you in deciding whether a patient will be appropriate for a student nurse.
- Obtain patient and family permission, as this may prevent early morning assignment changes because a patient refuses to have a student.

- Consider the specialty of your particular unit. Knowing the patient population will help determine when to make assignments. For example, if it is a surgical unit, you may want to make assignments later in the afternoon because patients may be admitted late to the unit after surgery. If you make an assignment too early, you may risk the problem of a patient being reassigned to a different unit or discharged.
- Be sure that students know who the charge nurse is in case the assignments need revision when faculty are not available. Establishing a protocol for this will lessen frustration among the staff.
- Always have a backup plan. Add a couple of extra patients to the assignment sheet in case something changes when faculty are not available. Create some backup observational assignments such as shadowing another health care provider such as a respiratory therapist or physical therapist. Create learning outcomes that focus on collaborative behaviors designed to provide patient-centered care.

experiences depends on the goals or expected outcomes of the program, the philosophy of the specific clinical teacher, the availability of resources in the clinical environment to assist students (e.g., to answer questions and provide guidance in patient selection), and facility policy.

Involvement of the clinical faculty is important when students select their experiences. For example, faculty serve as resource advisers and sources of emotional support, communicate goals, and intended outcomes, assist students in assessing the congruency between personal learning needs and course objectives, facilitate planning the experiences, collaborate with students as they strive to meet goals, and evaluate accomplishments (see Case Study 18.2).

Strategies for Implementing Clinical Assignments

Clinical assignments are an integral part of nursing practicum experiences. Several strategies for making clinical assignments have been adopted for clinical teaching. The traditional strategy is one in which nursing students are taught in a clinical setting with a varying faculty-to-student ratio. Ratios should be determined with an aim for facilitating optimum learning, knowledge of regulatory and agency requirements, and consideration of the workflow of the unit or agency. Most importantly,

---

CASE STUDY 18.2 Making Assignments

A faculty is teaching a group of 8 students on a 30-bed medical–surgical unit. This is their second clinical rotation. The clinical hours are from 7 am to 4 pm. This is the students second day on the unit and their first medical–surgical rotation in acute care. Students shadowed a nurse the first day at the medical–surgical unit to learn the unit routine and culture. The plan is to have each student take care of one of the patients they encountered during the shadowing experience. The faculty arrives at the unit to make assignments and finds the census is nine and four patients are scheduled to be discharged.

1. How should the faculty make assignments?
2. What learning activities can the faculty use to help students learn in this clinical environment?

---

consideration of patient safety and quality care is essential (Mella, 2021). From a student's perspective, this strategy involves the assignment of one student to one or two patients. The students assume responsibility for the nursing interventions needed in the care of the patient and should work collaboratively with the assigned staff nurse in planning, implementing, and evaluating nursing activities.

Alternatives to the traditional method of clinical assignment are dual and multiple assignments. The dual assignment strategy involves assigning two students to one patient. This alternative is useful when the level or complexity of care is beyond the capabilities of one student. Because students must work closely to implement care, collaboration and communication between the students are requisites for effective use of this strategy. Benefits of this strategy include improved time management, opportunities for collaboration and peer support, and fewer numbers of patients for which the faculty is responsible. When dual assignments are made, faculty have the responsibility of ensuring that each student understands his or her specific responsibility. For 2-day clinical rotations, roles may be reversed on the second day of care. Such reversal makes it possible for both students to direct care of the patient.

As with dual assignments, the roles of each student must be clearly defined. Adequate time must be made available for collaboration and discussion among students and faculty. There is a lack of current evaluation and research addressing learning outcomes related to the multiple assignment model, and the use of this model may increase with the growing scarcity of clinical sites. Clinical faculty should create a systematic plan for evaluating the efficacy of the multiple assignment strategy so adjustments can be made as needed.

Establishing a process for communicating patient assignments is the responsibility of the clinical teacher. The clinical teacher should work with the unit leader to determine preferred process to assure nursing staff responsible for each patient's care can determine if a student is assigned for patient care. Communicating what roles and tasks the student will be assuming is critical to assure patient care is safe and delivered according to standards of practice. The clinical teacher should also assure the nursing staff are provided with updates regarding the patient status and response to treatment throughout the clinical day. The students should always report off to the assigned staff nurse when leaving the unit.

In summary, faculty, staff, and students play a significant role in determining assignments. Assignments are made by balancing a number of factors, including course objectives, learner needs, skill level, complexity of the clinical environment, and patients' acuity.

CONDUCTING CLINICAL CONFERENCES

Clinical conferences are group learning experiences that are an integral part of the clinical experience. The use of clinical conferences in nursing is common and the standards that addressing debriefing in simulation can be applied to clinical conferences. Conferences can provide meaningful learning experiences and excellent opportunities for students to bridge the gap between theory and practice. Through conferences students can develop clinical reasoning and clinical decision-making skills and acquire confidence in their ability to express themselves with clarity and logic (Vezeau, 2016).

Successful clinical conferences are planned and should be flexible to accommodate group reflection related to serendipitous learning experiences. Plans for conferences should take into consideration the curriculum and the learner. An identification of the purpose, topic, process, and discussion strategies should be clarified before the conference. Methods to assess how and if clinical conferences are addressing course and program outcomes are essential if the teacher is to be instrumental in bridging the gap between theory and clinical practice (Vezeau, 2016).

Types of Conferences

The conferences can include preclinical, midclinical, and postclinical conferencing. As a result of advancing technology, conferences may take place through electronic media and online. As such, the rules and regulations related to HIPAA and the Health Information Technology for Economic and Clinical Health Act apply to clinical groups that use clinical conferencing by electronic media, and compliance with program agency policy is essential. Student groups must be aware of maintaining patient confidentiality as the group presents patient data by electronic means. Using this form of conferencing is a means of using technology while supporting the needs of students. Some may be doing clinical assignments at different sites, and electronic conferencing brings students together where debriefing can occur without having to travel to a central location.

Traditional Conferences

Preclinical, midclinical, and *postclinical conferences* by nature are small-group discussion periods that immediately precede, occur during, or follow a clinical experience. Each provides opportunities for discussion. In preclinical conferences, students share information about upcoming experiences, ask questions, express concerns, and seek clarification about plans for care. Preclinical conferences also provide opportunities for faculty to correct student misconceptions, identify problem areas, assess student thinking, and identify student readiness to implement care. Preclinical conference provides opportunity for the clinical teacher to facilitate anticipatory thinking which allows the student to identify what concerns they should be exploring (Tanner et al., 2022).

In contrast to preclinical and postclinical conferencing, midclinical conferencing is another form of gathering students together to provide some form of midclinical debriefing. Conducting a midclinical conference may be particularly useful when the clinical experience lasts for 12 hours. This gives students an opportunity to gather to share pertinent patient information and plan for further interventions, which may include patient teaching and discharge planning. This midclinical conference time also may help students collectively evaluate the efficacy of prior patient interventions. This exchange of data, in the form of a midconference, is a method of imparting knowledge and sharing common data with the intent of positively affecting patient care.

Postclinical conferences provide a forum where students and faculty can discuss the clinical experiences, share information, analyze clinical situations, clarify relationships, identify problems, ventilate feelings, and develop support systems. In postclinical conferences, there is interaction between the teacher and the students that offers both a medium for learning and an exchange resulting in meaningful experiences.

Online Conferences

Online conferencing that occurs before or after clinical experiences can assist students to come together in a virtual environment to exchange ideas, solve problems, discuss alternatives, and acquire information about issues of clinical care that occurred before or during the clinical experience. The COVID-19 pandemic prompted the use of online conferences to include both synchronous and asynchronous formats (Petrovic et al., 2020). A recent literature review (Petrovic et al., 2020) found online postconferences provided ample opportunity for students to connect theory with practice, engage in reflection, and consider how clinical learning impacts future clinical practice. Online postconferences allow faculty to provide feedback effectively and promote meaningful reflection on the feedback provided. Peer dialogue and learning are enhanced with online postconferences, and targeted discussion related to clinical reasoning can be provided by asking students to reflect and describe their thinking and reasoning. Fatigue was identified as an issue negatively impacting face-to-face postconference at the end of a long clinical day (Petrovic et al., 2020). Scheduling a synchronous online postconference or using a synchronous format can mitigate this challenge. There is lack of strong evidence in literature establishing the impact of face-to-face postconference as a foundational clinical education practice (Petrovic et al., 2020). Without an established baseline, it is difficult to compare the outcome of face-to-face postconferences with online postconferences (Petrovic et al., 2020).

Student and Faculty Roles During Conferences

Both students and faculty have specific roles in conferences. Students should be made aware of their role as active participants. As such, they should defend choices of care, clarify points of view, explore alternatives, and practice decision

making. A student may also assume the role of group leader. Faculty serve as conference facilitators by supporting, encouraging, and sharing information; posing questions and asking for alternative hypotheses; giving feedback; helping students identify patterns; and guiding the debriefing process. As conferences are facilitated, efforts should be made to ask higher-level questions that assist students in applying knowledge to clinical situations (Petrovic et al., 2020; Vezeau, 2016). Conferences also provide opportunities for students to apply group processes and develop team-building skills.

Evaluating the Conferences

Conferences should be evaluated to determine their effectiveness and goal accomplishment. The teacher should obtain and provide feedback regarding the extent to which goals were accomplished, the effectiveness of the teaching methods or strategies, and the degree of learning achieved. The data from the evaluation can be used for planning future conferences.

In summary, traditional and online conferences play a significant role in facilitating students' learning. Conferences afford opportunities for enhancing critical thinking, clinical reasoning, and decision-making skills; for creating new meaning for care issues; and for enhancing group process and team-building skills. Successful conferences are planned and accommodate evolving situations and student learning style and preferences (Vezeau, 2016). Identifying the purpose, selecting topics, selecting teaching methods, and conducting and evaluating these methods are all inherent in planning.

COMPLEMENTARY CLINICAL EXPERIENCES

Nursing Grand Rounds

The practice of nursing grand rounds is a teaching strategy that uses the patients' bedside for direct, purposeful experiences. These experiences may involve demonstration, interview, or discussion of patient problems and nursing care. Rounds also afford an excellent opportunity for the exchange of ideas about patient care situations, which may involve clinical faculty, students, and staff.

The use of rounds as a teaching strategy requires planning. Planning includes obtaining permission from the patient and providing information about the nature of the rounds and the role the patient will play. After the session, patient participation should be acknowledged and some form of debriefing should occur, including planning for subsequent rounds.

Concept-Based Learning Activities

Concept-based learning activities are a type of experience used recently in clinical education (Gonzalez, 2018; Nielsen, 2016). This learning activity is designed to develop deep learning and pattern recognition of a particular health problem or medical diagnosis. Concepts are identified for students to study in the context of the patient care environment. Fluid and electrolytes is an example of a concept students may explore. Each student completes an in-depth assessment of a patient with a fluid and electrolyte problem. The pathophysiology, treatment, pharmacology, and patient response to care are explored. The faculty facilitates comprehensive discussion of each case and directs discussion, so students begin to see the similarities and differences between each patient in an effort to begin to identify salient findings related to each case. The faculty help students identify unexpected findings in the patients' situation related to the concept being studied and help students recognize current or potential complications that need to be addressed. Students are not responsible for care but need to address any safety issues that emerge as they are assessing their assigned patient. This activity allows the student to engage in critical thinking about the concept being studied without the distraction of attending to tasks associated with general patient care (Nielsen, 2016). Communicating the focus of this assignment and learning activity with staff are essential to avoid misunderstanding of the student's role in the unit (Nielsen, 2016).

Written Assignments

Written assignments generally complement clinical experiences and are considered to be useful as they facilitate development of critical thinking and clinical reasoning and reflection that connect classroom content to clinical practice. Such assignments may include short papers, clinical reasoning papers, nursing care plans, clinical logs, journals, and concept maps. Written assignments provide opportunities for students to reflect on clinical experiences, communicate with the teacher, identify mistakes and negative experiences, and learn from these experiences. See Box 18.6 for possible journaling questions.

Point-of-Care Technology and Mobile Health

Nurses are increasingly using handheld devices, electronic health records, and other point-of-care technologies in the clinical setting, and faculty must provide opportunities for students to become familiar with their use. Simulated electronic health records can be embedded in clinical simulations as preparation for their use in the clinical agency or as a substitute for learning when agency policy precludes students' use of them in the agency. Smartphones equipped with reference software enable access to clinical information; care plans; and nursing, procedure, and evidence-based practice guidelines and can provide access to skills videos and patient teaching materials (Firth, 2022). Increasingly, nurses are using

---

BOX 18.6   Sample of Journaling Questions

- How did you feel about your clinical day?
- What was the best part of your clinical day?
- What did you feel most confident about?
- If you could do your clinical day over, what would you do differently?
- What were you most concerned about as related to your patient's care?
- What did you learn today that can apply to future patients with similar problems?
- What do you need to learn more about?
- Describe interactions with other professions. What went well? Describe how the interaction was or was not patient centered.
- Describe any patient quality or safety issues you had to address or manage. What goals do you have for your next clinical day?

software applications ("apps") on a smartphone to diagnose, monitor, and teach patients in community-based settings; students must have experience using these point-of-care and mobile health technologies as well. Kenny et al. (2020) found students' anxiety decreased and confidence increased when they were allowed to use mobile technology such as smartphones during clinical learning experiences. See Chapter 21 for information about policies for using technology in clinical settings.

MODELS FOR TEACHING IN THE CLINICAL ENVIRONMENT

Several models for clinical education are used to educate nursing students. These models, alternatives to the traditional model, include preceptorship, associate model, paired model, academia–service partnerships, and adjunct faculty joint appointments. These models have evolved to increase capacity for clinical placements, facilitate development of competency for today's practice, manage faculty shortages, prepare graduates to be competent for practice, and foster closer ties with clinical agencies (Forber et al., 2016). Given the diversity of health care settings, faculty shortage, and the need for reduced faculty-to-student ratios, new models serve to enhance effective student learning, facilitate development of clinical skills, and promote role development. Comparing the outcomes of various models of clinical education is challenging as there is a lack of evidence demonstrating the traditional apprenticeship approach results in desired learning outcomes and attainment of clinical competency (Leighton et al., 2021).

Preceptorship

Preceptorship is a teaching model in which the student is assigned to a nurse who serves as a preceptor. Preceptors are experienced nurses who facilitate and evaluate student learning in the clinical area during a specified time while balancing clinical role responsibilities (Griffiths et al., 2022). Their role is intentionally implemented in conjunction with other responsibilities related to patient care in the clinical environment. The preceptor model is based on the assumption that

a consistent one-on-one relationship provides opportunities for socialization into practice and bridges the gap between theory and practice. The preceptor model may be used at several levels. The use of preceptorships is ubiquitous as a model for graduate students in AP programs (McQueen et al., 2018; Pleshkan & Hussey, 2020). Preceptorships are considered particularly useful for senior-level students as a strategy to better prepare graduates who are work ready on completion of their prelicensure program (Chicca & Shellenbarger, 2021). Use at these levels provides opportunities for students to synthesize theoretical knowledge and apply information, including evidence-based research, in the practice environment. This method is also an excellent way for students to practice collaboration and socialize in the profession.

Theoretically, the preceptor provides one-on-one teaching, guidance, and support and serves as a role model. Typically, the preceptor faculty and student form a triad to facilitate the student's acquisition of clinical competencies. The preceptor and student meet before the first clinical experience to discuss learning styles and goals for competency attainment and the desired outcome of the clinical experience. Although faculty have ultimate responsibility for the course and students' learning outcomes, the student and preceptor are empowered to conduct formative and summative evaluations of the student's clinical performance and learning outcomes. The student should assume a proactive role, not only as a student but also as a member of the health care team. The preceptor assumes responsibilities as a clinical teacher, mentor, and role model, and faculty serve as a role model, facilitator, and a consultant for the preceptor and the student (Chicca & Shellenberger, 2020b).

Preceptors are expected to be clinical experts, willing to teach, and able to teach effectively (Griffiths et al., 2022). Benefits that have been derived from preceptorships include enhanced ability to apply theory to practice, improvement in psychomotor skills, increased self-confidence, and improved socialization.

In a preceptorship, the role of the nursing faculty transitions from direct instruction to an emphasis on facilitation and evaluation. Preceptors and faculty must work in a close relationship. Faculty provide the link between practice and education. In providing this link, faculty monitor how well the student completes assignments and meet course outcomes. Evaluation is a collaborative responsibility of faculty, students, and preceptors, but most nurse practice acts require the faculty to assume accountability for evaluating the student's attainment of learning outcomes.

Preceptors are critical for assuring the NP students are providing patient care that meet course outcomes. Faculty are the liaison between the school and the preceptor and must provide adequate oversight and supervision to assure the learning environment is optimum and meets the students' needs. Preparing preceptors for their role with NP students is the responsibility of faculty. Preceptor education focuses on role expectations, coaching and teaching strategies, policy, and course outcomes. Studies show preceptor training improves the clinical environment for both students and preceptors (Davis et al., 2021; Perryman, 2022). Academic-practice partnerships are another strategy purported to increase the number of available clinical sites and preceptors for NP programs (Padilla & Evans-Krieder, 2020; Padilla & Evans-Krieder, 2022). Preceptor orientation, support, and ongoing education were shown to be critical elements for positive experiences and successful clinical learning for AP programs (McQueen et al., 2018).

The use of preceptors requires planning to ensure an understanding of their role. Ideally, this is facilitated through strategically planned orientation and follow-up sessions; some schools of nursing offer workshops or courses to orient preceptors to their role (Wu et al., 2020). These sessions provide a forum for sharing information related to the philosophical perspectives of preceptorship, expected outcomes, teaching strategies, and methods of evaluation and are critical for all levels of preceptorships. Preceptor orientation should also address strategies to reduce bias and racism in the clinical environment (Johnson et al., 2021). Preceptor training should include bias awareness which may include lectures, discussions, and case studies designed to help preceptors identify bias

and strategies for intervening if incidents of racism or bias occur (Johnson et al., 2021). The training should address the potential for bias in student evaluations and provide strategies for giving objective, unbiased feedback (Johnson et al., 2021).

The value of the preceptor model is generally related to providing students with a sense of independence for patient care and the ability to develop a professional identity. Preceptors and clinical agencies also value the preceptor model because preceptors develop additional skill sets related to teaching and the clinical agency benefits from hiring a well-prepared graduate. Assuring faculty, students, and preceptors, all understand their own roles and responsibilities is necessary for a successful clinical experience (Chicca & Shellenbarger, 2020b).

Paired Model

The paired model is designed to pair a student and a staff nurse for a practicum experience. It is an alternative to the one-patient, one-student model and is a variation of the preceptor model. This model is often used in combination with the Dedicated Education Model and in community-based setting such as an ambulatory care center or clinic (Hill et al., 2020). During the course, each student has a specified number of days in a paired relationship. The remaining time is spent acquiring experiences by using the traditional model. The staff nurse plans the learning experience, and the faculty member oversees the experiences while creating a learning environment for students. However, most of the faculty member's time is spent in the traditional role with other students who have not been paired. To enhance the effectiveness of the paired model, it is essential that the staffing pattern be evaluated before assignments are made.

Academia–Service Partnerships

The clinical teaching partnership is a collaborative model shared by service and academic settings to enhance mutual goals of developing nurses who are competent for practice and creating safe practice environments. Partnerships are also formed to create new models of clinical instruction and increase student and faculty capacity in nursing programs (Gilliss et al., 2021). Although these partnerships take different forms, they are established collaboratively and result in redesigned clinical education experiences for students and faculty and for the nurses at the clinical agency. Academic and service partnerships are a promising framework to address the nursing faculty shortage and ensure new graduates develop new competencies needed to function as leaders and as members of an interprofessional team and that they can function to full scope of their educational preparation (Robertson et al., 2021).

Academic partnerships provide an infrastructure for developing shared goals related to creating optimum CLEs that support students, faculty, and agency nursing staff and organizational mission. Clinical residency training for NPs is an outcome of academic-practice partnerships and allows academic units and clinical agencies to pool resources and strengthen nursing in both settings (Gilliss et al., 2021).

Wros et al. (2015) report that students in their partnership model were better integrated into the clinical setting and gained an understanding of health care environments that focus on underserved populations in community-based settings. The model involves a faculty in residence who is assigned a provider role in a community-based setting. The faculty is assigned a caseload of patients and oversees the continuity of care as students rotate to the site and participate in health teaching and care coordination activities. Initial findings indicate that in a positive CLE, underserved client health outcomes improve and students participate in a meaningful clinical experience.

Graduate nurse AP programs rely on academic-practice programs as the demand for primary care providers increases and enrollment grows in these programs. Academic-practice partnerships will expand as AP nurses provide care in hospitals, clinics, retail pharmacies, school-based care clinics, long-term care, and in occupational health (DeBiase et al., 2022; Gilliss et al., 2021; Robertson et al., 2021). As academic-practice partnerships increase and expand in scope, faculty must take the time to participate in policy development, designing meaningful and innovative clinical learning experiences, ongoing assessment, and preceptor development (Spector et al., 2021). Working collaboratively with practice partnerships provides opportunity to create models of care designed to prepare advance practice students to practice at the full scope of their licensure (Nahm et al., 2022).

Dedicated Education Units

Dedicated education units (DEUs) are an example of academic-practice partnerships. DEUs are patient care environments where academic institutions and health care organizations partner to provide students with quality clinical experiences. The partners collaborate to transform patient care units into environments designed to support learning experiences for students and staff nurses while continuing the critical work of providing quality care to the patient population served by the organization (Rusch et al., 2018). DEUs originated in acute care environments and have expanded to include other health care agencies such as home health, long-term care, and community agencies (Morgan et al., 2019). Multiple studies found that the DEU model facilitates stronger relationship building between nurses in academia and practice, and students report significantly more positive learning experiences compared with traditional clinical placement experiences (Musallam et al., 2021). DEUs facilitate positive student outcomes to include (a) improved clinical self-efficacy and confidence, (b) teamwork and collaboration skills, (c) development of nursing knowledge and competency, and (d) increased student satisfaction (Musallam et al., 2021). Successful DEUs require ongoing collaboration from both the academic and practice partnership and can potentially have a positive impact on student satisfaction and nursing staff serving as mentors and preceptors (Lapinski & Ciurzynski, 2020).

Adjunct Faculty

Adjunct faculty are health care professionals who are employed in the service setting and have a part-time academic appointment. Adjunct faculty may assume various roles, including those of preceptor, clinical teaching associate (CTA), mentor, guest lecturer, and supervisor. These individuals may also collaborate on research projects.

Faculty who are appointed in an adjunct capacity are registered professional nurses or professionals who are experts in areas such as clinical practice, research, leadership, management, legislation, and law. Robust orientation and faculty development that address competencies related to the clinical teaching role should be provided for adjunct faculty (McPherson, 2019). As the nursing faculty shortage becomes a prominent challenge, experts posit increased reliance on adjunct faculty for clinical instruction (McPherson, 2019). Orientation for adjunct faculty should include assuring they incorporate strategies to coach the students in developing clinical reasoning (Tyo & McCurry, 2019)

Residency Models

New graduates are expected to demonstrate entry-level competency at graduation, yet research reveals gaps in their ability to apply nursing knowledge and make sound clinical judgments (Kavanagh & Sharpnack, 2021; Rush et al.,

2019). Nurse residency programs support professional transition into practice and have been shown to improve new nurse retention (Cantrell et al., 2022). Accreditation and regulatory standards have been developed for this approach to residency.

Studies have been conducted to examine the outcomes of nurse residency programs (Laflamme & Hyrkas, 2020). The findings indicate nurse residency programs increase overall confidence and competence particularly in the ability to organize, prioritize, communicate effectively, and provide leadership (Laflamme & Hyrkas, 2020; Spector et al., 2018). Residency programs have a statistically positive influence on nurse retention rates, reduce errors, lower stress levels of new graduates, and improve job satisfaction (Makic et al., 2022; Spector et al., 2018). Further research is needed to determine the influence of postgraduate nurse residency programs on patient outcomes (Makic et al., 2022).

▌ CHAPTER SUMMARY: KEY POINTS

- There are several models for teaching in the clinical environment such as using preceptors or pairing students with nurses. Faculty should consider characteristics of the students, available resources, and course learning outcomes when designing clinical learning experiences.
- Mastery learning is a sound pedagogical approach to facilitate clinical competency.
- Clinical learning environments may include laboratory, acute care, transitional, and community sites, including homeless shelters, clinics, schools, camps, and social service agencies.
- The clinical nurse educator should evaluate the clinical environment to determine if it facilitates learning.
- The faculty is responsible for assuring the clinical environment is inculsive and is free from bias or racism.
- Faculty must have in-depth knowledge of teaching behaviors that facilitate students' learning and development, have complete knowledge

of the culture of the practice area, and must remain clinically competent. The NLN Core Competencies for Nurse Educators provide guidance for professional development.
- Simulation, virtual simulation, telehealth, and other technology is creating a new model for clinical nursing education.
- Academic-practice partnerships will continue to promulgate in response to changing health care, the faculty shortage, and in response to the scarcity of traditional acute care clinical learning environments.
- The Future of Nursing 2020–2030 report will influence clinical learning to include experiences that address the Social Determinants of Health.
- Empirical research on the effectiveness of various models of teaching in the clinical environment has been sparse; there is a need for further evaluation of and research about these models in terms of their effectiveness on student learning and preparation for the workforce.

REFLECTING ON THE EVIDENCE

1. Choose a set of clinical teaching strategies for a group of students. What do you need to consider about the student, the setting, and the patients to make this decision? What evidence for practice will you draw on to make your decision?

2. What is the role of virtual teaching and learning activities in clinical teaching? Can clinical practice be learned in a fully online course?

3. What is the state of science about clinical teaching? What research questions are being asked? What research methods are being used? What variables are included in the studies?

4. What clinical teaching strategies are evidenced based? Which strategies require additional evidence of their effectiveness?

REFERENCES

American Association of Colleges of Nursing. (2021). *The essentials: Core competencies for professional nursing education.* https://www.aacnnursing.org/Portals/42/AcademicNursing/pdf/Essentials-2021.pdf

Badowski, D. M., Rossler, K. L., & Gill-Gembala, L. (2019). Telehealth simulation with motivational interviewing: Impace on learning and practice. *Journal of Nursing Education, 58*(4), 221–224. https://doi.org/10.3928/01484834-20190321-06.

Benner, P., Sutphen, M., Leonard, V., & Day, L. (2010). *Educating nurses: A call for radical transformation.* Jossey-Bass.

Bowles, W., Buck., Brinkman, B., Hixon, B., Guo, J., & Zehala, A. (2022). Academic-clinical nursing partnership use an evidence-based practice model. *Journal of Clinical Nursing, 31*, 335–346. https://doi.org/10.1111/jocn.15710.

Buerhaus, P., & Yakusheva, O. (2022). Six part series on value-informed nursing practice. *Nursing Outlook, 70*, 89. https://doi.org/10.1016/j.outlook.2021.10.005.

Cant, R., Ryan, C., & Cooper, S. (2021). Nursing students' evaluation of clinical practice placements using the clinical learning environment, supervision and nurse teacher scale: A systematic review. *Nurse Education Today, 104*, 104983. https://doi.org/10.1016/j.nedt.2021.104983.

Cantrell, F. L., McKenzie, K., & Hessler, K. (2022). Task layered clinical orientation for new graduate registered nurses. *Journal for Nurses in Professional Development, 38*(2), E13–E18. https://doi.org/10.1097/NND.0000000000000841.

Chicca, J., & Shellenbarger, T. (2020a). Fostering inclusive clinical learning environments using a psychological safety lens. *Teaching & Learning in Nursing, 15*, 226–232. https://doi.org/10.1016/j.teln.2020.03.002.

Chicca, J., & Shellenbarger, T. (2020b). Implementing successful clinical nursing preceptorships. *Nurse Educator, 45*(4), E41–42. https://doi.org/10.1097/NNE0000000000000750.

Chicca, J., & Shellenbarger, T. (2021). Preparing, maintaining, and evaluating remote preceptorships: Considerations for nurse educators. *Teaching and Learning in Nursing, 16*, 396–400. https://doi.org/10.1016/j.teln.2021.04.006.

Cook, C. (2016). A "toolkit" for clinical educators to foster learners' clinical reasoning and skills acquisition. *Nursing Praxis in New Zealand, 32*(1), 28–37.

Coyne, E., Calleja, P., Forster, E., & Lin, F. (2021). A review of virtual-simulation for assessing healthcare students' clinical competency. *Nurse Education Today, 96*, 104623. https://doi.org/10.1016/j.nedt.2020.104623.

Davis, L., Fathman, A., & Colella, C. (2021). An immersive clinical experience to create sustainable clinical learning opportunities for nurse practitioner students. *Journal of the American Association of Nurse Practitioners, 33*(1), 66–76. https://doi.org/10.1097/JXX.0000000000000297.

Davis, R. G., & Wood, F. (2022). Cultivating clinical judgment in pharmacological decision-making through reflection on practice. *Journal of Nursing Education, 61*(3), 143–146. https://doi.org/10.3928/01484834-20221128-10.

DeBiase, V. M., Coburn, C. V., More, L., & Parsons, L. (2022). Changing landscapes: Academic-practice partnerships in evolving ambulatory care settings-Part 1. *Nursing Economics, 22*(2), 98–303.

Dickison, P., Haerling, K. A., & Laster, K. (2019). Integrating the national council of state boards of nursing clinical judgment model into nursing educational frameworks. *Journal of Nursing Education*, 58(2), 72–78. https://doi.org/10.3928/01484834-20190122-03.

Doherty, C. L., Fogg, L., Bigley, M. B., Todd, B., & O'Sullivan, A. L. (2020). Nurse practitioner student clinical placement process: A national survey of nurse practitioner programs. *Nursing Outlook*, 2020, 55–61. https://doi.org/10.1016/j.outlook.2019.07.005.

Donovan, L. M., Strunk, J. A., Lam, C., Argenbright, C., Robinson, J., Leisen, M., & Puffenbarger, N. (2022). Enhancing the prelicensure clinical learning experience. *Nurse Educator*, 47(2), 108–113. https://doi.org/10.1097/NNE.0000000000001085.

Drees, J. (2020, June 22). 30% of Johns Hopkins in-person visits will convert to telehealth post pandemic, CEO says. *Becker's Hospital Review*. https://www.beckershospitalreview.com/telehealth/30-of-johns-hopkins-in-person-visits-will-convert-to-telehealth-post-pandemic-ceo-says.html.

Eckhoff, D., Diaz, D., & Anderson, M. (2022). Using simulation to teach intraprofessional telehealth communication. *Clinical Simulation in Nursing*, 67, 39–48. https://doi.org/10.1097/NHH.0000000000001061.

Epp, S., Reekie, M., Denisen, J., de Bosch Kemper, N., Wilson, M., & Marck, P. (2022). An innovative leap: Embracing new pedagogical approaches for clinical education. *Journal of Professional Nursing*, 42, 168–172. https://doi.org/10.1016/j.profnurs.2022.07.005.

Eppich, W., & Cheng, A. (2015). Promoting excellence and reflective learning in simulation (PEARLS): Development and rationale for a blended approach to health care simulation debriefing. *Simulation in Healthcare*, 10(2), 106–115. https://doi.org/10.1097/SIH.0000000000000072.

Firth, K. H. (2022). How technology can aid in competency-based nursing education. *Nursing Education Perspectives*, 43(1), 67–68. https://doi.org/10.1097/01.NEP.0000000000000934.

Fogg, N., Kubin, L., Wilson, C. E., & Trinka, M. (2020). Using virtual simulation to develop clinical judgment in undergraduate nursing students. *Clinical Simulation in Nursing*, 48, 55–58. https://doi.org/10.1097/NHH.0000000000001143.

Foisy-Doll, C., & Leighton, K. (2018). *Simulation champions: Fostering courage, caring, and connection*. Wolters Kluwer.

Forber, J., DiGiacomo, M., Carter, B., Davidson, P., Phillips, J., & Jackson, D. (2016). In pursuit of an optimal model of undergraduate nurse clinical education: An integrative review. *Nurse Education in Practice*, 21(2016), 83–92. https://doi.org/10.1016/j.nepr.2016.09.007.

Foster, M., Lioce, L., & Adams, M. (2021). Telehealth in nursing education: A systematic review. *Journal of Nursing Education*, 60(11), 633–635. https://doi.org/10.3928/01484834-20210913-06.

Ganotice, F. A. Jr, Chan, C. S., Chan, E. W. Y., Chan, S. K. W., Chan, L., Chan, S. C. S., Lam, A. H. Y., Leung, C. Y. F., Leung, S. C., Lin, X., Luk, P., Ng, Z. L. H., Shen, X., Tam, E. Y. T., Wang, R., Wong, G. H. Y., & Tipoe, G. L. (2022). Autonomous motivation predicts students' engagement and disaffection in interprofessional education: Scale adaptation and application. *Nurse Education Today*. https://doi.org/10.1016/j.nedt.2022.105549

Giddens, J., Douglas, J. P., & Conroy, S. (2022). The revised AACN essentials: Implications for nursing regulation. *Journal of Nursing Regulation*, 12(4), 17–22.

Gigli, K. H., & Gonzalez, J. D. (2022). Meeting the need for nurse practitioner clinicals: A survey of practitioners. *Journal of the American Association of Nurse Practitioners*, 34(8), 991–1001. https://doi.org/10.1097/JXX.0000000000000749.

Gilliss, C. L., Poe, T., Hogan, T. H., Intinarelli, G., & Harper, D. C. (2021). Academic/clinical integration in academic health systems. *Nursing Outlook*, 69, 234–243. https://doi.org/10.1016/j.outlook.2020.09.002.

Goers, J., Mulkey, D., & Oja, K. (2022). A call to reform undergraduate nursing clinical placements. *Nursing Outlook*, 70, 371–373. https://doi.org/10.1016/j.outlook.2022.01.006.

Gonzalez, L. (2018). Teaching clinical reasoning piece by piece: A clinical reasoning concept-based learning method. *Journal of Nursing Education*, 57(12), 727–735. https://doi.org/10.3928/014834-20181119-05.

Gonzalez, L., & Kardong-Edgren, S. (2017). Deliberate practice for mastery learning in nursing. *Clinical Simulation in Nursing*, 13(1), 10–14. https://doi.org/10.1016/j.ecns.2016.10.005.

Gonzalez, L., Nielsen, A., & Lasater, K. (2021). Developing students' clinical reasoning skills: A faculty guide. *Journal of Nursing Education*, 60(9), 485–493. https://doi.org/10.3928/01484834-20210708-01.

Gonzalez-Pascual, J. L., Lopez-Martín, I., Saiz-Navarro, E. M., Oliva-Fernandez, O., Acebedo-Esteban, F. J., & Rodríguez-García, M. (2021). Using a station within an objective structured clinical examination to assess interprofessional competence performance among undergraduate nursing students. *Nurse Education in Practice, 56*, 103190. https://doi.org/10.1016/j.nepr.2021.103190.

Griffiths, M., Creedy, D., Carter, A., & Donnellan-Fernandez, R. (2022). Systematic review of interventions to enhance preceptors' role in undergraduate health student clinical learning. *Nurse Education in Practice, 62*. https://doi.org/10.1016/j.nepr.2022.103349.

Havola, S., Koivisto, J. -M., M€akinen, H., & Haavisto, E. (2020, September). Game elements and instruments for assessing nursing students' experiences in learning clinical reasoning by using simulation games: An integrative review. *Clinical Simulation in Nursing, 46*(C), 1–14. https://doi.org/10.1016/j.ecns.2020.04.003.

Hayden, J. K., Smiley, R. A., Alexander, M., Kardong-Edgren, S., & Jeffries, P. R. (2014). The NCSBN national simulation study: A longitudinal, randomized, controlled study replacing clinical hours with simulation and prelicensure nursing education. *Journal of Nursing Regulation, 5*(2 Suppl), S3–S40. https://doi.org/10.1016/S2155-8256(15)30062-4.

Hill, R., Woodward, M., & Arthur, A. (2020). Collaborative learning in practice (CLIP): Evaluation of a new approach to clinical learning. *Nurse Education Today, 85*. https://doi.org/10.1016/j.nedt.2019.104295.

INACSL Standards Committee. (2021). Onward and upward: Introducing the Healthcare Simulation Standards of Best Practice™. *Clinical Simulation in Nursing, 58*, 1–4. https://doi.org/10.1016/j.ecns.2021.08.006.

Jesse, M. A. (2021). An update on clinical judgment in nursing and implications for education, practice, and regulation. *Journal of Nursing Regulation, 12*(3), 50–58.

Johnson, R., Browning, K., & DeClerk, L. (2021). Strategies to reduce bias and racism in nursing precepted clinical experiences. *Journal of Nursing Education, 60*(12), 697–701. https://doi.org/10.3928/01484834-20211103-01.

Jones-Schenk, J. (2021). Redesigning clinical learning. *The Journal of Continuing Journal in Nursing, 52*(9), 402–403. https://doi.org/10.3928/00220124-20210804-03.

Kavanagh, J. M., & Szweda, C. (2017). A crisis in competency: The strategic and ethical imperative to assessing new graduate nurses' clinical reasoning. *Nursing Education Perspectives, 38*(2), 57–62. https://doi.org/10.1097/01.NEP.0000000000000112.

Kavanagh, J. M., & Sharpnack, P. A. (2021). Crisis is competency: A defining moment in nursing education. *OJIN: The Online Journal of Issues in Nursing, 26*(1). https://doi.org/10.3912/OJIN.Vol26No01Man02. Manuscript 2.

Laflamme, J., & Hyrkas, K. (2020). New graduate orientation evaluation: Are there any best practices out there? *Journal for Nurses in Professional Development, 36*(4), 199–212. https://doi.org/10.1097/NND.0000000000000642.

Lapinski, J., & Ciurzynski, S. (2020). Enhancing the sustainability of a dedicated education unit: Overcoming obstacles and strengthening partnerships. *Journal of Professional Nursing, 36*, 659–665. https://doi.org/10.1016/j.profnurs.2020.09.007.

Leighton, K., Kardong-Edgren, S., McNelis, A. M., Foisy-Doll, C., & Sullo, E. (2021). Traditional clinical outcomes in prelicensure nursing education: An empty systematic review. *Journal of Nursing Education, 60*(3), 136–142. https://doi.org/10.3928/01484834-20210222-03.

Li, Y. Y., Au, M. L., Tong, L. K., Ng, W. I., & Wang, S. C. (2022). High-fidelity simulation in undergraduate nursing education: A meta-analysis. *Nurse Education Today, 111*. https://doi.org/10.1016/j.nedt.2022.105291.

Mann, C., & De Gagne, J. C. (2017). Experience of novice adjunct faculty: A qualitative study. *The Journal of Continuing Education in Nursing, 48*(4), 167–174. https://doi.org/10.3928/00220124-20170321-07.

Marion-Mantins, A. D., & Pinho, D. (2020). Interprofessional simulation effects for healthcare students: A systematic review and meta-analysis. *Nurse Education Today, 94*(104568). https://doi.org/10.1016/j.nedt.2020.1404568.

Makic, M. B. F., Casey, K., Oman, K. S., & Fink, R. M. (2022). Developing the graduate nurse residency: An oral history with Dr. Colleen Goode and Dr. Mary Krugman. *The Journal of Continuing Education in Nursing, 53*(4), 171–177. https://doi.org/10.3928/00220124-20220311-07.

McGaghie, W. C. (2020). Mastery learning: Origins, features and evidence from the health professions In W. C. McGaghie, J. H. Barsuk, & D. B. Wayne (Eds.), *Comprehensive healthcare simulation: Mastery learning in the health professions*. Springer.

McKay, M. A., Pariseault, C. A., Whitehouse, C. R., Smith, T., & Gunberg Ross, J. (2022). The experience of baccalaureate clinical nursing faculty transitioning to emergency remote clinical teaching during the COVID-19 pandemic: Lessons for the future. *Nurse Education Today, 111*. https://doi.org/10.1016/j.nedt.2022.105309.

McNelis, A. M., Ironside, P. M., Ebright, P. R., Dreifuerst, K. T., Zvonar, S. E., & Conner, S. C. (2014). Learning in practice: A multisite, multimethod investigation of clinical education. *Journal of Nursing Regulation*, 4(4), 30–35. https://doi.org/10.1016/S2155-8256(15)30115-0.

McKenna, L., Cant, R., Bogossian, F., Cooper, S., Levett-Jones, T., & Seaton, P. (2019). Clinical placements in contemporary nursing education: Where is the evidence? *Nurse Education Today*, 83, 104202. https://doi.org/10.1016/j.nedt.2019.104202.

McPherson, S. (2019). Part-time clinical nursing faculty needs: An integrated review. *Journal of Nursing Education*, 58(4), 201–206.

McQueen, K. A., Poole, K., Raynak, A., & McQueen, A. (2018). Preceptorship in a nurse practitioner program: The student perspective. *Nurse Educator*, 43(6), 302–306. https://doi.org/10.1097/NNE.0000000000000498.

Mella, A. J. (2021). An integrative review on selecting assignments for undergraduate nursing students in the clinical setting. *Nurse Education Today*, 107. https://doi.org/10.3928/01484834-20190321-03.

Metzger, I., Anderson, R. Funlola, A., & Ritchwood, T. (2020). Healing interpersonal and racial trauma: Integrating racial socialization into trauma-focused cognitive behavioral therapy for African American youth. *Child Maltreat*, 26(1):17–27. https://doi.org/10.1177/1077559520921457.

Morgan, J. L., Weierbach, F. M., Sutter, R., Livsey, K., Goehner, E., Liesveld, J., & Goldschmidt, M. K. (2019). New Education Models for Preparing Pre-licensure Nursing Students with Enhanced Skills upon Entering Community-based Nursing Practice. *Journal of Professional Nursing*, 35(6), 491–498. https://doi.org/10.1016/j.profnurs.2019.05.004.

Musallam, E., Alhaj, A., & Nicely, S. (2021). The impact of dedicated educational model on nursing students' outcomes. *Nurse Educator*, 46(5), E113–ED116. https://doi.org/10.1097/NNE.0000000000001022.

Nahm, E.-S., Mills, M. E., Raymond, G., Costa, L., Chen, L., Nair, P., Seidl, K., Day, J., Murray, L., Rowen, L., Kirschling, J., Daw, P., & Haas, S. (2022). Development of an academic-partnership model to anchor care coordination and population health. *Nursing Outlook*, 70, 193–203. https://doi.org/10.1016/joutlook.2021.09.005.

National Academies of Sciences, Engineering, and Medicine. (2021). *The future of nursing 2020–2030: Charting a path to achieve health equity*. The National Academies Press. https://doi.org/10.17226/25982.

National Council of State Boards of Nursing. (2022). The NCSBN 2022 environmental scan: Resiliency, achievement, and public protection. *Journal of Nursing Regulation*, 12(4), S1–S56. https://doi.org/10.1016/S2155-8256(22)00015-1.

National League for Nursing (NLN). (2022a). *Certified academic clinical nurse educator examination candidate handbook*. https://www.nln.org/awards-recognition/certification-for-nurse-educators-overview/cne-cl/Certification-for-Nurse-Educatorscnecl/cne-cl-handbook

National League for Nursing (NLN). (2022b). *NLN core competencies for academic nurse educators*. https://www.nln.org/education/nursing-education-competencies/core-competencies-for-academic-nurse-educators

National Task Force. (2022). Standards for quality nurse practitioner education, A report of the national task force on quality nurse practitioner education (6th ed.). https://www.aacnnursing.org/-Portals/42/CCNE/PDF/NTFS-NP-Final.pdf

Nielsen, A. (2016). Concept-based learning in clinical experiences: Bringing theory to clinical education for deep learning. *Journal of Nursing Education*, 55(7), 365–371. https://doi.org/10.3928/01484834-20160615-02.

Noone, J. (2022). Creating inclusive learning environments: Challenging and changing the paradigm. *Journal of Nursing Education*, 61(3), 115–116. https://doi.org/10.3928/01484834-20220215-01.

Oermann, M. H. (2021). COVID-19 disruptions to clinical education. *Nurse Educator*, 45(1). https://doi.org/10.1097/NNE.0000000000000947. 1–1.

Padilla, B. I., & Kreider, K. E. (2020). Communities of practices: An innovative approach to building academic-practice partnership. *Journal for Nurse Practitioners*, 16, 308–311. https://doi.org/10.1016/j.nurpra.2020.01.017.

Padilla, B. I., & Kreider, K. E. (2022). The added value of clinical faculty in building effective academic-practice partnership. *Journal of the American Association of Nurse Practitioners*, 34(2), 66–76. https://doi.org/10.1097/JXX.0000000000000644.

Perryman, K. W. (2022). Nurse practitioner preceptor education to increase role preparedness. *Journal of the American Association of Nurse Practitioners*, 34(5), 763–768. https://doi.org/10.1097/JXX.0000000000000702.

Petrovic, K. A., Hack, R., & Perry, B. (2020). Establishing meaningful learning in online nursing postconferences: A literature review. *Nurse Educator*, 45(5), 283–287. https://doi.org/10.1097/NNE.000000000000762.

Pleshkan, V., & Hussey, L. (2020). Nurse practitioners' experiences with role transition: Supporting the learning curve through preceptorship. *Nurse Education in Practice*, 42. https://doi.org/10.1016/j.nepr.2019.102655.

Porter, K., Jackson, G., Clark, R., Waller, M., & Stanfill, A. G. (2020). Applying social determinants of health to nursing education using a concept-based approach. *Journal of Nursing Education, 59*(5), 293–296. https://doi.org/10.3928/01484834-20200422-12.

Pusey-Reid, E., & Blackman-Richards, N. (2022). The importance of addressing racial microaggression in nursing education. *Nurse Education Today, 114,* 105390. https://doi.org/10.1016/j.nedt.2022.105390.

Rambur, B., Palumbo, V., & Nurkanovic, M. (2019). Prevalence of telehealth in nursing: Implications for regulation and education in the era of value-based care. *Policy, Politics, & Practice, 20*(2), 64–73. https://doi.org/10.1177/1527154419836752.

Rauch, L., & Malloy, S. (2020). Home hospitals: Maximizing nursing student clinical placements. *Journal of Nursing Education, 59*(5), 269–273. https://doi.org/10.3928/01484834-201200422-06.

Reising, D. L., James, B., & Morse, B. (2018). Student perceptions of clinical instructor characteristics affecting clinical experiences. *Nursing Education Perspectives, 39*(1), 4–9. https://doi.org/10.1097/01.NEP.0000000000000241.

Rim, D., & Shin, H. (2021). Effective instructional design template for virtual simulations in nursing education. *Nurse Education Today, 96,* 104624. https://doi.org/10.1016/j.nedt.2020.104624.

Robertson, B., McDermott, C., Star, J., & Clevenger, C. K. (2021). The academic-practice partnership: Educating future nurses. *Nursing Administration Quarterly, 45*(4), E1–E11. https://doi.org/10.1097/NAQ.00000000000487.

Rusch, L., Beiermann, T., Schoening, A. M., Slone, C., Flott, B., Manz, J., & Miller, J. (2018). Defining roles and expectations for faculty, nurses, and students in a dedicated education unit. *Nurse Educator, 43*(1), 14–17. https://doi.org/10.1097/NNE.0000000000000397.

Rush, K. L., Janke, R., Duchscher, J. E., Phillips, R., & Kaur, S. (2019). Best practices of formal graduate transition programs. *International Journal of Nursing Studies, 94,* 139–158. https://doi.org/10.1016/j.ijnurstu.2019.02.010.

Rutledge, C. M., O'Rourke, J., Mason, A. M., Chike-Harris, K., Behnke, L., Melhado, L., Downes, L., & Gustin, T. (2021). Telehealth competencies for nursing education and practice: The four P's of telehealth. *Nurse Educator, 46*(5), 300–305. https://doi.org/10.1097/NNE.0000000000000988.

Sanko, J., Mckay, M., Shekhter, I., Motola, I., & Birnback, D. J. (2020). What participants learn, with, from and about each other during interprofessional encounters: A qualitative analysis. *Nurse Education Today.* https://doi.org/10.1016/j.nedt.2020.104387.

Saunders, R., Dugmore, H., Seaman, K., Singer, R., & Lake, F. (2018). Interprofessional learning in ambulatory care. *The Clinical Teacher, 16,* 41–46.

Sebach, A. (2022). Psychometric testing of a toll assessing nurse practitioner clinical educator competence. *Journal for Nurse Practitioners, 18,* 217–220. https://doi.org/10.1016/j.nurpra.2021.11.010.

Shellenbarger, T., & Sebach, A. M. (2022). Development of psychometric testing of the academic clinical nurse educator skill acquisition tool. *Nursing Education Perspectives, 43*(4), 217–221. https://doi.org/10.1097/01.NEP.0000000000000956.

Shorey, S., & Ng, E. D. (2021). The use of virtual reality simulation among nursing students and registered nurses: A systematic review. *Nurse Education Today, 98,* 104662. https://doi.org/10.1016/j.nedt.2020.104662.

Simmons, B. (2010). Clinical reasoning: Concept analysis. *Journal of Advanced Nursing, 66*(5), 1151–1158. https://doi.org/10.1111/j.1365-2648.2010.05262.x.

Sommer, S., Johnson, J., Clark, C., & Mills, C. (2021). Assisting learners to understand and incorporate functions of clinical judgment in practice. *Nurse Educator, 46*(6). https://doi.org/10.1097/NNE.0000000000001020. 373–372.

Spector, N., Blegen, M. A., Silvestre, J., Barnsteiner, J., Lynn, M. R., Ulrich, B., & Alexander, M. (2018). Transition to practice study in hospital settings. *Journal of Nursing Regulation, 5*(4), 24–38. https://doi.org/10.1016/S2155-8256(15)30031-4.

Spector, N. M., Buck, M., & Phipps, S. (2021). A new framework for practice-academic partnerships during the pandemic and into the future. *American Journal of Nursing, 121*(4), 39–44.

Subke, J., Downing, C., & Kearns, I. J. (2020). Practices of caring for nursing students: A clinical learning environment. *International Journal of Nursing Sciences, 7,* 214–219. https://doi.org/10.1016/j.ijnss.2020.03.005.

Tanner, C. A. (2006). Thinking like a nurse: A research-based model of clinical judgment in nursing. *Journal of Nursing Education, 45*(6), 204–211.

Tanner, C. A., Messecar, D. C., & Deelawska-Elliott, B. (2022). Evidence-based practice In L. Joel (Ed.), *Advanced practice nursing: Essentials for role development fifth edition.* FA Davis.

Thomas, L. J., & Asselin, M. (2018). Promoting resilience among nursing students in clinical education. *Nurse Education in Practice, 28*(2018), 231–234. https://doi.org/10.1016/j.nepr.2017.10.001.

Tyo, M. B., & McCurry, M. K. (2019). An integrative review of clinical reasoning teaching strategies and outcome evaluation in nursing education. *Nursing Education Perspectives*, 40(1), 11–17. https://doi.org/10.1097/01.NEP0000000000000375.

Vezeau, T. M. (2016). In defense of clinical conferences in clinical nursing education. *Nurse Education in Practice*, 16(1), 269–273. https://doi.org/10.1016/j.nepr.2015.10.006.

von der Lancken, S., & Gunn, E. (2019). Improving role identity by shadowing interprofessional team member in a clinical setting: An innovative clinical education course. *Journal of Interprofessional Care*, 33(5), 464–471. https://doi.org/10.1080/13561820.2018.1538940.

Walker, L. E., Cross, M., & Barnett, T. (2019). Students' experiences and perceptions of interprofessional education during rural placement: A methods study. *Nurse Education Today*. https://doi.org/10.1016/j.nedt.2018.12.012.

Whitcomb, J., Stanley, L., Valentine, K. L., Bush, H., Wetsel, M. A., Mejia, S., Parker, V., Higgs, L., McFarlane, A., Gonzales, L., Farmer, K., Mayfield, M., & Garrison, A. (2022). A commitment to caring when preparing the bedside nurse: Evaluating perceived quality across university academic and clinical learning environments. *International Journal for Human Caring*, 26(1), 3–15. https://doi.org/10.1891/HumanCaring-D-20-00065.

Williams, E., Presti, C. R., Rivera, H., & Agarwal, G. (2020). Preparing students for clinical practice: The impact of a TeamSTEPPS® interprofessional education session. *Nurse Education Today*. https://doi.org/10.1016/j.nedt.2019.104321.

Wros, P., Mathews, L. R., Voss, H., & Bookman, N. (2015). An academic-practice model to improve the health of underserved neighborhoods. *Family Community Health*, 38(2), 195–203. https://doi.org/10.1097/FCH.0000000000000065.

Wu, X. V., Chi, Y., Chan, Y. S., Wang, W., Ang, E. N. K., Zhao, S., Sehgal, V., Wee, F. C., Selvam, U. P., & Devi, M. K. (2020). A web-based clinical pedagogy program to enhance registered nurse preceptors' teaching competencies—An innovative process of development and pilot program evaluation. *Nurse Education Today*, 84. https://doi.org/10.1016/j.nedt.2019.104215.

Yoder, C. M., & Pesch, M. (2020). An academic-fire department partnership to address social determinants of health. *Journal of Nursing Education*, 59(1), 34–37. https://doi.org/10.3928/01484834-20191223-08.

Zeydani, A., Atashzadeh-Shoorideh, F., Abdi, F., Hosseini, M., Zohari-Anboohi, S., Skerrett, V. Effect of community-based education on undergraduate nursing students' skills: a systematic review. *BMC Nurs*. 2021 Nov 18;20(1), 233. https://doi.org/10.1186/s12912-021-00755-4.

19

Teaching and Learning Using Simulations

Susan Gross Forneris, PhD, RN, CNE, CHSE-A

Simulation technology and pedagogy in nursing education continues to evolve, pushing the boundaries of experiential learning. Nursing education has moved from the first patient simulator, "Mrs. Chase," delivered to the Hartford Hospital Training School for Nurses in 1911, to the use of high-fidelity manikins along with artificial intelligence and virtual reality. Simulation experiences no longer involve simply teaching and practicing psychomotor skills. Simulation is an evidence-based contextual-learning teaching strategy that facilitates experiential learning and fosters critical thinking and clinical reasoning (Franklin & Blodgett, 2020; Morse et al., 2020). Effective facilitation and debriefing of the simulation experience provide an opportunity for educators to be meaning makers.

In today's complex, fast-paced health care environment—with the demands of high-quality, effective patient care and the growing lack of clinical placements for nursing students—simulation has become an effective teaching strategy that can replicate practice situations. Simulation offers nurses, students, and health professionals the opportunity to learn in situations that are comparable to actual patient encounters within a controlled learning environment allowing for the transfer of content knowledge to realistic patient interactions (Lioce, 2020). Clinical simulation technology is becoming increasingly more realistic, and nursing programs make substantial investments in equipment and learning space. As simulations and related teaching and learning strategies move into nursing programs and evidence supports clinical simulations

as an alternative to actual clinical experiences, nurse educators must be prepared to teach using this methodology.

This chapter discusses simulations as an experiential, student-centered pedagogical approach. The chapter begins with an overview of types of simulation—the purposes, challenges, and benefits of clinical simulations—and concludes with a review of evidence-based simulation used throughout nursing curricula. The chapter emphasizes (1) the types of clinical simulations being developed and implemented in nursing programs; (2) considerations for thoughtful integration of simulation into nursing curricula; (3) evaluation of simulation learning; (4) simulation and debriefing theory that provides a foundation for steps to consider when developing and using simulations; and (5) the recent evidence in nursing education literature that supports the use of simulation in our contemporary teaching and learning environments.

DEFINITION AND NOMENCLATURE FOR SIMULATION

Simulation is

> *"A technique that creates a situation or environment to allow persons to experience a representation of a real event for the purpose of practice, learning, evaluation, testing, or to gain understanding of systems or human actions.*
>
> ***Healthcare Simulation Dictionary, Society for simulation in Healthcare. (Lioce, 2020, p. 44)"***

Examples of simulation use include performing basic life support on a patient simulator to manage a cardiac arrest and providing nursing care to a patient simulator or simulated patient (SP) experiencing shortness of breath. Simulations are used when real-world training is too expensive or is not available, occurs rarely, or puts participants (or patients) at unnecessary risk. Simulations provide the opportunity for students to apply their knowledge within their scope of practice, think critically, problem-solve, make clinical judgments, and care for diverse patients in a nonthreatening, safe environment. Incorporating simulations into a nursing curriculum as a teaching and learning strategy offers nurse educators the opportunity to support learners' educational needs by providing them with an interactive, experiential instructional strategy.

Simulation Nomenclature
Fidelity Versus Realism
Fidelity, or the realism of simulations, is described along a continuum—from low fidelity to high fidelity—relative to the degree to which they approach reality. There are various types of simulations. The terms used to describe various aspects of the simulation experience are described here. The simulation nomenclature matrix is categorized by types of *fidelity*. Fidelity is the ability of the simulation experience to mirror reality. The higher the level of fidelity, the more realistic the experience. An important point to remember is that *realism* is interpreted by the learner. Therefore the educator must carefully consider the use of the learning environment, tools, and other resources to enhance fidelity. See Table 19.1 for differentiation of levels of fidelity.

Fidelity is categorized into three different dimensions: *conceptual fidelity*—details within the simulation scenario are aligned and make sense to the learner (e.g., O_2 saturation levels match the respiratory effort displayed by the patient simulator or simulated patient); *physical/environmental fidelity*—details of the physical space where the simulation scenario unfolds take into account the type of environment, noise, smells, use of manikins versus an SP, and other props; and *psychological fidelity*—details within the simulation experience are structured to evoke the emotions, beliefs, and self-awareness of the participants (INACSL Standards Committee, Watts, et al., 2021).

Simulation Modalities
The structure of the simulation is determined by the simulation scenario learning outcomes. The simulation is formatted using the modality that will best help learners achieve the outcomes. A modality is the specific platform upon which the simulation will be experienced. Modalities encompass a simulated clinical immersion, an *in situ* simulation, computer-assisted simulation, virtual reality, and procedural simulations. These modalities are further enhanced by using standardized patients, manikins, partial task trainers, haptic devices, avatars, etc. For example, the use of partial task trainers such as a body part, plastic model, or partial manikin is used to assist students to practice a psychomotor skill such as catheterization or insertion of a nasogastric tube, or with haptics that evoke physical sensation such as practicing an intubation. Manikin simulators, such as VitalSim Kelly, may be used to help learners achieve the skills of a physical assessment; manikin simulators, such as a SimMan, that provide the objective physiologic

TABLE 19.1 **Levels of Fidelity**		
Low Fidelity	**Medium Fidelity**	**High Fidelity**
• Case studies to educate students about patient situations • Role playing • Task trainers	• Technologically sophisticated 2-dimensional, focused experience • Solve problems, perform skills, and make decisions during the clinical scenario	• Involves full-scale, high-fidelity human patient simulators, virtual reality, or standardized patients • Extremely realistic and provide a high level of interactivity and realism for the learner

responses (e.g., blood pressure, pulses, blinking eyes, sweating, etc.) may be used to immerse the participants in a mock code situation or a simulated live birth. See Table 19.2 for a comparison of modalities relative to levels of fidelity.

Differentiating Simulation Modalities/Learning Environments

Research in the use and effectiveness of simulation has broadened since 2016, moving to higher levels of evidence (e.g., beyond measures of confidence and satisfaction) (Jeffries, 2016, 2022). Emphasis is now focused on how simulation-based education impacts learning, practice behaviors and change in patient outcomes. There continue to be a variety of technology-based simulations to support student and novice nurses, such as computer-based interactive simulations or virtual screen-based simulations and virtual reality. In addition to types of simulations categorized by the equipment or manikin used, there are simulations categorized by the type of pedagogy used when implementing the simulations. These types of simulations are described in the following sections.

Hybrid Simulation

A hybrid simulation is the combination of a standardized patient and the use of a patient simulator in one scenario to depict a clinical event for the learner. For example, the simulation scenario may begin with the student performing a health history on a standardized patient who has just arrived in the emergency department after having been involved in a motor vehicle accident. As the case evolves, the simulator plays an active role in the scenario by enabling clinical symptoms (e.g., drop in heart rate or blood pressure) that provide the objective physiological responses to reflect reality. This is a hybrid simulation because both a live standardized patient (i.e., patient providing the history) and a simulator (i.e., simulator displaying objective vital signs, etc.) are used in the experience. A common hybrid simulation in obstetrics involves a low-fidelity task trainer with a standardized patient for simulations of normal birth or complications such as shoulder dystocia. This can be done with a standard actor and the pelvis of a birthing simulator or with the use of the Mama Natalie, which is a low-cost, wearable device that can manually deliver a baby and placenta and simulate postpartum complications. Another approach to hybrid learning is the use of QR (quick response) codes (a contemporary 2-dimensional bar code) that can be placed on the manikin or the simulated patient and scanned, producing an immediate link to a website or online content area and providing more detailed information to assist learners for more interaction during the scenarios or specifically with interactive skills practice (Herrington & Wang, 2017).

Unfolding Case Simulations

Another type of simulation is the unfolding case. Unfolding cases evolve over time in an unpredictable manner. An unfolding case may include three to four events that build on each other, providing students an opportunity to plan care across a clinical event, a hospitalization, a care transition, or the life span (Hobbs & Robinson, 2022; Moench, 2019). Unfolding cases can be used to meet a variety of learning goals:

1. To demonstrate hierarchal order so the learner can follow the progression of a health problem and the related nursing care. For example, the first scenario demonstrates the patient being admitted with a head injury caused by a fall; the learner must conduct a focused neurological assessment. The unfolding case leads to a second scenario in which the patient experiences specific neurological signs (e.g., severe headache, widening pulse pressure); the learner must use additional assessment skills. The third case occurs postcraniotomy and involves care of the patient after the subdural hematoma is removed.

2. To visualize and prioritize the hospital trajectory and care of a patient that progresses. For example, the patient is admitted through the emergency department, with the learner performing an assessment. The second scenario depicts the patient being admitted to the progressive care unit, and the third scenario is designed for the learner to prepare the patient with discharge instructions.

TABLE 19.2 Simulation Modalities and Levels of Fidelity

Low Fidelity	Medium Fidelity	High Fidelity	SPs: Standardized/Simulated Patients
Manikins: Partial Task Trainer/Static Manikins	**Manikins: Moderate-Fidelity Simulators**	**Manikins: High-Fidelity Simulators**	**SPs: Standardized/Simulated Patients**
• Most common • Meant to represent a body part or structure • Examples: Arm for blood pressure	• Offer more realism than static, low-fidelity manikins • Vital signs present—breaths sounds, heart sounds, pulses	• Most realistic simulated patient experience • Cosmetic fidelity and response fidelity • All vital signs, breathing, talking, blinking, responding	• Real-life person trains to consistently portray with realism a patient or other individual with a specific condition

Low Fidelity		Medium Fidelity		High Fidelity		SPs	
PROS	**CONS**	**PROS**	**CONS**	**PROS**	**CONS**	**PROS**	**CONS**
• Focused technical skills/practice • Less expensive	• Lack of realism • Acontextual	• Good for deeper subject matter and review of competencies	• Limited functionality	• Increased levels of realism • Respond to learners physiologically	• Expensive • Regular maintenance required	• Trained to portray broad range of cases to match student level • Trained to perform learner assessment	• Expensive relative to dedicated staff/equipment

Virtual Environments
• Involve the use of software developed to simulate a subject or situation

PROS
• Test a variety of knowledge, skills and abilities like critical thinking
• Learners can use anytime, anywhere
• Can include elements of real time
• Can include game-based approaches that are responsive to the learner; can incorporate teamwork and collaboration across geographical location

CONS
• Scenarios are built to represent one specific environment and can't be modified
• Support needed
• Quality of graphics for realism vary 2D versus 3D

Virtual Environments: Haptics
• Involve a touch sensation as feedback to the learner or player in a virtual environment
Examples include: virtual intubation; surgical tools

PROS
• Realism is enhanced

CONS
• Limited to task training
• Expensive

3. To provide the learner with a view of care transitions, showing the effect of the health disruption or disease process and nursing interventions required for a particular patient. For example, the first scenario depicts a hospitalized patient newly diagnosed with chronic obstructive pulmonary disease (COPD). The second scenario progresses to the patient having compromised gas exchange related to COPD and being managed at an ambulatory care center. The third scenario depicts end-stage disease with a focus on end-of-life care with hospice care.

4. To serve as a mechanism to include a variety of important assessments and findings where one event leads to another. For example, the first scenario focuses on hypotension and subtle findings of sepsis and the second scenario centers on the critically ill patient with sepsis and hypotension.

Several organizations have developed unfolding case studies related to particular topics that are available at no cost to faculty. Unfolding cases that focus on populations who may be at risk and address the complexity of decision making about their care can be found at the National League for Nursing (NLN) site at http://www.nln.org/professional-development-programs/advancing-care-excellence-series. Unfolding cases or related to patient safety can be found at the Quality and Safety Education for Nurses (QSEN) site at https://qsen.org/tag/case-studies/.

Simulated Participants

Simulation can involve the use of human role players who will interact with the learner in a variety of ways. These individuals commonly have been called standardized patients or SPs. Human role players can also portray family members or other members of the health care team who interact with the learner, expanding the SP role to a simulated participant. The Association for Standardized Patient Educators (ASPE) published the ASPE Standards of Best Practice that provide an understanding of the nature, scope, and function of those portraying roles (Lewis et al., 2017). The terms *standardized patient* and *simulated patient* are used interchangeably and define the individuals who are portraying the role of a patient in a realistic and repeatable way. However, standardized patients conduct their role in a "standard or replicable" manner to give each learner the same consistent experience and for reliability when evaluating physical assessment skills, history taking, communication techniques, patient teaching, and types of psychomotor skills or objective structured clinical examinations (OSCE). ASPE recommends the use of simulated participant or simulated patient to refer to the use of a live person in the simulation scenario that is not to be specifically trained to conduct their role in a standard or replicable manner (see ASPE at https://www.aspeducators.org/).

In Situ Simulations

In situ simulation is a type of simulation that involves training performed in a real-life setting where patient care is commonly provided (Wang & Podlinski, 2021). The aim of this type of simulation is to achieve high fidelity by performing the simulations in actual clinical settings, blending and providing both a clinical and learning environment. Typically, the simulation-based experiential learning focuses on interdisciplinary professional teams. Practicing professionals are well versed in their particular field, possess a fair amount of experience, and prefer their learning to be problem centered and meaningful to their professional lives. Adults learn best when they can immediately apply what they have learned. Traditional teaching methods (e.g., a teacher imparts facts to the student in a unidirectional model) are not particularly effective in adult learning because it is important for adults to make sense of what they experience or observe.

Extended Reality (XR) Simulation and Digital Platforms

Simulations can also take place in virtual environments. The term extended reality (XR) simulation is now considered an umbrella term that encompasses virtual reality (VR); virtual reality simulation (VRS); augmented reality (AR); and mixed reality (MR). They are differentiated as follows: VR is defined as the use of technology to create a 3D environment; augmented reality AR is described as the projection of digital content directly into a learners environment; MR blends the digital content with the learner's environment in such a way that interaction is possible; and VRS includes the use of a scenario operationalized in a virtual environment (Aebersold & Dunbar, 2021). The Society for Simulation in Healthcare (SSIH) dictionary defines XR and is fast becoming the category that best represents these media.

> *XR is a fusion of all the realities – including AR. VR. And MR – which consists of technology-mediated experiences enabled via a wide spectrum of hardware and software, including sensory interfaces, applications, and infrastructures. XR is often referred to as immersive video content, enhanced media experiences, as well as interactive and multidimensional human experiences. (Lioce, 2020, p. 20)"*

Virtual reality simulation programs can be hosted online and accessed using a choice of navigable software using learning objectives that vary from highly focused technical skills training to broader, case-based patient scenarios that require critical thinking and clinical decision making. Increasing development in virtual patient simulation has evolved to more robust interaction between the learner and the virtual patient (i.e., avatar) and the environment through a digital media platform. In these virtual simulated worlds, users can explore, meet other users, socialize, participate in individual or group activities, and create services for one another or travel throughout the world. The software is a 3-dimensional modeling tool that attempts to depict reality for the users (Aebersold & Dunbar, 2021).

Software programs that replicate clinical practice and respond to learner interactions (i.e., VRS); provide written feedback to the learner with suggestions and evidence as feedback. Some popular virtual simulation software products available for online nursing education are Sentinel U, Shadow Health, and vSim for Nursing. Simulation is based on the theory of deliberate practice and engages students with the opportunity to repeat an activity continually to achieve mastery. Simulation through game-based learning can be independently performed or moderated, and this type of simulation helps prepare students for the clinical setting and allows the learner to make decisions and interact

with a patient with real-time response in a safe learning environment.

There is a growing body of evidence surrounding the use of virtual simulation in nursing education. Lea (2020) reported that 65% of schools of nursing use some form of virtual simulation or adaptive technology. Aebersold et al. (2018) used a tablet-based program for learners to practice nasogastric tube insertion. The technology incorporated augmented reality with findings supporting those learners demonstrated higher competency than learners trained using traditional methods. A strong trend in nursing education in the use of virtual products to immerse learners is supported by the increases in cognitive scores seen in recent evidence by Kyaw et al. (2019). This systematic review and metaanalysis across health care education found improvement in postintervention knowledge scores compared to traditional learners (Kyaw et al., 2019). Nursing education is now studying the use of these technologies (Wüller et al., 2019).

Simulation: A Teaching and Learning Strategy

Purpose of Simulations

Clinical simulations in nursing education can be used for many purposes, for example, as a teaching strategy or for assessment and evaluation or as an avenue to encourage interprofessional education (IPE). Students can be immersed in a simulation where they can actually portray the primary nurse, a newly employed nurse in orientation, or whatever role within the scope of nursing practice that the learner is assigned. As programs of nursing adjust their curricula to meet the demands and changes in nursing practice that limit clinical environment spaces for teaching and learning, simulation must be thoughtfully and intentionally integrated to achieve student and program learning outcomes.

Simulations as Experiential Learning

The use of simulation corresponds with a shift from an emphasis on teaching to an emphasis on learning in which the faculty facilitate learning by encouraging students to discover, or construct, knowledge and meaning (e.g., active learning approaches; see also Chapter 16). Simulation is an example of active learning whereby students become the center of the teaching and are engaged in the experience as opposed to merely consuming the information. Simulation is experiential learning that allows for situated cognition—or learning in context—a concept at the forefront of contemporary educational reform (Argawal, 2019; Roth & Jornet, 2013). Contextualized learning brings classroom and clinical together; simulation engages learners with diverse perspectives to reflect and reframe the understanding of practice, bringing thinking and doing together.

When making a shift in approach from a focus on teaching to a focus on learning, student learning outcomes serve as the framework for the development of specific learning activities. For example, both nursing students and novice nurses entering professional practice find it difficult to transfer theoretical knowledge into clinical practice. The use of simulation allows students to experience the application of theory in a safe environment where mistakes can be made without risk to patients.

The use of highly realistic and complex simulations may not always be an appropriate educational approach. In some situations, beginning students can use low-fidelity simulations to work on attainment of foundational skills, including effective communication with patients, psychomotor skill performance, and basic assessment techniques. With task trainers or standard manikins, students can practice procedural skills and caregiving in a safe environment that allows them to make mistakes, learn from those mistakes, and develop confidence in their ability to approach and communicate with patients in the clinical setting. In addition, students benefit from the opportunity to work with technologically sophisticated equipment, such as clinical information systems and hemodynamic monitoring systems, in the educational setting before encountering such equipment in the clinical setting.

Advanced practice nursing students benefit from high-fidelity simulations that are complex, realistic, and interactively challenging experiences that support them in developing and practicing leadership abilities, teamwork, and decision-making skills (Nye, 2020). With patient simulators or standardized patients, for example, students can practice complex assessment skills in their area of clinical practice (Ndiwane et al., 2017). Faculty can create scenarios and program equipment to simulate acute care situations (Keiser & Turkelson, 2019) and on-call situations (Griffith et al., 2019; Kelly at al., 2019; Woroch et al., 2018). Simulations are also appropriate to prepare psychiatric nurse practitioners. As students respond to these more complex situations, they demonstrate their abilities to establish priorities, make decisions, take appropriate action, and work successfully as part of a team (Reising et al., 2017).

Simulations Used for Assessment and Evaluation of Learning

Given the widespread use of simulations, there is also the potential for using simulations for assessment and evaluation of student learning. Using simulation for assessment and evaluation of learning should be integrated into the larger process of planning, implementing, assessing, and evaluating learning. Faculty should identify the purpose of the assessment or evaluation early in the process to ensure that the evaluation is relevant and evaluates the learning outcomes for which it is intended. Although more traditional forms of assessment continue to be employed—for example, pretesting and posttesting using multiple-choice tests and Next Gen test item types—simulation-based assessments are being used increasingly in the evaluation process, both in a formative manner, as part of an educational activity or training, and in a summative manner, as part of a graduation or certification process.

When simulations are being used for assessment or evaluation, the activities fall into two broad categories—"low stakes" and "high stakes" situations—depending on the significance of the evaluation (Oermann et al., 2016a). Low-stakes assessments are formative learning experiences in which the simulation is used by the learner and faculty to mark progress toward personal, course, or program learning goals. Faculty can use low-stakes simulation as a summative evaluation (i.e., providing a grade that reflects achievement of learning). High-stakes assessments are a type of summative evaluation, but the difference is in consequence to the learner. It is a *pass/fail* outcome with no opportunity for the learner to remediate. Thus high-stakes activities provide a high-risk evaluation and include licensing and certification examinations, credentialing processes, and employment decisions (Hunsicker & Chitwood, 2018; INACSL Standards Committee, McMahon, et al., 2021; Oermann et al., 2016a,b). Simulation technologies used for assessment range from case studies and standardized patients (e.g., OSCEs) to haptic task trainers and high-fidelity human simulators.

As with any type of assessment, faculty must consider the issues of validity and reliability (Holland et al., 2020). For assessments in low-stakes or learning situations, construct and concurrent validity should be addressed. *Construct validity* is the degree to which an assessment instrument measures the dimensions of knowledge or skill development intended. *Concurrent validity* is determined by evaluating the relationship between how individuals perform on the new assessment (in this case a simulation) and how they perform on the traditional (standard) assessment instrument. An assessment with high concurrent validity, for example, is one in which the learner's simulator assessment score is comparable to his or her score when performing the same examination on a standardized patient scored by using a checklist.

Predictive validity is required for simulations used in assessments in which licensure, certification, or employment is at stake. Determining predictive validity in high-stakes assessment is a complex process. Predictive validity is the extent to which performance on a particular simulation predicts future performance, such as clinical decision making or psychomotor skills. Evaluating predictive validity requires that, in addition to current performance, the clinical skill or decision making of specific individuals be tracked over time. There has been little research and evidence-based information specifically focused on quantifying the effect of simulation-based assessment activities on student or practitioner learning.

Simulations also are being used to assess and evaluate students' clinical skill competencies and clinical decision-making capabilities. OSCEs are clinical examinations that vary in format but mostly include a set period for the student to assess and interact with a standardized patient

and an actor or actress hired to portray a certain type of patient with a specific diagnosis and clinical symptoms. The use of OSCEs has been popular since the early 1970s, when they were introduced to nursing education as a means of assessing clinical skills. Advanced practice nursing education continues to explore the use of OSCEs to determine if a learner can demonstrate identified competencies in a simulated environment (Nye et al., 2019). Prion and Haerling (2020) reviewed the history of simulation evaluation in nursing education using Kirkpatrick's Levels of Evaluation as an organizing framework. Kirkpatrick's (1994) levels of evaluation provide a conceptual model that differentiates evaluation in simulation across four levels. (1) Reaction: evaluation of learner feelings and reactions; (2) Learning: evaluation of achievement of knowledge, skills, abilities; (3) Behaviors: evaluation of learner direct application of learning in practice; and (4) Results: evaluation of learning that changes patient outcomes. They conclude that evaluation of outcomes in simulation learning environments is necessary at all levels of evaluation across the nursing education continuum.

When using simulations as an assessment mechanism, the nurse educator should also consider the improvement in the use of standardized patients, the sophistication of computer-based evaluation techniques, the use of newer physiological electromechanical manikins, and the fidelity of immersive haptic devices. Because of these advances, nurse educators are now better able to assess learning, promote a better educational effort, improve academic courses and programs, and ultimately prepare students to provide quality, competent, and safe patient care. In a later section of this chapter, there is a further discussion of evaluation of simulation in nursing education, specifically evaluation of simulation design, facilitation, learning outcomes, and programs.

Simulations Used in Interprofessional Education

Conventionally, nursing and other health care education as a whole is delivered on a uniprofessional basis, eliminating the reality of everyday interprofessional collaborative clinical practice. Interprofessional education (IPE) is bridging that gap. (See Chapter 11.) There are many advantages of using simulations to promote IPE and interprofessional practice (IPP), including breaking down both real and perceived barriers between different clinical aspects, enhancing interprofessional cohesiveness and awareness, and providing an opportunity to develop mutual respect among members of an interdisciplinary team. Debriefing discussions highlight the importance and value of IPP, especially when the debriefing is well contextualized and facilitated through exposure to realistic scenarios (Iverson et al., 2018; Poore & Cooper, 2020; Tankimovich et al., 2020).

Simulations in the Classroom

With the COVID-19 pandemic, nursing education has undergone extraordinary transformation. Simulation as a teaching and learning strategy has become essential in assisting faculty to pivot from face-to-face to virtual teaching and learning. This section discusses how high-quality simulation as a teaching and learning strategy employed using the standards achieves best practices in teaching and learning.

The pandemic brought to reality what nurse educators now realize is essential: the importance of creating and implementing teaching methodologies that replace inactive, traditional classroom learning environments. For example, employing virtual simulation can easily bring clinical context to a classroom (virtual or face-to-face) or provide an opportunity to unfold clinical encounters in real time. Educators organize students into small groups to discuss the patient encounter being unfolded on the large classroom screen in real time. Faculty pause the patient encounter for students to decide on next steps for the simulated care situation. This process encourages their use and application of the content knowledge assigned for that class period as they together work in context and build on the simulation story with the educator guiding the classroom conversation. Expanding the use of simulation in the classroom for virtual concept mapping provides another opportunity for learning how to examine nursing care holistically. As educators guide their classroom conversation, they are role modeling their thinking strategy, thereby demonstrating how an expert nurse would think through the patient care situation, uncover

areas of unknowing, use resources, etc. Learners explain their decision making and the basis for their actions (Forneris & Fey, 2021).

Nurse educators have used low-fidelity simulation, such as manikins, role play, and case studies, as a teaching–learning strategy for decades. The introduction of high-fidelity simulation (in the form of affordable, portable, and versatile human patient simulators) in the late 1990s transformed health care education and is now one of the foundational strategies in the preparation of health care professionals not only for teaching but also for assessment and evaluation, development of interprofessional team skills, and clinical substitution, and to make up for missed experiences.

Simulations Used for Clinical Substitution and Clinical Make-up

A landmark multisite study conducted by the National Council of State Boards of Nursing (NCSBN) explored the clinical competency of new graduates on their transition to practice based on their participation in either a control group, a group that substituted 25% of real clinical hours for simulation, or a group that substituted 50% of their clinical hours for simulation (https://www.ncsbn.org/685.htm). The study report stated:

> *"This study provides substantial evidence that up to 50% simulation can be effectively substituted for traditional clinical experience in all prelicensure core nursing courses under conditions comparable to those described in the study. These conditions include faculty members who are formally trained in simulation pedagogy, an adequate number of faculty members to support the student learners, subject matter experts who conduct theory-based debriefing, and equipment and supplies to create a realistic environment. Boards of Nursing (BONs) should be assured by nursing programs that they are committed to the simulation program and have enough dedicated staff members and resources to maintain it on an ongoing basis. Hayden et al. (2014, p. S38)"*

The NCSBN convened an expert panel to evaluate the study findings, previous research, and the INACSL *Standards of Best Practice: Simulation*™ to create guidelines for the use of simulation in prelicensure programs. These guidelines provide faculty and program directors with evidence-based information to inform preparation and planning for use of simulation in nursing programs (Alexander et al., 2015; NCSBN, 2015). These findings are significant for the nurse educator community because too often quality clinical sites are difficult to find; health care agencies are limiting the amount of practice and procedures students can actually perform in the clinical setting; and the client census is diminishing in the acute care settings such that clinical experiences are limited and focus only on the acute care population.

The NCSBN outlines the following guidelines for boards of nursing to use in evaluating the readiness of prelicensure nursing programs to use simulation to substitute for traditional clinical experiences. These guidelines are also for use by nursing education programs to assist them in establishing evidence-based simulation programs (https://www.ncsbn.org/9535.htm).

Before using simulation as a teaching/learning strategy, guidelines include the following:

1. Commitment has been obtained from the school supporting the use of simulation.
2. Appropriate facilities are available to conduct simulation to include educational and technological resources to achieve learning outcomes.
3. Faculty and simulation laboratory support staff are qualified to facilitate and debrief simulations.
4. Faculty are prepared to lead simulations.
5. The program has processes in place to guide best practice in the use of simulation, which includes use of a theory-based debriefing method, training and evaluation of faculty facilitating simulation and debriefing, and evaluation methods for simulation learning.

The COVID-19 pandemic has challenged nursing education to meet student learning outcomes targeted at enhancing knowledge, skills, and abilities while providing direct patient care. With many health care settings off access to students in health care disciplines, simulation has been the relied-upon teaching and learning strategy to get learners the hands-on nursing practice needed to achieve program outcomes. Outside of the pandemic, the growth in nursing education research looking at the efficacy of simulation beyond the teaching of psychomotor skills is well documented (Smiley, 2019; Waxman et al., 2019). Simulation has now been supported as a viable teaching and learning strategy with modalities that include interactive manikins for physical assessment, standardized patients for communication skill enhancement, and use of virtual reality and screen-based simulation for clinical reasoning (Aebersold, 2018; Bradley et al., 2019). Simulations continue to be used, outside of the pandemic for schools of nursing to assist in the difficulty of finding quality, appropriate clinical sites, particularly in specialty areas such as pediatrics or maternal health (Karding-Edgren et al., 2020)

Surveys of Boards of Nursing (BON) in the United States show growth in the adoption of simulation to replace actual clinical experiences (Cipher et al., 2020; Smiley, 2019). In 2008 Nehring (2008) reported that only 17 jurisdictions out of 61 allowed simulation as a substitute. In 2014, that number had increased to 47 out of 61 (Hayden et al., 2014). While the pandemic increased that number further with temporary orders by many jurisdictions, simulation as a replacement for clinical hours continues to vary (Bradley et al., 2019; Smiley, 2019). Recent research is advancing the science supporting substitution of simulation as a viable clinical replacement with evidence of improving clinical reasoning (Sullivan et al., 2019).

Now more than ever, simulation is being sought to assist nurse educators with clinical time referred to as "off-campus" clinical for actual experiences in health care institutions and "on-campus" clinical when the clinical experience is obtained in the simulation laboratory. Simulations are also being used for "clinical make-up" days for those students missing clinical because of illness, weather, or other unforeseen causes. There can be an entire "clinical day" set up in the simulation laboratory for clinical hours. Some nurse educators use virtual simulations (computer-based learning) that have a debriefing component and scoring to meet clinical makeup hours when needed and when the content fits with the curriculum needs.

CHALLENGES AND BENEFITS OF USING SIMULATIONS

Simulation can offer nurse educators and health care providers a significant educational method that meets the needs of today's learners by providing them with interactive, practice-based instructional strategies. Implementing and testing the use of simulations in educational practice has both challenges and benefits.

Most of the challenges of using clinical simulations center on educators' preparation for using simulations and interprofessional simulations. See Table 19.3.

Thoughtful Integration of Simulation into the Curriculum

Using simulations as a teaching–learning strategy requires advance planning. Planning should consider the need for resources, thoughtful integration into nursing curricula, preparation of the student, and faculty development.

Resources

Operationalizing simulation requires physical space and equipment, the use of different types of simulation equipment and technology (such as manikins, virtual reality, video conference

TABLE 19.3 Benefits and Challenges of Simulation	
Benefits	**Challenges**
Active Involvement of Students in Their Learning Process	
• Immersed in the context of learning. • Use of content knowledge to think through the challenges presented in the learning activity—moving thinking to a higher order. • Decision-making and critical thinking skills are reinforced.	• Importance of fidelity and a fiction contract for learners to suspend disbelief. • Learner psychological safety to share thinking behind action. • Faculty experience in both role modeling and eliciting critical thinking.
More Effective Use of Faculty in the Teaching of Clinical Skills and Interventions	
• Opportunity to observe students more closely. • Allow students to demonstrate potential more fully. • Opportunity to uncover student thinking and understanding.	• Faculty expertise and clear understanding of performance indicators relative to simulation learning outcomes. • Creating a psychologically safe environment for learners to feel comfortable making mistakes. • Using dialog versus monologue (lecture) during debriefing.
Increased Student Flexibility to Practice Based on their Schedules	
• Ability to access simulation (i.e., virtual or lab) independently. • Ability to practice both synchronously and asynchronously with peers/instructors for extra reinforcement. • Ability to revisit a skill several times in an environment that is safe, nonthreatening, and conducive to learning.	• Providing support for learner engagement to assist with independent learning. • Staffing and scheduling for resources to support simulation outside of lab/classroom activities.
Improved Student Instruction	
• Better consistency of teaching. • Increased learner satisfaction in both the classroom and the clinical setting. • Opportunity for safer, nonthreatening practice of skills and decision making. • State-of-the-art learning environment.	• Faculty and staff development on best practice in use of simulation as a teaching/learning strategy.

TABLE 19.3 **Benefits and Challenges of Simulation—cont'd**	
Benefits	**Challenges**
Effective Competency Check for Undergraduates, New Graduates, or New Nurses Going Through Orientation	
• Provides a competency check of the participants' knowledge, skills, and problem-solving abilities in a nonthreatening, safe environment.	• Faculty and staff development on best practice in use of simulation as a teaching/learning strategy. • Faculty development in best practices in evaluation of learning and performance of learners, facilitators and the simulation program.
Correction of Errors Discussed Immediately	
• Immersed in a learning experience, with debriefing immediately after the encounter. • Unfolds thinking and rationale behind actions taken or not taken. • Provides a clear understanding of how knowledge or lack of knowledge informed their reasoning.	• Faculty development in best practices in prebriefing and debriefing simulation learning activities.
Standardized, Consistent, and Comparable Experiences for All Students	
• Use of consistent, standardized teaching activities. • Ability to assure all learners experience an important clinical event, assessment activity, or another essential clinical learning encounter.	• Faculty development in standards of best practice in simulation facilitation.
Opportunities for Collaboration and IPE	
• Provides opportunity for knowledge and understanding of other professionals' roles and skills that all students in a clinical course can experience.	• Faculty development in standards of best practice in simulation enhanced interprofessional education (IPE).

technology [e.g., Skype, Zoom], and electronic health records), faculty, and support staff. Staffing of simulation requires careful consideration of all the staffing necessary to deliver simulation using best practice standards (Farina & Bryant, 2020). With simulation used extensively during the COVID-19 pandemic, faculty now understand the dedicated resources needed to deliver effective simulation move far beyond the use of a mannikin, a room, and one dedicated faculty. It requires a team approach to deliver effective simulation with careful planning of the necessary faculty and resource/rooms to accommodate learners across a program of study (Blodgett et al., 2018; Howard, 2019). Careful consideration must be made to the scheduling and availability of the faculty facilitating/debriefing the simulation, simulation space, availability of debriefing rooms, staff ready

for staging areas quickly to keep the simulation schedule on track, etc. and the necessary budgets for staffing and supplies (Blodgett et al., 2018; Zamora, 2019). The physical space must be large enough to accommodate teaching and learning activities, office space for faculty and staff, storage space, debriefing space, and, if used, space for video recording. Well-resourced spaces may mimic an acute care setting or operating room suite. Resources also include support staff who assist faculty in managing the equipment and supporting the audiovisual and simulator technology.

Curriculum Considerations

A needs assessment and analysis should be performed to understand the intricacies of the curriculum in general and how the specific courses intersect with each other. Examining specific course content and the clinical site placements gives a broad overview of the types of experiences students are exposed to and how objectives are met. Consideration should be given to the need for all learners to have the experience in managing common clinical situations (i.e., low acuity/high frequency versus high acuity/low frequency). This would mean that faculty should use patient experiences for commonly occurring health problems versus only providing simulation for high-acuity patients experiencing stroke or heart attack (Peddle et al., 2020). Further examination of QSEN competencies, national patient safety goals, the NCSBN Licensure Examination blueprint, the Institute of Medicine Initiatives, and standardized testing results can help design and pattern content for simulation. In thinking *who* the learners are, *why* they learn, *what* they learn, and *how* they learn, a schematic design for each course can be developed to determine how the goals of theory, simulation, and clinical are interconnected and where simulation would be appropriate—both inside the classroom (virtual simulation) or in the simulation laboratory.

Preparing the Learner

Simulation is likely a learning strategy that is a new experience for the student. An important first step in successfully preparing the student for simulation is prebriefing. Prebriefing in simulation is an orientation to the simulation learning experience. Thoughtful time spent with the learners before engaging in the simulation helps set the stage for successful achievement of learning outcomes (INACSL Standards Committee, McDermott, et al., 2021; Rudolph et al., 2014). Prebriefing activities include reviewing learning outcomes; creating a "fiction contract" (i.e., agreement that the learner will accept the level of fidelity in the simulation and fully participate despite the setting "not being real"); and orienting participants to the equipment, environment, manikin, roles, etc.

The main purpose of prebriefing is to establish a psychologically safe environment for the learner. Setting the stage for a psychologically safe learning environment begins before the learning experience (Daniels & Onello, 2017). Psychological safety refers to the learners' perception of the learning environment and the potential risks for interpersonal interaction. Faculty must be intentional about setting the stage for a safe learning encounter, yet they cannot dictate the nature of safety; the learner must perceive the space as safe. Faculty are called to create a learning space that provides an opportunity for the learner to take risks with the learning encounter respecting that mistakes will be made and these will be met with open, honest conversation and multiple perspectives of thought. Preparing the student also includes orienting the student to the use of the equipment and to their role as an active and engaged learner. Students must understand the learning goals, what assignments they should complete or information to have at hand during the simulation, how the simulation relates to the reality of clinical practice, and the significance of the debriefing session. If the simulation is being used for assessment or evaluation, faculty must be transparent about this and provide an opportunity for students to become familiar with and use the equipment before the evaluation performance. Clarity surrounding the rubrics that will be used to evaluate performance is critical (Daniels & Onello, 2017).

Faculty Development

As teachers and learners move away from content-laden curricula to curricula that emphasize experiential learning, it is critical that nurse educators have the requisite knowledge and skills to use simulation to its full potential (National League for Nursing, 2015a).

Educators prepared for the use of simulations are essential to the success of integrating simulations across the curriculum. However, unlike the traditional classroom setting, the faculty role when using simulations is no longer teacher centered but is student centered, with the educator assuming the role of a facilitator in the student's learning process. The educator's role during the simulation process varies. Lioce et al. (2018) discuss the evolution of the faculty role in simulation. No longer is it acceptable to have only one person manage all the varied roles required to deliver best practices in simulation. Additional consideration should be given depending on whether the simulation is being conducted for learning or evaluation purposes. Educators must provide learner support as needed throughout the simulation and facilitate or guide the debriefing at the conclusion of the experience. If the simulation is being conducted for evaluation purposes, the teacher's role changes to that of an observer and rater/grader. Boards of Nursing (BONs) across the country continue to set guidelines and regulations for the use of traditional clinical experiences. With the advances being made in the use and evidence of simulation in nursing education, BONs are challenged to develop guidelines that allow for schools of nursing to substitute traditional clinical with simulation. Criteria that are now being included are: (1) percentage of clinical replacement; (2) ratio of simulation to clinical hours; (3) definition of simulation; and now (4) simulation educator requirements. The International Association for Clinical Simulation and Learning (INACSL) has a Simulation Regulations Committee that provides information on the above criteria (INACSL, 2020). Thirty BONs have now established simulation regulations (Bradley et al., 2019; Waxman et al., 2019).

When using simulations for the first time, faculty must feel comfortable with the simulations they are using. Faculty development on simulation pedagogy and debriefing is essential (NLN, 2015a, 2015b). Faculty may require assistance with simulation design, use of the technology, and setting up equipment for the activity. Faculty development is also needed to maintain fidelity in the design, implementation, and evaluation of simulation programs. Operationalizing critical thinking learning within the simulation and structured debriefing requires facilitation skill.

Simulation is an active, experiential teaching strategy, and consideration of the following for faculty development is also necessary for delivering best practice simulation:

1. A firm foundation in experiential learning
2. Clear learning objectives for the simulation experience
3. A detailed design, taking into account that an educator facilitates learning (versus tells the learner)
4. Sufficient time for learners to experience the simulation, to reflect on the experience, and to make meaning of the experience
5. Faculty development in the area of simulation pedagogy; the teaching strategy is student centered, which is a paradigm shift in teaching for many
6. Strategic ways to quantify and document clinical simulation hours toward licensure or certification
7. When using IPE simulation, there must be alignment of student clinical placements across the professions; preparation of all faculty and preceptors involved; commitment from all professions to making IPE experiences a priority; and adequate financial, human, and space resources (see also Chapter 11)

Schools of nursing have found it helpful to send faculty to an orientation course or develop their own orientation to develop faculty for using simulations in their teaching. These courses include information about simulation selection and use, curriculum integration, the role of the facilitator, and how to conduct the debriefing. Faculty experience a simulation firsthand as they participate in these courses. (See Case Study 19.1.)

CASE STUDY 19.1 Facilitating Simulation in a Nursing Program Orienting Faculty to Using Simulation

The lead faculty for a nursing program's committee on simulation curriculum integration is preparing to increase the use of simulation throughout the curriculum. The faculty member has been involved in the use of simulation for about 2 years and is an advocate of simulation as a teaching/learning strategy. During the past year, the nursing department has seen a greater rate of faculty turnover and many of the faculty seasoned in the use of simulation have retired. The faculty is planning to develop an orientation program for new faculty. The faculty decides to begin with a foundational review of simulation practices using the Healthcare Simulation Standards of Best Practice (International Nursing Association for Clinical Stimulation and Learning, n.d.).

Using the INACSL Standards cited above:

1. What should the faculty include in an orientation plan for the newly employed faculty?
2. What pedagogical approaches should the faculty include in the plan?
3. What experiential activities will facilitate the new faculty's understanding of simulation?
4. How should the faculty document the new faculty's attainment of the competencies attained in the orientation program?

OPERATIONALIZING SIMULATION

Simulations should be carefully planned. The process of selecting, designing, implementing, and evaluating a simulation to support learning in nursing education is best done using a systematic, organized approach. To help nursing educators and researchers in this developmental process, a simulation theory (Jeffries, 2022) was developed to identify the components of the process and their relationship to guide the design, implementation, and evaluation of these activities.

Once the simulation is designed, faculty members are ready to implement it into the nursing course. The following guidelines may be useful to educators implementing simulations into their nursing courses:

1. Make sure specific objectives match the implementation phase of the simulation. When faculty design a simulation, the objectives and nature of the simulation should be clearly defined for the students and facilitator. Furthermore, if the simulation is designed, for example, around the care of an insulin-dependent patient, then the scenario should be created using problems typically encountered and the problem-solving skills needed for that patient's care. The simulation should focus on the objectives and not on potential comorbidities or extraneous issues.

2. Set a time limit for the simulation and the debriefing encounter and then adhere to it. Too often, instructors observe that in simulations students are immersed for a specific time limit but are not able to accomplish all of the assessments and interventions the instructor had desired. At times instructors may let the scenario proceed beyond the specific time frame, but if the simulation is scheduled for 20 minutes, the encounter needs to be 20 minutes. If students do not achieve the objectives desired, the reflective observation time can be spent on their experiences and the meaning they make of them.

3. Implement an appropriate orientation of students to the simulation labs where they will be interacting with the simulators. This is an important step to help eliminate the anxiety and fear of the unknown associated with initial exposure to simulation as a whole. It is also important to engage in a confidentiality agreement with the students that makes debriefing a safe environment for students and faculty and, lastly, implement a fiction contract where students are expected to treat the simulation environment as they would a true clinical encounter.

4. In undergraduate nursing programs, it is advisable to make assignments so that students know their specific roles during the simulation. Unless developing or testing team leadership skills, students need roles (e.g., nurse, observer, family member) assigned before encountering the simulation to bring organization to the experience. If roles are not assigned, students waste time trying to decide what role to play. In advanced practice nursing programs, role delineation may be handled by the students. It is conceivable that advanced practice nurses can come together to determine specific roles and responsibilities. This may also be a good topic to investigate during debriefing.

5. Avoid interrupting the simulated encounter when students are trying to problem-solve on their own. In simulation, the learners function as professionals, not as students, so they are asked to step beyond their comfort zone and interact in the scenario without someone directing them on how to act. Facilitators should observe a simulation remotely, either behind a one-way mirror or via closed-circuit television, so students cannot see facial expressions, hear comments, or see nonverbal gestures. It is best for faculty to conduct the simulation debriefing immediately after the simulation event. If this is not done in the immediacy of the simulation, actions taken or not taken can be forgotten or confused with other scenarios.

6. Involve a limited number of learners in the simulation experience in addition to one or two observers or recorders of the encounter. Typically, two to six students are each assigned a role in the simulation experience. The roles within the simulation need to be identified before and recognized during the simulation. For example, students can wear name tags or labels and appropriate clothing for particular

roles or have certain props available to help delineate the roles. When an educator has more students than are needed to participate in the simulation, these students can be assigned an observer role.

7. Ensure that the simulation is appropriate for the learners' skill levels and cognitive ability. Although a prominent design feature when developing simulations is fidelity, simulations need to be realistic to the degree that matches the learning level of the student group. Early on in exposure to the simulation environment, students benefit from scenarios that are comparable to their didactic learning. Low- or medium-fidelity manikin and standardized patients with basic care needs offer opportunities to focus on basic skill and knowledge acquisition. Failure and anxiety in the simulation scenario can occur when the simulation objectives include skills or competencies students have not learned (e.g., IV management before IV curriculum or altered cardiac or lung sounds before cardiac or lung modules). As exposure to the simulated environment increases, learners benefit from a higher level of complexity and a mix of fidelity, including challenges found in a complex environment such as simulated emergent events that involve critical thinking, active interaction, teamwork, and collaboration with the health care team to achieve a common goal. Simulations assist students at the application level of learning to practice their decision-making, problem-solving, and team member skills in a nonthreatening environment. The environment needs to be sufficiently realistic to allow for suspension of disbelief so that students can make the transition of knowledge from theory to practice. In simulation there is no "pretend." All necessary equipment should be available and standards and protocols should be followed to mimic the clinical setting. If a patient is to take a medication, the proper steps for administration should be used.

8. When planning to incorporate simulations into the course or curriculum, ensure that faculty development is included in the planning. Faculty need to know how to conduct a simulation and a debriefing session to achieve the desired outcomes with the teaching–learning strategy. Faculty need to be prepared to design and conduct simulations in the educational setting before they are actually placed in the learning laboratory or clinical practicum with students in a simulation situation. All faculty members using this type of strategy in their classroom or clinical instruction need to be aware of and clear about the purpose of the simulation activity. At the end of the simulation, all instructors need to include a clear summary and highlights, particularly if there are several educators using the same simulation in a course. Discussion about simulations and how to implement them and clarity on learning outcomes for the simulation are needed and must be agreed on by faculty before implementation of the simulation. Clear delineation of the objectives of the scenario and the debriefing model should be followed by all facilitators. A predesigned concept map for each scenario can help guide facilitators for consistent debriefing. (See Case Study 19.2.)

Evaluation of Simulation in Nursing Curricula

Simulation learning activities can be evaluated in several ways; (1) learner outcomes; (2) simulation experience/design; and (3) facilitation/debriefing. Learner evaluation can be evaluated formatively or summatively, as previously discussed earlier in this chapter. To evaluate the design and development of simulations created by nurse educators, Jeffries (2022) developed the Simulation Design Scale (SDS). The purpose of this tool is to provide the educator with information and feedback that can be used to improve the simulation design and implementation. The SDS is a 20-item tool that the learner completes after participating in a simulation to provide feedback on whether the intended simulation design features were present. Table 19.4 briefly describes the five components of the SDS.

Evaluation of the Implementation Phase

When simulations are implemented, particular components need to be included to ensure a good learning experience, student satisfaction, and good learner performance. According to Chickering and

---

CASE STUDY 19.2 Integrating Simulation Into a Curriculum

Faculty teaching in a fundamentals course wish to integrate a simulation to help students conduct a physical assessment. The faculty review the simulation and related learning outcomes. (see below).

Simulation Learning Outcomes
1. Conduct a head-to-toe assessment of the patient
2. Use appropriate evidence-based tools to complete an overall assessment and assess for confusion
3. Identify critical assessment findings
4. Discuss pertinent assessment findings and relate which findings are commonly found in the older adult patient
5. Use SBAR techniques when communicating with other members of the health care team

Simulation
Patient is an 84-year-old Caucasian female who lives alone in a small home. She has one daughter, who is 50, lives nearby, and is the patient's major support system. Her current medical problems include: hypertension, glaucoma, osteoarthritis of the knee, stress incontinence, osteoporosis, and hypercholesterolemia. Objectives for this scenario include the identification and use of appropriate assessment tools for older adults with confusion, recognition of an elevated blood pressure, and notification of primary care provider using SBAR format.

1. What steps should the faculty take to integrate this simulation into the course?
2. What preparations will be helpful to the faculty?
3. How should the faculty prepare the students?
4. What implementation strategies will be helpful?
5. How could faculty determine the effectiveness of using this simulation?

Gamson (1987, 1991), incorporating the Principles of Best Practice in Education assists educators to implement quality teaching activities and improve student learning. As a component of the simulation theory (Jeffries, 2022), educational practices are evaluated using the Educational Practices in Simulation Scale (EPSS) (Jeffries, 2022). The EPSS is a 16-item tool that the learner completes after a simulation. The best practice elements being evaluated in the EPSS are active learning, diverse ways of learning, high expectations, and collaboration, as shown in Table 19.5.

Evaluation of Learning Outcomes

As discussed previously, learning outcomes can be measured through low-stakes and high-stakes simulations. Outcomes are defined for the learning activity and can be measured by a well-designed clinical simulation. Research in this area is growing as educators measure the outcomes of the simulation activity, desiring to close the knowledge and skills gap within academe and practice (Prion & Haerling, 2020)

The Simulation Theory

The NLN Jeffries Simulation Theory (Fig. 19.1) assists educators by outlining the steps of simulation development, providing a consistent and empirically supported model to guide the design and implementation of simulations and the assessment of learning outcomes when using simulations (Jeffries, 2022). Within the theory, seven concepts that underpin the design, facilitation, and evaluation of simulation are outlined (Jeffries et al., 2022).

When developing the scenario, the design features are considered within the development process. For example, problem-solving components are considered in the scenario progression writing. Faculty can consider one or two problem-solving components designed in the scenario to be implemented by the novice students and three or four decision-making components for the more advanced student, perhaps to facilitate and emphasize prioritization at this level. After the simulation template is completed, it is advised that the scenarios be peer reviewed by content experts to ensure that evidence-based practices are being

TABLE 19.4 Simulation Design Scale: Components

Component	Description
Objectives/information	Clear objectives and time frame for the simulation are needed by students before the simulation begins. Information needs to be provided on what learners need to know and what they are expected to learn.
Student support	Student support is offered before, during, and after a simulation. Support includes providing information and direction to the student prior to the simulation. During the simulation, cues can be provided to the students participating in the simulation via a lab test, a chest X-ray (CXR) report, a phone call from a physician or a nurse manager, or in other ways. After a simulation, support is provided during the debriefing. Students find the debriefing part of the simulation a most important aspect; instructors are helpful when they correct misinformation or inappropriate actions that happened in the scenario, in addition to emphasizing components that should have been done but were not or areas of nursing care that were done well.
Problem-solving/ complexity	The simulation needs to be designed with problem-solving components embedded in the scenario or case that is written. The level of problem-solving needs to be considered (e.g., simple tasks and decisions if students are in a fundamentals course versus more complex problem-solving if students are in an upper-level course and six months from graduating).
Fidelity	A simulation should be designed to be as close an approximation as possible to the real event or activity that is being developed to promote learning. A realistic, simulated clinical situation requires three elements: (1) relatively little information should be available initially; (2) students should be allowed to investigate freely, employing questions in any sequence; and (3) students get important clinical information over time during the simulation.
Guided reflection/ debriefing	Guided reflection reinforces the positive aspects of the experience and encourages reflective learning, which allows the participant to link theory to practice and research, think critically, and discuss how to intervene professionally in complex situations. At the end of the session, the group should discuss the process, outcome, and application of the scenario to clinical practice and review the relevant teaching points. The last step in the simulation activity is to share and generalize information with the students.

From Jeffries, P. R. (2012). *Simulations in nursing education: From conceptualization to evaluation.* The National League for Nursing. Used with permission.

incorporated into the scenario and to confirm accuracy and that the content is up to date. Finally, the scenario must be pilot tested with targeted end users so that educators can ensure that the scenario is at the correct level for the learner and can review the scenario for sufficient decision-making points and cues to engage the students in the simulation. A simulation template used as a guide to developing clinical simulations can be found on the Simulation Innovation Resource Center (SIRC) website at http://sirc.nln.org/.

Evidence-Based Debriefing and Reflection

Debriefing is one of the key design features to consider when operationalizing a simulation (see Fig. 19.1). Debriefing is a process by which educators facilitate learners' reflection or reexamination of clinical encounters (Morse et al., 2020). Facilitators face challenges in debriefing, including blame setting for performance, statements such as "this wouldn't happen in real clinical," learners who are open with dislike of the learning environment, and learners who are hostile and defensive or who are

TABLE 19.5   Educational Practices in Simulation Scale

Components	Description	Examples
Active learning	Through simulation, learners are directly engaged in the activity and obtain immediate feedback and reinforcement of learning. Learning activities can range from simple to complex. Case scenarios, simulation of real-life clinical problems requiring assessment and decision-making skills, role-playing with actors, and critiquing one's or a peer's videotape of a selected skill performance are examples of methods faculty can use to promote active learning. Such active and interactive learning environments encourage students to make connections between concepts and engage them in the learning process.	In a case scenario in which an intubated patient is restless, agitated, and coughing, affecting his oxygenation status, students can be asked to select the most appropriate intervention and describe the rationale for the intervention. The patient simulator can support more complex active learning strategies because the opportunity allows students to assess a critical health incident (e.g., collapsed lung or status asthmaticus) through the measurement of physiological parameters and communication with the "patient," perform on-the-spot planning for quick and appropriate nursing interventions, and obtain a real-time response by the simulator for realistic evaluation and further intervention.
Diverse ways of learning	Simulations should be designed to accommodate diverse learning styles and teaching methods and allow students and groups with varying cultural backgrounds to benefit from the experience.	Design a scenario that has visual, auditory, and kinesthetic components. For example, use a monitor or lab reports (visual), program a patient simulator conversation about his symptoms (auditory), and require a procedure to be done (kinesthetic).
High expectations	High teacher expectations are important for students during a learning experience because expecting students to do well becomes a self-fulfilling prophecy. Students should set goals with faculty and seek advice on how to achieve those goals. When both faculty and students have high expectations for the simulation process and the outcomes, positive results can be achieved.	Set up a scenario with multifaceted patient problems for the learner who needs to be challenged and needs to advance to the next level of knowledge and skills. Nurses can be pushed to expand their competency levels and empowered to achieve greater learning in a safe learning environment.
Collaboration	Collaboration is pairing students in a simulation to work together. Roles are assigned so that students jointly confirm assessments, make decisions about interventions, and evaluate outcomes.	An example of collaboration is assigning a student the role of primary nurse and a third-year medical student the role of primary physician. Place the two students in a setting where they will be confronted with a deteriorating patient for whom decisions need to be made, interventions need to be performed immediately, and assessments need to be done quickly and accurately.

From Jeffries, P. R. (2012). *Simulations in nursing education: From conceptualization to evaluation.* The National League for Nursing. Used with permission.

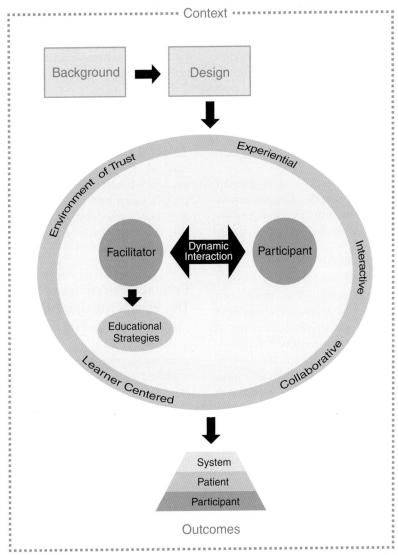

FIG. 19.1 Diagram of NLN Jeffries simulation theory. (From Jeffries, P. R. (Ed.). (2016). The NLN Jeffries simulation theory. National League for Nursing. Used with permission.)

self-critical and defeated based on performance. These issues can be avoided with a thoughtful pre-briefing, as described earlier. Facilitators provide a safe, nonjudgmental environment and coach students to reflect on what they saw, heard, and experienced.

Three core concepts provide a foundation for understanding the nature of debriefing: conceptualizing learning as meaning making, the cognitive strategy of being critical, and engaging learners through purposeful learning conversations (Forneris & Fey, 2020). The challenge with debriefing is to shift the emphasis from delivering content to guiding the use of content through a process of thinking. It is a conversation that moves from *let me show you how to do this* to *tell me how you understand this*. Debriefing in the context of simulation involves moving beyond the simple application of facts and rules to a process of sense making. Inherent in sense making is the learners' ability to organize the contextual elements of the surroundings. This requires reflection, perspective taking, and examining one's biases and beliefs to understand the whole of the situation—to be truly *critical*. Critical pedagogy, although not new, is the philosophical foundation that underpins and guides many contemporary teaching strategies, such as debriefing, that use reflection as a core attribute. (See Chapter 14.)

Debriefing encompasses the cognitive domain assessing knowledge, the kinetic domain assessing skill and action, and the affective domain—or how the learner felt or interacted with the patient or other staff.

The role of faculty in facilitating debriefing is to support participants in the reflection process. Objectives of debriefing include the opportunity for the learners to describe what the experience was like for them; this can involve a release of emotional tension about the experience, a guided review of the patient and objectives, the identification and sorting of thinking, and reinforcement of teaching and correction of misconceptions. Debriefing is an opportunity to reference real-life experiences, normalize behaviors, and acknowledge emotions. These conversations take more time and should be well planned and structured. In the use of theory-based debriefing, debriefing should be twice as long as the scenario time and involve active participation from all learners (caregivers to observers).

The NCSBN guidelines recommend that faculty who are facilitating and debriefing simulation be educated in a theory-based debriefing method. Theory-based debriefing methods are varied, and several models are used in the simulation setting (Dreifuerst, 2012; Eppich & Cheng, 2015; Rudolph et al., 2006; Waznonis, 2014). The NLN's (2015b) vision statement, *Debriefing Across the Curriculum*, recommends that faculty use evidence-based resources to develop their skills in debriefing. In an effort to assist faculty development in the ability to guide a reflective conversation, Forneris and Fey (2017a, 2017b) developed *The NLN Guide for Teaching Thinking* (Table 19.6). It is a learner-centered approach involving a three-part conversation structure: *Context, Content, and Course. The NLN Guide for Teaching Thinking* lays a foundation for Socratic inquiry. Educators can build on this three-part conversation structure when implementing a theory-based debriefing method (Forneris & Fey, 2017a, 2017b).

The Debriefing Assessment for Simulation in Healthcare (DASH) tool is designed to evaluate and develop the debriefing skills of the facilitator. This tool evaluates the facilitators' ability to conduct debriefings after specific behaviors. It is an evidence-based tool designed according to how people learn and change in experiential learning and was vetted by an expert panel at Harvard (https://harvardmedsim.org/debriefing-assessment-for-simulation-in-healthcare-dash/).

Evidence-Based Use of Simulation Throughout Nursing Education

Simulations can be integrated into nursing courses, laboratory experiences, and clinical courses to promote more active and experiential learning within nursing education. With increasing use, thoughtful integration of simulation into the curriculum is the necessary and agreed-upon approach as opposed to having only one or two experiences in a program of study (Leighton, 2018). Thoughtful integration of simulation into the curriculum is interpreted as assessing how and where simulation would enhance achievement of student learning outcomes. "Low acuity–high frequency" is a curricular planning strategy. Faculty can use nursing practice standards, the NCLEX blueprint, patient safety goals, etc., to identify common, fundamental, low-acuity yet frequently occurring care situations (e.g., hypoglycemia, respiratory distress) that all students should be competent to manage as they enter professional practice. Simulation provides the opportunity for *every student* to experience the same encounter. Faculty can also modify the simulation to increase its complexity so that students can identify what happens when signs and symptoms change or are missed at the basic level and how that informs changes in acuity care management. The reverse strategy of low frequency–high acuity (e.g., mock codes) can also be an effective curricular

TABLE 19.6   Critical Conversations: The National League for Nursing Guide for Teaching Thinking

Guided Questions for the Learner	Directions for the Guide
Context	**Identify Patient's Story**
• How did caring for this patient/family make you feel? • Who is this patient? • What are your main concerns?	• Uncover the thinking and emotions. • Describe the patient care story. • Determine if all important aspects of the situation have been identified.
Content	**Understand and Guide Thinking**
• I saw... • I think... • I wonder... • Describe what you were thinking about during your experience. • What sources of knowledge influenced/should have influenced your thinking? • How have past experiences helped you to make sense of the current situation?	• Use concrete objective data to clarify perspective. • Discuss your impressions of their thinking. • Provide your perspective based on past experience. • Relay strategies that have worked in the past. • Understand the knowledge guiding their thinking.
Course	**Integrate into Practice**

• Set immediate course:
  • So based on... what are your next steps going forward?
• Set long-term course:
  • How would the care differ if you... compare and contrast care situations (e.g., patient age change, setting change)
• What will you do differently moving forward?
	• Discuss how this experience might influence thinking and practice going forward.
	• Discuss the aspects of this situation that affected learning and will help them to remember this experience.

From Forneris, S., & Fey, M. (Eds.). (2017). *Understanding the NLN guide for teaching thinking. Critical Conversations: The NLN guide for teaching thinking* (pp. 1–11). National League for Nursing. Used with permission.

integration strategy (Tagliareni & Forneris, 2016). Integrating unfolding cases in simulation, as discussed previously, has the potential to transform traditional teacher-centered classrooms into interactive, engaging learning environments.

Faculty have integrated simulations in a variety of courses. Beroz (2016) used multipatient clinical simulations in a senior leadership course to better prepare and facilitate new graduates' transition to clinical practice. The multipatient simulation was developed using three evidence-based, peer-reviewed medical–surgical scenarios. Two of the scenarios were at the basic level and the third was more complex. Using the Seattle University Simulation Evaluation Tool (SUSET) (Mikasa et al., 2013), the students were evaluated for their level of performance with assessment/intervention/evaluation, critical thinking/decision making, communication/collaboration, direct patient care, and professionalism. Data analysis revealed that 25% of these students were unable to use surveillance skills to identify subtle cues to patient complications. The study concluded that integrating multipatient simulations as a teaching–learning strategy may improve surveillance and ultimately decision making.

During the COVID-19 pandemic, telesimulation was used not only for health care but incorporated as a means of clinical experience for learners. Telesimulation is "a process by which telecommunication and simulation resources are utilized to provide education, training, and/or assessment to learners at an offsite location" (Papanagnou, 2017, p. 137). With the need to reach rural health care and limitations to manage highly acute patients, not only has telehealth provided an avenue for access to care but it can be effectively used when social distancing prevents live face-to-face simulation experiences. An example of one such study involved the use of telesimulation to provide nurses with just-in-time education on ventilator strategies (Naik et al., 2020). The simulation incorporated learner prep work on ventilator management. Learners then attended a virtual synchronous online simulation. As learners, they formed the care team with the goal of managing a patient experiencing respiratory distress. The simulation was managed by a sim operator using a tablet to control the manikin with the ability to display the ventilator settings on the screen. Throughout the simulation, images of the manikin and vital signs monitor were available to the learners. The learners were expected to manage the ventilator settings based on the vital signs, lung compliance, ventilator pressure, and arterial blood gas values. When debriefing learners in this experience, they reported being able to accomplish the same learning outcomes as if they were in person because of their ability to similarly manage ventilator settings remotely (Naik et al., 2020).

Foronda et al. (2016) used vSim for Nursing in a mixed-methods study to understand students' experiences managing acute medical–surgical patients. They concluded that the learning experience was very positive for students and can extend the classroom experience as content preparation to enhance and reinforce learning.

CHAPTER SUMMARY: KEY POINTS

- Educators use simulations to enhance learning outcomes and promote safe patient care environments—thoughtful integration into nursing curricula to achieve student learning outcomes should always be considered.
- Nursing education literature now supports how simulation design and implementation practices assist in achieving learning outcomes as well as enhancing clinical reasoning. Ongoing research is needed for nursing organizations, commissions of higher education, accrediting bodies, academic institutions, and schools of nursing to continue to support, approve, and operationalize simulation at all levels of nursing education.
  - Educators and researchers must join forces to develop more rigorous research studies testing simulation outcomes.
  - National, multisite simulation studies by nurse educators are currently being conducted to enhance understanding of the educational usefulness of nursing simulations.
    - When simulations are used as a teaching–learning intervention, are learning outcomes improved?
    - How can simulations be used to prepare for or replace clinical experience?
    - How does the use of simulations contribute to advancing nursing into the next generation?
    - How does the use of simulation contribute to a change in patient care outcomes?
- Educators need to make certain they develop the teaching and learning skills for using simulation and debriefing and stay informed about the possibilities of simulations, their usefulness in enhancing student education, and the progress of educational research efforts conducted on using simulation in nursing education.

REFLECTING ON THE EVIDENCE

1. What evidence is available on the effectiveness of using simulation in support of learning?
2. When using a simulation theory, how would you construct a research project to test the framework?
3. Identify three research questions that might be addressed when studying reflective observation.
4. What is the optimal balance of simulated versus actual clinical practice in nursing education?

REFERENCES

Aebersold, M., & Dunbar, D. M. (2021). Virtual and augmented realities in nursing education: State of the science. In T. A. (2021). Schneidereith (Ed.), *Annual review of nursing research: Healthcare simulation* (39, pp. 225–242). Springer Publishing.

Aebersold, M., Voepel-Lewis, T., Cherara, L., Weber, M., Khouri, C., Levine, R., & Tait, A. R. (2018). Interactive anatomy-augmented virtual simulation training. *Clinical Simulation in Nursing*, 15, 34–41. http://doi.org/10.1016/j.ecns.2017.09.008. https://doi.org/10.1891/9780826166340.

Alexander, M. A., Durham, C. F., Hooper, J., Jeffries, P. R., Goldman, N., Kardong-Edgren, S., & Tillman, C. (2015). NCSBN simulation guidelines for prelicensure nursing programs. *Journal of Nursing Regulation*, 6(3), 39–42. https://doi.org/10.1016/S2155-8256(15)30783-3.

Argawal, P. K. (2019). Retrieval practice and Bloom's Taxonomy: Do students need fact knowledge before higher order learning? *Journal of Educational Psychology*, 111(2), 189–209.

Beroz, S. T. (2016). Exploring the performance outcomes of senior-level nursing: Students in a multiple-patient simulation. *Nursing Education Perspectives*, 37(6), 333–334. https://doi.org/10.1097/01.NEP.0000000000000045.

Blodgett, N. P., Blodgett, T., & Kardong-Edgren, S. E. (2018). A proposed model for simulation faculty workload determination. *Clinical Simulation in Nursing*, 18, 20–27. https://doi.org/10.1016/j.ecns.2018.01.003.

Bradley, C. S., Johnson, B. K., Dreifuerst, K. T., White, P., Conde, S. K., Meakim, C. H., Curry-Lourenco, K., & Childress, R. M. (2019). Regulation of simulation use in United States prelicensure nursing programs. *Clinical Simulation in Nursing*, 33, 17–25. https://doi.org/10.1016/j.ecns.2019.04.004.

Chickering, A. W., & Gamson, Z. F. (1987). Seven principles for good practice in undergraduate education. *AAHE Bulletin*, 39(7), 3–7.

Chickering, A. W., & Gamson, Z. F. (1991). Applying the seven principles for good practice in undergraduate education. *New Directions for Teaching and Learning*, 47, 5–12.

Cipher, D. J., LeFlore, J., Urban, R. W., & Mancini, M. E. (2020). Variability of clinical hours in prelicensure nursing programs: Time for reevaluation. *Teaching and Learning in Nursing*, 23, 41–46. https://doi.org/10.1016/j.teln.2020.05.005.

Daniels, A., & Onello, R. (2017). Psychological safety. In S. F. Forneris & M. Fey (Eds.), *Critical conversations: The NLN guide for teaching thinking* (pp. 13–26). National League for Nursing.

Dreifuerst, K. T. (2012). Using debriefing for meaningful learning to foster development of clinical reasoning in simulation. *Journal of Nursing Education*, 51(6), 321–333. https://doi.org/10.1016/j.ecns.2016.01.009.

Eppich, W., & Cheng, A. (2015). Promoting excellence and reflective learning in simulation (PEARLS): Development and rationale for a blended approach to health care simulation debriefing. *Simulation in Healthcare*, 10(2), 106–115. https://doi.org/10.1097/SIH.0000000000000072.

Farina, C. L., & Bryant, K. (2020). Simulation-based Operations. *Annual Review Nursing Research*, 39(1), 181–200. https://doi.org/10.1891/0739-6686.39.181.

Forneris, S. G., & Fey, M. (2017a). *Critical conversations: The NLN guide for teaching thinking*. National League for Nursing.

Forneris, S. G., & Fey, M. (Eds.). (2017). *Understanding the NLN guide for teaching thinking. Critical conversations: The NLN guide for teaching thinking* (pp. 1–11). National League for Nursing.

Forneris, S. G., & Fey, M. K. (Eds.). (2021). *Critical conversations Vol. 2: Moving from Monologue to Dialogue*. National League for Nursing.

Foronda, C. L., Swoboda, S. M., Hudson, K. W., Jones, E., Sullivan, N., Ockimey, J., & Jeffries, P. R. (2016). Evaluation of vSIM™ for nursing: A trial of innovation. *Clinical Simulation in Nursing*, 12(4), 128–131. https://doi.org/10.1016/j.ecns.2015.12.006.

Franklin, A. E., & Blodgett, N. P. (2020) Simulation in undergraduate education. *Annual Review Nursing Research*, 39(1), 3–31. https://doi.org/10.1891/0739-6686.39.3.

Griffith, P. B., Kelly, M. M., & Becker, D. (2019). On-call simulation for adult gerontology acute care nurse practitioner students: A comparative descriptive study. *Journal of the American Association of Nurse Practitioners*, 1–12. Advance online publication. https://doi.org/10.1097/JXX.0000000000000355

Hayden, J. K., Smiley, R. A., Alexander, M. A., Kardong-Edgren, S., & Jeffries, P. R. (2014). The NCSBN National SImualtion Study: A longitudinal, randomized, controlled study replacing clinical hours with simulation in pre-licensure nursing education. *Journal of Nursing Regulation*, 5(Suppl), s3–s40. https://doi.org/10.1016/S2155-8256(15)30062-4.

Herrington, A., & Wang, C. (2017). QR codes and augmented reality: What are they and how can I use them in the nursing classroom?

Hobbs, J. R., & Robinson, C. (2022). Learning and transfer effects of an unfolding case study in an adult health nursing course. *Nursing Education Perspectives, 43*(1), 47–48. https://doi.org/10.1097/01.NEP.0000000000000801.

Holland, A., Tiffany, J., Blazovich, L., Bambini, D., & Schug, V. (2020). The effect of evaluator training on inter and intra-rater reliability in high stakes assessment in simulation. *Nursing Education Perspectives, 41*(4). https://doi.org/10.1097/01.NEP.0000000000000619.

Howard, V. M., Leighton, K., & Gore, T. (2019). Simulation in healthcare education. In R. Nelson & N. Staggers (Eds.), *Health informatics: An interprofessional approach* (2nd ed., pp. 454–471). Elsevier.

Hunsicker, J., & Chitwood, T. (2018). High-stakes testing in nursing education: A review of the literature. *Nurse Educator, 43*(4), 1. https://doi.org/10.1097/NNE.0000000000000475.

INACSL Standards Committee, McDermott, D. S., Ludlow, J., Horsley, E., & Meakim, C. (2021). Healthcare Simulation Standards of Best Practice™ prebriefing: preparation and briefing. *Clinical Simulation in Nursing, 58*, 9–13. https://doi.org/10.1016/j.ecns.2021.08.008.

INACSL Standards Committee, McMahon, E., Jimenez, F. A., Lawrence, K., & Victor, J. (2021). Healthcare Simulation Standards of Best Practice™ evaluation of learning and performance. *Clinical Simulation in Nursing, 58*, 54–56. https://doi.org/10.1016/j.ecns.2021.08.016.

INACSL Standards Committee, Persico, L., Belle, A., DiGregorio, H., Wilson-Keates, B., & Shelton, C. (2021). Healthcare Simulation Standards of Best Practice™ facilitation. *Clinical Simulation in Nursing, 58*, 22–26. https://doi.org/10.1016/j.ecns.2021.08.010.

INACSL Standards Committee, Watts, P. I., McDermott, D. S., Alinier, G., Charnetski, M., Ludlow, J., Horsley, E., Meakim, C., & Nawathe, P. A. (2021). Healthcare Simulation Standards of Best Practice™ simulation design. *Clinical Simulation in Nursing, 58*, 14–21. https://doi.org/10.1016/j.ecns.2021.08.009.

Iverson, L., Bredenkamp, N., Carrico, C., Connelly, S., Hawkins, K., Monoghan, M. S., & Malesker, M. (2018). Development and assessment of an interprofessional education simulation to promote collaborative learning and practice. *Journal of Nursing Education, 57*(7), 426–429. https://doi.org/10.3928/01484834-20180618-08.

Jeffries, P. (2012). *Simulation in nursing education: From conceptualization to evaluation* (2nd ed.). Lippincott Williams & Wilkins.

Jeffries, P. R. (Ed.). (2016). *The NLN Jeffries simulation theory* (1st ed.). National League for Nursing.

Jeffries, P. R. (Ed.). (2022). *The NLN Jeffries simulation theory* (2nd ed.). National League for Nursing.

Jeffries, P. R., Rodgers, B., & Adamson, K. A. (2022). NLN Jeffries simulation theory: Brief narrative description. In P. R. Jeffries (Ed.), *NLN Jeffries simulation theory* (2nd ed., pp. 45–49). National League for Nursing.

Keiser, M. M., & Turkelson, C. (2019). Using simulation to evaluate clinical performance and reasoning in adult-geriatric acute care nurse practitioner students. *Journal of Nursing Education, 58*(10), 599–603. https://doi.org/10.3928/01484834-20190923-08.

Kelly, M. A., Blunt, E., & Nestor, K. (2019). After-hours/on-call simulation in primary care nurse practitioner education. *Clinical Simulation in Nursing, 26*, 49–53. https://doi.org/10.1016/j.ecns.2018.05.002.

Kirkpatrick, J. (1994). *Evaluating training programs: The four levels*. Bernett-Koehler.

Kyaw, B. M., Saxena, N., Posadski, P., Vseteckova, J., Nikolaou, C. K., George, P. P., Divakar, U., Masiello, I., Kononowicz, A. A., Zary, N., & Car, L. T. (2019). Virtual reality for health professions education: Systematic review and meta-analysis by the digital health education collaboration. *Journal of Medical Internet Research, 21*(1), 312959.

Lea, M. (2020). How virtual training is set to change nursing education. https://healthtechmagazine.net/article/2020/05/how-virtual-training-set-change-nursing-education

Leighton, K. (2018). Curriculum development in nursing simulation programs. In C. Foisy-Doll & K. Leighton (Eds.), *Simulation champions: Fostering courage, caring and connection* (pp. 397–428). Wolters Kluwer.

Lewis, K. L., Bohnert, C. A., Gammon, W. L., Holzer, H., Lyman, L., Smith, C., Thompson, T. M., Wallace, A., & Gilva-McConvey, G. (2017). The association of standardized patient educators (ASPE) standards of best practice (SOBP. *Advances in Simulation, 2*(1). https://doi.org/10.1186/s41077-017-0043-4.

Lioce, L. (Ed.). (2020). *Healthcare simulation dictionary—Second edition*. Agency for Healthcare Research and Quality; September 2020. AHRQ Publication No. 20-0019. https://doi.org/10.23970/simulationv2

Lioce, L., Graham, L., & Young, H. M. (2018). Developing the team: Simulation educators, technical, and support personnel in simulation. In C. Foisy-Doll & K. Leighton (Eds.), *Simulation champions: Fostering courage, caring, and connection* (pp. 429–444). Wolters Kluwer.

Mikasa, A., Cicero, T., & Adamson, K. (2013). Outcome-based evaluation tool to evaluate student performance in high-fidelity simulation. *Clinical Simulation in Nursing, 9*(9), e361–e367. https://doi.org/10.1016/j.nepr.2020.102818.

Moench, B. (2019). *Unfolding case studies to develop clinical forethought in novice nursing students.* QSEN Institute. https://qsen.org/using-unfolding-case-studies-to-develop-clinical-forethought-in-novice-nursing-students/

Morse, K. J., Fey, M. K., & Forneris, S. G. (2020). Evidence-based debriefing. *Annual Review Nursing Research, 39*(1), 129–148. https://doi.org/10.1891/0739-6686.39.129

Naik, N., Finkelstein, R., Howell, J., Rajwani, K., & Ching, K. (2020). Telesimulation for COVID-19 ventilator management training with social-distancing restrictions during the Coronavirus pandemic. *Simulation and Gaming, 51*(4). https://doi.org/10.1177/1046878120926561.

National Council of State Boards of Nursing. (2015). National simulation guidelines for pre-licensure nursing programs. https://www.ncsbn.org/9535.htm

National League for Nursing. (2015a). A vision for teaching with simulation. http://www.nln.org/docs/default-source/about/nln-vision-series-(position-statements)/vision-statement-a-vision-for-teaching-with-simulation.pdf?sfvrsn=2

National League for Nursing. (2015b). Debriefing across the curriculum. http://www.nln.org/docs/default-source/about/nln-vision-series-(position-statements)/nln-vision-debriefing-across-the-curriculum.pdf?sfvrsn=0

Ndiwane, A. N., Baker, N. C., Makosky, A., Reidy, P., & Guarino, A. J. (2017). Use of simulation to integrate cultural humility into advanced health assessment for nurse practitioner students. *Journal of Nursing Education, 56*(9), 567–571. https://doi.org/10.3928/01484834-20170817-11.

Nye, C. (2020). State of simulation research in advanced practice nursing education. *Annual Review Nursing Research, 39*(1), 33–51. https://doi.org/10.1891/0739-6686.39.33.

Nye, C., Campbell, S. H., Francher, S., Short, C., & Thomas, M. (2019). The use of simulation in advanced practice nursing programs: A North American perspective. *Clinical Simulation in Nursing, 26,* 3–10. https://doi.org/10.1016/j.ecns.2018.09.005.

Oermann, M. H., Kardong-Edgren, S., & Rizzolo, M. A. (2016a). Towards an evidence-based methodology for high-stakes evaluation of nursing students; clinical performance using simulation. Teaching and Learning. *Nursing, 11*(4), 133–137. https://doi.org/10.1016/j.teln.2016.04.001.

Oermann, M. H., Kardong-Edgren, S., & Rizzolo, M. A. (2016b). Summative simulated-based assessment in nursing programs. *Journal of Nursing Education, 55*(6), 323–328. https://doi.org/10.3928/01484834-20160516-04.

Peddle, M., Livesay, K., & Marshall, S. (2020). Preliminary report of a simulation community of practice needs analysis. *Advances in Simulation, 5,* 11. https://doi.org/10.1186/s41077-020-00130-4.

Poore, J. A., & Cooper, D. D. (2020). Interprofessional simulation: From the classroom to clinical practice. *Annual Review Nursing Research, 39*(1), 106–125. https://doi.org/10.1891/0739-6686.39.105.

Prion, S., & Haerling, K. (2020). Evaluation of simulation outcomes. *Annual Review Nursing Research, 39*(1), 149–180. https://doi.org/10.1891/0739-6686.39.149.

Reising, D. L., Carr, D. E., Gindling, S., Barnes, R., Garletts, D., & Ozdogan, Z. (2017). Team communication influence on procedure performance: Findings from interprofessional simulations with nursing and medical students. *Nursing Education Perspectives, 38*(5), 275–276. https://doi.org/10.1097/01.NEP.0000000000000168.

Roth, W. M., & Jornet, A. (2013). Situated cognition. *WIREs Cognitive Science, 4,* 463–478. https://doi.org/10.1002/wcs.1242.

Rudolph, J. W., Raemer, D. B., & Simon, R. (2014). Establishing a safe container for learning in simulation: The role of the presimulation briefing. *Simulation in Healthcare, 9*(6), 339–349. https://doi.org/10.1097/SIH.0000000000000047.

Rudolph, J. W., Simon, R., Dufresne, R. L., & Raemer, D. B. (2006). There's no such thing as "nonjudgmental" debriefing: A theory and method for debriefing with good judgment. *Simulation in Healthcare, 1*(1), 49–55.

Smiley, R. A. (2019). Survey of simulation use in prelicensure nursing programs: Changes and advancements, 2010–2017. *Journal of Nursing Regulation, 9*(4), 48–61. https://doi.org/10.1016/S2155-8256(19)30016-X.

Sullivan, N., Swoboda, S. M., Breymier, T., Lucas, L., Sarasnick, J., Rutherford-Hemming, T., Budhathoki, C.,

& Kardong-Edgren, S. (2019). Emerging evidence toward a 2:1 clinical to simulation ratio: A study comparing the traditional clinical and simulation settings. *Clinical Simulation in Nursing, 30,* 34–41. https://doi.org/10.1016/j.ecns/2019.03.003.

Tagliareni, E., & Forneris, S. (2016). Sim beyond the Sim Lab (white paper). http://www.nln.org

Tankimovich, M., Swail, J., & Hamburger, M. (2020). Nurse practitioner and medical students' perceptions of teamwork before and after a standardized patient pilot simulation. *Nursing Education Perspectives, 41*(3), 171–173. https://doi.org/10.1097/01.NEP0000000000000503.

Wang, C., & Podlinski, L. (2020). Hospital-based simulation. *Annual Review Nursing Research, 39*(1): 83–103. https://doi.org/10.1891/0739-6686.39.83.

Waxman, K. T., Bowler, F., Forneris, S. G., Kardong-Edgren, S., & Rizzolo, M. A. (2019). Simulation as a nursing education disruptor. *Nursing Administration Quarterly, 43*(4), 300–305. https://doi.org/10.1097/NAQ.0000000000000369.

Woroch, R. A., Alvarez, D. V., Yingling, C. T., & Handrup, C. T. (2018). Family nurse practitioner/psychiatric mental health nurse practitioner collaboration in drug-seeking telephone triage simulation in an advanced practice registered nurse curriculum. *Clinical Simulation in Nursing, 18,* 14–19. https://doi.org/10.1016/j.ecns.2018.01.002.

Wüller, H., Behrens, J., Garthaus, M., Marquard, S., & Remmers, H. (2019). A scoping review of augmented reality in nursing. *BMC Nursing, 18*(1), 19. https://doi.org/10.1186/s12912-0190-0342-2.

Zamora, Z., Shedd, J., & Kittipha, P. (2019). Budget friendly simulation for clinical nursing education: Putting it all together. *Nursing Education Perspectives, 40*(2), 123–124. https://doi.org/10.1097/01.NEP.0000000000000357.

20

Using Technology to Facilitate Learning in the Classroom[*]

Karen H. Frith, PhD, RN, NEA-BC, CNE

Learning is the acquisition of knowledge, skills, and values, and the role of faculty is to facilitate learning and the development of learners (National League for Nursing [NLN], 2021). Historically, the role of the faculty had been to deliver information to students in a classroom. Each student's role was to pay attention to the faculty and receive wisdom. This approach is inadequate because of the vast amount of knowledge and the pace of knowledge changes: no one person can be the sole source of information. Nursing faculty are responsible for facilitating learning for today's domain knowledge and developing information literacy skills for the future. Faculty have many choices to facilitate learning by using educational technology or adapting technology for educational purposes. As faculty use their creativity to develop well-planned learning experiences, nursing students engage more with the subject matter and their peers (Smart et al., 2020).

This chapter focuses on using technology in the classroom to facilitate learning. While specific technology will be described, the emphasis will be on the pedagogical selection of technology to meet student learning outcomes. The chapter offers specific suggestions for effective ways to use the technologies to engage students in learning and teach them about nursing practice in a complex, patient-centered, and technology-rich health care environment.

CALL FOR TECHNOLOGY IN HIGHER EDUCATION

When educators use technology to teach, they can expose students to the larger world, make learning more interesting, and provide learning experiences outside of the traditional lecture approach. Until recently, there has been fragmented evidence in nursing on the effect of technology and learning modalities (traditional, online, or hybrid) on pass rates for the National Council Licensure Examination-Registered Nurse (NCLEX-RN). Spector et al. (2020) conducted a quantitative study of annual reports from 43 boards of nursing over 5 years and found that programs using hybrid modality had significantly higher NCLEX-RN pass rates (80% or higher) than either traditional or fully online modalities. While modality alone does not account for the differences in pass rates, it is worth considering that the use of technology in hybrid modalities influences this important student learning outcome.

The United States (US) Department of Education set a goal for faculty in "higher education and post-secondary [to] use technology to design learning experiences that better support and enable student learning, while building and using evidence to improve and evolve their instructional approach over time" (Office of Educational Technology, 2017, p. 24). This goal clearly shows the national call for the use of education technology, not just because it is available but because technology creates innovations in pedagogy, assessment of student learning outcomes, and evaluation of teaching practices.

The COVID-19 pandemic changed the face of nursing education abruptly, requiring faculty to

---

[*]The author acknowledges the work of Brent Thompson, PhD, RN in the previous editions of the chapter.

use many technologies for the classroom, lab, and clinical settings to keep students progressing in their programs of study. The sudden change to online education pushed faculty into learning technology skills. Faculty have continued to use their skills for on-campus and hybrid nursing courses (EDUCAUSE, 2021). Out of necessity, faculty innovated nursing education using technology (Fogg et al., 2020; Horvath et al., 2020; Lubarsky & Thomas, 2021; Williamson et al., 2021).

EDUCATIONAL FRAMEWORKS AND PEDAGOGICAL INNOVATIONS

The way faculty teach over the past three decades has been influenced by changes in higher education, the increasing availability of learning technology, emerging evidence from nursing education research, and the COVID-19 pandemic, as discussed above. The most sweeping change in higher education occurred in the early 21st century when online education became possible through the internet. The faculty who were early adopters of online education used the technology tools available at the time—primarily text-based materials. Critics of online education complained that text-heavy online courses functioned asynchronously as independent studies and lacked interaction with students. Today, faculty who teach online education can use asynchronous or synchronous strategies, or a combination of both. The necessity of reaching online learners created the need for technology that could also connect faculty and students with live video streaming, such as Zoom. Many other educational technologies are on the market to help faculty to bring learners into an active role. However, it is important for faculty to select technology based on its contribution to the learning experience; faculty can use learning theories and frameworks to guide their decisions.

Theories and Frameworks for Using Technology

One of the most impactful theories is the Community of Inquiry (CoI) framework because of its emphasis on people engaging with one another in the learning process (Castellanos-Reyes, 2020). The CoI is a collaborative-constructivist framework showing three critical elements, namely cognitive presence, social presence, and teaching presence. Research using the CoI framework shows that teaching presence positively influences cognitive and social presence. Intuitively, the findings make sense. Faculty use teaching strategies to create the learning context; these strategies cause learners to be passive when listening to lectures or active when problem solving. For example, students can construct knowledge by unfolding cases and concept maps for brainstorming nursing interventions, both of which create a cognitive presence. For students to experience social presence, faculty set up strategies, such as private groups on social media, that let students get to know one another. Although the CoI framework guides online education, it still informs pedagogical decisions in the classroom. When used effectively, faculty can shift their role to a guide, coach, and facilitator of learning. (See Chapter 16 for other strategies to promote engaged learning.)

Digital materials are ubiquitous on the internet, smart devices, learning management systems (LMSs), simulation laboratories, and classrooms. The selection of teaching strategies that use digital materials can be daunting. However, frameworks such as the cognitive learning theory, the cognitive load concept, and metacognition are informative. Cognitive theory focuses on how a stimulus is processed in the working memory and later retained in long-term memory (Schneider et al., 2022). Many times, the stimulus, including images, animations, and videos, can be helpful in gaining the attention of learners. However, in some cases, the stimuli in digital materials can overload learners' ability to focus on the most important information; this problem is called cognitive overload (Skulmowski & Xu, 2022). Used in combination with metacognitive approaches such as asking questions, giving students an opportunity to use information to solve an authentic problem, encouraging students to think aloud, and requesting students to do self-reflection on what they learned, faculty can use educational technology effectively to facilitate deep learning (Schneider et al., 2022).

The Office of Educational Technology, in its 2017 report, strongly signaled the need for technology in teaching. The report lists three rationales for the use of technology in collegiate education. These rationales clearly show the shift to student-centered teaching practices.

- "Technology can provide instructors with the means of creating active learning environments that connect students with content in different ways" (Office of Educational Technology, 2017, p. 28).
- "Instructors can use technology-enabled tools to provide personalized and connected experiences to all students" (Office of Educational Technology, p. 30).
- "Learning experiences enabled by technology should be accessible for all learners, including those with special needs" (Office of Educational Technology, p. 55).

Pedagogical Innovations

The rise of online education and its accompanying technology has led to teaching innovations called the *flipped* classroom. The term flipped is used because the traditional lecture method presented to students, followed by homework, is reversed (Njie-Carr et al., 2016). In the flipped classroom, faculty provide preparatory material for the classroom session, such as narrated presentation slides, videocasts, and podcasts to present course concepts; they assign reading materials and case studies. Faculty even give quizzes before class to assist students with metacognition (Njie-Carr et al.). Students engage in learning through activities that practice the application of the course material and receive feedback about their progress in attaining the learning outcomes set for the class. In the flipped classroom, students use digital devices to access information and participate in learning activities with peers and monitor their progress throughout the course. Learning assessment is aided by tools such as testing software in LMSs and audience response systems (ARSs) that record individual student responses to questions.

ASSESSMENT OF STUDENT LEARNING OUTCOMES AND FACULTY TEACHING PRACTICES

Accreditation standards in the nursing discipline mandate that faculty assess student learning outcomes (Accreditation Commission for Education in Nursing [ACEN], 2020; Commission on Collegiate Nursing Education [CCNE], 2018; National League for Nursing [NLN], 2023). The easiest way to think about teaching and assessment is that they are complementary—the faculty design the teaching strategies and assessment methods to determine if students achieve learning outcomes. The most important learning outcome in nursing is competency to practice as nurses. Faculty can use technology to accurately assess student learning outcomes before, during, or after courses are complete (Office of Educational Technology, 2017). Three principles of student assessment bear out the rationale for using technology in the assessment of student learning outcomes:

- "Technology enables assessment to be done through formative learning activities" (Office of Educational Technology, 2017, p. 40).
- "Instructors can use data gathered about student learning to provide targeted interventions and tailored feedback" (Office of Educational Technology, p. 25).
- "Technology-enabled assessments can allow more precise measurement of student learning against clearly mapped competencies" (Office of Educational Technology, p. 39).

Faculty should also assess their teaching practices at regular intervals. Through this assessment, faculty gain insights into the effectiveness of teaching strategies to achieve the desired student outcomes. Technology can elevate the practice of teaching because faculty can simultaneously use it to teach and collect data on student engagement and student outcomes. The Office of Educational Technology cites three principles of using technology to elevate the practice of teaching in higher education.

- "Instructors and institutions can use student learning data to evaluate the efficacy of new teaching practices or new technologies (Office of Educational Technology, 2017, p. 27)."
- "Institutions can foster ongoing professional learning for instructors that supports them in developing their skills as users of technology for teaching in online and blended environments and enhances their knowledge of research-supported teaching practices (Office of Educational Technology, p. 34)."

• "Institutions can create new career ladders for faculty and instructors who master technology in teaching (Office of Educational Technology, p. 35)."

PREPARATION FOR USING TECHNOLOGY IN THE CLASSROOM

Student Readiness

Most nursing students have grown up in a digital world and are accustomed to instantaneous entertainment and information. This generation of students has been called *digital natives* because of their familiarity with technology. Many nursing faculty are digital immigrants, meaning they were born before the internet and mobile apps were widely available. Despite these generational differences, it is essential for nursing faculty not to confuse technological familiarity with expertise or wisdom about how to use technology in the learning process. Faculty who facilitate learning in the classroom also need to make the reasons for using technology clear: students need to know the technology-enhanced learning activity will give them new knowledge, skills, or attitudes necessary for their future roles.

Orientation to technology and support while completing an activity is necessary for student readiness (Smart et al., 2020). While students come to class with one or more of their own devices, such as laptops, tablets, e-book readers, and smartwatches, they need assistance in becoming competent in using instructional technology delivered on various devices (Smart). They also need to be proficient in file management, word processing, the LMS, communication software, learning resources provided by the nursing program, and internet-based or mobile technologies used in nursing education or health care delivery (Smart). Technologist specialists or faculty can provide orientation or develop a required course, including computer literacy, information literacy, and nursing informatics. Another strategy is just-in-time video help guides for students when support is needed. Quick response (QR) code technology provided by faculty gives students access to help guides easily using a smartphone QR code reader (Karia et al., 2019)

Students accept technology as part of their everyday lives. Gaddis (2020) reported that 93% of students surveyed about educational technology were optimistic about the effects on their learning. Most said technology created more access to materials anywhere and was an efficient way to study. Students also reported that technology created more interaction between their classmates and faculty. However, faculty must carefully design technology instruction for student satisfaction and acceptance of the technology (Silva et al., 2019).

Faculty Preparedness

Changes in nursing education require a change in the role of the faculty. To create technology-enhanced learning activities, faculty must learn to use standard educational technology in new ways and learn new technologies. Most colleges and universities will have centralized or decentralized faculty support for teaching using technology. Centralized technology specialists are likely responsible for the LMS, institutional software licenses, instructional design support, and training for faculty. In cases where faculty support is in departments, a single person or small team will provide instructional design support and training on instructional software for faculty. Departments may use faculty superusers of instructional software or testing software. Ultimately, though, it is the responsibility of nursing faculty to reach out for help to designated faculty or staff in their departments, colleges, or universities. The faculty must also read about current technology trends in nursing education journals and attend conferences that focus on using technology in teaching to become or maintain effective teaching strategies in nursing.

Technology Support

Faculty and students need technology support all day, every day, regardless of location. Some institutions require the registration of devices before providing technical support permitting wireless access. Faculty need to know how to access support for classroom technologies before using the hardware and software in the classroom. Prior to use, faculty should practice connecting projectors, using sound amplification of computer presentations or videos, using a microphone, raising or lowering a screen, and controlling the room lights and any other technologies such as smartboards or ARSs.

Mobile Technology in Classrooms

Having mobile devices in the classroom changes the teaching and learning environment. Students, on average, connect two devices to campus Wi-Fis (Gierdowski et al., 2020). Creating learning experiences that require students to use mobile devices (laptops, tablets, or smartphones) in class improves student information literacy and the ability of students to become lifelong learners. Faculty must be engaged in program-level decisions about using mobile technology in classrooms to ensure consistency across courses in a curriculum.

Requiring Student Use of Mobile Devices

Some nursing programs require students to own laptops, tablets, or smartphones. Faculty will need to inform students before admission to the nursing program and provide the minimum standards for devices. Students prefer using their own devices in class (Gierdowski et al., 2020); therefore, faculty should be flexible and avoid selecting a particular device type or brand. Fortunately, most software programs work with Apple's iOS™, Microsoft Windows™, and Google's Android operating systems.

There are two issues to consider when instituting a mobile device requirement for students: (1) devices can be expensive; and (2) faculty may lack familiarity with the technology for teaching or be unwilling to change teaching and learning methods. Nursing programs need to address the issues before adopting a requirement for mobile devices. Program directors must consider how to provide training for faculty and students, particularly if testing software is used.

Students should have an opportunity to practice with the device and the software before using it in the classroom or clinical settings. The classroom is the best place for students to learn how to use mobile resources for providing patient care. Faculty can create situations for students, either individually or in small groups, to use resources for planning patient care. (See Box 20.1.)

Electronic Device Policies

Faculty may be reluctant to permit device use in classrooms because they anticipate students will

---

BOX 20.1 Suggestions for Using Mobile Devices in Technology-Enhanced Classrooms

- When learning pharmacology, have students use a drug guide to explain why a particular drug would be prescribed. Have students explain the benefits, risks, and administration considerations.
- Create a vocabulary quiz in which students find the meaning of a word using their mobile dictionary.
- Present a short case study and have students use their resources to develop the needed assessments, nursing diagnoses, and interventions.
- Present laboratory findings for a case study. Have students use their mobile laboratory value guide to evaluate the meaning of the values and develop needed nursing care.
- When discussing a nursing procedure, have students search the literature for evidence-based practice research on that procedure. Ask students to compare the literature with what is seen at their clinical agencies.
- Give students drug calculations with metric conversions. For example, present a patient case with their weight in pounds, then have students convert the weight to kilograms. Students can then apply the weight to an mg/kg drug-dosing calculation.
- Present case assessments that are aided using clinical calculators for findings such as body mass index, Glasgow Coma Scale, and pregnancy due dates.

---

be distracted by social media apps and internet searching (Burnsed, 2016). Therefore, nursing programs need to have clear policies about using electronic devices in classrooms. These policies should be broad enough to cover present and future technologies, have clear statements of expectation, and outline violation consequences. Classroom electronic device policies are generally tailored to prevent classroom disruptions and academic integrity violations. Here is an example of a device use policy: "The use of laptops and tablets is acceptable in class for class-related activities only. Students found to be using electronic devices for activities not related to the class will be asked to discontinue its use" (The University of Alabama in Huntsville College of Nursing, Fall 2021 Syllabus Template). Other essential policies relate to testing; for example, "Exams will be taken on personal laptops. A laptop, Ethernet cable, power cord, and security screen are required. Chromebooks, tablets (e.g., iPad), Microsoft Surface, and Linux computers are incompatible. No other electronic devices are allowed, including smartphones, smartwatches, smart glasses during the testing period." (The University of Alabama in Huntsville College of Nursing, Fall 2021 Syllabus Template). Students can use those devices to cheat on exams or take videos and photos of exam items.

THE TECHNOLOGY-ENHANCED CLASSROOM

Technology can enhance the teaching/learning environment by enriching the content with different modes such as audio and video recordings, animations, games, virtual reality experiences, and many other methods (Krautscheid, 2021). These multimodal resources can bring authentic situations to the learning experience wherein students engage in thinking, acting, and reflecting on action. The technology-enhanced classroom can improve student engagement, increase the amount of feedback for learning, and provide opportunities for the application of course concepts to clinical experiences (Lin, 2019; Logan et al., 2020; Sailer & Sailer, 2021; Tseng et al., 2021). The following sections will describe the approaches for creating a technology-enhanced classroom, including the physical space, cloud space, devices, and instructional software.

Physical Learning Space for a Technology-Enhanced Classroom

Unlike traditional classrooms with a teaching podium at the front of the classroom and chairs set in rows for the students, a fully technology-enhanced classroom can be designed with movable chairs and tables for students to work in teams or alone as needed. The classroom can have wall-mounted screens, smartboards, and writing surfaces distributed around the room for student and faculty use. The classroom can also support video conferences or telehealth experiences. Even though the flexibility of the moveable tables seems consistent with active learning approaches, research on the effect of physical layouts of classrooms on student engagement and satisfaction is mixed

(Clinton & Wilson, 2019; Jarocki, 2019; Swart & MacLeod, 2021). Some studies found that movable tables create better learning spaces, but expensive classroom redesigns might not be needed if the faculty use multimodal technology approaches in pedagogically sound methods with mobile technologies (Swart & MacLeod).

Cloud-Based Space for a Technology-Enhanced Classroom

Learning Management Systems

Many institutions purchase or use open-source LMSs to integrate technology into classrooms, providing all-in-one solutions for storing course materials, managing grades, communicating with students, giving quizzes, and submitting assignments. An LMS can also track students' progress toward mastery of established learning outcomes. The LMS's online collaboration tools can help students connect with each other and the faculty between class meetings. An essential aspect of the LMS is that the faculty control access by restricting the information to authorized users. This restricted access protects the integrity of the course materials and student privacy.

Cloud Storage Systems

Cloud-based solutions for higher education are available from major technology companies such as Google for Education™, Microsoft Teams™, and Amazon Web Services™. Often, colleges and universities contract with a technology company to provide email, video conferencing, and storage space. Faculty use these services to design collaboration in their courses using shared documents in Google Drive™, Box, Microsoft OneDrive™, or Dropbox™. Some LMSs have integrated cloud storage systems, giving flexibility to faculty for their courses.

Equipment for Technology-Enhanced Classrooms

Technology-enhanced classrooms must have an internet connection using either ethernet or Wi-Fi connection. The connection to the internet using ethernet is the most stable. However, a Wi-Fi connection is a cheaper method of making a connected classroom. Wi-Fi has limitations in the number of simultaneous connections and classroom coverage. When students use Wi-Fi for the first time, the faculty or technical support personnel provide the Wi-Fi name and password. If the institution has an agreement with Eduroam, students and faculty will have access to the internet at their universities and over 10,000 other locations worldwide. Eduroam is a global hotspot service for colleges, universities, and research centers and is free to students and faculty (Eduroam global site, 2021). The service is secure and convenient: the same username and password connect students using Eduroam at their home and other campus locations.

Once connected to the internet, faculty will display presentations, websites, and software from laptop or desktop computers. Classrooms often have projectors or video monitors already installed, but it is important to know how to connect to the projector. The two main connectors are the older video graphics array (VGA) video cable with an attached audio cable or the newer high-definition multimedia interface (HDMI) that can transmit video and sound. The HDMI cable transmits higher-quality video and sound, so faculty should use it if the computer has an HDMI port. The HDMI will automatically format the video display and control the sound volume to the projector or monitors.

Audience Response Systems

Audience response systems (ARSs) are interactive devices for use in classrooms or conferences. The use of ARS increases student engagement and satisfaction; it also improves the metacognition of students, an important skill to improve the learning process (Papadopoulos et al., 2019). Each student has a radio transmitter with an individual identifier or uses a smartphone to connect to the ARS. When faculty ask a question, students press responses on the remote system. The receiver gathers the responses, passes them on to the preinstalled software on the presenter's computer, and displays the results to the faculty and students. ARSs can be used to poll for opinions, pose multiple-choice questions, administer a graded quiz, or take attendance. An anonymous ARS may reduce student anxiety about selecting the wrong answer to a faculty's questions. See Box 20.2 for other suggestions on using ARSs.

> ### BOX 20.2   Using Audience Response Systems
>
> - Be sure all faculty know how to incorporate audience response systems (ARSs) questions into lectures. Encourage faculty to practice before using it in a live classroom.
> - If students must purchase an ARS transmitter, they expect it to be used regularly. Make it part of most classes.
> - If ARS transmitters are required, establish consequences for failure to bring it to class.
> - Show questions at regular intervals to keep students engaged.
> - Improve student reasoning skills by asking students to explain their answer before revealing the classroom tally.
> - Vary the timing of asking questions. Questions do not have to be done at the end of every lesson concept. Showing questions later in the class or even another day helps students test their retention of knowledge.
> - Provide sample exam questions. These help students learn how to approach questions and learn how to reason when taking the actual exam.

Curating Learning Objects for Classroom Instruction

A starting point for facilitating learning with technology is curating learning objects such as images, videos, animations, and games. Fair use rules of US copyright law allow learning objects to be used in face-to-face instruction or online through a password-protected LMS. Learning objects with a Creative Commons license are free to use. The faculty member is responsible for understanding the different options within the Creative Commons license and adhering to the restrictions. More information can be found at https://creativecommons.org/.

Faculty can start searching for learning objects in existing curated repositories using a federated search of 15 OER repositories with the Mason OER Metafinder (https://oer.deepwebaccess.com/oer/desktop/en/search.html). If faculty need to browse for learning objects, open repositories are free and easy to use. Multimedia Educational Resource for Learning and Online Teaching (MERLOT) is one of the most comprehensive repositories with nearly 100,000 learning objects, all free for registered users (MERLOT, 2021). MERLOT uses content editors in their disciplines to provide expert reviews and conduct peer reviews of the learning objects. Users of MERLOT can browse by discipline and types of learning objects and apply filters to find highly rated learning objects designed for collegiate students. Other curated repositories include Open Educational Resources (OER) and Openly Available Sources Integrated Search (OASIS).

Images

Time spent searching and finding realistic images, informative figures, and educational graphics can pay off in the classroom. Faculty can present abstract concepts such as cellular anatomy, the function of organ systems, and pathophysiology in more understandable ways with images. Google Image searches (https://www.google.com/imghp?hl=en) quickly retrieve relevant images in seconds. Faculty can use a filter to get images with Creative Commons licenses. Image repositories relevant to nursing include MedPix (https://medpix.nlm.nih.gov/home); PHIL, the Public Health Image Library from the Centers for Disease Control and Prevention (https://phil.cdc.gov/); and National Library of Medicine digital collections (https://collections.nlm.nih.gov/).

Streaming Videos and Animations

Streaming videos and animations can convey psychomotor skills, emotional situations, and patient care situations. In the psychomotor domain, watching the steps of a procedure enhances the learning of those steps. In the cognitive domain, unique animations of concepts such as those presented by the Khan Academy designed for nursing students can also aid learning (https://www.khanacademy.org/). Because a video can create an authentic patient context, faculty can use these learning objects as a case study or part of an unfolding case in the classroom. Faculty can find streaming videos on common video sites such as YouTube and Vimeo, but they are also available commercially from nursing care video providers. A potential difficulty with streaming videos is that the loss of internet access prevents the video from playing.

Some streaming videos can be downloaded and saved to a USB memory stick when the internet is unavailable or is not of high enough speed for streaming.

Games

Students love games! Students are familiar with the competitive nature of games and enjoy winning digital badges or small prizes. Faculty use games to set goals, nudge students through paths, give feedback, and reinforce good performance (Krath et al., 2021). Depending on the complexity of the digital game, students can pursue goals and make decisions; the game presents results based on decisions made. For example, faculty adapted the idea of escape rooms for their classroom or remote instruction (Diaz et al., 2021; Evans et al. 2020; Kubin, 2020; San Martin et al., 2021; Vestal et al., 2021). The rooms require students to find clues, which reinforce knowledge. Unlocking the escape room requires students to correctly analyze clinical data, which improves their clinical judgment skills. Faculty can create game shows such as *Jeopardy, Who Wants to Be a Millionaire, Family Feud*, and *Wheel of Fortune* by using templates for presentation software. These templates can be found by searching the internet.

Social Media

Social media are forms of electronic communication used to create online communities and share information. Social networking and media are prevalent; millions visit sites such as Facebook, Twitter, Instagram, TikTok, LinkedIn, Pinterest, YouTube, and personal blogs. Faculty can use social media for health-related postings as a springboard for discussions on health care issues, health policy, patient teaching, and alternative treatments. A study on pharmacology education for nurses compared learning outcomes and satisfaction with content shared via Facebook and email. There were no differences between knowledge levels, but nurses preferred delivery on social media (May et al., 2021). Even though faculty can use social media in teaching, they should attend to potential risks, including misinformation and privacy violations (Edwards & Roland, 2019; Steers & Gallop, 2020).

Creating Content for Students

Presentation Software

Presentation software, such as Microsoft PowerPoint, Apple Keynote, Google Slides, and Prezi, has become commonplace in nursing classrooms. Before using presentation software, it is vital to consider the learning outcome and the best use of the presentation. Will the "slides" be used to provide a script for the faculty? Will they be used to assist in the student's learning of new concepts? Will they be used to facilitate or organize note-taking? Will they be shared with students before class to aid their preparation? Are they being used to facilitate learning for students with learning style preferences for visual learning? Will they be used to guide student interaction?

Developing and using effective presentations requires careful planning. Common errors include too much text per slide, too many slides for the length of the presentation, and color or font choices that decrease legibility. A good rule of thumb is "less is more." Images help visual learners by keeping them focused on key concepts. Presentations should be organized around the learning outcomes and build on previous learning, communicate the main points of nursing concepts, and connect new content to clinical contexts.

Faculty sometimes make the mistake of reading from slides. This approach is boring to students and, in some cases, is perceived as insulting. Faculty can rehearse presentations to ensure they finish within the allotted time. Ideally, faculty should rehearse in the room to check the projection and lighting. Faculty can then determine the clarity of slides, color contrasts, and text clarity and look for words that could be removed or reduced to short phrases.

Faculty need to plan the background and text colors to be contrasting so that words are legible in the different lighting conditions. Slides with a dark background should have text colors of contrast, such as white or yellow. White background with dark black or primary color text is often readable in a room where the lights are on for students to take notes and interact.

Presentation slides can include images, videos, and graphs. Faculty can find images and video clips using filters on search engines. Videos demonstrating assessment techniques, equipment operation, and therapeutic communication can be embedded into a presentation slide. Embedding videos into presentations avoids issues with internet connections or unwanted advertisements playing before the selected video. Also, faculty can trim downloaded videos to the desired portion of the video using simple video editors. An MP4 file dropped into a presentation slide will have a controller for starting and stopping. Such files will significantly increase the presentation file size and prevent sharing with students via email.

Although digital presentations are often considered a low-impact teaching strategy, the software can facilitate higher-order learning when used appropriately. Faculty can embed interactive activities into the presentation software to achieve higher-order thinking. Faculty can embed case studies with questions, knowledge checks, and NCLEX-style questions to prepare students for classroom tests, licensing exams, or certification exams. When faculty give feedback combined with class discussion, the case studies or questions can develop clinical judgment skills. The faculty can unfold a case using short video, audio, or text with relevant images. Students then work through the case as a class or in smaller groups. Faculty can develop short questions to check students' knowledge throughout the presentation using online software such as Kahoot! or Mentimeter™. The NCLEX-style questions can be placed directly in the presentation software, and answers scored immediately with ARSs. Other content creation applications that nurse educators can use include Animoto, a drag-and-drop video maker (https://animoto.com/); Glogster (https://edu.glogster.com/), an online poster tool; Powtoon (https://www.powtoon.com/), an animation software; Voki (https://www.voki.com/), an avatar creator; and WebQuest (http://webquest.org/), an inquiry-oriented lesson plan. These approaches bring students into an active role during class rather than a passive one of listening or note-taking. Additional information about developing presentations and using presentation software is presented in Box 20.3.

BOX 20.3   Developing and Using Presentation Software

Developing the Presentation
- Use dark text on a light background; it is easier to see in a classroom with lights on.
- Use large fonts (24 points or larger) of a sans-serif font such as Arial, Helvetica, or Calibri.
- Label each screen to keep students prompted about the current topic.
- Limit punctuation (e.g., periods at end of lines).
- Avoid use of all capital letters; they are difficult to read.
- Use pictures to illustrate concepts rather than words wherever possible.
- Avoid using "clip art": it has become cliché and is rarely helpful.
- Video and audio clips are helpful. Avoid unnecessary sound effects.
- Avoid unnecessary animations or transitions unless needed.
- Fewer words and larger text improve learning. Slides are prompts and organizers, not scripts.
- Use charts to present data but keep them simple and illustrative of a major point or concept.

- Add interactive questions or unfolding case studies to engage the audience.
- Distribute the slides ahead of time by creating a handout of three to six slides per page and saving in PDF format. Students will be able to take notes and not need presentation software to view.

Rehearsing the Presentation Before Class
Position the screen in the middle of the classroom and the podium to the right of the screen. Arrange seats so that all students can view the screen. Test readability by standing in the back of the room with the lights on as they would be in the class.
- Obtain and test the needed passcodes for Wi-Fi access.
- Test internet links to web pages.
- If using linked video or audio clips, test the sound system and set at an appropriate volume.
- Check spelling and grammar. Use the built-in checkers.
- Time the presentation but realize that the actual class can take more time if there are questions.

Live Capture

Live capture provides faculty with a way to record lectures for nonsynchronous use. The technology can be simple or require production staff. Some classrooms have automated systems that the instructor can start themselves. The system then video-records the instructor and anything written on presentation software or a whiteboard. This system allows for demonstrations that could not be done with an audio-only podcast. Lecture capture in nursing education can be used for remote viewing by students in online sections, students absent from class, or students who wish to review the presentations.

Krautscheid (2021) described an innovation in technology allowing lecture capture away from a podium, called untethered lecture capture. The faculty use an iPad™ and a wireless receiver to mirror the iPad on video monitors. The wireless setup provides several advantages: (1) giving faculty the ability to move among students, (2) capturing presentations and whiteboard drawings, (3) annotating ability using an iPad pen, and (4) enlarging images or media for better screen viewing (Krautscheid). After the class, the faculty save

the file and upload it to their YouTube channel, add closed captioning, and then create a link to the video in the LMS.

Podcasts

Podcasts are compressed audio files distributed via the internet. Although podcasts have become less popular because of lecture capture, faculty can use software to record lectures and distribute the audio files to students. As a compressed file (usually in the MP3 format), an audio file can be quickly transmitted and takes up little space, even recordings several hours long. Students can listen to podcasts on their computers, smartphones, tablets, and cars using Bluetooth technology connecting to their smartphones. Podcasts are beneficial to students who lack access to broadband internet services because of the small file size.

Faculty can prepare podcasts for students in advance of the class or replace classroom lectures or discussions, which is part of the flipped classroom strategy discussed earlier. Podcasts can also help keep students up to date when circumstances such as illness or weather interfere with class

---

BOX 20.4 Making Podcasts

- Use a laptop or dedicated MP3 recorder.
- Use a good-quality microphone.
- Save files in MP3 format, mono, and 64 to 128 kilobytes per second (kbps) to save space without hurting audio quality. Lower kbps will save space but can reduce listenability of the recording.
- Give the file a meaningful name when saving to help identify the recording (e.g., Class 5-Postop-Feb28-2019.mp3).
- State learning outcomes and expectations at the beginning of the podcast.
- Keep podcast segments short; listener attention span is approximately 10 minutes.
- Create interactivity by posing questions or asking the student to perform a task or write an answer to a question.

---

attendance. Many students use podcast recordings of lectures they attended to review the content and their notes.

Most laptops and computers have a microphone and recording capability. Although no extra equipment is required, the sound quality can be poor. It is best to use a good-quality microphone held near the mouth while speaking. A gaming headset with a microphone is an excellent and moderately priced choice for high-quality voice recording. These pieces of equipment reduce ambient noise and create more clear recordings.

The distribution of podcasts can be public or private. Podcasts for public use require proper formatting and publicly accessible server space. If the files are for local use, complex formatting is not necessary. The simplest distribution method is to use the document-posting feature of an LMS. See Box 20.4 for suggestions for making and using podcasts.

Shared Documents

Wikis are online spaces where users can type, edit, or review a document (Microsoft, Inc., 2018). Wikis were designed to facilitate collaboration to produce content representing the group's consensus. While wikis are used less often today, collaborating in digital documents continues to be an effective way to engage students in problem-solving or creating academic products. For example, faculty who teach evidence-based practice could assign groups of students to develop evidence tables for research on interventions to improve the mobility of older adults using shared documents such as Google Sheets. Another use for shared documents is to have groups contribute concept maps to plan for an older adult who experienced a fall with injuries. Students learn by identifying resources needed to support the content, adding relevant content, and critiquing information added by other students. There are myriad other possible uses for shared documents in nursing, such as community assessments, debates on ethical issues, in-depth case studies on patients with complex health problems, and student-created study guides. Shared documents can help students connect, learn to critique the work of others, and learn how to justify an opinion or clinical decision.

Software for Teaching

Educational Software Packages

Software programs created for nursing education are commercially abundant. One segment of the education software market focuses on managing data such as immunizations, background checks, clinical scheduling, preceptor certification, evaluations, student e-portfolios, and curriculum mapping. Another market segment focuses on computer-based testing, proctoring and identification authentication systems, management of subjective assessment rubrics, objective structured clinical exams (OSCEs), and curriculum mapping.

Textbook publishers often provide a suite of educational software accompanying electronic textbooks (e-books). Educational software suites typically are in a publisher's password-protected portal. Students can use powerful search engines to find videos, animation, images, case studies, and reference materials in the publisher's titles. This access to educational resources adds value to the student learning experience. Some e-books can be highlighted and annotated; students share the annotations as part of their study groups. Faculty might opt for open-source e-books to reduce textbook costs for students. Most university libraries provide libguides with links to e-books in their holdings and online e-book repositories.

Licensure and certification exam preparation companies provide curricular reviews, testing, and remediation. In most cases, the software benchmarks the testing results to provide students and faculty information about expected performance on the NCLEX or certification exams in nurse practitioner programs. Finally, software programs made to augment simulation experiences, provide experience with electronic health records, and provide virtual clinical experiences are described in Chapter 19.

Reference Software

Electronic references include drug information, laboratory test norms, medical terminology dictionaries, nursing diagnoses, and evidence-based practice guides. Students with mobile versions of these references can have them where they go. The cost of references is equivalent to the print version. Applications such as the Skyscape Nursing Constellation or Unbound Medicine's Nursing Central have references and tools available for the iOS and Android operating systems. Other products, such as PEPID and Epocrates, provide searchable references useful for clinical. Electronic drug guides can be updated daily via the internet. Information on new drugs, black box warnings, or banned drugs is immediately available. The drug guides often have additional features, such as pill identifiers, drug dosage calculators, and drug interaction checkers. Evidence-based practice guides are also handy resources for students enrolled in advanced practice programs. All reference packages can be licensed to students through the bookstore or directly from a vendor for a certain period. Selecting reference software in a campus bookstore as a required resource allows students to purchase software through financial aid. The length of the license can vary from months to years. Most titles can still be used on a mobile device after the subscription ends, but they will no longer be updated unless students renew them after graduation.

Mobile Health Applications (M-Health Apps)

Health-related software for smartphones, smartwatches, and computers available from iTunes and Google Play Store has exploded over the past 5 years. Over 100,000 m-health apps are free or very low cost (Statista, 2021a, 2021b). Faculty can consider using m-health apps in their courses to teach topics such as health promotion, self-management of chronic diseases, and caregiver support. Assignments such as a comparison of features in m-health apps for diabetes, for example, can help students become better consumers of m-health apps and better serve as patient educators.

Many m-health apps are specifically designed for health care professionals. These include clinical calculators, health assessment tools, specialized reference tools, electrocardiographic monitoring, blood testing, and glaucoma screening. Clinical calculators are used for determining a child's growth percentile and the insulin needs of a patient with diabetes or converting units of measurement. Assessment tools can speed assessment of patients using validated tools such as a pain scale, neurologic assessment, functional ability, or behavior assessment.

The selection of an app for student use requires several steps. First, faculty should download and try several similar apps and evaluate their quality, ease of use, and applicability to the classroom or clinical experience. Faculty then must verify that the reference material used in the application is recent and peer reviewed. The faculty's decision for purchase can also consider cost, including licensing or subscription fees, and the benefit that students will derive from its use. Faculty who select an m-health app need to make sure it is available for Android and iOS. (See Case Study 20.1.)

CASE STUDY 20.1   Collaborative Learning Using Technology

Faculty teaching in a medical-surgical course want students to develop clinical judgment during a classroom activity on the concept of perfusion. The faculty want students to collaborate so that students learn from each other. The faculty select a virtual patient encounter from a vendor that requires students to conduct an admission assessment, do a medication reconciliation, develop a problem list, and prioritize nursing actions. The faculty plan to use this activity as formative assessment of the students' understanding of the perfusion concept.

1. The classroom is tiered with fixed seats and tables for 60 students. How can the faculty create a learning experience in this physical space?
2. What technologies can be used to create a small group experience?

FUTURE TECHNOLOGIES OF NURSING EDUCATION

Faculty who require students to use technology as part of the learning process prepare students for the emerging health care ecosystem of digital health, the Internet of Medical Things (IoMT), telehealth, and personalized health. These skills will become requisite to nursing practice soon. Virtual and augmented reality will likely be planned simulation experiences for students in highly resourced nursing programs where experimentation is encouraged before the technologies become more widely used. While it is difficult to predict future technologies successfully, there are some clear trends (see Box 20.5).

PUTTING IT ALL TOGETHER

Lecture-only approaches lead to memorization instead of applying knowledge to patient care. When faculty create learning outcomes that require higher-order thinking and application to practice in the classroom, they will use the affordances of the technology rather than letting the technology dictate learning outcomes. Educational technology, such as lecture capture, narrative presentations, and podcasts, allows flipping the classroom where lecture or review happens before students attend a class period and become active participants in the learning process.

The exponential growth of health care information requires students to learn how to locate and use new information. Faculty can help students learn how to use emerging health care technologies for health assessment, patient teaching, and evidence-based practice. Faculty who teach students to use electronic resources also prepare them to learn after graduation. Using m-health apps simultaneously gives students a valuable practice tool in the classroom and clinical settings. Solving real-world problems collaboratively also prepares students for practice in teams of health care professionals. (See Case Study 20.2.)

BOX 20.5   Emerging Technologies for Nursing Education

- Augmented Reality: Mobile devices can place three-dimensional images of objects in the device's camera image. Objects such as equipment or virtual patients can be superimposed into a real place.
- Virtual Reality: Using 3-D viewing glasses, a 3-dimensional virtual world can be explored by the user. The virtual world can be manipulated through gestures and actual movement through space.
- Natural User Interface: Using haptic (also called tactile) feedback to user to "feel" objects. Can be used in simulations of procedures with virtual or simulated patients.
- Next-Generation Learning Management Systems (LMSs): LMSs with more customizability, learning assessment tools, gamification, and analytics.
- Internet of Medical Things (IoMT): The IoMT is greater interconnection of objects with the internet. Sensors can track students' locations or activities, facilitate group learning, or maintain inventory of supplies in the laboratory.
- Artificial intelligence applied to big data, clinical decision support tools, and m-health apps.

CASE STUDY 20.2   Student Use of Technology

Pharmacology faculty want students to apply their knowledge of medications to patient teaching. The student learning outcomes for a module on anticoagulants are: (1) Identify the indications for anticoagulant use, (2) Discuss the mechanisms of action, (3) Describe the side effects, and (4) Create a safety plan for patients taking an anticoagulant. The faculty decide to design an active learning strategy to meet the learning outcomes. They break the class into groups of students with instructions to create patient education focused on a single class of anticoagulants. Group 1 decides to create an advertisement for direct thrombin inhibitors using video, and Group 2 wants to create a podcast to teach about coumadin. Group 3 decides to make a voiceover presentation software to teach about heparin, and Group 4 selects factor Xa inhibitors and decides to make an infographic.

1. What concerns might the faculty have about students' use of technology?
2. What planning steps should the faculty require students to take?
3. What strategies could the faculty use to support students while they create their projects?
4. What categories could be developed in a grading rubric that could fairly assess the achievement of student learning outcomes?

CHAPTER SUMMARY: KEY POINTS

- Faculty are expected to facilitate learning and the development of learners into competent nurses.
- The use of educational technology is recommended to engage students, assess learning,

and evaluate the effect of teaching on student learning outcomes.
- Faculty who use technology prepare students to be competent nurses and lifelong learners in complex, technology-dense health care systems.

REFLECTION QUESTIONS: USING TECHNOLOGY TO FACILITATE LEARNING

1. Design an ideal technology-enhanced classroom. What elements are important to you and your students?
2. Many nursing faculty may not be well versed in the use of technology in the classroom. What are your expectations of a new member of the faculty regarding their use of technology in their teaching? What plan is in place to assist new faculty to learn about technologies and how to apply them in pedagogically sound approaches?
3. Locate the technology and social media policies at your school. How is it communicated to students? What consequences are in place

for students who do not observe the policy? How does this policy relate to other policies at your school that guide ethical, legal, and moral behavior of students and faculty?
4. What are the facilitators and barriers you face in implementing technology in nursing education?
5. What new health care or learning technologies have been in the news recently? How will they affect your classroom teaching?
6. Virtual reality technologies are becoming available in nursing education. How should faculty evaluate the usefulness of this technology to teach nursing concepts and clinical judgment?

REFERENCES

Accreditation Commission for Education in Nursing [ACEN]. (2020). *ACEN accreditation manual.* https://www.acenursing.org/acen-accreditation-manual/

Burnsed, R. R. (2016). Differences between faculty and students' perceptions of the disruptiveness of electronic device usage in the classroom. *ProQuest,* 1–83. 10191965.

Castellanos-Reyes, D. (2020). 20 years of the Community of Inquiry Framework. *TechTrends, 64*(4), 557–560. https://doi.org/10.1007/s11528-020-00491-7.

Commission on Collegiate Nursing Education [CCNE]. (2018). *Standards for accreditation of baccalaureate and graduate nursing programs.* 1–32.

Clinton, V., & Wilson, N. (2019). More than chalkboards: Classroom spaces and collaborative learning attitudes. *Learning Environments Research, 22*(3), 325–344. https://doi.org/10.1007/s10984-019-09287-w.

Diaz, D. A., McVerry, K., Spears, S., Díaz, R. Z., & Stauffer, L. T. (2021). Using experiential learning in escape rooms to deliver policies and procedures in

academic and acute care settings. *Nursing Education Perspectives, 42*(6), E168–E170. https://doi.org/10.1097/01.NEP.0000000000000691.

EDUCAUSE. (2021). *2021 EDUCAUSE Horizon Report.* https://library.educause.edu/-/media/files/library/2021/4/2021hrteachinglearning.pdf?la=en&hash=C9DEC12398593F297CC634409DFF-4B8C5A60B36E

Eduroam global site. (2021). https://eduroam.org/

Edwards, S., & Roland, D. (2019). Learning from mistakes on social media. *Emergency Medicine Journal, 36*(8), 453–455. https://doi.org/10.1136/emermed-2019-208501.

Evans, J. J., Wiles, L. L., Tremblay, B., & Thompson, B. A. (2020). Behind the scenes of an educational escape room: Using an immersive gaming experience as a learning strategy. *AJN American Journal of Nursing, 120*(10), 50–56. https://doi.org/10.1097/01.naj.0000718636.68938.bb.

Fogg, N., Wilson, C., Trinka, M., Campbell, R., Thomson, A., Merritt, L., Tietze, M., & Prior, M. (2020). Transitioning from direct care to virtual clinical experiences during the COVID-19 pandemic. *Journal of Professional Nursing, 36*(6), 685–691. https://doi.org/10.1016/j.profnurs.2020.09.012.

Gaddis, M. L. (2020). Faculty and student technology use to enhance student learning. *International Review of Research in Open & Distance Learning, 21*(4), 39–60.

Gierdowski, D., Brooks, D., & Galanek, J. (2020). *EDUCAUSE 2020 Student Technology Report: Supporting the whole student.* https://www.educause.edu/ecar/research-publications/student-technology-report-supporting-the-whole-student/2020/technology-use-and-environmental-preferences

Horvath, C., Everson, M., Goode, V., & Schoneboom, B. A. (2020). Innovation during disruption: Implementing a nurse anesthesiology educational program during a pandemic. *Maryland Nurse, 21*(5), 12–14.

Jarocki, Z. (2019). It looks nice, but does it work? Using student learning outcomes to assess library instructional spaces. *Performance Measurement & Metrics, 20*(3), 213–218. https://doi.org/10.1108/PMM-08-2019-0039.

Karia, C. T., Hughes, A., & Carr, S. (2019). Uses of quick response codes in healthcare education: A scoping review. *BMC Medical Education, 19*(1), 456. https://doi.org/10.1186/s12909-019-1876-4.

Krath, J., Schürmann, L., & von Korflesch, H. F. O. (2021). Revealing the theoretical basis of gamification: A systematic review and analysis of theory in research on gamification, serious games and game-based learning. *Computers in Human Behavior, 125.* https://doi.org/10.1016/j.chb.2021.106963.

Krautscheid, L. (2021). Untethered lecture capture: Stimulating educational affordances through technology-enhanced teaching. *Nursing Education Perspectives, 42*(6), E176–E178. https://doi.org/10.1097/01.NEP.0000000000000771.

Kubin, L. (2020). Using an escape activity in the classroom to enhance nursing student learning. *Clinical Simulation in Nursing, 47,* 52–56. https://doi.org/10.1016/j.ecns.2020.07.007.

Lin, Y. -T. (2019). Impacts of a flipped classroom with a smart learning diagnosis system on students' learning performance, perception, and problem solving ability in a software engineering course. *Computers in Human Behavior, 95,* 187–196. https://doi.org/10.1016/j.chb.2018.11.036.

Logan, R. M., Johnson, C. E., & Worsham, J. (2020). The sandbox: Development and implementation of a technology-enhanced classroom. *Nursing Education Perspectives, 41*(5), E50–E51. https://doi.org/10.1097/01.NEP.0000000000000522.

Lubarsky, S., & Thomas, A. (2021). Thinking inside the box: Using old tools to solve new problems in virtual learning. *Medical Education, 55*(1), 108–111. https://doi.org/10.1111/medu.14388.

May, C. C., Mahle, J., Harper, D., & Smetana, K. S. (2021). Pharmacy-based nursing education utilizing a social media platform. *Critical Care Nursing Quarterly, 44*(4), 360–367. https://doi.org/10.1097/CNQ.0000000000000372.

Multimedia Educational Resource for Learning and Online Teaching [MERLOT]. (2021). https://www.merlot.org/merlot/

Microsoft, Inc. (2018). *Create and edit a wiki.* https://support.microsoft.com/en-us/office/create-and-edit-a-wiki-dc64f9c2-d1a2-44b5-ac59-b9d535551a32

National League for Nursing [NLN]. (2021). *Nurse educator core competencies.* http://www.nln.org/professional-development-programs/competencies-for-nursing-education/nurse-educator-core-competency

National League for Nursing [NLN]. (2023). *Standards of Accreditation.* https://cnea.nln.org/standards-of-accreditation

Njie-Carr, V., Ludeman, E., Lee, M., Dordunoo, D., Trocky, N., & Jenkins, L. (2016). An integrative review of flipped classroom teaching models in nursing education. *Journal of Professional Nursing, 33*(2), 1–12. https://doi.org/10.1016/j.profnurs.2016.07.001.

Office of Educational Technology. (2017). *Reimagining the role of technology in higher education.* Office of Educational Technology. https://tech.ed.gov/highernetp/.

Papadopoulos, P. M., Natsis, A., Obwegeser, N., & Weinberger, A. (2019). Enriching feedback in audience response systems: Analysis and implications of objective and subjective metrics on students' performance and attitudes. *Journal of Computer Assisted Learning, 35*(2), 305–316. https://doi.org/10.1111/jcal.12332.

Sailer, M., & Sailer, M. (2021). Gamification of in-class activities in flipped classroom lectures. *British Journal of Educational Technology, 52*(1), 75–90.

San Martin, L., Walsh, H., Santerre, M., Fortkiewicz, J., & Nicholson, L. (2021). Creation of a "patient" hospital escape room experience to reduce harm and improve quality of care. *Journal of Nursing Care Quality, 36*(1), 38–42. https://doi.org/10.1097/NCQ.0000000000000485.

Schneider, S., Beege, M., Nebel, S., Schnaubert, L., & Rey, G. D. (2022). The Cognitive-Affective-Social Theory of Learning in digital Environments (CASTLE). *Educational Psychology Review, 34*(1), 1–38.

Silva, I., Ângelo, J., Santos, F., Lumini, M. J., & Martins, T. (2019). Satisfaction and usability of an information and communications technology in nursing education: A pilot study. *Revista de Enfermagem Referência*, 4(21), 143–150. https://doi.org/10.12707/19013.

Skulmowski, A., & Xu, K. M. (2022). Understanding cognitive load in digital and online learning: A new perspective on extraneous cognitive load. *Educational Psychology Review*, 34(1), 171–196.

Smart, D., Ross, K., Carollo, S., & Williams-Gilbert, W. (2020). Contextualizing instructional technology to the demands of nursing education. *CIN: Computers, Informatics, Nursing*, 38(1), 18–27. https://doi.org/10.1097/CIN.0000000000000565.

Spector, N., Silvestre, J., Alexander, M., Martin, B., Hooper, J. I., Squires, A., & Ojemeni, M. (2020). NCSBN regulatory guidelines and evidence-based quality indicators for nursing education programs. *Journal of Nursing Regulation*, 11(2, Supplement), S1–S64. https://doi.org/10.1016/S2155-8256(20)30075-2.

Statista. (2021a). *Healthcare apps available Apple App Store 2021*. Statista. https://www.statista.com/statistics/779910/health-apps-available-ios-worldwide/

Statista. (2021b). *Healthcare apps available Google Play 2021*. Statista. https://www.statista.com/statistics/779919/health-apps-available-google-play-worldwide/

Steers, M., & Gallop, S. (2020). Ethical tipping point. *Nursing*, 50(12), 52–54. https://doi.org/10.1097/01.NURSE.0000694768.02007.f1.

Swart, W., & MacLeod, K. (2021). Evaluating learning space designs for flipped and collaborative learning: A transactional distance approach. *Education Sciences*, 11. https://eric.ed.gov/?q=collaborative+learning+classroom+design&id=EJ1300959.

Tseng, L., Hou, T., Huang, L., & Ou, Y. (2021). Effectiveness of applying clinical simulation scenarios and integrating information technology in medical-surgical nursing and critical nursing courses. *BMC Nursing*, 20(1), 1–14. https://doi.org/10.1186/s12912-021-00744-7.

The University of Alabama in Huntsville College of Nursing, *Fall 2021 Syllabus Template*, Huntsville, AL.

Vestal, M. E., Matthias, A. D., & Thompson, C. E. (2021). Engaging students with patient safety in an online escape room. *Journal of Nursing Education*, 60(8), 466–469. https://doi.org/10.3928/01484834-20210722-10.

Williamson, K. M., Nininger, J., Dolan, S., Everett, T., & Joseph-Kemplin, M. (2021). Opportunities in chaos: Leveraging innovation to create a new reality in nursing education. *Nursing Administration Quarterly*, 45(2), 159–168. https://doi.org/10.1097/NAQ.0000000000000464.

21

Teaching and Learning at a Distance[*]

Barbara Manz Friesth, PhD, RN

Teaching and learning at a distance has become increasingly common within higher education. Students welcome the flexibility that distance education can provide them, allowing them to balance school more easily with other life responsibilities. Regardless of what type of nursing program faculty teach in, the likelihood is high that they will use technology to teach their students from a distance at some point in their career. When designed and implemented using evidence-based teaching-learning strategies, distance education can be very effective in enabling students to meet their educational goals.

Distance education is broadly defined as students receiving instruction through the use of technology in a location other than that of the faculty, with the technology being used to support regular and substantive interaction between students and faculty. The separation of teacher and student can be as close as within the same community or campus or as far away as across states or continents.

There are numerous terms used nearly synonymously for distance education including: online, e-learning, blended, hybrid, decentralized, and distributed learning (Downs, 2017). Definitions of these terms vary and best practice is to understand the definitions for distance education used within your university- or college-level system, as they are responsible for adhering to state and national accrediting agencies. Accrediting bodies and regulatory agencies may also have differing definitions for distance education methods, many based upon some percentage of distance-delivered content. However, distance technology can be categorized into two major modes of course delivery: synchronous and asynchronous. Synchronous delivery allows faculty and students to simultaneously engage in real-time communication across geographic distances. Asynchronous course delivery allows students the flexibility to access the learning materials at a time and place that is most convenient to them. Many courses are designed to use both synchronous and asynchronous forms of distance technology, allowing students to have the opportunity for real-time communication as well as the convenience of flexible access.

With the onset of the COVID-19 global pandemic, many faculty were suddenly thrust into the world of distance education as social distancing restrictions were put in place. The pandemic exposed students and faculty to distance education on a scale never before experienced. While the shift to distance learning was quick and unexpected for many, it allowed learning to continue during the pandemic disruption. Many faculty and students were exposed to the potential benefits of teaching and learning with distance technology, and it is likely that they will view this technology as an acceptable way to teach and learn even as normal on-campus schedules have returned. While it remains to be seen how the pandemic will affect this desire for more flexible schedules and online preferences in the future, preliminary reports indicate a continued preference for more flexibility in instruction (Johnson et al., 2021). It is important

[*]The author acknowledges the work of Julie McAfooes, MS, RN-BC, CNE, ANEF, FAAN, who wrote "Teaching and Learning in Online Learning Communities" in the previous edition.

to distinguish, however, that emergency remote learning is not the same product as well thought out and designed online or other means of distance learning (Hodges et al., 2020).

The pandemic is not the sole reason for the increase in the use of distance technology in higher education. Data analyzed from the Integrated Postsecondary Education Data System (IPEDS) prior to the pandemic showed the rate of growth in distance education continued to increase, despite decreases in higher education in general (Seaman et al., 2018). Most students taking distance courses were doing so within their own state (Seaman et al., 2018). Increasingly, students want to learn in more convenient and flexible programs that allow them to maximize their time and meet other life commitments (Adams Becker et al., 2017).

There are other potential benefits to the use of distance education. For example, distance education offers the ability to educate and bring increased numbers of health care practitioners to rural and underserved areas. By educating those who already live in rural areas, there may be a greater likelihood that they will remain and practice in their hometowns after completion of their studies. In a recent study to investigate workforce demands of nurse practitioners (NP) in rural areas, nearly 80% of respondents elected to work in rural areas because they were from rural areas (Toerber-Clark et al., 2021).

Another potential advantage of distance education is that it may be used to ameliorate the current nursing faculty shortage. This trend is expected to worsen in the coming years with advancing faculty age and looming retirements (Rosseter, 2019). Distance education programs, however, offer a means to reduce the faculty shortage by connecting faculty with desired expertise to programs and students wherever they may be located. Distance technology makes it possible to connect specific student learning interests with faculty expertise despite the distance between the two (National Advisory Council on Nurse Education and Practice, 2021).

Distance education delivery systems that encourage innovation and flexibility have the potential for maximizing use of institutional infrastructure, improving access to credit courses, and providing consistency for learning at multiple locations. Carefully designed courses and programs that utilize distance education require faculty development, resources, and planning to be successful. The purpose of this chapter is to describe the various forms of distance education technology and the resources and elements necessary to successfully plan and implement high-quality distance education.

THE USE OF DISTANCE LEARNING TECHNOLOGIES

The options of available delivery systems to implement distant academic courses or continuing education opportunities have become increasingly diverse and are frequently defined by cost, administrator and faculty knowledge, acceptance, and readiness. Additionally, computers, mobile devices, and computer-based communication systems continue to have a positive and dramatic effect on teaching and learning, thus becoming invaluable tools for distance instruction. Faculty must become proficient and comfortable with the use of technology and teaching at a distance in their practice and as educators (Matthias et al., 2019).

Distance education delivery systems are undergoing rapid change. In most cases, technologies have merged with others to form a blend of delivery or are being replaced by new and innovative delivery options. Obsolescence of existing media within the next 5 to 10 years will be commonplace, as technologies continue to evolve. However, the concepts related to leading, planning, using, supporting, administering, and evaluating student learning in distance education environments remain applicable. The virtual classroom, defined for this purpose as the learning environment occurring wherever the student can access information, has become more common as colleges and universities endeavor to offer efficient and effective higher education opportunities to students at any place and at any time.

Online education is continuing to grow at a rate that is faster than the overall higher education market in general (Seaman et al., 2018). Following their 2009 landmark metaanalysis comparing traditional and distance learning modalities, the US

Department of Education (DOE) concluded that distance modalities were at least equivalent to traditional face-to-face courses and that blended or hybrid approaches that use a combination of online and face-to-face formats may produce the best outcomes overall.

While large-scale metaanalyses have offered support for the use of distance education in general, few large-scale studies have focused exclusively on the equivalency of instruction in nursing specifically. One recent scoping review focused specifically on nursing education evaluated blended learning in undergraduate education (Leidl et al., 2020). The review found that a wide variety of topics on nursing were being taught with a blended approach, that student engagement was enhanced, learning outcomes were at least equivalent to traditional methods, with learners expressing satisfaction. Although the literature that was drawn from for the review was significantly smaller than the DOE metaanalysis, given the focus on nursing education, the researchers' conclusion was that online or blended instruction was at least equivalent and had additional positives related to engagement and satisfaction.

There are a variety of learning technologies that can be used to deliver distance education. For example, synchronous video technologies offer one way to deliver blended or hybrid courses to students at a distance without requiring the time and expense associated with travel to the host site. The use of blended approaches in higher education has increased and is expected to continue to grow as faculty use instructional strategies that capitalize on the types of learning activities and experiences that students can engage in online versus face to face (Seaman et al., 2018). The technologies available today offer a wide variety of strategies for delivering blended approaches at a distance.

Use of distance learning technologies requires planning and development of materials long before the course begins (Hodges et al., 2020). State-of-the-art resources for faculty development of instructional materials must be available. Training and support for faculty to develop and use the new technology must be present. In addition, support for students must be provided in the use of the technology. With proper resources for development and support, faculty can deliver distance-accessible programs that meet the educational needs of students enrolled in online courses.

The use of online course management software, commonly called *learning management systems* (LMSs), has facilitated the building of online learning communities. LMSs provide an instructional environment that incorporates a support system for course management. This includes course information and content, announcements, communication for synchronous and asynchronous collaboration, and assessment and evaluation of student learning. The LMS used in conjunction with synchronous and asynchronous strategies opens the realm of possibilities for connecting students with faculty and peers and providing media-rich content in an online learning community.

With the shift toward computer-based instruction, the number of courses offered exclusively in the form of face-to-face instruction is decreasing substantially. However, many courses offer a blended or hybrid approach with other technologies such as videoconferencing, audio conferencing, video streaming, podcasting, and other specialized web-based computer applications to offer a blend of synchronous and asynchronous learning experiences. Some technologies use *synchronous* technologies, or technologies that connect people simultaneously (at the same time). Other technologies use *asynchronous* approaches, allowing learners to access materials without the constraints of a specific time or place. This chapter covers selected strategies used in educating students who are geographically dispersed and separated from the faculty and both synchronous and asynchronous approaches. An overview of delivery systems, their advantages and disadvantages, and other pertinent information specific to each medium are also presented in Table 21.1.

SYNCHRONOUS LEARNING TECHNOLOGIES

With expected continued growth in the blended format of higher education programs, there is a growing need to use technology to provide face-to-face interactions for students at a distance.

TABLE 21.1	**Instructional Delivery Systems**		
Type	**Advantages**	**Major Disadvantages**	**Costs Related to Technology**
Institutionally based dedicated video conferencing systems	• Highest quality audio and video • Easy to use • Multiple sites possible • Students may attend in group or from home depending on their preference	• Requires hardware at all remote sites • Requires technical support at all remote sitesNo ability to provide spontaneous breakout sessions for small group work	• Expensive, with need for specialized hardware • Hardware units required at host and all remote locations-Support staff at host and remote locations
Computer-based video-conferencing systems (two-way)	• Interactive video from multiple participants	• Finite limit to number of participants • Video quality may decrease with increased number of participantsHigh-speed internet required for all participants	• Institutionally purchased software • Cost of computer, web camera, headset with mic, and access to high-speed internet for both host and recipients • Support for audio and video difficulties
Webinar	• Real-time video over internet to personal computers	• One-way video • Response may be audio or instant message • High-speed internet required for all participants	• Institutionally purchased software • Cost of computer, web camera, headset with mic, and access to high-speed internet for host • Recipients require computer and high-speed internet
Individual or small group web conferencing	• Very low-cost or free software • Easy to install and use	• Limited to one-on-one participation or to very small number of interactive video participants	• Often free software options available
Audio conferencing	• Learner centered • Low cost • Can be taught from or received at any location that has telephone or high-speed internet access	• Calls may be joined from remote classrooms or homes • Styles of class presentation may need to be altered • Visual learners and students with hearing limitations may be at a disadvantage	• Long-distance telephone toll charges • Audio conferencing equipment at receive sites if more than one student is enrolled • Service provider fees
Podcast, enhanced podcast, vodcast	• Learner centered • Access anywhere • Real-time and any time delivery • Engaging across learning styles • Portable • Inexpensive	• Requires smartphone or another mobile device to use in mobile format • Need for faculty to learn new technology • Potential compatibility issues across platforms	• High-speed internet access • Personal player or computer required • Production staff salaries

Synchronous technologies offer a way to deliver blended courses to students at a distance without requiring travel to the host site. Synchronous video technologies discussed in this chapter include institutionally based dedicated video conferencing systems, computer-based videoconferencing solutions, and one-on-one or small group video web conferencing programs. Synchronous audio-only technologies include audio conferencing over either existing telephone lines or Voice over Internet Protocol (VoIP) systems. VoIP is essentially a telephone connection that uses a computer or hardware and the internet to digitally transmit the call.

Audio Conferencing

Some distance teaching universities and colleges incorporate audio conferencing in a blended manner with other technologies, such as webinars, where additional materials may be presented visually over the internet. Use of audio-only technologies aids learners who may live in remote or rural areas with poor options for high-speed internet or broadband connection. Existing phone conferencing services may be used for the audio conferences and some LMSs have VoIP audio conferencing capabilities built into their software. Freely available software such as Skype and Google Hangouts can also be used as well.

If the chosen blend of instruction does not include a visual component, photographs or a video of the instructor and students may be shared by electronic or other means at the beginning of the course. In addition, students should be encouraged to identify themselves and their location when they speak during the audio class sessions to facilitate a feeling of classroom community. For the best audio experience, students should be instructed to use a headset with a built-in microphone. Participants not currently speaking should be asked to "mute" their lines to eliminate distractions and extraneous noises during the conference call. Activities that provide opportunity for some student socialization should also be incorporated in early class sessions at the same time that students are provided orientation to the use of the technology. Because the teacher is unable to identify nonverbal cues,

teaching strategies should include more questioning to determine class understanding of content being addressed. Methods of drawing students into discussion should be planned and appropriately incorporated into classes throughout the course. One common strategy to engage students at remote sites is to call on students on a rotational basis.

Institutionally Based Dedicated Classroom Videoconferencing Systems

Many educational institutions have created classrooms and conference rooms dedicated to high-quality internet-based solutions. These rooms utilize multiple microphones and specialized cameras for the highest possible audio and high-definition video to support synchronous learning. Some systems have manual controls over the cameras, while higher-end systems will utilize technology to geolocate the speaker in the room and autofocus on one or more individuals who are actively speaking. These specialized rooms may be connected to other similar rooms at various locations across the state, country, or literally anywhere around the world.

Video output from the conference is typically displayed using large flat-panel high-definition televisions, visually connecting learners across distances. The video output from the conference can be customized to display one or multiple parties on the screen. When using a single-view option of remote sites, the system will automatically switch to active video signals to display the site that is currently speaking. Another important feature of these dedicated video conferencing systems is sophisticated audio handling. The dedicated units use echo cancellation technology, which eliminates problems where the remote parties may hear their own voices speaking back to them over the system (echo) and reverberation or audio feedback. These institutionally based units have the highest quality audio and video available on the market today and are typically very easy to use. Most institutionally based systems also allow remote participants to join using videoconferencing software and their personal computer with camera and microphone.

The major advantage of using institutionally based dedicated video conferencing systems is the exceptionally high quality of the video. State-of-the-art systems use high-definition video and enable participants to see facial expressions and body language, which is particularly important in courses that use any role playing or student presentations. The major disadvantage is that managing large groups, or the ability to view large groups of students, can be difficult, and the video connection requires good broadband connectivity for all participants.

Computer-Based Videoconferencing Systems

For institutions that are unable to leverage regional and institutionally based video conferencing units where the target students are located, computer-based conferencing offers a convenient and easy-to-access alternative for distance students. Institutionally focused videoconferencing software allows connection of two or more individuals simultaneously. These services are typically provided by "cloud-based" companies that use the internet to provide videoconferencing solutions to institutions that do not want to maintain or provide the hardware to provide videoconferencing locally.

Computer-based videoconferencing systems represent an area of rapid growth, with new products and features coming to market often. Due to this rapid growth in use, many learners have had previous personal experience with these systems. Examples of such software include Webex, GoTo Meeting, Microsoft Teams, and Zoom. Some videoconferencing software requires installation of software on each participant's part, whereas others are strictly web-based applications and require no installation to join. Computer-based videoconferencing systems are often being built directly into institutionally deployed LMSs.

Each individual who is connecting to the videoconference does so via a computer connected to high-speed internet. Participants may receive audio and video from other participants, but they must also have a web camera to share their own video. To avoid audio feedback problems, participants should be encouraged to use a headphone with a built-in microphone and to mute their audio when not speaking.

Although it is possible to see all participants who have web cameras, the actual size and quality of the video may vary greatly based on the number of participants and the quality of each person's bandwidth. The ability to switch between speakers and view multiple participants concurrently varies somewhat across systems. As many students may opt to turn off the video to preserve bandwidth or to not be viewed by their faculty and peers, it is important for faculty to share expectations with students about whether the use of video is expected during class.

Most computer-based videoconferencing software has a number of features that can be used to support classroom learning. For example, collaboration among students can be encouraged through the ability to share desktops, thus sharing presentations or papers from either the host or participant computers. Many systems also have polling software and instant messaging or chat functions available. Videoconferences can be recorded and made available for students to view later or for students who miss a particular class session to review later. Some of the systems permit students or faculty to create breakout group areas, allowing for small group collaboration among participants working on group projects. Content experts can also easily be invited to join the course from a distance to share their knowledge and interact with learners. In addition to videoconferencing for face-to-face class sessions, office hours may be scheduled using the software, thus enabling a face-to-face interaction for students desiring to take advantage of such support. If the videoconferencing software is being used to support synchronous meetings in an otherwise asynchronous course, it is important for faculty to plan ahead and establish dates for synchronous class meetings at the beginning of the course so students can plan their schedules.

Another version of videoconferencing is "webinars," which are typically one-way broadcasting of actual video. The software used to deliver webinars is the same as that used for web conferencing, and the capabilities of displaying slides and desktop applications are similar. There are several advantages of webinars over interactive two-way video conferences. One advantage is the possible number of participants. Because video is broadcast in only one direction, broadband limitations are generally not affected by multiple participants, and it is possible to have more than 100 participants in any given webinar. Participants may still engage during live sessions but will do so via polling mechanisms, chat, and audio only. Webinars still require high-speed internet access, although a web camera is not necessary for participation at remote locations. The obvious disadvantage to webinars is the loss of face-to-face interaction with the remote sites.

Individual or Small Group Videoconferencing

Although many institutions may subscribe to professional-level web conferencing software solutions, software also exists for connecting one on one or in small groups for a free, or very little, cost. Examples of this software include Skype, FaceTime, and Google Chat. Most of these videoconferencing solutions are offered as a free download with the creation of an account for their service. The software is easy to use and requires either a smartphone or a computer with a web camera, headphones with microphone, and high-speed internet access.

Most of these types of software also allow for instant messaging and a "status indicator" to let people know if you are available for videoconferencing or messaging. Although not designed to allow numerous video connections at one time, such software is a cost-effective way to enable one-on-one, face-to-face interactions between faculty and students or between small student groups. Such software may be used to facilitate face-to-face tutoring sessions or to bring groups together for project work across geographical locations. Instructors can also use the software to host office hours with students by posting their availability to students and being available at specified times each week. Some of the software allows for desktop sharing, but overall, the robustness of sharing features is limited compared with institutionally focused web conferencing solutions. Nonetheless, given the inexpensive cost to use these products, these tools offer a valuable way to connect with students.

Support and Strategies for Synchronous Connections

Each synchronous connection medium has identifiable differences specific to the technology, but the similarities of required support for planning and implementing use of the technology in the classroom and online represent the major focus. Virtual classroom teaching requires faculty to carefully plan the best strategies for learning over a distance. Within this overall process, students must be oriented to the technology and clear expectations must be communicated to the learners. Student outcomes can be influenced by both the process and the content of learning. Clear and concise orientation is an important step toward improved academic self-concept. A summary of adapted teaching strategies specifically for teaching with synchronous technology is provided in Table 21.2.

As with other instructional delivery strategies, synchronous systems of instruction require marketing, site selection, effective communication, and ongoing course coordination to be managed efficiently. Faculty and administrators must work together closely to ensure that these components of the total educational plan are in place.

Selection of a Synchronous System

The selection of any video conferencing solution for a given institution will vary based on existing resources and the student population. Whether there are already existing regionally based video conferencing units in the locations desired will affect the decision. Collaborative relationships or rental of remote equipment is also possible in some cases. The regional video conferencing model gives remote students a chance to get to know others geographically close to them because they come together in remote classrooms. In rural areas or areas with poor broadband access, videoconferencing units located at regional hospitals or small-town libraries may be one way to accommodate access to the virtual synchronous classroom, particularly when students do not have access to broadband in their homes.

TABLE 21.2 Adapting Teaching Strategies for Use With Synchronous Technologies	
Teaching Strategies Used in Courses Delivered by Synchronous Technology	**Adapted Teaching Strategies**
Lecture Provides an efficient method of presenting factual information in a short period.	• Present key concepts in short minilectures (10–15 min) or podcasts interspersed with feedback, interaction, questioning, and application opportunities. • Engage learners with key concept material through self-assessment strategies, reflection, advanced organizers. • Enhance minilectures with web- and computer-based materials and other media such as presentation software, video, and computer graphics. • Coach guest speakers to design interactive presentations, with ample opportunity for question–answer exchanges with learners.
Discussion Provides a student-centered learning environment. Facilitates a collaborative learning process. Engages learners in active learning. Provides an opportunity for critical inquiry.	• Elicit multiple perspectives, points of view, and experiences for learners to reflect on. • Preassign individuals to give specific reports to enhance discussion. • Call on students frequently; establish a dialogue between learners at various reception sites. • Allow sufficient time for learners to respond to questions and enter the discussion, encouraging all sites to participate • Ask high-level questions that require students to compare, apply, synthesize, hypothesize, or evaluate. • Repeat and rephrase question while waiting for students to prepare a response. • Encourage participation from learners by effectively using camera to engage in eye contact with learner and focus on those speaking.
Interview Experts or clients bring additional information or viewpoints to the class in an interview format.	• Prerecord segments with expert "live" for web-based question and answer exchanges or have expert available by telephone. • Moderator should summarize and clarify key points and keep interview timely and on point.
Panel Discussion Facilitates the introduction of a wide range of informed opinions in an efficient manner.	• Learners should be prepared by previous assigned learning activities. • Ensure that panel members understand their role on the panel and what they are to contribute to the discussion. Three or four panel members are optimum. Choose panelists with differing viewpoints or areas of expertise. Keep presentations short so that all panel members have sufficient time to present their information. Conduct a rehearsal with the panel before class as needed. • Panel members can be geographically dispersed and live or online, but be sure to include all panel members in discussion. • Moderator's summaries are crucial to identifying important points and keeping panel members to the allotted time so that all have an opportunity to speak.

TABLE 21.2   Adapting Teaching Strategies for Use With Synchronous Technologies—cont'd

Teaching Strategies Used in Courses Delivered by Synchronous Technology	Adapted Teaching Strategies
Role Playing Encourages simulated decision making, collaboration, and engagement.	• Role-playing scenario can be prerecorded and shown during class; consider using groups at different reception sites. • Role playing can be used to follow up on a previous assignment, such as "What would you do in this situation?" • Prepare learners ahead of time because there is less spontaneous activity than in a face-to-face classroom. • Keep role-playing segments short so that students from all sites can react and respond. • Debrief the role-playing scenario with discussion to emphasize key learning, reflection, feelings, etc.
Learning Circles, Discussion Groups, and Study Groups Facilitates discussion in larger classes Provides opportunity for practical work sessions in a collegial and collaborative environment. Encourages participation and active learning and builds group rapport within the class.	• Use technology that supports the formation of synchronous or asynchronous groups; divide class into groups of 5–10 for discussion purposes. In classes with large groups of students, break the students into smaller groups and ask each group to select a "reporter" to present the group's work. • Use team-building skills to develop collaborative learning. • Give groups explicit instructions as to the task to be accomplished, such as "develop one question" or "agree on one disadvantage." Keep instructions clear and simple. • Use with problem-based learning and team-based learning scenarios. • Have groups report back during videoconference class time.
Question and Answer Provides feedback to faculty and learner. Stimulates discussion. Engages learners in class.	• Participants should be encouraged to make note of questions or comments as the class proceeds so that they are ready to respond. • Respect for individuals' questions is essential; provide the opportunity through asynchronous discussion forum, chat function, live stream, or 800 number to answer questions from individuals who did not have a chance to participate during the class session.
Case Study/Simulation Helps individuals to weigh and test values, separate fact from opinion, and develop critical thinking skills.	• Case studies should be available to learners in advance of class so that the learners can review and prepare individual or group responses. • If oral case studies are presented, they can add a change of pace; keep these short (5–10 minutes) so that others in the group can assimilate the details. • Incorporate presentation software, video clips, or other media to enhance case study presentation; encourage learners to do the same to enhance their responses to the case study.

Continued

TABLE 21.2	Adapting Teaching Strategies for Use With Synchronous Technologies—cont'd
Teaching Strategies Used in Courses Delivered by Synchronous Technology	**Adapted Teaching Strategies**
Debate Clarify points and positions. Helpful for values clarification and developing critical thinking and communication skills. Supports learning in the affective domain.	• Plan ahead and give clear directions. • Have groups develop criteria for evaluating presentations. • Be sure learners at all sites can hear points; repeat as needed. • Can preassign positions to be debated to specific groups.
Multimedia, Graphics, Slides Provides visual clarity and a close-up view of selected material.	• Keep graphics simple. • Use the "horizontal" or "landscape" aspect. • Use a large font size. • Use contrasting background and foreground (blue, gray, and pastel are best as background colors).

In areas where students do have access to high-speed internet, use of a computer-based video-conferencing solution offers great flexibility for access to the virtual classroom. Many institutions subscribe to a particular product, and use of the institutionally available product will be most cost effective. It is important to note that the quality of the video may not result in the ability to see facial expressions and detail, but it will provide some of the benefits of a face-to-face interaction. When thinking about videoconferencing, one must consider the potential number of students expected at remote sites and select a product with capabilities to accommodate concurrent anticipated usage. With large numbers of participants, switching to a webinar format may be preferred, however, this option must be weighed against the loss of two-way interactive video.

One area of considerable growth has been the ability to connect handheld mobile devices such as smartphones and other tablet devices to web conferences. The ability to join mobile devices is significant, as research indicates that students are likely to own at least two internet-capable devices, one of which is a smartphone (Gierdowski, 2019). Given the complexity of the number and types of devices students may own, it is important to consider a device-agnostic or flexible platform that will accommodate a wide variety of brands, operating systems, and models. (See Case Study 21.1.)

CASE STUDY 21.1   Evaluating Videoconferencing Technology

A university currently delivers the MSN program to only one of the campuses within a four campus system. There is a need for more advanced practice nurses throughout the state, and the decision has been made to begin offering the MSN program to the three other campuses. Faculty endorsed the decision to begin offering the MSN program in a hybrid format to the other three campuses utilizing videoconferencing technologies.

1. What additional information is needed to evaluate potential videoconferencing solutions?
2. What hardware and software might you recommend for the videoconferencing?
3. What additional resources might be needed as you transition to delivering the program across all four campuses?

ASYNCHRONOUS LEARNING TECHNOLOGIES

Although there is increased growth in use of a variety of synchronous technologies, asynchronous technologies have also grown and become more interactive. Asynchronous technologies do not require the student to be tied to a specific time or place, hence offering the greatest flexibility in scheduling and participation in course materials. A variety of audio-only and video-enhanced technologies exist to deliver content and materials to students on their own schedule.

Podcasts

A popular tool for receiving streaming media over the internet is a podcast. *Podcast* was a term originally derived from Apple's portable music player, the iPod, and involved the broadcast of audio that could be subscribed to and automatically downloaded to a computer. Now the term *podcast* typically refers to any type of audio programming that can be automatically downloaded to a computer or mobile device. The most common file type for distribution of audio-only podcasts is the MP3 format. Students subscribe to a particular podcast with software either in their LMS or other freely available programs to automatically receive the new files.

One popular form of podcasting is to capture live, face-to-face lectures. An easy way for faculty to capture lectures for podcasting is with portable flash memory audio recorders that record directly in the MP3 format. The recording can be made at a low bit-per-second rate (32 kbps is recommended) that reduces file size without much compromise in audio quality. The use of a lapel microphone will help ensure higher audio quality. It is important to state the name and date of the class at the beginning to help students know the topic of the audio file. These files require no postrecording processing except for changing the name of the file. Files can be uploaded to a course LMS or can be emailed directly to students.

Advantages of this style of podcasting include making content available for additional student review to increase the understanding of difficult concepts and allow additional note-taking time for items missed during class. An archive of lectures can be created and used for inclement weather dates or in case of faculty illness for future classes. The major disadvantage of this form of podcasting is that it does not foster active learning, and some students may perceive an opportunity to miss class periods. Strategies such as using interactive learning activities in class that build on concepts introduced in the podcast can help discourage this behavior. Another disadvantage of this form of podcasting is that it does not add any additional information to the class.

Another form of podcasting involves replacing lecture time with prerecorded podcasts. A relatively newer phenomenon of "flipped" classrooms may use podcasts to deliver course content outside of the classroom. For more in-depth information on the flipped classroom, please refer to Chapter 16.

The podcasting of supplementary materials to students is another strategy in the use of podcasting. This allows students to explore topics in greater depth and extend their learning beyond what was received in the classroom. Ideas for podcasting include addressing most common questions from the week, bringing guest lecturers to students, producing a weekly review of topics, or creating a "precast" of materials before class to allow better preparation for in-class periods.

Enhanced Podcasts and Video Podcasts

Enhanced podcasts are audio podcasts that include still images that are synced with the audio narration. One common format of an enhanced podcast in education is presentation-style slides with voiceover narration. The slides and audio are synced together, delivered via the distribution feed, and made playable on computers and some mobile devices.

A video podcast, or *vodcast*, is a podcast that includes video. This video may include enhanced material, such as slides with synced narration, but typically it includes live-action film of the speaker or speakers. Vodcasts may be used to provide content, give instructions or expectations for assignments, clarify content, or provide feedback. Lecture capture as a vodcast is the most frequently requested technology by undergraduate students (Galanek & Brooks, 2019). Vodcast files tend to be relatively large, and therefore careful attention should be given to whether video is a necessary component to the delivery of the material. If video is essential, editing and breaking clips into shorter segments (less than 5–10 minutes) is desirable to limit the size of the file download. The size of the playback window can also be reduced to make smaller file sizes for distribution.

Podcast and Vodcast Creation Tools

Simple audio-only files are easy to capture and may be created with a variety of portable recorders. For the most professional results, the use of a soundproof booth and special microphone will result in the best sound quality, but at a minimum, use of a good microphone in a quiet room will result in much higher quality sound. Editing of audio files can be done with software such as GarageBand (Mac platform) or Audacity (Mac or PC) that is available free via the internet.

Creation of vodcasts involves cameras to capture the live video and postproduction software to edit the video. Video may be captured simply by using a smartphone or built-in web cameras or may be done with professional video cameras and microphones. Use of professional equipment will result in higher-quality audio and video in the final product. Software needed to edit and process such files includes Adobe Premiere, Adobe Rush, and iMovie. If extensive editing of video files is required, it is recommended to have support staff who are skilled in the use of such software provide assistance in this area, as learning to use video editing software with proficiency can be time consuming. Similar to enhanced podcasts, it is important to understand the user group when making vodcasts available and either provide multiple file formats or target those most used by the student group.

TEACHING AND LEARNING IN THE ONLINE ENVIRONMENT

The online courses and programs offered in higher education today are just as likely to attract students who are living on campus as those who live at a distance. Students desire the flexibility of attending courses that do not require them to be in a specific geographical location at a specific time. Online learning allows students to learn at a place and time that is convenient to them with access to online tools and resources. In some cases the students and faculty may meet entirely online in an asynchronous manner; in other cases, the course may have a blended or hybrid delivery design, combining synchronous

and asynchronous learning experiences. Engaging successfully in online learning requires faculty and students to reconceptualize their roles as teachers and learners in the teaching-learning process.

Faculty Role in Online Learning

The faculty's role as an educator undergoes a change when teaching online courses. First, real-time, face-to-face interaction with students becomes more limited, with many interactions occurring asynchronously. Most importantly, in online courses the educator is less likely to be the primary source of information for students. Instead, the educator's role becomes one of facilitating students' learning experiences. Students assume more responsibility for identifying their own learning needs and being self-directed in how they choose to meet identified learning outcomes. For some faculty new to online teaching, this results in feeling a loss of control over the learning process. Teaching online may require faculty to rethink long-held beliefs about the role of the educator in the teaching–learning process and explore new paradigms of teaching.

Becoming a "facilitator" of learning, however, does not lessen the need for the educator or the importance of the educator's role in the learning process. The educator retains responsibility for identifying the expected outcomes of the course, designing learning activities that will promote active student involvement in the learning process and higher-order thinking, and evaluating student performance. Facilitating online discussion is another important role for faculty who are teaching online. Faculty should encourage peer interaction rather than student–instructor conversation. There should be variety in the types of discussion, which may include reflection, critical thinking, and postclinical conferencing. Clear grading rubrics to evaluate discussion provide timely feedback to students so that they will know whether they are achieving the desired learning outcomes.

Managing Online Discussion

Managing asynchronous online discussion so that it remains interactive, student driven, and on topic is an important aspect of the faculty's role as a facilitator of student learning. Faculty should strive to serve as discussion facilitators, encouraging students to engage with the course content and their peers. At times the educator may find it necessary to change the direction of the discussion or to correct any factual errors students may have made in their postings; however, faculty should strive to avoid dominating the conversation. Successful management of asynchronous discussion requires the educator to clearly identify desired learning outcomes related to the discussion and to ensure that all students are participating in the course activities.

Because online courses promote student flexibility and convenience in learning, students tend to access the course materials, post comments, and send emails to faculty at all hours of the day, 7 days a week. As a result, time management may become an issue for faculty teaching online courses because of the amount of student communication generated within the course. The communication generated by students in online courses can be overwhelming if the educator has not given some prior thought to how to manage it. That is why it is essential to implement time management strategies before the course begins. By having a plan in place, faculty can respond to student comments in a timely manner without becoming overwhelmed.

Some strategies for managing online communication that have proven helpful include (1) deciding how quickly to respond to student inquiries (e.g., within 48 hours) and informing students of this time frame so that they will know when to anticipate an answer; (2) establishing individual student electronic file folders in which to retain a record of course communication; (3) capitalizing on the communication options available within the LMS (videoconferencing, messaging, chat, and email); (4) establishing "electronic" office hours to interact with students; and (5) creating and saving standardized responses to the most commonly asked questions that can be quickly accessed and individualized for students. Faculty may also find it helpful to "block out" scheduled amounts of time each week to devote to the online course.

Another means of managing online discussion is to have students provide peer feedback to postings in the discussion forums. Students can critique posted assignments, lead and summarize group discussions, and participate in collaborative group learning activities. Students can also be responsible for synthesizing and analyzing the responses in the forum, thus providing faculty and classmates from other groups an opportunity to respond to summarized work. Faculty can appoint and rotate student discussion leaders to provide opportunities for all students to experience a leadership role. Not only do these techniques foster timely feedback and reduce sole reliance on the faculty for feedback, but they also promote active learning. It is not desirable for faculty to respond to every comment made by students in online discussion. Faculty should focus their comments on emphasizing or summarizing key concepts, encouraging participation, providing constructive feedback, and acknowledging students' efforts. These strategies also work to effectively manage discussion in classes that have larger enrollments.

Managing Large Enrollments in Online Courses

Educator shortages, increased student enrollment, and pressures to admit additional students to nursing programs have led to faculty teaching classes with larger enrollments, including online courses. Although there is no evidence to indicate that student satisfaction and the quality of teaching and learning is less in larger classes, faculty are responsible for ensuring quality learning experiences in their courses and need to consider strategies for facilitating learning when course enrollment increases.

What constitutes a large class? The answer to this question depends on the nature of the content being taught, with foundational content lending itself more to larger class sizes than upper-level and graduate courses. While there is very little empirical literature to support appropriate class sizes for distance education, Taft et al. (2019) examined the literature in regard to class sizes in online courses and subsequently proposed that large enrolling courses were ones with 40 or more learners, medium to large were those with 31–39 learners, medium were those with 24–30 learners, small to medium were courses with 16–23 learners, and small were those with less than 15 learners. While this large synthesis of existing literature on enrollment sizes helps to clarify numbers across many institutions, ultimately, policies regarding class sizes vary widely among institutions.

When teaching an online course with larger enrollments, faculty must ensure that the course and educational practices are designed to promote and maximize higher-order learning. For courses that have enrollments surpassing 15 students, faculty may find it more effective to divide the students into smaller learning groups to promote interactions among students and faculty. Assignments should be carefully designed and selected to foster engagement and higher-order learning and promote application of course concepts. The use of grading rubrics also makes expectations clear to students, increasing the likelihood of them successfully completing assignments and making it easier for faculty to evaluate learning outcomes.

DESIGNING ONLINE COURSES AND LEARNING ACTIVITIES

Offering a course or academic program fully or partially online provides faculty with an opportunity to reconceptualize the way the course or program is designed and sequenced. Course design influences how students learn and how well the course influences time on task and productive use of students' learning time. Ideally, faculty have access to course design specialists such as instructional designers, graphic artists, and web technicians. Ultimately, however, faculty are responsible for the design and integrity of courses that are moved to a distance-accessible format and must be aware of course design basics.

Evaluation of students using methods other than testing has spurred the popularity of grading rubrics. A rubric should not be added as an afterthought when creating an assessment activity, but rather, it should be integrated during the development process. Use of universal program-wide rubrics for discussion forums can reduce faculty time for grading, clarify learner expectations, and improve overall quality of postings (McKinney, 2018).

Nurse educators should develop their online courses according to theories of teaching and learning and instructional design (see Chapters 14 and 16). These theories suggest that students learn when they actively engage, interact in a social and applied context, and reflect on their practice.

When developing online courses, faculty first need to consider whether the course, the course content, and the needs of the students can be best met in a fully online course; in synchronous or asynchronous modes; or with a mix of online activities, on-campus meetings in a classroom or laboratory setting, use of videoconferencing, or clinical practice settings. At this time, faculty also need to consider what learning or course management tools and online resources are available or need to be acquired to support the pedagogical goals.

Course development should also be guided by frameworks and models that ensure attention to all steps of the teaching–learning process (see Chapters 10, 14, and 16). Course development should also be guided by the use of good practices in education, such as high expectations, active learning, feedback, interaction with faculty, interaction with classmates, time on task, and respect for diverse ways of learning (Chickering & Gamson, 1987).

Basic Principles of Course Design

Attending to the following course design principles can help faculty design effective online courses. It is suggested, however, that faculty work with an instructional design team when designing online courses for the first time.

1. *Start with the learner.* The student is the focal point for designing online courses. Educators must assess student learning styles, learning needs, current knowledge, motivation, and adaptive needs (see Chapter 2). Although not all students prefer learning online or have well-developed self-directed learning skills that are essential to success in an online or hybrid format, most students can adapt and draw on strengths and resources that facilitate their learning when online coursework is required. Faculty should also understand the learner's technology skills and provide learner support and adequate resources, particularly when online courses are offered for the first time.

2. *Define learning outcomes, objectives, and competencies.* Specifying learning outcomes is a curricular process and should be completed within the context of course and curriculum development (see Chapter 10). Outcomes in all domains of learning can be facilitated within online courses, and the course design can accommodate a variety of learning domains and levels within the domains.

3. *Organize content into short, logical units such as lessons or modules.* Courses designed for the classroom are typically planned for the semester and class hour schedule of the institution. With web-based courses, however, there is more flexibility in scheduling, and thus the content can be organized with additional attention to pedagogical principles. Storyboards and course plans facilitate the organization of modules and courses. Each unit should include an overview, outcomes, learning activities, readings and assignments, and evaluation.

4. *Provide students with opportunities to practice and apply course principles in context.* Set expectations and objectives with higher order action verbs on Bloom's taxonomy to assist the students in moving from comprehension to synthesis and evaluation and to connect the learning to clinical practice (See also Chapter 27).

The course should begin by establishing clear and high expectations. These are communicated in the full syllabus. Learning activities should require active learning and participation—interaction with the content, course, classmates, and teacher. A variety of learning activities such as debates, games, concept maps, WebQuests, case studies, questions, treasure hunts, or written work such as papers, reflective journaling, and projects engage the student in active learning. Most nursing textbook publishers have created virtual environments and interactive learning activities that accompany the textbook; faculty can integrate these rich resources into the course design to provide students with opportunities for active and self-directed learning.

Assignments that foster active learning at higher levels are those that promote analysis or critique of a concept. These include concept clarification, case studies, and debates. Identifying a challenging clinical problem or ethical health care issue and having students brainstorm solutions or debate the pros and cons of a given solution to the problem are other examples of higher-level discussion techniques that promote discussion and interaction. It is relatively easy for students to identify real-life issues in nursing practice that can be used to generate online discussion. See Box 21.1 for

---

BOX 21.1   Discussion Forums

Introductions
Introduce yourself: Tell us where you work, why you are taking this course, and anything else you want us to know about you!

Module 1: Focus on the Learner
Post a description of your learners, how you will assess their needs, and what support they need in your web course.

Module 2: Debate
Question: Should all nursing courses be designed to be offered only on the internet? Participants with last names A–M will argue the affirmative; participants with last names N–Z will argue the negative. Participant with first last name starting with the letter A, summarize the affirmative; person with first last name starting with the letter Z (or last of alphabet) summarize the negative.

Module 3: Treasure Hunt
In this course, find the various strategies used to inform learners about the course expectations and learning outcomes to be attained. Post your findings and comment on the value of each strategy.

Module 4: Round Robin
Post a response to the question, "How can we assist learners in web courses to obtain feedback?"

Module 5: Chat Summary
Summarize the work of your chat room discussion.

Module 6: 1-Minute Paper "Online Learning Communities"
Write a "1-minute paper" describing what helped you become a member of the online learning community in this course.

Module 7: Muddiest Point
What is still not clear to you at this point in the course? Post your questions and all (faculty and participants) will try to clear up your muddiness.

Student Lounge
This is the place to kick back and relax.

Question Office
Post your questions about the course content, process, or technical aspects here. Answers will be provided within 24 hours.

examples of discussion forums showing the use of a variety of teaching–learning strategies used to promote active learning.

Students must receive feedback while they are learning. Feedback in online courses can include acknowledgment, for example, by recognizing that students have submitted work; information, by giving information or direction; and evaluation such as making judgments about students' work and offering information for improvement. Feedback can come from students themselves, classmates, and the faculty. Feedback can include the use of automated responses and computer-graded practice tests. Self-graded case studies are simple ways for students to check their own progress. Peer review on written work or small study and discussion groups provides students an opportunity to learn from each other. Faculty must provide feedback at every step of the learning process by monitoring student work, correcting errors, and providing examples of expected outcomes. The faculty role also includes developing the students' own capabilities for self-reflection.

Interaction is essential in online learning. Students must have opportunities to work with each other, share ideas, collaborate, and work in groups. When students work together, there is a sense of social presence and being connected to the course. The isolation often attributed to online courses can be overcome by course design that encourages interaction. As noted earlier, faculty, too, must be actively engaged and "present" in the course by responding to students' questions, providing feedback, and establishing a collegial learning environment. Faculty can demonstrate caring by providing feedback, responding to students in a timely fashion, and conveying a sense of empathy. Videoconferencing, messaging, email, and comment features built into most modern-day LMSs can all be used to facilitate interaction and collaboration.

Respecting Diverse Ways of Learning

Online courses must also be designed to respect the diversity of ways in which students learn and the diversity of the learners themselves. This occurs by providing options for participating in the course, for ways of learning course material, and for assessing and evaluating learning outcomes. Because of the increasing racial, ethnic, generational, and language diversity of students in nursing schools, faculty must also design courses and communicate expectations for respecting differences of opinion and ways of learning.

1. *Create assessment, evaluation, and grading plans.* The evaluation and grading criteria should be clearly stated. A variety of strategies for assessment and evaluation can be adapted for use in online learning environments (see Chapter 24). These include tests, case studies, simulations, journals, debates, discussions, and portfolios. Many classroom assessment techniques (CATs) have been modified as "e-CATs" and are effective for both students and faculty to assess learning (see Chapters 16 and 24). Evaluation strategies should be selected to provide formative feedback to students while they are learning and to evaluate learning outcomes at the end of the module, lesson, or course. The faculty must indicate the grading plans and guidelines to the student at the outset of the course.

2. *Use graphic design principles.* Course design is improved by the use of colors, fonts, and visual images. The use of colors and fonts must meet design standards, and the use of images must not infringe on copyright; faculty are well served by working with design experts. The course designer should integrate media such as videos, audio, and visuals thoughtfully.

3. *Respect copyright laws.* Because of the easy availability of graphics, text, and video media, it is tempting to include many of these resources in online courses. Faculty and instructional designers, however, must work within the guidelines of the US Copyright Act and the Technology, Education, and Copyright Harmonization Act (TEACH Act). Faculty must be familiar with these laws and consider that copyright works can be used only for educational purposes, for "fair use," and with permission of the copyright holder.

Creating Community

The absence of face-to-face communication in the online community has led to faculty needing to use specific strategies to overcome the sense of distance and create a learning environment in which students feel connected and have a sense of the presence of each member. At the beginning of each course, the educator can establish a learning community through activities that promote personal student interaction and allow the class to get acquainted with each other as individuals.

Using a video introduction from the faculty and each member of the class during the first week of the course in combination with an ice-breaker is a simple activity to promote engagement and foster a sense of community (Center for Innovative Teaching and Learning, n.d.). Establishing a discussion forum that can be used by students to ask course questions and promote student dialogue without faculty presence can also be helpful in promoting a learning community. Establishing office hours using videoconferencing is another way to foster student success and community.

Promoting Civility

Several factors have contributed to a growing concern about incivility in general and in nursing education in particular. Although incivility is subjective, identifying behaviors that represent incivility help faculty recognize it and how to take action to avert it.

Many of the behaviors that signal incivility in face-to-face classrooms are not present in the online learning environment, with one notable exception—online discussion. Students accustomed to posting their candid thoughts on social media may have few inhibitions about posting in a similar manner on discussion boards and forums. There are some steps faculty can take to promote civility in online discussions. Rules and guidelines can describe what is acceptable discourse and what is out of bounds. Many programs have adopted netiquette policies that students are expected to follow (Sanderson et al., 2020). Those who do not adhere to these may face point deductions on grading rubrics or other sanctions from the program.

Faculty also need to be self-aware regarding how their comments are perceived by students who may claim that their aggressive replies were in response to negative faculty remarks. Avoid escalating the situation, especially in group discussions. Offer to take the conversation "offline" and call the student to have a synchronous conversation. Consider asking a neutral third party to attend the call to act as a witness or perhaps a mediator. See Chapter 15 for an in-depth discussion on managing student incivility.

CLINICAL TEACHING AND THE ONLINE ENVIRONMENT

Although the clinical practice experiences with clients required in nursing cannot be provided online, the tools and strategies that are the strengths of distance learning can be used to support clinical experiences for students and nurses. Several types of clinically focused courses lend themselves to being offered in an online or hybrid environment. For example, in a physical assessment course, students can access online resources to learn concepts related to performing clinical skills and practice clinical decision-making skills that are the expected outcomes for the course, then transfer that knowledge to application in the clinical setting. Faculty can use email, chat, and discussion forums to link students to their instructors, classmates, preceptors, expert nurses, health care professionals, and clients in the broader community of professional practice.

In the clinical teaching environment, the knowledge learned in the didactic course is applied. Here apprenticeship strategies, use of preceptors, and interaction with colleagues facilitate knowledge transfer. The online learning environment can also be used for preconference and postconference discussions associated with a particular clinical experience, thus facilitating both preparation for the clinical experience and postexperience reflection and journaling. For courses in which students are dispersed throughout a range of clinical experiences, the online environment provides an ideal setting for bringing students together to share experiences and apply content to demonstrate attainment of clinical learning outcomes.

Increasingly, the online learning environment has become a resource environment for students and practicing nurses. Here, links to research findings, evidence for practice, and access to information about drugs and therapeutic interventions provide the basis for informed practice. As students acquire the skills, knowledge, and values of the profession rather than memorize facts, access to online resources by way of mobile devices will become increasingly important.

Clinical Technologies and Telehealth

Just as education underwent a shift to online or distance learning in the spring of 2020, so did much of health care shift to virtual delivery, escalating the need for telehealth skills (Rutledge & Gustin, 2021). Telehealth involves the use of electronic communication equipment to share clinical and health-related information. Telehealth nursing is the use of these electronic communication devices and equipment to deliver, manage, and coordinate nursing care from a distance (Adzhigirey et al., 2019). Similar technologies that are used to provide care and monitoring to remote locations might also be used to monitor students at remote sites or to connect with preceptors in rural areas (Zournazis & Marlow, 2015).

Simulations have also been found to be effective in giving APRN students experience with telehealth and technology (Cassiday et al., 2020). Such technologies include video and audio conferencing, computers, and specialized remote monitoring equipment. Remote teleprecepting has also been used to facilitate clinical placements; however, attention to privacy and security issues must be addressed in advance to ensure integrity of the clinical encounters (Guenther et al., 2021).

ACADEMIC INTEGRITY IN ONLINE COURSES

Academic integrity must be observed and protected in the online community and in the classroom. Concern about the reported lapses in academic integrity in higher education has prompted faculty to reconsider how to manage plagiarism and cheating on tests in their on-campus and online classrooms.

Plagiarism involves using the work of another without attributing credit to the original author. Internet-based companies advertise "assistance" for nursing students that ranges from selling papers to logging in with the student's credentials to take tests, make posts, and submit assignments.

Large enrollment nursing programs are vulnerable targets for companies who make a profit from nursing students looking for quick and effortless ways to purchase work and pass courses.

Faculty have a responsibility to assist students in learning the conventions of citing published work and to proactively offset the potential for plagiarism. Simple measures include developing an honor code or academic integrity attestation statement, requiring students to submit copies of all cited references, selectively altering assignments each semester, and choosing assignments that can be completed only by using original work such as a care plan for a specific patient. See Box 21.2 for an example of an academic attestation statement.

Plagiarism detection software (e.g., Turnitin) allows faculty to check students' written work for similarities to other student papers or published works. Various options exist for setting up plagiarism software such as Turnitin to submit files and generate reports on the amount of similarity that is detected among internet sources and student repositories for previously submitted work. Many LMSs have plagiarism detection software built into their systems. Faculty and students may possess personal accounts for such software or may rely on institutional access to the service.

BOX 21.2 **Academic Attestation Statement**

Students may check that they have read the statement or may type it into a text box. Failure to complete this can range from no action to barring access to the course content or course failure.

I acknowledge that I am responsible for fully complying with all aspects of academic integrity, including the prevention of plagiarism, while a student at [_____]. I understand that I will be held accountable for all violations of the academic integrity policy and that a lack of knowledge or understanding of the policy does not constitute a defense for violations.

[Name]

Include directions, links to the academic integrity policy, deadline for completion, and how to ask any questions about the policy.

While Turnitin and similar software applications are tools that assist faculty to detect plagiarism, they do not definitely determine whether cheating has occurred. Faculty need to be trained on how to interpret similarity reports to screen out false positives, such as long titles, references, verbiage on forms, and other words that will match but do not indicate plagiarism.

Faculty also have a responsibility for creating a culture of academic integrity through test security. As in the classroom, methods for ensuring test security can be simple and low cost or they may be complicated and involve additional human and fiscal resources. Easy-to-manage security in online tests includes having students log in with a user name and password, using timed tests, adding new questions to each test, giving "open book" tests, and using test software features to randomize test questions and answers or generate alternative versions of examinations.

A persistent concern is that online students may ask others to take tests on their behalf. One approach is to require online students to take high-stakes examinations at a nearby campus, or at test proctoring centers. Although this assures that the test-taker is the actual person completing the examination, barriers include the need to schedule, travel, and pay for this service.

Many institutions are increasingly turning to remote proctoring software and services that provide live proctoring to ensure student identity and test security. Although effective, this labor-intensive approach can be cost prohibitive. In response, companies such as Examsoft offer automated digital remote proctoring. Students download software to computers with webcams that monitor their identities throughout test-taking. These online proctoring solutions allow students to take examinations anytime, anywhere, and, if allowed, on-demand. But students complain that the intrusive nature of software adversely affects test performance (Singer, 2015). Still, the pressure on institutions to verify student identity and prove the legitimacy of the online degrees they award is so great that they believe the benefits outweigh the concerns.

Programs that rely on student evaluations to assess faculty performance may find faculty who are reluctant to pursue potential academic integrity cases lest students give them poor marks. Also, onerous procedures for processing these cases can be a deterrent to action. A culture of integrity should encourage faculty to report suspected cheating, not deter it. Those who employ a progressive approach to sanctions need a method to track cases, especially in programs where the faculty are unaware of a student's prior performance. Nursing programs need to foster a culture of integrity through a comprehensive approach that addresses all aspects of cheating and ways to prevent its root causes. See Table 21.3 for factors contributing to academic dishonesty and ways to reduce its occurrence. See Chapter 3 for further discussion of academic dishonesty issues.

REGULATORY INFLUENCES ON DISTANCE EDUCATION

There are numerous regulatory influences on the delivery of online and distant learning. At the federal level, the DOE has state authorization policies that are tied to Title IV funding. Distance programs, which include online education, must demonstrate compliance with laws in each state in which they operate or their students are not eligible for federal grants and loans.

Most states have established guidelines for the delivery of distance education through the government bodies that regulate higher education, which include state boards of nursing (BONs). At times, there is conflict between a state's board of education and board of nursing in terms of what each requires for approval of distance education programs. This can cause confusion for a nursing program that must satisfy both. There can be wide variation in the regulations among the boards of education and nursing within a state. In addition, there is variation in the regulations among the BONs in the United States. The National Council of State Boards of Nursing (NCSBN) examined the regulations for distance education among the BONs and found inconsistencies in requirements (Lowery & Spector, 2014).

The NCSBN (Lowery & Spector, 2014) noted that cross-state online education has expanded

TABLE 21.3 Factors that Contribute to Academic Dishonesty and Approaches to Reduce Them

Contributing Factors to Cheating	Approaches to Reduce Them
Ignorance of what constitutes cheating and the policies governing cheating.	Develop clear policies on academic integrity that describe what constitutes cheating Publish or link to these policies to increase their visibility in places such as the course syllabus, course catalog, student handbook, and other locations. Remind students about academic integrity policies on assignment guidelines. Require students to sign or type an attestation statement that they are aware of the policies on academic integrity. Consider gating the online course so that content is not revealed until the student completes the attestation. Integrate content on integrity into the curriculum that highlights the need for academic integrity.
Inadequate time to complete assignments.	Create milestone assignments for large projects that result in smaller deliverables that may be submitted throughout the course. Suggest homework that describes formative benchmarks for assignments that should be completed in the weeks before the due date, and urge students to avoid procrastination. Teach time management techniques that help students find a work–life–school balance. Publish the estimated amount of time students will likely need to complete an assignment.
Ill-prepared academically to complete assignments.	Provide tutoring services on subjects that are challenging for students to master. Offer tutoring at times that are convenient for students. Assess students to discover those who may need remedial courses in subjects like math or English and offer courses that will help students improve in these subjects.
Difficulty with understanding English.	Develop assistance for nonnative English speakers who grasp the content, but have problems expressing their thoughts in English through writing.
Tempted by enablers who provide the means to cheat.	Communicate to well-intentioned peers that enabling cheating by providing answers, papers, and posts to other students does not help them and violates academic integrity policies. Create academic integrity policies that address consequences for those who enable cheating.

rapidly in nursing education. But there have been barriers. Institutions that want to offer nursing courses to residents in states outside of their home states may be required to work with multiple state regulators to meet varying requirements. Some states require that faculty hold licenses only in the home state where the program is located. Others require that faculty also be licensed in the host states where the students reside and participate in clinical studies. Sometimes these requirements change depending on whether the course taught is a didactic or clinical course. Other differences pertain to the qualifications, licensing, and monitoring of preceptors. Online programs find that they may be blocked from offering programs to students in a particular state because they cannot satisfy every board's conflicting requirements. The National Council for State Authorization Reciprocity Agreements (NC-SARA, n.d.) was established in 2013 to help its member states expand the educational offerings to residents of its states, reduce costs and barriers to access to programs across state lines, and improve the quality and coordination of distance programs nationwide. NC-SARA is a private, nonprofit organization administered by four regional education compacts and is voluntary for states and institutions that are accredited by an agency recognized by the US Department of Education. NC-SARA has resulted in more effective, efficient, and uniform delivery of online education throughout the member states. At the writing of this book, more than 2,200 institutions in 49 states, the District of Columbia, Puerto Rico, and the Virgin Islands have been accepted into SARA (NC-SARA, n.d.).

In addition to federal and state regulatory higher education issues, nursing also faces regulatory compliance with state BONs. Although there is agreement among BONs that clinical faculty must be licensed in the state(s) where students are located and doing their practicums, there is less consensus currently around whether didactic-only instructors must also be licensed in every state (NCSBN, 2015). In addition, it has been noted that BONs want to know when students from out-of-state programs are engaged in clinical experiences within their state. The compact nursing license has addressed some of the licensing issues across states who offer compact licensure (Oyeleye, 2019); however, the issue remains complex and fluid. For most recent information, it is best to consult the state board of nursing in question, as well as the NCSBN website, for the most recent information on the status of compact nursing licensure.

INSTITUTIONAL PLANNING FOR DISTANCE EDUCATION AND ONLINE LEARNING

When an institution makes the decision to engage in distance education, including online education, many issues must be considered. To successfully plan, implement, and evaluate distance education, institutions and individual programs must identify how the government and accrediting organizations will influence their decisions. Even if institutions plan to primarily serve their on-campus student population with online learning opportunities, the same issues are relevant.

Institutions must identify the needed infrastructure for distance education, how it will be sustained, and how faculty and student development and support needs will be met. It is common for planning committees consisting of administrators, technology staff, student support personnel, and faculty to be charged with addressing and monitoring these issues. The various perspectives of each of these individuals are important when designing a model for distance and online education that can be sustained within the institution. Policies and procedures specific to distance or online education may need to be developed within the institution.

Before implementing online education, the institution and program need to give some consideration to how offering online courses or programs fits with the mission of the institution. Administrators and faculty should be clear about the forces driving the desire to deliver online education. Is the institution or nursing program interested in primarily serving and retaining the current student population or in extending course or program offerings to a wider target audience, maybe even serving a global market? An understanding of the reasons for engaging in online education will help guide marketing decisions.

Before an online course or program is developed, if the intent is to increase market outreach, it can be helpful to conduct an environmental scan to gauge the market and identify which other universities are offering online education and the nature of the courses offered online. What niche does the proposed course or program fill that is not being met by another institution? A needs assessment can also be conducted among prospective students to identify the level of interest in enrollment in an online course or program and the reasons for their interest in online education, in addition to the level of computer skills and availability of internet access present within the targeted population. Having this information before an online offering is planned can help ensure that the learners' educational needs will be met.

Institutional Planning and Commitment

At the institutional level, decisions must be made about the institution's commitment to distance education, including online education in terms of human, fiscal, and physical resources. Organizational and administrative infrastructure, funding sources, technology support services, and student support services are areas that will need to be addressed. For example, who within the institution's organizational structure will provide administrative oversight for the development, implementation, and evaluation of online education? Does the institution already employ the technical and instructional design personnel needed to provide course design and delivery support, or will additional positions need to be created and funded? A decision will also need to be made as to which of these services will be centralized within the institution or decentralized to the respective academic units.

How the development, implementation, and evaluation of online courses and programs will be funded is another crucial area in which decisions will need to be made. Although many online nursing programs are initially developed with the use of grant funds, it is important that sustainability of grant-funded initiatives be addressed. It is likely that student technology fees or distance education fees will need to be assessed in addition to tuition fees to sustain online education within the institution. If such technology or distance education fees are collected by the institution, further decisions will need to be made about how the funds will be dispersed across the academic and service units within the institution.

Reliable and effective technology support for faculty and students is essential for delivering quality asynchronous and synchronous distance education. As mentioned previously, a decision will need to be made about which technology support services will be centralized within the institutional structure and which will be decentralized in the individual schools and programs. A combination of centralized and decentralized support may be a more effective support model. Outsourcing support services is another option to be considered and may be more economically feasible depending on the extent of technology expertise that already exists within the institution.

The level and extent of technology support that the institution will provide to faculty and students will also need to be determined. Many institutions have found it necessary to provide round-the-clock support services to faculty and students to limit undue frustration and "down time" related to technology issues. Faculty and student satisfaction with online learning and learning from a distance is frequently related to their satisfaction with technology support services.

The acquisition and maintenance of the hardware and software necessary to support online education and facilitate access is another area that must receive serious institutional attention. Are the institution's current computer network system and bandwidth capable of providing online access to large numbers of simultaneous users with speed and reliability, or are upgrades required? Do faculty have convenient access to the hardware and software needed to support teaching online? Is there a plan to replace computer hardware and software on a regular schedule in faculty offices and student computer clusters to maintain access to adequate technology resources? Do students have access to broadband internet services in their geographical region? If not, online courses will have to be developed with these bandwidth constraints in mind, and content delivery options that require large amounts of bandwidth, such as video streaming, will need to be minimized or avoided.

The institution will also need to consider the means by which ongoing faculty and student development for teaching and learning with technology will be provided. Faculty development issues that will need to be addressed include intellectual property policies and ownership of any developed online courses; policies related to providing additional compensation and release time, if any, for faculty who design and teach online courses; and the amount and type of resources that will be provided to help facilitate faculty designing online courses and transitioning to online teaching. The institution or program may also wish to consider questions about what the average student enrollment numbers should be in online courses. Student development issues are primarily related to ensuring that students have the technology access and skills needed to participate in online learning and facilitating student transition to online learning.

Adequate institutional planning to address questions similar to those raised in the preceding paragraphs is essential to ensuring the success of any distance education efforts. It is also important that an institutional infrastructure be established that allows for such planning efforts to be ongoing and include input from all stakeholders, as constant advancements in educational technology will need to be monitored for the institution to stay current and informed about developing trends in online education.

Faculty Development and Support

The advances in educational technology have changed the way that teaching and learning occur. Faculty who are expert teachers in the classroom may find themselves in the role of a novice when teaching online.

Faculty who are facing the transition from in-class to online teaching need to reconsider their role in the learning process and redesign their pedagogical strategies to facilitate student learning. Faculty development needs encompass the following areas: instructional design and course development, technology management, workload and time management, role reconceptualization, student learner development, student–faculty interactions and socialization, and assessment and evaluation of learner outcomes.

Before faculty begin any online course development, it is important to assess their knowledge and comfort level regarding conversion of traditional classroom courses into online courses and identify what level of instructional design support will be needed. Developing expertise in online teaching is usually a gradual learning process for faculty and initially may be intimidating even for experienced faculty. Scheduling an ongoing series of educational sessions focused on such topics as technology and time management, developing online courses that promote active learning and foster student–faculty interactions, and evaluating learner outcomes throughout the academic year can help faculty acquire the knowledge and skills necessary to successfully design and teach online courses.

Learner Development and Support

Introducing distance and online education into a program will have a major effect on the delivery of learner support services, especially if the introduction of online education affects more than just a few individual courses. All aspects of the institution's student support services will ultimately be affected and need to be reconsidered to best serve the needs of students who are geographically distant from the campus and those who are on campus. It is a requirement of national higher education accrediting bodies, and nursing accrediting bodies, that the academic support services for online students be similar to those available for on-campus students. Student support that will need to be reconsidered and redesigned for students who enroll in distance education programs includes academic advising, tutoring, financial aid, library, and bookstore services. Ensuring that all online experiences are accessible to students with disabilities is another important institutional consideration. The admission and registration processes may also need to be restructured so that students who live at a distance will be able to accomplish these tasks without being physically present on campus.

The decision to deliver online education will also result in the need for the institution to make financial decisions regarding tuition costs and any additional student technology or distance education fees. Many universities or colleges automatically charge students on-campus usage fees, such as activity fees and parking fees. Will these fees be waived for students who have never come to campus? These decisions and others related to the delivery of student support services will require the consideration and collaboration of numerous departments in the institution so that students will have a quality learning experience.

Faculty should proactively address the development needs of students engaging in online learning. Learners who are new to online learning frequently need some initial guidance on how to manage their time when they are taking online courses. The relatively independent nature of online education requires students to understand that they are assuming responsibility for their own learning to an extent to which they may be unaccustomed. They are moving from the structure of the traditional classroom to a more unstructured learning environment that does not necessarily include the physical, face-to-face presence of faculty and peers and the weekly time commitment to attend class. Some students may assume that an online course will be "easier" than a traditional course, a notion that is usually quickly dismissed after the course begins and they become overwhelmed with the independence that an online course allows them in managing their own time to meet their learning needs. It is easy for students to undeestimate the amount of self-direction and self-pacing needed to be successful in online learning.

Faculty can help students by clearly identifying expectations for participation and due dates for assignments. If weekly online discussion is expected, this should be stated in the course syllabus. During the first 2 to 3 weeks of the course, those students who are not participating in the course should be actively sought out. The lack of participation is likely a result of technology issues or the inability to be self-directive in learning. Reaching out to the student at this critical point in the course may make a difference in whether the student will be successful in completing the course.

Content Ownership

Technology has made the duplication, distribution, and display of copyrighted material quick and easy. But just because it is possible does not make it legal. Stakeholders including faculty, librarians, and content developers need to understand the laws governing the inclusion of copyrighted material in online courses.

There are four types of intellectual property: copyright, trademark, patent, and trade secret. Online courses are influenced the most by copyright law because it covers the rights to duplicate, distribute, derivate, display, and perform content directly, digitally, or through telecommunications. A copyright pertains only to the expression of an idea, such as a video or written work, and not the idea itself. One way to avoid copyright infringement is to transform the presentation of an idea.

Education enjoys a Fair Use Exemption for the reasonable use of copyrighted materials. Four factors are considered when determining whether an exemption applies. Market effect favors an exemption for nonprofit educational institutions because for-profit colleges and universities may be viewed as selling online courses for financial gain.

The Face-to-Face Teaching Exemption and TEACH Act allow for nonprofit educational institutions to digitally transmit copyrighted work provided the amount is comparable to that typically displayed in class and other conditions are met. It is imperative that faculty and students be made aware of copyright laws and violations so that they can be avoided.

A copyright does not mean that a work cannot be inserted into a course. Permission to use copyrighted material may be obtained from the copyright holder. Some agreements will include requirements such as posting the owner's name and copyright status. Others will want payment for the use of the content. Some institutions may be willing to remit a one-time fee but avoid paying royalties because of the tracking, accounting, and ongoing costs involved. Institutional librarians are invaluable resources in determining fair use and acquiring educational content that can be made accessible to all students.

Online courses combine content developed by faculty, third parties, and educational institutions. Copyright or ownership of the content depends on contracts and licensing agreements among the parties involved and on laws that govern intellectual property and education use. Traditionally, the college or university offers online courses to defined groups of students who have been registered and authenticated and are affiliated with the institution.

Students in these online courses own the intellectual property that they contribute in the form of papers and discussion posts.

EVALUATION OF STUDENT LEARNING OUTCOMES

Ongoing evaluation of student learning outcomes provides the best measure of learning success and will provide faculty with information to improve teaching strategies and the use of technology for distance learning. Both formative and summative evaluation of distance education delivery systems should occur. Formative evaluations are extremely important for the success of both the instructor and the student in distance learning environments. These evaluations can be used to determine student understanding of the content and instructor effectiveness. Simply asking the student, "What have you liked the most so far in this class?" or "What have you liked the least so far in this class?" is an effective way to obtain valuable feedback. Summative evaluations can also be done at the end of the course using a variety of online survey technologies. More in-depth information related to formative and summative evaluation can be found in Chapter 23.

Peer evaluation of the course by other educators familiar with the technology being used and blended learning environments is important. Peer evaluation may occur at the local level by individuals from the school or institution or through a program such as Quality Matters. Quality Matters is a nationally recognized review process that uses evidence-based standards for online and blended courses and certifies peer evaluators. These peer evaluators may conduct peer reviews of both online and blended courses, using an evidence-based rubric (Quality Matters, n.d.).

Student and faculty perceptions of the technology and delivery efficacy should be explored, in addition to the rate of student success within the course. Reasons for student attrition should be researched and strategies designed to address any negative trends.

Evaluation data should also include the cost of the course to the university or college. Factors considered will include salaries or wages for faculty, technicians, site coordinators, and other support staff; equipment, hardware, and software; potential lease fees for facilities and communication systems; travel costs for faculty; mailing or courier charges; and other resources needed for course implementation. All expenditures must be evaluated against the income generated through tuition and provided by other financial support sources.

PROGRAM EVALUATION IN DISTANCE EDUCATION

Program evaluation and accreditation in general is addressed in Chapters 27 and 28. Some differences or additional considerations regarding program evaluation and accreditation for distance education will be addressed here. First and foremost in evaluation and accreditation standards is the issue of student authentication and verification—that the student enrolled in the program is the one being assessed and evaluated in the course. The Higher Education Opportunity Act of 2008 requires programs that deliver distance-accessible courses to have verification procedures in place to ensure that the student who is admitted to a program and attending a distance-accessible course is the same individual (WCET, n.d.). Currently a secure login and passcode are acceptable methods of identification, but many universities are adopting additional measures such as proctored assessments, biometric identification, or the use of webcams for monitoring classwork or examinations.

From a nursing program accreditation standpoint, two of the three major accrediting agencies, namely the National League for Nursing Commission for Nursing Education Accreditation (NLN CNEA, 2021) and the Commission on Collegiate Nursing Education (CCNE, 2018), require that all standards are met regardless of program delivery method. The Accreditation Commission for Education in Nursing (ACEN, 2020) stipulates similar criteria to traditionally delivered programs, but they also have a policy that spells out more explicitly some of their definitions around distance education and critical elements to be included in a self-study under their criteria.

Special consideration of all the evaluation criteria should be examined in light of a distance-delivered program. For example, when examining resources related to a distance-delivered program, one must be able to demonstrate that the technology infrastructure is sufficient to support learners at a distance. Students enrolled at a distance must also have access to resources such as student support services, a library, and learning resources. Evaluation of the adequacy of fiscal resources to support distance education is also a necessity. Ensuring that faculty have had development in best practices for teaching at a distance is also a special consideration when considering evaluation of a distance-accessible program. These are just a few examples of special consideration when evaluating programs delivered at a distance, but the big take-away message is that the programs must meet the same standards regardless of delivery method (see Case Study 21.2).

> ### CASE STUDY 21.2   Converting to an Online Program
>
> Based on a needs assessment, there appears to be strong demand for converting an existing face-to-face RN-BSN program to an online program. The assessment supports conversion of most courses to a fully online and asynchronous format. To date, only a couple of the faculty in the institution have taught online courses, with a few more faculty having experience with hybrid or blended delivery of courses.
>
> 1. What resources do you anticipate would be needed to support faculty development for online education? What are existing resources within your unit or campus? What additional resources might be needed?
> 2. What would be a reasonable timeline for conversion of courses to an online format? Are there any regulatory hurdles to address in the conversion to an online program?
> 3. How would you evaluate success of the conversion?

CHAPTER SUMMARY: KEY POINTS

- Demand for distance and online education is expected to continue to increase as students welcome the flexibility and convenience these learning modalities provide.
- Distance education is broadly defined as students receiving instruction mediated through the use of technology in a location other than that of the faculty, with the technology being used to support regular and substantive interaction between students and faculty.
- Distance education may be provided through synchronous or asynchronous delivery methods. Synchronous delivery allows faculty and students to simultaneously engage in real-time communication across geographic distances. Asynchronous course delivery allows students the flexibility to access the learning materials at a time and place that is most convenient to them.
- Technology is continuously evolving, providing better options for reaching learners at a distance via both synchronous and asynchronous technologies.
- It is essential that nursing faculty have the skills to engage learners with state-of-the-art distance technologies.
- In online courses, the educator's role shifts from being the students' primary source of information to one facilitating students' learning experiences.
- For faculty to deliver quality, effective distance and online education, faculty development needs encompass the following areas: instructional design and course development, technology management, workload and time management, role reconceptualization, student learner development, student–faculty interactions and socialization, and assessment and evaluation of learner outcomes.
- Delivery of courses and programs from a distance requires institutional commitment, resources, and support.
- It is a requirement of national higher education accrediting bodies, and nursing accrediting bodies, that the academic support services for distance education students be similar to those available for on-campus students.
- Regardless of delivery modality, student and program outcomes must be demonstrated through ongoing evaluation strategies.

▮ REFLECTING ON THE EVIDENCE

1. Given your institutionally provided resources, what additional resources would be needed to convert your existing face-to-face courses to a hybrid format?
2. Design opportunities in your curriculum for your learners to utilize telehealth technologies.
3. What support structures must be in place to assist learners who are taking courses fully online or at a distance?
4. How will you evaluate your distance or online program outcomes? How will you evaluate your learners at a distance?

REFERENCES

Accreditation Commission for Education in Nursing. (2020). *ACEN accreditation manual.* https://www.acenursing.org/acen-accreditation-manual/

Adzhigirey, L., Berg, J., Bickford, C., Broadnax, T., Denton, C., Leistner, G., McMenamin, J., Nims, P., Smedley, L (2019). *Telehealth nursing: A position statement.* https://www.americantelemed.org/wp-content/themes/ata-custom/download.php?id=3444

Cassiday, O., Nickasch, B., & Mott, J. (2020). Exploring telehealth in the graduate curriculum. *Nursing Forum, 56,* 228–232.

Center for Innovative Teaching and Learning, Indiana University (n.d.). https://citl.indiana.edu/teaching-resources/guides/icebreakers.html

Chickering, A., & Gamson, Z. (1987). *Seven principles of good practice in undergraduate education.* Johnson Foundation.

Commission on Collegiate Nursing Education. (2018). *Standards for accreditation of baccalaureate and graduate nursing programs.* https://www.aacnnursing.org/Portals/42/CCNE/PDF/Standards-Final-2018.pdf

Downs, L. (2017). *What is distance education?—Definitions and delineations.* https://wcet.wiche.edu/frontiers/2017/11/07/what-is-distance-education-definitions-and-delineations/

Hodges, C., Moore, S., Lockee, B., Trust, T., & Bond, M. (2020). *The difference between emergency remote teaching and online learning.* https://er.educause.edu/articles/2020/3/the-difference-between-emergency-remote-teaching-and-online-learning

Galanek, J., & Brooks, D. (2019). *Enhancing student academic success with technology: What students want from their instructors (in their own words).* https://www.educause.edu/ecar/research-publications/enhancing-student-academic-success-with-technology/what-students-want-from-their-instructors

Gierdowski, D. (2019). *ECAR study of community college students and information technology, 2019.* https://www.educause.edu/ecar/research-publications/ecar-study-of-community-college-students-and-information-technology/2019/device-access-ownership-and-importance

Guenther, J., Branham, S., Calloway, S., Hilliard, W., Jiminez, R., & Merrill, E. (2021). Five steps to integrating telehealth into APRN curricula. *The Journal for Nurse Practitioners, 17,* 322–325.

Johnson, N., Seaman, J., & Veletsianos, G. (2021). *Teaching during a pandemic: Spring transition, fall continuation, winter evaluation.* https://www.bayviewanalytics.com/reports/teachingduringapandemic.pdf

Leidl, D., Ritchie, L., & Moslemi, N. (2020). Blended learning in undergraduate nursing education—A scoping review. *Nurse Education Today, 86,* 1–9.

Matthias, A., Gazza, E., & Triplett, A. (2019). Preparing future nurse educators to teach in the online environment. *Journal of Nursing Education, 58*(8), 488–491.

McKinney, B. (2018). The impact of program-wide discussion board grading rubrics on student and faculty satisfaction. *Online Learning, 22*(2), 289–299. https://doi.org/10.24059/olj.v22i2.1386.

National Advisory Council on Nurse Education and Practice (NACNEP). (2021). *Preparing nurse faculty, and addressing the shortage of nurse faculty and clinical preceptors.* National Advisory Council on Nurse Education and Practice 17th Report to the Secretary of Health and Human Services and the U.S. Congress. https://www.hrsa.gov/sites/default/files/hrsa/advisory-committees/nursing/reports/nacnep-17report-2021.pdf

National Council for State Authorization Reciprocity Agreements (n.d.). https://nc-sara.org/about-nc-sara.

National League for Nursing Commission for Nursing Education Accreditation. (2021). *Accreditation standards for nursing education programs.* https://irp.cdn-website.com/cc12ee87/files/uploaded/CNEA%20Standards%20October%202021.pdf

Oyeleye, O. (2019). The nursing licensure compact and its disciplinary provisions: What nurses should know. *Online Journal of Issues in Nursing, 24*(2), 1–11.

Quality Matters. (n.d.). https://www.qualitymatters.org

Rutledge, C., & Gustin, T. (2021). Preparing nurses for roles in telehealth: Now is the time!. *The Online Journal of Issues in Nursing, 26*(1). Manuscript 3.

Sanderson, C., Cox, K., & Disch, J. (2020). Virtual nursing, virtual learning. *Nurse Leader, 18*(2), 142–146. https://doi.org/10.1016/j.mnl.2019.12.005.

Seaman, J., Allen, I., & Seaman, J. (2018). *Grade increase: Tracking distance education in the United States.* https://www.bayviewanalytics.com/reports/gradeincrease.pdf

Singer, N. (2015, April 5). Online test-takers feel anti-cheating software's uneasy glare. *New York Times.* https://www.nytimes.com/2015/04/06/technology/online-test-takers-feel-anti-cheating-softwares-uneasy-glare.html.

Taft, S. H., Kesten, K., & El-Banna, M. M. (2019). One size does not fit all: Toward an evidence based framework for determining online course enrollment sizes in higher education. *Online Learning, 23*(3), 188–233. https://doi.org/10.24059/olj.v23i3.1534.

Toerber-Clark, J., Jamison, M., & Scheibmeir, M. (2021). Workforce demands of rural nurse practitioners: A descriptive study. *Online Journal of Rural Nursing and Health Care, 21*(1). https://doi.org/10.14574/ojrnhc.v21i1.656%C2%A0.

WCET. (n.d.). *Student identity verification.* https://wcet.wiche.edu/policy/student-identity-verification/

Zournazis, H., & Marlow, A. (2015). The use of video conferencing to develop a community of practice for preceptors located in rural and non traditional placement setting: An evaluation study. *Nurse Education in Practice, 15*, 119–125.

22

Introduction to the Evaluation Process

Judith A. Halstead, PhD, RN, CNE, ANEF, FAAN

One of the most important responsibilities nursing faculty have in their faculty role is that of evaluation. The faculty's primary involvement with evaluation takes place when they are evaluating student learning. The evaluation of student performance in classroom and clinical settings is the sole responsibility of the faculty. However, the faculty's responsibility for evaluation extends beyond evaluating student learning. Faculty also hold the responsibility for evaluating how effectively the program is meeting expected program outcomes in all aspects of the program's operation. For example, the evaluation process is applied to meeting program outcomes related to student learning, the curriculum and effectiveness of teaching–learning strategies, faculty productivity, adequacy of program resources, student support services, adequacy of technology and instructional resources, and other program elements specific to the program's mission and goals.

Faculty are accountable to many stakeholders including students, peers, administrators, employers, regulatory agencies and accrediting bodies, and, ultimately, society for the effectiveness of the nursing program in producing well-prepared graduates. Participating in the evaluation process requires faculty to demonstrate an ongoing commitment to creating an organizational culture of continuous quality improvement within the program.

The purpose of this chapter is to present an overview of the evaluation process by which nursing faculty can evaluate the various elements of the nursing program, analyze and use the data

to review outcomes and support program decision making, make changes as needed, and report results to stakeholders. The chapter provides an introduction to evaluation and delineates a step-by-step evaluation process for faculty to use to determine program effectiveness. Also, this chapter provides information about the use of evaluation models; selection of instruments; data collection procedures; and the means to interpret, report, and use findings to support program decision making. This chapter provides a foundation for understanding the evaluation process upon which subsequent chapters discussing specific evaluation activities and strategies are based.

EVALUATION DEFINED

Evaluation is a broad term that describes the process of determining value, worth, or quality; Stufflebeam and Coryn (2014) assert that "... evaluations essentially involve making value judgments" (p. 8). These value judgments are based on carefully collected and analyzed data. In nursing education, evaluation is a systematic, ongoing process that begins with faculty specifying expected or desired program outcomes with associated benchmarks to be achieved and providing opportunity to attain the expected outcomes. The evaluation process further consists of measuring achievement of expected outcomes by collecting and analyzing data about progress toward attaining the expected outcomes and ends with an evaluation or a judgment about the extent to which preestablished benchmarks associated with the expected outcomes have been met. The evaluation process is applied to measuring systematic program outcomes, such as those related to curriculum and teaching effectiveness, faculty, aggregate student achievement (graduation rates, licensure or certification pass rates, employment rates), and adequacy of program resources. The evaluation process is also applied when measuring student achievement of individual student learning outcomes in classroom and clinical settings at the course and program levels.

Evaluation involves gathering, analyzing, and placing a value on data gathered through one or more measurements. The analyzed data are disseminated to appropriate stakeholders and used by faculty to inform future program decision making, whether the decisions are being made about the achievement of program outcomes or individual outcomes, such as student or faculty outcomes. Evaluation is a process of making judgments using preestablished criteria or benchmarks that have been selected and communicated to stakeholders before their use. In nursing education, faculty engage in the evaluation process for numerous reasons. For example, faculty evaluate students' achievement of learning outcomes in the cognitive, psychomotor, and affective domains in both classroom and clinical settings; determine the effectiveness of teaching and learning strategies and adequacy of instructional resources and technology; evaluate the effectiveness of student support systems; and measure the achievement of program curricular outcomes.

Evaluation is also a professional activity that educators undertake to reflect on their own performance in the faculty role—teaching, scholarship, and service, as defined by institution and program mission—and the quality of the support provided to assist them in achieving their goals. Participating in evaluation activities and making decisions based on sound evaluation data to improve practice is a professional responsibility (Stufflebeam & Coryn, 2014) and is considered to be a core competency of nurse educators (National League for Nursing, 2019). Evaluation can be further defined by the time frame in which it is conducted: formative or summative.

Formative Evaluation

In *formative evaluation*, the judgment about the outcome or performance is conducted while the event being evaluated is occurring. Formative evaluation focuses on determining progress being made toward achievement of benchmarks associated with program goals and outcomes, student learning outcomes, course, and end-of-program curriculum outcomes. Formative evaluation provides the opportunity for feedback and improvement and is considered to be proactive by design, providing guidance for improving outcomes of the event (Stufflebeam & Coryn, 2014). The aim of formative evaluation is to monitor progress toward outcome achievement (e.g., in student learning, implementing new teaching–learning strategies, or in curriculum development and revision activities) and make ongoing adjustments to ensure the desired end result is attained.

One advantage of formative evaluation is that the events being evaluated are current, thus possibly increasing accuracy and preventing distortion by time. Examples of areas where formative evaluation can be of value to faculty are when results can be used to monitor and improve student performance before a course has concluded and final grades assigned and program effectiveness can be monitored by faculty to determine if program changes are performing as planned. Disadvantages of formative evaluation include prematurely drawing conclusions before the activity (classroom or clinical performance, program implementation changes) is completed and not being able to see the outcomes before judgments are made. Formative evaluation can also be intrusive and interrupt the flow of outcomes. There is also the possibility of providing a false sense of security when formative evaluation produces positive feedback, but the resulting outcomes are not as positive as predicted earlier in the evaluation process.

Summative Evaluation

Summative evaluation, on the other hand, refers to data collected at the end of the activity, instruction, course, or program. Summative evaluation is the process of evaluating outcomes and determining if they have been met as intended. The focus of summative evaluation emphasizes what is or was, and the extent to which outcomes and benchmarks were met for the purposes of accountability, such as resource allocation, assignment of grades (students), merit pay or promotion (faculty), or program accreditation. Summative evaluation is most effectively used to measure student learning outcomes at the end of a module, course, or program. Summative evaluation of individual student learning outcomes in a course usually results in assignment of a final grade. Summative evaluation of aggregate student achievement of program outcomes (i.e., NCLEX or certification pass rates, graduation rates, employment rates) can be used to measure effectiveness of the curriculum.

Summative evaluation is also beneficial for determining whether the intended outcomes related to any program initiative (e.g., curriculum revision, policy implementation, faculty development efforts, resource allocations, instructional technology adoption) have been achieved.

The advantages of performing an evaluation upon full implementation of the planned initiative are that all work has been completed, and the findings of the evaluation demonstrate the extent to which the intended outcomes were met. The major disadvantage of summative evaluation is that it is performed at the end of the implementation phase when it may be too late to modify strategies and possibly affect the outcomes in a positive manner.

Assessment

Assessment in the educational environment refers to the collection and analysis of data with the purpose of improving performance elements associated with specified outcome criteria. Assessment data are used to determine progress and provide guidance toward attaining the desired outcomes. Findings from assessment activities are diagnostic and are used for improvement, not to assign value or judgment to the element being assessed. For example, faculty can use assessment data to gain insight into the effectiveness of teaching-learning strategies and the impact on student learning or to coach and guide students to competency or mastery. Although similar to formative evaluation in that one of the purposes of assessment is to monitor progress toward outcome achievement, the focus of assessment is on improving the teaching and learning experience. Assessment is primarily an interactive process between students and faculty with the goal of improving learning outcomes and teaching effectiveness. However, assessment data can also be used to identify stakeholder needs and improve outcomes of other program elements such as student support services, faculty productivity, or adequacy of instructional resources.

Grading

Grading involves quantifying data from student work and assigning a value. The value is expressed as a "grade," or representation of the value of the student's work. Final grades, grades obtained at the end of the course of study, typically are required in academic programs and are used to communicate the student's achievement of expected learning outcomes as determined by the faculty to the student, the university, and the public. Grading criteria must be made evident to the student before the onset of the learning experience and the assignment of grades. These grading criteria are published, typically in course syllabi, for both grading assignments and calculating a final course grade.

PHILOSOPHICAL APPROACHES TO EVALUATION

Conducting an evaluation begins with understanding one's philosophy or values and beliefs about evaluation. Philosophical beliefs are reflected in a person's attitudes and behaviors. The philosophical beliefs a teacher holds about evaluation influences how evaluations are conducted, when evaluations are conducted, what methods are used, and how results are interpreted.

In nursing education, evaluations or judgments are made about performance (students and faculty), program effectiveness (curriculum), instructional resources and technology, or instruction (course, faculty). Evaluation activities in nursing education are conducted from various perspectives, and these perspectives influence outcomes. Therefore evaluators should be aware of their philosophical perspectives as they relate to and influence the decisions they make about the evaluation process.

Several philosophical perspectives tend to influence evaluation. Educators who rely on goals, objectives, and outcomes to guide program, course, or lesson development will likely have an *outcomes* approach to evaluation. The merits of the activity or program are largely indicated by the success of students demonstrating expected learning outcomes. A *service* orientation toward evaluation emphasizes the student learning process and includes self-evaluation, thus assisting educators to make decisions about learners and the teaching–learning process. Although all evaluation involves judgment, the evaluator with a *judgment* perspective focuses on establishing the worth or merit of the employee, student, product, or program. Others have a *research* orientation to evaluation and emphasize precision in measurement and statistical analysis to gain a general understanding of why students and programs do or do not succeed. The focus in this perspective is on tools, methods, and designs as they relate to validity and reliability of instruments. Yet another orientation is the *constructivist* view, which emphasizes the values of the stakeholders and builds consensus about what needs to be changed. Although faculty, in their role as evaluators, use a combination of these perspectives, one is likely dominant, and faculty should be aware of the perspective they bring to the evaluation process because their philosophical orientation toward evaluation will guide the evaluation process and influence outcomes. More importantly, results should be used by faculty for program improvement and ultimately to facilitate the academic success of students.

THE EVALUATION PROCESS

Evaluation is a systematic process that involves a series of actions (see Box 22.1).

The steps can be modified depending on the purpose of the evaluation, what is being evaluated (e.g., students, instruction, program, or system), and the complexity of the elements being evaluated.

Identifying the Purpose of the Evaluation

The first step in the evaluation process is to identify the purpose of the evaluation. What

---

> **BOX 22.1   Steps to the Evaluation Process**
>
> - Identifying the purpose of the evaluation
> - Determining when to evaluate
> - Selecting the evaluator
> - Choosing an evaluation framework or model
> - Selecting an evaluation instrument
> - Collecting data
> - Interpreting data
> - Reporting the findings
> - Using the findings
> - Considering the costs of evaluation

> **BOX 22.2   Purposes of Evaluation**
>
> - Facilitate learning—or change behavior of an employee or student
> - Diagnose problems—identify learning deficits, ineffective teaching practices, curriculum deficits, resource inadequacies, etc.
> - Make decisions—assign grades, determine performance raises, offer promotion or tenure, allocate resources, revise policies
> - Improve products—revise curriculum, add/delete course content, modify teaching strategies, improve student support resources
> - Judge effectiveness—determine whether program goals, outcomes, or benchmarks are being met
> - Appraise cost effectiveness—determine whether a program, instructional strategies, faculty/student support services, etc., are sustainable

questions about the element under review do the faculty want to have answered? What information do faculty need to make informed decisions about the program and its stakeholders? These questions may be broad and encompassing, as in program evaluation, or focused and specific, as in the classroom assessment or performance evaluation of students. See Box 22.2 for the purposes of evaluation. Regardless of the scope of the evaluation, the purpose or reason for conducting an evaluation should be clear to all involved in the process. Case Study 22.1 addresses the importance of identifying evaluation purpose and related questions when developing an evaluation plan.

A nursing program has been experiencing declin-
ing NCLEX-RN pass rates for the past 2 years, with
scores falling below the national average. If the trend
is not reversed within the next year, the state board
of nursing has indicated that the program will face the
potential of being placed on probation. The board of
nursing has requested that the program submit an
evaluation plan for improving the NCLEX pass rates.
The faculty are unsure of how to start the process of
developing and implementing an evaluation plan.

1. How can the evaluation process be used to support
   the program in addressing this challenge?
2. What would be the identified purpose of the evaluation plan? What questions might faculty want to
   seek answers to as they consider how to develop
   the evaluation plan?

Determining When to Evaluate

The evaluator must also weigh each evaluation
activity and determine when it is most appropriate to conduct the evaluation. Typically, the use of
both formative and summative evaluation methods can provide informative data and lend respective strengths to the evaluation plan.

In determining when to evaluate, the evaluator
must also consider the frequency of evaluation.
Evaluation can be time consuming, but frequent
evaluation can be beneficial and necessary in many
situations. For example, frequent evaluations are
important when the learning process is complex
and unfamiliar to the learners or when the risk
of failure is high and it is helpful to anticipate
potential problems to minimize failure. Finally,
important decisions require frequent evaluations.
Box 22.3 identifies additional situations in which
it may be helpful to conduct frequent evaluations.

Selecting the Evaluator

The evaluator is an important element in the evaluation process. Selecting an evaluator involves
deciding who should be involved in the evaluation
process and whether the evaluator chosen should
be internal or external to the program, or a combination of both (external evaluator). The advantages and disadvantages of using internal and
external evaluators are discussed below.

- Complex learning scenarios
- Desire to detect emerging trends
- Problems are anticipated
- Problems are identified
- High risk of failure for the individual or program
  exists
- Poor outcome could lead to serious consequences
- Major program changes have recently been
  implemented

Internal Evaluators

Internal evaluators are those directly involved
with the learning, course, or program element to
be evaluated, such as the students, faculty, administrators, or staff. Many stakeholders may have a
vested interest in the outcomes of the evaluation
process and can be selected to participate. There
are advantages and disadvantages associated with
internal evaluators, and often several evaluators
are helpful to obtain the most accurate and objective data.

Advantages of using internal evaluators include
their familiarity with the institution and program,
the context and purpose of the evaluation activity and the standards (benchmarks) being evaluated, cost-effectiveness, and the potential for less
disruptive evaluation. Additionally, the findings
of evaluation can be acted upon more quickly
and disseminated for prompt faculty review and
consideration.

Disadvantages of using internal evaluators
include the potential for bias, control of evaluation,
and reluctance to share controversial findings.
When internal evaluators are chosen and used, it
is important to note their position in the organization and responsibility and reporting lines to avoid
potential conflicts of interest.

External Evaluators

External evaluators are those not directly involved
in the events being evaluated. They are often
employed as consultants. State regulatory agencies
(boards of nursing) and national accrediting bodies are other examples of external evaluators. The
advantage of external evaluators is that they are
less likely to demonstrate bias, are not involved in

> **BOX 22.4   Questions to Ask When Selecting an Evaluator**
>
> - What is the evaluator's philosophy regarding evaluation? What is the evaluator's experience with evaluating the elements under review?
> - What methods or instruments does the evaluator use? Have experience with?
> - Is the evaluator responsive to the client's needs?
> - Does the evaluator communicate well with others?
> - Does the evaluator provide feedback to stakeholders using constructive, supportive strategies?

organizational politics, may have expertise in the element being evaluated or a particular type of evaluation, and do not have a stake in the results. Disadvantages of using external evaluators include expense, unfamiliarity with the institution and program context, and potential time and travel constraints. Because evaluators are so critical to the evaluation process, faculty should select evaluators carefully. Box 22.4 identifies questions to ask when selecting an evaluator.

Choosing an Evaluation Framework or Model

The use of an evaluation framework or model can help ensure that a comprehensive evaluation process is designed and implemented. An evaluation model represents the ways by which the variables, items, or events to be evaluated are arranged, observed, or manipulated to answer the evaluation question. A model serves to clarify the relationship of the variables to be evaluated and provides a systematic plan or framework for the evaluation.

Using an evaluation model has several advantages. A model makes variables explicit and often reflects a priority about which variables should be evaluated first or most often. A model also provides structure that is visible to all concerned; the relationships of parts are evident. Using an evaluation model helps focus the evaluation activity and keep the evaluation efforts on target to address the necessary elements. Finally, a model can be tested and validated.

Evaluation models for nursing education may be found in education, nursing, or business literature or may be developed by nurse educators for a specific use. An evaluation model should be selected according to the demands of the evaluation question, the context, and the needs of the stakeholders. Commonly used evaluation models in nursing education are noted here; specific applications of evaluation models in systematic program evaluation can be found in Chapter 26.

Program evaluation and *accreditation models* often have been adopted from higher education. Common models include Chen's theory-driven model, which directs the variables to be measured (Chen, 2004); Stufflebeam's (1971) model, which organizes the variable to be evaluated as context, input, process, and product; and naturalistic models such as those proposed by Lincoln and Guba (1985), which involve the participation of stakeholders in determining consensus about what needs to be changed (see Chapter 26).

Adoptions of innovations and *change models* focus on the extent to which learning or use of a teaching–learning strategy has been integrated into practice. These models can be used to guide change and to evaluate process and outcome. Kirkpatrick and Kirkpatrick's (2014) model evaluates four levels of change: reaction, learning, behavior, and results. The first two levels (reaction and learning) indicate time and resources devoted to teaching and learning, and levels three and four (behavior and results) reveal the lasting educational outcomes. See Chapter 11 for the application of the model to interprofessional education. Rogers' (2003) model of adoption of innovations provides a framework for understanding how innovations are diffused through an organization. Adoption of an innovation, such as a new curriculum or new teaching strategy, depends on the nature of the innovation, the communications within the organization, the time span, and the social system. Rogers (2003) notes that not all persons involved in the adoption of a change do so at the same time and offers a continuum to indicate that there will be a range of adopters, from those who are early adopters to those who are later adopters, described as laggards.

Quality assurance or *total quality improvement models* are also used in nursing education. One example is the use of Quality Matters (2022) to evaluate online courses (see Chapter 21). This group has developed benchmarks for online courses with rubrics used to assess standards for the design of online courses. Courses are reviewed by trained reviewers.

Selecting an Evaluation Instrument

After an evaluation model has been selected, and the variables to be evaluated and their relationship to each other have been identified, the evaluator then selects evaluation instruments that can be used most easily to obtain the relevant data. Data collected may be quantitative or qualitative. The selection of evaluation instruments is determined by the evaluation question and the evaluation model.

Types of Instruments

Many instruments are available for measurement and can be found by doing a literature review. To use a published instrument, faculty must contact the publisher and obtain permission.

Questionnaire. A *questionnaire* is a type of instrument in which the respondent provides written answers to questions using a provided form. The questionnaire is usually self-administered. Questionnaires are cost effective and can provide anonymity to the respondent but may lack substance. Questions must be clear, concise, and simple and lack bias (Polit & Beck, 2021). This type of instrument is often used to measure qualitative variables, such as feelings and attitudes. Questionnaires can also be used to measure stakeholders' level of satisfaction with the nursing program's effectiveness, such as students, alumni, employers, and clinical practice partners.

Interview. An *interview* involves direct contact with individuals participating in the evaluation and can be conducted with an individual or in focus groups. Exit interviews, for example, are often conducted as a faculty member leaves the school of nursing or as students graduate. Interviews can be used to elicit both qualitative and quantitative data. Faculty, students, or external evaluators may be assigned to collect the data. The interview should be scheduled at a time that is convenient for both the interviewer and the participant. It is important that the interviewers have no perceived or actual conflict of interest with the variables and participants being evaluated. It

is also important that both the interviewer and the participant understand the purpose and focus of the interview, and how any findings will be used and disseminated by the program.

The interviewer should provide a quiet, private environment within which to conduct the interview. A participant may respond more openly if he or she feels that the conversation will be private and confidential. The participants should be made aware of the anonymity and confidentiality of the interview responses. If the interview is being recorded or if the information is going to be directly associated with the identity of a specific participant, written permission should be obtained before beginning the interview (Adams, 2015; Stufflebeam & Coryn, 2014). An objective outline should be created and followed during the interview, and notes should be kept in a file. Great care must be taken to avoid personalizing the information. One negative aspect of interviews is that they can be time intensive; it is recommended that they be conducted in less than 50 minutes (Stufflebeam & Coryn, 2014). Additional guidelines for conducting successful interviews are to avoid using jargon and keep questions relatively short, establish rapport with the participants before engaging in more substantive questioning, remain neutral and nonjudgmental, and approach positive questions first before seeking information on areas for improvement or other more negatively toned questions (Adams, 2015).

Rating Scale. A *rating scale* is used to measure an abstract concept on a descriptive continuum. The rating scale is designed to increase objectivity in the evaluation process. Rating scales work well with norm-referenced evaluation, although they are not the best tools to use for this type of evaluation. Grades can easily be assigned to the ratings.

Checklist. A *checklist* is two-dimensional in that the expected behavior or competence is listed on one side and the degree to which this behavior meets the level of expectation is listed on the other side. With a detailed checklist of items and well-defined criteria being measured, the evaluator can easily identify expected behaviors or acceptable competence. This type of instrument is useful for formative and summative evaluations. A checklist can be used to evaluate a student's performance of clinical procedures. The steps to be followed can be placed in sequential order and the observer can then check off each action that is taken or not taken.

Attitude Scale. An *attitude or social psychological scale* measures the respondent's perceptions or opinions about a subject at the time he or she answers the question. Such scales create a numerical score continuum upon which the respondent's feelings can be measured (Polit & Beck, 2021), thus gathering quantitative data about individuals' varying degrees of perceptions or attitudes on a given topic.

Several types of attitude scales are commonly used in nursing education evaluation. The most popular is the Likert scale, typically in the form of a 5- to 7-point scale. In a Likert scale, statements are used to express an opinion on a particular issue. Each statement represents a construct of the issue being measured. Participants are asked to indicate the degree to which they agree or disagree with the statement. Equal numbers of positively and negatively worded items should be used to prevent bias in the responses.

Semantic differential is another type of scale used to measure attitude. An example of a semantic differential scale is a *bipolar scale*, which is used to measure the reaction of the participant. Each item on the scale is followed by bipolar adjectives such as good–bad, active–passive, or positive–negative. The number of intervals between each adjective is usually odd, so the middle interval is neutral. A list of five to seven intervals is adequate. Analysis is performed by adding values for each item, which is similar to what is done with the Likert scale. The reader is referred to statistical textbooks for further discussion on the most appropriate means by which to analyze Likert scale data.

Portfolios. A portfolio is used to provide evidence of the achievement of program learning outcomes through the collection of artifacts documenting the student's learning throughout the program. An artifact is the outcome of a learning experience and may take the form of a written assignment, PowerPoint presentation, concept map, care plan, and so on. A guide for collection of artifacts is provided to students at the start of their program to facilitate successful portfolio documentation. Portfolios are stored either electronically or in an organized paper version. Often reflections are added to each artifact to show how the artifact met program learning outcomes. Reflections enhance student learning and ensure progress toward meeting program learning outcomes.

Reliability and Validity of Evaluation Instruments Used in Nursing Education

When any instrument is used, its validity and reliability for evaluation needs to be determined. Special procedures can be used to determine reliability and validity of instruments used for clinical evaluation, program evaluation, and examinations given to measure classroom achievement. Determining the reliability and validity of specific evaluation strategies is discussed in appropriate chapters of this book. A general overview of the concepts of validity and reliability is provided here.

Validity. The validity of an instrument can be defined as the extent to which the instrument measures what it is intended to measure (Polit & Beck, 2021) and that faculty are in fact collecting and analyzing the results they intend to measure. An instrument must be valid for faculty to make appropriate interpretations of the findings (McDonald, 2018). Measurement validity, particularly in the area of educational assessment and evaluation, has attributes of relevance, accuracy, and utility. *Relevance* of an instrument is achieved when the instrument measures the educational objective as directly as possible. The instrument is *accurate* if it is measuring the educational objective precisely. The instrument has *utility* if it provides formative and summative results that have implications for evaluation and improvement. As a result, valid evaluation instruments have relevance for the program and can provide meaningful results to support faculty decision making as they consider making program changes.

Although there are several types of validity, measurement validity is viewed as a single concept. Content-related evidence, criterion-related evidence, and construct-related evidence are considered to be categories of validity (McDonald, 2018). For the most accurate interpretation of data, evidence from all validity categories is ideal, as it raises the degree of support for validity. The validity of an instrument can best be determined when faculty understand the nature of the content and specifications in the evaluation design, the relationship of the instrument to the significant criterion, and the constructs or psychological characteristics being measured by the instrument.

Content-related evidence refers to the extent to which the instrument is representative of the construct (subject matter or behavior) being evaluated. Content-related evidence is particularly important to establish for the evaluation of student learning using clinical evaluation instruments and classroom tests. For example, with classroom tests, the following question is raised: "Does the sample of test questions represent the content taught in the course?" In clinical evaluation, the question posed is: "Does the clinical evaluation instrument measure attitudes, behaviors, and skills drawn from the domain of being a nurse and represent the student performance outcomes expected at this level of the program?"

Criterion-related evidence is used to relate the outcomes of one instrument to the outcomes of another. In this sense, it is used to predict success or establish the predictability of one measure with another one, either concurrently or in the future. Criterion-related evidence is established by using correlation measures. There are two means by which to establish criterion-related evidence: concurrent validity and predictive validity. *Concurrent validity evidence* is the correlation of one score with another measure that occurs at the same time. One common example of concurrent validity is the correlation of clinical course grades with didactic course grades. Concurrent validity of the instrument is said to occur, for example, when there is a high correlation between clinical evaluation and examination scores in a class of students. *Predictive validity evidence*, on the other hand, is a correlation of one score or measure that predicts future measures obtained after completion of the event or intervention, such as a test, course, or lesson (Polit & Beck, 2021). For example, there may be predictive validity between students' program admission tests and future academic performance in the program. Another

example of predictive validity is the correlation between grade point average and scores on licensing or credentialing examinations. When there is a high positive correlation between the grade point average and the examination score, there is said to be criterion-related evidence.

Construct-related evidence is defined as determining that the measure being used is really measuring what is intended to be measured and not some other unrelated variable. Construct-related evidence is used to infer the relationship of a test instrument to the variable that is being measured but cannot be directly observed (Polit & Beck, 2021). For example, how well does an instrument actually measure (operationalize) the theoretical construct of the clinical reasoning of students or is it measuring some other unrelated concept?

Reliability. Reliability is the extent to which an instrument (self-report examination, observation schedule, or checklist) is dependable, precise, predictable, and consistent. Reliability is the degree to which test scores are free from errors of measurement. Reliability refers to the consistency by which the instrument yields similar results upon repeated administrations. Reliability answers the question: "Will the same instrument yield the same results with different groups of students or when used by different raters?"

Several types of reliability—stability reliability, equivalence reliability, and internal consistency reliability—are relevant to evaluation instruments and achievement examinations. *Stability reliability* of an instrument is the perceived consistency of the instrument over time. An assumption of stability in results is assumed. *Equivalence reliability* entails the degree to which two different forms of an instrument can be used to obtain the same results. For example, when two forms of a test are used, both tests should have the same number of items and the same level of difficulty. The test is given to the group at the same time as the equivalent test is given or the equivalent test is administered at a later date. *Internal consistency reliability* is associated with the extent to which all items on an instrument measure the same variable and with the homogeneity of the items. This reliability is considered only when the instrument is being used to measure a single concept or construct at a time. Because the validity of findings is threatened when an instrument is unreliable, faculty should use measures to ensure instrument reliability.

Collecting Data

The next step of the evaluation process is use of the evaluation instrument to gather data. Although the instrument will determine to some extent what data are collected and how, several other factors should be considered at this time. These include the data collector, the data sources, amount of data, timing of data collection, and informal versus formal data collection.

Data Collector

Consideration must be given to who is collecting the data. For example, the evaluator who gathers the data might be the faculty responsible for evaluating the clinical performance of the students. In other situations, students or research assistants may administer instruments. Data collectors should be oriented to the task and the data-collecting procedures being used. Interrater reliability must be ensured when more than one person is collecting data.

Data Source

When designing the evaluation activity, the evaluator must identify sources from which the data will be collected. Will the data be observed (as in clinical evaluation), archived (as when grade point average is obtained from student records), or reported (as obtained from a longitudinal questionnaire of graduates)? If records were in need to be accessed to collect data, it is important to verify that permission will be granted to access the records.

Amount of Data

The amount of data to be collected must also be determined and specified. All data may be collected or a sample may be sufficient, but a decision must be made. For example, in clinical evaluation or classroom testing it is impossible to collect data about each instance of clinical performance or knowledge gained from the classroom experience. In this instance a sampling procedure is used and guided by the clinical evaluation protocol, blueprint, or plan for the classroom test. It

is important to note that if a sampling plan is to be used, the criteria for the data to be sampled must be clearly established at this stage of the evaluation process, to ensure consistency in the data collection process.

Timing of Data Collection

When is the best time to collect the data? An understanding of the context of the evaluation is essential. Should the data be collected at the beginning, middle, or end of the activity being evaluated? When gathering data from students, it is important to allow adequate time and to gather data when students are able to give unbiased responses. For example, course evaluation data collected immediately after test results have been given may not yield the most reflective responses.

Formal Versus Informal Data Collection

Decisions about use of formal and informal data must also be made. Data can be obtained in a formal manner, such as by using a structured evaluation tool. Data can also be collected through the use of informal methods, such as in the form of spontaneous comments made by program stakeholders. Although informal data collection methods can yield informative data, disadvantages to relying on informal methods are that it is unsystematic, can lead to inadequate or biased data, and ultimately lacks validity (Stufflebeam & Coryn, 2014). The evaluator must decide whether both formal and informal data will be used in the plan.

Interpreting Data

The interpretation step of the evaluation process involves translating data to answer the evaluation questions established at the beginning of the process. This includes putting the data in usable form, organizing the data for analysis, and interpreting the data against preestablished criteria. When interpreting the data, the context, frame of reference, objectivity, and legal and ethical issues must also be considered.

Frame of Reference

Frame of reference refers to the reference point used for interpretation of data. In nursing education, the frame of reference is particularly important to consider when evaluating such program elements as the effectiveness of academic policies and aggregate and individual student performance. Two frames of reference are discussed here: norm-referenced interpretation and criterion-referenced interpretation.

Norm-Referenced Interpretation. *Norm-referenced interpretation* refers to interpreting data in terms of the norms of the group of individuals being evaluated. The scores of the group form a basis for comparing each individual with the others. In norm-referenced evaluation, there will always be an individual who has achieved at the highest level and one who has achieved at the lowest level.

Norm-referenced interpretation permits evaluators to compare achievement of students in several ways. Students in the same group can be compared and ranked. Students can be compared with students in another group or class section or with national group norms, as in the case of licensing examinations or nursing specialty certification examinations. Consequently, an *advantage* of norm-referenced interpretation is the ability to make comparisons within groups or with external groups and to use the data for predictive purposes, such as admission criteria. A *disadvantage* of norm-referenced interpretation is the focus on comparison, which may foster a sense of competitiveness among students.

Criterion-Referenced Interpretation. In *criterion-referenced interpretation* results are judged against preestablished criteria and reflect the degree of criteria attainment. Criterion-referenced interpretation is typically used in competency-based learning models in which the goal is to assist the learner to achieve competence in or mastery of specified learning outcomes. Because students are evaluated on the basis of their achievement of the outcomes and not compared with each other, all students can achieve competence.

The *advantages* of criterion-referenced interpretation include the following: emphasis on mastery and the potential for all learners to achieve competence, increased learner motivation, sharing and collaboration among students, and ability to give clear progress reports to learners. *Disadvantages*

of criterion-referenced interpretation include the inability to compare students with each other or with other groups.

Issues of Objectivity and Subjectivity

The issues of objectivity and subjectivity in evaluation always arise when data are interpreted. Different evaluators can look at the same data yet render different interpretations (judgments). The differences may be a result of evaluator bias or degrees of difference in objectivity. In some ways, faculty need to accept that there is a certain amount of subjectivity in evaluation; after all, this is "evaluation" and not "measurement." However, faculty should recognize subjectivity and the role it may play in interpretation of findings.

Legal and Ethical Considerations

There may be legal aspects involved in the interpretation of findings. Legal consideration is particularly important in the area of student rights. How and to whom will the results of evaluations be shared? What data about students can be collected? Does the evaluation process and the nature of the data being collected require the protection of human subjects? Who is affected by the evaluations? Will there be moral or ethical dilemmas in reporting the data? How will they respond to the results? What effect will evaluation have on a student or faculty, a program, or a curriculum? Data should only be collected if it is meaningfully aligned with the purpose and context of the evaluation activity. See Chapter 3 for additional discussion of legal and ethical aspects of evaluating students' academic and clinical performance. Case Study 22.2 addresses a faculty's concern with participating in the evaluation process due to concerns with how the data will be used.

Reporting the Findings

In this step of the evaluation process, the results of evaluation are communicated to appropriate stakeholders. Factors to consider when findings are reported include who will receive the findings and when and how to report the findings.

CASE STUDY 22.2 Improving Evaluation Processes

A nursing program has just completed an accreditation evaluation visit in which the program was cited for lacking a systematic evaluation plan. The accrediting body noted that data was sporadically collected and frequently not analyzed and findings were not used to guide program decision making. The nursing faculty have historically been reluctant to participate in evaluation efforts, citing faculty workload and concerns that data will be used to change how they teach their courses and negatively impact their performance reviews. The accrediting body has given the program 12 months to address the ineffective evaluation process currently in place within the program.

1. What steps can be taken by the program to develop a culture of continuous quality improvement in which faculty participate in the evaluation process and use data to inform their decision-making?
2. What strategies can be implemented to increase faculty comfort with participating in the evaluation process?

Who Receives the Findings?

The evaluator must know to whom the data should be reported and be transparent about the reporting process. Typically, both the persons and group being evaluated and those requesting the evaluation receive the evaluation reports. Issues of reporting and confidentiality should be established at the outset of evaluation. Confidentiality of the report must be maintained. Only those persons designated to receive the report should do so. The evaluator should destroy any unneeded background information after the report is completed.

In reporting findings, it is also important to consider the recipient of the report. What will the recipient want and need to know? For example, students receiving a test grade are usually prepared only to understand the grade, not the complex methods that were used to determine the grade or the item analysis statistics. If the report is focused on a curriculum review that indicates changes may be needed in how the curriculum is implemented, how is this likely to affect the faculty who teach in

the curriculum? Preparing the recipient(s) for the evaluation report may also be helpful if the recipient does not have adequate background information to receive and understand the context of the report.

When to Report Findings

The timing of the report is also crucial. There tends to be a readiness to know the results of evaluation, and if the report of results is delayed, the recipients may lose interest. For example, students prefer having immediate results and can have increased anxiety or lose interest if results are delayed. The timing of the report may also be based on when information is needed, for example, at the end of the semester when grades are to be reported to the registrar.

How to Report Findings

Evaluation reports can take many forms. They may be written or oral, formal, or informal. An example of an informal evaluation is talking with the student about his or her performance in a clinical experience, without a structured evaluation. This type of evaluation is far from ideal and may leave the student and the instructor without objective criteria and a sense of fairness. In the event that the student should fail the course, the instructor is not able to defend the decision without formal documentation of the evaluation.

In a formal report, statistical analysis of the data will be accessible along with a discussion of the findings. Specific methods of reporting findings related to student performance and program evaluation to students, faculty, administrators, and external audiences are discussed in subsequent chapters.

Using the Findings

Evaluation is a mutual effort between the evaluator and the individual, group, or program being evaluated. Although using the findings is the last, and often forgotten, step of the evaluation process, all parties have a responsibility to review and use the findings to inform future decision making about sustaining and improving the program's effectiveness.

To use the evaluation findings effectively requires purposeful, strategic planning. Four perspective strategies are purpose, people, planning, and presentation. The *purpose* of the evaluation must be understood by all stakeholders. For evaluation findings to be successfully used, the *people* involved in the evaluation should be included in the process. The main strategy in promoting evaluation is *planning* the activities and disseminating the evaluation information. Considering the preparation and *presentation* of the evaluation report to the stakeholders (those who will use and be affected by the report) is a priority. The report should be in a format that is easily understood, and graphs and other visual aids should be used as needed.

Evaluation results can be used in a variety of ways. Common uses in nursing programs are to measure student learning outcomes and assign grades; revise teaching/learning strategies, courses, and curricula; revise program policies or student support services; and demonstrate program effectiveness in achieving desired outcomes.

Several ways to improve the use of the evaluation process are as follows:

1. Involve those potentially affected by the results in designing the evaluation plan.
2. Engage all stakeholders in the evaluation process.
3. Report findings in a timely manner.
4. Make realistic recommendations that can be used to support the program's continuous quality improvement efforts.
5. Develop a plan for how to share and disseminate the evaluation findings with the appropriate individuals.
6. Encourage the recipient(s) to consider ways in which to change behavior as appropriate in response to evaluation findings.
7. Establish trust and share sensitive findings in a constructive manner, being careful to avoid fault finding.
8. Place findings in context. Encourage the recipients to consider what the findings mean and how they can be used in their own setting.

Considering the Costs of Evaluation

The evaluation process requires the nursing program to have the fiscal and human resources required to implement the plan successfully and to also address any concerns the findings may reveal with program effectiveness. Program administrators and faculty need to carefully consider the costs associated with the chosen evaluation strategies and ensure that adequate resources are available. Addressing the following questions can help identify the potential costs associated with any proposed evaluation plan:

- What fiscal or human resources (e.g., fees, evaluation materials, faculty and staff time) are associated with the proposed evaluation plan?
- How much faculty and/or staff time will be required to develop and administer tools, analyze and interpret data, and report results to stakeholders? Will implementation of the evaluation process require any dedicated personnel positions to manage the process?
- How much time will be required of those being evaluated to complete survey tools or be interviewed? Will the time commitment be a potential constraint to participation in the process?
- If the results of the evaluation process indicate changes in curriculum, policies, or procedures are desirable, will the program have the resources to respond with the needed changes?
- How will the organizational culture be nurtured to encourage faculty, staff, and students to engage in ongoing continuous quality improvement efforts and be active participants in any evaluation efforts?
- If evaluation feedback indicates that stakeholder needs are not being met at acceptable levels, is the program prepared to allocate resources to address the issues?
- When the evaluation of individual student performance indicates that students are not meeting expected learning outcomes, what resources can the program make available to support student success?

BOX 22.5   Internet-Based Resources Related to Evaluation

- Society for College and University Planning—http://www.scup.org/.
- Integrated Postsecondary Education Data System (IPEDS)—http://nces.ed.gov/ipeds/
- The National Center for Education Statistics (NCES), US Department of Education, is the primary federal entity for collecting and analyzing education-related data—http://nces.ed.gov/
- The National Postsecondary Education Cooperative promotes the use of quality postsecondary data at the federal, state, and institution levels to support policy development—http://nces.ed.gov/NPEC/
- The Education Resources Information Center (ERIC), sponsored by the US Institute of Education Sciences within the US Department of Education—http://eric.ed.gov/
- Council for Higher Education Accreditation—http://www.chea.org
- *PROGRAM-Based Review and Assessment: Tools and Techniques for Program Improvement.* http://www.umass.edu/oapa/sites/default/files/pdf/handbooks/program_assessment_handbook.pdf
- Basic Guide to Program Evaluation—https://managementhelp.org/evaluation/program-evaluation-guide.htm

---

CHAPTER SUMMARY: KEY POINTS

- Evaluation is a means of appraising data or placing a value on data gathered through one or more measurements.
- The evaluation process is used to determine nursing program effectiveness in meeting expected program outcomes, including but not limited to those related to student learning outcomes, curriculum, teaching/learning strategies, faculty outcomes, and resources.
- Faculty are responsible for participating in the evaluation process and using the findings to guide program decision making.
- Evaluation of expected program outcomes is an ongoing systematic process best accomplished within a culture of continuous quality improvement.
- The evaluation process involves a systematic series of actions starting with establishing a clear purpose for the evaluation and encouraging the participation of affected stakeholders.
- Evaluation models or frameworks can be used to guide the process, choice of instruments, data collection methods, and reporting procedures.
- Evaluation findings should be disseminated to affected stakeholders and addressed with transparency in a constructive, supportive manner.
- Faculty should be prepared to address any issues or concerns identified through the evaluation process with a goal of sustaining or increasing the effectiveness of the nursing program in the preparation of qualified graduates.
- See Box 22.5 for websites that are useful resources for additional information on the evaluation process.

REFLECTING ON THE EVIDENCE

1. What philosophical beliefs do you have about the evaluation process, especially as applied to evaluating student learning outcomes? Consider the teaching-learning strategies that you currently use in the classes you teach. How are those teaching-learning strategies influenced by your philosophical beliefs about evaluation?
2. Think about the organizational culture present in your nursing program. To what extent can you identify a commitment to continuous quality improvement (CQI) as applied to the evaluation of your program's identified outcomes? What could be done by the program's administration and faculty to further strengthen this commitment to CQI?
3. In your faculty role, in what ways do you contribute to the evaluation process used to measure the effectiveness of the nursing program in achieving expected program outcomes?

REFERENCES

Adams, W. C. (2015). Conducting semi-structured interviews. In K. E. Newcomer, H. P. Hatry, & J. S. Wholey (Eds.), *Handbook of practical program evaluation* (4th ed., pp. 492–505). Jossey-Bass.

Chen, H. T. (2004). A theory-driven evaluation perspective on mixed methods research. *Research in the Schools*, 13(1), 75–83.

Kirkpatrick, J. D., & Kirkpatrick, D. L. (2014). *The Kirkpatrick Four Levels: A fresh look after 55 years—1959–2014.* Kirkpatrick Partners. https://www.kirkpatrickpartners.com/Our-Philosophy/The-Kirkpatrick-Model.

Lincoln, Y. S., & Guba, E. G. (1985). *Naturalistic inquiry.* Sage.

McDonald, M. E. (2018). *The nurse educator's guide to assessing learning outcomes.* Jones & Bartlett Learning

National League for Nursing. (2019). *The Scope of Practice for Academic Nurse Educators and Academic Clinical Nurse Educators* (3rd ed.). Author.

Polit, D. F., & Beck, C. T. (2021). *Essentials of nursing research: Appraising evidence for nursing practice.* Lippincott Williams & Wilkins.

Quality Matters. (2022). *Why quality matters.* Retrieved from https://www.qualitymatters.org/why-quality-matters/process.

Rogers, E. M. (2003). *Diffusion of innovations* (5th ed.). Free Press.

Stufflebeam, D. L. (Ed.). (1971). *Educational evaluation and decision-making.* Peacock.

Stufflebeam, D. L., & Coryn, C. (2014). *Evaluation theory, models, & applications.* Jossey-Bass.

23

Strategies for Evaluating Learning Outcomes

Jane M. Kirkpatrick, PhD, RN, ANEF and Diann DeWitt, PhD, RN, CNE

The purpose of this chapter is to explore a variety of strategies that faculty can employ to assess and evaluate student learning outcomes. Uses, advantages, disadvantages, and issues related to each strategy are discussed. Included are ways to select strategies, improve their validity and reliability, and increase the effectiveness of their use.

Never has there been a greater challenge to the evaluation process. Priorities for nursing education are continually informed by national trends. New essentials for nursing education from The American Association of Colleges of Nursing (2021) and the National League for Nursing (2012) have embraced the work of the Institute of Medicine's (2011) *Future of Nursing* report. The Campaign for Action (2021) and the call from the National Academy of Medicine's (2021) report, *The Future of Nursing 2020–2030: Charting a Path to Achieve Health Equity*, are bringing additional influences to nursing curricula. The 2016 Interprofessional Education Collaborative (IPEC) core competencies are currently under review with an expected new publication date of 2023. The National Council of State Boards of Nursing has a next-generation licensing exam scheduled for release in 2023 that emphasizes clinical judgment competency via case studies (National Council of State Boards of Nursing, 2021; Sturdivant & Allen-Thomas, 2022). These curricular influences bring strong emphasis on outcomes such as leadership, diversity, social determinants of health, and the impact of policy on health and healthcare. Many competencies have elements of the affective domain. As educators work to develop deep learning and reflective practice skills in students, they continue to explore ways that the student learning outcomes can be evaluated (Masuku et al., 2021). Multiple measures are especially important when evaluating complex competencies such as those that require higher-order thinking (Oermann et al., 2022; Ying, 2020). Acknowledging that lifelong learning is essential in the nursing profession requires engaging learners in the evaluation process to enhance their self-assessment skills (Cardwell, 2020). Involving students in the evaluation process can help them develop their character in such a way to create a socially responsible professional (Masuku et al., 2021).

ASSESSMENT AND EVALUATION

Just what is the difference between assessment and evaluation? In many instances, it seems that these two terms are interchangeable, but there are distinct differences. *Assessment* involves obtaining information about teaching and learning for the purpose of improvement. The information collected may be quantitative and/or qualitative. The process of assessment requires faculty to first make clear the expectations and quality of performance expected—think student learning outcomes. From there, decisions are made on the strategies to best assess the learning outcomes, followed by the collection, analysis, and interpretation of student work. Information gained from assessment provides evidence about current learning and then is used to promote further learning (Oermann & Gaberson, 2021; Oermann et al., 2022). Normally, assessment is conducted while learning, or the course or program is ongoing, and changes and improvements can be made.

Evaluation, on the other hand, refers to making judgments as to whether the student has achieved the specified learning outcome (Oermann & Gaberson, 2021; Oermann et al., 2022). This usually occurs at the end of learning, courses, or programs. Evaluation can be formative or summative. *Formative evaluation* occurs while learning is taking place; opportunity for feedback and improvement is implicit. *Summative evaluation* is more holistic and considers all the aspects that have led to attaining outcomes. Summative evaluation marks the end of the particular teaching–learning process and leads to a judgment, often expressed as a grade. In clinical disciplines, faculty must evaluate student attainment of course outcomes and defined program competencies to ensure that graduates are prepared for safe practice.

SELECTING EVALUATION STRATEGIES

The strategies discussed in this chapter provide faculty with a variety of techniques to use to assess and evaluate student learning outcomes. Several of the strategies discussed may also be familiar as teaching strategies. The idea of adapting a teaching strategy for use in evaluation allows students to practice and receive formative evaluation in the same process by which they ultimately will experience summative evaluation. Although most strategies can be used for both formative and summative evaluation, some strategies are better suited to a formative experience, whereas others are clearly more effective in determining final outcomes of learning and assigning grades.

The major reason for faculty to consider a variety of strategies is to better evaluate (1) all the domains of learning (including the affective domain), (2) higher levels of the cognitive domain (e.g., analysis, synthesis, creation), (3) critical thinking and clinical reasoning, and (4) students' preparation for licensing or certification examinations. By providing a more authentic evaluation wherein the student is asked to perform or demonstrate the learning in a way that is closely related to the ultimate performance required in the real world, the faculty will gain richer and deeper evidence of student achievement (Jeffries, 2021; Killam & Camargo-Plazas, 2021).

In selecting evaluation strategies, the philosophy of the faculty regarding accountability and responsibility for learning and desired program outcomes should be considered. If a program goal is to create a graduate who is a self-directed, lifelong learner, then the strategies for teaching and learning should enhance this skill development. Many of the strategies discussed in this chapter are compatible with active learning techniques. For example, critical reflections, short essays, and guided writing assignments encourage students to interact with the material in a different way than if they were learning the material for a multiple-choice test.

Evaluation strategies are not without challenges. Major challenges include (1) the time it takes to use the strategy for both the students and the faculty and (2) difficulty in establishing validity and reliability of data-gathering instruments and methods. To avoid some of the pitfalls associated with these strategies, and to gain the greatest reward from evaluation efforts, faculty should:
1. Clearly delineate the *purpose* of the evaluation.
2. Consider the *setting* in which the learning and evaluation will take place.
3. Choose the best evaluation *strategy* for the purpose.
4. Determine the *procedure* for the strategy selected.
5. Establish the *validity* and *reliability* of the strategy.
6. Assess the overall *effectiveness* of the process.

Purpose

The purpose of evaluation is to ascertain that students have achieved their potential and have acquired the knowledge, skills, and abilities set forth in learning activities, courses, and curricula. The instructional goals and course outcomes and objectives indicate the type of behavior (cognitive, affective, or psychomotor) to be assessed or evaluated. The learning experiences should be designed to have relevance to the students. The evaluation activity should carry value in the overall grading system. Finally, the grading criteria should be shared with the students before evaluation occurs.

Setting

Another critical factor to consider is the setting in which the instruction and evaluation will occur. Most faculty are comfortable with evaluation in traditional classroom settings, but with the expansion of either completely online instruction or hybrid (blended) instruction, new issues emerge for both faculty and students in these environments. (See Chapter 21 for additional discussion of best practices in distance and online learning.) Most of the strategies discussed in this chapter can be used in an online community. For example, a threaded discussion can be used for reflection, critique, or even as a forum for verbal questioning. Concept maps are available in electronic formats. Students or faculty can maintain an electronic portfolio representative of student work throughout the course or program. When considering assessment or evaluation strategies in an online environment, the faculty needs to be sure the technology is relevant for the purpose and must build in learning time for both students and faculty to become proficient in the use of the technology (Oermann et al., 2022). Bearman et al. (2020) discuss the need for universities to prepare students for the realities of a digital work world and caution that simply putting an "e" before an assessment is not an adequate approach.

The expansion of interprofessional education (IPE) creates new opportunities to collaborate with educators from other professions. Gleason et al. (2021) propose that interprofessional practice in diagnostic processes empowers nurses toward achieving safer patient outcomes. The National Center for Interprofessional Practice and Education provides a variety of resources and tools relevant to assessment and evaluation on its website: https://nexusipe.org/. Clearly identified shared competencies (IPEC, 2016) are crucial to the evaluation of IPE. As with any team-teaching effort, consistent application of criteria is essential. Evaluation strategies discussed in this chapter are appropriate for all professions.

Choice of Strategy

When choosing the best strategy for the purpose, faculty must weigh the advantages and disadvantages of each strategy. Faculty should also consider time for preparation, implementation, and grading. Other issues, such as cost, may also be determining factors. Faculty must decide how often to evaluate, who will evaluate, and how the students will be prepared for the evaluation. When selecting an evaluation strategy, it is imperative that students have ample opportunity to practice in the way in which they will be tested.

Procedures

Although procedures for using evaluation strategies vary, any procedure selected must be well planned. The strategy should be pilot tested before it is fully implemented. This process will help prevent unexpected difficulties, and it allows for refinement and quality improvements before full-scale implementation. It is also important to delineate the responsibilities associated with the methods used. For example, in the case of portfolio evaluation, a decision must be made about whether students or faculty will collect and keep the work. Another area of concern is the environment in which the evaluation will take place. Because of the anxiety and stress associated with the process of being evaluated, faculty must attempt to provide an atmosphere conducive to the process. Appropriately used humor may help place students at ease.

Validity and Reliability

The issues of validity and reliability are critical, especially when the purpose is for evaluation. In Chapter 22, the terms *validity* and *reliability* are defined and described. For the purposes of this chapter, specific examples are given to clarify the establishment of validity and reliability when non-multiple-choice evaluation methods are used.

In determining validity, faculty must ask whether the technique is appropriate to the purpose and whether it provides useful and meaningful data (Miller et al., 2013). Faculty must consider the fit of the strategy with the identified objectives. In other words, does the strategy measure what it is supposed to measure? For instance, if the objective for an assignment is for the student to demonstrate skill in written communication, evaluating student performance through oral questioning will not provide valid data. Similarly, at the nursing department level, faculty should coordinate strategies across the curriculum to evaluate achievement of nursing program outcomes such as evidence-based practice, clinical judgment, and communication. It can be a challenge to develop sound criteria for evaluation that accurately reflect the specified outcomes, objectives, and content.

To establish *face validity*, faculty must seek input from colleagues by asking questions such as, "Do these criteria appear to measure the specified objectives?" In addition, obtaining the opinion of other content experts can assist in determining whether there is adequate sampling of the content (*content validity*). These traditional approaches to establishing validity are being replaced by a unitary concept, based on several different categories of evidence (e.g., face-related evidence, content-related evidence). The evidence available to establish validity determines whether validity is considered low, medium, or high (Miller et al., 2013).

Once evaluation criteria are developed, it is essential to establish their reliability or the ability to be dependable in measuring the desired learning outcome. Frequently, evaluation criteria are placed in rubrics as a way of articulating the grading scale for assessment criteria. A commonly used method for establishing reliability of an evaluation rubric is to have two or more instructors independently rate student performance using the agreed-on criteria for sample work. Ratings are correlated to establish *interrater reliability* (IRR), which is expressed as a percentage of agreement between scores. When agreement is less than 80%, faculty should continue to refine the specificity and clarity of each criterion to come to a stronger agreement of 80% or greater (Gray & Grove, 2021). An example of using criteria to establish IRR is provided in Box 23.1.

It is especially important to establish IRR when multiple faculties are grading the same assignment. Belur and associates (2021) studied IRR for systematic reviews in crime prevention. Their exploration reported coding behavior changes both between and within individuals over time thus emphasizing the importance of testing IRR at regular intervals (Belur et al., 2021). This highlights the need for regular establishment of IRR for both teaching teams and individual faculty when using rubrics for grading.

BOX 23.1 Example of Using Criteria to Establish Interrater Reliability

Procedure:
Develop criteria and apply them to sample work.
Have two or more observers independently rate performance and then correlate.
The formula for % interrater reliability is as follows:

number of rater agreements ÷ total number of possible rater agreements

Example: Three raters evaluate written communication using the following 4 criteria:
1. Clear expression of ideas
2. Logical flow and organization
3. Correct use of syntax, grammar, American Psychological Association format
4. Incorporation of research findings

Rating:
- Item 1: Two agree and one does not
- Item 2: All three agree
- Item 3: Two agree and one does not
- Item 4: All three agree

Interraterater reliability:

10 (rater agreements) ÷ 12 (total possible agreements) = 10/12 = 0.83 or 83% (>80% is good)

Adapted from Gray, J. R., & Grove, S. K. (2021). Burns and Grove's the practice of nursing research (9th ed.). Elsevier.

A multiplicity of evaluation strategies can provide a more complete picture of student's abilities and therefore contribute to the trustworthiness of the process. It is a serious limitation to rely on a single strategy. Each strategy has limitations and issues that can influence the reliability, validity, and appropriateness of the strategy for given student populations. Using multiple strategies provides a more robust and accurate framework for making decisions.

Effectiveness

After the evaluation strategy is implemented, it is essential to determine its overall effectiveness and the potential issues that can arise related to the implementation of the strategy. Some questions faculty should ask include: Was the strategy an effective use of resources (e.g., student and faculty time and financial resources)? Were there adequate data to determine whether the learning outcome was met? Are there any problems with the implementation of the technique? What revisions are necessary? Would the faculty consider this strategy to be a good choice for future use?

MATCHING THE EVALUATION STRATEGY TO THE DOMAIN OF LEARNING

Educators must also be mindful of the domain of learning being evaluated. A full discussion of the domains of learning can be found in Chapter 10 and teaching strategies are found in Chapter 16. Cognitive learning has five categories (1) remembering, (2) understanding, (3) applying, (4) analyzing, (5) evaluating, and (6) creating (Anderson & Krathwohl, 2001). The taxonomy of the affective domain as applied to nursing has five behavioral categories: (1) receiving, (2) responding, (3) valuing, (4) organization of values, and (5) characterization by a value or value complex (Anderson & Krathwohl, 2001). The psychomotor domain is characterized by (1) imitation, (2) manipulation, (3) precision, (4) articulation, and (5) naturalization (Anderson & Krathwohl, 2001). Assessing cognitive learning is typically accomplished with quizzes and tests (see Chapter 24) along with other written assignments. The higher levels of the cognitive domain require more creativity to assess and may be integrated in a larger assignment where multiple learning outcomes are evaluated. Assessment in the psychomotor domain may be part of a skills checklist. However, use of simulations and simulated patients and ultimately clinical practice (see Chapter 19) integrates psychomotor skills with cognitive and occasionally the affective domain. For example, knowing how to perform a procedure is the psychomotor component; the why and when of performing the procedure is from the cognitive domain; and the valuing of patient preferences demonstrates the affective domain.

When evaluation strategies are used to collect data for grading purposes, it is imperative that the grading requirements be communicated to the students before they complete the assignment. Information about grading criteria is typically provided to students in the course syllabus. Other methods, such as checklists, guidelines, or grading scales, can be used as well.

Affective Domain Focus

Evaluating the affective domain is challenging, yet particularly important, in nursing. For that reason, this section expands on evaluation of this domain. Development of the affective domain is progressive and can be tied to clinical reasoning. Because of the progressive nature of development, formative evaluation across the curriculum may be most appropriate, with a summative evaluation at the time of graduation. Many of the evaluation strategies listed in this chapter can be adapted for the affective domain. For example, using the concept of cultural competency, formative and summative evaluation can be planned throughout the curriculum. At the beginning level, students may be expected to become self-aware using exploration of their own cultural and health care practices and values. A midprogram outcome could focus on student awareness of the cultural orientation of the patients under their care. At graduation, the expected outcomes (including knowledge, skills, and attitudes) would be to act in a culturally sensitive manner when providing care to all patients and demonstrate the ability to advocate for an individual patient's unique needs.

The explosion of new knowledge and the challenges of how to insert additional content into an already full curriculum may result in losing instructional time dedicated to the affective domain. Olantunji (2014) and Ondrejka (2014) suggest that colleges and universities tend to overemphasize the cognitive domain, with a resultant neglect of the affective domain, and propose that regaining a balance between the cognitive and affective domain during the educational experience would increase the quality of the graduates. Donnelly et al. (2020) found that 360° video in the operative setting assisted in developing the affective learning domain for nursing and medical students with additional benefits in assessing this realm.

Multiple strategies can be used to evaluate the affective domain. Ying (2020) recommends that selected assessment strategies align well with the learning outcomes to respect the resource expenditure for both learner and evaluator. By again considering the example of acquiring cultural sensitivity, faculty might consider using written papers with the purpose of having students first identify their own cultural background and then develop a critical analysis of an interaction in caregiving with a patient of another culture. Critiquing impact of a health care policy on individuals in the cultural community of interest rounds out the assessment. The use of media (e.g., digital video recording, photography, webpage development, or even a collage) to demonstrate key concepts and values held by a given culture is another method that can be used. These learning activities not only encourage self-awareness and recognition of the values and value conflicts in areas in which judgments must be made, but also can help students appreciate the implications of how respect and caring are communicated in various cultures. The evaluation criteria for these activities must emphasize the desired outcome. For example, if the selected strategy is a written assignment, overemphasis on process (such as writing style) may negate the importance of students' insights and self-awareness.

Other areas within the nursing profession that lend themselves well to evaluation in the affective domain include, but are not limited to, socialization to the roles of the nurse, developing a professional identity, appreciating the roles of other health care professionals, caring for patients who are dying, meeting spirituality needs, working with sexuality concerns, and appreciating the impact of culture and public policy on health and health care delivery for individuals and communities. The Quality and Safety Education for Nurses (QSEN) competencies specifically focus on attitudes and knowledge and skills needed by nurses (Cronenwett et al., 2007). QSEN exemplars take a defined concept and list outcomes for associated knowledge, skills, and attitudes. For example, an attitudinal competency identified in the category of patient-centered care is "Value seeing health care situations 'through patients' eyes" (http://qsen.org/competencies/pre-licensure-ksas/). McCoach et al. (2013) provide in-depth direction on instrument development for educators and employers who wish to better measure the affective domain. They address how constructs such as values and self-efficacy relate to success in either academic accomplishment or corporate quality and performance. The website of the National Center for Interprofessional Practice and Education provides information about various tools that can be used to evaluate interprofessional collaborative practice learning outcomes (https://nexusipe.org/advancing/assessment-evaluation).

USING RUBRICS AS CRITERIA FOR GRADING PERFORMANCE

Rubrics are rating scales used to determine performance. Rubrics not only provide exquisite clarity of the grading criteria but also provide a mechanism to inform students about grading expectations. The two basic types of rubrics are *holistic* and *analytic*. The holistic approach is based on global scoring, often with descriptive information for each area based on a numerical scoring system, whereas analytic scoring involves examining each significant characteristic of the written work or portfolio. For example, Stanley et al. (2020) suggest that evaluation of writing, organization, ideas, and style may be judged individually according to analytic scoring. The global method seems more suitable for summative evaluation, whereas the analytic method is useful in providing specific feedback to students for the purpose of formative evaluation, and ultimately, performance improvement. Less common are three additional types of rubrics: generic, specific, and qualitative (Stanley et al., 2020). See Box 23.2 for an example of a holistic grading rubric and Table 23.1 for an example of an analytic grading rubric.

Regardless of the type, rubrics are composed of four parts: (1) a task description (the assignment), (2) a scale, (3) the dimensions of the assignment, and (4) descriptions of each performance level. The first portion of a rubric contains a clear description of the assignment and should be matched to the learning outcomes of the course. The next part of the rubric is a scale to describe levels of performance. Such a scale may include levels such as "excellent," "competent," and "needs work." The dimensions of the assignment appear in the third part of rubric development, where the task is broken down into components. Finally, differentiated descriptions of each performance level are explicitly identified. Rubrics thus provide clarity of

BOX 23.2   Example of Holistic Grading Rubric

"A" Grade

The final course *synthesis paper* clearly defines a researchable problem; the search strategy provides sufficient relevant data for understanding the problem; the coding sheet is focused and guides the analysis of the data; issues of reliability and validity are identified; the literature is synthesized, rather than reviewed or summarized; the paper concludes with recommendations based on the research synthesis. The paper is written using the IUSON writing guidelines.

Participation in discussions and learning activities integrates course concepts and reflects critical thinking about research synthesis. Participation is thoughtful, respectful, informed, and substantiated. Peer review of the synthesis paper reflects the reviewers' understanding of the synthesis process, provides practical suggestions, and is presented in a collegial manner.

Dissemination of the research synthesis findings includes a written *plan for publication* and an oral *presentation* to faculty and classmates. The plan for publication includes thoughtful selection of a journal; draft of a query or cover letter; and, if the paper needs revisions to suit publication guidelines, a statement about revisions needed that matches the journal publication guidelines. The professional presentation is well organized, is supported by visual aids (e.g., PowerPoint slides), and uses professional communication style to suit the audience.

"B" Grade

The final *synthesis paper* clearly defines a researchable problem; the search strategy yields mostly relevant data for understanding the problem; the coding sheet lacks one or more important data points or does not reflect the scope of the problem statement; issues of reliability and validity are unclear; the review of literature is primarily synthesis with minimal summary; the paper concludes with mostly appropriate recommendations. The paper is free of major errors in grammar or style.

Participation in discussions and learning activities usually integrates course concepts and reflects critical thinking about research synthesis. Participation is helpful but may not contribute substantially to the focus of the course. Peer review of the synthesis paper does not include relevant aspects of the peer review checklists or overlooks areas in which feedback is needed.

Dissemination of the findings of the research synthesis includes a written *plan for publication* and an oral *presentation* to faculty and classmates. The plan for publication includes appropriate selection of a journal; the drafts of the query or cover letter are generally appropriate to the situation; general revisions are noted but do not consider manuscript guidelines of the journal. The professional presentation is fairly well organized; the visual aids (e.g., PowerPoint slides) enhance the presentation; the presentation is delivered with consideration for the audience.

"C" Grade

The final *synthesis paper* has an ill-defined problem; the search strategy yields irrelevant or tangential data for understanding the problem; the coding sheet is not well focused or neglects key variables or includes irrelevant variables; issues of reliability and validity are not identified or are ignored; the review is more summary than synthesis; the paper does not include recommendations or includes recommendations that are not drawn from the data. There are substantial errors in grammar or writing style.

Participation in discussions occurs on an irregular basis and is not grounded in course concepts, comments do not reflect critical thinking, and there are breaches of course norms and etiquette. Peer review of the synthesis paper does not provide substantive or helpful feedback to classmates; significant aspects of the peer review checklist are ignored.

Dissemination of the research synthesis findings includes a written *plan for publication* and an oral *presentation* to faculty and classmates. There is no plan for publication or the journal selected is not appropriate for the content of the paper; the drafts of the query or cover letters are not clearly written and do not capture the attention of the reader; there is no clear understanding of the revisions needed of the paper for the style requirements for the selected journal. The professional presentation is not well organized; visual aids (e.g., PowerPoint slides) or the visuals do not clarify or highlight key points of the presentation; the presentation exceeds time limits or is not suited to the audience. The presenter is unable to answer audience questions, if any, about the material.

IUSON, Indiana University School of Nursing.

TABLE 23.1 Example of a Shared Online Analytic Rubric for Evaluation of a Group Presentation

Group Presentation Rubric

	Excellent	Good	Fair	Poor
	40 pts	30 pts	20 pts	10 pts
Organization	Excellent	Good	Fair	Poor
	Presentation was very organized and was very easy to follow. Transitions between group members were well planned and executed cleanly.	Presentation was fairly organized and pretty followable. Transitions might have been slightly discontinuous but did not take away greatly from the overall presentation.	Presentation was not clearly organized. Transitions between members were jumpy or awkward.	Presentation lacked organization. Poor transitions between group members and individual parts. Presentation lacked order and was very difficult to follow.
Teamwork/ participation	Excellent	Good	Fair	Poor
	The group worked very well with each other, and the presentation was shared equally among the group members.	The group worked well with each other and communicated well. Some members participated slightly more than others.	The group communicated relatively well, with a few lapses in the presentation; some students dominated the presentation and others did not participate much.	Group did not work well together. There were obvious miscommunications and lapses in the presentation.
Content	Excellent	Good	Fair	Poor
	Group members had a strong hold on the content, and the content was thoroughly addressed. No mistakes were made with regard to content knowledge.	Most of the group members had a solid understanding of the content. Content was missing minor elements or contained minor errors.	Group members had only a superficial understanding of content. Several mistakes were made during the presentation.	Group members had little to no understanding of the content addressed in the presentation.
Visual aid(s)	Excellent	Good	Fair	Poor
	Visual aids used were used effectively throughout presentation. Group members used visual aids as a supplement, not as a crutch.	Visual aids used were somewhat effective but were not used consistently throughout presentation.	Visual aids used did not support verbal presentation. They lacked information, or group members read from them.	Visual aids were not used at all.

Retrieved from http://www.rcampus.com/indexrubric.cfm

expectations to assist students in the successful completion of assignments, making grading of these assignments more objective for the faculty. Lee and associates (2021) describe the psychometric testing of a clinical reasoning assessment rubric (CRAR) for nursing students. The process used is an excellent example of the laborious, yet vital process of establishing reliability and validity for rubrics used in nursing education. According to the literature review by Nkhoma et al. (2020) rubrics "…benefit students in learning and achieving better results as well as how they assist teachers and educators in making accurate assessments about their students' performance" (p. 239). More recently, there is evidence that students co-creating rubrics benefit both the student and teacher (Kilgour et al., 2020). Specifically, students report better understanding of the assessment process and teachers report a positive impact on student perspectives related to rubrics (Kilgour et al., 2020).

The Association of American Colleges and Universities (AACU) has developed the Valid Assessment of Learning in Undergraduate Education (VALUE) initiative, a set of standardized rubrics to evaluate multiple skills, such as reasoning, critical thinking, and written work, across a university or college (McConnell et al., 2019). The 16 rubrics are viewed as both an alternative to standardized testing for the evaluation of student learning outcomes and as a way of communicating criteria associated with achievement and student success. These rubrics are not designed for individual grading, but rather for use at the program and university levels. The AACU has a database in which student work can be deposited and scored using the VALUE rubrics (https://www.aacu.org/value/rubrics). (See Case Study 23.1.)

EVALUATION STRATEGIES FOR LEARNING OUTCOMES

Nursing faculty have a multitude of available strategies to evaluate student learning. This section identifies several strategies known to be effective in nursing. Table 23.2 provides an overview of these strategies.

CASE STUDY 23.1 Developing Rubrics

The teaching team in an undergraduate clinical course is implementing a verbal patient care plan during post-conference time. There are multiple sections of this course and six faculty. They are very excited about this as it will save time for the students and faculty. The process will display how the students are thinking and faculty are able to provide rapid, relevant feedback. The challenge is how to consistently implement this assessment in the multiple sections with multiple faculty.

1. What type of rubric will be most appropriate for scoring the oral patient care plan presentation?
2. What elements should the teaching team consider when developing the rubric?
3. What process should the teaching team use to ensure interrater reliability across the faculty?

Portfolios
Description and Uses

Portfolios, at the most basic level, are collections of student work. Although the medium most widely used in the past for portfolios has been print, electronic portfolios, commonly called *e-portfolios*, have flooded higher education, including nursing education. Farrell (2020) traces the history of portfolio development from paper to electronic formats noting that after 2000 when technology became widespread, portfolios became an integral part of higher education around the world. There has been research that supports the impact of portfolios on student learning in the last decade (Farrell, 2020). The Association of American Colleges and Universities (AAC&U) has identified e-Portfolios as high-impact practice (HIP) and devotes a website (Publications on e-Portfolio: Archives of the Research Landscape—PEARL) to research studies related to e-Portfolios.

The e-portfolio experience has been shown to be most effective when students have a clear understanding of the technology and have an appreciation for the relevance of using this method of evaluation (Kahn, 2019; Lu, 2021). Kahn (2019) supports that e-Portfolios are a high-impact practice (HIP) for teaching, learning, and assessment especially when skills are taught throughout the curriculum that aid students to reflect upon their learning.

	Domain/ Assessment	Possible			
Technique	**Purpose**	**Applications**	**Advantages**	**Disadvantages**	**Issues**
Portfolio (paper and electronic)	High-level cognitive Affective Psychomotor (if video) Formative Summative	Placement in program of study For evidence of progress Outcome measure for individual or program Marketing tool for job placement Demonstration of professional development	Broad sample of student work Documents progress Identifies student strengths and weaknesses Critical thinking with student reflection If e-portfolio, is easier to make updates and convenient for online programs	Time for collection and grading Need storage space Not direct observation Limited reliability Additional expenses with electronic portfolios Time needed for learning	Ownership responsibility for collection Nonselective vs. selective portfolio Are you assessing process or product? Deciding on the format for organizing the portfolio
Role play	Cognitive Affective Psychomotor Formative	Formative feedback for psychomotor skills, communication techniques, problem-solving skills	Active participation of student Stimulates creativity Variables can be controlled Can repeat Provides practice in peer review skills	Immediate feedback may not be possible Self-consciousness of participant	Takes time to build comfort with technique Need familiarity with material
Reflection	High-level cognitive Affective domain Formative Summative (for trending)	Self-assessment Integration of learning can be demonstrated Appropriate for assessing the higher-level cognitive skills; critical thinking can be assessed	Active student involvement Encourages students to form connections within and between content Assists students to practice self-assessment based on criteria Encourages recognition of learning in students' life experience	Time consuming for both students and faculty Student frustration with lack of clarity of assignment	Grading criteria can be developed jointly Requires a high degree of trust Students will need orientation to this process May want to consider anonymous grading

TABLE 23.2 Overview of Evaluation Strategies

Continued

TABLE 23.2	**Overview of Evaluation Strategies**—cont'd				
Technique	**Domain/ Assessment Purpose**	**Possible Applications**	**Advantages**	**Disadvantages**	**Issues**
Paper	High levels of cognitive and affective domains Formative Summative	Critical thinking skills Writing skills Development of arguments Synthesis of ideas	More in-depth information in area of interest A public work to be assessed Writing is the scholarly model for self-expression	Time for both faculty and student Subjectivity in grading Limited sample of ability	Reliability Grading criteria
Essays	High levels of cognitive and affective domains Formative Summative	Critical thinking skills Free form Demonstrate problem-solving abilities, decision making, and rationale Analysis	Shorter than a paper Assess recall and synthesis at one moment rather than at several times Creativity Easy to construct and administer	Less sample of content and ability Time to write and time to grade	Reliability Grading criteria Clarity of questions Use a test plan to better cover content
Oral (verbal) questioning	All ranges of cognitive domain Affective domain Formative Summative	Evidence of thinking process with "why" and Socratic questioning Evidence of verbal skills Defense: determines content mastery and evidence of synthesis	Quick to prepare Inexpensive Opportunity for student to receive immediate corrective feedback Works well for nonlinear ideas	Can be perceived by students as threatening Bias of evaluator	Must determine the difference between questions for teaching vs. evaluation Criteria for assessment should be established before use Can be subjective
Concept mapping	All ranges of cognitive domain Affective Formative	Concepts expressed in a visual way Shows relationships between and among topics	Works well for students who are highly visual in their orientation Computer-based tools available for electronic submissions	Can be frustrating to concrete thinkers Time required to master electronic format	Reliability Grading criteria must be defined Takes time to grade Allow for student creativity

	Domain/				
Technique	**Assessment Purpose**	**Possible Applications**	**Advantages**	**Disadvantages**	**Issues**
Audio and video recording	All ranges of cognitive domain Affective domain Video gives evidence of psychomotor domain Formative Summative	Verbal skills Interviews Group discussion Video captures nonverbal performance	Provides evidence when presence of faculty may be intrusive or when faculty are unable to be present Relatively inexpensive Permanent record Evidence can be replayed Works for self-assessment	Limited by mode of recording May be difficult to get quality recording of each group member Requires time to listen Expense and maintenance of high-quality equipment	Requires consent Student should be aware of how the recording will be used Must determine whether entire recording or a sampling of it will be assessed Confidentiality of patient data is critical
Patient simulation	Psychomotor High-level cognitive Affective	Safe practice environment for psychomotor skills Preparation for clinical Alternative for clinical Screen-based does not require actual presence at site	Active involvement of students and faculty Team interaction Mimics real world	Expensive Specially trained personnel, including faculty Small numbers of active students per scenario Training persons for patient role Extra coordination for IPE	Integration into the curriculum Selection of scenarios Opportunity to practice before evaluation Equipment maintenance Faculty education/ training Personnel needs Efficient scheduling of students
Service-learning	Higher levels of cognitive domain Affective domain Formative Summative	Evidence of complex communication and problem-solving skills; teamwork, if group project	Authentic learning and assessment; effect on student, preceptor, and community; student exposure to diverse and/or underserved populations	Time to coordinate with students, agency personnel; risk that expectations of students and agency for scope of project are not alike	Assessment should include outcomes for student learning, preceptor and agency satisfaction, and effect on targeted community Group grade may not take into account individual effort

TABLE 23.2   Overview of Evaluation Strategies—cont'd

Further, assessing e-Portfolios allows insights into how students learn and the learning outcomes attained (Kahn, 2019). Lu (2021) reviewed the theoretical and research literature related to e-Portfolios concluding that they are high-impact tools documenting student's achievement over time and maintains that educators should integrate the portfolio over the student's entire educational process. Similarly, Tan et al. (2022) reviewed portfolios of medical students and recommend that creating micro-competency milestones across the program is useful in documenting achievement of knowledge, skills, and attitudes relevant to professional identity formation. They noted that the meaningfulness of the portfolio linked to the effectiveness of formative evaluation and contributed to a larger summative evaluation method (Tan et al., 2022).

Regardless of the format, portfolios are used to obtain a broader sample of student accomplishment and for a variety of purposes. They can be used (1) as proof of achievement in a class, (2) as an outcome measure of a program, (3) as a marketing tool for job placement, (4) for student placement in a program of study, (5) to support student learning, or (6) as evidence of professional development or lifelong learning.

The purpose of the portfolio needs to be clearly established before work is collected for inclusion. Portfolios for student *assessment* are a collection of student work within the course or program of study that is designed to demonstrate *progress* of the learning. The learning outcomes help in determining the specific materials to be included in the portfolio. Decisions need to be made on whether the portfolio is for formative or summative evaluation or both. The work and assignments to be included, the timing of the collection of the assignments, and whether the grading remarks will be included in the portfolio are also decisions that need to be made. *Nonselective portfolios* are collections of all student work for a specified period. The focus of these is more on formative evaluation of student progress. A compilation of certain completed works of students is frequently referred to as a *selective portfolio*. A selective portfolio often contains works that are the best efforts of the student and are usually part of a summative evaluation.

Evaluation of the portfolio may occur during the course or plan of study (formative) or at the end (summative). A comprehensive portfolio may be used to demonstrate the acquisition of competencies during a program of study (Kahn, 2019; Lu, 2021) and may be used in the clinical setting. It is important that clearly established criteria be identified for the assessment, evaluation, or grading of the portfolio. These criteria need to be shared with students at the onset of the process.

Students may be required to *critique* their *progress* as the portfolio develops during the course, clinical placement, or plan of study. When clearly delineated criteria are used, this exercise engages students in self-assessment and critical reflective skills that more effectively prepare them for real-world practice. Parker and McMillan (2020) created a survey that assisted MSN students to identify their character strengths as a basis for further development. Using an e-portfolio provided the students with a format in which to showcase the development of their soft skills (such as teamwork and communication) in the clinical practice arena (Parker & McMillan, 2020).

Stec and Garritano (2016) examined the use of e-portfolios in a Doctor of Nursing Practice (DNP) program as a means to evaluate student achievement of program objectives. They suggest that to effectively incorporate portfolios as a measure of program outcomes, there must be consistency in how the portfolio is organized, that the standards for achievement of outcomes are clearly defined, and that documentation is well structured.

Portfolios used as an *outcome measure of a program* can include selections of student work acquired throughout the curriculum. Samples of these portfolios can be used to evaluate student progress in an area such as writing skills to provide feedback about the effectiveness of the program (Stec & Garritano, 2016).

Digital badges are another electronic method to demonstrate specific competency acquisition (Noyes et al., 2020). The digital badge can be linked to the student's electronic resume or portfolio. An employer can open the badge to view criteria for the badge and samples of work accomplished. In some geographical areas, jobs for new graduates are competitive, and an outstanding portfolio may assist to secure employment.

A portfolio or dossier may be useful when applying to academic institutions for advanced education. Portfolios are a method of demonstrating prior learning and experience.

Portfolios are often used in nursing programs for advanced placement of students. The portfolio is a compilation of objective evidence demonstrating expertise and skills acquired through prior learning, practice experience, or both. Guidelines for compiling and assessing such portfolios must be clearly delineated. Examples of documentation that may be included in this type of portfolio include (but are not limited to) a resume, performance evaluation, course syllabi or outlines, and evidence of professional activity and certification.

Faculty may use portfolios when they are seeking promotion or demonstrating evidence of impact for performance evaluations. Guidelines for construction of such portfolios usually include evidence and assessment of teaching, scholarship, and service, although specific requirements differ among institutions.

Advantages

Portfolios provide a broad sample of student work and can show evidence of progress or accomplishment, especially as they are linked to program outcomes or competency. Identification of student strengths and weaknesses in formative evaluation allows students to make improvements. Student reflection on the work in a portfolio can stimulate deeper thinking and provide evidence of the developing affective domain. Using portfolios for advanced placement in programs enables students to receive credit for previous experience and reduces repetition of content. The e-portfolio provides increased access by both students and faculty and allows large amounts of data to be gathered, increasing the comprehensiveness of the data. The e-portfolio lends itself well to online courses and programs.

Disadvantages

Although collection of the portfolio data is not time consuming, the main disadvantage associated with portfolios is the time needed to provide feedback and grades. In addition, it is challenging and takes time for faculty to determine validity and reliability for the established grading criteria or rubrics. If e-portfolios are used, additional resources may be needed, such as the expense of software licensing or online storage and time for faculty and students to learn the technology.

Issues

Major issues related to student portfolios are ownership of the portfolio, responsibility for collection, fair grading, use of nonselective versus selective portfolios, and the format used to organize the portfolio. Both paper and electronic formats may be used. When a portfolio is used for classroom or program assessment or evaluation, the faculty must determine the purpose of the portfolio (e.g., to assess writing skills or critical thinking), which works will be collected, who is responsible for maintaining the portfolio, what criteria will be used to assess the collection, the scoring method, and timing of feedback.

When a portfolio is used for program evaluation purposes, faculty buy-in and adequate faculty development are key to success (Kahn, 2019; Stec & Garritano, 2016). These authors emphasize the need to clarify faculty role expectations for development and participation in the portfolio review process, institution of reward structures to recognize faculty service provided, and the development of tools that adequately reflect the program outcomes as necessary for successful implementation of the portfolio for program assessment. This strategy of program evaluation can influence and support organizational culture change.

Critical Reflection

Description and Uses

The development of self-assessment skills is key to student success and is an essential component of professional development. The use of reflection is frequently incorporated into learning strategies (e.g., service-learning, interpretation of case studies, written work, debriefing from simulation and clinical experiences) to assess the development of leadership, cultural and social awareness, and learning outcomes from the affective domain. Reflection is also a technique that may enhance the development of shared mental models among members of an interprofessional team. Shared mental models are defined as "the knowledge framework of the relationships between the task the team is engaged in and how the team members will interact" (Lioce, 2020, p. 42). The concept of reflective practice has developed from the work of Schön (1983) who determined two kinds of reflective thinking: The first occurs in the moment and can be characterized by the phrases "thinking on one's feet" or "mindfulness." The second is reflection after the fact. Both of these reflective activities are important for practicing health professionals. Engaging learners in assessment and evaluation is encouraged (Cardwell, 2020; Masuku et al., 2021). Self-monitoring of clinical practice (paying attention to clinical actions while in the moment, purposely examining the effect of one's actions, and using these insights to improve future thinking, clinical reasoning, and practice) should be cultivated by students in nursing, as well as medicine and other health care professions (National Academy of Medicine, 2021; Park et al., 2022). The purpose of self-reflection is to create a more thoughtful, self-aware, and reflective practitioner who will ultimately contribute to improved quality of care. There is a collaborative nature of learning and assessment between faculty and learners that takes place in critical reflection. Masuku et al. (2021) suggest this collaborative accountability promotes active engagement of the learner in the process and lends itself to the promotion of deep learning, critical thinking, and personal claiming of the knowledge.

The use of reflection encourages the students to fully consider a question, an experience, or a thesis, and to process their thoughts. The reflection itself may be implemented through a variety of techniques such as short (one- to two-page) papers, progressive journaling, or oral questioning and discussion with individuals or in groups. Reflections allow faculty to evaluate the level of understanding, guide students in the awareness of their mental models, and help students expand critical thinking skills as part of their professional development (formative evaluation). Journaling can be a strategy for reflection and can be organized as preclass (preparing for the class), intraclass (as a result of activities conducted during the class or clinical experience), and postclass (such as a homework reflection where examples may be used to demonstrate understanding of key concepts). Lee et al. (2021) found through their systematic review, that reflection via structured debriefing following simulation, attributed to learning, critical thinking, clinical reasoning, clinical judgment, and in some cases improved motivation. Macartney et al. (2021) found that using critical reflection following a video simulation was positively perceived by students as enhancing their clinical reasoning processes. Brown et al. (2022), in their systematic review, found that journaling promoted clinical judgment skills and emotional competency.

Assessment of reflection is based on an educational connoisseurship model, in which students become connoisseur critics. According to Eisner (1985), a connoisseur is able to appreciate and distinguish the important from the trivial. Although students may not have enough experience to be true connoisseurs, the faculty member can role model and coach students to develop these skills. Bevis and Watson (1989), in a modification of Eisner's work, identified six levels of critiquing: looking, seeing, perceiving and intuiting, rendering, interpreting meaning, and judging. These steps include identifying an event, viewing it with a focus, interpreting the event on a personal level (complete with value clarification), and discerning the significance of the event. Evaluation criteria can be built around these steps. Flournoy and Bauman (2021) propose that students' reflective practices can become a method to establish achievement of program outcomes. This expands beyond classroom and clinical grading purposes, to the outcomes-based evaluation of the entire program; more on program outcomes evaluation in Chapter 26.

Advantages

As a strategy, reflection provides an opportunity to examine critical thinking and values awareness. Reflection, in whatever form it takes, helps demonstrate these insights to the faculty.

Reflection can be done in oral form or written form, and easily lends itself to online formats. Learning outcomes from the affective domain can be assessed using critical reflection. Sequential reflections provide evidence of learning over time and students can view their progress toward course and program outcomes. Feedback on reflective practices can serve as both formative and summative evaluation. It is important that faculty provide clarity on the purpose of the evaluation.

Disadvantages

The use of critical self-reflection for evaluation requires time for both students and faculty. Students may experience initial frustration if the scope of the assignment is not well defined, and the skills required for critiquing are not practiced. Park et al. (2022) concluded in their longitudinal study of self-reflection with medical students that faculty support on approaches to self-reflection as well as explanation of the value of this practice in professional development was integral to growing student skill and appreciation for self-reflection practice. The process used to grade the critique must be clearly defined. For this type of assignment, the grading may be less focused on form and more focused on the insights. Defining the criteria for evaluation and clearly communicating them is essential (Masuku et al., 2021), and there is still work to be done to develop rubrics for evaluation that are valid and reliable (Brown et al., 2022).

Issues

Students must be oriented to the elements that are essential to a high-quality reflection. The authors' initial experience with reflection found that students spent the majority of a written reflection assignment describing the event or incident, providing minimal analysis. If the purpose of the reflection activity is to provide evidence of analysis and application, then the assignment and grading criteria need to be structured for this. A three-part journal framework can accomplish this goal. The first section is for description of the event, the second section requests the student to demonstrate an understanding of the concepts by applying the content from the course to the experience, and the third section asks the student to apply the understanding gained from the analysis to a future professional experience. The grading criteria should be weighted to reflect the importance of the desired outcome.

Time involved for both students and faculty is an issue. Developing thoughtful reflections, regardless of format, requires a time commitment on the part of students. Those who procrastinate may not obtain the benefits of the exercise. For example, some students may complete all journal entries at once, losing the opportunity for growth and self-awareness. For faculty, reading, viewing, and responding can be a lengthy process. For example, if reflections are assigned in the framework of a sequential journal or blog framework, faculty must decide whether they are going to read each entry for evaluation purposes or take a sample.

The purpose of the assignment must be clearly established, and students need mentoring in the process of self-reflection for its full benefits to be realized. Establishing grading criteria before students complete the assignment will help convey outcome expectations. Joint development of the criteria for grading with students is a technique to engage them in the process and identify the value of the activity. Faculty feedback should also be of a critically reflective nature and may be most effective as a formative evaluation. The use of anonymity could be appropriate for grading this kind of assignment because it can enhance objectivity on the part of the evaluator and minimize student fears that can inhibit honesty and creativity.

In critical reflection, the relationship of the student and faculty changes to shared power in the learning environment. The faculty–student relationship becomes more collegial, and a high level of mutual trust and desire to grow is essential. It is also imperative that the philosophy of the school and faculty support the practice of critical reflection. Students should also know who will view their reflections. If peers will view the reflections (e.g., via threaded discussions, group synthesis), the amount of self-disclosure students choose to provide may be affected. Confidentiality for the student reflection is an important consideration.

Papers and Essays

Description and Uses

Papers and assigned essays or essay questions on examinations can be used to demonstrate organizational skills, critical thinking, clinical reasoning, and written communication while encouraging creativity. *Papers* are written reports, whereas *essays* are free-form responses to open-ended questions. Students are encouraged to be creative in responding to essay questions. Both papers and essays can measure both the affective domain and higher levels of the cognitive domain.

Providing feedback to written student reflections can take several forms. Although computer programs are currently available to provide automated instruction and feedback to improve writing skills of college students (Roscoe et al., 2017); critique of higher-order skills requires thoughtful responses by faculty. Effective assessment includes feedback about the student's efforts; individualized and clearly expressed comments that focus on the work—not the student as an individual; and concern for the student's learning. Faculty comments should focus on the learning to be obtained from the assignment. Beccaria et al. (2019) found that online "just in time" tutoring feedback to support essay writing of first-year baccalaureate nursing students resulted in improved essays that reflected deeper learning. Mitchell et al. (2020) conducted a qualitative systematic review of nursing students' responses to academic writing. They found that writing assignments aid in developing professional identity; however, when writing mechanics were excessively accentuated, there was a negative impact on student learning and engagement (Mitchell et al., 2020). This emphasizes the need to change focus from "mechanical-technical to transformative writing" so that formative feedback can help engage students and positively impact the final product (Mitchell et al., 2020, p. 1). Seven components for responding to writing identified by Beach and Marshall (1991) provide a classic framework for faculty responses to written work and are described in Box 23.3.

BOX 23.3 Seven Components for Responding to Written Work

1. **Praising:** providing positive reinforcement for students
2. **Describing:** providing "reader-based" feedback about one's own reactions and perceptions of the students' responses that imply judgments of those responses
3. **Diagnosing:** determining the students' own unique knowledge, attitudes, abilities, and needs
4. **Judging:** evaluating the sufficiency, level, depth, completeness, validity, and insightfulness of a student's responses
5. **Predicting and reviewing growth:** predicting potential directions for improving student responses according to specific criteria and reviewing progress from previous responses
6. **Record keeping:** keeping a record to chart changes across time in student's performance
7. **Recognizing/praising growth:** giving students recognition and praise for demonstrating growth

Excerpt from Beach, R. W., & Marshall, J. D. (1991). *Teaching literature in the secondary school* (pp. 211–212). Harcourt Brace & Company.

Advantages

In-depth information can be obtained through the writing of papers. This helps students clarify their own thinking about topics and learn to write better. Papers are a public work and can be assessed by others in the profession. Writing papers requires students to integrate their ideas with those found in other sources. Similarly, essays are useful for assessing higher-level cognitive skills such as analysis and synthesis.

Using essay questions in a testing environment has the advantage that essay questions are easier to construct than multiple-choice examination questions. It is important to make the essay question clearly understood and focused; providing the grading criteria to students will help them allocate their response time more effectively during the testing session. Essay tests can demonstrate the ability of the student to synthesize material they have learned and convey their ideas clearly without the benefit of resources.

Disadvantages

The major disadvantage of papers for both students and faculty is the amount of time involved in writing and grading. Faculty can become distracted from the content of the paper when a student exhibits poor writing skills. As well, faculty feedback may be more focused on supporting the grade assigned even when faculty states their belief that the purpose of feedback is to improve students' skill acquisition. Providing constructive comments can be accomplished through facilitative comments by posting questions versus being authoritative. Davis (2009) suggests using the question "What do you hope your reader will understand your thesis to be?" instead of a directive statement such as "State your thesis more clearly" (p. 328). Faculty should also avoid the temptation to rewrite the paper while they are grading. An essay test may involve less sampling of the content than a multiple-choice examination.

Issues

Reliability in grading papers is an issue. Reliability can be increased by having clearly established grading criteria and having more than one person grade the paper. This is especially important for papers that receive low or failing grades. Anonymous grading can increase the objectivity of the grader. Faculty should determine the assessment plan based on the purpose of the paper and desired outcomes. For example, if the purpose is to demonstrate critical thinking and creativity, the format of the paper may have less value in the total grade of the paper. Alternatively, if the purpose is for the student to demonstrate scholarly writing, evaluation may emphasize the format and style of writing.

Writing a clear and focused essay question can be a challenge for faculty. The question needs to be stated in such a way that the scope is clear to the students. It is also important to follow a test plan when essay tests are constructed so that the content is adequately sampled. Before grading an essay examination, faculty must establish clear grading criteria. When more than one person is grading, IRR needs to be established. Time required to answer the essay should be determined. Davis (2009) suggests providing approximately twice the amount of time for students to provide their answer in a testing environment as it takes for the faculty member to write out the answer to the essay.

Concept Mapping

Description and Uses

Concept, *mind*, and *nursing process mapping* are all descriptive terms applied to a strategy in which students express concepts and their relationships in a visual format. It is based in constructivist learning theory and is an active learning strategy that has been in use for several decades (Krieglstein et al., 2022; Novak & Gowin, 1984). Concept mapping can assess and evaluate both progress of learning and how well a student understands a topic (Bank & Daxburger, 2020; Kapuza et al., 2020; Kroeze et al., 2021). This strategy is a visual means for students to demonstrate the relationships of ideas. The choice of concepts to be mapped can be provided by the faculty or generated by the students. The structure of the map may vary. Computer-based tools are increasingly available and useful for online learning and evaluation. Using electronic maps allows each piece of the concept map to be hyperlinked to a resource. This application of concept mapping is called a *concept resource map*. Examples of concept mapping are provided in Fig. 23.1.

Nursing faculty can use concept mapping to assess student understanding of the underpinnings and factors that guide the delivery of patient care as well as factors influencing leadership decisions and quality improvement initiatives. Complex maps can incorporate multiple patient problems, allowing students to demonstrate the interrelationship of the problems to patient care. Multiple studies in the literature from nursing, medicine, education, and other disciplines over the past decades attest to the positive effect of concept maps on student learning. Lafave et al. (2021) found that concept maps were an effective tool for students to demonstrate their grasp of evidence-informed practice. Krieglstein et al. (2022) note that concept mapping uses both verbal and visual channels of information processing, thereby decreasing the risk of cognitive overload.

The process of creating and evaluating concept maps is time consuming for both students and

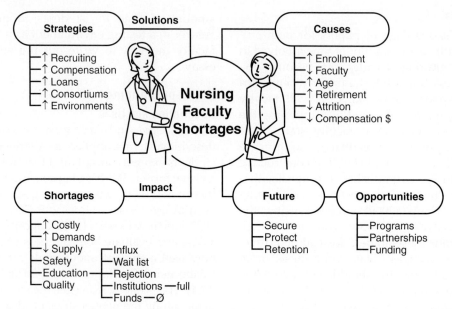

Strategies — Solutions
- ↑ Recruiting
- ↑ Compensation
- ↑ Loans
- ↑ Consortiums
- ↑ Environments

Nursing Faculty Shortages

Causes
- ↑ Enrollment
- ↓ Faculty
- ↑ Age
- ↑ Retirement
- ↓ Attrition
- ↓ Compensation $

Shortages — Impact
- ↑ Costly
- ↑ Demands
- ↓ Supply   — Influx
- Safety   — Wait list
- Education   — Rejection
- Quality   — Institutions — full
              — Funds — Ø

Future
- Secure
- Protect
- Retention

Opportunities
- Programs
- Partnerships
- Funding

FIG. 23.1 Concept map created to analyze the nursing faculty shortage. (Courtesy Carolyn Low, RN-BSN Graduate of Colorado Christian University.)

faculty; therefore, the application of concept mapping may be underutilized in large lecture courses (Bank & Daxburger, 2020). In their study to determine if there was synergy in combining concept mapping and retrieval strategies to enhance learning, O'Day and Karpicke (2021) noted that students spent significantly more time with the material when doing concept mapping as compared to a free-form retrieval practice. However, they found that the learning retention from concept maps did not exceed that gained from retrieval or the combination of both concept maps and retrieval.

When using concept mapping for evaluation, the purpose of the assignment drives the scoring criteria. For example, criteria may include such things as the number of nodes and number of relationships tied to the nodes, the clarity of the organizational structure, accuracy of relationships, and categorization of content. It is possible to have students self-assess, or peer assess concept maps as a way of building the professional skills of self-assessment and peer assessment. This would best serve as a formative evaluation and require guidance and practice. Establishing clear criteria and IRR is essential for summative evaluation. Bank

and Daxburger (2020) developed a rubric based on three criteria: concepts, prepositions connecting the concepts, and visual appearance as part of a final evaluation in a science course. The work to automate concept map grading is promising and may ultimately minimize instructor time required for providing feedback (Bank & Daxburger, 2020; Hubal et al., 2020; Kroeze et al., 2021).

Advantages

Concept maps serve to stimulate and demonstrate metacognition, thinking about how you think. This skill contributes to awareness of how information is used in critical decision making and is essential for health care clinicians (Hubal et al., 2020). Mapping also lends itself well to evaluation, especially in determining the way students grasp the relationship of their knowledge. Having students verbally explain the concept map to faculty can add clarity to the relationships expressed by the lines on the concept map. Concept mapping requires students to demonstrate cognitive synthesis skills with a minimum amount of writing. Mapping also allows faculty to gain insight into the way students assimilate new information and how students are connecting the material.

Disadvantages

Time is required to prepare students who are unfamiliar with concept maps. Reading and responding to concept maps can take faculty time away from other activities. Concept maps on the same topic can vary and may be large and difficult to follow. It can also be more challenging to interpret the student's intent because only key words and phrases are used. In a handwritten format, it is possible that the artistic ability and overall appearance and readability of the map could influence faculty. To help avoid subjectivity in evaluation, inter- and intrarater reliability must be established. Tools, such as rubrics, need to have established validity and reliability. For digital concept maps, special software is required. Time required for both students and faculty to learn the program needs to be acknowledged.

Issues

The faculty must teach students how to successfully create a map and allow them practice in completing maps before using this as an evaluation strategy. By practicing the mapping strategy as an in-class learning experience, the students will have a greater familiarity with the process (Bank & Daxburger, 2020). Small groups can work on a concept map during class time and then share their maps with peers. Using an evaluation rubric to provide peer feedback not only provides the students an opportunity to practice the skill of providing feedback but also familiarizes them with the expectations of the assignment. Special software can improve the capabilities of concept mapping in an electronic environment. Software to support concept mapping does add a learning curve for students. Regardless of the method used to construct the map, a limitation of mapping is the challenge of uncovering the rationale for the relationship of ideas. One way of addressing this limitation is to use the map as the focus for a faculty–student conference, by face-to-face or digital modality. The grading of the exercise could easily become subjective unless there are clear criteria for grading. These criteria must be defined for the students before submission of their work. Faculty need to establish the validity and reliability of their tools for this evaluation.

Oral Questioning

Description and Uses

In the quest to assess the student's ability to think critically and develop clinical reasoning skills, faculty have historically used oral questioning. At the graduate level, oral questioning is used for the defense of the dissertation and thesis. In this process, the student must demonstrate a working knowledge of the discipline and the ability to express arguments orally. The answers to these questions demonstrate the knowledge, skills, and attitudes held by the student.

For health professions, the use of oral questioning during clinical learning is designed to assess all levels of the cognitive and affective domains and to provide evidence of critical thinking. Questions can solicit comparisons, priorities, and rationale. During a questioning session, students can be asked to elaborate and justify their responses. Questioning as a formative technique can be sequenced to move the student from a basic level (factual information) to a higher cognitive level (clarifying relationships).

A high degree of trust and sense of collaboration for learning growth in the relationship of faculty and learner is a key for success in this method. The Socratic questioning strategy is one model of questioning (Abou-Hanna et al., 2021; Dewald, 2020). By leading the student with questions that do not provide direct information to the learning at hand, the faculty member guides the student through questioning to discover the answer or to recognize the gaps in knowledge that need to be resolved in order to answer the question. For examples of Socratic questioning, see Box 23.3. For examples of how Bloom's taxonomy can be used to generate questions, see Box 23.4.

Faculty should explain the purpose and value of oral questions and communicate respect during the process. Faculty skill in helping students build on their prior knowledge with questions that create a learning challenge typically promotes student engagement (Thammasitboon & Brand, 2021). Providing the opportunity for students to think on their feet is preparation for the reality of the clinical work environment. Socratic questioning can also be applied in the online environment (Dewald, 2020). It is again important to keep the questioning relevant and respectful of student time.

BOX 23.4 Examples of Questions to Assess Students' Ability to Use Knowledge in the Cognitive Domain

Remember
Define _____.
List the five principles for _____.
Based on your assignment, what do you recall about _____?

Understand
Explain the meaning of _____.
Tell me in your own words what is meant by _____.
Which of the examples demonstrates _____?

Apply
What is a new example of _____?
How could _____ be used to _____?
Show how this information could be graphed.

Analyze
What are the implications of _____?
What is the meaning of _____?
What are the key components of _____?

Evaluate
Explain the effectiveness of this approach.
Which solution would you choose? Justify your opinion.
What are the consequences of _____?

Create
What are some possible solutions to the problem of _____?
From this information, create your own model of _____.
Suppose you could _____. How would you approach _____?

Cognitive taxonomy dimensions based on Krathwohl, D. R. (2002). A revision of Bloom's taxonomy: An overview. *Theory into Practice, 41*(4), 212–218. Adapted from Hansen, C. (1994). Questioning techniques for the active classroom, and King, A. Inquiry as a tool in critical thinking. In D. F. Halpern (Ed.), *Changing college classrooms: New teaching and learning strategies for an increasingly complex world* (pp. 13–38, 93–106). Jossey-Bass.

Advantages

Oral questioning is inexpensive, requires no special equipment, and can be quickly developed by faculty. During oral questioning, it is possible to give immediate feedback to the student, which makes this an excellent option for formative evaluation.

Disadvantages

Students may feel highly stressed by the experience. Abou-Hanna et al. (2021) reported that 39% of medical students in their study felt humiliated when they did not answer correctly; however, only 5% of the students thought faculty asked questions with the purpose of humiliating. They found that faculty underestimated the value students placed on probing questions. Unless the session is recorded, there is no permanent record of it. The evaluator may be biased by a variety of factors during the evaluation. For example, if the student performs well at the beginning of the session and the performance deteriorates as the session progresses, the earlier performance may be biased by what occurred subsequently. It is imperative that the criteria for evaluation be fully developed before the questioning session. Establishing reliability of an oral examination requires extra effort on behalf of the faculty.

Issues

Using questions for evaluation must be distinguished from using questions to encourage active student learning. Avoid fact-only, as well as leading or loaded questions. Consider giving students a minute to write down an answer. This can minimize the stress of a questioning session. It is important for faculty to avoid interrupting the student as an answer is being given. Oral feedback from the teacher to the student, especially when correcting the student, needs to have as its primary focus the purpose of improving future performance. That makes this technique most suited as an evaluation strategy. Not all faculty are well trained in this technique. The criteria for evaluation must be established before the session with the student. Because of the lack of a permanent record of the interaction, risk of subjectivity is greater in this kind of evaluation.

Audio and Video Recording
Description and Uses

Audio recording can be used to evaluate communication skills, group process, clinical caregiving simulations, and interviewing skills. Audio recording allows the evaluator to focus on verbal communication without other distractors. Video recording captures a more complete essence of the competencies being evaluated. For example, evaluation of psychomotor skills and aspects of clinical reasoning can be demonstrated in the video capture. Faculty must determine at the outset if audio and video recording is used as an assessment to provide feedback to students for performance improvement (formative) or if their performance is being evaluated and graded (summative).

Using a video recording device to document student performance can be a means of evaluating several performance parameters. Video of student performance is useful for evaluating communication skills because it picks up the student's actual words as well as inflections and body language. The live-action feature of the video recording also provides evidence of the sequencing of student actions in hands-on skill performance. This method works well for skill validation and is very useful for students to self-assess their performance using a rubric. Video recording student skill performance provides a visual capture of their actions and may assist them in making improvements. Fieler (2020) incorporated video recording of students completing physical assessment and compared self-assessment with those who did not have a video recording of the exam. The results indicate that students with no video may overestimate their level of competence, thus supporting the use of video in skill attainment (Fieler, 2020). Jonassen and Yarbrough (2021) incorporated smartphones to record indwelling urinary catheter placement by students in the lab. The student and peer dyads used self-reflection and feedback from each other to make improvements as well as decrease anxiety (Jonassen & Yarbrough, 2021).

The video capture has been long used for debriefing after simulations. Basic video recording equipment has become inexpensive; high-quality cameras are included in most cell phones, tablets, and computers. Comprehensive audio and video capture equipment specifically designed to link with high-fidelity simulation can be very expensive. More recently, there are commercially available collaborative, multimedia slide shows that hold images, documents, and videos and allow people to navigate pages and leave comments in five ways—using voice (with a microphone or telephone), text, audio file, or video (via a webcam). These programs interface with learning management systems and allow students to demonstrate a variety of skills.

Advantages

Obtaining audio recording equipment is inexpensive. Most digital cameras, cell phones, tablets, and computers have audio and video recording capabilities and are fairly inexpensive. In the case of audio recording, the presence of the microphone may be less threatening to the student than use of a video camera or direct faculty observation. Video recording works well for evaluation of mastery, particularly with psychomotor skills. These techniques allow students to practice and record their skills in private, listen to or view and critique their own performance, and even rerecord the procedure until they are satisfied with the performance before submitting it for a grade.

This strategy affords flexibility in scheduling for both students and faculty. Faculty can conduct a secondary analysis of the recording if necessary. With both audio and video recording, faculty can assess student performance with patients without being intrusive in the dynamic of the student–patient relationship.

Disadvantages

It can be difficult to distinguish individual voices in a group of participants when listening to an audio recording. One suggestion is to have each group member state his or her name at the beginning of the recording so that voices can be identified. In addition, communication has both verbal and nonverbal components. Thus, one limitation of audio recording as a strategy is that only the verbal components of the skill can be evaluated.

A certain level of competence is required in knowing how to position video equipment correctly to secure quality visual and audio recording. The skill of the cameraperson and the camera angle can affect the quality of the recording. It may be necessary to use small microphones to adequately secure the audio components. More expensive options are commonly found in high-fidelity simulation rooms, where video cameras may be mounted in multiple sites throughout the room and inputs from each camera are synchronized in a control room. Extra technical personnel are usually needed to maintain the equipment. If patients are involved, their consent is required. Requirements of the Health Insurance Portability and Accountability Act of 1996 (HIPAA) privacy rules are of concern whenever there is use of digital data from patients; therefore, protocols should be in place to maintain security. Students should be educated about the uses of the recordings, especially the issues surrounding confidentiality of the materials, and sign agreements indicating their understanding.

The experience of being recorded can cause stress to some students who may feel self-conscious about being "on camera." However, in some cases, the stress level may be lower than that experienced with direct observation by the faculty member. If patients are also being video recorded, explanations of expectations should be provided, and consent obtained before the recording begins. Evaluators need good observational skills.

Issues

The protocol for scoring must be determined before this strategy is instituted. Students need an opportunity to practice with the strategy before it is used in the assignment of a grade. A decision needs to be made about whether the entire recording or a sampling will be used for evaluation. Confidentiality and the need to obtain consent from all individuals who are included in the recording is an issue. HIPAA guidelines are required for digital patient data.

Role Play

Description and Uses

In role play, the learner portrays a specific individual and is generally given much freedom to act out that role spontaneously. Role play is particularly appropriate for objectives related to developing interpersonal relationships with patients, peers, and other health care providers (Oermann & Gaberson, 2021). The role-playing process provides a live sample of human behavior that serves as a vehicle for students to (1) explore feelings; (2) gain insight into their abilities, values, and perceptions; (3) develop their problem-solving skills and attitudes; and (4) explore subject matter in different

ways. Role playing affords students the opportunity to apply content in a relevant, everyday context that promotes deeper learning and may exceed a traditional approach (Vizeshfar et al., 2016). This may provide a rationale for the use of role playing in simulation. Role-playing in the classroom encourages active participation whether the student is part of the role play or observing the interactions. Nemec et al. (2021) provide a helpful guide for implementing role-playing in the nursing classroom as an active learning strategy that promotes the development of clinical reasoning skills.

More recently, gaming that includes varying degrees of virtual reality (VR) are being explored in nursing education. Ma et al. (2021) used computer role-playing games (CRPGs) with resultant improvement in nursing student empathy. McEnroe-Petitte and Farris (2020) reviewed the literature about gaming in nursing and concluded that it is very useful to promote student engagement; however, outcome measures were not assessed. Chen and associates (2020) conducted a metaanalysis that found increased knowledge with VR but no statistical differences in skills, satisfaction, confidence, or performance time. It is evident that additional research is needed to explore student learning outcomes from using all types of gaming in nursing education.

The time for role play can vary according to the time available and the complexity of the role play situation. The student is informed of the concept or role to be performed and given time to be creative in its presentation. The content, not the performance ability, should be assessed. The content and process can be assessed for use of communication techniques. Role reversal is used in situations in which the purpose is to change attitudes. This facilitates an understanding of opposing beliefs. On termination of the role play, the student observers analyze what occurred, what feelings were generated, what insights were gained, why things happened as they did, and how the situation is related to reality.

Advantages

Situations can be structured or prepared as open-ended responses. After students critique the role play, the process can be repeated. Role play affords the opportunity for students to practice peer review. This technique actively involves the students and fosters creativity.

Disadvantages

Role play can be awkward for the faculty and student if it is not practiced before the time of assessment or evaluation. Immediate feedback is difficult to provide if many groups are performing at the same time.

Issues

Using role play as a teaching mode before its use in evaluation assists students and faculty to become familiar with the technique and material; however, all that could happen cannot be anticipated. Students need to be informed in advance about the use of this technique for assessment. It may take time and experience to build comfort with this technique.

Patient Simulation

Description and Uses

Simulation is the creation of a representation or model that allows students to experience an imitation of a real-life situation with the purpose of practice, learning, evaluation, testing, or to gain understanding of systems or human actions (adapted from Lioce, 2020). In nursing, simulations provide a safe practice environment for student learning, assessment, and evaluation (Dreifuerst et al., 2021a). The continuum of simulation ranges from role playing to high-fidelity, computer-supported simulation that uses realistic mannequins and computer-driven equipment to closely replicate real-life clinical situations.

Use of standardized patients (individuals who are trained to act as patients) is another form of role playing used to evaluate student performance in simulations. The objective structured clinical examination (OSCE) has been implemented in nursing at both the undergraduate and graduate levels to determine clinical competency. Studies have shown that faculty and students agree this is a realistic way to assess clinical ability (Vincent et al., 2022). Students have a positive response to this approach and improved self-efficacy was noted with graduate students following their experiences (Montgomery et al., 2021).

The use of virtual reality, "any learning that is offered in a reality that is not the current physical environment" (Dreifuerst et al., 2021b, p. 240) is expanding. It can be 2- or 3-dimensional, depending on available equipment. These screen-based simulations can be quite robust; some tracking participants' responses and providing prompts and feedback. The National Council of State Boards of Nursing study on simulation demonstrated that undergraduate students could experience up to 50% of clinical instruction via simulation (Hayden et al., 2014). Simulation is heavily relied upon due to increasingly limited clinical resources, and challenges created by the COVID-19 pandemic, when simulation became an essential method to continue nursing education experiences during clinical site and campus closures (Dreifuerst et al., 2021b; Shea & Rovera, 2021). The process of assessment and evaluation is tied to debriefing. Lioce (2020, p. 15) defines debriefing as "a session after a simulation event where educators/instructors/facilitators and learners reexamine the simulation experience for the purpose of moving toward assimilation and accommodation of learning to future situations." A structured debriefing was found to be most effective (Lee et al., 2021). Arrogante et al. (2021) found that using simulation as a formative assessment was more positively received by students than its use as evaluation. Reliability and validity of assessment instruments are important, especially when simulation is used for summative purposes. Faculty need to consider the most appropriate way to assess and evaluate clinical learning. Both faculty and students need to be clear about the purpose of the simulation. For example, distinguishing simulation used for assessment (feedback for improvement) from use for evaluation and grading is important.

Advantages

Standardized patients and low-fidelity and high-fidelity simulation provide safe environments to assess and evaluate skills that are essential for quality nursing practice. Low-fidelity simulations can allow the opportunity for students to practice psychomotor skills in a more authentic environment. For example, instead of setting up individual stations where students validate their ability to perform procedures, a more authentic simulation involves new orders on a given patient that requires performance of the skills in the context of patient care. The combination of video recording with simulation provides opportunities for debriefing with students and for faculty to establish IRR when evaluating the simulations. Faculty must carefully consider if these situations are appropriate for evaluation or better used to help students learn. Timing in the semester may dictate the choice. In addition to assessing skill performance and demonstration of higher order thinking skills of an individual student, simulations also allow for assessment of team and interprofessional interaction. High-fidelity simulations have been used for IPE to improve communication and teamwork across disciplines. Students and faculty alike find the simulated patient care environment interesting and stimulating. Again, faculty must be thoughtful in their decision to use simulations for grading and evaluation in these situations.

Disadvantages

The main disadvantage of using high-fidelity simulations for evaluation is the time and expense involved. Although equipment cost is decreasing, it remains rather high for the initial purchase. Another disadvantage is that simulations can only accommodate a small number of active participants at a given time. Similarly, disadvantages of using standardized patients include the training required, the expense involved, and increased faculty workload for evaluation. Arrogante et al. (2021) found that using simulation as a formative assessment was more positively received by students than its use as a summative assessment. Students cited limited time and anxiety in the summative evaluation. The authors recommended increased student orientation and experiences with simulation prior to its use as a summative evaluation. Establishing IRR for faculty who debrief and assess student performance is essential. Bradley et al. (2021) established that the Debriefing for Meaningful Learning Scale is a valid and reliable tool and provides a method to establish faculty IRR for debriefing. Schaye et al. (2022) validated the revised-IDEA assessment tool to build a shared mental model for feedback on clinical reasoning in the admission notes of medical school residents and fellows. They plan to develop an algorithm for an automated feedback program with this tool as a way of improving timeliness and decreasing faculty workload in providing feedback. Lewallen and Van Horn (2019) and Lee et al. (2021) noted in their respective systematic reviews of clinical evaluation and debriefing methods that very few valid and reliable tools were available to evaluate the construct of clinical competency or best methods to conduct debriefing. Both propose standardized evaluation tools should be tested with large numbers of students for validity and reliability.

Issues

Major issues related to using simulation as an evaluation strategy include but are not limited to selection of scenarios, opportunity for practice before evaluation, maintenance of equipment, adequate technical support, faculty education and training, personnel needs, and efficient scheduling of students. The format of the scenario for evaluation should match the format used for practice. There is a need for ample opportunity for student practice and receipt of formative feedback before using simulation for summative evaluation. This assists the students to become more comfortable with the simulated environment before they receive a grade (even if it is satisfactory or unsatisfactory).

Using reliable and valid instruments for evaluation and ensuring IRR for those providing debriefing and assessment of their use is another issue. The International Nursing Association for Clinical Simulation and Learning (INACSL) has standards addressing all components of simulation. The standards for debriefing are especially relevant to this discussion (INACSL, 2021). Time for faculty development and training is another consideration.

The efficient scheduling of students for evaluation must be addressed as simulations only accommodate a small number of active participants, whether simulations are used as a teaching, assessment, or evaluation strategy. Scheduling interprofessional simulated experiences has the additional challenge of layering student schedules from multiple disciplines. When collaborative partnerships have been developed between practice and academia for shared simulation equipment and space, scheduling issues may again be complicated, such as priority for the use of the

CASE STUDY 23.2 Choosing an Assessment Strategy for a Simulation Using an Interprofessional Partnership

To meet the interprofessional partnership competencies related to teamwork, communication and conflict resolution, senior capstone students are completing a simulation. The team is comprised of students from nursing, medicine, pharmacy, nutrition, and social work. The case centers around a homeless veteran admitted from the ED in diabetic ketoacidosis (DKA). Choose an assessment strategy to determine how the students meet the following competencies:

1. Which assessment strategy will determine how students meet the following competency?
"Evaluate effectiveness of interprofessional communication tools and techniques to support and improve the efficacy of team-based interactions." (AACN, 2021, p. 42)
2. Which assessment strategy will determine how students are meeting the following competency?
"Engage health and other professionals in shared patient-centered and population-focused problem solving." (IPEC, 2016, p. 14)
3. What challenges might arise from developing an assessment strategy for an interprofessional partnership?

equipment, technical support, and use of personnel to administer the simulation. When large numbers of students must complete a simulated evaluation over the course of several days, there is a risk of losing the security of the exam. One way to address this is by having multiple simulation scenarios that test the same competency. (See Case Study 23.2.)

Service-Learning

Description and Uses

Many college campuses have embraced community engagement as part of their engagement mission as evidenced by their participation in organizations such as Campus Compact (https://compact.org). Service-learning, either as the framework for a course or as a component within a course, creates ways of engaging students with the community, and creating opportunities for civic engagement while also learning professional skills. Service-learning experiences can meet curricular goals to develop civic and community engagement (see also Chapter 12 and 13).

A service-learning project can take multiple forms. It can be designed as an individual project where one student works on a project that meets a need for an agency (e.g., developing an in-service for a nursing unit on a given topic) or it may be a group project wherein several students work together (e.g., developing and carrying out a health fair for senior citizens at a community center), or may be part of an international study abroad program (e.g., an interprofessional group working to provide clean water for a community in a developing country). Zhu et al. (2022) found in their systematic review of research in service-learning with nursing students that students increased their appreciation of cultural issues and contexts. They also found that students gained skills in leadership and collaboration.

Venter (2020) proposes a synergy between appreciative inquiry (AI) and service-learning that enhances engagement, relationships among team members, and leads to meaningful actions. Using formative evaluation strategies such as an appreciative inquiry (AI) reflection at least once with a service-learning group at the midpoint of the project can be useful in addressing challenges that arise in the teams. Timing of the AI reflection midway through the project allows the group to adjust their processes and helps with self-awareness.

Typically, a final group presentation or report is submitted for evaluation and grading. An example of a rubric for a group presentation is in Table 23.1. Rodriguez-Nogueria et al. (2020) determined that physiotherapy students experienced gains in social–emotional skills of empathy, inclusivity, and collaboration in clinical practice as well as an appreciation of their abilities to handle the stress as a result of a semester-long service-learning project. They used three reflective sessions as well as a personal reflective journal for the evaluation process. Naumann et al. (2021) found that students from four different professions reported gains in their value of teamwork for patient care and better appreciation of the contribution of other professions to improve outcomes of diabetic patients because of a service-learning project. They also noted that students valued the authenticity of the learning experience and thought it was best suited for the later part of their learning program.

Advantages

A service-learning project has relevance for the students because the learning experience is authentic and based in a real-world situation. Seating the learning in the context of reality exposes students to situations they may encounter after graduation, and it allows them the opportunity to find their way while still having the support of faculty. Through service-learning students may have first-hand experience with health care disparities, work with communities whose culture is different from their own and learn at a personal level the way community organizations interface with health care. Service-learning projects provide students the opportunity to better understand the needs of individuals and communities. The fit with the national emphasis of nurses working to improve the health of the nation is clear. Service-learning can contribute to positive visibility for the school when contributions provided by the service-learning projects meet needs of the community. Evaluations from service-learning projects may also contribute to documenting program outcomes for cultural and social sensitivities as well as interprofessional competencies and leadership skills.

Disadvantages

Time for faculty to manage service-learning projects can be viewed as a disadvantage because out-of-class time is required to meet with the agencies, arrange the experiences, and follow up regularly with students and agencies. It takes care to be sure that the expectations of the agency are in concert with the expectations of the faculty for the learning requirements and that evaluation criteria align with both sets of expectations. Faculty may need to help students clarify and resolve conflicts with agencies and within groups. There is also a risk that the student group may fall short of the expectation of the agency and the reputation of the school could be jeopardized in the community.

Issues

The ultimate question becomes how to evaluate the learning that takes place. Again, the faculty must focus on the desired learning outcomes. For example, if the primary purpose is to help students learn to work in teams, evaluation strategies that emphasize growth in self-awareness, communications, and conflict resolution are appropriate.

When working on an interprofessional service-learning project, faculty need to collaborate to ensure that the project meets course outcomes for each profession. Scheduling of group meetings may be a challenge across professions. A variety of strategies may be used for evaluation. It is common to have reflections or papers as a means to consider the outcomes. Group work or teamwork can be triangulated by looking at individual and group reports in addition to observation by the faculty and the agency staff. In some cases, students may be asked to provide peer review.

Evaluation processes should be shared with students prior to the experience. Agencies, preceptors, and students are all sources of evaluation data. Standardization of evaluation is important to better demonstrate the effect of service-learning on student learning outcomes and ultimately on the profession. Organizing, supervising, and evaluating service-learning activities requires time from the faculty to develop, nurture, and maintain relationships with the community partner.

CHAPTER SUMMARY: KEY POINTS

- Using more than one strategy will more fully demonstrate student outcome achievement.
- When using any evaluation strategy, students should have the opportunity to practice before the activity is used for grading.
- The strategies addressed in this chapter include portfolios, reflections, papers, essays and essay tests, concept mapping, oral questioning, audio and video recordings, simulations, role play, and service-learning.

- To select the best strategy, faculty members must consider the purpose and setting; the time required for preparation, implementation, and grading; the cost; and the advantages and disadvantages of each strategy.
- Although it requires time, energy, and persistence to plan evaluation of student achievement of learning outcomes, the effort ultimately benefits students and the patients they are preparing to serve.
- Faculty who implement evaluation strategies will continue to increase the evidence base for best practices and contribute to the scholarship of teaching.
- The findings from the use of assessment and evaluation strategies can be used for a variety of purposes:
  - to provide feedback to the learner and to revise instruction and learning activities.
  - as evidence of critical thinking, clinical reasoning, and therapeutic communication as a part of the systematic program assessment plan.
  - evidence of individual faculty effectiveness in teaching.
- As nursing education meets current challenges, the refinement of assessment and evaluation strategies will continue to expand in tandem with the development of teaching strategies, thereby contributing to the ever-increasing quality of education for nurses of the future.

REFLECTING ON THE EVIDENCE

1. How might you assess student appreciation of the culture of poverty and its impact on population health and associated health care policy implications?
2. Your course uses a group project to meet specific outcomes. Using the information in this chapter, determine a plan to assess the acquisition of teamwork and problem-solving skills. In addition, you would like to assess the individual effort of the group members to the product.
3. Choose a learning experience that is employed in your course and select a way to use the principles of assessment discussed in this chapter to evolve the learning experience into an assessment strategy.
4. The graduate nursing course you are teaching has the following learning outcome:
   - Appraise scientific evidence as a tool in advocating for a vulnerable population.

   Develop a plan to evaluate this course's student learning outcome based on ideas from this chapter.

REFERENCES

Abou-Hanna, J., Owens, S., Kinnucan, J., Mian, S., & Kolars, J. (2021). Resuscitating the Socratic method: Student and faculty perspectives on posing probing questions during clinical teaching. *Academic Medicine, 96*(1), 113–117. https://doi.org/10.1097/ACM.0000000000003580.

American Association of Colleges of Nursing. (2021). *The essentials: Core competencies for professional nursing education*. https://www.aacnnursing.org/AACN-Essentials

Anderson, L. W., & Krathwohl, D. R. (Eds.). (2001). *A taxonomy for learning, teaching, and assessing: A revision of Bloom's taxonomy of educational objectives.* Pearson.

Arrogante, O., Gonzalez-Romero, G., Lopez-Torre, E., Carrion-Garcia, L., & Polo, A. (2021). Comparing formative and summative simulation-based assessment in undergraduate nursing students: Nursing competency acquisition and clinical simulation satisfaction. *BMC Nursing, 20*(92). https://doi.org/10.1186/s12912-021-00614-2.

Bank, C. -G., & Daxburger, H. (2020). Concept maps for structuring instruction and as a potential assessment tool in a large introductory science course. *Journal of College Science Teaching*, *49*(6), 65–75. https://www.nsta.org/journal-college-science-teaching/journal-college-science-teaching-julyaugust-2020/concept-maps.

Beach, R., & Marshall, J. (1991). *Teaching literature in the secondary school*. Harcourt.

Bearman, M., Dawson, P., Ajjawi, R., Tai, J., & Boud, D. (2020). *Re-imagining university assessment in a digital world*. Springer.

Beccaria, L., Kek, M., & Huijser, H. (2019). Using "just in time" online feedback to improve first year undergraduate nursing students' essay writing performance. *Journal of University Teaching & Learning Practice*, *16*(4), 2019. https://ro.uow.edu.au/jutlp/vol16/iss4/7.

Belur, J., Tompson, L., Thornton, A., & Simon, M. (2021). Interrater reliability in systematic review methodology: Exploring variation in coder decision-making. *Sociological Methods & Research*, *50*(2), 837–865. https://doi.org/10.1177/0049124118799372.

Bevis, O. M., & Watson, J. (1989). *Toward a caring curriculum: A new pedagogy for nursing*. National League for Nursing.

Bradley, C. S., Johnson, B., & Dreifuerst, K. T. (2021). Psychometric properties of the revised DML evaluation scale: A new instrument for assessing debriefers. *Clinical Simulation in Nursing*, *56*, 99–107. https://www.nursingsimulation.org/article/S1876-1399(21)00047-5/fulltext.

Brown, L., Briscoe, G., & Grabowsky, A. (2022). The influence of journaling on nursing students: A systematic review. *Journal of Nursing Education*, *61*(1), 29–35. https://doi.org/10.3928/01484834-20211203-01.

Campaign for Action. (2021). *Campaign for action dashboard*. https://campaignforaction.org/resource/campaign-dashboard-indicators

Cardwell, L. (2020). Engaging learners in the evaluation process. *Continuing Education in Nursing*, *51*(4). https://doi.org/ezproxy.lib.purdue.edu/10.3928/00220124-20200317-02.

Chen, F. -Q., Leng, Y. -F., Ge, J. -F., Wang, D. -W., Li, C., Chen, B., & Sun, Z. -L. (2020). Effectiveness of virtual reality in nursing education: Meta-analysis. *Journal of Medical Internet Research*, *22*(9). https://www.jmir.org/2020/9/e18290.

Cronenwett, L., Sherwood, G., Barnsteiner, J., Disch, J., Johnson, J., Mitchell, P., Sullivan, D. T., Sullivan, D. T., & Warren, J. (2007). Quality and safety education for nurses. *Nursing Outlook*, *55*(3), 122–131. https://doi.org/10.1016/j.outlook.2007.02.006.

Davis, B. G. (2009). *Tools for teaching* (2nd ed.). Jossey-Bass.

Dewald, R. J. (2020). How would Socrates enhance online learning in nursing education. *Nursing Education Perspectives*, *41*(4), 253–254. https://doi.org/10.1097/01.NEP.0000000000000582.

Donnelly, F., McLiesh, P., & Bessell, S. (2020). Using 360° video to enable affective learning in nursing education. *Journal of Nursing Education*, *59*(7), 409–412. https://doi.org/10.3928/01484834-20200617-11.

Dreifuerst, K. T., Bradley, C. S., & Johnson, B. K. (2021a). Debriefing: An essential component for learning in simulation pedagogy. In P. R. Jeffries (Ed.), *Clinical simulations in nursing education: From conceptualization to evaluation* (3rd ed., pp. 45–68). Wolters Kluwer.

Dreifuerst, K. T., Bradley, C. S., & Johnson, B. K. (2021b). Using debriefing for meaningful learning with screen-based simulation. *Nurse Educator*, *46*(4), 239–244. https://doi.org/10.1097/NNE.0000000000000930.

Eisner, E. (1985). *The educational imagination* (2nd ed.). Macmillan.

Farrell, O. (2020). From portafoglio to eportfolio: The evolution of portfolio in higher education. *Journal of Interactive Media in Education*, *2020*(1), 19. https://doi.org/10.5334/jime.574.

Fieler, G. (2020). Utilization of video for competency evaluation. *Nursing Education Perspectives*, *41*(4), 255–257. https://doi.org/10.1097/01.NEP.0000000000000645.

Flournoy, E. L., & Bauman, L. C. (2021). Collaborative assessment: Using self-assessment and reflection for student learning and program development. *The Canadian Journal for the Scholarship of Teaching and Learning*, *12*(1). https://doi.org/10.5206/cjsotl-rcacea.2021.1.14207.

Gleason, K., Harkless, G., Stanley, J., Olson, A., & Graber, M. (2021). The critical need for nursing education to address the diagnostic process. *Nursing Outlook*, *69*(3), 362–369. https://doi.org/10.1016/j.outlook.2020.12.005.

Gray, J. R., & Grove, S. K. (2021). *Burns and Grove's The practice of nursing research* (9th Ed.). Elsevier.

Hayden, J. K., Smiley, R. A., Alexander, M., Kardong-Edgren, S., & Jeffries, P. R. (2014). The NCSBN national simulation study: A longitudinal, randomized, controlled study replacing clinical hours with simulation in prelicensure nursing education. *Journal of Nursing Regulation*, *5*(2), S3–S40. https://doi.org/10.1016/S2155-8256(15)30062-4.

Hubal, R., Bobbitt, L., Garfinkle, S., Harris, S. C., Powell, B. D., Oxley, M. S., Anksorus, H. N., & Chen, K. Y. (2020). Testing of a program to automatically analyze students' concept maps. *Pharmacy, 8*(4), 209. https://doi.org/10.3390/pharmacy8040209.

INACSL Standards Committee, Decker, S., Alinier, G., Crawford, S. B., Gordon, R. M., & Wilson, C. (2021, September). Healthcare Simulation Standards of Best Practice™ the debriefing process. *Clinical Simulation in Nursing, 58*, 27–32. https://doi.org/10.1016/j.ecns.2021.08.011.

Institute of Medicine. (2011). *The future of nursing: Leading change, advancing health.* The National Academies Press. https://doi.org/10.17226/12956.

Interprofessional Education Collaborative (IPEC). (2016). *Core competencies for interprofessional collaborative practice: 2016 update.* Interprofessional Education Collaborative. https://www.ipecollaborative.org/ipec-core-competencies.

Jeffries, P. R. (Ed.). (2021). *Clinical simulations in nursing education: From conceptualization to evaluation* (3rd ed.). Wolters Kluwer.

Jonassen, S., & Yarbrough, A. (2021). Integrating technology in skills lab: Using smartphones for urinary catheter validation. *Journal of Professional Nursing, 37*, 702–705. https://doi.org/10.1016/j.profnurs.2021.04.005.

Kahn, S. (2019). Transforming assessment, assessing transformation: ePortfolio assessment trends. In S. P. Hundley & S. Kahn (Eds.), *Trends in assessment: Ideas, opportunities, and issues for higher education (Chapter 9).* Stylus Publishing LLC.

Kapuza, A., Koponen, I. T., & Tyumeneva, Y. (2020). The network approach to assess the structure of knowledge: Storage, distribution and retrieval as three measures in analyzing concept maps. *British Journal of Educational Technology, 51*(6), 2573–2590. https://doi.org/10.1111/bjet.12938.

Kilgour, P., Northcote, M., Williams, A., & Kilgour, A. (2020). A plan for the co-construction and collaborative use of rubrics for student learning. *Assessment in Higher Education, 45*(1), 140–153. https://doi.org/10.1080/02602938.2019.1614523.

Killam, L. A., & Camargo-Plazas, P. (2021). Revisioning assessment and evaluation in nursing education through critical caring pedagogy: Using authentic examinations to promote critical consciousness. *Advances in Nursing Science, 45*(1), E15–E30. https://doi.org/10.1097/ANS.0000000000000382.

Krieglstein, F., Schneider, S., Beege, M., & Ray, G. D. (2022). How the design and complexity of concept maps influence cognitive learning process. *Education Technology Research Development* https://doi.org/10.1007/s11423-022-10083-2.

Kroeze, K. A., Van Den Berg, S. M., Veldkamp, B. P., & De Jong, T. (2021). Automated assessment of and feedback on concept maps during inquiry learning. *IEEE Transactions on Learning Technologies, 14*(4), 460–473. https://doi.org/10.1109/TLT.2021.3103331.

Lafave, L. M. Z., Yeo, M., & Lafave, M. R. (2021). Concept mapping toward competency: teaching and assessing undergraduate evidence-informed practice. *Competency Based Education, 6*(2). https://doi.org/10.1002/cbe2.1242.

Lee, J., Park, C. G., Kim, S. H., & Bae, J. (2021). Psychometric properties of a clinical reasoning assessment rubric for nursing education. *BMC nursing, 20*(1), 177. https://doi.org/10.1186/s12912-021-00695-z.

Lewallen, L., & Van Horn, E. (2019). The state of the science on clinical evaluation in nursing education. *Nursing Education Perspectives, 40*(1), 4–10. https://doi.org/10.1097/01.NEP.0000000000000376.

Lioce, L. (Ed.). (2020). *Healthcare simulation dictionary* (2nd ed.). Agency for Healthcare Research and Quality Publication. No. 20-0019. https://doi.org/10.23970/simulationv2.

Lu, H. (2021). Electronic portfolios in higher education: A review of literature. *European Journal of Education and Pedagogy, 2*(3), 96–101. https://ej-edu.org/index.php/ejedu/article/view/119/57.

Ma, Z., Huang, K. T., & Yao, L. (2021). Feasibility of a computer role-playing game to promote empathy in nursing students: The role of immersiveness and perspective. *Cyberpsychology, Behavior, and Social Networking, 24*(11), 750–755. https://doi.org/10.1089/cyber.2020.0371.

Macartney, M. J., Pathmavathy, N., & Cooper, J. (2021). Student nurse perceptions of video simulation and critical reflection for developing clinical-reasoning skills: A cross cohort study. *Student Success, 12*(1). https://doi.org/10.5204/ssj.1653.

Masuku, M. M., Jili, N. N., & Sabela, P. T. (2021). Assessment as a pedagogy and measuring tool in promoting deep learning in institutions of higher learning. *International Journal of Higher Education, 10*(2), 274–283. https://doi.org/10.5430/ijhe.v10n2p274.

McCoach, D. B., Gable, R. K., & Madura, J. P. (2013). Defining, measuring, and scaling affective constructs: *Instrument development in the affective domain* (3rd ed.). Springer.

McConnell, K. D., Horan, E. M., Zimmerman, B., & Terrel, L. (2019). *We have a rubric for that: The VALUE approach to assessment*. Association of American Colleges and Universities.

McEnroe-Petitte, D., & Farris, C. (2020). Using gaming as an active teaching strategy in nursing education. *Teaching and Learning in Nursing*, 15(1), 61–65. https://doi.org/10.1016/j.teln.2019.09.002.

Miller, M. D., Linn, R. L., & Gronlund, N. E. (2013). *Measurement and assessment in teaching* (11th ed.). Prentice-Hall.

Mitchell, K. M., Blanchard, L., & Roberts, T. (2020). Seeking transformation: How students in nursing view their academic writing context—A qualitative systematic review. *International Journal of Nursing Education Scholarship*, 17(1). https://doi.org/10.1515/ijnes-2020-0074. 20200074.

Montgomery, A., Chang, H., Ho, M., Smerdely, P., & Traynor, V. (2021). The use and effect of OSCES in post-registration nurses: An integrative review. *Nurse Education Today*, 100. https://doi.org/10.1016/j.nedt.2021.104845.

National Academy of Medicine. (2021). *The future of nursing 2020–2030: Charting a path to achieve health equity*. The National Academies Press. https://doi.org/10.17226/25982.

National Council of State Boards of Nursing (NCSBN). (2021). *Next generation NCLEX project*. https://www.ncsbn.org/next-generation-nclex.htm

National League for Nursing. (2012). *Outcomes and competencies for graduates of practical/vocational, diploma, baccalaureate, master's practice doctorate, and research doctorate programs in nursing*. Wolters Kluwer.

Naumann, F., Mullins, R., Cawte, A., Beavis, S., Musial, J., & Hannan-Jones, M. (2021). Designing, implementing and sustaining IPE within an authentic clinical environment: the impact on student learning. *Journal of Interprofessional Care*, 35(6), 907–913. https://doi.org/10.1080/13561820.2020.1837748.

Nemec, R., Brower, E., & Allert, J. (2021). A guide to implementing role-play in the nursing classroom. *Nursing Education Perspectives (Wolters Kluwer Health)*, 42(6), E163–E164. https://doi-org.ottawa.idm.oclc.org/10.1097/01.NEP.0000000000000678.

Nkhoma, C., Nkhoma, M., Thomas, S., & Le, N.Q. (2020). The role of rubrics in learning and implementation of authentic assessment: A literature review. In M. Jones (Ed.), *Proceedings of InSITE 2020: Informing Science and Information Technology*. http://proceedings.informingscience.org/InSITE2020/InSITE2020p237–276Nkhoma6195.pdf

Novak, J. D., & Gowin, D. B. (1984). *Learning how to learn*. Cambridge University Press.

Noyes, J. A., Welch, P. M., Johnson, J. W., & Carbonneau, K. J. (2020). A systematic review of digital badges in health care education. *Medical Education*, 54(7), 600–615. https://doi.org/10.1111/medu.14060.

O'Day, G. M., & Karpicke, J. D. (2021). Comparing and combining retrieval practice and concept mapping. *Journal of Educational Psychology*, 113(5), 986–997. https://doi.org/10.1037/edu0000486.

Oermann, M., De Gagne, J., & Phillips, B. (2022). *Teaching in nursing and the role of the educator* (3rd ed.). Springer.

Oermann, M. H., & Gaberson, K. B. (2021). *Evaluation and testing in nursing education* (7th ed.). Springer.

Olantunji, M. O. (2014). The affective domain of assessment in colleges and universities: Issues and implications. *International Journal of Progressive Education*, 10(1), 101–116.

Ondrejka, D. (2014). *Affective teaching in nursing: Connecting to feelings, values, and inner awareness*. Springer.

Park, K. H., Kam, B. S., Yune, S. J., Lee, S. Y., & Im, S. J. (2022). Changes in self-reflective thinking level in writing and educational needs of medical students: A longitudinal study. *PLoS One*, 17(1), e0262250. https://doi.org/10.1371/journal.pone.0262250.

Parker, F. M., & McMillan, L. R. (2020). Using e-portfolio to showcase and enhance soft skill reflection of MSN students. *Journal of Nursing Education*, 59(5), 300. https://doi.org/10.3928/01484834-20200422-16.

Rodriguez-Nogueira, O., Moreno-Poyato, A., Alvarez-Alvarez, M., & Pinto-Carral, A. (2020). Significant socio-emotional learning and improvement of empathy in physiotherapy students through service-learning methodology: A mixed methods research. *Nurse Education Today*, 90. https://doi.org/10.1016/j.nedt.2020.104437.

Roscoe, R. D., Wilson, J., Johnson, A. C., & Mayra, C. R. (2017). Presentation, expectations, and experience: Sources of student perceptions of automated writing evaluation. *Computers in Human Behavior*, 70, 207–221. https://doi.org/10.1016/j.chb.2016.12.076.

Schaye, V., Miller, L., Kudlowitz, D., Chun, J., Burk-Rafel, J., Cocks, P., Guzman, B., Aphinyanaphong,

Y., & Marin, M. (2022). Development of a clinical reasoning documentation assessment tool for resident and fellow admission notes: A shared mental model for feedback. *Journal of General Internal Medicine*, 37(3), 507–512. https://doi.org/10.1007/s11606-021-06805-6.

Schön, D. A. (1983). *The reflective practitioner: How professionals think in action*. Basic Books.

Shea, K., & Rovera, E. (2021). Preparing for the COVID-19 pandemic and its impact on a nursing simulation curriculum. *Journal of Nursing Education*, 60(1), 52–55. https://doi.org/10.3928/01484834-20201217-12.

Stanley, D., Coman, S., Murdoch, D., & Stanley, K. (2020). Writing exceptional (specific, student, and criterion-focused) rubrics for nursing studies. *Nurse Education in Practice*, 49. https://doi.org/10.1016/j.nepr.2020.102851.

Stec, M., & Garritano, N. (2016). Portfolio implementation as a means for achievement of standards. *The Journal for Research and Practice in College Teaching*, 1(2), 1–6.

Sturdivant, T., & Allen-Thomas, K. (2022). Teaching with a PURPOSE: An NGN approach to clinical education and assessment. *Teaching and Learning in Nursing*, 17(1), 7–10. https://doi.org/10.1016/j.teln.2021.10.004.

Tan, R., Ting, J. J. Q., Hong, D. Z., Lim, A. J. S., Ong, Y. T., Pisupati, A., Chong, E. J. X., Chiam, M., Lee, A. A. I. A., Tan, L. H., Chin, A. M. C., Wijaya, L., Fong, W., & Krishna, L. K. R. (2022). Medical student portfolios: A systematic scoping review. *Journal of Medical Education and Curricular Development*, 9, 1–15. https://doi.org/10.1177/23821205221076022.

Thammasitboon, S., & Brand, P. L. (2021). The physiology of learning: Strategies clinical teachers can adopt to facilitate learning. *European Journal of Pediatrics*, 181, 429–433. https://doi.org/10.1007/s00431-021-04054-7.

Venter, K. (2020). An appreciative leadership integrated service-learning praxis framework for positive organisations or institutions. *AI Practitioner: International journal of appreciative inquiry*, 22(1). https://doi.org/10.12781/978-1-907549-42-7-10.

Vincent, S. C., Arulappan, J., Amirtharaj, A., Matua, G. A., & Hashmi, I. A. (2022). Objective structured clinical examination vs traditional clinical examination to evaluate students' clinical competence: A systematic review of nursing faculty and students' perceptions and experiences. *Nurse Education Today*, 108, 105170. https://doi.org/10.1016/j.nedt.2021.105170.

Vizeshfar, F., Dehghanrad, F., Magharei, M., & Sobhani, S. M. (2016, March). Effects of applying role playing approach on nursing students' education. *International Journal of Humanities and Cultural Studies*, 5(2). http://www.ijhcs.com/index.php/ijhcs/index.

Ying, J. (2020). Embedding and facilitating intercultural competence development in internationalization of the curriculum of higher education. *Journal of Curriculum and Teaching*, 9(3). https://doi.org/10.5430/jct.v9n3p13.

Zhu, Z., Xing, W., Liang, Y., Hong, L., & Hu, Y. (2022). Nursing students' experiences with service-learning: A qualitative systematic review and meta-synthesis. *Nurse Education Today*, 108. https://doi.org/10.1016/j.nedt.2021.105206.

24

Using Classroom Tests to Evaluate Student Attainment of Learning Outcomes

Diane M. Billings, EdD, RN, ANEF, FAAN

Evaluating student learning is a significant aspect of the faculty role, one that ensures the students' ability to provide safe nursing care and determines progression throughout the academic program. Both commercial and faculty-made classroom tests are frequently used to make decisions about students' potential success and ultimately about their attainment of program and course learning outcomes. Because tests can sample a large body of knowledge and are easy to administer, they are used in most academic programs to determine course grades and progression throughout the program. Thus, faculty have an ethical and professional responsibility to ensure that the tests they develop and grades they assign are valid, reliable, and fair.

Although developing classroom tests seems like a relatively straightforward task, it is, in fact, an involved process and one that takes time to develop. Moran et al. (2022) in a national study of faculty test-taking abilities found that few faculty are actually prepared to write test questions and recommend developing an evidence-based item writing process and related school policies. Moore (2021) found that evidence-based testing practices such as using a blueprint, writing questions to test course learning outcomes and higher-order thinking and judgment skills, and using item analysis procedures to revise test questions were observed more often by experienced faculty who had 5 or more years of experience than by those who were identified as having less than 5 years of experience. In this chapter, readers will learn seven evidence-based steps to follow when evaluating students' attainment of course learning

outcomes using teacher-made classroom tests. The steps include planning the test; using a test blueprint; writing test items and obtaining peer review; administering the test and maintaining test security; analyzing test results; conducting a posttest review with course faculty and students; and assigning grades.

PLANNING THE TEST

Developing or using a test that is valid (representative) and reliable (consistent) requires much thought and planning. Before planning the test, faculty must review all aspects of the teaching–learning cycle (writing student competencies and learning outcomes, providing instruction followed by active learning, ensuring all students have attained the learning outcomes through practice and assessment, and finally, developing and administering the test). At this time, faculty must ensure that the test to be developed links to the preceding steps of the teaching–learning cycle.

During the planning stage, faculty must make thoughtful and informed decisions about the test design, administration, and use of the test results. These decisions must be based on evidence, follow best practices, and be made *before* the test is administered and graded. Also, information about the test and grading scale must be posted in the information about the course evaluation methods in the course syllabus before faculty administer the test(s). This section discusses the plans that are considered before developing the test: determining the purpose of the test, understanding the type of test (criterion-referenced versus norm-referenced tests), developing a test blueprint, choosing item types, writing test items, and improving the reliability and validity of a test.

Purpose of the Test

Tests in nursing education are given for a variety of reasons, and faculty must first determine how the test will be used. If using an already developed test, it will also be important to understand the validity and reliability and other metrics of the test because test results have significant consequences for evaluating learning and determining students' admission, progression, and graduation.

Tests Used to Determine Admission, Progression, and Graduation

One of the first tests nursing students may encounter is one of those used for admission. Although there are a variety of standardized college admissions tests such as the Scholastic Aptitude Test (SAT) and the Graduate Record Exam (GRE) that may be required for admission to the college or university, faculty are reconsidering the usefulness of these tests for determining the potential for success in their program. In prelicensure programs, many schools use a battery of tests specifically designed to test basic academic skills of nursing students. Faculty must continually monitor the contribution of standardized tests to the overall student recruitment and admission practices at their school.

Standardized tests are also used, particularly in prelicensure nursing programs, to monitor students' progress throughout the program and as an exit examination at the end of the program that may be used to determine whether the student graduates. Because the decisions made based on these tests have serious consequences for the student admitted and progressing through the program, these tests are referred to as *high-stakes* tests (National League for Nursing, 2021). When using commercially developed tests that are used primarily for high-stakes evaluations, faculty must consider the ethical and legal aspects of using these tests in addition to the cultural and socioeconomic diversity of the students who will be taking the tests. For example, faculty must consider the implications for students when standardized tests

are used to determine progression or graduation for students who have paid tuition, demonstrated attainment of learning on teacher-made tests, and demonstrated requisite knowledge, skills, and attitudes in clinical practice. Some schools use the results of commercially available achievement exams to gauge their students' achievement against national norms for that test and use the information for curriculum planning and not for decisions about course grades. Faculty can develop or revise policies about how to use the results to promote learning; ensure fairness about decisions affecting admission, progression, and graduation; and satisfy concerns from students and external program review agencies.

Tests Used to Determine Readiness or Placement or as Advance Organizers

If the test is to be given *before* instruction as a pretest, the test may be used to determine readiness (the grasp of prerequisite skills needed to be successful) or placement (the level of mastery of instructional objectives). Administering a test that is similar to a unit or final examination can also serve as an "advance organizer" to alert students to significant content that should be learned and will be subsequently tested.

Tests Used to Improve Learning (Practice Tests)

During instruction, tests may be used as an *assessment* strategy for students to practice taking the type of question that will appear on the test. Here, tests are used as formative evaluation of learning or as a diagnostic tool to identify problems with understanding the course concepts or in answering a particular type of test question.

Faculty can use practice tests in several ways. The practice test question can be embedded in pre/post and during classroom activities such as adding test questions to a PowerPoint presentation, having students work in small groups to answer a case study, collaborate in a team to answer test questions as they might appear on an exam, or take short quizzes after each class session. Faculty can also place practice test questions in a learning management system and either assign the students to take the test and award minimal points for completing the assignment or make the use of the practice test questions optional. Sartain and Wright (2021) found that frequent quizzing improved students' test scores when using practice tests after short presentations of information in an online or on-campus classroom setting using a lecture or narrated PowerPoint presentation as a teaching–learning strategy.

Another approach to including practice tests in a learning setting is to use computerized adaptive quizzing programs. Adaptive quizzes are tailored to the students' learning needs by determining a baseline of student abilities, and as the student answers more questions correctly, the difficulty of the question is increased until the student attains a preset level of mastery. In a review of literature about testing effects, Binks (2017) found that testing improves learning when the test requires students to apply information rather than recognize it. Similarly, Tu et al. (2017) found that test-enhanced learning, the use of testing with feedback after instruction, was effective, particularly for low-scoring students. Additionally, adaptive quizzing systems used for formative testing can improve student learning and reduce course failure (Simon-Campbell & Phelan, 2016) and improve end-of-program examination scores (Presti & Sanko, 2010). With the wide availability of test banks, such as those that accompany textbooks, and the ease of creating tests in a test-authoring component of a learning management system, faculty can use tests as a way for students to practice and assess their own learning.

Types of Tests Used to Determine Grades

The most common use of tests is to assign grades. In this situation, tests serve as a way of evaluating learning outcomes and provide summative evaluation of learning on which grading decisions may be based.

Criterion-referenced tests. Criterion-referenced tests are those that are constructed and interpreted according to a specific set of learning outcomes (McDonald, 2018). This type of test is useful for measuring mastery of subject matter. An absolute standard of performance is set for grading purposes. Typically, nurse educators tend to use criterion-referenced tests because the goal of nursing education is for all students to attain mastery of the content. For example, criterion-referenced tests are frequently used to ensure safety in areas such as drug dosage calculation, in which the absolute standard of performance may be set as high as 100%, regardless of the performance of other students.

Norm-referenced tests. Norm-referenced tests are those that are constructed and interpreted to provide a relative ranking of students (McDonald, 2018). This type of test is useful for measuring differential performance among students. A relative standard of performance is used for grading purposes. Standardized tests such as the SAT and GRE are examples of norm-referenced tests.

USING A TEST BLUEPRINT

A test blueprint (table of specifications, test map, test grid, test plan) is a visual representation of the relationship of the test item to the course competency/learning outcome and the relative number of the items for each course competency. The purpose of the test blueprint is to ensure that the test serves its intended purpose by representatively sampling the intended course competencies/learning outcomes and instructional content.

The first step in developing a test blueprint is to review *course competencies/student learning outcomes* and determine which competencies are to be evaluated using a test. At this time, faculty should identify at which level of the cognitive domain the student is expected to attain the competency and link the test question to that level of the domain. The test question must align with the course competency, and in some instances faculty may determine that the course competency needs to be revised to more accurately define the expected level of the competency the student is to attain. Bloom's taxonomy has been used as a guide for developing and leveling course competencies and thus also serves as a guide for linking the level of the learning outcome to the level of the test question (Anderson & Krathwohl, 2001). Although the cognitive components of the affective and psychomotor domains can be evaluated using tests, tests have most often been used to determine achievement of outcomes in the revised six levels of Bloom's cognitive domain (see Chapter 10).

The NCLEX licensing examinations place emphasis on cognitive processing skills used by nurses, such as critical thinking and clinical judgment (Dickison et al., 2017), and tests that are being used to prepare students to take licensing examinations should develop test items that evaluate learning at higher levels of the cognitive domain. This is vital because higher-level skills are more likely to result in retention and transfer of knowledge, and they will assist in preparing students for the licensing and certification examinations that test primarily at the levels of application and above.

The second step in developing a test blueprint involves *determining the instructional content to be evaluated and the weight to be assigned to each area*. This can be accomplished by developing a content outline based on lesson, unit, or course learning outcomes. Faculty can develop a simple blueprint with a two-way grid that includes the competencies, content, and number of questions about each content area (Table 24.1). Some faculty prefer to use a comprehensive test blueprint based on the National Council of State Boards of Nursing (NCSBN) licensing examination blueprint. This blueprint identifies the number of questions per content area and information about the competency being tested, the level of the cognitive domain, the type of question, client needs category and related activity statement, and the integrated processes (Table 24.2). This type of blueprint ensures that both students and faculty understand what is being tested and how each question relates to all components of the licensing examination blueprint. Faculty can also *use the test blueprint to ensure the test evaluates intended learning outcomes and aligns with the teaching, learning, and practice activities.*

Selecting Item Types

Several types of items can be used to test attainment of learning outcomes. Items may be selection-type, providing a set of responses from which to choose, or supply-type, a constructed response type requiring the student to provide an answer. Common *selection-type* items include true–false, matching, multiple-choice, multiple-response, cloze, matrix, and ordered-response questions. *Supply-type* items include fill-in-the-blank, short-answer, and essay questions. If teaching prelicensure students, faculty should obtain current information on the types of test questions and examination format at the NCSBN (http://www.ncsbn.org).

The primary reason for choosing one type of item over another can be determined by answering the question: "Which type of item most directly measures the intended learning outcome?" Both selection-type and supply-type questions can be developed for all levels of the cognitive domain and to test critical thinking and nursing clinical judgment. Other factors may also influence the item-type selection. For example, a large class size may prohibit the use of supply-type items because of the time required for grading the test item.

Selecting Item Difficulty

Determining the item difficulty, the percentage of students who answered the question correctly primarily depends on the purpose and type of the test. If the purpose of the test is to evaluate

TABLE 24.1 **Sample Test Blueprint Using Learning Outcomes and Content Topics**					
Learning Outcome	**Topic A**	**Topic B**	**Topic C**	**Topic D**	**Topic E**
Assess client for side effects of medications	Question 1		Question 2		Questions 3, 4, 5
Assess client's heart sounds		Question 6			
Develop a care plan for a client with heart disease	Question 7	Question 8		Question 9	Question 10

TABLE 24.2 Sample Test Blueprint Using Elements of the NCLEX-RN Licensing Exam Blueprint

Concept/ Competency	Learning Outcome	Client Need	Activity Statement	Integrated Process	Level of Cognitive Domain	Question Type	Question Number
Infection control	Develop a plan for isolating a group of clients with a communicable disease	Safe, effective care environment	Apply principles of infection control	Nursing process	Create	Multiple response	1

learning to assign a grade, the test should be moderately difficult and distinguish the students who have learned the content from those who have not. If the test is a criterion-referenced test, difficulty should match the level of the learning that reflects the skills to be mastered. For some questions, therefore, the item may be an "easy" item if all students are expected to answer it correctly. Norm-referenced tests involve eliminating easy items and using average-difficulty items to maximize the differences among students.

Determining Number of Items

Determining the number of items to include on a test depends on the number of competencies/learning outcomes to be evaluated. Although test reliability increases with the number of test items, the number of test items is limited by many practical constraints. For example, more selection-type items than supply-type items can be answered in a given period. Similarly, items that require higher-level thinking skills and solving mathematical problems take more time to answer than those that require lower-level skills.

Determining Time Allocation

A general, but not evidence-based, guide for planning the time it will take for students to complete the test is to allow 1 minute for questions that require a shorter amount of reading or calculation time. For tests with greater difficulty and longer questions, such as multiple-response type questions, the time allocation may need to be longer,

approximately 1.5 minutes per question. In practicality, the time available for a classroom test (usually a class session) may determine the number of items on the test.

Faculty should also consider the numbers of culturally and linguistically diverse students and students requiring accommodations in the class and create a supportive test-taking environment by allowing sufficient time for all students to process the question and respond to the answer options. In one study, Birkhead (2018) allowed an extension to the testing time and gave students the option of arriving 30 minutes prior to the scheduled start of the test. This extra time alleviated students' test anxiety and provided additional time for students with learning disabilities and students whose native language was not English. This testing procedure did not adversely affect program outcomes such as graduation and passing the licensing exam.

WRITING TEST ITEMS AND CONDUCTING A PEER REVIEW OF TEST ITEMS

Most types of test items used by nurse educators involve a *scenario*, a description of a nursing care situation that requires students to interpret data such as findings from a health history and physical assessment, nurses notes, or laboratory results and make a clinical judgment about the client's needs, develop a plan, and evaluate outcomes of nursing care; a *stem*, or question; and a set of *answers*, or options, one or more of which are correct and others that are incorrect (*distractors*). See Box 24.1 for general guidelines for writing test items.

Faculty should use a variety of types of questions on each test and select the type of question based on the best fit to assess or evaluate a learning outcome and to prepare students for taking each type of question that is used on a licensing or certification examination. The definitions, advantages, disadvantages, guidelines for writing, and an example of each of these types of test items follow.

Item Types
Multiple-Choice Items
A multiple-choice item consists of a scenario, which provides data about a client situation and cues to which the test-taker must respond; a stem, which is the question; and answers, one of which is correct and three of which are incorrect (distractors). Multiple-choice items, when carefully constructed, can measure critical thinking, nursing clinical judgment, and higher levels of the cognitive domain.

Multiple-choice items allow the faculty to sample a large amount of content in a single test. Test items can be scored easily and objectively. Scores on multiple-choice tests are less influenced by guessing than are scores on true–false tests. These items are versatile because they can measure learning of several levels of cognitive processes. On the other hand, writing items with plausible distractors can be time consuming. These items may discriminate against the creative, verbal student. Scores can be affected by students' reading ability and the instructor's writing style. This item type can raise the score of the student who can recognize rather than produce the correct answer.

BOX 24.1 Guidelines for Writing Test Questions

Scenario
1. Present a single, realistic clinical encounter that requires the student to make nursing clinical judgments.
2. Provide cues about the environment/setting, client and client's symptoms, data from the chart, and time frame of the clinical encounter that require the test-taker to analyze data, set priorities, make clinical judgments, and evaluate outcomes. Include relevant and irrelevant data to test students' ability to differentiate significant data but, at the same time, avoid unnecessary information or excessive descriptive information.
3. Specify age, gender, ethnicity, race, or clinical setting only when essential to answering the question.
4. Do not use names for clients.

Stem
1. Poses the question; write as a complete or incomplete sentence; can ask for priorities such as what the nurse should do *first*.
2. Should be clear enough to answer without looking at the options.
3. Write the stem in a precise manner. If it is too complex, the student will spend too much time trying to decipher it.
4. State the stem in a positive rather than a negative manner. Highlight (underline, italicize, or use bold font for) key words such as *first* and *next*.

5. Use action verbs that are consistent with the cognitive process being measured. The cognitive level of the question must match the learning outcome it is being used to evaluate.
6. Avoid clue words in the stem.
7. Keep as much information in the stem to avoid repeating it in the options.
8. Write the stem using active voice.
9. Use precise terms and measurements; avoid words such as *frequently, often*, and *some*.

Correct and Incorrect Answers
1. Keep all options grammatically consistent with the stem to avoid giving clues to the correct answer.
2. Arrange the answers/options in either alphabetical or numerical order.
3. Keep the answers the same length.
4. Make all the incorrect answers reasonable and homogeneous.
5. Use only one best answer on which all authorities would agree.
6. Avoid the use of "all of the above" or "none of the above." Students can often guess the correct answer with only partial knowledge. Multiple response-type questions can be used to evaluate students' ability to cluster data.
7. All answers must be plausible.

Example. An older adult is admitted to the hospital because of severe diarrhea. The client is thirsty and skin turgor is poor. The blood pressure is 92/64 and pulse is 100. The serum sodium (Na^+) level is 165 mmol/L. The nurse should include which priority in the care plan?
1. Protect the skin from friction.
2. Increase fluids.
3. Prevent excoriation of the rectal area.
4. Place the client on "falls alert."

Multiple-Response Items

A multiple-response item tests the student's ability to choose more than one item that answers the question. For example, if the item is testing the student's ability to determine if a nursing action was effective (evaluate an outcome), there may be more than one piece of information that relates to the effectiveness of the action. Multiple-response items have a scenario, stem, and answers; however, there are 5 to 10 answers and the answers are written so that at least one answer is correct and others are incorrect. Students are instructed to choose all correct responses ("select all that apply") and must select *all* of the correct responses to receive credit for the question. Another way of scoring the responses is to frame the question by indicating how many responses to select (*select n*). In this case, the item is scored by awarding one point for all correct answers and deducting a point for all incorrect answers. Items that are scored by awarding and deducting points may require specialized scoring procedures that not all computerized test-authoring programs may have.

Example. The nurse is implementing a medication safety teaching plan for an older adult. Which statements by the client indicate that the teaching has been effective? "I will..." (Select all that apply.)
1. "...throw away any medications I am no longer using."
2. "...have my prescriptions filled at different pharmacies to get the best price."
3. "...tell my physician about any nonprescription medications I am taking."
4. "...crush any medications that I have difficulty swallowing."

5. "...take all of my medications with food to avoid stomach upset."
6. "...report possible side effects of my medications to my physician."

Chart and Exhibit Questions

These questions determine the test-taker's ability to seek and use data presented on a client's chart or health record. The data is presented from one or more chart "tabs": prescriptions, history and physical, laboratory results, imaging results, flow sheets, intake and output, medication administration records, nurses' progress notes, and vital signs. When the test is administered by computer, the test-taker will be required to search for the chart tabs in a way that simulates search through a client's chart or computerized health record. The question may be similar to a multiple-choice question with four responses, with one correct response, or a multiple-response question with more than four options that asks the test-taker to "select all that apply" or select "n."

Chart and exhibit questions test the ability to consider which data are needed for nursing care and to test in higher levels of cognitive domain. These questions require test-takers to use data to make nursing clinical judgments, develop a plan of care, and evaluate outcomes of nursing care. These questions also simulate obtaining data from a client's chart and can ascertain whether test-takers know what data to obtain and where on a chart to find it. Faculty can make these test items realistic by obtaining information from actual client records and clinical situations and modifying the information to protect client information.

Example. A parent has brought a 4-month-old to the immunization clinic. The nurse is reviewing the immunization record on the progress notes (see Progress Notes.)

Progress Notes

11/1/2015	1-month well-child visit; administered HepB #1
12/3/2015	2-month well-child visit; administered DTaP #1, IPV #1

The infant will receive which immunization(s) at this visit? (Select all that apply.)
1. DTaP #3
2. HepB #2
3. IPV #2
4. MMR #1
5. Varicella

Drag and Drop Questions

These questions require the test-taker to drag (using a mouse for computer-administered tests as used in licensing or certification exams; or placing the answer in the correct order or space using a paper and pencil exam) an item of information from one column to another column. The test question may ask the test-taker to put steps of a procedure in order or to move from a list of possible nursing actions to a list of correct nursing actions for the particular client scenario.

Other Item Types

Nurse educators may also use other item types on their classroom tests and quizzes. *True–false* tests can be used to assess or evaluate student's ability to remember and understand nursing information such as a side effect of a drug or a step of a procedure. These questions align with learning outcomes in the lowest levels of the cognitive domain and are more useful on a quiz. *Fill-in-the-blank* questions or short-answer questions may be useful to determine student's ability to recall information or calculate drug doses, intravenous infusion rate, or input/output. These "supply-type" questions can include a scenario and a stem, but the test-taker must supply the answer. This type of question requires the student to apply information to a particular situation. Faculty can use *essay questions* to evaluate students' ability to analyze data and create nursing care plans and reports. Essay tests typically require short answers to one question, These items must be hand-graded and require faculty time to grade, and in the case of an essay test, faculty may need to develop a grading rubric.

Next Gen NCLEX Questions

The NCSBN continually updates and tests new types of items that best evaluate test-takers' knowledge of nursing practice and safe client care. As of Spring 2023, the licensing examinations for registered nurses and licensed practical nurses will include three new item types, six question types that test the students' ability to make clinical judgments, and three scoring models. Detailed information about the Test Plan (2023) and writing and scoring test questions can be found on the NCSBN website at https://ncsbn.org/exams/testplans.page.

Item types. There are three item types: the case study and stand-alone items, bow-tie, and trends. The *case study* is a set of six questions that are based on a clinical scenario that follows the six steps of the NCSBN Clinical Judgment Measurement Model (CJMM): recognize cues, analyze cues, prioritize hypothesis, generate solutions, take actions, and evaluate outcomes. *Bow-tie questions* include the six steps of the CJMM in one item. The item includes a scenario and answers that require the test-taker to move (drag) answers from one column to another. *Trend questions* use any item type and ask the test-taker to interpret data over time that has been recorded on a chart or flow sheet.

Question types. The items use a variety of question types: (1) *extended multiple response*, which has more options than the traditional multiple response and in which students select one or more answers from a list and using partial credit scoring; (2) *extended drag and drop*, in which students move answers from one list of options to the correct location in another list, such as moving a list of assessment findings to a list of assessment findings that require immediate follow-up; (3) *cloze* (drop down) in which the test-taker selects the answer from a "drop-down" by "clicking" the mouse to highlight the item(s) selected from a list that may be placed in a table or chart; (4) *enhanced hot spot/highlighting*, in which the test-taker highlights by clicking on predefined words or phrases that answer the question stem; and (5) *matrix/grid*, which involves looking at items in a matrix/table and clicking on the radio buttons that answer the question. For example, the question in the matrix may ask the student to choose from a list of potential orders and click to identify if the order is anticipated, nonessential, or contraindicated.

Scoring models. The Next Gen NCLEX questions use three different scoring models. In 0/1 scoring, one point is awarded for each correct response. In +/− scoring, one point is awarded for each correct response and one point is deducted for an incorrect response. In the Rational Scoring Model, points are awarded when *both* responses are correct.

Reviewing Test Items for Accuracy, Potential Bias, and Readability

After test items have been developed, it is necessary to review and edit them before placing them in a test bank or in an exam. Faculty should review each item for accuracy, bias, and readability.

At this stage, peer review of test items by colleagues with content knowledge and test item writing skills is helpful. Hensel and Billings (2022) developed and tested a peer review form for writing Next Gen NCLEX-style questions. Faculty who were oriented to using the peer review form and process were able to provide actionable feedback using a blind review process. Additionally, faculty who provided peer review also improved their own test item writing skills. See Box 24.2 for guidelines for editing a test.

Accuracy

Faculty should review each item to be sure it is accurate in terms of the content, use of charts, tables, or images, and the answer. Writing a rationale and identifying a source for both the correct and incorrect answers is one way to document the accuracy of the test item.

Bias

Students of equal ability should have an equal probability of correctly answering a test item. If systematic differences in responses to an item exist among members of particular groups, independent of total scores, then the item may be biased. Bosher (2003) classifies potential areas of bias in test items into four categories of bias: test-wise flaws, irrelevant difficulty, linguistic bias, and cultural bias. *Test-wise flaws* are those errors in items that provide cues to the correct answer within the item or test itself. These flaws potentially provide an unfair advantage to students with more test-taking experience or training and to native English speakers who can more easily recognize grammatical and

---

BOX 24.2   Guidelines for Editing a Test

1. Do items align with student learning outcomes and the test blueprint?
2. Are items stated in a precise manner? Are the items written using short, simple, direct sentences?
3. Is there one best answer for each item (except for multiple-response items)?
4. Does each item stand alone?
5. Are sentence construction and punctuation correct?
6. Have stereotyping, prejudices, and biases been eliminated?
7. Have "slang" or words with several meanings been eliminated?
8. Does the question eliminate gender bias, such as referring to the nurse as "she"? or not using the patient's preferred pronouns?
9. Has the use of humor been avoided?
10. Has extraneous information been deleted?
11. Has a colleague reviewed the test?
12. Is the placement of correct options varied so that there is no obvious pattern?
13. Is the terminology used on the test the same as it has been used in the classroom and in reading assignments?
14. Does the layout of the test on the page facilitate easy reading of the question? Is there sufficient "white space"? Is the entire question on the same page (no page breaks within the scenario, stem, and options)?

---

other cues. Items with *irrelevant difficulty* may be missed for reasons related more to format than to content. This type of bias can occur from writing, unclear stems, providing superfluous information, or using negative phrasing. *Linguistic complexity*, grammatical errors, and inconsistent word use also may result in biased items. *Linguistic modification* involves writing short and clearly understood questions (Abedi, 2014). Faculty can reduce the reading load of test items by eliminating irrelevant information, using simple words, and using short sentences. Faculty also should avoid using idioms or "slang" that may only be understood by certain groups of students. Faculty can also reduce linguistic load in test questions by using the present tense and active voice.

Faculty must also guard against *cultural bias* when constructing test items (Bias Free Guidelines, American Psychological Association [2020]; Inclusive Language Guidelines, American Psychological Association [2021]). These items depend on culturally specific knowledge and should not be used unless cultural practices *per se* are the domain of the question. The guidelines for writing items are designed to avoid bias.

Readability of Test Items

Test items must be written at the level of reading comprehension of the test-taker. Readability refers to the semantic and syntactic complexity of the test item. There are several tests of readability such as the Lexile Framework, Fry, and the Flesch–Kincaid readability tests. Word processing software also have simplified versions of readability tests. If interested, faculty can obtain a rough estimate of readability of their tests using one of these programs. NCSBN uses grade reading levels linked to the Lexile scale to determine readability of their licensing examination. The readability level for the Practical Nurse examination does not exceed eighth-grade reading level; the reading level for the Registered Nurse examination does not exceed a tenth-grade reading level.

If the test is to be administered by a computer, the faculty and instructional designer must also consider perceptual readability, which includes elements such as the screen position, screen color, and font size. Most colleges and universities follow Americans with Disabilities Act (ADA) guidelines for readability of computer screens. The NCSBN assumes that the candidate can read text presented on a computer screen. Candidates who do have difficulty with reading computer screens and have a documented disability can request an accommodation from their state board of nursing.

Test Banks and Test-Authoring Systems

Faculty should attempt to create a large pool of questions from which the items for a specific test can be drawn. Although it is time consuming to amass a large number of questions, the effort is rewarded by being able to administer different versions of the test or to generate a "makeup" test for students who were not able to take the test at a regularly scheduled time. Having the test items available in a word processing file makes revision of the test easier. All test files should be secured in password-protected areas of a file server accessible only by the faculty.

Many textbook publishers provide test items at no cost to faculty adopting their texts. Often these test items are written to test specific knowledge presented in the various chapters of the textbook, are written at lower levels of the cognitive domain, contain item writing flaws, and do not test critical thinking or nursing clinical judgment skills. If using these test items, faculty must review them for alignment with their student learning outcomes and test blueprints. Faculty can revise questions from test banks to test at higher cognitive levels, to test nursing clinical judgment skills, and to meet the needs of a particular course.

The task of creating test items can be simplified by using computerized test development software that typically is included as a component of a learning management system. This software can facilitate test development by creating a collection of test items (test bank) from which faculty can select appropriate questions according to the test blueprint. Alternative forms of tests can also be generated because the item pool can be large enough so that questions can be selected randomly. Some test-authoring software can be used for online testing in a computer classroom or on the internet, thus simplifying the test administration process.

Assembling a Test

Once the items are written and edited, they must be assembled into a test, to administer either online or in the classroom using a printed version of the test and a scantron answer sheet (and alternative versions of the same test if using this strategy to maintain academic honesty). This step includes arranging the items, writing test directions, reproducing the test (if printed for distribution in the classroom), and administering the test.

Arranging Items Within the Test

Unless using test-administration software in which items will be randomly generated, faculty can determine how the test items should be arranged on the test. It may be helpful to place several easy questions at the beginning of the test to reduce student anxiety and increase student confidence. To enhance thought tracking, group items that test similar concepts. These principles for arranging items on a test also should be observed when creating an alternative version of the test.

Formatting the Test and Writing Test Directions

Considering the design format of the test makes the test easier for students to read. When designing a test to be administered in the classroom or testing center with paper tests and scantron score sheets, use standard font and type size. Pay attention to layout so that the test item is not split between two pages. Use white space to separate items and avoid visual overload. Double-check that the items are numbered consecutively. Print the test on one side only. Similar design considerations are used if the test is to be administered online in a test authoring/administration system. Additionally, format the font and layout to conform with ADA guidelines and other guidelines from the campus or school of nursing.

Test directions should be self-explanatory and include the following information:

1. *Purpose of the test:* This may not need to be included if it has been addressed earlier in the instructional process.
2. *Time allotted to complete the test:* This information allows the students to pace themselves when responding to items.
3. *Basis for responding:* This provides the students with information necessary to choose the appropriate response (e.g., "choose only one answer"; "matching options can be used more than once").
4. *Recording answers:* Answers may be recorded in a variety of ways to expedite grading (e.g., recording answers on a computer sheet using a No. 2 pencil, marking an X through the correct answer on a separate answer sheet for stencil grading, marking answers directly on the test booklet in the left column).
5. *Guessing:* Encouraging the students to answer all questions prevents the inflation of scores of students who take the risk to make a guess.

6. *Value/points assigned to items:* This information allows the students to effectively plan the use of their time.
7. *Academic honesty policy:* Some faculty cite the policy or remind students of the policy. Faculty may also ask the students to sign that they are complying with the policy.

ADMINISTERING THE TEST AND MAINTAINING TEST SECURITY

Tests can be administered in the classroom using a test booklet and answer sheet, online in a proctored computer testing center, or remotely with students at a remote testing site or at their own computers. Regardless of where the exam is administered, the faculty have responsibilities to ensure the environment is conducive to test taking, students' needs for accommodation have been met, and the test questions are protected before, during, and after administering the exam.

Establishing a Comfortable and Secure Test Environment

The physical environment for administering the test should be selected so that students have a quiet and comfortable place to take the test conducive to the task. In a classroom, this includes adequate lighting, a comfortable temperature, sufficient workspace, and minimal interruptions. To reduce student anxiety, the faculty member should maintain a positive, nonthreatening attitude and avoid unnecessary conversation before and during the test. Some faculty teach students anxiety reduction strategies such as meditation, deep breathing, and using positive self-talk, and start the class with a few minutes of silence for students to settle in.

Students should review the policies that faculty will use when proctoring the test to maintain a quiet and secure environment. For example, students should not ask the faculty for clarification of questions during the test, or if the faculty suspects students are cheating, they may be asked to sit in a different part of the room.

When administering the test in an online environment, faculty must determine whether the test will be administered in a proctored testing center in the school of nursing or on the campus or if the test will be administered to students on their own computer and during a specified period. When taking the test on a computer, the student should have a comfortable chair, desk, computer, and sufficient space to provide privacy. If allowed, students may bring scratch paper and a pencil to the environment.

Accommodations for Test Taking

Students with disabilities or circumstances that require special consideration may request accommodations for test taking (see also Chapter 4). Considerations may be given for the following reasons: allowing extra time for taking the test, needing additional or extra time for rest breaks, requiring adaptations for using a computer such as reading a computer screen (need for increased font size or color change) or for use of a trackball mouse, having hearing or other auditory disabilities, having visual or eyesight difficulties (such as requiring Braille or large print), requiring a quiet space with limited distractions, having a reader to read or record test-taker responses, needing a sign language interpreter, or having a medical device in the room.

At a college or university, the policies for accommodations for classroom tests are established by the faculty and made public. Students must have documented need for accommodations on file with the office that deals with ADA compliance (see Chapter 4) and follow established procedures for implementing the request for accommodation for taking a test. For other tests, such as licensing examinations or certification examinations, the policies are set by the test administration service (state board of nursing in the case of the PN or RN licensing examination) and the test-taker must make the request in writing and have a letter from an appropriate health professional confirming the diagnosis or disability. Approval or disapproval of these requests can be determined based on the effect the disability has on the candidates' ability to practice nursing in the state.

Maintaining Academic Honesty During the Test

Faculty have a responsibility to maintain a secure test environment and ensure that all students follow the academic honesty policy at their institution (Palmer et al., 2016). In the classroom, the most effective strategy to prevent cheating is to use an adequate number of proctors, 1 for every 15 students. (See Box 24.3 for suggestions for maintaining a secure test environment and academic integrity.)

Tests are increasingly being administered remotely at the student's home or work or at a remote testing site using remote proctoring tools. There are several options for remote proctoring depending on the level of security needed. For high-stake tests, Furby (2021) recommends using a live online proctoring service and, for midstakes tests, an automated proctoring system, and, if the students can be trusted to complete the exam independently, using an honor system. Challenges to remote proctoring include the students' ability to learn how to install and use the proctoring software, making accommodations for students with disabilities, and ensuring adequate exam security (Furby, 2021). See Chapter 21 for additional information about maintaining security for online tests.

Security of the Test and Test Bank

Most faculty maintain a bank of test questions from which they draw questions for a specific test. Faculty must ensure that the test bank is maintained on a secure file server and not on a faculty or staff desktop computer. Security must also be maintained for tests that are stored inside a learning management system.

Faculty should also be aware that students have access to many test questions that are available on websites and are also available for purchase. Students also use study questions provided as electronic resources that accompany textbooks. To guard against student access to these readily available sources of questions, faculty must ensure that they are using original or revised test questions that align with the teaching–learning cycle. (See Case Study 24.1.)

BOX 24.3 Maintaining Test Security and Academic Integrity

Before Administering the Test

1. Understand the campus' and school of nursing's policies for dealing with suspected cheating. Be familiar with the student handbook and appeals processes.
2. Communicate expectations for academic honesty in writing in academic policies, in each course syllabus, in class several days before the examination, and again before administering the examination. Explain how the test will be proctored and what will happen if cheating is suspected—for example, there will be two proctors who will walk around the room, and if cheating is suspected, the proctor will move those students to another part of the classroom. If administered in an online environment, will video cameras be used to proctor the test?
3. Administer fair tests, use a test blueprint, and provide students an opportunity to practice taking tests similar to the one that is used to assign grades.
4. Teach student anxiety management strategies such as deep breathing and positive self-talk.
5. Maintain test security (e.g., lock up copies of the test or place on a secure file server). For paper and pencil tests, number tests and answer sheets and, if practical, place the student's name on the test and answer sheet. Make sure all copies of tests are returned before students leave the classroom.
6. Develop alternative forms of the test for each examination.
7. Modify the test each time the test is given.

During the Test

1. Have students sign an honor pledge that has been written on the test (or precedes an online test) that the work during the test is their own.
2. In large classes where faculty may not know all of the students, require students to present identification before taking the examination.
3. Require that book bags, cell phones, and items of clothing such as hats in which "cheat sheets" can be stored be brought to the front of the room.
4. Proctor students consistently throughout testing; have at least two proctors in the room while students are taking the test. Proctors should move around the room and monitor student behavior. Have a clear plan about how proctors are to manage cheating when it is observed or suspected.
5. Designate special seating arrangements (e.g., have an empty chair between students; have students sit in an assigned order).
6. When cheating is suspected, move the involved students to another area of the room. Inform students before the test if this is the plan for managing suspicious behavior.
7. Communicate with the course coordinator or department chair if cheating is suspected.

CASE STUDY 24.1 Maintaining Academic Honesty and Test Security

A faculty member is to proctor a 50-item test. The students will have 1 hour to complete the test. Seventy students are taking the test in a 100-seat amphitheater-style classroom. After the administration of an examination, two students report that they observed two students who were cheating by looking at each other's answer sheets.

1. What should the faculty do?
2. How should the faculty respond to the students who reported the incident?
3. What measures can the faculty take to prevent cheating incidents during the next test?

Collaborative Testing

Collaborative testing is a particular assessment or evaluation strategy faculty can use to promote learning, develop critical thinking and clinical judgment skills, improve test scores, and develop teamwork skills (Phillips et al., 2019; Reid & Hofstetter, 2020). Students work in groups of two or more to take the test. In one approach, the student team collaborates to answer the questions and all students in the group receive the grade achieved by the group. Using a two-stage approach, faculty structure the test so that each student first completes the test and receives a grade for the individual effort, and then takes the test several hours or days later in a group; the student's grade is then calculated by combining scores or using the average of the two scores. Grades can also be calculated by adding extra points to individual scores if the collaboration resulted in a better test score for the group. Collaborative testing can also be used during a posttest review in which students take the test in groups and discuss the answers, but they are not graded. Groups can be configured randomly or by assigning a mix of high-performing and low-performing students to each group. Riley et al. (2021) found that prelicensure students' scores increased when the test was used in a collaborative group. Because the test is easily available for all students, faculty must monitor student use and ensure that all tests have been returned to the faculty.

ANALYZING TEST RESULTS

Once the test has been administered and scored, faculty should review the results using concepts of measurement and data analysis. On the basis of these findings, faculty assign grades. Faculty at most schools of nursing have access to test scoring services that calculate test statistics and provide item analysis. Although there may be a fee associated with the service, the data provided by test scoring services are helpful, particularly for the first few times the test is used. Faculty should seek the assistance of these services and the consultation that can be obtained at testing centers.

Concepts of Measurement

A variety of metrics are used to determine the effectiveness of a test. These include validity, reliability, and measures of central tendency.

Validity

The concept of validity refers to the appropriateness, meaningfulness, and usefulness of inferences made from test scores. Validity is the judgment made about a test's ability to measure what it is intended to measure. This judgment is based on three categories of evidence: content-related, criterion-related, and construct-related.

Content-related patterns of evidence should show that the test adequately samples relevant content. In nursing education, the relevant content is defined by nurse educators, the course, and the profession. Some examples of content-related evidence of validity are correspondence of the test content with the following:
1. The test blueprint
2. Professional judgments of peers
3. Core material as defined by professional organizations
4. Standards of care as defined by agencies and professional organizations

Criterion-related patterns of evidence should show that the test adequately measures performance, either concurrently or predictively. The performance must be compared with some criterion variable. Nurse educators may use performance on the licensing examination (NCLEX-RN or NCLEX-PN) as the criterion variable (pass or fail).

Construct-related patterns of evidence should show a relationship between test performance and some "quality" to be measured. This is a broad category of evidence that must include specifics about the test (from the content and criterion categories) in addition to a description of the quality or construct being measured.

Some of the factors that may adversely affect test validity are unclear directions, inconsistent or inadequate sampling from the table of specifications, poorly written test items, and subjective scoring (McDonald, 2018). Careful preparation of the test can improve test validity (Box 24.4).

Reliability

Reliability refers to the ability of a test to provide dependable and consistent scores. A judgment about reliability can be made based on the extent

---

BOX 24.4   Improving Test Validity

- Use a test blueprint.
- Develop test items based on common nursing practice.
- Base test items on standards of care.
- Develop test items using evidence for best nursing care practices.
- Conduct peer review of blueprint and test questions.

to which two similar measures agree. Reliability is a necessary but not sufficient condition for validity. However, reliability may be high even with no validity. Nurse educators must look for evidence to judge tests as both reliable and valid.

Among the factors that may adversely affect test reliability are insufficient length and insufficient group variability. For the purpose of increasing reliability, a minimum test length of 25 multiple-choice questions with an item difficulty sufficient to ensure heterogeneous performance of the group is sufficient for classroom testing. See Box 24.5 for ways to improve test reliability.

Reliability could be measured by giving the same test to the same group and noting the correspondence (test-retest method) or by giving "equivalent" tests to the same group. Both of these methods have major disadvantages for classroom testing and are not generally used by nurse educators. Reliability can be measured with a single test administration by using either the split-half or internal consistency method. The split-half method separately scores responses to odd and even questions and then compares the "odd-question" score with the "even-question" score. The internal consistency of a test can be calculated by using one of the Kuder-Richardson (KR) formulas (McDonald, 2018). Most test scoring programs supply a test reliability coefficient as part of the results.

Reliability is measured on a scale of 0 to 1.00. A reliability coefficient of 1.00 represents 100% correspondence between two tests or measures. Many standardized tests have reliability coefficients of 0.9 or higher. These tests with high reliability are often norm referenced, have high variability among the test-takers, and are administered to large numbers of students. Classroom tests in nursing typically do not attain such high coefficients because of using mastery testing for small

numbers of students. Acceptable reliability for nursing tests is 0.6 (Magaldi et al., 2018).

Test Statistics

Various test statistics can be calculated, generated by test-authoring software, or reported from computer scoring services. These statistics help faculty interpret test results and provide data for item revision. Test grading software typically provides students' raw and percentage scores, individual student reports, and test statistics such as central tendencies and test reliability indices in addition to item analysis data.

Raw Score

The raw score is the number of test questions answered correctly. Raw scores are the most accurate test scores but yield limited information. A frequency distribution can be used to arrange raw scores to create class intervals. If tests are scored by computer, a frequency polygon is likely. The percentage score compares the raw score with the maximum possible score.

Central Tendency

Central tendency is a descriptive statistic for a set of scores. Measures of central tendency include the mean, median, and mode. The mean (or average) has the advantage of ease of calculation. The mean is calculated as the sum of all scores divided by the total number of scores.

The median divides the scores in the middle (i.e., 50% of scores fall below the median and 50% of cores are above the median). The median is a better measure of central tendency than the mean if the scores are not normally distributed.

Variability

Variability refers to the dispersion of scores and is thus a measure of group heterogeneity. Variability of scores affects other statistics. For example, low variability (homogeneity of scores) will tend to lower reliability coefficients such as the Kuder-Richardson coefficient. Relative grading scales are most meaningful when they are applied to a wide range of scores. Mastery tests, by design, may show little variability. As groups of students progress in a nursing program, there may be less

---

BOX 24.5 Improving Test Reliability

- Increase number of test items.
- Improve discrimination levels.
- Increase number of test-takers (<25 decreases reliability).
- Increase variability of scores (mastery tests have low variability).

variability in scores because of attrition of students (failure or withdrawal from the program).

Range

The range is the simplest measure of variability and is calculated by subtracting the lowest score from the highest score.

Standard Deviation

The standard deviation (SD) of scores is the average distance of scores from the mean. The higher the SD, the more variability there is in the test scores. The SD is the best measure of variability.

Normal Curve

The normal curve is a theoretical distribution of scores that is bell shaped and symmetrical. The mean, median, and mode are the same score on a normal curve. Also, for a normal curve, 68% of scores will fall within $\pm 1\,SD$ of the mean and 95% of scores will fall within $\pm 2\,SDs$ of the mean. This distribution may be used in assigning grades.

Standard Error of Measurement

The standard error of measurement is an estimate of how much the observed score is likely to differ from the "true" score. That is, the student's "true" score most likely lies between the observed score plus or minus the standard error. The standard error of measurement is calculated by using the SD and the test reliability.

Item Difficulty

The item difficulty index (P value) is simply the percentage correct for the group answering the item. The upper limit of item difficulty is 1.00, meaning that 100% of students answered the question correctly. The lower limit of item difficulty depends on the number of possible responses and is the probability of guessing the correct answer. For example, for a question with four options, $P = 0.25$ is the lower limit or probability of guessing. An item difficulty index of greater than 0.80 indicates low difficulty; an index of 0.30 to 0.80 indicates medium difficulty; and that less than 0.30 indicates high difficulty (Tarrant & Ware, 2012). McDonald (2018) recommends keeping the P values of the items in the range of 0.70 to 0.80 to help

ensure that questions separate learners from nonlearners (a good discrimination index). Clifton and Schriner (2010) recommend using 0.50 as a quick reference point, with low limits at 0.30 and high limits at 0.80. Some items may be slightly easier or more difficult, however, and faculty can determine the range of difficulty that is appropriate for their students and tests.

Item Discrimination

Item discrimination, the item discrimination index, refers to the way an item differentiates students who know the content from those who do not. Discrimination can be measured as a point biserial correlation. The point biserial correlation compares each student's item performance with each student's overall test performance. If a question discriminates well, the point biserial correlation will be highly positive for the correct answer and negative for the distractors. This indicates that the "learners," or the students who knew the content, answered the question correctly and the "nonlearners" chose distractors. An index of greater than 0.40 indicates excellent discrimination; an index of 0.30 to 0.39 indicates good discrimination; an index of 0.15 to 0.29 is satisfactory; an index of less than 0.15 indicates low discrimination; and an index of 0 indicates that there is no discrimination (Tarrant & Ware, 2012). If the item difficulty index is either too high or too low, the discrimination index is attenuated. The discrimination index is maximized when the item difficulty is moderate ($P = 0.5$). Ultimately, test reliability depends on item discrimination. Inclusion of mastery-level material on a norm-referenced test tends to lower test reliability because that item tends to be answered correctly by many students and will thus be a poor discriminator.

Distractor Evaluation

In addition to the evaluation of the correct answer to an item for a positive point biserial correlation, each distractor should be individually evaluated. Effective distractors should appeal to the nonlearner, as indicated by negative point biserial correlation values. Distractors with a point biserial correlation of zero indicate that students did not select them and that they may need to be revised or replaced with a more plausible option to appeal to students who do not understand the content. Distractors that were not selected increase the chances that a student could have obtained the correct answer by guessing. One way to develop appealing distractors is to periodically ask open-ended questions to determine the most common errors in thinking. Distractors for questions with numerical answers may need to be worked out by following the most typical mistakes that students make.

CONDUCTING THE POSTTEST REVIEW

After faculty have obtained the item analysis for the test, the course faculty should meet and discuss the findings from the analysis. Faculty do not post grades until they have considered the results of the item analysis. After posting grades, faculty conduct a posttest review with the students either individually or in groups.

Posttest Review With Course Faculty

After obtaining the item analysis from their test scoring service, all course faculty, even if they did not contribute items to the test, meet to discuss the results of the item analysis. Faculty should discuss each test item and consider the reliability (Kuder–Richardson reliability coefficient), validity (use test blueprint, course learning outcomes), mean, SD, range for the test, and the difficulty and discrimination for each item. These data points should be considered in the context of the purpose of the test and course and lesson learning outcomes.

When each item has been reviewed, faculty can identify any issues with the test items such as a mistake in identifying the correct answer when submitting the test for scoring, the item was too difficult, the content the item tested was not taught in class, or the wording of the question was confusing. If any of these issues are *identified from the data*, faculty can consider removing the flawed item or accepting more than one answer and rescoring the test *before* giving the results of the exam to the student (Magaldi et al., 2018). When there are issues with the questions and exam scores are lower than expected, faculty can consider giving the students the benefit of the doubt by adding the standard error of measurement to all student scores. (See Case Study 24.2.)

When the posttest review reveals that a substantial number of students did not pass the test or obtained scores lower than is usual in the course, faculty may be tempted to discard quite a few

---

CASE STUDY 24.2 Test Item Analysis

Four course faculty are conducting a posttest review session. They are reviewing the item analysis below (mean = 82; Standard Deviation = 1.5; Kuder-Richardson Reliability Coefficent 0.75).

Question	Percentage Choosing Each Alternative (Item Difficulty)				Correlation of each Alternative With Total Score (Item Discrimination)			
	A	B	C	D	A	B	C	D
1	3.84	57.69	15.38	23.0	0.07	0.23-	0.34-	0.00
4	0.00	88.46	11.53	0.00	0.00	0.50	0.50-	0.00
9	79.92	19.23	3.84	0.00	0.45	0.44-	0.09-	0.00
17	88.46	0.00	0.00	11.5	0.13	0.00	0.00	0.13-

1. How should the faculty interpret the mean and standard deviation for this test?
2. Which items are too easy? Too difficult?
3. Which item indicates there may be an issue with the test item?
4. What action should the faculty consider?
5. Which questions should the faculty prioritize for revision?
6. What data should faculty use to make this recommendation?
7. What concerns might the faculty have about the number of students who did not pass the test?
8. What actions should the faculty consider?

questions or consider allowing students to take a quiz or write a paper to improve their scores. While these options deal with the issue of low test grades, they do not keep the focus on the *reasons* for low test scores. At this point, faculty need to consider the quality of the questions and possible revisions to the test item, increasing the assessment opportunities for students such as taking ungraded practice tests, and ensuring that the teaching and testing are aligned. The test must not be used again until faculty have attended to the underlying reasons for low test scores. (See Case Study 24.3.)

CASE STUDY 24.3 Improving Learning and Testing

Two course faculty are teaching fundamentals of nursing course and are reviewing the results of the first exam. They have administered a 50-item test that test course learning outcomes at application levels of the cognitive domain and above. The test items are based on course learning outcomes. The faculty shared the blueprint with the students. There are 30 students in the course. The mean for the test was 65 and 18 students did not obtain a passing score.

1. What strategies to improve the pass rate should the faculty consider?
2. What are possible explanations for the results of the item analysis?

Revising Test Items

Developing a valid and reliable test is an ongoing process. It is helpful to revise the test immediately after administering it while faculty can recall items and student responses to them. Item revision should be conducted after item analysis. One way to analyze items for revision is to use a test item analysis form (Fig. 24.1) in which the result of item analysis for each question is entered in the form.

Items to be considered for revision should include those with the following statistical characteristics:

1. Items with P (item difficulty) values that are too high, above 81% (easy), or too low (difficult), below 69%.
2. Correct answers with low positive or negative point biserial values (>0.30 is ideal).

Those items falling outside of the "ideal" range, as seen in the outlined area in Fig. 24.1 (items 2, 18, 26, 1, 7,13, 22, 30, 8), should be considered for revision. The ideal range in this figure shows that the item had an item discrimination index of above 0.30 and was of average difficulty (70%–80%). Items that are either too easy or too difficult or do not discriminate between high-performing and low-performing students and fall at the extremes of the form should receive priority for revision. The most effective items in the example shown in Fig. 24.1 are item numbers 3, 5, 25, and 27; other

Test   2
Date 3/08

P (Item Difficulty) / D (Item Discrimination)	>.50	.40–.49	.30–.39	.20–.29	.10–.19	.01–.09	Negative	Total
Very difficult $P=50\%$ or less								
Difficult $P=51\%–69\%$	20	10	4	2, 18, 26				6
Average $P=70\%–80\%$	3, 5, 25, 27	9, 14, 19, 24	12, 16, 17, 23, 29					13
Easy $P=81\%–100\%$			6, 8, 11, 15, 21, 28	1, 7, 13, 22, 30				11
Total number of items	5	5	12	8				

X   75
KR   .75
SD   3.7
SEM 2.8

FIG. 24.1 Sample test item analysis form for a 30-item test.

test items in the ideal range are also acceptable and would not need revision. Quite a few of the items on this test were in the easy range, but items 6, 8, 11, 15, 21, and 28 had acceptable discrimination indexes. Faculty must consider the context of the test when making decisions about revising test items.

Other considerations for revising test items include those questions that were scored incorrectly, items not written clearly or noted by students who did not understand the question because of linguistic or cultural bias or were not aligned with the teaching–learning process of having clear learning outcomes, clarity of instruction, and opportunity for practice with feedback.

Magaldi et al. (2018) recommend developing a document to guide the posttest review discussion. Additionally, the discussion among the faculty may indicate that faculty development for writing high-quality test items and understanding item analysis procedures may be helpful.

Posttest Review With Students

Once faculty have returned exam results to the students, it is important to review the test with the students. This can be done individually, in small groups during office hours, or with the entire class while ensuring security of the exam. Faculty should identify each student who did not attain an acceptable test score and ensure that the student has had an opportunity to review the exam and make plans for improvement.

Before scheduling the posttest review, faculty should establish ground rules for the review that will be observed by all faculty in the course and academic program. Ground rules include: (1) the purpose of the review is to help students learn the content; (2) test scores/grades will not be changed; (3) students can learn metacognitive strategies to improve their studying and test taking abilities.

One effective strategy to help students develop metacognitive skills for test taking is to teach the student to use *exam wrappers*. An exam wrapper is the use of a questionnaire that reveals to students why they may not have answered questions correctly and how they can develop study skills and metacognitive thinking abilities to improve their

test taking abilities (Schuler & Chung, 2019). Using the questionnaire, students answer questions about their study habits (time spent studying, class attendance, methods used, studying alone or in a group, or test review session) and reasons for not answering the question correctly (did not understand the question; did not know the answer, did not understand the terms used, "read into" the question, changed answers, rushed to complete the exam). Using an exam wrapper involves a three-step process in which students answer the list of questions before seeing their test score and predict how well they did on the exam; next, students review their test for items they missed and possible reasons for their score; and last, develop an action plan for improvement. (Williams, 2021). Outcomes from student use of exam wrappers vary but may include improved study habits and test taking skills, development of test metacognition, and higher test scores (Sethares & Asselin, 2021). While the use of exam wrappers is a helpful study aid, some students still prefer talking with their faculty.

ASSIGNING GRADES

The last step of the test development process is to assign grades. In the academic setting, assignment of grades may be guided by the institution's grading policy, but the course evaluation plan and grading scale must be posted in the syllabus for each course. Principles of good grading include the following:

1. Informing students of the specific grading criteria at the beginning of the course (stated explicitly in the syllabus)
2. Basing the grades on learning outcomes (not factors such as attendance or effort)
3. Gathering sufficient data (amount and variety) for the assignment of a valid grade
4. Recording data collected for grading purposes quantitatively (e.g., 89%, not B+)
5. Applying the grading system equitably to all students
6. Keeping grades confidential
7. Using statistically sound principles for assigning grades

Grading Scales

The two basic methods for assigning grades are the absolute and the relative ("curved") scales (described in the following sections). Typically, in nursing the absolute scale is used as schools of nursing emphasize "mastery" of course concepts and intend that all students master course concepts. Students may experience the use of the relative grading scale in prenursing courses.

Absolute Scale

An absolute grading scale rates performance relative to a standard (McDonald, 2018). The student's earned points are compared with the total possible points and are expressed as a percentage earned. The standard should be included in the syllabus at the beginning of the course. Theoretically, all students could receive an A (or an F) with this scale. In reality, the dispersion of the grades depends on the difficulty of the tests. See Table 24.3 for an example of an absolute grading scale.

Relative Scale

A relative grading scale rates students according to their ranking within the group. To assign grades in this system, faculty record scores in order, from high to low. Grades may then be assigned by using a variety of techniques. One method is to assign the grades according to natural "breaks" in the distribution. This method has the disadvantage of being subjective. A better method of assigning grades based on a relative scale is to use the test statistics to create a "curve":

1. Decide whether to use the mean or the median as the best measure of central tendency. If the mean and median are approximately the same,

use the mean. If the distribution is skewed, use the median.

2. Determine the SD. The C grade will be set as the mean plus or minus one-half of the SD (encompassing 40% of the scores). See Table 24.4 for an example of a relative grading scale.

Table 24.5 shows a comparison of the grades assigned to the raw scores with the absolute and relative grading scales described.

Relative grading scales may also be developed by using linear scores such as z scores or t scores. Assuming a normal curve, a t score of 50 would be assigned a grade of C. Computer grading

TABLE 24.3 Sample Absolute Grading Scale

Percentage Correct	Assigned Grade
90–100	A
80–89	B
70–79	C
60–69	D
<60	F

TABLE 24.4 Sample Relative Grading Scale

Grade	Calculation	Example	Range
A	>Upper B	>45.5	>45.5
B	Upper C +1 SD	40.5 + 5	40.6–45.5
C	Mean ± 0.5 SD	38 ± 2.5	35.5–40.5
D	Lower C –1 SD	35.5–5	30.5–35.4
F	<Lower D	<30.5	<30.5

TABLE 24.5 Comparison of Grades Assigned by Three Methods

Raw Score	Percent Score	Grade (Absolute)	Grade (Relative)
49	98	A	A
45(2)	90	A	B
42(2)	84	B	B
40	80	B	C
39(3)	78	C	C
38(4)	76	C	C
37	74	C	C
35(2)	70	C	D
34(3)	68	D	D
33	66	D	D
30	60	D	F
28	56	F	F

programs that calculate grades according to absolute or relative scales are available. Many experts in assessment and grading do not recommend the use of relative grading scales (Haladyna, 2004; McDonald, 2018).

Grading Standards, Grade Inflation, Grade Indexing, and the Meaning of Grades

Periodically, faculty, administrators, boards of trustees, or consumers raise questions about the relative meaning of grades and potential or actual grade "inflation." Some possible causes for grade inflation are improved academic readiness of admitted students; student retention programs; competency-based assessments; competitive admission standards; a student population of older, mature, and career-directed students; and pass–fail grading systems.

Grade indexing involves indicating how many students in a given course or section of a course received grades that equaled or exceeded the grade of a given student. This index may appear on the student's transcript.

Grades also have meaning for students. In a study using Heideggerian hermeneutic phenomenology approach to interviewing nursing students in undergraduate and graduate nursing programs, Poorman & Mastrovovich (2019) found that students "needed" to get an A in every course. Often the expectation of the ability to attain an A and the reality of not achieving that grade did not match, and that students were more interested in the grade than learning the course concepts.

Nursing faculty must articulate a consistent philosophy about fair and equitable testing and grading and develop policies that communicate expectations to students. Faculty must also continually strive to administer valid and reliable tests that measure students' attainment of course and program competencies.

CHAPTER SUMMARY: KEY POINTS

- Because students take tests to determine admission, progression, and graduation, faculty have an obligation to ensure that the tests they develop and administer in their courses evaluate program and course outcomes and are valid, reliable, and fair. Using a planning process ensures that faculty are using best practices as they develop classroom tests.

- Planning, the first step in developing a test, involves identifying the purpose, developing a test blueprint, and determining the type, difficulty, and number of test questions

- Faculty must write test items that evaluate student attainment of a program or course competency. The item must be written at the same level of the domain as the program or course competency. All items should be easy to read, avoid bias, and follow diversity, equity, and inclusion guidelines for writing test items.

- Administering tests involves creating a safe and secure environment for the student, allowing accommodation when requested by the student, and maintaining test security.

- Faculty can use a test scoring service to provide data about the validity and reliability of the test as well as statistics such as mean, median, standard deviation, item difficulty, effectiveness of distractors, and discrimination index. The data provide information for making decisions about scoring the test and revising test items.

- All course faculty should participate in a posttest review of the test to consider the results of the item analysis and review these data in the context of the course, students, and the test itself. Faculty may make decisions to eliminate a test item or award selected points and rescore the test before returning the test to the student.

- Faculty also conduct a posttest review with students in small groups, with the entire class or in a private meeting with students. Prior to reviewing the test results with students, faculty establish norms and policies such as confidentiality of the test must be observed and test results will not be changed. The purpose of the review is to help students learn the correct answer and also to understand why they did not answer the question correctly, as well as to understand why they chose the incorrect answer. Using exam wrappers is one strategy to help students develop metacognitive strategies for taking tests.

- Faculty assign grades as the last step of a test development process. Faculty can use several grading methods and scales but must post the information in the syllabus.

■ REFLECTING ON THE EVIDENCE

1. Compare course learning outcomes with the test blueprint and the test used to determine the extent to which students attained the outcomes. How well do the course learning outcomes, test blueprint, and the actual test items align? Do the test items test a particular learning outcome? What is the level of the cognitive domain in which the learning outcome is written? What is the level of the cognitive domain of the related test question?

2. What is your philosophy of testing? What are the pros and cons of using tests as the primary or only way of obtaining data to assign a grade to the student?

3. What are the benefits of developing a test blueprint? Should the blueprint be given to the students? If so, when and how?

REFERENCES

Abedi, J. (2014). Linguistic modification, part I: Language factors in the assessment of English language learners: The theory and principles underlying the linguistic modification approach. In National clearinghouse for English language acquisition. http://www.ncela.us/files/uploads/11/abedi_sato.pdf

American Psychological Association. (2020). *Bias free guidelines.* https://www.apa.org/about/apa/equitydiversity-inclusion/language-guidelines.pdf

American Psychological Association. (2021). *Inclusive language guidelines.* https://www.apa.org/about/apa/equitydiversity-inclusion/language-guidelines.pdf

Anderson, L. W., & Krathwohl, D. R. (2001). *A taxonomy for learning, teaching, and assessing: A revision of Bloom's taxonomy of educational objectives.* Longman.

Binks, S. (2017). Testing enhances learning: A review of the literature. *Journal of Professional Nursing,* 34(3), 205–210. https://doi.org/10.1016/j.profnurs.2017.08.008.

Birkhead, S. (2018). Testing off the clock: Allowing extended time for all students on tests. *Journal of Nursing Education,* 57(3), 166–168.

Bosher, S. (2003). Barriers to creating a more culturally diverse nursing profession: Linguistic bias in multiple-choice nursing exams. *Nursing Education Perspectives,* 24(1), 25–34.

Dickison, P., Luo, X., Woo, A., Muntean, W., & Bergstrom, B. (2017). Assessing higher-order cognitive constructs by using an information-processing framework. *Journal of Applied Testing Technology,* 17(1), 1–19.

Furby, L. (2021). Remote proctoring: What is the takeaway from the student perspective? *Nursing Education Perspectives,* 42(4), 267.

Haladyna, T. M. (2004). *Developing and validating multiple-choice test items* (3rd ed.). Lawrence Erlbaum.

Hensel, D., & Billings, D. M. (2022). Creating a peer review process for faculty-developed next generation NCLEX items. *Nurse Educator* https://doi.org/10.1097/NNE.0000000000001322.

Magaldi, M., Kinneary, M., Colalillo, G., & Sutton, E. (2018). A guide to postexamination analysis, using data to increase reliability and ensure objectivity. *Nurse Educator,* 44(2), 61–63.

McDonald, M. E. (2018). *The nurse educators' guide to assessing learning outcomes* ((4th ed.). Jones & Bartlett.

Moore, W. (2021). Does faculty experience count? A quantitative analysis of evidence-based testing practices in baccalaureate nursing education. *Nursing Education Perspectives,* 42(1), 17–21.

Moran, V., Wade, H., Moore, L., Israel, H., & Bultas, M. (2022). Preparedness to write items for nursing education examinations: A national survey of nurse educators. *Nurse Educator,* 47(2), 63–68. https://doi.org/10.1097/NNE.0000000000001102.

National League for Nursing. (2021). The fair testing imperative in nursing education: A living document from the NLN, revised. *Nursing Education Perspectives, 42*(1), 66.

Palmer, J. L., Bultas, M., Davis, R. L., Schuke, A. D., & Fender, J. B. (2016). Nursing examinations: Promotion of integrity and prevention of cheating. *Nurse Educator, 41*(4), 180–184. https://doi.org/10.1097/NNE.0000000000000238.

Phillips, T., Munn, A., & George, T. (2019). The impact of collaborative testing in graduate nursing education. *Journal of Nursing Education, 58*(6), 357–359.

Reid, D., & Hofstetter, A. (2020). Collaborative 2-stage testing in nursing education. *Nurse Educator, 45*(3), 159.

Riley, E., McCormack, L., Ward, N., Renteria, F., & Steele, T. (2021). 2-Stage collaborative testing results in improved academic performance and student satisfaction in a PreLicensure Nursing Course. *Nurse Educator, 46*(4), 261–265.

Sartain, A., & Wright, V. (2021). Effects of frequent quizzing on exam scores in a Baccalaureate Nursing Course. *Nursing Education. Perspectives, 42*(1), 39–40.

Schuler, M., & Chung, J. (2019). Exam wrapper use and metacognition in a fundamentals course: Perceptions and reality. *Journal of Nursing Education, 58*(7), 417–421.

Sethares, K., & Asselin, M. (2021). Use of exam wrapper metacognitive strategy to promote student self-assessment of learning. *Nurse Educator, 47*(1), 37–41.

Simon-Campbell, E. L., & Phelan, J. (2016). Effectiveness of an adaptive quizzing system as an institution-wide strategy to improve student learning and retention. *Nurse Educator, 41*(5), 246–251. https://doi.org/10.1097/NNE.0000000000000258.

Tarrant, M., & Ware, J. (2012). A framework for improving the quality of multiple-choice assessments. *Nurse Educator, 34*(3), 109–113.

Test Plans. (2023). National council of state boards of nursing. https://ncsbn.org/exams/testplans.page

Tu, Y. C., Lin, Y. J., Lee, J. W. & Fan, L. W. (2017). Effects of didactic instruction and test-enhanced learning in a nursing review course. *Journal of Nursing Education, 56*(11), 683-687. https://doi.org/10.3928/01484834-20171020-09

Williams, C. (2021). Exam Wrappers: It is time to adopt a nursing student metacognitive tool for exam review. *Nursing Education Perspectives, 42*(1), 51–52.

25

Clinical Performance Evaluation

Christine L. Hober, PhD, RN-BC, CNE and Wanda
Bonnel, PhD, RN, APRN, ANEF

Evolving health care demands, coupled with increasing patient acuity and findings from studies that identify gaps in newly employed nurses' abilities to make effective clinical judgments, are driving changes in how faculty evaluate students' clinical performance. Furthermore, revision of accreditation standards, redefined program outcomes, and reimagined evaluation strategies all require faculty to reconsider how to best evaluate students' attainment of clinical knowledge, skills, and abilities. As students, faculty, and clinical partners come together to establish a culture of safety and quality patient care, evaluation of student clinical performance is assuming greater significance. This chapter identifies best practices for clinical performance evaluation, including the evaluation process, models, methods, strategies, and instruments that faculty can use to evaluate students' attainment of clinical practice outcomes.

CLINICAL PERFORMANCE EVALUATION

The purpose of evaluating clinical performance is to determine that students have attained program and course outcomes and are adequately prepared for practice (Lee, 2021; Lewallen & Van Horn, 2019). Clinical performance evaluation provides information to the student about performance and provides data that may be used for individual student development, assigning grades, and making decisions about the curriculum. As faculty prepare to evaluate students' clinical performance, they must consider the timing of the evaluation, the culture in which evaluation takes place, respecting students' rights, ensuring equity in evaluation, and

observing the ethical and legal principles when conducting the evaluation and assigning grades.

Differentiating Formative and Summative Evaluation

Clinical performance evaluation involves both facilitating learning (*formative* evaluation) and evaluating the attainment of learning outcomes (*summative* evaluation and grading). Faculty should orient students to these terms and clarify for students when each of these occurs, for example, noting whether a simulation is being assessed as a formative learning activity or if it is to be evaluated for successful outcomes completion. Timely feedback to students from faculty, both ongoing and formally scheduled, decreases the risk of unexpected evaluation results.

Formative evaluation, also known as assessment, or practice with feedback and opportunity to improve, focuses on the process of student learning and development during the clinical activity. Formative evaluation can assist in diagnosing student problems and learning needs. Ongoing formative evaluations keep students and faculty aware of the progress toward attainment of learning outcomes and promote opportunities for goal setting. This early intervention by a faculty member may provide needed direction for improvement and prevent a student from receiving an unsatisfactory evaluation of clinical performance. Appropriate feedback enables students to learn from their mistakes and allows for growth and improvement in behavior.

Summative evaluation, on the other hand, occurs at the conclusion of a specified clinical activity to determine and document student accomplishment and assign a grade. Summative evaluation attests to competency attainment or meeting of designated objectives and provides information to the student about their performance. Summative evaluation also provides data for faculty as they make decisions about the curriculum and the need for coursework that prepares students for success in clinical courses.

Ensuring Fairness and Equity

Providing fair and reasonable clinical evaluation is one of the most important and challenging aspects of the faculty role. Faculty must discern whether students can think critically within the clinical setting, make nursing clinical judgments, maintain a professional demeanor, interact appropriately with patients, prioritize problems, have basic knowledge of clinical procedures, and complete care procedures correctly. All the while, faculty need to minimize student anxiety within the complex health care setting so that student clinical performance and not extraneous factors, such as anxiety or fatigue, are being observed.

At the same time, students have the right to a reliable and valid evaluation process that assesses achievement of course outcomes and competencies. Evaluations must be fair and evaluation strategies used equitably for all students. Quality practice includes multidimensional evaluation with diverse evaluation methods completed over time, seeking student growth and progress. All evaluations should respect students' dignity and self-esteem.

Maintaining Just Culture

It is also important that faculty consider the concept of "just culture" related to clinical evaluation. It is important because it means blame is not automatically put on the individual if an error occurs but rather addresses potential health care system flaws as well. Faculty help analyze an unsafe student versus an unsafe health care system. This approach includes determining questions to help identify if an individual is at fault for an error or if it is more of a systems-related problem. For example, instead of losing clinical points for an honest mistake, the student might participate in debriefing and help others learn by analyzing what happened and why (Walker et al., 2019).

Observing Students' Rights

There are both ethical and legal issues relevant to privacy of evaluation data that can affect the student, faculty, and institution. Before conducting clinical evaluations, faculty must determine who will have access to data. In most cases, detailed evaluative data are shared only between the faculty member and the individual student. Program policy should identify who additionally may have access to the evaluation and how evaluative information will be stored and for how long. Evaluative data should be stored in a secure area.

As designated by the Family Educational Rights and Privacy Act (FERPA), students 18 years of age or older or in postsecondary schools have the right to inspect records maintained by a school (U.S. Department of Education, 2014). A school's program materials such as catalogues and handbooks can be tools to ensure the creation of reasonable and prudent policies that are in compliance with legal and accrediting guidelines. Additionally, anecdotal notes, text-based summaries of student performance, should be objectively written. Privacy of written anecdotal notes, computer documents, and mobile device notes also needs to be maintained. Inadequate security of this information could lead to a breach of student privacy.

The need to protect patient privacy can also become an issue, particularly when evaluating students' use of electronic health records. Faculty need to be familiar with the guidelines and procedures that clinical agencies have developed for students and faculty to access needed patient care documents. Ongoing discussions about students' electronic record use and its role in evaluation are important to future clinicians. If clinical access to electronic health records is limited, another way to evaluate the student's ability is to provide simulations using commercial academic products designed to teach about the electronic health record. At a time when it is critical for learning documentation for safe, quality care, Winstanley's (2017) descriptive study of nurse faculty supported that electronic health records provide students opportunities to increase their familiarity, comfort, and expertise with documentation before they transition into practice. Additional legal considerations are discussed in Chapter 3. Box 25.1

BOX 25.1 Quick Tips for Clinical Evaluation

- Define clearly knowledge, skills, and abilities, that students will need to demonstrate.
- Use multiple sources of data for evaluation.
- Be reasonable and consistent in evaluation of all students.
- Use formative mini-evaluations and suggest minor, easy corrections at the time they are needed.
- Present feedback and evaluation in nonjudgmental language, confining comments to a student's behavior.
- Provide evaluation "sandwiches," commenting first on a strength, then on a weakness, then on a strength of the student's behavior.
- Carry an anecdotal record or mobile device equivalent for each student, maintaining privacy of data.
- Make specific notes, focusing on specific details of a student's behavior.
- Document student patterns of behavior over time through compilation of records.
- Invite students to complete self-assessments and summarize what they have learned.
- Help students prioritize learning needs and turn feedback into constructive challenges with specific goals for each day.

---

provides some "quick tips" to be considered at the beginning of the evaluation process.

Using Models/Frameworks With Clinical Performance Evaluation

Clinical evaluation can be guided by models or frameworks. Typically, models/frameworks emphasize a particular aspect of clinical practice, such as clinical judgment or patient safety, and, as such, can be integrated into a curriculum or course evaluation plan, linked to appropriate teaching strategies that help students attain the related learning outcomes, and related instruments used as the primary evaluation or along with course evaluation instruments developed by faculty.

Clinical Judgment Models

Recent studies (Kavanagh & Sharpnack 2021; Kavanagh & Szweda, 2017) and reviews of literature (Klenke-Borgmann et al., 2020) have revealed that newly employed nurses account for a high percentage of patient care errors, often caused by the inability to make effective clinical judgments. Because of these findings, the National Council of State Boards of Nursing (NCSBN), Nursing Accrediting Agencies, and schools of nursing are revising program outcomes and competencies and developing teaching and evaluation strategies to ensure that graduates of nursing programs are better prepared to make clinical judgments. Thus, faculty are considering a variety of models/frameworks that facilitate the teaching and evaluation of clinical judgment and integrating them into clinical evaluation practices.

National Council of State Boards of Nursing clinical judgment measurement model. Motivated by findings from studies that indicate new graduates account for high percentages of patient errors (Kavanagh & Sharpnack 2021; Kavanagh & Szweda, 2017), the NCSBN has developed a measurement model with new item types that will be used on the NCLEX licensing exam to test students' ability to make clinical judgments. This model (Dickison et al., 2017) has six sequential steps that are embedded in nursing practice when making clinical judgments. The steps include (1) recognizing cues; (2) analyzing cues; (3) prioritizing hypotheses; (4) generating solutions; (5) taking action; and (6) evaluating outcomes.

Tanner's clinical judgment model. Developed by Tanner (2006), the clinical judgment model includes four aspects: noticing, interpreting, responding, and reflecting. The noticing phase encompasses what the nurse sees in the situation, while interpreting involves understanding the situation sufficiently to be able to determine how the patient is responding. In the final aspect, the nurse reflects-in-action while considering the patients' response and reflects-on-action to determine the outcomes as a result of nursing actions. The Lasater Clinical Judgment Rubric is an instrument based on Tanner's model that faculty can use to guide evaluation of students' clinical performance related to making clinical judgment as well as the other aspects of Tanner's model.

Quality and safety model. The Quality and Safety Education for Nurses model focuses on patient-centered care, teamwork and collaboration, evidence-based practice, quality improvement, safety, and informatics. Cronenwett et al. (2007) describe the knowledge, skills, and abilities required to provide high-quality and safe patient care. Valid clinical evaluation instruments have been developed based on this model for both prelicensure and advanced practice nurses (APNs) (Altmiller, 2017; Altmiller & Dugan, 2020). As Lewallen and Van Horn (2019) discussed, evaluating nursing students' clinical competence, accurately defined and efficiently measured, requires reliable and valid instrumentation

A national model for clinical performance evaluation. Inconsistency of clinical evaluation methods, safe practice outcomes, and the need to clarify communication to stakeholders about health care providers' role has prompted discussion among several health professions. To address these gaps, medicine and pharmacy have identified national standards, known as Entrustable Professional Activities, that are addressed in the curriculum of these programs and evaluated prior to graduation, thus ensuring graduates of these programs have attained the requisite curricular competencies. Preliminary discussions of using national standards for nursing in the same way are underway. Developing national standards in nursing would require agreement on specific nursing outcomes/competencies and be followed by the development of reliable and valid evaluation instruments (Wilson et al., 2021). Competency-based education can lead to a common outcome language for the discipline, promoting enhanced communication and teamwork to minimize errors (Kavanagh & Sharpnack, 2021).

CLINICAL EVALUATION OF STUDENTS: THE PARTICIPANTS

Clinical evaluation is complex. Although faculty have primary responsibility for evaluating students' clinical performance, gaining multiple individuals' perspectives or a team approach enhances the evaluation as designated others contribute to student evaluation. Participants can include the faculty, interdisciplinary staff, preceptors, student's peers, and patients. When using a variety of persons who are contributing to student evaluation, it will be important that each

person is familiar with the course and the learning outcomes and be oriented to approaches for providing fair and equitable evaluations (Johnson et al., 2021).

Faculty

Faculty are the primary participants in evaluating students' clinical abilities because they are knowledgeable about the purpose of the evaluation and the learning outcomes and competencies that will be used to judge each student's performance. This clarity of purpose provides direction for selection of evaluation tools and processes.

Initial faculty challenges in completing clinical evaluations include factors such as faculty value systems, the number of students supervised, and availability of reasonable clinical opportunities for students. Faculty need to be aware of their own value systems to avoid biasing the evaluation process. When faculty are supervising a group of students in the delivery of safe and appropriate nursing care, faculty can only sample student behaviors. Limited sampling of behaviors or individual biases may result in an inaccurate or unfair clinical evaluation. Because of these limitations, faculty use a variety of evaluation methods to capture the broader picture of student competence. Faculty strive to identify equitable assignments and can consider evaluation input from other sources with potential adjunct evaluators, including nursing and health care staff and preceptors, students' own self-evaluations, peer evaluators, and patients.

Students

Completion of self-assessments by students not only provides data, as part of the evaluation process, but also can be a learning experience for the students. Student self-evaluation provides a starting point for reviewing, comparing, and discussing evaluative data with faculty. Initial student involvement in self-assessment tends to facilitate student behavior changes and provides a positive environment for learning and improvement. Participation in their own evaluation also empowers students to make choices and identify their strengths. Self-assessments are further discussed later in this chapter as a component of self-evaluation and self-reflection.

Nursing Staff

New models for clinical education (see Chapter 18), including dedicated units with entire patient care nursing staff engaged in educating students, dedicated preceptors, interprofessional teams, and academies to support clinical teaching, emphasize the need to focus on engaging nursing staff and a variety of health care professionals as part of the clinical evaluation team. Nursing staff can provide input to the evaluation process and a perspective of working with the student. Even with newer clinical evaluation models, these team members often have limited experience with clinical evaluation; faculty should orient those involved in evaluation to their role with staff expectations in the evaluation process clearly articulated. This includes determining whether staff feedback should be provided directly to the student only or shared with faculty as well. One of the disadvantages of including nursing personnel and others in the evaluation process is that expectations in the clinical area may differ from course performance objectives. Sharing course objectives, expectations of students, and clinical evaluation forms with staff promotes an evaluation partnership. Although contributing to student evaluation is time consuming for busy nurses, this may be part of a nurse's career development or joint appointment responsibilities.

Preceptors

Preceptors have a specified role in modeling and facilitating clinical education for students. Typically, the preceptor, student, and faculty form a triad with regular times established for discussing progression toward course outcomes. Preceptors should be oriented to the nursing school's evaluation plan. While the faculty assumes responsibility for assigning the final grade, roles should be clarified, indicating whether the preceptor will be asked to provide occasional comments, to report only incidents or concerns, or to complete a specific evaluation form. Adequately preparing adjunct evaluators for their role, specifying clinical activities to evaluate, and guiding them in using tools such as rubrics for student feedback includes addressing specifically the importance of supportive preceptors and safe clinical environments in reducing bias and racism in nursing precepted clinical experiences (Johnson et al., 2021). These authors note that engaging and orienting preceptors to the use of fair and equitable clinical evaluation principles can promote dignity, respect, and safety for all parties. Preceptors also have indicated the need for faculty support, especially when students are unprepared for clinical (Ong et al., 2021).

Student Peer Evaluators

Peer evaluation can help students develop collaborative skills, build communication abilities, and promote professional responsibility. Students have described value in peer review roles but also indicate the need for faculty support and clear guidelines for the review. Because there is debate about the appropriateness of having student peers act as evaluators in the clinical setting, student peers should only evaluate competencies and assignments that they are prepared to judge. A potential disadvantage is that peers may be biased in providing only favorable information about student colleagues or may have unrealistic expectations of them. Providing students with this peer evaluation opportunity and then appropriately weighting the contribution can be a reasonable practice. Interprofessional education competencies call for peer feedback as a key concept in preparing for interprofessional practice. Peer review, an important component of team and group work, includes learning to share thoughtful, objective critique against standards such as rubrics. Providing student peers opportunities to critique and give feedback to each other can also be a team learning opportunity. Faculty can help students appreciate the importance of peer review, use basic rubrics, and practice professional peer communication.

Patients

Patients provide data from the consumer viewpoint. Patient satisfaction is considered an important marker in quality health care and can be considered as part of student evaluation. Judgments about student performance are made from patients' personal experiences and data should be weighted for their value. Patients often have positive comments to make about their students, which can be positive for the students to hear. While not a new focus, the importance of engaging patients in their health gains attention as an essential component of safe, quality care (Quality and Safety Education for Nurses Institute, 2021). Particularly as health care moves to incorporate patients into stronger team member roles, their perceptions of student care can add value.

CLINICAL EVALUATION STRATEGIES AND INSTRUMENTS

Clinical performance evaluation measuring outcomes that adequately prepare prelicensure nurses for practice is indicated (Lewallen & Van Horn, 2019; Wilson et al., 2021). Faculty are encouraged to use a standardized, systematic clinical evaluation instrument and documented process that demonstrate student attainment of specified competencies to ensure graduates are prepared for work across all health care settings (Wilson et al., 2021).

A variety of evaluation strategies and instruments can be used to measure learning in the clinical setting and should be incorporated in clinical evaluation, including evaluating cognitive, psychomotor, and affective behaviors as well as affective domain abilities such as the development of a professional identity, cultural competence, and ethical comportment. The goal of evaluation is an objective report about the extent to which students have met course learning outcomes and demonstrate competency in clinical performance. Faculty need to be aware that potential exists for evaluation of students' clinical performance to be subjective and inconsistent. Even with "objective" instruments based on measurable and observable behavior, subjectivity can still be introduced into a tool that is viewed as objective. Faculty should be sensitive to the forces that contribute to the subjective side of evaluation as they strive for fairness and consistency (Kavanagh & Szweda, 2017).

While good evaluation principles apply across student program levels, additional considerations exist when evaluating students who are preparing for advanced practice roles (APN). Different from undergraduates, these students often use a precepted practicum at a distant site. This approach often involves a three-way evaluation combining information about attainment of learning outcomes from faculty, student, and preceptors. Students, for example, record data about patients seen in software programs such as Typhon. Preceptors and faculty often complete clinical rubrics related to observations and assignments. Another approach to evaluation is to incorporate standardized patients and advanced clinical simulations. Students must also use self-assessment skills and reflection to judge their clinical practice performance. In an evaluation of student self-assessments of their recorded videos, Fieler (2020) noted that the mean self-assessment score for those reviewing their videos suggested enhanced student objectivity in scoring compared with those students who did not use video recordings.

Fair and reasonable evaluation of students in clinical settings requires use of appropriate evaluation instruments that are efficient for faculty to use (National League for Nursing, 2020). The instrument used to measure clinical learning and performance should have criteria that are consistent with course objectives and the teaching institution's purpose and philosophy Butts (2022). Evaluation instruments should show progression of student competency not only across semesters but across the curriculum. Faculty teams should be engaged in ongoing discussions about the instruments they choose to use and their purposes. Faculty must make decisions about using these instruments according to their purpose for clinical evaluation. The best tools are reliable clinical tools that guide in determining how well students meet objectives, verify their competency as safe practitioners, and allow opportunities for formative and summative feedback.

Primary strategies for the evaluation of clinical practice include (1) observation, in person and virtually, (2) written communication, (3) oral communication, (4) simulation, and (5) self-evaluation. Because clinical practice is complex, a combination of methods used over time is indicated and helps support a fair and reasonable evaluation. See Table 25.1 for a summary of common strategies and clinical evaluation tools by category.

TABLE 25.1   Sample Evaluation Strategies and Tools by Category (Which Can be Used In Person or Virtually)

Observation	Anecdotal notes Rubrics Checklists Rating scales
Written	Charting and progress notes Concept maps Care plans Process recordings Written tests Web-based clinical assignments
Oral	Student interviews and case presentation Clinical conferences (face-to-face or video)
Simulations	Interactive multimedia patient simulators Role play and clinical scenarios Standardized patient examinations
Self-evaluation	Reflective journals and logs Rubric self-evaluations Videotaped self-assessments Clinical portfolios

Evaluation Strategies: Observation

Observation is the method used most frequently in clinical performance evaluation. Student performance is compared to clinical competency expectations as designated in course objectives. Faculty observe and analyze the performance, provide feedback on the observation, and determine whether further instruction is needed. Video recordings can also be used as an observation strategy. As noted, continuing issues in clinical evaluation include wide variability in clinical environments, increasingly complex patients, and more diverse students.

Advantages of observation include the potential for direct visualization and confirmation of student performance, but observation can also be challenging. Factors that can interfere with observations include lack of specificity of the particular behaviors to be observed; an inadequate sampling of behaviors from which to draw conclusions about a student's performance; and the evaluator's own influences and perceptions, which can affect judgment of the observed performance (Oermann & Gaberson, 2021).

Faculty should seek tools and strategies that support a fair and reasonable evaluation. The more structured observational tools are typically easy to complete and useful in focusing on specified behavior. Although structured observation tools can help increase objectivity, faculty judgment is still required in interpretation of the listed behaviors. Problems with reliability are introduced when item descriptors are given different meanings by different evaluators. Faculty training can help minimize this problem.

Instruments to Track Clinical Observation Evaluation Data

An abundance of information must be tracked in clinical observation. Faculty can benefit from systems to help document and organize this information. Faculty can carry copies of evaluation instruments and anecdotal records or can consider the use of mobile devices to help facilitate retrieval and use of clinical evaluation records. A variety of strategies exist for using mobile devices in the clinical setting. In graduate clinical programs, for example, students typically document their own patient logs electronically, as one component of competency evaluation. Common methods for documenting observed behaviors during clinical practice include anecdotal notes, checklists, rating scales and rubrics, and videotapes.

Anecdotal notes. Anecdotal or progress notes are objective written descriptions of observed student performance or behaviors. The format for these can vary from loosely structured "plus–minus" observation notes to structured lists of observations in relation to specified clinical objectives. Serving as part of formative evaluation, as student performance records are documented over time, a pattern is established. This record or pattern of information pertaining to the student and specific clinical behaviors helps document the student's performance pattern for both summative evaluation and recall during student–faculty conference sessions. The importance of determining which clinical incidents to assess and the need to identify both positive and negative student behaviors are noted.

Checklists.   Checklists are lists of items or performance indicators requiring dichotomous responses such as satisfactory–unsatisfactory or pass–fail (Table 25.2). A checklist is an inventory of measurable performance dimensions or products with a place to record a simple "yes" or "no" judgment. These short, easy-to-complete tools are frequently used for evaluating clinical performance. Checklists, such as nursing skills check-off lists, are useful for evaluation of specific, well-defined behaviors and are commonly used in the clinical simulated laboratory setting. Rating scales and rubrics, described in the following paragraph, provide more detail than checklists concerning the quality of a student's performance.

Rating scales and rubrics.   Rating scales incorporate qualitative and quantitative judgments regarding the learner's performance in the clinical setting (Box 25.2). A list of clinical behaviors or competencies is rated on a numerical scale such as a 5-point or 7-point scale with descriptors. These descriptors take the form of abstract labels (such as A, B, C, D, and E or 5, 4, 3, 2, and 1), frequency labels (e.g., *always, usually, frequently, sometimes,* and *never*), or qualitative labels (e.g., *superior, above average, average,* and *below average*). A rating scale provides

TABLE 25.2 **Example of Checklist Items**					
	Midterm/ Formative			**Final/ Summative**	
Professional Domain	Satisfactory	Unsatisfactory	Not Observed	Satisfactory	Unsatisfactory
Practices within legal boundaries according to standards.					
Uses professional nursing standards to provide patient safety.					
Follows nursing procedures and institutional policy in delivery of patient care.					
Displays professional behaviors with staff, peers, instructors, and patient systems.					
Demonstrates ethical principles of respect for person and confidentiality.					
Participates appropriately in clinical conferences.					
Reports on time; follows procedures for absenteeism.					

BOX 25.2   Example of Rating Scale Items and Format

Instructions: On a scale of 1 to 5, rate each of the following student behaviors:

(Rating Code: 1 = marginal; 2 = fair; 3 = satisfactory; 4 = good; 5 = excellent; NA = not applicable)

1. Serves as patient caregiver (independence when providing patient care, timely completion of all patient care).
2. Functions in the role of team member.
3. Uses correct procedure when performing nursing interventions.
4. Relates self-evaluation to clinical learning objectives.
5. Displays positive behavior when given feedback.

---

the instructor with a convenient form on which to record judgments indicating the degree of student performance. This differs from a checklist in that it allows for more discrimination in judging behaviors as compared with dichotomous "yes" and "no" options.

Rubrics, considered a type of rating scale, help convey clinically related assignment expectations to students. They provide clear direction for graders and promote reliability among multiple graders. They can support accurate, consistent, and unbiased ratings as well as tracking and monitoring progression over time. The detail provided in a rubric grid allows faculty to provide rapid and informative feedback to students without extensive writing (Quality Matters, 2021). Students can use these tools for self-assessments and participate in peer assessments to promote learning.

Typical parts of a rubric include the task or assignment description, breakdown of assignment parts, and some type of scale with performance level descriptors. Skill-based rubrics can provide students with direction in their skill practice and learning. Serving as a scoring guide, rubrics help focus on expectations for best practices in completing skills and improve communications.

Rubrics play a prominent role in evaluating clinical judgment in the American Association of Colleges of Nursing (2022) toolkit of resources,

Clinical Judgment Concept Across Domains. For example, the Lasater Clinical Judgment Rubric (Lasater, 2007) is a featured evaluation tool. Based on Tanner's model, Lasater (2007, 2011) further developed a clinical judgment tool focused on these four broad phases and further delineated them with 11 dimensions that describe a trajectory of clinical judgment development in prelicensure students. This rubric may be useful in guiding student reflection on their clinical experiences during debriefing, clinical conferences, or journaling activities and as a basis for giving students' feedback on their thinking as expressed in these activities (Lasater & Nielsen, 2009). Lee (2021) reviewed 20 studies specific to evaluating clinical judgment, finding that the Lasater Clinical Judgment Rubric had value in clinical evaluation but noted that, as with using all evaluation instruments when more than one person is using the instrument in a course with different sections of students, issues such as inter- and intrarater reliability must be considered.

Video recordings as source of observational data. Another method of recording observations of a student's clinical performance is through videos. Often completed in a simulated setting, videos can be used to record and evaluate specific performance behaviors relevant to diverse clinical settings. Advantages associated with videos include their valuable start, stop, and replay capabilities, which allow an observation to be reviewed numerous times. Videos can promote self-evaluation, allowing students to see themselves and evaluate their performance more objectively. Videos also give faculty and students the opportunity to review the performance and provide feedback in determining whether further practice is indicated. As the Harris et al. (2019) survey of nurse practitioner students and faculty who participated in remote clinical site evaluations reported, the method not only removed distance evaluation barriers but also provided an efficient mentoring and monitoring option with favorable experiences for both students and faculty.

Videos are particularly popular for simulation debriefing as well as evaluation in distance learning situations. Videos can also be used with rating scales, rubrics, checklists, or anecdotal records to organize and report behaviors observed in the videos. As the Fieler (2020) study reported, video recordings can support learner self-assessment and accountability to improve clinical competency evaluation while also helping eliminate bias between learner and evaluator.

Additionally, an approach to involving students as observers in evaluation is to engage them in observing and evaluating online clinical videos such as the National Institutes of Health Stroke Scale (NIHSS, 2021) training. In this example, video cases were developed based on needed competencies for appropriate use of the Stroke Scale. Students complete testing specific to these competencies as they refer to the online video cases. This approach allows students to participate in a type of standardized testing. There may be additional opportunities for students to observe videos as components of clinical evaluation, for example, critique of online videos developed by faculty or others.

Evaluation Strategies: Student Written Communication

Use of written communication, whether paper-based or electronic, enables the faculty to evaluate clinical performance by assessing students' abilities to translate what they have learned into the written word. Review of student nursing care plans or written notes allows faculty to evaluate students' abilities to communicate with other care providers. Through writing assignments, students can clarify and organize their thoughts. Additionally, writing can reinforce new knowledge and expand thinking on a topic.

Reflective Writing

Reflective writing assignments, appropriately designed, can help faculty observe students move from telling or describing data to translating information to knowledge. Smith, using guided reflective writing based on the clinical judgment model, found support from both students and faculty in its learning value. Beginning faculty guides for helping to develop and evaluate students' clinical reasoning skills have been developed (Gonzalez et al., 2021). Evaluation and grading of reflective writing focuses on the quality of the content and student ability to communicate information and ideas in written form. The rater can determine the student's perspectives and gain insight into

the "why" of the student's behavior. A scoring tool such as a rubric with specified objectives for a designated assignment can promote consistency and efficiency in grading specified assignments (Quality Matters, 2021).

Patient Progress Notes and Electronic Health Record Documentation

The use of electronic text–based communication in the changing health care system is increasing, with the ability to write cogent nursing and clinical progress notes an important clinical skill. Reviewing student documentation provides faculty with an opportunity to evaluate students' ability to process and record relevant data. Students' skills in using health care terminology and documentation practices can be examined and critical thinking processes can be demonstrated in these notes. With the focus on electronic records as a tool in patient safety, orienting students to these tools and evaluating students' skill in this area is essential. In some clinical practice settings, there may be limited student access to electronic health records or unfamiliar electronic systems; faculty can use clinical lab settings and simulations to first engage students in learning to use academic electronic health records and then evaluate their documentation using case studies. Developing ongoing strategies with clinical agency partners may be needed to continue evaluation of students' electronic documentation abilities as they advance in clinical patient care.

Concept Maps

Concept maps are another tool for evaluating students' ability to document thinking processes and allow students to create a diagram of patient needs and nursing responses, including relationships among concepts. These tools can help students visualize and organize patient-specific data relevant to diagnostic work and nursing and medical diagnoses. Concept maps can serve as worksheets for students and serve as organizing tools for documentation (Schuster-McHugh, 2020). Faculty can evaluate students' understanding of concepts and relationships among relevant concepts and assist in clarifying students' misconceptions. These tools also provide faculty with opportunity to complete a quick review of students' thinking patterns, particularly as they are making clinical judgments, and determine further learning needs before students provide direct patient care. In today's complex health care world, concept maps may better represent care processes than more traditional linear models of documentation. Concept maps, further discussed in Chapter 24, can provide a useful tool for evaluating students' abilities to synthesize concepts in care of specific patients. Gonzalez et al. (2021) in a review of the literature found conceptual approaches such as concept maps useful in assessing and evaluating clinical judgment.

Nursing Care Plans

Nursing care plans allow faculty to evaluate students' ability to determine and prioritize care needs according to understanding and interpretation of individual patients' health care problems. Historically, nursing care plans have been used by students to document clinical thinking processes. Some programs report replacing or combining detailed clinical care plans with concept maps or clinical journals and logs to help students clarify the interrelationship of patient problems. While debate exists about the value of the traditional nursing care plan, the value of tools that help nursing students gain skills for critical judgment and that promote patient safety are well accepted. Long-term care settings, for example, emphasize the need to continue teaching and evaluating care plans as integral to the team approach for enhancing the client experience.

Process Recordings

Process recordings have been used to evaluate the interpersonal skills of students within the clinical setting. This form of evaluation requires students to write down their patient–nurse interactions and self-evaluate the communication skills they used. A type of self-reflection, process recordings provide a form of student self-evaluation that allows students to analyze their own interactive behavior, enabling them to better identify the strengths and weaknesses of their interpersonal communication.

Written or Electronic Testing Formats

Written testing is frequently used to assess students' basic knowledge for problem solving and decision making in clinical practice. Various test formats (true–false, multiple choice, matching, short answer, essay) can be incorporated into preclinical or postclinical conferences to gauge students' understanding of specific concepts. (See Chapter 24 for information about writing test questions.)

Written Work in Learning Management Systems

Written evaluation can also include web-based clinical evaluation formats. For example, faculty can implement postclinical conferences or lead clinical case discussions within online learning management systems (see Chapter 21). Within online learning systems, students can submit electronic clinical logs to document patterns of ages and diagnoses of their patients. Opportunities exist for faculty to provide rapid feedback to students on written clinical papers, threaded discussion boards, or e-journals. Although not limited to students at a distance, web-based strategies are especially popular for clinical evaluation of students in geographically diverse settings. They may be useful as well for clinical conferences and student evaluation in community health courses with clinical coursework in diverse community settings.

Evaluation Strategies: Oral Communication Methods

Communication and information sharing are common nursing tasks and important nursing skills. Oral communication strategies such as student interviews, case presentations, and clinical conferences provide evaluative opportunities. These can be used to assess the student's ability to verbalize ideas and thoughts clearly. In addition, these strategies allow faculty to assess a student's critical thinking skills and pose questions to elicit more complex forms of thinking. Evaluation strategies identified as oral or verbal communication methods are described in the following paragraphs.

Questions, Prompts, and Case Presentation

Questioning is a strategy in which faculty ask questions and students respond. These question-and-answer sessions can be used to assess student learning and provide feedback, and also, in evaluation mode, to provide faculty with the opportunity to probe for more detail from students and determine thinking and judgment processes. Faculty can focus on asking "higher-order" questions, moving beyond just factual recall, to better promote student critical thinking. Student case presentations, such as "bullet-point" summaries of patient problems and care strategies, assist students in developing concise presentation skills. Prompts are specific questions used to elicit information. When used as evaluation, faculty can judge the students' knowledge and judgment process skills. Case presentations, while often used in teaching, can also be used to evaluate the students' abilities to organize and evaluate care for a patient. Rubrics are useful tools for evaluating students' presentation of a case.

Clinical Conferences

Clinical conferences provide opportunities for students to integrate theory and practice in terms of their own clinical experiences. Questions, reflections, and discussions within conferences encourage critical thinking and allow for peer feedback. Debriefing of clinical experiences, similar to the debriefing of simulations, provides students with opportunity to reflect and further cement learning. As students debrief, they gain opportunity to assess what happened during their clinical care, compare this to accepted criteria, and consider how well they did. Conferences provide an opportunity for faculty to gauge students' abilities to analyze data and critique plans. The multiple student participants in clinical conferences enable faculty to evaluate more than one student at a time. Asking students to engage in goal setting for further learning is another important component of clinical conference debriefing (Bonnel et al., 2019). When facilitating a clinical conference, faculty must inform students if the focus is on teaching and learning (formative evaluation) or on evaluation (judging and grading).

Interprofessional conferences are another form of clinical conference in which the process of problem-solving and decision-making is a collaborative effort of the group. Involving multiple health care disciplines, evaluation is concerned with the student's active participation within the group

and abilities to present ideas clearly in terms of the care plan for the patient. Increased focus on interprofessional education makes this an important time to address student abilities to clearly communicate and collaborate in problem solving with team members. While students may find a degree of risk involved with sharing their knowledge and being evaluated critically by other disciplines, gaining these competencies facilitates development of mutual respect and supports interprofessional communication.

Evaluation Strategies: Clinical Simulations, Role Play, Case Studies, and Standardized Patient Examinations

Simulations

Simulations can range from simple case role plays to interactions with complex electronic manikins and virtual approaches. Through simulations, an instructor can identify specific clinical objectives to be demonstrated and focus on student cognitive and psychomotor behaviors defined for the case. Simulations help to create a safe environment for student learning. Benefits of simulations include skill validation in a standardized setting with no risk to actual patients. With the changing health care setting, students will likely not have opportunities to care for all types of patients in the various clinical settings for which they will be responsible after graduation. Teaching pattern recognition with case studies and scenarios in safe, structured learning environments is becoming an increasingly important strategy. Case studies typically serve as the basis for simulations and problem-based learning to enhance concept application, reflection, and clinical judgment (see Chapter 19). Learning can then be transferred to specific patients and settings. Sample approaches to simulations include technology-based patient simulations, role play and clinical scenarios, and standardized patient examinations.

Technology-Based Evaluations—Patient Simulations

Rapidly advancing technologies provide additional opportunities for clinical evaluation, including virtual case-based simulations and high-fidelity simulations. Virtual case-based simulations, with similarities to high-fidelity simulation, include web-based avatars in online simulated settings. Avatars, a type of on-screen representation of students placed in virtual health care settings, provide a semirealistic learning experience for students to assume nursing roles, interact with a virtual patient, and make care decisions. Through the use of interactive multimedia, these nursing case studies can be presented in a safe setting without clinical environmental distractions, or the risk involved in student clinical decision making, and thus used for clinical performance evaluation in a structured environment.

High-fidelity patient simulators as mechanisms to document student competencies are taking on increasing importance in today's health care settings. Research findings regarding high-fidelity simulations as both teaching and evaluation tools are becoming increasingly available. Faculty should clarify for students whether a simulation activity is formative (for teaching purposes) or summative (for outcomes evaluation). Further discussion of simulations as a form of clinical evaluation can be found in Chapter 19.

Debriefing and feedback to students, as formative evaluation, are considered to be critical elements in the teaching–learning process with high-fidelity patient simulations (see Chapter 19 for debriefing guidelines). These debriefing sessions provide opportunity for students to gain insight into their performance and consider opportunities for improvement.

The potential for simulation as a summative evaluation tool has been studied, with emphasis on the need for well-designed and facilitated scenarios, as well as valid and reliable evaluation instruments if the simulation is to be used for high-stakes testing and evaluation. Building on National League for Nursing (2020) fair testing principles, faculty must ensure that students have had adequate exposure to simulation prior to a summative evaluation (see Chapter 19).

Role Play, Case Studies, and Clinical Scenarios

Role play provides an opportunity for students to try out new behaviors, simulating aspects of nursing care in relation to clinical practice. As students implement the roles called for in specified case studies (or scripts for role plays), they gain opportunities to practice competent nurse interactions and behaviors. Students practice interpersonal communication skills and gain opportunity to observe, evaluate, and provide feedback to each other.

Just as role play engages students, so too can case studies or clinical scenarios. Written clinical cases or clinical scenarios, or those created with audio or video clips, provide students the opportunity to review an approach to a clinical scenario and actively learn while faculty facilitate the procedure. As students identify cues and analyze cases, clinical judgment and its evaluation can begin in the classroom. The potential for diverse cases, relevant to a majority of nursing arenas, can be used as evaluation in a variety of settings, including online. An advantage that these methods offer is a readily available means of evaluating specific clinical practices without having to wait for a similar opportunity to arise in the clinical setting. Clinical scenarios can be economically beneficial in the educational setting with large groups of students.

Additionally, case studies of clinical scenarios, with their applications focus, can help students prepare for the Next Gen NCLEX (Caputi, 2019). Examples and resources for unfolding cases that might be used in the evaluation phase are provided by the Quality and Safety Education for Nurses (QSEN, 2021) and the National League for Nursing Unfolding Cases (http://www.nln.org/acesxpress/).

Standardized Patient Examinations

Standardized patient examinations, sometimes referred to as *objective structured clinical examinations* (OSCEs), are another way to evaluate competencies in clinical education. These OSCEs involve actors or "pretend patients" in a created environment designed to simulate actual clinical conditions. A simulation center, modeled as an authentic clinical environment with standardized patients, can provide a safe setting in which to observe and document student competencies. OSCEs can be used to increase the independence of students' practice and enhance their understanding. In the safe, controlled environment of the lab, students can be evaluated on designated criteria (Aronowitz et al., 2016; Phillips et al., 2020). In a pilot evaluation of feasibility of OSCEs for an advanced practice nurse program with 28 nurse practitioner students, the use of OSCEs demonstrated improved clinical competence and confidence (Hickey, 2021).

Standardized patients can provide feedback (formative evaluation) to students and help ensure competence before students are evaluated or begin practice in the complex "real" world settings. Potential exists for multiple evaluators to observe and test students in the performance of numerous skills during brief examination periods. The OSCE process, considered an acceptable and powerful approach in clinical performance evaluation, allows rapid feedback to students about attainment of learning outcomes. Many programs use the OSCE as a learning tool with formative feedback. Students have reported learning and satisfaction with the standardized patient experience (Phillips et al., 2020). If the OSCE is used as high-stakes testing, faculty must consider the implications of this evaluation, and as discussed earlier, prepare the students.

Evaluation Strategies: Self-Reflection, Self-Evaluation, Portfolios, Journals, Logs

Self-Reflection and Self-Evaluation

Reflecting on one's practice is an integral component of clinical learning. Reflection, considered to be an introspective process with self-observation of one's thoughts and feelings, provides opportunity to consider and make sense of experiences. Potential outcomes of reflection include new perspective on experience, change in behavior, readiness for application, and commitment to action. (See Chapter 16.)

Self-evaluation and self-reflection are related concepts. In *self-evaluation* students complete criteria-based assessments using self-reflection. Self-evaluation against a standard is one way to assist students to gain lifelong learning skills. In self-evaluation, students describe and make qualitative judgments about specified experiences, helping balance the quantitative nature of evaluation with qualitative data. Self-evaluation against a rubric or standard can be a significant student

learning tool, helping students examine their progress, identify their strengths and weaknesses, and set goals for improvement in the areas indicated. It can also help faculty better understand student attitudes and values as well as thinking processes.

Self-reflection provides students with an opportunity to think about what they have learned and promotes becoming reflective clinicians. Clinical reasoning depends on both cognitive and metacognitive (thinking about one's thinking) skill development. There are different ways to incorporate reflection into clinical practice, including preactivity, during the activity, and postactivity. As faculty consider reflection as an important tool for clinical evaluation, continued focus is needed on being precise and thoughtful about approaches, including purposes and the key elements students are being asked to reflect on. Box 25.3 provides sample reflective prompts based on the Tanner's (2006) Clinical Judgment Model (Smith, 2021). Self-assessment provides students with opportunity to

---

BOX 25.3 Sample Reflective Prompts for Clinical Judgment Based on Tanner's (2006) Clinical Judgment Model

1. **Noticing:** Describe what you noticed about your patient immediately. Describe what you noticed as you spent more time with the patient and possibly their family.
2. **Interpreting:** What did your observations during the clinical experience lead you to believe about your patients? What was the priority of care? What additional information was needed to provide patient care? What resources supported your interpretation?
3. **Responding:** After consideration of your clinical experience, what were the goals for your patient? What interventions did you complete during the clinical experience to support these goals? How did you support therapeutic communication with your patient?
4. **Reflecting:** What are other possibilities for supporting this patient? In what ways did Noticing, Interpreting, Responding, and Reflecting help improve your patient care?

Modified from Smith, T. (2021). Guided reflective writing as a teaching strategy to develop nursing student clinical judgment. *Nursing Forum, 56*(2), 241–248.

review their progress against a rubric or standard, identify weaknesses as well as strengths, and set goals for improving their clinical learning.

A potential disadvantage of self-evaluation is that students may not be honest about their level of self-understanding in an effort to protect themselves against potential criticism. The ability to critically reflect on individual performance may be influenced by the maturity and self-esteem of the student. Students are more likely to share summaries and reflections with faculty if a foundation of trust has been established. If self-evaluation begins at the onset of the students' clinical experience, students can benefit from examining their ongoing progress. Through the teacher–student interaction process, observations and perceptions can be shared, student strengths and weaknesses can be discussed, and self-evaluation strategies can be improved. Student–teacher relationships can become stronger and more constructive as students progress.

Portfolios

Portfolios provide students opportunity to assemble evidence that documents different types of learning, providing opportunity for a holistic approach to evaluation (Kaplan et al., 2013). Described as collections of evidence prepared by students, they provide a collage or album of student learning rather than a one-time snapshot. Portfolios allow integration of a number of assessments and can help provide progressive documentation of specified clinical learning outcomes (see Chapter 24). Reflective portfolios are designed to help students consider their progress in clinical learning and also help faculty understand students' clinical learning processes. Faculty can provide portfolio guidelines that help students organize their portfolio components and incorporate reflective summaries. Portfolios can help students learn strategies for documenting clinical competencies as a part of lifelong learning, including clinical specialties. For example, related to psychiatric nursing education, a descriptive study supported that students made professional progress in both practice and theory after using e-portfolios to document competencies gained. When portfolios are well implemented, they can be both practical and effective in helping students take learning responsibility and supporting their professional development.

Journals and Logs

Journals and logs are, in essence, written dialogues between the self and the designated reader. These written dialogues provide opportunity for students to share values and critical thinking abilities. Journals give students the opportunity to record their clinical experiences and review their progress. This enables students to consider areas of needed improvement and work on problems and clinical performance weaknesses. The concepts of *clinical logs* and *journals* are sometimes used synonymously, but clinical logs can vary in the amount of detail, ranging from a listing of types of patients and noted student care roles to a more detailed log with a reflection on each patient care experience. A guided reflection, such as one providing reflective prompts based on a clinical judgment model, provides clear direction for helping students describe their clinical thinking. In Smith's (2021) qualitative study focusing on early and completing undergraduate student perceptions of reflective clinical logs, students described more active learning and thinking about their actions and processes with use of a detailed reflective clinical log.

Faculty should provide specific guidelines as to the amount of detail required in clinical journals or logs and provide clear guidelines as to how (or if) journals or logs will be graded, providing students a rubric as guidance. Faculty feedback about student self-reflections provides opportunity for further dialogue on learning experiences. Self-reflection and self-evaluation can become part of the process for lifelong, self-directed learning.

CLINICAL EVALUATION PROCESS

Before the evaluation process begins, faculty and students need a clear understanding of the outcomes to be attained at the culmination of the experience. Clinical evaluation is a systematic process that can be considered as having three consecutive phases: (1) preparation, (2) clinical activity phase, and (3) final data interpretation and feedback. A listing of sample tasks within each phase and the roles faculty will assume during each phase are provided in Box 25.4. Additional discussion of selected points in each phase follows. (See Case Study 25.1.)

BOX 25.4 Role of Faculty Evaluator during the Evaluation Process

Phase I: Preparation

Determine objectives and competencies. Identify evaluation methods and tools. Choose clinical site.

Orient students to the evaluation plan. Focus on objectivity in evaluation.

Phase II: Clinical Activity

Orient students and staff to the student role. Provide students with clinical opportunities. Ensure patient safety.

Observe and collect evaluation data from multiple perspectives. Provide student feedback to enhance learning.

Document findings and maintain privacy of records. Contract with students regarding any deficiencies.

Phase III: Final Data Interpretation and Presentation

Interpret data in fair, reasonable, and consistent manner. Assign grade.

Provide summative evaluation conference (ensure privacy and respect confidentiality).

Evaluate experience.

CASE STUDY 25.1 Orienting a New Faculty to the Evaluation Process

A faculty who is a course coordinator for a medical–surgical nursing course is orienting a newly employed faculty to teaching in the clinical setting. The newly employed faculty has worked as a unit manager for a medical–surgical unit at Hospital X but will be teaching first-year students at Hospital Y.

1. What should the course coordinator include in an orientation plan for the new faculty about the clinical evaluation process?
2. What should the newly employed faculty know about each phase of the evaluation process?
3. What aspects of the newly employed faculty's previous experience as a unit manager might influence their evaluation of first year students?

Preparation Phase
Choosing the Clinical Setting and Patient Assignment as Part of the Evaluation Process

Faculty are responsible for providing each student with ample opportunities to achieve course objectives and must give careful attention to choosing a clinical site that will give students these opportunities. Especially when traditional clinical settings will be the evaluation site, advance planning is needed. Even in the ideal clinical setting, daily variability exists in terms of patients, providers, and the activity level of the unit, which can complicate evaluation. In addition to student unit assignments, specific patient clinical assignments should also be considered as part of a fair evaluation. This includes both the types of patients assigned to students and the duration of clinical assignments.

Teaching and learning in a natural setting provide unique challenges for both students and faculty. Negotiating the balance between student independence and supervision is complex. Faculty must provide adequate supervision to ensure safe delivery of care with the welfare and the safety of patients as the first priority but are also challenged by being a guest in the clinical setting and communicating with the staff.

Before the clinical experience begins, faculty must develop criteria for what is considered unsafe or inappropriate behavior and what consequences will occur if such behavior is observed. Policies related to safety and incident reporting, both in academia and clinical agencies, should be considered. The faculty must be prepared to remove a student from the clinical setting if the student is not adequately prepared to provide safe nursing care; students have the right to know the standard used for safe practice and evaluation. Ongoing dialogue with academic and clinical partners is indicated.

Communication between faculty and students before the clinical experience begins is essential, including orientation to the grading process. Students should be given an orientation to the clinical facility and to the policies and procedures that will apply to the clinical experience. Unit orientations, as well as orientation to evaluation methods, are important in decreasing the anxiety that can hamper student clinical performance.

Students and faculty are essentially visitors in an established system, and the status of student comfort and support in the clinical environment should be considered in evaluation as well. The importance of a positive clinical learning environment for student learning is clear; students should have opportunity to share with faculty their evaluation of the clinical setting. A sample form for student evaluation of a clinical setting is provided in Box 25.5.

Determining the Standards and Evaluation Tools

Faculty have the responsibility for choosing the appropriate methods and tools for evaluation of the learners' clinical performance. Specific evaluation instruments chosen will be the means of documenting and communicating judgments made about student performance. These tools should document performance expectations relevant to course objectives and be practical and time efficient.

The concepts of interrater reliability (whether results can be replicated by other raters) and content validity (whether a tool measures what is desired) at a minimum should be considered in selection of a specific clinical evaluation instrument. See Chapter 23 for further discussion of reliability, interrater reliability, and validity.

Faculty should work together to determine or develop tools that reflect the increasing complexity of competencies required as students progress from program beginners to graduating seniors and to promote consistency from course to course. Inconsistencies in evaluation can result if each course coordinator develops course tools independently.

BOX 25.5   Student Evaluation of Clinical Setting

Name of Agency
Specific Unit
Designated Preceptor

Directions
Please respond to the following statements with the rating that best describes your opinion.
A. Strongly Agree
B. Agree
C. Disagree
D. Strongly Disagree
  Please qualify any rating of C or D with comments or suggestions. Your ratings and written comments will be used to determine clinical placement for future students and may be shared with individuals in the setting but only in summary form.

Application of Course Material
  1. The staff facilitated my ability to meet clinical objectives.
  2. I was able to meet the objectives of this course in this setting.

Population/Patients
  3. Patients presented clinical problems appropriate to the objectives of this course.

  4. Culturally diverse patients (e.g., cultural, social, economic) were available in the setting.

Health Professionals
  5. Nurse managers, staff nurses, and support staff were available to me to answer questions.
  6. The nursing staff were positive role models.
  7. Nurses demonstrated professional relationships with other health care professionals.

Physical Environment
  8. The setting was conducive to working with patients and other health care team members.
  9. Space was available for conferences with faculty and other students.

Overall Impression of Setting
  10. I have a positive impression of the quality of care provided in this setting.
  11. I would recommend this setting for future students taking this course.
  12. How could your clinical experience have been improved in this clinical setting?
  Please share any additional comments and suggestions.

Adapted with permission from a form used by Fort Hays State University, Department of Nursing.

Clinical Activity Phase

In both obtaining and analyzing clinical evaluation data, faculty need to make professional judgments about the performance of students, being aware of the subjective nature of evaluation. To prevent biased judgments, faculty need to be aware of the factors that can influence decision making and must actively use strategies to prevent biases (see Case Study 25.2). Strategies that can help support trustworthiness of the clinical evaluation data include the following:

- Have specified objectives or competencies on which to base the evaluation.
- Use multiple strategies and combined methods of evaluation for compiling data.
- Include both qualitative and quantitative measures.
- Determine a practical sampling plan and evaluate students over time.
- Provide clear scoring directions for tools to promote consistency between raters in collection and interpretation of data.
- Orient faculty in use of specific clinical evaluation tools and approaches for consistency and fairness in grading.

CASE STUDY 25.2 Evaluating a Student Who Is Not Making Progress in the Course

A faculty is preparing to hold mid-term conferences with students. One of the students appears to have "borderline" clinical skills and is not attaining all course objectives. The faculty is reviewing the data in order to provide a fair and helpful mid-term evaluation.

1. What should the faculty consider to prevent bias and guide the student toward attainment of course outcomes?
2. What are the issues involved in this situation?
3. What resources could the faculty use to prepare for the mid-term conference?
4. What feedback will be most helpful to the student at this time?
5. What are the legal and ethical implications of this situation?

- Be aware of common errors such as the halo effect (assuming that of assuming that behaviors are positive behaviors).
- Incorporate teacher self-assessment of values, beliefs, or biases that might affect the evaluation process (Oermann & Gaberson, 2021).

Final Data Interpretation and Presentation Phase

Clinical Evaluation Conference

The findings of the clinical evaluation are usually shared with the student individually at the end of the clinical experience or course. No surprises should be presented at this time. The timely feedback from the earlier formative evaluation should provide students with information sufficient to prepare them for this evaluation. A student's self-evaluation is often submitted before the evaluation conference and discussed at this time.

Evaluation results are commonly reported in both written and oral forms. Often, the primary evaluation tool is presented to show student improvement and specifically recall incidents. The faculty should clarify initially that the purpose of the conference is to provide information on the student's clinical performance. The results should be explained, giving specific incidents in which the student had difficulties, excelled, performed adequately, or improved. In addition, the faculty member needs to assist the student in establishing ongoing learning goals. Finally, the faculty member needs to summarize the conference, ending on a positive or encouraging note.

The environment in which the evaluation conference takes place should be comfortable for the student, and privacy should be maintained. An hour during which the student is responsible for patient care or directly after a tiring clinical experience is not the most conducive time for a conference. An appointment during office hours away from the clinical site provides a more comfortable and private setting for students to listen to constructive criticism or encouraging comments. In a study of students' perceptions of grades, student stress was a common theme. Authors discussed the importance of faculty considering the power of their words as well as the value of orienting and mutual discussions related to the concept of grading (Poorman & Mastorovich, 2014).

Student Response

The student's response to the faculty evaluation can vary. Typically, a student perceives the results as fair if his or her own appraisal is congruent with that of the faculty. A student self-evaluation submitted before the conference helps faculty gain insight into student perceptions and can give faculty time to prepare a response. However, an important way to ensure congruent results is for faculty to provide the student with a sufficient number of formative evaluations and time to reflect on their own performance. Faculty need to be sensitive to the student's needs, emphasizing the student's strengths as well as weaknesses and encouraging goals and aspirations.

Working With Students Who Are Not Safe or Not Attaining Course Competencies

Dismissing an unsafe student from clinical practice. Faculty must immediately identify student behaviors that are unsafe for patient care such as lack of preparation, violence, or substance abuse. A well-developed syllabus that outlines policies and expected clinical norms can minimize students' anxieties and support positive behaviors (Clark, 2017). A broad and thorough policy that allows for safe and appropriate actions to protect both the patient and the student is indicated. Clear policies help prevent arbitrary or capricious responses to an incident. O'Connor (2014) summarizes key points related to the student who is unsafe to care for patients, noting that safety of the patient is the first priority in removing a student but that faculty have an obligation to ensure that all students are returned to an area of safety as well. For the student unprepared to care for an assigned clinical patient, faculty should refer to school policies addressing the issue. The first step is to remove the student from the situation and from the patient if the student is in a patient care situation. The next step is to discuss the behavior with the student and determine what action should be taken next. In some instances, the student may be having a health problem and should be referred immediately for diagnosis and treatment; in other situations the student may not be prepared to provide patient care and needs further preparation before taking care of patients. The final step is to document the incident and report it to the appropriate administrators.

Supporting at-risk students. Developing a positive learning environment is a basic step in promoting positive, supportive student learning relationships. Students have a right to expect respect. Frequent formative feedback that points out areas in which students need to improve and specific ways to achieve clinical goals promotes positive learning opportunities and minimizes potential legal risks.

Faculty discussions can help clarify definitions of safe and unsafe clinical practices. Having clear policies and guidelines provides direction for working with students who are not attaining course outcomes (Clark, 2017). Minimum patient safety competencies can be observed, checked off, and documented in the learning lab. School policies can indicate minimum safety competencies that need to be achieved in the learning laboratory before a student moves into the actual clinical setting. Students' behaviors that put patients at safety risk also typically put students at risk for failing.

Supporting at-risk students also involves ensuring that clinical experiences take place in an environment of a culture of safety or just culture. For example, students might want to avoid disclosing mistakes, such as medication errors, if there were concerns such as grade retaliation. Just culture and the culture of safety involve discussion and learning from mistakes rather than being punitive (Walker et al., 2019).

When faculty notice that a student is not attaining course outcomes, it is important to first document the behavior, communicate with the student, and provide support. The following guidelines can be used when faculty determine that students are not attaining course outcomes or clinical practice competencies.

- Ensure that students understand the criteria such as written course objectives or competency statements and course evaluation plan.
- Document the student's behavior. Faculty can use clinical evaluation instruments and anecdotal records to document a pattern of behaviors.

- Discuss the behavior with the student and identify expected behaviors.
- Develop a learning improvement plan or contract. Faculty must identify expectations as to what specific student behaviors need to occur for passing status to be achieved, how often the student will be observed, and how often evaluation conferences will be held. An annotated record of each counseling session and student evaluation should be signed by both the student and the faculty member and maintained by the faculty member.
- Follow written procedure from school handbooks; be familiar with student appeal processes (see Chapter 3).

Assigning a Failing Grade

When students are not demonstrating safe clinical practice, faculty are faced with making a decision to give a failing grade. Faculty may be reluctant to assign this grade and may consider not failing a student, known in the literature as "failing to fail" students who are not meeting clinical competencies. Faculty often feel challenged in assigning failing grades, including having emotional responses and anxiety as to whether their evaluations were correct.

Multiple authors address challenges related to the decision to assign a failing grade to students who are not meeting course outcomes. The challenges may include not having enough evidence, fear of reprisals from students, unclear policies for giving a failing grade, and limited or no administrative support Butts (2022). In a study of the psychometric properties of the *Gut Feelings Scale*, Hussein et al. (2021) addressed an instrument developed to help quantify faculty "intuition" when students are not attaining clinical course outcomes. This instrument is designed to help faculty document concerns relevant to student patterns of lacking clinical judgment or necessary actions and was determined to have reliability and validity.

Support from the university or college is essential when performance is determined to be unsatisfactory, and the administration should be notified of impending problems early in the grading process. Cassidy et al. (2017) conducted interviews and focus groups with 38 clinical faculty and found that if those who were assigning failing grades were to be comfortable with this task, they needed acknowledgment from colleagues and organizational entities that their decisions would be supported. Couper's (2018) national survey of 390 faculty included similar themes of needing to feel supported by administration when assigning a failing grade.

In a scoping review of the literature, Lewis (2020) found that while students who fail and repeat a course may have poorer outcomes, opportunities exist for supportive interventions. The author describes the situation as a systems issue with implications for all involved.

When a fair judgment is made that a student's performance is unsatisfactory or failing, strategies should be used to avert interpersonal or legal problems. Assigning a failing grade requires having clear program policies such as a student appeal process (see Chapter 3) and a clear chain of command for communicating problems that includes reporting to the course leader, department chair, dean, legal department, and university administrators.

Once the decision to assign a failing grade is made, communication with the student is essential. Documentation from formative evaluation conferences and student contracts can provide support for this decision. Published school policies and procedures involving appropriate administrators should be followed, including documentation that decisions were made carefully and deliberately.

Addressing student reactions to receiving a failing grade. Final evaluations that result in unsatisfactory or failing performance require special tact and concern. Faculty need to share specific findings that resulted in a student not meeting the expected clinical objectives and student contracts not fulfilled need to be identified. Students will need time to process the information and should not feel rushed. Faculty need to listen attentively, with a strong show of concern and support, to the student's perceptions. The student may need time to reflect and return for another conference after adjusting to the facts.

The student who has received a failing grade may react in a variety of ways. Caring faculty will recognize these behaviors and provide empathetic support. Students may respond with denial, providing their own perception of how a specified incident did or did not occur and offering excuses. Faculty need to steer the conversation to the student's not meeting the clinical course objectives and provide support for the student's emotional needs. A student may attempt to bargain for a passing grade. Faculty need to stand firm and focus on the evaluation results. As the reality of the loss is recognized, the student may respond with despair, confusion, lack of motivation, indecision, and tears. Faculty should provide support, listen attentively, and generally convey caring behaviors; in some instances, faculty may also need to recommend professional counseling. The student may come to terms with the outcome and begin to make plans for the future. Assistance from the faculty in considering further options is often sought by the student. Faculty can be prepared to provide information about any program options that are available to students who fail a clinical course. How well the student adapts to the final evaluation typically depends on how well he or she has been prepared for the results.

In other situations, the student may respond with anger. The student may become demanding or accusing and may have the potential to become violent. In this case, faculty need to take steps to ensure their own safety and that of the student. Faculty should not take the anger personally but provide guidance about feelings and focus on the anger as a part of loss. When potential exists for incivility at conferences, being prepared with and implementing broad communication scripts may help deal with actual or potential conflict situations (Clark, 2017).

Additionally, an established grievance policy should be available. Both students and faculty share responsibility for knowing about and appropriately employing such a policy. Students have a right to respond appropriately to grievances. See Chapter 3 for further discussion of legal issues.

EVALUATION OF THE EVALUATION EXPERIENCE

After the final student conference, the student and faculty need to evaluate the entire experience as a whole. The clinical site is evaluated to determine how well it meets the learning and practice needs of the students. Was the philosophy of the staff congruent with that of the faculty and students? Were the students given the opportunity to meet all objectives? As these questions are answered, the preparation phase for evaluation begins again. A continuous quality improvement process for clinical evaluation should be considered, with attention given to structure (appropriate evaluation tools with appropriate clinical environment and patient care opportunities), process (appropriate plans for sampling and evaluating clinical behaviors and for sharing feedback and results of evaluation), and outcome (satisfactory evaluative outcomes indicating safe, competent graduates). Additionally, faculty can question evaluation practices, including new approaches that further incorporate students' perspectives.

While this chapter focuses on clinical performance evaluation in more traditional clinical laboratory and health care settings, the same type of evaluation concepts and principles will extend to changing clinical settings and strategies. Clinical performance evaluation is important to patients' safety, students' skills and confidence, and assurances to the public that the school of nursing is graduating well-prepared students. While recent experience with the pandemic and a new emphasis on student competencies require new clinical approaches, strategies, and instruments, good evaluation principles still apply.

CHAPTER SUMMARY: KEY POINTS

- Especially in times of changing clinical contexts, best clinical evaluation practices include multidimensional evaluation with diverse evaluation methods completed over time, seeking student growth and progress.

- National nursing organizations and other entities are redefining expectations for clinical competencies for students in all academic programs.
- Tested models, strategies, and instruments are central to best evaluation practices.

- Advances in technology are promoting new opportunities for clinical performance evaluation including virtual case resources and simulations.
- Clinical performance evaluation provides students with opportunity for critical reflection and self-assessments using clinical standards.
- Formative assessments can help faculty and students identify student learning needs and prepare for summative evaluations.

- An appropriate summative evaluation process sets the stage for productive assessment of student competence and further learning.
- A systems approach, including appropriate policies and administrative backing, is needed for supporting faculty in documenting a student's earned unsatisfactory clinical evaluation.

REFLECTING ON THE EVIDENCE

1. What is your current process for completing a clinical evaluation? In what ways do you incorporate multiple clinical indicators into evaluation (e.g., data from interview, observation, and document review)? How do you then synthesize these diverse pieces of clinical evaluation data?
2. What are your concerns about the transition to practice gap? How do you see the national discussion of expected program competencies impacting this transition? What are the benefits and the challenges to development of national standards rather than individual program-based models of clinical evaluation?
3. What are the benefits of tools such as rubrics in the clinical evaluation documentation process? How does your faculty team currently use these tools? Are there ways you could expand or improve the use of these tools? In what ways do these approaches improve your efficiency and effectiveness in clinical evaluation?
4. In what ways is formative evaluation or feedback different from summative evaluation? How do you currently provide formative feedback to students?

5. What process do you use to identify/help students who are struggling to attain course competencies or at risk of failing? What strategies can be used to help identify and guide students who may be underperforming?
6. How do you use student reflection to inform evaluation? In what ways do you use reflective prompts to engage students in self-evaluation? What strategies do you use to challenge students to self-reflect and set further learning goals? How can these strategies contribute to active learning and clinical judgment?
7. In what ways can the clinical team be engaged to promote a positive evaluation environment? In what ways do "system factors" in the academic and practice settings impact the student grading process? In what ways does supporting a *just culture* for improvement factor in?
8. In what ways do you incorporate ongoing quality improvement in clinical evaluation? In what ways does your faculty team work together in determining best evaluation processes? What types of meetings and orientations do you use to monitor this process? As you list the steps and tools you use, what are your recommendations for ongoing quality improvement?

REFERENCES

Altmiller, J. (2017). Content validation of a quality and safety education for nurses-based clinical evaluation instrument. *Nurse Educator*, 42(1), 23–27. https://doi.org/10.1097/NNE.0000000000000307.

Altmiller, G., & Dugan, M. A. (2020). Content validation of the quality and safety framed clinical evaluation for nurse practitioner students. *Nurse Educator*, 46(3), 159–163. https://doi.org/10.1097/NNE.0000000000000936.

American Association of Colleges of Nursing (AACN) (2022). *Clinical judgment concept across domains*. https://www.aacnnursing.org/AACN-Essentials/Implementation-Tool-Kit

Aronowitz, T., Aronowitz, S., Mardin-Small, J., & Kim, B. (2016). Using Objective Structured Clinical Examination (OSCE) as education in advanced practice registered nursing education. *Journal of Professional Nursing, 33*(2), 119–125. https://doi.org/10.1016/j.profnurs.2016.06.003.

Bonnel, W., Smith, K., & Hober, C. (2019). *Teaching with technologies in nursing and health professions: Strategies for engagement, quality, and safety* (2nd ed.). Springer.

Butts, P. (2022). Clinical eval in prelicensure baccalaureate nursing programs: A qualitative descriptive study. *Nursing Education Perspectives, 43*(1), 14–18. https://doi.org/10.1097/01.NEP.0000000000000863.

Caputi, L. (2019). Reflections on the next generation NCLEX with implications for nursing programs. *Nursing Education Perspectives, 40*(1), 2–3. https://doi.org/10.1097/01.NEP.0000000000000439.

Cassidy, S., Coffey, M., & Murphy, F. (2017). Seeking authorization. A grounded theory exploration of mentors' experiences of assessing nursing students on the borderline of achievement of competence in clinical practice. *Journal of Advanced Nursing, 73*(9). https://doi.org/10.1111/jan.13292.

Clark, C. (2017). An evidence-based approach to integrate civility, professionalism, and ethical practice into nursing curricula. *Nurse Educator, 42*(3), 120–126. https://doi.org/10.1097/NNE.0000000000000331.

Couper, J. (2018). The struggle is real: Investigating the challenge of assigning a failing clinical grade. *Nursing Education Perspectives, 39*(3), 132–138. https://doi.org/10.1097/01.NEP.0000000000000295.

Cronenwett, L., Sherwood, G., Barnsteiner, J., Disch, J., Johnson, J., Mitchell, P., Taylor Sullivan, D., & Warren, J. (2007). Quality and safety education for nurses. *Nursing Outlook, 55*, 122–131. https://doi.org/10.1016/j.outlook.2007.02.006.

Dickison, P., Luo, X., Woo, A., Muntean, W., & Bergstrom, B. (2017). Assessing higher-order cognitive constructs by using an information processing framework. *Journal of Applied Testing. Technology, 17*(1), 1–19.

Fieler, G. (2020). Utilization of video for competency evaluation. *Nursing Education Perspectives, 41*, 255–257. https://doi.org/10.1097/01.NEP.0000000000000645.

Gonzalez, L., Nielsen, A., & Lasater, K. (2021). Developing students' clinical reasoning skills: A faculty guide. *Journal of Nursing Education, 60*(9), 485–493. https://doi.org/10.3928/01484834-20210708-01.

Harris, M., Rhoads, S., Rooker, J., Kelly, M., Lefler, L., Lubin, S., Martel, I., & Beverly, C. (2019). Using virtual site visits in the clinical evaluation of nurse practitioner students. *Nurse Educator, 45*, 17–20. https://doi.org/10.1097/NNE.0000000000000693.

Hickey, M. (2021). OSCEs as a method of competency evaluation in a primary care NP program. *Nurse Educator, 46*(5), 317–321. https://doi.org/10.1097/NNE.0000000000000951.

Hussein, M., McLarnon, M., & Fast, O. (2021). Psychometric testing of a theory-based measure to evaluate clinical performance of nursing students. *Nursing Education Perspectives, 42*(6), 358–364. https://doi.org/10.1097/01.NEP.0000000000000888.

Johnson, B., Browning, K., & DeClerk, L. (2021). Strategies to reduce bias and racism in nursing precepted clinical experiences. *Journal of Nursing Education, 60*(12), 697–702. https://doi.org/10.3928/01484834-20211103-01.

Kavanagh, J., & Sharpnack, P. (2021). Crisis in competency: A defining moment in nursing education. *Online Journal of Issues in Nursing, 26*(1). https://ojin.nursingworld.org/MainMenuCategories/ANAMarketplace/ANAPeriodicals/OJIN/TableofContents/Vol-26-2021/No1-Jan-2021/Crisis-in-Competency-A-Defining-Moment-in-Nursing-Education.html.

Kavanagh, J., & Szweda, C. (2017). A crisis in competency: The strategic and ethical imperative to assessing new graduate nurses' clinical reasoning. *Nursing Education Perspectives, 38*(2), 57–62. https://doi.org/10.1097/01.NEP.0000000000000112.

Klenke-Borgman, L., Cantrell, M. A., & Marianai, B. (2020). Nurse educators' guide to clinical judgment: A review of conceptualization, measurement, and development. *Nursing Education Perspectives, 41*(4), 215–221.

Lasater, K. (2007). Clinical judgment development: Using simulation to create an assessment rubric. *Journal of Nursing Education, 46*(11), 496–503. https://doi.org/10.3928/01484834-20071101-04.

Lasater, K. (2011). Clinical judgment: The last frontier for evaluation. *Nurse Education in Practice, 11*(2), 86–92. https://doi.org/10.1016/j.nepr.2010.11.013.

Lasater, K., & Nielsen, A. (2009). Reflective journaling for development of clinical judgment. *Journal of Nursing Education, 48*, 40–44. https://doi.org/10.3928/01484834-20090101-06.

Lee, K. (2021). The Lasater clinical judgment rubric: Implications for evaluating teaching effectiveness. *Journal of Nursing Education, 60*(2), 67–73. https://doi.org/10.3928/01484834-20210120-03.

Lewallen, L., & Van Horn, E. (2019). The state of the science on clinical evaluation in nursing education. *Nursing Education Perspectives, 40*(1), 4–10. https://doi.org/10.1097/01.NEP.0000000000000376.

Lewis, L. (2020). Nursing students who fail and repeat courses: A scoping view. *Nurse Educator, 45*(1), 30–34. https://doi.org/10.1097/NNE.0000000000000667.

National Institutes of Health Stroke Scale (NIHSS), (2021). *Online training.* American Heart Association. https://learn.heart.org/lms/nihss.

National League for Nursing (NLN). (2020). *Fair testing guidelines for nursing education.* http://www.nln.org/docs/default-source/advocacy-public-policy/fair-testing-guidelines2e88c-c5c78366c709642ff00005f0421.pdf?sfvrsn=2

O'Connor, A. B. (2014). *Clinical instruction and evaluation* (3rd ed.). Jones & Bartlett.

Oermann, M., & Gaberson, K. (2021). *Evaluation & testing in nursing education* (6th ed.). Springer.

Ong, S., Darryl, W., Goh, L., & Lau, Y. (2021). Understanding nurse preceptors' experiences in a primary health care setting: A descriptive qualitative study. *Journal of Nursing Management, 29,* 1320–1328. https://doi.org/10.1111/jonm.13272.

Phillips, T., Munn, A., & George, T. (2020). Assessing the impact of telehealth objective structured clinical examinations in graduate nursing education. *Nurse Educator, 45*(1), 17–20. https://doi.org/10.1097/NNE.0000000000000729.

Poorman, S., & Mastorovich, M. (2014). The meaning of grades: Stories of undergraduate, master's, and doctoral nursing students. *Nurse Educator, 44*(6), 321–325. https://doi.org/10.1097/NNE.0000000000000627.

Quality and Safety Education for Nurses Institute. (2021). *Quality and Safety Education for Nurses (QSEN) project.* http://qsen.org/about-qsen/

Quality Matters (QM). (2021). *QM rubrics and standards.* https://www.qualitymatters.org/research/curated-research-resources

Schuster-McHugh, P. (2020). *Concept mapping: A clinical judgement approach to patient care* (5th ed.). F.A. Davis.

Smith, T. (2021). Guided reflective writing as a teaching strategy to develop nursing student clinical judgment. *Nursing Forum, 56*(2), 241–248. https://doi.org/10.1111/nuf.12528.

Tanner, C. A. (2006). Thinking like a nurse: A research-based model of clinical judgment in nursing. *Journal of Nursing Education, 45*(6), 204–211.

U.S. Department of Education. (2014). *The Family Educational Rights and Privacy Act. Uninterrupted scholars act guidance.* https://studentprivacy.ed.gov/resources/uninterrupted-scholars-act-guidance

Walker, D., Altmiller, G., Barkell, N., Hromadik, L., & Toothaker, R. (2019). Development and validation of the just culture assessment tool for nursing education. *Nurse Educator, 44*(5), 261–264. https://doi.org/10.1097/NNE.0000000000000705.

Wilson, R., Wilson, B., & Madden, C. (2021). Creating a national standard for prelicensure clinical evaluation in nursing. *Journal of Nursing Education, 60*(12), 686–689. https://doi.org/10.3928/01484834-20211004-01.

Winstanley, H. D. (2017). *A qualitative descriptive study exploring associate degree nursing faculty's experiences teaching electronic health record systems use. KU Med Center Dissertations and Theses.* http://hdl.handle.net/1808/27045.

26

Systematic Program Evaluation

Peggy Ellis, PhD, RN

Program evaluation is a systematic assessment and analysis of all components of an academic program through the application of evaluation approaches, techniques, and knowledge to improve the effectiveness of the program in reaching its goals. A program evaluation plan is a document that serves as the blueprint for seeking information in a systematic fashion that helps judge the worth or effectiveness of a specific program. The evaluation plan describes the goals, the methods used, the frequency, and the individual or group responsible for each component of the evaluation along with the expected results or the desired goals of each component. The evaluation plan should be designed for use in all program levels including clinical doctoral programs. Although existing accrediting bodies do not currently evaluate PhD programs in nursing that are not clinical doctorates, use of an evaluation plan for assessing quality is an important aspect of program quality improvement. Quality indicators, expected outcomes, and curricular elements are identified and accessible online for use in the evaluation of PhD nursing programs (American Association of Colleges of Nursing [AACN], 2010).

The purpose of this chapter is to provide information on why and how to conduct comprehensive evaluation of nursing education programs. Background information about program evaluation and its benefits is followed by a description of the processes of conducting a program evaluation.

PURPOSES AND BENEFITS OF PROGRAM EVALUATION

The purpose of a comprehensive, systematic evaluation of a program is to determine the extent to which all activities for an academic program meet the established desired goals or outcomes. Evaluation is important for all programs, regardless of whether they are accredited. Program evaluation is conducted for all levels of educational programs from licensed practical or vocational nurse to doctor of nursing practice and doctor of nursing philosophy (PhD). Program evaluation determines the effectiveness of the program and informs decisions related to program improvements. Program evaluation may be developmental, designed to provide direction for the development and implementation of a program, or outcome-oriented, designed to judge the merit of the total program being evaluated. It examines whether a program is being delivered and implemented as planned and if the outcomes are as intended. It should be adaptable and responsive so that it creates a continuous feedback loop in the process (Jager et al., 2020). Specific purposes of program evaluation are to:

1. Determine how various elements of the program interact and influence program effectiveness.
2. Determine the extent to which the mission, goals, and outcomes of the program are realized.
3. Determine whether the program has been implemented as planned.

4. Provide a rationale for decision making that leads to improved program effectiveness.
5. Identify what resources are needed and how those resources can be used most efficiently to improve program quality and effectiveness.

RELATIONSHIP OF PROGRAM EVALUATION TO ACCREDITATION

Accrediting bodies exert considerable influence over nursing programs. Accrediting and approval bodies including the state board of nursing, professional nursing organizations, accrediting bodies for nursing, such as the Commission of Collegiate Nursing Education (CCNE), the National League for Nursing Commision on Nursing Education Accreditation (NLN CNEA), and the Accreditation Commission for Education in Nursing (ACEN). Regional accrediting bodies for universities are involved in ensuring that standards are met and quality is maintained (see Chapter 27). Nursing programs have historically depended on accreditation processes to guide program evaluation efforts. Some nursing programs do not fully engage in program evaluation until preparation of the self-study for an accreditation site visit has begun. However, to fulfill its purposes, program evaluation must be a continuous activity regardless of accreditation. Program evaluation built solely around accreditation criteria may lack examination of some important elements or understanding of the relationship between elements that influence program success. Although the use of only accreditation criteria may not consider some elements of what might influence program effectiveness, building the assessment indicators identified by these bodies into the evaluation process ensures ongoing attention to state and national standards of excellence.

HISTORICAL PERSPECTIVE

The earliest approaches to educational program evaluation were based on Ralph Tyler's (1949) behavioral objective model. Tyler's behavioral objective model was a simple, linear approach that began with defining learning objectives, developing measuring tools, and then measuring student performance to determine whether objectives had been met. Because evaluation occurred at the end of the learning experience, Tyler's approach was primarily summative. Formative evaluation, which includes testing and revising curriculum components during the development and implementation of educational programs, became popular during the 1960s and continued into the 1970s.

Outcomes assessment became the focus of educational evaluation in the 1980s. In 1984 the National Institute of Education Study Group on the Conditions of Excellence in American Postsecondary Education endorsed outcomes assessment as an essential strategy for improving the quality of education in postsecondary institutions (Ewell, 1985). By the mid-1980s the regional accrediting agencies began mandating outcomes assessment in their accreditation criteria (Ewell, 1985). By the early 1990s the National League for Nursing Accrediting Commission (NLNAC) added assessment of learning outcomes to its accreditation criteria. The Commission on Collegiate Nursing Education (CCNE) also included outcomes assessment in its initial accreditation standards, first published in 1997. Both organizations continue to require outcomes assessment. The United States Department of Education emphasizes outcomes, particularly outcomes pertaining to progress and graduation rates. In the past decade most of the nursing literature related to program evaluation has focused on specific elements of program evaluation rather than on comprehensive evaluation.

PROGRAM EVALUATION MODELS

Evaluation Models

Models provide an organizing or systematic approach to overall program evaluation. Box 26.1 provides a summary related to evaluation models and frameworks used in the past. Although it may be helpful to use a specific model to increase the effectiveness and efficiency of the program evaluation, most of these models are no longer commonly used in nursing education. Many of them are complex and difficult to apply. Baccalaureate nursing education programs are not required to use a

BOX 26.1 Evaluation Models

Models provide an organizing or systematic approach to overall program evaluation. It may be helpful to use a specific model to increase the effectiveness and efficiency of the program evaluation. Nursing faculty often do not subscribe to one model of evaluation more than others. However, the following models are commonly found in nursing program evaluation.

Scriven's Goal-Free Evaluation Model
Scriven's model was developed in the 1960s. It provides a broad perspective of evaluation and introduced the ideas of "formative" and "summative" evaluation. The model suggests that the evaluation of goals is unnecessary. The model measures outcomes or the actual effects of the program against the identified needs. Processes, procedures, outcomes, and unanticipated effects, both positive and negative, are examined. Scriven encourages the use of an outside, objective evaluator to avoid bias. The outside evaluator is used to learn about the program and its results with no knowledge of the goals of the program. This method encourages an assessment of both intended and unintended outcomes and broad range of outcomes (Scriven, 1991).

Stake's Countenance Model
Stake's model was introduced in the 1960s and describes three components: antecedents, transactions, and outcomes. *Antecedents* refer to things that existed before the instruction occurred such as an individual's readiness and ability to learn. *Transactions* include the instructional methods and processes involved in the teaching. *Outcomes* are the products that result from the antecedents and transactions. It was introduced in 1967 and emphasizes description and judgment. This model takes into account the stakeholders such as students and teachings, the educational experiences, and the outcomes (Stravropoulou & Stroubouki, 2014).

Tyler's Behavioral Objective Model
Tyler's Behavioral Objective Model was developed in the 1930s and is based on what the faculty would like students to achieve at the end of a course or program, or the determination of the objectives. The model also asks what experiences are needed to reach the objectives, how the experiences can be organized, and how faculty can determine whether the objectives have been met. The educational objectives should be derived from the assessment of society, the learners,

and the subject matter to be mastered. The experiences are prescribed by the faculty. However, Tyler recognized that those experiences are not totally under the control of faculty; they are influenced by the perceptions, interests, and previous experiences of the student. The defined objectives are then used as a benchmark against which it can be determined whether the student learned what was intended (Lunenburg, 2011).

Stufflebeam's Context, Input, Process, and Product Model
Stufflebeam's model originated in the late 1960s and is used as a guide for formative and summative evaluations. The CIPP model is a systems model with the acronym representing *context evaluation, input evaluation, process evaluation*, and *product evaluation*. Context evaluation looks at the context of the program being evaluated. During this stage, the evaluator looks at needs, problems, assets, and opportunities. This information is used to define goals, priorities, and desired outcomes. Input evaluation identifies a potential plan for achievement of the goals and examines what might be used to implement that plan. During this stage, alternative approaches are considered along with possible action plans and staffing plans. The budget needed to meet the needs and achieve the goals is identified and resources are allocated through grants or other mechanisms available. Process evaluation involves the implementation of the plan or instructional strategies and the judgment of program performance and interpretation of outcomes. Product evaluation is the assessment of the outcomes and the determination of whether the targeted outcomes were met. Going through this process will help answer the questions of whether the plan is succeeding or has succeeded, and what needs to be done or changed to reach the proposed goals. This model emphasizes improvement and corrections for problems within a program (Stufflebeam, 2003).

Deming's Continuous Quality Improvement Model
The CQI process was developed by W. Edwards Deming in the 1950s. This evaluation model is seen as a continuous process that is embedded in the culture of the school and its day-to-day work. It should be seen as a natural part of everyday routine. It is described as consisting of four phases: plan, do, study, and act. These phases represent a continuous cycle

Continued

BOX 26.1   Evaluation Models—cont'd

of activities. *Plan* includes the development of goals and objectives to identify the desired outcomes of the program. Data collection is the *do* phase. The analysis or *study* of data occurs to determine whether the program is performing as planned or where and how the program needs improvement or change to reach the intended outcomes. *Act* involves making the changes indicated in the analysis. Then the cycle starts all over so that a continuous process of plan, collect data, analyze, and make changes can occur (Brown & Marshall, 2008).

In all models, a commonality is the cycle of defining where you are headed, how you will get there, an analysis of whether you got there or what is the result, and what you should do next. It is always important to then redo the cycle so that you are continually evaluating and improving. Fig. 26.1 depicts this cycle.

Chen's Theory-Driven Model

Chen's model was introduced in 1980 and provides a framework that identifies the elements of the program, provides the rationale for interventions, and describes the causal linkages between the elements, interventions, and outcomes. Chen's theory calls for the study of the design and conceptualization of an intervention, its implementation, and its utility, then using models to guide the formulation of questions

and data gathering to discover the cause of intended and unintended outcomes (Chen, 1990).

Kirkpatrick's Four-Level Model

Kirkpatrick's model was developed more than 50 years ago and reflects his belief that evaluation should be comprehensive and identify the strengths and weaknesses of the program. His model is designed to evaluate outcomes from a variety of perspectives such as students, employers, and faculty. Outcomes should be evaluated across a variety of levels and phases. The four levels are: reaction, learning, behavior, and results. Reaction includes the perspectives of students related to courses, instructors, and whether or not outcomes are met. This does not ensure that learning has occurred but offers feedback from the perspective of the student. The learning level assesses whether learning has actually occurred through the use of assessment methods such as testing, simulations, exercises, and so forth. Behavior involves the assessment of practical skills or application of learning. The results level includes the assessment of the student's success on the job. This may include evaluations from employers, entrance into graduate programs, and more. This level refers to how the education actually translated to practice and the effects of the education on practice (DeSilets, 2018).

theory-driven approach to evaluation. Currently, most schools use nursing accreditation criteria as a framework to develop an evaluation plan that is systematic and comprehensive.

In all evaluation models, a commonality is the cycle of defining what is to be evaluated, how the evaluation will be conducted, a report of the findings, and recommendations for subsequent revisions. It is always important to repeat the cycle to ensure continual improvement. Fig. 26.1 depicts this cycle.

Regardless of the model or theory used, program evaluation is needed to make valid decisions about the program, the curriculum, and the improvements needed to offer high-quality programs. The evaluation plan can be divided into areas so that all aspects of the program are examined and analyzed to support program improvement decisions.

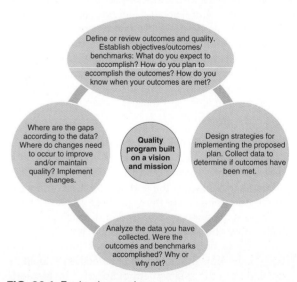

FIG. 26.1 Evaluation cycle.

Although the evaluation plan is important to the continued process, the use of assessment data to guide change involves the commitment of faculty to collect and examine the data and decide what and how to make improvements based on that data.

DEVELOPING A CULTURE OF EVALUATION AND CONTINUOUS QUALITY IMPROVEMENT

A culture of continuous quality improvement is important to the effectiveness and success of the program and school. One of the most important things a nurse educator can do is to ensure that the program(s) are vital, contemporary, and effective in providing a quality education. However, it is easy to put off the data collection and review needed for a thorough and consistent evaluation of the program(s). With all the responsibilities facing the daily lives of faculty, not much time is available for the tasks involved with this undertaking. Faculty need to be clear about the process, the importance of program evaluation, and the improvements that can be accomplished with the findings of the data obtained and analyzed. It is not just for accreditation and is not necessarily an indication of failure of the faculty. It is a matter of uncovering what might be working well or not working as well as had been hoped to provide a quality education. The evaluation plan is meant to guide this evaluation and provide the ability, through data collection and analysis, to provide a quality education. If the process is described clearly within the evaluation plan including what data are collected, who is responsible for collecting the data, how often the data is collected and reviewed, and what are the expected findings, it can provide a roadmap for those activities and become a way of life for faculty. Once faculty see the usefulness of the process in improving the program(s), a routine can be established. Engaging the faculty and staff in the process of evaluation helps them feel an ownership in the process and the outcomes of the process (Gualdron & Parker, 2021).

PROCESS OF DEVELOPING A PROGRAM EVALUATION PLAN

A program evaluation plan is important for the program or school but how is a plan developed? The plan is not required to be in a table; however, it is easier to follow in a table format. First, a decision needs to be made about the organizational structure of the plan. Will accreditation standards be used or some other structure? If the accreditation standards are not used, there must be a strategy to incorporate the evaluation of those standards within the plan in order to help with addressing required accreditation criteria. If the accreditation standards are used, other professional guidelines and standards, such as State Board of Nursing regulations and rules, should also be included. Consider what questions need to be asked and answered. Are there other stakeholder groups (i.e., students, employers, clinical agencies, et al.) who should be included in the process? Decisions should be able to be made about what data/evidence will be most important and accurate in determining whether a criteria has been met or, if not, where is the gap. What is that data/evidence and how can it be obtained, considering the resources available? Who should be responsible for collecting and analyzing that data/evidence?

The evaluation plan should include columns that designate: (1) what data is used to evaluate the element/standard or defined area and how the data is collected; (2) who is responsible for collecting and reviewing the data; (3) what is the timeline or frequency of data collection and evaluation; and (4) what are the expected outcomes for that area. This provides clarity in the process. It may be helpful to also include columns stating whether the expected outcomes were met and what action was taken as a result of that determination.

Make the process as clear as possible within the plan. Allow for all faculty to have input into the decisions needed to design an efficient and effective process. These considerations will provide for a quality evaluation plan that is owned by the faculty and result in a useful program evaluation. Remember that even the evaluation plan should be assessed at regular time intervals in order to make sure it is serving the program and faculty well and providing the answers necessary to determine program quality.

PROGRAM EVALUATION

The Program Evaluation Plan

The program evaluation plan provides a road map for organizing and tracking evaluation activities. This plan is a systematic and written document that contains the evaluation framework, activities for gathering and analyzing data, responsible parties, time frames, accreditation criteria and standards, and the means for using information for program decisions and improvement. The program evaluation plan provides the mechanism for maintaining continuous evaluation of program effectiveness.

Accrediting agencies require a systematic evaluation plan. Some may mention specific components that are needed in the plan. Accrediting agency guidelines may be good to reference as the evaluation plan is developed. Each program offered by the school must be addressed in an evaluation plan. It is not necessary to have separate evaluation plans for each program, although if that is the school's choice, it is acceptable. It is clearer, easier, and more consistent to have one evaluation plan that addresses each program when needed. Some parts of evaluation may have the same benchmarks/expected outcomes for all programs. However, each program should be addressed separately within the evaluation plan if the expected outcomes are different.

Table 26.1 provides a sample evaluation plan that demonstrates how all elements of the program

---

TABLE 26.1   Sample Evaluation Plan

School of Nursing Evaluation Plan

- The evaluation plan should be based on the individual school's resources and what the faculty defines as expected outcomes. What is provided is only an example.
- Standards and Key Elements used in this example are taken from Commission of Collegiate Nursing Education (Amended 2018), Standards for Accreditation of Baccalaureate and Graduate Nursing Programs.

Standard I. Program Quality: Mission and Governance

The mission, philosophy, goals, and expected aggregate student and faculty outcomes are congruent with those of the parent institution, reflect professional nursing standards and guidelines, and consider the needs and expectations of the community of interest. Policies of the parent institution and nursing program clearly support the program's mission, goals, and expected outcomes. The faculty and students of the program are involved in the governance of the program and in the ongoing efforts to improve program quality.

Key Elements	Input/Process	Evidence	Responsible Person/Group	Time Frame	Expected Outcomes
1-A The mission, goals, and expected program outcomes are: • congruent with those of the parent institution • reviewed periodically and revised as appropriate	• Philosophy and mission of the university • Five dimensions of the university • Philosophy and mission of SON	• Documents— reviewed and updated • Minutes indicate review and revision, if necessary, of the mission, goals, and expected outcomes.	• General Faculty Assembly (GFA) • Respective Program Directors and Program Coordinators • Dean, Associate Deans, and Faculty from respective programs	• Every five years or as needed. • Date for review: • 2025, 2030, 2035	• There is congruence between the university philosophy, and the philosophy, goals, and expected outcomes of the programs in the SON.

TABLE 26.1 Sample Evaluation Plan—cont'd

Key Elements	Input/Process	Evidence	Responsible Person/Group	Time Frame	Expected Outcomes
1-B The mission, goals, and expected program outcomes are consistent with relevant professional nursing standards and guidelines for the preparation of nursing professionals.	• Goals and expected program outcomes for the SON • Societal trends • Health care environment • Strategic plan **Most current version of Professional Standards and Guidelines including:** • The Essentials of Baccalaureate Education for Professional Nursing Practice and tool Kit (2008) • The Essentials of Master's Education in Nursing (2011) • The Essentials of Doctoral Education for Advanced Nursing Practice (2006) • The Research Focused Doctoral Program in Nursing: Pathways to Excellence (2010) • National Task Force on Quality Nurse Practitioner Programs (2016) "Criteria for Evaluation of Nurse Practitioner	• Documents—reviewed and updated • Minutes indicate review and revision, if necessary, of the mission, goals, and expected outcomes related to professional standards and guidelines.	• General Faculty Assembly (GFA) • Respective Program Directors and Program Coordinators • Dean, Associate Deans, and Faculty from respective programs	• Every five years or as needed. • Date for review: • 2025, 2030, 2035.	• There is congruence between the SON goals and current professional standards and guidelines.
1.C The mission, goals, and expected outcomes reflect the needs and expectations of the community of interest.	• Community of interest meetings • Community of interest surveys	• Community of interest committee meeting minutes • Community of interest survey results and comments	• Respective Program Directors and Program Coordinators • Dean, Associate Deans, and Faculty from respective programs	• Every five years. • Date for review: • 2023, 2028, 2038.	• Changes made in the SON philosophy, goals, and expected outcomes of the programs or changes made in the curriculum are evidenced in the SON minutes.
1.D The nursing unit's expectations for faculty are written and communicated to the faculty and are congruent with institutional expectations.	• University Faculty Handbook • SON Faculty Handbook • Faculty orientation agenda	• Comparison of University Faculty Handbook statement of faculty expectations and SON Faculty Handbook faculty expectations.	• Dean and Associate Deans • Faculty evaluation tool • Faculty surveys	• Annually	• There is congruence between university faculty expectations and SON faculty expectations. • Faculty are evaluated based on expectations. • Faculty surveys reflect faculty's awareness of expectations.

Continued

TABLE 26.1   Sample Evaluation Plan—cont'd

Key Elements	Input/Process	Evidence	Responsible Person/Group	Time Frame	Expected Outcomes
1.E Faculty and students participate in program governance.	• Faculty and student surveys • Committee rosters • SON Bylaws that include committee structure, purposes, and membership • Committee reports to General Faculty Assembly • University Faculty manual	• Minutes of committee meetings indicating attendance. • Faculty and student surveys indicating knowledge of committee membership requirements. • SON Bylaws stating eligibility of membership on committees.	• Dean • Associate Deans/Program Directors/Option and Specialty Coordinators • Faculty Association • Faculty	• SON Faculty Manual is reviewed at least annually. • Ballot for SON committee membership is distributed and committee membership roster is posted annually. • Bylaws are reviewed every 5 years: 2024, 2029, 2034.	• There is evidence in meeting minutes of students and faculty attending University and SON committees. • 100% of full-time faculty members participate in SON governance and/or university governance and committees.
1.F Academic policies of the parent institution and the nursing program are congruent and support achievement of the mission, goals, and expected program outcomes. These policies are: • fair and equitable; • published and accessible; and • reviewed and revised as necessary to foster program improvement.	• Academic policies such as grading, progression, and admission • Statement of student rights and responsibilities • Student grievance and appeals policies	• University catalogs • Websites • SON student handbooks • Course syllabi	• Program committees • Program Directors • Specialty coordinators	• Annually	• Policies are communicated to students. • Policies are fair and equitable, accurate and up to date in publications. • Students know where policies are published.

TABLE 26.1 Sample Evaluation Plan—cont'd					
Key Elements	Input/Process	Evidence	Responsible Person/Group	Time Frame	Expected Outcomes
1.G The program defines and reviews formal complaints according to established policies	• Student handbooks • University catalog		• Dean • Associate Deans • Faculty • Grievance Committee		• Definition of a formal complaint is available in SON student handbook and University Catalog. • Grievance policies are communicated to students. • Policies are fair and equitable, accurate and up to date in publications. • Students know where policies are published.
1.H Documents and publications are accurate. A process is used to notify constituents about changes in documents and publications.	• University catalog • University website • SON website • SON student handbooks • Course syllabi • Recruitment documents	• Policies are reviewed for accuracy on all sites where they are available.	• Associate Deans • Dean • Faculty	• Annually	• Policies are accurate. • Students and faculty are informed of changes.

evaluation plan may be articulated, including the program's theoretical elements, assessment activities, responsible parties, time frames, and related accreditation criteria. There are a variety of approaches to the evaluation plan. This example is based on CCNE Standards and Key Elements from 2018. This is not required but is helpful when preparing for accreditation through CCNE. However, the most current National League for Nursing Commission on Nursing Education Accreditation (NLN CNEA) Standards can be used or any standards that faculty choose as along as the standards for accreditation used by the chosen accrediting organization are all addressed. This example illustrates the important components of the plan. The expected outcomes are influenced by the specific program or school, the resources available for that program or school, and the individual aspects of the program(s) and school. The evidence used by the program or school and the person or group responsible to demonstrate the standard are also based on the individual program or school, the organizational structure, the expected outcomes, and what is available to demonstrate that the standard is met. Therefore, what is provided in the example evaluation plan may be different for each program/school. For the remaining evaluation components presented in this chapter, only examples of theoretical elements and methods for gathering and analyzing assessment data related to the review of expected and actual outcomes are provided. The theoretical elements and assessment strategies that are suggested here are not all-inclusive but may assist nursing faculty in further development of their own program theory and program evaluation plan.

Mission and Goal Evaluation

Program evaluation must begin by determining that the appropriate mission, philosophy, program goals, and expected outcomes have been defined. The mission and goals should be examined for agreement with the university's mission and goals. The expectations of both internal and external stakeholders must be considered. Internal stakeholders may include administrators, faculty, students, and university governing boards. External stakeholders may include religious organizations for private schools with religious affiliations, regional accrediting bodies, national discipline-specific accrediting bodies, state education commissions and boards of nursing, the legislature, the community, and professional organizations. There should be congruency between the expectations of stakeholders and the program's mission, philosophy, goals, and outcomes. For private institutions with religious affiliations, some perspectives may be prescribed and must be included in mission, philosophy, goals, or outcomes.

The mission of the nursing department or school should be congruent with the university's mission. Incongruence could indicate that the university would not be supportive of the nursing program. Comparison of key phrases or ideas in the department's mission with key phrases or ideas in the university's mission may be done to assess congruency between mission statements. The identification of gaps between the two mission statements provides information about areas where attention is needed. The assessment should be performed periodically and whenever changes are made to either mission statement.

There should be consensus among the faculty regarding the nursing school or department's mission and philosophy. A modified Delphi approach to determine the level of agreement among the faculty for each statement in the mission and philosophy is a useful strategy. The Delphi approach is useful for both the development and the evaluation of belief statements (philosophy). It gathers individual viewpoints and visions to reach a consensus. This approach allows for participants to be in multiple locations, and it can be done without the need for frequent face-to-face dialogue in a manner that protects the anonymity of participants. In this method, questionnaires that list proposition statements about each of the content elements of the belief statement are distributed. Respondents are provided with feedback about the responses after the first round of questionnaire distribution, and consecutive rounds may occur to determine the intensity of agreement or disagreement with the group median responses. The Delphi Method is helpful in allowing faculty to come to a consensus, however, the quality of the results is influenced by the number and background of the respondents (Niederberger & Spranger, 2020). In the evaluation of an established belief statement, the same process will provide data about which propositions continue to be supported, which propositions are no longer supported, and which propositions need to be openly debated. The result provides a consensus list of propositions that either support the belief statement as it is or suggest areas for revision. Chapter 7 provides further information on the development of a mission and philosophy.

All accrediting bodies have expectations related to mission, philosophy, program goals, and expected outcomes. Clear statements of mission, philosophy, and program outcomes are expected. For example, NLN CNEA and the CCNE include outcomes such as graduation rates, job placement rates, licensure and certification pass rates, and program satisfaction (CCNE, 2018; NLN CNEA, 2021). Expectations exist regarding congruency of the program's mission, goals, and outcomes with those of the parent institution, professional nursing standards and guidelines, and the needs of the community of interest.

Professional organization guidelines and standards may be considered in the program mission, philosophy, and goals. They may include but are not limited to the American Nurses Association (ANA), the AACN, the NLN, and the National

Organization of Nurse Practitioner Faculties. Other nursing organizations may be included as appropriate and as desired by the program faculty. Program goals and outcomes should be congruent with the chosen and required nursing organization standards and guidelines. Standards and guidelines that are often used include *ANA's Nursing: Scope and Standards of Practice, 4th Edition* (ANA, 2021) , the *Criteria for Evaluation of Nurse Practitioner Programs* (National Organization of Nurse Practitioner Faculties, 5th ed., 2016), the (Institute of Medicine IOM, 2016) *Assessing Progress on The Institute of Medicine Report on the Future of Nursing.*

Other important external stakeholders to consider in the development of the mission and goals include local constituencies, such as health care agencies, that provide clinical learning experiences or employ graduates of the program. A survey of current and potential employers of graduates will help faculty determine the knowledge and skill requirements of the marketplace and satisfaction with the program's graduates. Many nursing programs establish advisory committees to provide additional information and additional focus groups to add richness to the information. This information is used to ensure that program goals and outcomes are appropriate, to address marketplace needs, and to provide input for curriculum planning. They are also used to develop evaluation questions and tools for determining whether market needs are being met.

The mission and program goals should be clearly and publicly stated. Nursing schools that offer several different nursing programs will need to clearly articulate the purpose and program goals of each of the programs offered. Public announcement of the mission and program goals should be available through the internet and in printed program brochures and catalogs. Box 26.2 lists the theoretical elements for mission and goal evaluation.

Curriculum Evaluation

One of the most critical elements of program effectiveness is curriculum design. Curriculum design is a plan and process for putting together content, courses, and strategies for learning that is similar to an architectural blueprint. The curriculum design provides direction for both the content of the program and the teaching and learning processes

> ### BOX 26.2 Elements for Mission and Goal Evaluation
>
> - The mission of the nursing school or department is congruent with that of the university.
> - There is consensus among the faculty regarding the mission and philosophy.
> - There is congruency between the nursing mission, philosophy, conceptual framework, goals, and outcomes for each program.
> - There is congruency with professional nursing standards and guidelines as identified by the nursing program.
> - Expectations of the accrediting and approval bodies are known and considered in the program's mission, goals, philosophy, and outcomes.
> - The Nursing Program Advisory Committee and Community of Interest has meaningful input into program goals and outcomes.
> - Documents and publications accurately reflect the mission and goals.

involved in program implementation. It includes an organizing framework that provides logic for the arrangement of the curriculum elements. Curriculum content involves both discipline-specific knowledge and the liberal arts foundation. Faculty must determine their definition of the discipline of knowledge before the curriculum can be designed so that the courses selected will prepare the students for the practice of nursing. Faculty must also determine what ways of knowing, or methods of inquiry, are characteristic of the discipline and what skills the discipline demands. Program goals and outcome statements provide a guide for the development of the curriculum. The curriculum design and content should be congruent with the nursing program philosophy. The philosophy should define the concepts of person, health, nursing, and education. Those definitions provide some guidance for what should be in the curriculum and how it should be organized. The program goals link the mission and faculty belief statements (philosophy) to the curriculum design, teaching and learning methods, and outcomes. Consequently, the evaluation of the curriculum builds on the evaluation of mission and goals. More information on curriculum design can be found in Chapters 8, 9 and 10.

Evaluation of Curriculum Organization

Curriculum must be appropriately organized in a deliberate or structured manner to move learners along a continuum from program entry to program completion. The principle of vertical organization, or *scaffolding*, guides both the planning and the evaluation of the curriculum. Vertical organization provides the rationale for the sequencing or building of curricular content elements (Wijnen-Meijer et al., 2020). For example, nursing faculty often use depth and complexity as sequencing guides; that is, given content areas may occur in subsequent levels of the curriculum at a level of greater depth, breadth, and complexity. Faculty may also use a simple-to-complex model where the curriculum begins with what the faculty defines as simpler concepts and builds to more complex concepts. In evaluation of the curriculum, faculty must assess for increasing depth and complexity to determine whether the sequencing was useful to learning and progressed to the desired outcomes. Determination of whether course and level objectives demonstrate sequential learning across the curriculum during each semester can be used as a test of vertical organization. The analysis can be performed using Bloom's (1956) Taxonomy as a guide for determining whether objectives follow a path of increasing complexity. Bloom's Taxonomy was adapted to demonstrate the levels of learning and relate those levels to verbs. Fig. 26.2 is an example of Bloom's Taxonomy and the Learning Wheel.

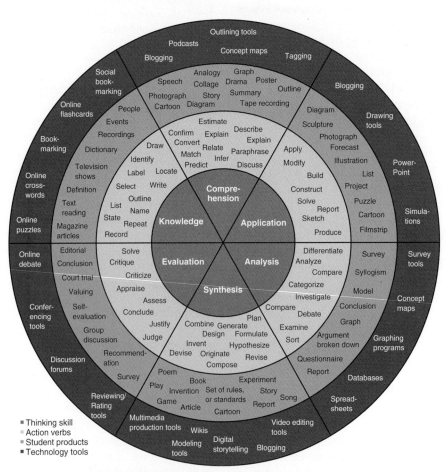

FIG. 26.2 Bloom's taxonomy and the levels of learning wheel. (Graphic created by Emily Hixson, Janet Buckenmeyer, and Heather Zamojski, 2011. Reprinted with permission of authors.)

The concept of sequencing related to the vertical organization helps guide the curriculum structure so that new information and experiences are not presented until existing knowledge has been assimilated. In other words, what prior knowledge must be present to provide a link for new knowledge in long-term memory? Often faculty believe everything needs to be learned at once. Of course, this is not possible. An appropriate question is: "What entry skills and knowledge does the student need as a condition of subsequent knowledge and experiences?" (Sar, 2022). How faculty answer this question will determine curriculum sequencing and implementation. The evaluation question would address the extent to which students have the entry-level skills needed to progress sequentially in the curriculum. This is a critical question in light of the changing profile of students entering college-level programs. It is often difficult to determine which prerequisite skills should be required for entry and which should be acquired concurrently. Computer skills are a good example. Students enter programs with varying ability in using computers. It is necessary to determine the prerequisite skills needed and the sequence in which advanced skills should be acquired during the program of learning.

The principle of linear congruence, sometimes called *horizontal organization* or *alignment*, assists faculty in determining the concurrent nature of courses during each semester or year level (Chen et al., 2015). This alignment means that the same concepts are built in more depth in each course or the direction of curricular elements is sideways, meaning they are introduced in one course and then continue in more depth in subsequent courses (Sar, 2022).

The principle of internal consistency is important to the evaluation of the curriculum. The curriculum design is a carefully conceived plan that takes its shape from what its creators believe about people and their education as defined in the program philosophy. The curriculum components must fit together to provide this consistency. Those components include: (1) program and course outcomes; (2) content, (3) teaching-learning strategies; and (4) assessment and evaluation of learning outcomes. Evaluation efforts should include examination of the extent to which the objectives and outcomes are linked to the mission and belief statements. Program objectives are consistent with the mission and philosophy. Level and course objectives then correspond to the program objectives. One method of assessing internal consistency is with the use of a curriculum matrix or map (Burwash & Snover, 2016). The curriculum map is a visual representation that lists all nursing courses and shows the placement of major concepts flowing from the program philosophy and conceptual framework. It demonstrates the relationship of the learning outcomes to the curriculum. This allows faculty to see where content is taught and whether there are gaps, redundancies, or inconsistencies. Curriculum mapping provides a broad picture of the curriculum and its components. It reveals gaps or redundancy in curricular content and its cohesiveness (Khailova, 2021) allowing faculty to make evidence-based decisions related to the curriculum. Some nursing programs use a specific conceptual framework that identifies essential program "threads" and provides further direction to curriculum development and implementation. Congruency between program threads, program goals, course objectives, and course content will also need to be assessed. Further information on curriculum development and curriculum frameworks can be found in Chapter 6.

Course Evaluation

Individual courses are reviewed to determine whether they have met the tests of internal consistency, linear congruence, and vertical organization. A triangulation approach to course evaluation is useful. This approach uses data from three sources—faculty, students, and materials review—to identify strengths and areas for change. Each course is evaluated to determine whether content elements, learning activities, assessment measures, and learner outcomes are consistent with the objectives of the course and the obligations of the course in terms of its placement in the total curriculum.

Faculty should clearly articulate the sequential levels of each expected knowledge and ability. Learning is scaffolded based on knowledge already attained by the student. It makes clear what the student should already know and allows the building of knowledge and the determination of teaching and learning strategies needed to move the student through the curriculum content. This also helps establish the evaluation criteria for determining that each stage of development has been achieved. This is important in relation not only to abilities or competencies specific to the discipline or major but also to the transferable skills acquired in the general education component of the curriculum. Some faculty achieve this by creating content maps for each major thread or pervasive strand in the curriculum with related knowledge and skill elements. The content maps chart the responsibility of each course in facilitating student progression to the expected program outcome and the relationship between the courses. The maps also provide a guide for the evaluation of whether the elements were incorporated as planned and not repeated unnecessarily.

Many tools are available to help with evaluation of teaching–learning strategies. Content and curriculum mapping, as discussed earlier in this chapter, is useful to determine content evaluation and course consistency. The achievement of course outcomes is also essential to course evaluation.

Evaluation of Support Courses and the Liberal Education Foundation

Liberal education is fundamental to professional education. Expected outcomes and structure for the liberal arts component of professional programs have received much attention in recent years. Liberal education is expected to provide students with a broad knowledge of the world in addition to the expert knowledge of nursing. It is intended to help students develop social and civic responsibilities in addition to intellectual and practical skills (Association of American Colleges and Universities, 2020). The goals of the liberal arts curriculum should be congruent with the university mission. Nursing faculty should work collaboratively with faculty across disciplines to ensure that the general education curriculum supports the expectations of a 21st-century liberal education.

Evaluation questions about general education courses should address the extent to which the courses selected enable student learning and contribute to the expected outcomes. They should also be examined for sequencing to ensure that the support and general education courses are appropriately placed to ground and complement the major. To develop evaluation questions related to the general education courses, faculty must first articulate what the rationale is for each course, what the expected outcomes are from the courses, and how the courses support the major and provide a broad, liberal education. External accrediting agencies also have expectations about liberal education. The ACEN, NLN CNEA, and the CCNE state that a liberal arts education provides a strong foundation for nursing. A liberal arts foundation enhances the knowledge and practice of a nurse. Box 26.3 provides a summary of the elements associated with curriculum evaluation.

When the expectations are clear, it is easier to select the measures needed to determine whether expectations have been met. Evaluation of the outcomes of the general education courses will be discussed in the section on outcomes.

Evaluation of Teaching Effectiveness

Evaluation of teaching effectiveness involves assessment of teaching strategies (including instructional materials), assessment of methods used to evaluate student performance, and assessment of student learning. Teaching strategies are

---

BOX 26.3 Elements of Curriculum Evaluation

- Course and level objectives demonstrate sequential learning across the curriculum that builds in depth and breadth (vertical organization).
- Course objectives are congruent with level objectives, which are congruent with the program goals (internal consistency).
- Course sequencing is defined with appropriate rationale for prerequisites and corequisites so that concepts build in depth (horizontal organization).
- Course content (coursework and clinical experiences) provides graduates with the knowledge and skills needed to fulfill course and level objectives, the program's goals, and defined competencies.
- Support courses enhance learning experiences and provide a foundation in the arts, sciences, and humanities.

effective when students are actively engaged, when strategies assist students to achieve course objectives, and when strategies provide opportunities for students to use prior knowledge in building new knowledge. Teaching effectiveness improves when teaching strategies are modified on the basis of evaluation data. See Chapter 16 for information on designing teaching strategies and student learning activities.

To demonstrate and document teaching effectiveness, faculty need multiple evaluation methods (Muñoz & Dossett, 2016). Evaluation methods may include student feedback about teaching effectiveness obtained through course evaluations and focus group discussions, feedback provided through peer review, formal testing of teaching strategies, classroom observations, and assessment of student learning.

Student Evaluation of Teaching Strategies

The institution or nursing department may develop course evaluations to obtain student feedback on teaching effectiveness. The advantage of internally developed evaluations is that they can be customized to the program. The primary disadvantage of internally developed tools is that they may lack reliability and validity. Standardized evaluation tools have documented reliability and validity and provide opportunities to compare results among and between academic programs, departments, schools with the institutional score, and a national benchmark. Examples of these include the Individual Development and Educational Assessment (IDEA), offered by the IDEA Center at Kansas State University, and the National Survey of Student Engagement, offered by the Center for Postsecondary Research and Planning. Articles related to this topic such as Guiding Learning and Assessment through Rubrics (2021) can be found on the IDEA website from Indiana University School of Education.

A focus group discussion with students can provide a qualitative assessment of teaching effectiveness. Focus groups provide an opportunity to obtain insights and to hear student perspectives that may not be discovered through formal course evaluations. The focus group leader should be an impartial individual with the skill to conduct the session. The leader should clearly state the purpose of the session, ensure confidentiality, provide clear guidelines about the type of information being sought, and explain how information will be used. Group leaders should solicit opinions from all participants, record all comments, and produce a formal report without listing specific names. The reliability and validity of information obtained from a focus group discussion is enhanced when the approach is conducted as research with a purposeful design and careful choice of participants. However, the danger is that students may not be willing to share negative aspects of the course or faculty because of the fear of the information not being confidential. It is important to develop a rapport between the focus group members and the interviewers so there is mutual trust and respect.

Peer Review of Teaching Strategies

Peer and colleague review may provide information on teaching effectiveness through classroom observation and assessment of course materials and can be either formative or summative. In this context, a peer is defined as another faculty member within the same discipline with expertise in the field; a colleague is defined as an individual outside of the discipline with expertise in the art and science of teaching. Peer review can serve to promote quality improvement of teaching effectiveness and as documentation for performance review. Before peer review is implemented, there is a need to be clear about what data will be gathered, who will have access to the data, and for what purposes they will be used. Faculty and administrators, as stakeholders in the endeavor, should collaborate to establish the norms and standards. Data from peer review may be used prescriptively to assist faculty in developing and improving teaching skills. At some point, peer review data may be needed for performance review and administrative decision making. Some schools require both classroom visits and opportunities to observe master teachers for all new faculty and periodic classroom visits for all faculty thereafter. In some schools, the observation of teaching is voluntary. The age of the classroom as the private domain of the teacher is disappearing rapidly, and both accountability and the opportunity to demonstrate the scholarship of teaching are causing colleges and universities to require increased documentation of teaching as a routine part of the evaluation process.

Although classroom observation has been used as a technique for the peer review of teaching for a number of years, the reliability and validity of this method has been suspect. Classroom teaching is just a part of the teaching role and teaching excellence as a whole. Observation of what happens in the classroom may not allow for evaluation of the faculty member's true ability to be a teacher. In addition, a peer as an evaluator may set up both the teacher and peer evaluator for bias. Neither may not want to have a frank discussion of weakness and what is needed for improvement. The validity and reliability of evaluation can be improved by examining the classroom through multiple visits. Syllabi, student ratings, contact time with students, and what goals were to be accomplished, among other defined activities can improve the validity of classroom observation. It is also important to establish clear, appropriate criteria in advance of the observation. The same criteria should be used for every faculty member with faculty involved in the development of the tool to be used. Before classroom teaching visits are made, the students should be advised of the visit and should be assured that they are not the focus of the observation. Peer reviewers should meet with the faculty member before the visit and review the goals of the session, what has preceded and what will follow the session, planned teaching methods, assignments made for the session, and an indication of how this class fits into the total program. This provides a clear image for the visitors and establishes a beginning rapport. Some faculty have particular goals for growth that can be shared at this time as areas for careful observation and comment. Finally, a postvisit interview should be conducted to review the observation and to identify strengths and areas for growth. This may include consultation regarding strategies for growth with the scheduling of a return visit at a later date. Many visitors interview the students briefly after the visit to determine their reaction to the class and to ascertain whether this was a typical class rather than a special, staged event. Unless there is a designated visiting team, the faculty member to be visited is usually able to make selections or at least suggestions about the visitors who will make the observation. Peer visits to clinical teaching sessions should follow the same general approach as classroom visits, although specific criteria for observation will be established to meet the unique attributes of clinical teaching and learning. An additional requirement is that the visitor be familiar with clinical practice expectations in the area to be visited.

Evaluation of Teaching and Learning Materials

The review of teaching and learning materials is another element of evaluation of teaching effectiveness that may be conducted through peer review. Materials commonly included for review are the course syllabus, textbooks and reading lists, teaching plans, teaching or learning aids, assignments, and outcome measures. In all cases, the materials are reviewed for congruence with the course objectives, appropriateness to the level of the learner, content scope and depth, clarity, organization, and evidence of usefulness in advancing students toward the goals of the course.

The syllabus is reviewed to determine whether expectations are clear and methods of evaluation are detailed. It is especially important that students understand what is required to "pass" the course. Grading scales and weighting of each of the evaluation methods used in the course should be explained.

In the review of textbooks for their appropriateness for a given course, multiple elements may be considered. The readability of a text relates to the extent to which the reading demands of the textbook match the reading abilities of the students. This assumes that the faculty member has a profile of student reading scores from preadmission testing. Readability of a textbook is usually based on measures of word difficulty and sentence complexity. Other issues of concern include the use of visual aids; cultural and sexual biases; scope and depth of content coverage; and size, cost, and accuracy of the data contained within the text. There are a variety of formulas to assess the readability of textbooks. Examples of these formulas can be found at https://readabilityformulas.com. Another factor of importance is the analysis of the textbook. This element relates to the organization and presentation of material in a logical manner that increases the likelihood of the reader's understanding of the content and ability to apply the content to practice. A review should determine the ratio of important and unimportant material and the extent to which important concepts are articulated, clarified, and exemplified. Do the authors relate intervening ideas to the main thesis of a chapter and clarify the relationships between and among central concepts? The ease with which information can be located in the index is important so that students can use the book as a reference. Because of the high cost of textbooks, it is useful to consider whether the textbook will be a good reference for other classes in the curriculum. A review of a textbook must also include consideration of whether the content has supported student learning. When student papers or other creative products are used for evaluation purposes, it is common to review a sample of these papers or products that the teacher has judged to be weak, average, and above average to provide a clearer view of expectations and how the students have met those expectations. This review provides an opportunity to demonstrate student outcomes. If a faculty member wants to retain copies of student papers and creative works to demonstrate outcomes, he or she should obtain informed consent from the students. Accrediting bodies often wish to see samples of student work, and faculty may use them to demonstrate learning outcomes for purposes of their own evaluation. Each student's identity should be protected and consent should be obtained.

The review of teaching and learning aids depends on the organization and use of these materials. The organization may be highly structured in that all faculty are expected to use certain materials in certain situations or sequences, or materials may be resources available to faculty and students for use at their discretion according to the outcomes they wish to achieve. Students may be expected to search for and locate materials, to create materials to facilitate their learning, or simply to use the materials provided in a prescribed manner. The emphasis will determine whether evaluation questions related to materials are based on variety, creativity, and availability or whether the materials have been used as intended. Regardless of the overall emphasis, teaching and learning materials should be evaluated for efficiency and cost-effectiveness. Efficiency can be evaluated by determining whether the time demands and effort required to use the materials are worth the outcomes achieved. Cost-effectiveness can be determined by considering whether the costs of the materials justify the outcomes.

Formal Measures for Evaluating Teaching Strategies

Formal, objective measures of teaching strategies may include experimental or quasiexperimental designs, with randomization of subjects and control of treatments. For example, a teacher may establish a control group and a treatment group to try different teaching techniques and to evaluate outcomes to prove or disprove a predetermined hypothesis. This technique is often used when there are multiple sections of a given course, although it can be accomplished within a section. A common method is to use the traditional strategy with the control group and the new strategy with the experimental group. A common examination or other assessment measure is used with both groups. Analysis may include checking for a significant difference in the scores of the two groups and checking areas in which the most questions were missed for congruence or no congruence between the two groups.

A weakness of some of these efforts is that they are context bound and not generalizable. A strength of these testing strategies is the provision of feedback of value to evaluation questions within a given curriculum.

Another measure for evaluating teaching strategies and assessing the value of courses in the curriculum is to have faculty complete a course report. The course report provides a record of the types of instructional methods used, the rationale for choosing these methods, and results of changes to these methods. Course reports can be reviewed annually through a peer review process or by program administrators. See Box 26.4 for a sample of a didactic course report for the evaluation of teaching strategies and Box 26.5 for a sample of a clinical course report for the evaluation of teaching strategies.

BOX 26.4 Example: Course Report for a Didactic Course

Program Evaluation Plan: Teaching Strategies Evaluation

The Program Evaluation Plan asks the following questions about teaching strategies and curriculum evaluation: (1) "Are we doing what we meant to do?" (2) "Are we doing the right things right?" This part of the program evaluation plan examines (a) teaching strategies, (b) the ability of chosen teaching strategies to accomplish course objectives, (c) opportunities to expand students' knowledge base, and (d) evaluation of student performance.

Teaching Strategies
1. Teaching strategies facilitate achievement of course objectives.
2. Rationale can be identified for all major teaching strategies.
3. Teaching strategies provide opportunities to use prior knowledge in building new knowledge.
4. Teaching strategies are modified based on evaluation data.

List Each Course Objective.

1. List the teaching strategies for each objective.
2. Identify the rationale for each strategy.
3. Identify how prior knowledge is used in building new knowledge. Examples of strategies include textbooks, assignments, presentations, homework, supplemental assigned readings, lectures, discussions in class or in online discussion forums, audiovisuals, group activities, guest speakers, web-based/web-supported courses, and others.
4. Describe the effectiveness of each strategy. Include student comments where appropriate. What will be changed the next time you teach this course?
5. Report on student evaluation of the course including course strengths and weaknesses.

BOX 26.5 Example: Course Report for a Clinical Course

Program Evaluation Plan: Teaching Strategies Evaluation
1. Teaching strategies facilitate achieving clinical objectives.
2. Rationale can be identified for all major teaching strategies.
3. Teaching strategies provide opportunities to use prior knowledge in building new knowledge.
4. Teaching strategies are modified based on evaluation data.

List Each Course Objective.

1. List the teaching strategies and types of clinical assignments used for each objective.
2. Indicate the rationale for each strategy.
3. Identify how prior knowledge is used in building new knowledge. Examples of strategies include daily data sheets, journaling, nursing process papers/care plans, instructor skill demonstrations (laboratory or clinical), student return demonstrations (laboratory), direct observations of skill performance and nursing care given, questioning, observational experiences, planned teaching projects, post conferences, role play activities, case studies, computer-based activities/study modules, math competency testing, skills testing in the laboratory, purposeful teaching assignments, and others.
4. Describe the effectiveness of each strategy. Include student comments where appropriate. What will be changed the next time you teach this course?

---

of the program of learning. Outcomes are used to provide students with an understanding of what they are to learn and to aid faculty in better assessing whether student learning occurred.

Both formal and informal methods may be used in the classroom to assess student progress and to evaluate the effectiveness of teaching strategies. Chapters 23, 24 and 25 discuss these methods in detail. Informal classroom assessment is useful to the teacher for determining how well students are learning. The teacher can use the data from the assessment to make changes to improve student learning as the course progresses. This form of classroom assessment is often not graded and is anonymous to allow for honest feedback.

Assessment of Student Learning

It is unacceptable to claim that teaching strategies are effective unless there is evidence that links the teaching transaction with student learning. Assessment within the classroom provides evidence for interim outcome evaluation. Interim evaluation refers to outcomes of specific learning episodes, course outcomes, or level outcomes as opposed to outcomes assessed at the conclusion

However, faculty also use more formal classroom assessments that are graded to get a feel for the quality of the teaching and determine how well the students are learning.

Students can use the formative assessment to set their own academic goals and to identify gaps between what they have learned and what the objectives say should be learned. This allows the student and teacher to focus on those gaps and to correct misconceptions, to evaluate study methods used, and to help prepare for future assessments (Rodriguez et al., 2021).

The use of formalized external testing in prelicensure programs is another option that assists in the evaluation of student learning. For example, several commercial testing products provide both content mastery and comprehensive predictor examinations that provide indicators of student learning. These assessments provide questions similar to those that students will experience on the licensure examination and provide faculty with feedback that indicates need for improvement in specific content areas. Faculty can then provide focused review of content in which students' scores were low. Tracking student scores in individual nursing courses also can be insightful in revising course content and curricula to improve student learning outcomes.

Evaluation of individual student performance must be effectively communicated to students. Documentation should provide evidence that evaluation leads to improvement in performance. This is especially important in clinical evaluation. Clinical evaluation tools should be congruent with course and program objectives. They should be designed to provide students with clear information about expectations. The evaluation tool should clearly demonstrate the student's performance and provide appropriate feedback regarding their performance and how it can be improved. The tools should also include information about how students responded to the feedback and how behavior changed.

Evaluating Student Performance Measures

In addition to documenting that teaching methods are effective, methods of evaluating student performance must be valid and reliable. Examinations are a common, cost-effective, and time-efficient method of testing knowledge acquisition both as students progress in a course and at the conclusion of the course and program. This format provides rapid, quantitative data for individual assessment and aggregate data for centralized evaluation. Other methods of evaluation are discussed in Chapters 23, 24 and 25.

Box 26.6 provides a summary of the elements associated with evaluation of teaching effectiveness. Box 26.7 provides an example of a course report related to student performance.

Evaluating Student Admission, Progression, and Graduation Policies and Procedures

The evaluation of admission, progression, and graduation (APG) policies and procedures begins with an examination of whether a sufficient number of qualified students are enrolled. Academic and demographic profiles of prospective students are important to consider. A first consideration is the mission and goals of the institution and school or department. If diversity is a goal, the selection of students will be different from schools where high selectivity is a goal. State and private schools may differ in the types of students they wish to attract. Trends in health care provide an important database for defining student enrollment goals. For example, health care reform has opened the market for nurse practitioners to the extent that many schools of nursing have targeted this population.

BOX 26.6 Evaluation of Teaching Effectiveness

- Students and faculty are satisfied with teaching strategies.
- Teaching strategies are modified based on evaluation data.
- Teaching strategies facilitate achieving course objectives.
- Teaching materials are effective and efficient.
- Evaluation of individual student performance is communicated to students and leads to improvement in performance.
- Methods of evaluating student performance are valid.

BOX 26.7   **Example: Course Report—Theory**

Program Evaluation Plan: Teaching Strategies Evaluation
Evaluation of Student Performance
1. Methods of evaluating student performance are valid and consistently applied.

Course Evaluation of Student Performance

Examinations	Data	Describe the effectiveness of these methods. Include student comments where appropriate.	What will be changed the next time you teach this course?
How do you use item analysis to improve your tests?	List range of KR 20 values on unit examinations, excluding the final examination. Range Fall Spring Summer (The KR20 has a normal range between 0.00 and 1.00 with higher numbers indicating higher internal consistency. You should not expect a score higher than 0.80 [commercially available tests will approach 0.95].)	Comment on the reliability of your tests, the difficulty level of the tests, and the ability of questions to discriminate between high/low achievers.	
What percent of the course grade is the final examination/assignment? (specify which)	Fall _____% Spring _____% Summer _____% _____examination _____assignment		
Is the final examination/assignment comprehensive?	Fall _____ yes _____ no Spring_____ yes _____ no Summer_____ yes _____ no		
How many students (number and percent of class) did **not** achieve an average examination score of 80%, but passed the course based on written assignments, homework, and/or student presentations?	Fall _____ % Spring_____ % Summer_____ %		

BOX 26.7 **Example: Course Report—Theory—cont'd**

Other Methods of Evaluation

What other methods of evaluation are used in this course?	_____ Written assignments _____ Student presentations _____ Homework _____ Blackboard discussion _____ Quizzes _____ Other (List ___)
Rubrics are used for all other graded work (yes or no). If no, what is used to determine validity and assure consistent application?	Yes No (explain)
Grading policies from the School of Nursing Policy Manual are followed in this course (yes or no). If no, describe what and why.	Yes No (explain)

External Measures of Student Performance (commercial products)

Identify Content Mastery Examination given in this course. What was the total number of students that took the Content Mastery Examination? What number and percent of class achieved the benchmark on the test? (Proficiency Level 2 and above)	Fall _____ Spring_____ Fall _____ % Spring _____ %	What did you learn from test analysis data	What (and why) will be changed the next time you teach this course?

Once a determination of the nature of the student to be recruited has been made, the methods of recruitment require attention. Marketing methods and materials should be reviewed in terms of access to catchment targets, clarity of the message delivered, and results of the effort. An entry inquiry as to the source of the student's information about the school is one way to determine the extent to which marketing materials influenced application decisions.

Admission policies should be clearly defined and support program goals. They should be reliable and valid with a goal of preventing unnecessary attrition while graduating students who are well qualified and who will ultimately pass licensing or certification examinations. Student profiles are an important way to track trends in the characteristics of students admitted to programs of learning. Many colleges and universities no longer require standardized entrance examinations related to basic skills, such as the Scholastic Aptitude Test (SAT) or discipline-specific tests and institutional examinations in mathematics, English, and reading skills. Grade inflation in both secondary and postsecondary schools has rendered transcript review a difficult measure of student ability. There are a variety of factors that contribute to success in prelicensure students. Factors such as GPA, grades in science courses, student coping strategies, student support provided by the university and the school of nursing, and an accurate view of nursing (Chan et al., 2019). Other factors such as income at poverty level and having English as a second language were even more important to academic success and passing the licensing examination. It may be helpful to use an overall profile of criteria to guide the selection of students who can successfully complete a nursing education program and who have attributes suited to the challenges of current health care delivery systems.

Admission policies should be evaluated for discriminatory elements. One must sort through those educational discriminators that ensure a fit between the student and the program of learning, and those that are clearly discriminatory from the perspective of social justice. For example, it is appropriate to require that students complete any remediation before admission to the program so they will have the basic skills necessary for success, especially if diversity is a goal. It is not appropriate and it is illegal to exclude students on the basis of gender, sexual orientation, religion, race, or ethnic origin.

Many states are increasing high school requirements with a concurrent shift in college entrance requirements. Individuals who perform evaluation reviews must keep abreast of these changes to maintain congruence and to determine what remediation programs may be needed for students who graduated from high school before the increased requirements were established. Plans must be in place to ensure communication of the changes in a timely fashion. Some programs find it useful to complete correlation studies to determine the relationship of admission criteria to such outcome measures as program completion or success on licensing or certification examinations after graduation. Although this approach does not measure the potential success of those not admitted, it may provide data about criteria that seem to have little relationship to success indicators.

Progression must be fair and justifiable, support program goals, and be congruent with institutional standards. For example, are there conditions for progression related to GPA at the end of each semester? If a student must drop out of school for any reason, what are the conditions and standards for return? Are they realistic? Are they known to the students? Do they apply equally to all students with exceptions made only in cases that are clearly exceptional?

Records of student satisfaction and formal complaints should be used as part of the process of the student dimension evaluation. An academic appeals process should be in place for students who wish to challenge rulings, and students should know how to find and use the process. Some form of due process should be in writing and in operation for the review of disputes regarding course grades or progression decisions. Whether these are discipline specific or campus specific is a function of the size and complexity of the institution. An annual review of appeals and the decisions regarding those appeals provides important information for making revisions to policies and processes that are in place or are needed. All stakeholders should participate in appeals reviews. Most programs have an appeals committee composed of both students and faculty with channels to administrative review.

An internal method of review is to survey or interview students who leave the program before graduating. An obvious data set is information about why students are leaving. Common reasons include academic difficulties or academic dismissal, financial problems, role conflicts, family pressure, military service, and health issues. An examination of the underlying reasons for leaving often suggests alternatives for intervention that reduces the attrition rate. These alternatives may relate to student services or specific program issues.

Some programs also gather data about antecedent events that may have influenced the potential to be successful in the program. The extent of data gathered depends on the goals of the review. Data that can be gathered from the student record are not included in the student survey. With the student's permission, data obtained from the record may include preentrance test scores, GPA, progression point at the time of withdrawal, specific course grades, and any history of withdrawals and returns. These data are extensive but can be used to develop a profile of the student who does not complete a program in an attempt to identify elements within the control of the school for potential intervention strategies. Including a control group of students who completed the program in the study gives more meaning to the findings by identifying success indicators and allowing for determination of significant differences between the two groups. Box 26.8 provides a summary of the elements associated with evaluation of APG policies and procedures. (See Case Study 26.1.)

BOX 26.8 Evaluation of Admission, Progression, and Graduation Policies and Procedures

- An adequate number of qualified students are recruited to maintain program viability.
- Admission policies are clearly defined, published, and support program goals.
- Progression policies are fair and justifiable, published, and support program goals.
- Records of student satisfaction and formal complaints are used as part of the process of ongoing improvement.
- Possible reasons for attrition are evaluated and addressed.

CASE STUDY 26.1 Student Licensure Exam Scores

Faculty are concerned that student licensure exam scores have decreased to unacceptable numbers over the last few years.

1. How should the faculty proceed to identify reasons for this change?
2. Once data is collected, what should be done with the results?
3. How should faculty use the data results?
4. How will faculty know if the decisions made are appropriate?
5. What next steps should faculty take?

Evaluation of the Faculty

There must be a sufficient number of qualified faculty to accomplish the mission, philosophy, and expected outcomes of the program. The nature of the program, the expectations of the parent institution, the number of students, and the requirements of accrediting bodies influence the desired number and qualifications of faculty. Qualifications of faculty may be measured from several perspectives such as credentials, diversity, and professional experience.

Qualifications of Faculty

Faculty should possess credentials appropriate to their teaching assignment, to the program levels in which they teach, and to the service and scholarship mission of the school. Faculty members' professional experience, education, and specialty certification should be congruent with their teaching assignments. Evaluation of the level of degree preparation of nursing faculty is related to the program level in which they teach. A master's degree in nursing is the minimum expectation for teaching in associate or baccalaureate degree programs. A doctorate in nursing, or a terminal degree in a related field with a master's degree in nursing, is the expectation for teaching in graduate programs. Many nursing schools also strive to have faculty with terminal degrees teaching in prelicensure nursing programs. The nursing profession has been challenged to meet these expectations partly because of the lack of nurses with terminal degrees. The AACN (2021) stated that only approximately 50% of nursing faculty are doctorally prepared. This report also identified that approximately 89.7% of unfilled nursing faculty positions are still seeking candidates with doctoral degrees in nursing or a related field (AACN, 2020). Enrollment in PhD programs focusing on research has declined 9.6% since 2014 (AACN, 2019). To address the shortage of nurses with terminal degrees, some nursing schools may provide additional incentives and support to faculty with master's degrees to assist them in pursuing their doctorates. In this situation, care must be taken to avoid "inbreeding," which may result in a disproportionate number of faculty with degrees from the same institution. Representation of a wide variety of educational institutions in the faculty profile demonstrates a commitment to diversity of ideas and openness to creative differences. "Inbreeding" of faculty may perpetuate the status quo.

Evaluation of faculty qualifications should also include the profile of faculty related to rank, classifications for tenure or non–tenure track appointments, and the balance of full-time and part-time positions. Assessment of the number and proportion of faculty for each level of rank provides a measure of faculty experience and expertise in their teaching role. If few faculty members within the school have achieved higher ranks, such as associate or full professor, there may be a lack of senior-level faculty or an inequity in nursing promotions compared with other academic units. In some universities, there are multiple categories of faculty, including non-tenure-track lecturers and clinical instructors, tenure-track faculty, and scientist tracks (see Chapter 1). In some universities, only tenure-track faculty may participate in the governance of the larger institution. Standing committees within both the school and the university may have criteria for rank and tenure as a condition of membership. A goal of full participation in governance issues at the university level can be compromised or enabled by the number of faculty eligible to participate. On the other hand, a faculty composed largely of tenured members could be a barrier to the recruitment of a more diverse faculty or a goal of increasing the number of faculty members with specific areas of expertise. The balance of full-time and part-time faculty is also of concern in ensuring adequate involvement in governance, meeting needs for academic advising, curriculum development, and program evaluation.

Setting goals for faculty qualifications allows the nursing school to measure progress in achieving those goals. Once the goals for qualified faculty have been identified, the faculty profile can be evaluated or analyzed in terms of those goals. Factors that may be interfering with the achievement of the goals will also need analysis. It is essential to track the profile of faculty and to examine reasons for faculty turnover. Control of the faculty profile is influenced not only by recruitment goals but also by faculty retention factors.

A factor related to both recruitment and retention of qualified faculty is the salary structure. If a goal of the school of nursing is to support quality programs and to achieve national stature, salaries must be competitive to attract the mix of faculty that promotes excellence. There are multiple sources for comparison of salaries. Internally, it is important to demonstrate that faculty salaries in nursing are congruent with those across the larger institution for comparable rank and productivity. External data are available from such sources as the AACN, the NLN, the American Association of University Professors, and regional groups such as the Big Ten universities. AACN provides salary information for full-time administrative and instructional nursing faculty, including mean and median salaries by rank and degree, and by region of the country (AACN, 2020–2021). The College and University Professional Association for Human Resources conducts an annual survey of faculty salaries for public and private institutions offering baccalaureate and higher degrees. The National Faculty Salary Survey for Four-Year Institutions provides salary data by discipline and rank (Bichsel et al., 2017). The results of this survey are available online. In addition, customized reports that sort data by variables such as region of the country, size of the institution's operating budget, and religious affiliation for private schools can be requested. Customized reports may provide a more accurate comparison in determining how faculty salaries compare with peer institutions. Some nursing schools may be able to obtain salary information by networking with a select cohort of peer institutions that agree to share data.

Faculty Development

Faculty development begins with orientation to the university or college, school, and department or division. In this orientation, faculty begin the process of socialization into the academy. They are introduced to the mission and goals of the institution and school at each level represented in the structure. Expectations are reviewed and any documents that will reinforce and guide movement toward those expectations are shared. For example, new faculty are usually given the institutional handbook that contains general policies and teaching, service, and research expectations. Support systems and personnel available to maintain them are introduced and a tour of the physical plant is conducted. More specific orientation occurs at each level. In addition to faculty development offerings at the campus and institutional levels, the school or department may offer a series of open and planned sessions for new and continuing faculty. The focus of the sessions may be related to common concerns, concerns identified through a needs analysis, or issues related to changes in the school. For example, many schools are offering regular sessions on the use of new technology as it is acquired. It may be necessary to offer faculty development related to policy changes, curriculum changes, or any other new development in the school or institution.

Once orientation is completed, faculty should receive ongoing support for professional development. Universities may have an office of research to assist faculty in research efforts or may have teaching centers or technology experts to assist faculty in their teaching role. Use of travel monies and planning that encourages faculty to attend conferences, seminars, and research colloquia are important parts of development and should be implemented and tracked as a part of the evaluation effort.

An increasing number of schools are developing mentoring programs that may provide generalist mentoring or specific mentoring in research and teaching. Mentoring is a multidimensional activity that consists of highly individualized dyadic processes and relationships. The ideal mentor is dedicated to helping the mentee develop in both a personal and professional way. The attributes of the mentor include characteristics such as good listener, approachable, accessible, credible, trustworthy, generous, and possessing qualities that the mentee wants to emulate (Eliades et al., 2017). The mentor and mentee develop a reciprocal relationship in which there is a knowledge differential between participants, and a relationship effect beyond the mentor relationship. Mentors listen, affirm, counsel, encourage, seek input, and help the novice develop status and career direction..

Whatever the view of the mentor, the role needs to be clear to the mentor and mentee and be flexible to allow for individualization. In large schools, the assignment of a mentor may occur at the department level. In smaller schools, the assignment is often the responsibility of a central administrator or a school committee of faculty. It is common for a senior faculty member to be assigned as a mentor for a period of 1 year, with continuing assignment based on individual need or the development plan. Each member of the mentoring dyad should evaluate the nature and effectiveness of the mentoring relationship at the end of the year or at regular intervals if the relationship extends beyond the year. The role of the mentor may vary by institution, but common functions include advice and counsel, review of course materials, observation of instruction, assistance in processing evaluation data, modeling master teaching, encouragement, and coaching.

Those who provide mentoring for research often assist the faculty member in accessing support systems on campus, identifying funding sources, and developing a research focus. The mentor can also serve as a resource as the mentee progresses in meeting promotion and tenure expectations. The purpose of the relationship is generally consultative and constructive; however, some schools may prefer a more directed, prescriptive approach, especially with new faculty. In an effort to create safety and opportunity for faculty development, the mentor does not become an evaluator.

Finally, larger schools may have their own department of continuing education. In those schools, one expectation of that department may be to participate in faculty development. Through continuing education, a department may offer a series of workshops related to teaching strategies, test construction, evaluation, or other issues of concern to faculty in general. These are usually open to others to create a more diverse mix of participants and to provide fiscal support to the department. Some continuing education departments assist faculty in hosting conferences related to their areas of expertise and cosponsor research colloquia or other events that serve faculty in their professional development and provide an opportunity for faculty to share their professional expertise as presenters.

Faculty Scholarship

Faculty achievements in scholarly activity should support program effectiveness. Many schools use Boyer's (1990) model of scholarship as a basis for evaluating faculty scholarship. Knowledge development (the scholarship of discovery) and the scholarship of teaching are essential to the academy, and they are an expectation for all faculty (see Chapter 1). Those who select research as their area of excellence will be measured against criteria established within the school or division. Those criteria will need to withstand the scrutiny of peer review both within and beyond the discipline. The *volume* of research and publications is less important than the *quality* of the effort. Some committees ask faculty to select two or three of their best research studies and best publications for review rather than submitting the entire body of work for review. This highlights the focus on quality. An additional expectation is that evidence of both external peer review and review by one's department chairperson be included in the work submitted for review. Selection of one's works for publication or presentation is evidence of its value to the reviewers. Where publications appear may also be of importance. Articles in refereed journals and journals held in high esteem in the discipline are considered evidence of quality review. Before publication, it is important to know the standards of the given institution. For example, some schools give greater weight to articles in refereed journals or to entire books compared with chapters in a book. Sole authorship versus joint authorship or placement in the listing of authors may be weighted as well. Invited works are often considered evidence of their value. Some institutions or disciplines also consider invited creative works such as radio or television productions, videotapes, musical scores, and choreography evidence of scholarship or excellence. Receipt of major awards and other forms of recognition as a leader in one's field provides compelling evidence of quality.

Funding for research, scholarly work, and special projects is widely accepted as evidence of scholarship. Weighting may be assigned on the basis of the source of the monies. External funding may be considered more valuable and weighted more heavily than internal funding. For example, funding from major foundations or federal programs may receive a more favorable review than several small grants from lesser known sources. Whether one is the principal investigator or a participant may be weighted in the review process. A growing value is attached to applied research that has meaning for a wider audience. Keys to the consideration of any scholarly endeavor are evidence of analysis and synthesis in studies grounded in theory, rather than simple descriptive studies. Variations occur according to the mission of the institution so that each school must determine criteria within the context of that mission. In the final analysis, scholarly works are best judged by one's intellectual peers.

The scholarship of application is demonstrated through professional practice and service. Practice as professional service is an area of emphasis in some institutions, whereas in other institutions, faculty believe it is not valued as highly as research. Again, evidence exists that more and more institutions are attempting to develop criteria to reflect scholarly service and to grant that service the recognition it merits. A common standard of evidence of scholarly clinical practice and clinical competence is national certification in one's field, especially for those faculty who wish to seek recognition and promotion in the clinical track. With some variation based on institutional mission, the focus on service is its connection to the faculty member's professional expertise. Internally, faculty may demonstrate service through participation and leadership in committees and projects within the department or division and, more broadly, at the campus or institutional level. Committees that affect decision making for innovative enterprises or improvement and policy development demonstrate thoughtful participation. Administrative appointments are generally accepted as evidence of professional service within the institution.

Beyond the institution, faculty may demonstrate service through practice and participation in professional, civic, and governmental organizations relevant to their expertise in a manner that reflects the application of knowledge and the extension and renewal of the discovery element of scholarship. Examples include providing technical assistance to an agency and analysis of public policy for governmental agencies or private organizations. Joint appointments or contracts with practice agencies that call on professional expertise are other examples. Certainly, faculty-run clinics are a strong example of such service. Some institutions place applied research in this category of review.

In addition to the listing and description of activities in the area of service, faculty are expected to have documented evidence of the merit or worth of that service. In this area as well, letters from external sources and awards based on service are evidence of merit. Within the institution, there is a need for more systematic feedback to those who provide valuable service. Often faculty receive perfunctory notes of thanks for service that do little to define the value of that service. A practice of thanking those who serve with comments about the special expertise provided and outcomes achieved as a result of that service is a valuable form of evidence.

The scholarship of integration is demonstrated through interdisciplinary research, interpreting research findings, and bringing new insight to the field of study. Presentations to the lay public that serve to advance public knowledge of discipline-related issues, development of new and creative teaching materials and modes of delivery, and professional presentations and publications are examples of integrative scholarship. The scholarship of integration may be evaluated by determining whether the activity reveals new knowledge, illuminates integrative themes, or demonstrates creative insight (Boyer, 1990).

It is not possible for a given faculty member to excel in all areas subject to review within the institution. The Boyer (1990) model attempts to respond to a need to look at scholarship differently and to provide multiple ways for faculty to demonstrate worthy productivity. Research and publication are important elements of the academy and are critical to comprehensive and research universities. Limiting the focus of faculty evaluation and reward decisions to a single area, however, discounts the valuable work of a diversified faculty. This very diversity and range of expertise enhances the reputation of an institution and enables the wise use of resources. The obligation of faculty is to provide evidence of scholarly productivity in one or more of the scholarship functions. Institutional leaders are obligated to enable that process and to reward positive outcomes.

Evaluation of Faculty Performance

Evaluation of faculty performance is intended to promote quality improvement. The focus of faculty performance evaluation is guided by the philosophy, mission, and goals of the parent institution and the school or division in which the nursing program is housed. Faculty evaluations may be structured against specific job descriptions related to classroom or clinical teaching assignments and include expectations for scholarship and service. Junior and community colleges and some colleges and universities focus heavily on the teaching and service mission of the institution within the community it serves. Faculty evaluation reflects this emphasis. Research universities share the teaching and service missions but include an emphasis on research and scholarship as well. Colleges and universities with religious affiliations may include expectations for church-related service in faculty review policies and standards.

The policy and process for faculty performance evaluation should be clearly communicated to faculty. A common approach is to require faculty to submit a yearly assessment of their performance during the preceding year and a development plan to the immediate supervisor that is consistent with the university and department missions and the department goals. Individual faculty goals may also be part of the development plan that includes the faculty member's goals and those identified by the supervisor. Goals can be short term and long term and should include strategies or activities planned to fulfill the goals and a timeline for completion. The goals and activities are not just related to teaching but may also be related to acquiring tenure and promotion. The faculty member's supervisor or administrator should have periodic meetings with the faculty to review progress on development goals.

The faculty member is expected to provide a self-evaluation at the end of the academic year that documents how performance and development goals were attained, what barriers blocked achievement of goals, and how these barriers will be overcome in the future so that performance will be improved. A portfolio process may also be used, in which the faculty member includes the development plan, self-evaluation, copies of student course evaluations, examples of scholarly work and service, or other artifacts that demonstrate faculty productivity. During the annual performance review, the supervisor reviews the faculty member's portfolio and provides written feedback on the faculty member's progress in fulfilling the job description and expectations. Depending on the processes used throughout the institution, performance evaluation may be done using standard forms with numerical rating scales. The use of standardized forms provides the opportunity to consistently analyze faculty performance across the unit and to determine whether the faculty demonstrates development needs in any one particular area. For example, if a number of new faculty are not performing well on a certain measure, additional orientation or training may be needed.

Peer review provides another component for the evaluation of faculty performance. Promotion and tenure review is a well-established form of peer review already in place in most institutions of higher learning. The criteria for the evaluation are developed by faculty and implemented through a faculty committee. Committee reviews usually are composed of both formative and summative evaluation procedures. A common practice is to review faculty at the midpoint of the probationary period, usually in the third year of appointment. A formative review may occur at regular intervals before the summative tenure review is conducted. Formative reviews allow the committee to provide advice to individual faculty members in preparation for the summative review that occurs near the end of the probationary period, usually the sixth year after initial appointment. In larger institutions, a primary committee of peers at the school or division level may do the initial review of a faculty member's final tenure portfolio, along with their recommendation regarding promotion or tenure, before it is forwarded to administration and a campus committee of peers and colleagues for further review. Final recommendations are submitted to institutional administration, the board of trustees, or other institutional governing body for final approval. Variations on this theme relate to the unique features of a given institution.

A common problem in higher education, especially in research-intensive universities, is the lack of evaluation plans and criteria for all classifications of faculty. Although the criteria and processes for promotion and tenure of tenure-track faculty are usually in place and subject to ongoing review and refinement, such criteria do not always exist for others beyond the routine annual review. Some schools have non-tenure-track faculty serving in lecturer, scientist, or clinical appointments who would benefit from the same careful delineation of criteria for systematic review of their roles consistent with their job descriptions and productivity expectations. Another group of faculty that requires evaluation and the opportunity to grow and develop is the part-time faculty cohort. Increasingly, expectations for annual review of part-time faculty with reappointment are contingent on favorable reviews. Adaptation of the tenure-track evaluation format can provide direction to create similar evaluative processes for non-tenure-track and part-time faculty.

External factors may influence elements of faculty evaluation. For example, external bodies such as state legislatures and education commissions may establish standards for accountability that must be met by all higher education programs in the state. A common example is in the teaching component of the faculty role. There are often mandates for faculty workload in terms of credit hours or classes taught. There are multiple ways to address this standard. Whatever productivity model is used, certain general standards apply. Faculty workloads should be designed to meet the mission and goals of the parent institution and the school or division and include those elements of the professional role of faculty emphasized by the institution (teaching, service, research). Although equity of workload expectations is an important standard, so is the flexibility to negotiate

BOX 26.9 Elements of Faculty Evaluation

- Faculty members are qualified and sufficient in number to accomplish the mission, philosophy, and expected outcomes of the program.
- Faculty receive orientation that prepares them to be successful.
- Faculty receive adequate support for professional development.
- Faculty achievements in scholarly activity support program effectiveness and the mission of the university.
- Evaluation of faculty performance promotes quality improvement.
- Aggregate and individual faculty outcomes demonstrate program effectiveness.

assignments to meet the needs of the school. Box 26.9 provides a summary of the elements associated with evaluation of the faculty.

Evaluation of Learning Resources

Classroom and laboratory facilities need to provide an effective teaching and learning environment to support program effectiveness. A review of instructional space includes evaluation of support space and a determination of whether classrooms are of sufficient size, number, and comfort to facilitate teaching and learning. Support space might include a learning resource center, a simulation laboratory, a computer cluster, and storage for instructional equipment and supplies. Additional support space may include lounges for students, staff, and faculty. In addition, office space, equipment, conference rooms, and space to support faculty teamwork and research are needed. Faculty need to have individual offices that have floor-to-ceiling walls to provide privacy for counseling, sensitive advisement, and evaluation conferences. Beyond these basic elements, space requirements are dictated by the mission and goals of the program. The space available should be congruent with the productivity expected of those who use the space, equipment, and supplies. This element is often reviewed through surveys of faculty, students, and staff. Another component of this review is documentation of holdings. It is important not only to have space and equipment needed to

accomplish the mission and program goals but also to know where it is located and how well it is maintained.

Clinical facilities should be evaluated to determine their effectiveness in providing appropriate learning experiences in relation to the mission and goals of the program. This evaluation includes consideration of the patients served by the facility. It is important to assess whether the patient population profile is consistent with the learning objectives of the program and whether the number of patients is sufficient to support the student population. It is equally important for the standard of care provided by the institution to be of high quality so that students will be socialized to high standards. One measure of quality is the accreditation of the facility. Another is the expert judgment of the faculty members who review the facility. The willingness of staff to interact with students in a facilitative manner is important, as is the skill of staff as role models. It is important to know how many other student groups are using the same facility and units within the facility and how easily reservations for these areas can be scheduled. Any special restrictions or requirements may influence decisions about use of the facility.

Evaluation of the clinical experience includes review of agency contracts. These contracts should be filed in a central location and should be reviewed on a regular schedule. The conditions of the agreement should be spelled out, with some standards required. For example, all contracts should include the process and time frame for canceling or discontinuing the contract with a clause that allows any students scheduled for that facility to complete the current course of study. It is also important that faculty maintain control of student assignments and evaluations within the framework of the agreed-on restrictions and regulations. A review of contracts by legal counsel will ensure that expert judgment has been applied to the legal parameters of the contract.

Some schools have developed and implemented faculty-run clinics that serve as learning sites for students. Reviews and contracts related to student learning in these clinics should be subject to the same evaluation as any other facility under consideration.

Instructional Technology

Information and instructional technology must be up to date and support the achievement of program goals. Productivity is directly related to the technology available to students and faculty, which enables them to meet their responsibilities and to create a dynamic learning environment. Outcome measures can be specifically stated in this area. For example, one might state that increasing numbers of faculty will incorporate virtual simulations into teaching methods until all faculty use virtual experiences to enhance student learning. Another outcome measure might state that virtual technology will be integrated throughout curricula by a stated target date. Assessment of virtual laboratory usage that includes frequency of use and type of learning experiences from simple to complex simulations can be completed. Faculty and student satisfaction with the virtual laboratory is another effective outcome measure. Technology needs should be linked broadly to the mission and goals of the school and specifically to the teaching, scholarship, and learning needs of faculty and students.

An assessment of student and faculty skills in the use of information technology at the time of admission or employment should be included. These data provide information for student and faculty development opportunities in the use of both software and hardware in the school itself and in resource facilities such as the library or a computer laboratory. Exciting advances have been made in instructional technology available for the teaching and learning of skills in nursing, but they require planning for availability of the equipment and software and preparation of faculty and students to use these resources. Creating a collaborative relationship with the information system's personnel is necessary to ensure an effective, ongoing dialogue between users of technology (faculty and students) and personnel who maintain the technology equipment.

Distance Education

Distance education is becoming more common in higher education and in nursing education. Distance education, in the context of course credit hour allocation and program review, is defined by various national and state commissions of higher education. Distance education is defined by the Distance Education Accrediting Commission (DEAC, 2021) as a program that occurs either online, through correspondence, or is internet based and has used technology to "meet the learning needs of a diverse, growing student population" (p. 6). Generally, if programs are delivered more than 50% via distance education methods, they are considered distance education programs. Some distance education programs use printed or electronic materials and meet face-to-face at specific intervals. When a program uses distance education for part or all of course delivery, the influence of this delivery mode on program outcomes, teaching–learning practices, and the use of technology and the teaching and learning quality that results must be considered in evaluation. Methods of data collection may need modification for distance education programs. Because students are not on-site, instructional strategies that are interactive and creative are needed. Evaluation methods will also need to be creative to assess student learning. Recruitment and retention of students requires special consideration in distance education because some students may lack the motivation or technological competence to be successful. Other aspects of program implementation that need special consideration for distance education include faculty development and support, student orientation and instruction on how to learn online, and learning resources and support services. The appropriate user support and technology, especially with internet delivery modes, must be available to sustain distance education. Costs associated with distance education should be considered in the financial analysis. (See also Chapter 21.)

Library Resources

Library resources must be sufficient to support the programs of learning offered by the institution and the school. Issues of concern in this evaluation include the holdings (books and journals), services, and rates of use. Faculty, students, and librarians are important stakeholders in this review, and each cohort often has a very different perception when the same questions are asked. There is controversy about the relative importance of on-site holdings and access to holdings through interlibrary loan and online databases. A core collection of holdings is crucial to students and faculty.

Various standards are used to measure the adequacy of library holdings. Some schools use published source lists as standards for library holdings. The *American Journal of Nursing* list of resources, based on an annual review of books, is often used as a standard. Some schools consider it important to include any required textbooks and required reading in the library holdings, at least at the undergraduate level. Graduate programs may require more extensive databases with access to more materials than undergraduate programs because of the scope of reading expectations. Faculty task forces are often assigned to review library holdings in relation to graduate education in specialty majors. Comparisons of the holdings of peer institutions with similar programs are sometimes used in these reviews. Some programs rely on the expertise of the faculty on the task force. Still others survey all faculty in the major for lists of holdings they consider to be critical. The aggregate becomes a point of reference for the review.

Library services are as important as the holdings and are usually assessed by a survey method. Evaluation of library services should occur on a consistent basis. Librarians, students, and faculty may indicate their views about services offered and the effectiveness of those services. Surveys may be internally developed and provide very specific information about library services. For example, an internal survey may review the interlibrary loan system to determine both satisfaction and levels of use related to the time frame for borrowing materials. This may be measured against an established goal, such as an average time of 1 week to secure a book. In addition to the quantitative data, an opportunity to comment on the best features and areas of concern related to library holdings and services often provides valuable qualitative data. Some libraries maintain specific use data by school or division. Others do not but can estimate whether a given group of students use the library facilities less, the same, or more than other students. Some libraries have very liberal hours and some do not. This may become an evaluation question, depending on the context.

> **BOX 26.10 Evaluation of Learning Resources**
>
> - Classroom and laboratory facilities provide an effective teaching and learning environment.
> - Clinical facilities provide effective, diverse learning experiences.
> - Information and instructional technology is up to date and supports achievement of program goals.
> - Library services and holdings are comprehensive and meet the needs of students and faculty.

Most libraries are able to make effective use of technology. The internet provides access to a wide variety of resources and access to full-text articles and copying services. This type of information, ubiquitous because of the internet, brings new opportunities and challenges to the provision of information resources to students over a wide geographical area. Those who make use of this opportunity will establish specific criteria for evaluation geared to access. It is important to identify and review the databases available to faculty and students and the methods used to orient them to the use of this service. Box 26.10 provides a summary of the elements associated with evaluation of learning resources.

Evaluation of Administrative Effectiveness, Structure, and Governance

The qualifications and leadership skills of program administrators are important to program effectiveness. Formal evaluation of administrators should occur annually or at regularly specified intervals. The specific evaluation of the administrator may include the extent to which the administrator guides the establishment of a clear mission and goals for the unit and the effectiveness with which the administrator represents the department or school, both internally and externally, and contributes to the reputation of the unit within and beyond the institution. Attention should be focused on the administrator's ability to raise funds and to allocate the budget in a fair and effective manner. Evidence of integrity and collegiality is an issue of concern, as are the leadership qualities of conflict resolution, decision making, motivation, and interpersonal skills.

Regardless of the university size and focus, evaluation of administrative effectiveness should be a collaborative process in which faculty members participate. Faculty members should have the opportunity to provide evaluative feedback on the performance of administrative faculty. This collaborative process can be replicated at various levels within the nursing school and the institution. For example, the responsibility for the evaluation of the nursing department chair may rest with the dean of the school; however, information from faculty members should be considered in that evaluation. This process may be repeated to the level of the vice president for academic affairs who evaluates the dean and who in turn receives evaluation feedback from the faculty. At all levels, input from supervisors and subordinates is taken into consideration as the faculty or administrator writes his or her own self-evaluation, identifying strengths, plans for improvement, and goals for the upcoming year. In addition to defining the appropriate process for performance review, faculty and administrators should reflect on the effectiveness of the process, including the utility of evaluation forms and the usefulness of evaluation in improving performance.

The use of standard assessment tools, such as those provided by the IDEA Center for the evaluation of department chairs and deans, is another means of obtaining feedback on administrative effectiveness. The advantage of these standardized tools is that they provide the opportunity to compare administrative performance with national benchmarks. The disadvantage of this approach is the cost.

In addition to effective leadership, the structure and governance of the department must provide effective means for communication and problem solving. Bylaws and written policies are two mechanisms for promoting effective department governance. The nursing school's bylaws should be examined for congruence with the constitution and bylaws of the larger institution and the structures included to facilitate faculty governance in relation to academic authority. For example, it is useful to do a comparative analysis of standing committees and the mission and goals of the school. Are the standing committees configured to address major issues related to faculty affairs, student affairs, curriculum, budget, and major thrusts of the mission? In universities with a school of law, consultation is often readily available to review the fit of the bylaws with parliamentary rules and congruence checks.

The extent to which stakeholders are included in the committee structures delineated in the bylaws is important as well. For example, are students represented on appropriate committees, and how are voting privileges defined? Whether the established mechanisms actually function in the manner described is another issue for evaluation. Minutes of all standing committees should be filed in a central location. These minutes should reflect membership, agenda items, salient discussions, and a precise statement of decisions made and actions taken. It is useful for evaluation follow-up to designate membership annually in the minutes of the first meeting of each committee. After each name, there should be an indicator of representation (e.g., faculty, student, alumni, consumer). In this way, one can track whether stakeholders indicated in the bylaws are in fact represented on designated committees. Representation is an intended means of integration of stakeholders, but attendance and participation are indicators of actual participation. Therefore attendance should be recorded for each meeting. Accreditation teams may review minutes for these elements and often track membership participation and decisions. Including tracking data is important. For example, the minutes of each meeting should state how decisions and documents are channeled for final decision making and what actions have been taken. If a curriculum committee recommendation was forwarded to the faculty council for deliberation and action, the date it was forwarded should be included. The minutes of the faculty council can then be tracked to ensure that the decision item moved forward in a timely fashion and what decision was made. Accurate record keeping facilitates evaluation tracking.

Policies should be evaluated for their effectiveness in supporting and guiding communication and decision making relevant to program implementation. Policies should be organized in a manual or file and should be available to all to whom they apply. Many schools provide all new faculty with an electronic or written policy manual and send updates to the manual on a regular basis. Students usually receive information related to relevant policies at an appropriate time. For example, some policies are included in the school catalog. Policies related to specific courses are usually included in course materials. An investigation of how policies are disseminated to those affected by the policies should be a part of the evaluation of policies. A mechanism should be in place to let the appropriate constituents know about changes in policies. Policies should be reviewed annually and updated regularly. The approval documentation that should be present on every policy will demonstrate that all stakeholders had input into their development and approval. Minutes of meetings of appropriate bodies will provide evidence of discussion and action by the stakeholders. Policies need to be clearly stated and widely communicated. Evidence that policies are not followed is cause for analyzing reasons and intervening accordingly. Box 26.11 highlights elements for the evaluation of administrators, organizational structure, and governance.

Evaluation of Fiscal Resources

Program effectiveness depends on the availability of adequate fiscal resources. The budget of the nursing unit (school or department) should be reviewed in relation to personnel, equipment and supplies, travel, and infrastructure. As a starting point, personnel salaries are reviewed in terms of supply and demand, and against guidelines for faculty and staff salaries at the university, plus regionally and nationally. For example, one may have indicated a desired mix of faculty to meet the mission and goals, but that mix depends on the fiscal ability to recruit and attract faculty to meet the mix outcome expectation. If a large percentage of the personnel budget is targeted for part-time faculty, it may be difficult to convert to full-time positions at a desired level to meet broad educational goals in terms of teaching, scholarship, and service. The data gathered in the comparative analysis of salaries noted previously will also have implications for the budget review. If salaries need to be upgraded or compression issues exist, there will be a need for a review of alternatives available to meet competing needs for fiscal support.

As technology advances, it becomes increasingly important to identify fiscal support for its use beyond the usual physical environment considerations noted in the physical space section. Although internal and external sources may be found for the acquisition of such technology, funding for maintenance and upgrading is an issue that requires attention. Many programs have received grants for technology hardware only to find that the monies for software, upkeep, and upgrading are not available in the budget. Careful record keeping provides a database for projecting future needs in this area and the cost–benefit evaluation of technology. Decisions must be made regarding the technology that will provide the greatest return for the investment involved. These data also provide supportive evidence when one goes in search of additional funding. Solid data make a stronger case than a wish list. Future acquisitions may depend in part on the data available about the effective use of existing technology. This is a multiple stakeholder issue.

Maintenance and extension of infrastructure needs require careful documentation as well. Records of such basic issues as heating, lighting, and telephone service provide trend data for projecting future needs. The need for building maintenance and expansion for new programs must be documented. Requesting funds without data will ultimately result in the need to make choices that may not be well grounded.

BOX 26.11 Evaluation of Administrators, Organizational Structure, and Governance

- Qualifications and skills of program administrators enhance program effectiveness.
- The structure and governance of the department or school provides effective means for communication, decision making, and problem solving.
- Nursing faculty participate actively in the nursing department/school and university governance system.
- There is an adequate number of qualified staff and professional personnel to support program effectiveness.

Funding for faculty development is important to faculty growth. Input from administration and faculty is needed to target the funds based on the mission and goals of the school and department. For example, if increased scholarship productivity is a goal, a percentage of this budget might be targeted for attending research conferences and giving presentations. A percentage might be targeted for conferences and presentations related to teaching and learning to advance excellence in teaching. Some schools designate some funds to enable students to participate in scholarly conferences or to present papers based on their student research efforts. Evaluation requires a review of the use of the monies for the designated purposes and follow-up in some cases to determine what benefit accrued to the school from the activities funded by the school. Some schools indicate the amount any one person can receive in a specified period and monitor this as an evaluation measure to foster equity.

Fiscal resources may also depend on the ability of the nursing school to seek and secure external funding. The size and nature of the parent institution and the school or division will guide outcome expectations in this area. Increasingly, schools are pressed to obtain external funding for programs and scholarship efforts. The sources of stable funding also influence this area. State schools have, in the past, assumed that they would receive their funding in thirds from the state, from tuition, and from external funding. State appropriations are decreasing in most states, and efforts are being made to control increases in tuition and fees to offset this loss. As a result, there is a greater need to establish clear goals for external funding and to measure progress in this area. Stated goals may be somewhat broad or very specific. For example, some schools may simply indicate that there will be evidence of increased external funding reviewed on an annual basis. In this scenario, any increase is evidence of success. Other schools may set specific goals such as indicating the percentage of increase expected every 1 or 2 years or a 5-year goal of an increase at a stated level with annual targets to achieve the long-term goal. Others indicate specifically where the increases should occur. For example, some schools indicate a desire to increase funding from specific sources such as the National Institutes of Health. These measures provide specific evaluation targets. Trend data over 5- and 10-year periods are useful for analysis of progress over time and as a database for future goals.

Another issue related to fiscal resources is development monies. Often resources must be provided to establish a fundraising program from which returns are expected. For example, many schools support a "friends of [discipline]" advisory group gathered to enable fundraising campaigns. The goals of the fundraising should be specified. Some believe that giving is more likely to occur when a specific project that is valued by potential donors is identified. Certainly, a percentage of monies should be designated to be used at the discretion of the school to advance goals, but targeted funding is also critical to success. Evaluation includes measuring the cost of the fundraising effort against resulting gains. Trend data are critical to this area. It is important to know not only the amount of giving but also the sources of those gifts and the relationship of those sources to marketing efforts.

Many schools have targeted financial incentive projects to encourage donors to engage in the educational mission. Examples include endowed chairs, centers of excellence, technology initiatives, faculty and student recognition programs, library enhancement, and programs for curricular innovations. Evaluation of the success of these initiatives reaches beyond the mere counting of dollars received. It should include the congruence of the initiative to the stated mission and goals, trend data with indicators of performance outcomes for the investment, comparisons with peer institutions, and analysis of the worth of the initiative in meeting the stated goals for that initiative.

The sources of funding are important for review as indicators for future efforts as well. Some schools have relied exclusively on alumni as a source for development monies. Others reach out to corporations and special interest groups. In nursing, for example, hospitals have often provided funding for initiatives of interest to future human resources. They are more likely to continue their interest if evaluation reports are created indicating the efficient and effective use of the monies provided. One of the elements of evaluation often overlooked in this area is the mechanism to inform donors of the outcomes achieved as a result of their generosity. This alone may affect future giving.

Another source of data for analysis and decision making is a review of the goals of funding groups and state initiatives that may have attached funding. When the goals and initiatives of external agencies are congruent with the mission and goals of the school, this may provide opportunities to apply for funds that will contribute to the desired outcome of increased external funding. These data are usually available through the parent institution, library searches, professional organizations, the office of research and development, or direct contact with the funding group.

Regardless of the sources of funding, nursing programs, like others in higher education, are facing greater expectations to be cost-effective. As colleges and universities face the need to increase quality and strengthen academic reputation, they also face state and national calls for financial accountability. Because academic programs are the primary driver of costs, it is logical that institutions of higher education examine the cost-effectiveness of academic programs. Nursing schools may find themselves participating in institutional program prioritization projects to examine cost-effectiveness. Large nursing schools with multiple nursing programs may need to conduct a school-based prioritization project to determine resource allocation among nursing programs. Other methods of allocating resources may include equal distribution across all disciplines or charging academic units with covering their own costs by generating their own revenue (Hnat et al., 2015). Regardless of the method of allocation, there should be a defined process.

An adequate number of qualified staff and professional personnel is necessary to support program effectiveness. The level of clerical and professional staff is important to all program levels as well. For faculty to meet the expectations of teaching, scholarship, and service, the support personnel available to them are critical. The nature of the institution and the mission and goals also influence the standards set in this area. Nursing schools with graduate programs, for example, consider the number of graduate assistants and research assistants to be an issue of importance and in some cases computer programmers and statisticians may be important to goal achievement. Faculty-to-staff ratios and satisfaction surveys to elicit administration, faculty, and staff perceptions

about the quality of this support provide baseline data for this review. The analysis of these data may suggest the need for further data to complete a full analysis.

Many institutions of higher education have central evaluation tools and processes for the evaluation of function and performance of professional and clerical staff. Others rely on school or departmental evaluation. Still others supplement the central evaluation process with unit-specific efforts. The scope of staff under review will vary widely according to the size and complexity of the school. In any event, the evaluation should focus on the job descriptions and expectations of the individuals under review and the extent to which the job responsibilities are met in terms of efficiency and effectiveness. As with all other areas of evaluation, the process should include feedback on strengths and areas for growth; the establishment of goals for growth should be appropriate to the evaluation findings. All subsequent evaluations include a review of progress toward the stated goals. A common problem encountered in staff evaluation is the finding that the role of the staff member has drifted, because of changing circumstances, from the job description. This may create tensions that negatively affect evaluation. It is therefore necessary to include a periodic review of the job description for congruence with ongoing expectations. Revisions should occur as needed and as a collaborative effort between the staff member and the appropriate supervisor. Box 26.12 provides a summary of the elements associated with evaluation of fiscal resources.

BOX 26.12 Elements of Evaluation of Fiscal Resources

- Faculty and staff salaries are commensurate with institutional, regional, and national salary guidelines.
- Budget supports technology and instructional innovations.
- There are fiscal resources to recruit and develop faculty and staff.
- Resources are available to faculty for development.
- There is a plan to raise funds from external sources, foundations, alumni, and friends.

Evaluation of Partnerships and Relationships With External Agencies

Program effectiveness is influenced by the relationship of the nursing program with outside agencies. For example, partnerships and collaborative arrangements with health care agencies are essential to providing needed educational experiences for students. One method of facilitating these relationships is establishing an advisory board that can provide a direct communication link with these important stakeholders. The composition of the advisory board should be evaluated to determine that its membership is appropriate. The purpose and functions of the advisory board should be communicated to members and reviewed periodically for clarity. Effectiveness of the board's function can be determined by surveying board members and nursing faculty regarding their perception of the board's effectiveness in fulfilling its purpose.

Many nursing programs have agreements with other educational institutions that provide mobility pathways for students to complete upper-level degrees. An articulation agreement may define special admissions policies and the type of transfer credits that will be accepted between a community college and a university. For example, an articulation agreement may involve the admission of students in an associate degree program to a baccalaureate degree program while they are enrolled in the associate degree program. The effectiveness of these articulation agreements and mobility plans can be evaluated by having both institutions review the transfer admission criteria for appropriateness. The nursing program accepting students should conduct a periodic audit of the transcript evaluation process to ensure that transcripts are being accurately evaluated. The final test of the effectiveness of an articulation agreement is an examination of enrollment and various outcomes. Does the agreement support enrollment goals? Are students in the mobility program successful? Comparison of progression, retention, and completion rates of the students in the mobility program with those of students in a more traditional program will provide baseline data from which to determine the effectiveness of the articulation program. Box 26.13 provides a summary

> ### BOX 26.13 Evaluation of Partnerships and External Agencies
>
> - Advisory board and other communities of interest provide effective communication links with important stakeholders to support program improvements and quality.
> - Articulation and other collaborative agreements are mutually beneficial, and written agreements meet requirements of both parties' organizations.

of the elements to consider when evaluating partnerships and relationships with external agencies associated with evaluation of the interorganizational dimension.

Evaluating Student Support Services

The evaluation plan should include elements of evaluating student support services before admission, while matriculating, and after graduation. If the program's relationship with prospective students is not satisfactory, students will be discouraged from pursuing admission. A positive relationship with prospective students begins when students receive current and accurate information about the program. Because of the cost of higher education, prospective students need accurate information about financial aid. Transcript evaluation needs to be accurate and performed in a timely manner for all transfer students. New student registration should be run efficiently and provide a welcoming atmosphere. The admission and registration process should occur efficiently in as little time and hassle as possible. Universities may lose students if there is frustration because of being sent from one place or person to another to get admitted and enrolled. After students are admitted and registered, they will need orientation to the nursing program. Orientation should provide information about nursing program policies, especially requirements for admission into clinical courses and academic progression policies.

Activities at program completion may influence the satisfaction of students and their ongoing relationship as alumni in addition to their success in achieving terminal outcomes. The nursing school may offer special workshops in preparing students for licensure examinations. Career services may provide assistance in résumé preparation and job searches.

Academic advising is an important factor in program effectiveness and influences student success from program entry through completion. Some institutions use staff-level student advisers to assist students with registration and ongoing advisement, whereas others assign students to faculty advisers. Programs to educate faculty in effective advising should be evaluated for their utility. Further analysis of advising effectiveness can be determined by surveying students regarding their level of satisfaction with advising. As a component of the advising system, academic advising records are created when a student enters the program. These records should provide a thorough and objective record of student advisement. An audit of student files may be done to determine that files are set up correctly and maintained accurately through program completion.

Other aspects of the immediate environment that influence program success include housing, health services, student academic support services, business office and registrar, and cocurricular activities. One method of evaluating these functions is through student satisfaction surveys. One survey commonly used to assess the engagement of students in support services and activities on campus is the National Survey of Student Engagement (Indiana University School of Education NSSE Institute, 2019). This survey examines student engagement in effective educational practices by measuring the amount of time students spend on educationally related activities and how institutions organize the curriculum and on-campus activities to encourage student participation in campus activities. Results are provided at an institutional level, and comparisons are made with national norms.

Box 26.14 provides a summary of the elements associated with evaluation of student support services.

Outcome Evaluation

The purpose of outcome evaluation is to determine how well the program has achieved the expected outcomes. This step of the evaluation plan may be integrated into the final semester courses or may

> ### BOX 26.14 Evaluation of Student Support Services
>
> - Prospective students receive current and accurate information about program options, admission criteria, and financial aid.
> - Student recruitment plans support admission for a diverse population of students.
> - Transcript evaluation is accurate and performed in a timely manner for all transfer students.
> - New student registration is run efficiently and provides a welcoming atmosphere.
> - Students receive adequate orientation to the program.
> - Services are in place to support an academically, linguistically, and culturally diverse group of students.
> - Academic advising is effective.
> - Advising records are accurate and maintained from program entry through program completion.
> - Support for student learning is adequate.
> - Students receive final preparation after program completion for licensure examinations.

be applied at exit and during alumni and employer follow-up studies. For each of the outcomes, a simple model provides a framework for assessment and evaluation. The behavior of interest must be clearly defined and the attributes of that behavior must be delineated with benchmarks set. Faculty must then determine what measures will be used to assess the behavioral attributes with rationale for the selected measures. Finally, faculty must demonstrate how the data from such assessment and evaluation measures will be or have been used to develop, maintain, or revise curricula. To achieve this final objective for outcome evaluation, it must be placed within the context of overall program evaluation. Outcomes assessment in isolation will not provide adequate direction for program revision. Nevertheless, outcome evaluation is critical in that it may be the primary measure by which external stakeholders judge the merit of the program.

Student Outcomes

Student outcomes are measured at multiple levels in the program of learning. Student learning outcomes deal with attributes of the learner that demonstrate achievement of program goals. Examples include critical thinking, communication, and therapeutic interventions. Other areas of measurement of learner outcomes occur at the course, clinical practice, and classroom levels. Assessment of learner outcomes at the broad program level usually involves aggregate data designed to examine general measures of learner success. At this level, one can communicate to the public the extent to which one is preparing well-educated and competent practitioners to meet the human resource needs of the community.

Of particular interest are the graduation and retention rates in each program within the school. A clear understanding of the graduation and retention rates will influence decisions about recruitment and retention methods in the future. The state is interested in the graduation rate from the perspectives of human resource flow and as a measure of return on investment in the educational program. Tracking graduation rates is a measure of the productivity of a program and may provide information about the program itself. A low graduation rate or high attrition rate can indicate problems with admission criteria, the curriculum, or teaching effectiveness and mentoring of students. It is useful to track the absolute attrition of individuals over time and to document the number of graduates compared with the number of program entrants by graduation year. This allows the program to track students who are readmitted and who eventually graduate. In programs with high numbers of adult students, there may be a larger number of students who leave the program because of family problems or job-related issues. They may return and graduate at a later date. Thus a given class, when defined by the admission enrollment, may have a lower attrition rate than a class defined by numbers admitted and numbers graduated in a defined expected time span for program completion.

Many programs use the pass rate on national licensing examinations or certification examinations as a measure of program success. The number of graduates licensed or certified to practice in a given area is seen as a measure of production of qualified human resources. Pass rates that are lower than the benchmark set by the school or set by approval or accreditation bodies may be an indication of an issue in the nursing program such as problems with the curriculum. However, variables other than the program of learning, such as individual preparation or test anxiety, may also influence a graduate's performance on the examination. Certainly, a school should be concerned if the pass rate falls below reasonable norms, and additional assessment measures should be initiated to attempt to determine what issues may be involved and what might be done to improve those concerns. There may be issues involved that are not under the control of the nursing program.

Employment rate is an aggregate measure of product demand. The extent to which the graduates are able to find employment may provide both marketing data and a broad measure of employer satisfaction with the product a program produces. Less information may be gleaned in a tight market in which demand exceeds supply. When the demand is high, employment rates may be more an indication of need than selective employment based on the quality of the applicant. When the supply exceeds the demand, the specific applicants the employer selects may provide stronger data. If the graduates of a given program are not in demand or are not marketable, the nursing program should be evaluated to determine whether the reason for the decreased marketability is related to the quality of the graduate and the curriculum. Obtaining data from potential and current employers may be useful. Ultimately, the viability of the program may be questioned.

Employer Outcomes: Graduate Employment Rates and Satisfaction

Employer surveys may provide a means to determine the extent to which the consumer believes the graduate of the program has the skills necessary to meet employment expectations. Feedback from employers provides useful data for program review. It is difficult to obtain good response rates from employer surveys. Brevity and ease of completion are key to a high response rate. This is of particular importance during a time of work redesign and increasing demands on employers in health care. Extensive survey tools designed for each program with long lists of questions about skills to which the individual is asked to respond are less likely to be completed. Respondents are more likely to reply to fewer questions that have been well developed to provide useful information. Other avenues for gathering data may be useful such as focus groups made up of employers.

Gathering data related to several areas are of particular interest. Brief demographic information about the nature of the agency is helpful in learning which settings use the program graduates. Expressed concerns or commendations may be specific to a given setting; therefore, it is important to look for themes from a variety of employers. It is useful to know whether an employer would hire more graduates of the program if they were available. When questions about satisfaction with particular abilities are asked, it is helpful to state them in broad terms rather than providing the traditional laundry list of individual skills. For example, data about satisfaction may be linked to the extent to which an employer believes the graduates of the program are able to problem-solve, think critically, resolve conflicts, communicate effectively, use resources efficiently, and perform essential psychomotor skills safely. These and other broad classifications of behaviors can be selected on the basis of program outcome expectations. Provision of space for comments allows for the addition of qualitative information and the opportunity to identify any specific areas of concern.

Another issue in many employer surveys is the identification of which stakeholders are in the best position to respond to particular questions. Although an administrator may be able to respond more quickly and accurately to demographic questions and inquiries about the number of graduates employed, he or she may not be in the best position to respond to questions about the skills and abilities of graduates. The administrator may respond according to perceptions based on factors other than direct observation. Some employers delegate completion of the survey. Therefore it is helpful to request information about the respondent in the cover letter that accompanies the survey. For example, one might ask for the title of the respondent as a guide for determining how likely he or she is to be in a position of interacting directly with graduates. Some schools send employer surveys to graduates and request that they forward the surveys to their immediate supervisors for completion. This practice is problematic in that it usually results in a low return rate and a completed survey often reflects a respondent's reaction to an individual graduate rather than the aggregate of program graduates he or she has observed. Box 26.15 provides an example of an employer survey and sample questions.

Another method of obtaining ongoing feedback about the graduates of a program is to establish an advisory committee of consumers from agencies that typically employ program alumni. Such committees often provide advice and counsel on multiple matters, but satisfaction with the product and advice about the changing needs of the marketplace are traditional agenda items for such a group.

Alumni Evaluation: Employment Rates and Profile

There are multiple avenues for obtaining alumni data. One approach is to survey students who are about to become alumni. The exit survey is a method of determining product satisfaction with a program just completed. At this point, students' perceptions are fresh in their minds. Through the exit survey, it is possible to learn which students have found employment at the time of graduation, follow up on entry data collected for comparison purposes, and identify students' perceptions about the strengths and weaknesses of the program they have just completed. An online survey generally has a higher return rate than a survey sent through the regular mail. The exit survey is usually done within 10 days of graduation and has the advantage of a higher return rate than surveys sent at a later time. A disadvantage is that the exiting students may not have had an opportunity to apply their education in a work setting, which may change their perceptions.

Another method commonly used for exit data is the focus group. A focus group provides an opportunity for a representative group of students in the graduating classes to reflect in more detail about their experiences. Selection of the moderator is important to the collection of rich and valid insights.

A first concern is that the moderator be skilled in group process and listening. The moderator

---

BOX 26.15 Example: Employer Survey

To improve the quality of our academic nursing program, your thoughtful and honest responses to this survey are very important to us. Darken the oval that corresponds to your response.

Section I: Program Goals	Poor	Fair	Good	Excellent
1. Example program goal #1: Value	0	0	0	0
2. Example program goal #2: Communicate	0	0	0	0

Section II: Components of Program Goals	Poor	Fair	Good	Excellent
3. Example: Manages an environment that promotes clients' self-esteem, dignity, safety, and comfort.	0	0	0	0
4. Example: Establishes and maintains effective communication with clients, families, significant others, and health team members.	0	0	0	0
5. Example: Promotes continuity of client care by utilizing appropriate channels of communication external to the organization.	0	0	0	0

Section III: Overall Satisfaction With Nursing Program	Poor	Fair	Good	Excellent
6. My overall satisfaction with this employee is:	0	0	0	0

Other Examples of Employer Survey Questions

7. What is your primary source of information about this graduate?

8. What are your recommendations for strengthening this nursing program?

9. What suggestions do you have to facilitate transition into the professional role?

10. What changes in the health care environment will affect the educational preparation of future graduates?

11. Other comments: Survey completed by: _____ Position _____

---

should have several questions prepared to guide the group discussion yet be able to respond to and facilitate group discussion when other relevant issues emerge. In an end-of-program focus session, more open-ended questions encourage free-flowing responses and invite the participants to provide the amount of information they wish. If specific types of information are desired, the questions may be more structured. The more structured the question, the more reliable the data, but the trade-off may be less richness of data. One may find it useful to begin with open and broad questions and follow up with more structured questions as the discussion unfolds.

If the focus group is conducted by someone the students view as a neutral person and if that person is able to facilitate equally the expression of opposing points of view, the participants are more likely to be open in their comments and the content is likely to be more valid. Focus groups have the advantage of providing qualitative data in more detail than is usually obtained in a written survey, but they have the disadvantage of being a representative group that may or may not provide the range of data that a full group survey would provide. Use of both a survey and a focus group may resolve this issue, but students may be reluctant to participate in more than one end-of-program evaluation effort when they are in the process of final examinations and end-of-semester evaluations. Timing is important in this effort.

Alumni surveys may be conducted at regular intervals to obtain long-term data about the products of an educational program. Data can be collected in a nonthreatening way and they are relatively inexpensive to administer. The timing of such surveys depends on the data desired, the size and complexity of programs in the school, and the cost–benefit ratio of the survey effort. It is common to complete at least 1-year and 5-year surveys. The information sought depends on the level of the program and the outcome measures for which data are sought. Alumni surveys can involve the use of a tool developed by the nursing program or can be done using a standardized tool such as that developed by Skyfactor. The advantage of a standardized tool is the ability to make comparisons to other schools nationwide and to accreditation standards. One approach is to provide a two-part survey in which one part is devoted to broad outcome measures and the graduates' perceptions of their general education experience on the campus. Questions on this survey may relate to perceptions about the extent to which they acquired skills such as critical thinking, and effective written and oral communication; gained an understanding of different cultures and philosophies; and developed a sense of values and ethical standards, leadership skills, an appreciation of the arts, an ability to view events and phenomena from different perspectives, and an understanding of scientific principles and methods. One can also learn about the alumni's view of services available across the campus and opportunities to interact with students and faculty across disciplines. An advantage to this survey is the opportunity to compare the responses of students across disciplines to determine relative experiences and perceptions.

The second component of an alumni survey is usually discipline specific. In addition to general demographic data, the survey seeks information about positions held (title, location, population served, salary), the extent to which alumni believe they were prepared to practice according to the program outcomes, their general satisfaction with the program and activities related to scholarship such as publications, presentations, certifications, and entering advanced educational programs. Graduate programs find data related to the scholarship of alumni to be particularly valuable.

When surveys are conducted, the questions should be considered carefully in terms of data that will be used in decision making. If surveys are concise and questions are clearly stated, responses are more likely to be received. As a rule, response rates will be improved if the survey does not take more than 10 minutes to complete. A high response rate increases the credibility of the data in reflecting the perspectives of the population surveyed. The survey can be sent through regular mail or online. Online surveys are cheaper to send; however, studies have demonstrated that mail surveys result in higher response rates (Guo et al., 2016). With the volume of e-mails sent, the message may be lost or ignored and there may be issues related to internet access or web navigation. Incentives used in e-mail or mail surveys have been shown to be effective in increasing response rates (Guo et al., 2016). The cover letter is an important element of the survey. The letter should be concise yet spell out the importance of the data to the educational program and the value placed on the input received from graduates. The more personalized the letter and the more professional the survey tool, the more likely it is that alumni will respond. The letter should also include a statement about confidentiality and the use of pooled or aggregate data in reports of survey findings to protect the anonymity of the respondents. Although it is useful to have several open-ended questions to obtain qualitative data, the simpler the tool is to complete, the more likely it is that respondents will complete the task. Well-designed questions, for which the respondent can check or circle an item or provide a number as a response, are more likely to be answered. Multiple mailing is another method of improving the return rate. There are several opinions about the best mailing sequence. One method is to send a second mailing or e-mail within 2 to 3 weeks of the first, with a second survey tool included in case the first mailing has been misplaced. If the survey is being sent through regular mail and cost is an issue, a reminder card may suffice. A third mailing in the form of e-mail or a postcard should occur between 10 days and 3 weeks after the second mailing, depending on the nature of the survey. Rewards can help with response rates. A small monetary reward or an opportunity to be entered into a lottery are commonly used strategies (Guo et al., 2016).

Box 26.16 provides an example of an alumni survey and sample questions.

BOX 26.16 Example: Alumni Survey

As a graduate of our nursing program, you are especially qualified to tell us what works well and what does not. We would like your input and would appreciate any suggestions that you might have. Would you please take a few minutes and complete this survey? The survey is completely anonymous.

Darken the oval that corresponds to your response.

Section I: Perceptions of Attainment of Program Goals. Indicate how well the program prepared you to fulfill the following program goals

	Poor	Fair	Good	Excellent
1. Sample program goal #1: Integrate ...	0	0	0	0
2. Sample program goal #2: Utilize ...	0	0	0	0
3. Sample program goal #3: Synthesize ...	0	0	0	0

Section II. Satisfaction With Nursing Courses. Indicate how well each course contributed to your attainment of program goals

	Course Not Taken— Does Not Apply	Poor	Fair	Good	Excellent
4. Sample Course A	0	0	0	0	0
5. Sample Course B	0	0	0	0	0
6. Sample Course C	0	0	0	0	0

Section III: Overall Satisfaction With BSN Nursing Program

	Poor	Fair	Good	Excellent
7. My overall satisfaction with the Nursing Program	0 0	0	0	0

Additional Example Survey Questions

8. What semester and year did you graduate or complete your program?

9. What I liked best about my program was:

10. One thing I believe should be changed is:

11. What suggestions do you have to facilitate transition from the student role to professional practice?

12. Additional Comments:

BOX 26.17 Elements of Outcomes Evaluation

- Students achieve all program goals and outcomes by graduation.
- Students achieve all technical competencies by graduation.
- The program has defined a benchmark for graduation rates.
- The program has defined a benchmark for first-time National Council Licensure Exam (NCLEX) passage rates and certification rates as appropriate.
- The program has defined a benchmark for employment rates.
- Students are satisfied with the overall quality of the program.
- Employers are satisfied with the performance of graduates.
- Other potential outcomes are identified and evaluated

Box 26.17 provides a summary of the elements associated with outcomes evaluation.

Improving Program Outcomes

For the purpose of determining how to improve the program's outcomes, faculty first must review each variable that contributes to program success. These can include:

1. Qualifications of students admitted to the program
2. Definition and implementation of progression policies
3. Quality of the curriculum
4. Quality of instruction
5. Evaluation methods used to determine students' knowledge, skills, and abilities
6. Student preparation for employment and employer satisfaction.

The program evaluation plan should be reviewed at regular intervals to determine that each of these variables is examined as part of the program evaluation plan. A similar process should be followed for all program outcomes. Mapping the relationship between and among variables may help clarify the role each variable has in influencing outcome achievement.

Potential variables should be reviewed annually and added to the evaluation plan as needed. Intervening variables may be identified through literature review, program evaluation reports, or internal studies. All variables need to be evaluated at some point in the program evaluation plan. Analysis of these variables will help define where to make program improvements so that benchmarks can be met.

INTERNAL PROGRAM EVALUATION

Some universities require programs to undertake an internal evaluation or review of their programs. The purpose of many internal program evaluations is to assess and improve the quality of programs and to determine whether they are helping accomplish the university's mission. The questions to be answered include: (1) How well are we doing what we say we are doing? (2) How do we support student learning? (3) How well are the academic programs relating to each other? (4) Is the university fulfilling its mission and achieving its goals? This process informs the university about successes and weaknesses in the programs so that improvements can be made. The assessments are generally made in a rotation so that each program is reviewed at a specific interval.

The internal evaluation process usually calls for a written, evidence-based self-study. The information is reviewed by a team from outside the department and at least one representative from the profession who is external to the school and can be an objective reviewer. The reviewers are responsible for synthesizing and making judgments about the program quality. Those judgments then lead to a list of recommendations for improvement. The availability of resources to accomplish the goals and recommendations is assessed along with the involvement of campus administrators, faculty, and the community in the program and its evaluation.

Although each institution may have a different process, many regional accrediting bodies require that institutions of higher learning conduct internal program evaluations (Middle States Commission on Higher Education, 2020).

COMPREHENSIVE PROGRAM EVALUATION

Overall program evaluation provides the opportunity to examine the program in its entirety and to make revisions to improve its effectiveness. Program evaluation seeks to ensure that program improvement occurs as a result of a comprehensive collection and analysis of data.

A comprehensive program evaluation plan should be developed and written and should include the following questions:

1. What areas should be evaluated?
2. How often should the evaluation occur?
3. Who is responsible for collecting and analyzing the data?
4. Who is responsible for making decisions based on the data?
5. What benchmarks is the program setting to show quality?

The areas to be evaluated include any potential intervening factors, and should designate what data will be collected and how the data will be collected. The accreditation standards are often used as a framework to help define intervening factors and to demonstrate that the standards are met. The evaluation plan should also be reviewed at regular intervals for completeness.

The time frame for evaluation of each area should be set. For example, the mission and goals of the program may only need to be evaluated on a cycle of every 3 or 5 years. This is generally often enough to evaluate something so all-encompassing that changing it would only occur very carefully. However, graduation rates and National Council Licensure Examination–Registered Nurse (NLCEX–RN) pass rates need to evaluated annually.

Someone should be designated as responsible for the data collection, analysis, and decision making related to each item in the evaluation plan. Things tend to be overlooked unless someone takes responsibility. The responsibility will lie with a committee or a person associated with a position. For example, evaluation of faculty often lies with the dean, whereas evaluation of the curriculum lies with the faculty or a faculty committee such as a curriculum committee.

Setting benchmarks provides a goal for which to aim. A benchmark is a quality designation that allows faculty to determine progress toward attainment of the goal. They should be set fairly high but not at an unattainable level. They should be reviewed at regular intervals and altered as appropriate. Examining other schools nationwide and trend data for some benchmarks may help faculty set the benchmark. For example, it may be unreasonable to set 100% pass rate as a benchmark for NCLEX–RN. However, after examining trend data, faculty may decide that 90% is an attainable benchmark that demonstrates quality.

Once the evaluation plan is developed, it should be implemented correctly. Identifying evaluation activities called for in the plan by responsible parties at the beginning of the academic year will help ensure that evaluation activities are completed. Entering the program evaluation plan into an electronic spreadsheet or database may assist faculty in determining responsible parties, activities, and time frames allowing the plan to be sorted into these categories. Preparation of a year-end report with all completed forms and data sets will help track implementation of evaluation activities.

A record should be maintained of the data collected, the analysis of the data, decisions made related to the data, and program changes resulting from evaluation activities. Analysis of the data may not always result in change. The ultimate decision may be to gather data for another year or to maintain what exists and reevaluate. However, any decision should be reported.

Actions taken to improve program quality can be summarized in a yearly report. This report will serve as a permanent record of the utility of the evaluation plan in bringing about program improvements. Faculty may want to review these summary reports, discuss strengths and limitations of the plan, and propose changes to improve the plan's effectiveness after they have reviewed year-end reports. Questions that will help guide this review include "Does the plan provide information when it is needed for decision making?" and "Do the faculty trust the information provided by evaluation strategies?"

Another important factor in the plan's effectiveness is the reliability and validity of evaluation tools. Reliability refers to the accuracy of measurement. Validity means that evaluation tools measure what they intend to measure. Internally developed measurement tools should be evaluated for reliability and validity at the time of their development. If faculty are unable to demonstrate reliability and validity of evaluation tools, they will not be able to trust the results of program evaluation activities. In addition, data need to be appropriately aggregated and trended over time to support decision making. Faculty should be cautious about making decisions based on limited data.

The evaluation of any education program is context specific. Consequently, the results of program evaluation may not be generalized to other programs. Nevertheless, nursing faculty should report successful strategies in program evaluation in the nursing literature. Nursing faculty across the nation may benefit from program evaluation research studies, such as those that report successful assessment strategies or provide insight about intervening variables for common program outcomes.

Box 26.18 provides a summary of the elements associated with comprehensive program evaluation.

Accountability for Program Evaluation

Responsibility for development and implementation of the program evaluation plan rests with the nursing administration and faculty. The process for development and implementation may vary across nursing schools, depending on such factors as the number of faculty in the nursing school and the institutional resources available to support the evaluation. In some schools, an evaluator position is created to manage program evaluation practices, including the development and implementation of the program evaluation plan. An office of evaluation may be necessary in large schools, providing support staff to coordinate data collection at multiple levels. A common approach in small- and moderate-sized nursing schools is to appoint a standing committee of faculty who provide leadership and coordination of evaluation efforts. Regardless of the plan, the nursing faculty must determine accountability for each element of the evaluation plan. Without clear accountability and firm time frames, it is easy for evaluation efforts to get lost in the press of daily demands on faculty and administration.

Another issue of concern is the reporting and recording of evaluation data. Information is of little value to decision making unless it is channeled to those who are responsible for making decisions. Careful attention to this issue not only increases the likelihood that decisions will be based on actual data but also facilitates analysis of the value of the data. Evaluation data also serve as a rich resource when responses to external reports and accreditation expectations are required. One of the dangers is data overload. Because data are used for making decisions, it is best to determine what information is necessary and what is interesting but not important. Over time, a goal of evaluation is to streamline the amount of data collected. Asking questions such as "Why do we need these data or information?" and "How will these data or information assist in making decisions for improvement?" will assist in eliminating data overload.

The location of evaluation information is also important. Access to the information increases the likelihood of its use. An official location for evaluation reports ensures that they can be found when they are needed. Advances in technology have made the development of computer databases an important source of information that can be accessed by multiple stakeholders from a central location or file server.

Finally, the outcome of evaluation efforts in terms of creating change is an element that is

---

BOX 26.18 Elements of Comprehensive Program Evaluation

- Assessment strategies are reliable and valid.
- Evaluation activities provide meaningful data for program improvement.
- The evaluation plan is reviewed and modified to improve its effectiveness.
- The evaluation plan is implemented as written; decisions are made and changes implemented related to the data collected.
- Data collected through the implementation of the evaluation plan are used to improve the program

sometimes omitted in record keeping. It is important to close the loop related to data collection and decision making. Accrediting bodies are as concerned about the actions that result from analysis of evaluation data as they are that a plan is in place. The best plan loses value if it does not create change when a need for intervention is indicated by the data. (See Case Study 26.2.)

CASE STUDY 26.2 **Evaluation Plan Based on Criteria From an Accreditation Body**

The dean at a new nursing program in a medium-sized university has asked the faculty to develop an evaluation plan for the undergraduate nursing program. The evaluation plan will be based on the criteria from the school's accreditation body. Decisions need to be made about what data should be collected in relation to the criteria and how it will be collected.

1. What should be considered in making these decisions?
2. What resources are available to collect the data?
3. What expected outcomes will be measured?
4. How will the data be used to measure the criteria and expected outcomes?

CHAPTER SUMMARY: KEY POINTS

- Program evaluation is a comprehensive, cyclic, and complex process.
- The evaluation process is used as a guide for improvement for nursing education programs.
- Use of a systematic approach to program evaluation increases the likelihood that all program elements will receive appropriate attention and that evaluation activities will lead to program improvement.
- The program evaluation plan serves as a road map to ensure that program evaluation activities are appropriately implemented.

- Development and implementation of a carefully designed program evaluation plan will support continuous quality improvement for nursing education programs.
- Program evaluation should include all aspects that might influence program quality.
- Revisions of the program are based on review of data collected to measure program quality and revisions in the program when indicated.

REFLECTING ON THE EVIDENCE

1. What is the relationship between program evaluation and a quality curriculum?
2. What models of evaluation are useful for nursing education and would be consistent with the philosophical base of the curriculum?
3. What aspects of the overall program should be evaluated and why?
4. What kinds of data should be evaluated, and how do you interpret that data?

5. Who should be involved in the evaluation process and why?
6. How can a systematic program evaluation be used in new program development?
7. What is the process for developing and implementing a comprehensive evaluation plan, and what should be included in an evaluation plan?

REFERENCES

American Association of Colleges of Nursing. (2010). *The research-focused doctoral program in nursing: Pathways to excellence.* https://www.aacnnursing.org/Portals/42/Publications/PhDPosition.pdf

American Association of Colleges of Nursing. (2019). *AACN annual report.* American Association of Colleges of Nursing. https://www.aacnnursing.org/Portals/42/Publications/Annual-Reports/Annual-Report-2019.pdf

American Association of Colleges of Nursing. (2020, September). *Nursing faculty shortage*. American Association of Colleges of Nursing. https://www.aacnnursing.org/news-information/fact-sheets/nursing-faculty-shortage

American Association of Colleges of Nursing. (2021). *PhD Education*. American Association of Colleges of Nursing. https://www.aacnnursing.org/Nursing-Education-Programs/PhD-Education

American Nurses Association. (2021). Nursing: Scope and standards of practice. https://www.nursingworld.org/nurses-books/nursing-scope-and-standards-of-practice-4th-edit/

Association of American Colleges and Universities. (2020, May 4). *What liberal education looks like: What it is, who it's for, and where it happens (e-title)*. https://secure.aacu.org/imis/ItemDetail?iProductCode=E-WHATLELL

Bichsel, J., McChesney, J., & Calcagno, M. (2017). Faculty in higher education salary report: Key findings, trends, and comprehensive tables for tenure track, non-tenure track teaching, and non-tenure track research faculty; Academic department heads; And adjunct faculty at four-year institutions for the 2016–17 academic year [Research report]. *CUPA-HR* https://www.cupahr.org/surveys/fhe4.aspx.

Bloom, B. S. (1956). *Taxonomy of educational objectives: The classification of educational goals. Handbook I: Cognitive domain*. McKay.

Boyer, E. L. (1990). *Scholarship rediscovered: Priorities of the professorate*. The Carnegie Foundation for the Advancement of Teaching.

Brown, J. F., & Marshall, B. L. (2008). Continuous quality improvement: An effective strategy for improvement of program outcomes in a higher education setting. *Nursing Education Perspectives, 29*(4), 205–211.

Burwash, S. C., & Snover, R. (2016). Up Bloom's pyramid with slices of Fink's pie: Mapping an occupational therapy curriculum. *The Open Journal of Occupational Therapy, 4*(4). https://doi.org/10.15453/2168-6408.1235.

Chan, Z. C. Y., Cheng, W. Y., Fong, M. K., Fung, Y. S., Ki, Y. M., Li, Y. L., Wong, H. T., Wong, T. L., & Tsoi, W. F. (2019). Curriculum design and attrition among undergraduate nursing students: A systematic review. *Nurse Education Today, 74*, 41–53. https://doi.org/10.1016/j.nedt.2018.11.024.

Chen, H. (1990). *Theory driven evaluation*. Sage.

Chen, H. C., O'Sullivan, P., Teherani, A., Fogh, S., Kobash, B., & Cate, O. (2015). Sequencing learning experiences to engage different level learners in the workplace: An interview study with excellent clinical teachers. *Medical Teacher, 37*, 1090–1097.

Commission on Collegiate Nursing Education (CCNE). (2018). Standards for accreditation of baccalaureate and graduate nursing education programs. https://www.aacnnursing.org/CCNE

DeSilets, L. D. (2018). An update on Kirkpatrick's model of evaluation: Part two. *Journal of Continuing Education in Nursing, 49*(7), 292–293. https://doi.org/10.3928/00220124-20180613-02.

Distance Education Accrediting Commission. (2021). The DEAC accreditation handbook. https://www.deac.org/UploadedDocuments/Handbook/DEAC_Accreditation_Handbook.pdf

Eliades, A. B., Jakubik, L. D., Weese, M. M., & Huth, J. J. (2017). Mentoring practice and mentoring benefit 6: Equipping for leadership and leadership readiness—An overview and application to practice using mentoring activities. *Pediatric Nursing, 43*(1), 40–42.

Ewell, P. T. (1985). *Introduction to assessing educational outcomes: New directions for Institutional research*. Jossey-Bass.

Gualdron, D. R., & Parker, K. (2021). Evaluation in health professions education: Enhancing utility and supporting innovation. *Clinical Teaching, 18*, 621–626. https://doi.org/10.1111/tct.13416.

Guo, Y., Kopec, J. A., Cibere, J., Li, L. C., & Goldsmith, C. H. (2016). Population survey features and response rates: A randomized experiment. *American Journal of Public Health, 106*(8), 1422–1426. https://doi.org/10.2105/AJPH.2016.303198.

Hnat, H. B., Mahony, D., Fitzgerald, S., & Crawford, F. (2015). Distributive justice and higher education resource allocation: Perceptions of fairness. *Innovative Higher Education, 40*(1), 79–93. https://doi.org/10.1007/s10755-014-9294-3.

Indiana University School of Education. (2019). *NSSE Annual Results 2019*. https://nsse.indiana.edu/research/annual-results/past-annual-results/nsse-annual-results-2019/index.html

Jager, F., Vandyk, A., Jacob, J. D., Meilleur, D., Vanderspank-Wright, B., LeBlanc, B., Chartrand, J., Hust, C., Lalonde, M., Rintoul, A., Alain, D., Poirier, S., & Phillips, J. C. (2020). The Ottawa model for nursing curriculum renewal: An integrative review. *Nurse Education Today*(87).

Khailova, L. (2021). Using curriculum mapping to scaffold and equitably distribute information literacy instruction for graduate professional studies programs. *The Journal of Academic Librarianship, 47*. https://doi.org/10.1016/j.acalib.2020.102281.

Lunenburg, F. C. (2011). Curriculum development: Deductive models. *Schooling*, 2(1), 1–17.

Middle States Commission on Higher Education. (2020). Standards for Accreditation and Requirements of Affiliation. https://www.msche.org/standards/

Muñoz, M. A., & Dossett, D. H. (2016). Multiple measures of teaching effectiveness: Classroom observations and student surveys as predictors of student learning. *Planning and Changing*, 47(3/4), 123–140.

National League for Nursing Commission on Nursing Education Accreditation (NLN CNEA). (2021). *Accreditation Standards for Nursing Education Programs.* https://cnea.nln.org/standards-of-accreditation

National Organization of Nurse Practitioner Faculties. (2016). Criteria for evaluation of nurse practitioner programs. https://www.nonpf.org/page/15

Niederberger, M., & Spranger, J. (2020). Delphi technique in health sciences: A map. *Frontiers in Public Health*, 8(457). https://doi.org/10.3389/fpubh.2020.00457.

Rodriguez, A. L., Gallardo, K., Tapia Ruelas, C. S., & Piza Gutierrez, R. I. (2021). Perceptions of formative assessment in secondary education: Beyond teaching styles. *The International Journal of Assessment and Evaluation*, 28(2). https://doi.org/10.18848/2327-7920/CGP/v28i02/35-51.

Sar, J. (2022). *Patterns of curriculum development.* https://www.academia.edu/25237982/Patterns_of_Curriculum_Organization

Scriven, M. (1991). Pros and cons about goal-free evaluation. *American Journal of Evaluation*, 12(1), 55–62. https://doi.org/10.1177/109821409101200108.

Stravropoulou, A., & Stroubouki, T. (2014). Evaluation of educational programmes—The contribution of history to modern evaluation thinking. *Health Science Journal*, 8(2), 193–204.

Stufflebeam, D. L. (2003). The CIPP model for evaluation. In T. Kellaghan & Stufflebeam, D. L. (Eds.), *International Handbook of Educational Evaluation.* Kluwer Academic Publishers.

Tyler, R. W. (1949). *Basic principles of curriculum and instruction.* University of Chicago Press.

Wijnen-Meijer, M., van den Broek, S., Koens, F., & Cate, O. T. (2020). Vertical integration in medical education: The broader perspective. *BMC Medical Education*, 20(1), 509. https://doi.org/10.1186/s12909-020-02433-6.

27

The Accreditation Process*

Laurie Peters, PhD, RN

Nursing program accreditation is a voluntary, ongoing, peer-review process provided by private, nongovernmental accrediting agencies. Accreditation is designed to ensure academic quality, promote excellence and integrity in nursing education, and create a culture of continuous quality improvement. The accreditation process determines the extent to which nursing programs demonstrate compliance with professional standards and criteria. Nursing programs must demonstrate that an ongoing, systematic process for program evaluation and improvement is in place, incorporating appropriate program outcome measures and utilization of data for evidence-based decision making for program improvement. Additionally, programs utilize the systematic evaluation process to demonstrate achievement of program outcomes and accreditation standards and criteria. A culture of continuous quality improvement promotes academic quality, identification of achievements and areas for improvement, and development of strategies and actions for improvement.

Programs granted initial and continued accreditation approval are responsible for maintaining compliance with current standards as defined by the accrediting agencies. The three nursing education accrediting agencies in the United States are the Accreditation Commission for Education on Nursing (ACEN), the Commission on Collegiate Nursing Education (CCNE), and the National League for Nursing Commission for Nursing Education Accreditation (NLN CNEA). All three accreditation agencies have been recognized by the US Department of Education (USDE) and are dedicated to maintaining quality nursing programs. In addition, there are also specialty nursing accrediting agencies. For example, the Accreditation Commission for Midwifery Education (ACME, n.d.) is recognized by the USDE as an accrediting agency for nurse-midwifery and midwifery education programs and the Council on Accreditation of Nurse Anesthesia Educational Programs (COA) is the accrediting agency for nurse anesthesia programs.

Nursing program accreditation and state board of nursing regulation are two distinct, independent processes. Boards of nursing are state-specific, governmental entities designed to protect public health, safety, and welfare. State boards of nursing monitor nursing practice and the quality of nursing education programs within their jurisdiction through established rules and regulations. Nursing programs must be approved by and comply with the state board's administrative code and submit annual reports addressing compliance with state regulatory standards. An accredited nursing program may lose its accreditation status and remain operational as accrediting agencies lack the authority to close a program. However, under their jurisdiction, state boards of nursing have the regulatory authority to close nursing programs found to be out of compliance with the board's rules, regulations, and administrative codes.

This chapter provides an overview of accreditation in the United States, the history of

*The author acknowledge the work of Michael Kremer, PhD, CRNA, CHESE, FNAP, FAAN, and Betty J. Horton, PhD, CRNA, FAAN in the previous edition of the chapter.

accreditation, and distinctions between institutional and programmatic accreditation. Nursing accreditation agencies and their guidelines for initial and ongoing nursing program accreditation are reviewed. This chapter also discusses elements of the accreditation process for nursing programs, including preparation of the self-study document, use of consultants, and the on-site visit.

ACCREDITATION IN THE UNITED STATES

Accreditation in higher education has existed in the United States since the late 19th century, starting with development of the first postsecondary accreditation associations. No singular authority exists in the United States providing centralized control over accreditation in higher education institutions and programs. Accreditation of postsecondary institutions and programs by recognized accrediting agencies was developed to "serve as a marker of the level of acceptable quality of educational programs and postsecondary schools" (Hegji, 2020). The goal of accreditation is to ensure that institutions and programs meet acceptable levels of quality. Accreditation is a process by which nongovernmental accrediting agencies grant accreditation to postsecondary institutions and programs found to meet or exceed the standards and criteria established by the accrediting agency. Programs granted initial and continued accreditation demonstrate a high level of educational quality to various communities of interest including students, families, and the general public. Accreditation enhances opportunities for institutional and program public and private funding and employment options for program graduates. Nursing program accreditation facilitates the transfer of academic credits between institutions, and for students, graduating from an accredited nursing program is a requirement for admission to many graduate programs.

History of Accreditation

Accreditation has evolved over the last 100 years to include provision of accreditation services not only in the United States but also, in some cases, in other countries. In the United States, accreditation has been described as changing from an "independent, collegial process by which higher education decides and evaluates academic quality on its own to a compliance-driven process" (Eaton, 2017, p. 1). Factors associated with this shift include: entities responsible for accreditation oversight; how *quality* is defined; defining what information is required and to whom accrediting agencies are responsible; and how accreditation agencies should function (Eaton, 2017). Following passage of the 1965 Higher Education Act, "Congress expanded the role of accrediting agencies by entrusting them with ensuring academic quality of the educational institutions at which federal student aid funds may be used subject to oversight by the federal government through the recognition process" (USDE, n.d.).

Accrediting agencies are accountable to various constituents including institutions, programs, students, the public, and government agencies. Subject matter experts develop the standards, policies, and procedures used by accrediting agencies for conducting peer reviews to determine the quality of higher education institutions and programs. Elements reviewed during the on-site evaluation include the program and institutional missions, vision and goals, financial resources, academic policies, curricula, and student support services to ensure sufficient quality, resources, and processes are in place to meet the institutional and program missions and goals. Nursing educators and administrators should maintain an understanding of current changes in accreditation standards and policies, ensuring that the appropriate structures, processes, and outcome variables used to assess program quality and improvement are in place.

Benefits of Accreditation

Institutions and programs granted accreditation approval demonstrate to the public and its constituents that high-quality educational standards have been met or exceeded. Accreditation provides formal recognition through a peer-review process for institutions and programs. The public is assured that accredited institutions and programs undergo extensive evaluation through a peer-review process and meet or exceed high-quality standards. Institutions and programs benefit from engagement in the self-evaluation and improvement process and enhanced credibility, and the potential to recruit nursing students and faculty. Eligibility for participation in federal financial aid programs is only available to students attending accredited institutions. Students graduating from accredited programs benefit from the ability to more easily transfer credits to other institutions and increased competitiveness in the job market. For the nursing profession, accreditation enhances the overall quality of care provided by graduates of accredited nursing programs.

Accreditation exists to ensure quality assessment and to assist with quality improvement. Accreditation can apply to institutions or programs, whereas certification and licensure are related to individuals. Accreditation does not ensure the quality of individual graduates but provides reasonable assurance of the context and quality of the education that is offered.

There are numerous benefits to program accreditation for the public, students, programs, and the profession.

The public receives:
- reasonable assurance of the external evaluation of a program and its conformity with general expectations in the professional field;
- identification of programs that have voluntarily undertaken explicit activities directed at improving their quality and their successful execution;
- improvement in the professional services available to the public resulting from modification of program requirements to reflect changes in knowledge and practice that are generally accepted in the field; and
- less need for intervention by public agencies in operation of educational programs because of the availability of private accreditation for the maintenance and enhancement of educational quality.

Student benefits include:
- reasonable assurance that the educational activities of an accredited program have been found to be satisfactory and meet the needs of students;
- assistance in transferring credits among programs and institutions; and
- a uniform prerequisite for entering the profession.

Programs accreditation provides:
- the stimulus needed for self-directed improvement;
- peer review and counsel provided by the accrediting agency;
- enhancement of their reputation, because of the public's regard for accreditation; and
- eligibility for selected governmental funding programs and private foundation grants.

Professions benefit from accreditation, which provides:
- a means for participation of practitioners in establishing the requirements for preparation to enter the profession; and
- a contribution to the unity of the profession by bringing together practitioners, educators, students, and communities of interest in an activity directed toward improving professional preparation and practice (COA, 2021).

Through the accreditation process, nursing programs ensure high-quality education through a culture of continuous quality improvement in the preparation of a nursing workforce able to meet the changing acute and long-term care needs in the United States and across the globe.

Accrediting Agency Recognition

External recognition of US accrediting agencies entrusted with the responsibility for providing institutional and programmatic accreditation is designated by the USDE and Council for Higher Education Accreditation (CHEA). Accrediting agencies granted recognition by the USDE and/or CHEA are considered to be reliable authorities for determining the quality of educational programs and institutions (Hegji, 2020). CHEA is a nongovernmental association providing recognition to institutional and programmatic accrediting agencies. The purpose of CHEA recognition is "to provide assurance to the public that accrediting organizations are competent to engage in quality review of institutions and programs based on the standards that CHEA has developed, which are presented in the CHEA Standards and Procedures for Recognition" (CHEA, 2021). CHEA's recognition process focuses on the quality of regional accreditors that accredit 2- and 4-year public and private colleges and universities; national faith-related accreditation agencies, which accredit nonprofit, degree-granting, religious, or doctrine-based institutions; and national career-related accreditors, which review single-purpose, for-profit, career-based institutions, and programmatic accreditors for specific programs and professions (USDE, n.d.). CHEA-recognized accrediting agencies must meet and remain in compliance with all current standards and requirements. The maximum term for CHEA recognition is 7 years, at which time accreditation organizations must complete a recognition review (CHEA, 2021).

USDE-recognized accrediting organizations must meet established policies and procedures. According to the USDE, "In order for students to receive federal student aid from the U.S. Department of Education (Department) for post-secondary study, the institution must be accredited by a 'nationally recognized' accrediting agency" (USDE, n.d.). The USDE and CHEA publish on their websites lists of recognized accrediting agencies considered to be "reliable authorities as to the quality of education or training provided by institutions of higher education" (USDE, n.d.).

IMPACT OF COVID-19 ON NURSING PROGRAM ACCREDITATION

The COVID-19 pandemic has significantly impacted schools and institutions, at times forcing closures of various durations worldwide. Initial and continued accreditation processes include a number of tasks necessary for demonstration of compliance with accreditation standards. The abrupt change in teaching modalities from classroom to online learning methodologies experienced by many programs limited their availability to prepare for accreditation reviews (Abdelhadi, 2020). As the pandemic continues in the United States and globally, higher education institutions and programs continue to identify the acute and long-term effects on education quality.

In 2020, nursing accrediting agencies responded by delaying on-site visits and/or opting for "virtual" reviews. Many programs established virtual "exhibit rooms" for document accessibility, incorporated virtual tours of campus and program facilities, and conducted interviews with faculty, students, administrators, and other communities of interest via internet technology applications such as Webex or Zoom. Nursing accrediting agencies provided information on their websites regarding changes in policies or procedures related to COVID-19. Examples include program guidance related to virtual site visits, frequently asked questions, and the use of distance technology during virtual accreditation visits. As the pandemic continues to unfold, it is important that program administrators remain current regarding accreditation guidelines and process updates provided by the USDE and nursing program accrediting agencies.

INSTITUTIONAL AND PROGRAMMATIC ACCREDITING AGENCIES

There are different categories of accrediting agencies, including institutional and programmatic accrediting agencies. Programmatic accrediting agencies accredit individual programs within the institution. In the United States, recognition of accrediting agencies is granted by the CHEA and/or the USDE. The CHEA "... recognizes institutional and programmatic accrediting organizations" focusing on "... higher education accreditation and quality assurance" (CHEA, n.d.-a). Accrediting agencies recognized by CHEA have standards and processes that "are consistent with the academic quality, improvement and accountability expectations that CHEA has established" (CHEA, n.d.-b). Institutions that house nursing programs may also possess institutional accreditation.

Institutional accreditation is granted to an entire institution, which includes all programs offered within the institution. CHEA also grants recognition to regional accrediting agencies which set the standards for institutional accreditation and monitor compliance with those standards. Six CHEA- and USDE-recognized regional accreditation organizations are: Accrediting Commission for Community and Junior Colleges (ACCJC); Western Association of Schools and Colleges (WASC); Higher Learning Commission (HLC);

Middle States Commission on Higher Education (MSCHE); New England Commission of Higher Education (NECHE); Northwest Commission on Colleges and Universities (NWCCU); Southern Association of Colleges and Schools Commission on Colleges (SACSCOC); and the Senior College and University Commission (WSCUC).

Programmatic accreditation is provided to discipline-specific programs and professional schools such as nursing, law, pharmacy, medicine, allied health, audiology, aviation, and engineering. The programmatic accreditation agencies for nursing programs are ACEN, CCNE, and NLN CNEA. In addition to these entities, there are advanced practice nursing accrediting agencies including the COA and the ACME.

The USDE provides oversight of accrediting agencies who serve as *gatekeepers* for institutions and programs who wish to participate in federal student aid programs. Grants, loans, and work-study programs authorized under Title IV of the Higher Education Act are the major source of federal student aid (Federal Student Aid [FSA], n.d.). Students seeking federal (and sometimes state) grants and loans need to attend a college, university, or program that is accredited by a nationally accrediting agency and recognized by the USDE for this purpose. In this regard, the USDE-recognized accreditation agency is considered a "Title IV gatekeeper" for federal funds (Hegji, 2019).

Many nursing students finance their educational costs through federal funds provided by institutionally accredited colleges and universities. Students participating in hospital-based or single-purpose freestanding nursing programs that are not institutionally accredited rely on approved USDE Category 3 programmatic accrediting to obtain federal financial aid. ACEN, COA, and ACME are examples of nursing program accrediting agencies recognized by USDE as Category 3 agencies. The nursing program accreditors CCNE and NLN CNEA are considered to be Category 2 accrediting agencies and, as such, do not serve as Title IV gatekeepers for federal student aid, instead relying upon the institution's accreditation by a USDE-recognized, institutional accrediting Title IV gatekeeper to serve that purpose.

OVERVIEW OF THE NURSING ACCREDITATION PROCESS

Nursing accrediting agencies typically follow a three-step accreditation model. The accreditation process starts with the program's self-analysis of compliance with accreditation standards which is then documented in the self-study report. The self-study document provides a systematic self-assessment of nursing program effectiveness, quality, and the extent to which the program's mission, goals, and outcomes are met. Supporting documents are provided as part of the self-study report demonstrating compliance with the accreditation standards and criteria. The self-study document is reviewed by peer evaluators including faculty members, administrators, and practitioners within the stated profession.

The second step in the accreditation process is an on-site visit conducted by peer evaluators to validate and clarify information contained in the self-study report, as well as to collect additional data. Document review and interviews with stakeholders are included in the on-site review. Basic components addressed in the accreditation process include measurable program outcomes, mission, goals and governance, organizational structures, administrators and faculty, students, academic support services, quality and adequacy of resources, policies and procedures, formal complaint mechanism, curriculum and evaluation processes, systematic program evaluation plan, and continuous quality improvement.

The third step involves review of the on-site team report by committees of the accrediting agency. Following the on-site visit and review of the self-study report and supporting information, peer evaluators submit an independent analysis of the program's compliance with accreditation standards to the accrediting agency. The decision-making body of the accreditation agency is composed of elected representatives who make the final decision to grant accreditation or deny accreditation, or place the program on probation. Accreditation agencies publish the accreditation actions taken by their board on their websites, as well as lists of accredited programs.

NURSING PROGRAM ACCREDITATION AGENCIES

The ACEN, CCNE, and NLN CNEA serve as the three accrediting bodies for nursing programs in the United States. A summary of each agency and their standards, criteria, and processes are provided in this section. The reader is advised to review each agency's website for the most current information.

Accreditation Commission for Education on Nursing

In 1996, the NLN approved the creation of the National League for Nursing Accreditation Commission (NLNAC) as an accrediting entity. The NLNAC changed its name in 2013 to the ACEN. The mission of ACEN is to support nursing education and practice, and the public, through its accreditation functions and "improvement of institutions or programs related to resources invested, processes followed, and results achieved" (ACEN, 2020). ACEN accredits nursing programs including clinical doctorate/DNP specialist certificates, master's/postmaster's certificates, baccalaureate, associate, diploma, and practical nursing programs. ACEN defines accreditation as a "voluntary peer-review, self-regulatory process by which non-governmental associations recognize educational institutions or programs that have been found to meet or exceed standards and criteria for educational quality" (ACEN, 2020). ACEN serves as a Title IV gatekeeper for programs eligible to participate in federal financial aid and is recognized by CHEA and the USDE.

ACEN is governed by a 17-member Board of Commissioners composed of elected individuals including nurse educators representing ACEN-accredited programs (11), public representatives (3), and commissioners representing nursing service (3). The ACEN Chief Executive Officer reports to the Board of Commissioners (ACEN, 2020). Decisions regarding accreditation status, policy, administration, and budget are the responsibility of the ACEN Board of Commissioners. The ACEN operations are supported by professional, administrative, and support staff; program evaluators; and committees. ACEN peer evaluators conducting the on-site visit include nurse administrators, nurse educators, and nurse clinicians who possess knowledge of postsecondary and/or higher education, curriculum, instructional methods, current issues and trends in health care, and nursing education and practice within the various types of nursing programs. Peer evaluators are selected based on defined criteria established by the ACEN and may be appointed to serve on various ACEN committees. Following the on-site visit, peer evaluators make recommendations to the ACEN Board of Commissioners for final accreditation decisions.

ACEN Standards and Criteria

ACEN accreditation standards and related criteria are provided for the various types of nursing programs it accredits and are published in the *ACEN Accreditation Manual: 2017 Standards and Criteria* (ACEN, 2020). The six ACEN standards address: (1) Mission and Administrative Capacity; (2) Faculty and Staff; (3) Students; (4) Curriculum; (5) Resources; and (6) Outcomes. A separate *Glossary* and *ACEN Accreditation Manual Supplement for International Programs* are available (ACEN, 2020).

Programs seeking initial accreditation approval by the ACEN are required to demonstrate compliance with all accreditation standards and substantial compliance with standards to receive continued accreditation. Nursing programs are expected to provide a summary of program strengths, areas needing development, and an action plan based on the standards and criteria. ACEN offers online asynchronous, self-paced courses including *Understanding and Applying the ACEN Standards and Criteria* and *Effectively Leading an ACEN Accredited Program*, available on their website at https://www.acenursing.org/.

ACEN Accreditation Process

ACEN follows a similar three-step accreditation model as discussed earlier in the chapter. The accreditation process includes determination of program eligibility and candidacy (for initial accreditation only), review of the program's self-study report, an on-site evaluation, a review of submitted materials by the Evaluation Review Panel (ERP), and a final review and accreditation decision by the ACEN Board of Commissioners.

Following program submission of their self-study report, an on-site evaluation is conducted by a team composed of professional peer evaluators from nursing education and practice. The team of peer evaluators verify congruence between the self-study and program practices and the extent to which the program is in compliance with the ACEN standards and criteria. Following the visit, a report is developed by the peer evaluators and submitted to the ACEN. A draft copy of the site visit report is sent to the program's nurse administrator for review and correction of any factual errors, which are documented on the *Nurse Administrator Response Form*. The final site visit report is emailed to the Nurse Administrator and the on-site peer evaluators.

ACEN's *ERP* consists of members appointed by the ACEN Board of Commissions. The ERP is responsible for conducting an independent analysis regarding the extent to which the program meets the ACEN standards and criteria through validation of the site visit report. During the ERP review, areas of agreement are identified in addition to areas in which a lack of clarity exists. A recommendation from the ERP is then made to the ACEN Board of Commissioners, which has the sole authority for determining the accreditation status of nursing program applicants.

Initial and Continuing Accreditation

Nursing programs seeking initial and continued ACEN accreditation must be approved by the state or county agencies that have legal authority for nursing education programs. Programs must also demonstrate their ability to meet all current eligibility and continued eligibility requirements of the ACEN. Eligibility requirements are available in the *ACEN Accreditation Manual—Policy 3* (ACEN, 2020).

To initiate the ACEN initial and continuing accreditation process, official authorization must be submitted by the Chief Executive Officer of the governing institution and the nursing program administrator. Eligibility for ACEN accreditation begins with submission of a *Candidacy Eligibility Application* (CEA) and supporting documents (ACEN, 2020). Once program eligibility is determined, programs provide a signed Authorization

for Candidacy form and have up to 1 calendar year to begin the candidacy process. Candidacy eligibility applications for programs in the United States and international programs are located on the ACEN website at https://www.acenursing.org/candidacy/. Program administrators must submit state board of nursing approval documentation, fees, and information related to the governing institution, faculty, curriculum, and resources. Once candidacy status is established, the nursing program has 2 calendar years to schedule an initial accreditation visit. Failure to comply with accreditation standards and criteria may result in denial of accreditation. The next review process is 5 years from the accreditation cycle resulting in the ACEN Board of Commissions' approval of initial accreditation. Programs unable to demonstrate compliance with all accreditation standards may be denied initial accreditation, which can be appealed following established ACEN policies and procedures (ACEN, 2020).

ACEN-accredited nursing programs are scheduled for reevaluation at specified intervals to ensure ongoing compliance with ACEN Standards and Criteria. The ACEN website (https://www.acenursing.org/) provides various online resources for programs including (but not limited to) the ACEN Accreditation Manual and Glossary, forms, and resources regarding preparation of the self-study report, on-site visit, reporting substantive changes, and continuing education. Programs preparing for a continuing accreditation site visit may request an *Advisory Review* by an ACEN staff member who provides feedback on draft program documents.

Programs seeking continued accreditation must be in compliance with all ACEN standards and criteria. The maximum accreditation term is 8 years (ACEN, 2020). Continuing accreditation with conditions or warnings is designated to programs for noncompliance with one or more accreditation standards. Nursing programs facing possible denial or revocation of accreditation can appeal those decisions. ACEN provides a 30-day timeframe to initiate the appeal of an adverse accreditation decision (ACEN, 2020). An Appeals Committee reviews all materials relevant to the accreditation decision and testimony presented at an appeal hearing where representatives of the nursing program, including the program administrator, may present evidence. The appeal panel decision ranges from affirmation of the adverse decision, amendment, or remanding the decision to the Board of Commissioners. All ACEN accreditation decisions are made available to the USDE, state boards of nursing, and the public. The ACEN website provides extensive information to guide nursing programs in every aspect of the accreditation process.

Commission on Collegiate Nursing Education

In 1998, the American Association of Colleges of Nursing (AACN) created the Nursing Education Accreditation Commission (NEAC) for the sole purpose of accrediting baccalaureate and higher-degree nursing programs including master's degree (MSN) and Doctor of Nursing Practice (DNP). The NEAC was subsequently renamed the *CCNE*. The CCNE is an autonomous accrediting agency of the AACN recognized by the USDE for accreditation of baccalaureate, master's, DNP, postgraduate advanced practice registered nurse (APRN) certificate programs, and entry-to-practice nurse residency programs, including distance education programs throughout the United States. Standards for accreditation of nurse practitioner fellowship/residency programs were approved by CCNE in 2020, with procedures for accreditation approved in 2021. CCNE standards, procedures, and resources are located on the AACN website (AACN, n.d.).

The mission and purpose of the CCNE focus on contributing to public health improvement and promotion of quality and integrity in nursing programs through accreditation processes identifying effective educational practices. CCNE does not provide Title IV gatekeeping functions for the programs it accredits. Accreditation activities are founded on the following principles and core values:
- Foster trust in the process, in CCNE, and in the professional community.
- Focus on stimulating and supporting *continuous* quality improvement in nursing education programs and their outcomes.
- Be inclusive in the implementation of its activities and maintain openness to the *diverse*

institutional and individual issues and opinions of the community of interest.
- Rely on review and *oversight* by peers from the community of interest.
- Maintain *integrity* through a consistent, fair, and honest accreditation process.
- Value and foster *innovation* in both the accreditation process and the programs to be accredited.
- Facilitate and engage in *self-assessment*.
- Foster an educational climate that supports program students, graduates, and faculty in their pursuit of lifelong learning.
- Maintain a high level of *accountability* to the public served by the process, including consumers, students, employers, programs, and institutions of higher education.
- Maintain a process that is both *cost effective* and *cost accountable*.
- Encourage programs to develop graduates who are *effective professionals and socially responsible* citizens.
- Ensure *autonomy and procedural fairness* in its deliberations and decision-making processes.

CCNE is governed by a 13-member Board of Commissioners composed of faculty members from CCNE-affiliated programs (3); chief nurse administrators (3); practicing nurses (3); public members (2); and professional members affiliated with employers of health care professionals (2). The CCNE Executive Director reports to the CCNE Board of Commissioners.

The Board is the final authority on all accreditation and policy decisions. The CCNE committees include the Accreditation Review, Report Review, Entry-to-Practice Residency Accreditation, Substantive Change Review, Budget, Nominating, Entry-to-Practice Nurse Residency Program Standards, and Nurse Practitioner Residency/Fellowship Standards Committees. CCNE staff members provide support for all board and standing committee activities in addition to administration of accreditation processes and procedures. CCNE on-site evaluators consist of professionals from nursing education and practice. All individuals selected as CCNE evaluators are required to participate in the CCNE evaluation training program. Training for education and residency evaluators is conducted separately.

CCNE Standards, Key Elements, and Elaborations

The CCNE *Standards for Accreditation of Baccalaureate and Graduate Nursing Programs* (CCNE, 2018) are utilized to evaluate the quality of nursing education programs. The four standards for baccalaureate and graduate nursing programs representing broad statements of expected institutional performance are:

- Program Quality: Mission and Governance.
- Program Quality: Institutional Commitment and Resources.
- Program Quality: Curriculum and Teaching-Learning Practices.
- Program Effectiveness: Assessment and Achievement of Program Outcomes.

A separate set of accreditation standards is used for nurse residency programs addressing program delivery, institutional commitment and resources, curriculum and assessment, and achievement of program outcomes. The *Key Elements* associated with each standard provide direction in meeting the overall standard. *Elaborations* are provided for each key element and are used to help clarify and interpret each key element. A list of *Supporting Documents* is provided at the end of each standard to be incorporated into the self-study document or made available for review during the on-site evaluation. During the self-assessment, nursing programs are expected to address strengths, challenges, and an action plan for improvement for each standard, providing evidence of the program's ongoing improvement processes. CCNE provides self-study workshops, webinars, videos, FAQs, and a CCNE Online Community with accreditation overviews, updates, and guidance about the CCNE accreditation process.

CCNE-accredited programs or those seeking initial accreditation must comply with current standards and key elements. In April 2021, the AACN membership approved *The Essentials: Core Competencies for Professional Nursing Education* (AACN, 2021). This document describes a new competency-based model of nursing education quality for entry- and advanced-level nursing education programs and incorporates 10 domains and 8 concepts for nursing practice (AACN, 2021). The new 2021 *Essentials* provides curricular content and expected competencies for graduates for baccalaureate, master's, and DNP programs. Programs seeking initial accreditation or continued accreditation by CCNE should visit the AACN website for additional information and resources regarding implementation of the 2021 *Essentials*.

CCNE Accreditation Process

The nursing program conducts an in-depth self-assessment resulting in development of a self-study report used to demonstrate compliance with CCNE's accreditation standards and key elements. Program strengths, areas for improvement, and action plans for continuous quality improvement are identified in the self-study. An on-site visit is conducted by a team of peer evaluators who validate information provided in the self-study report through document reviews; interviews with administrators, faculty, students, and other constituents; and review of the program's continued self-improvement processes. Peer evaluators consist of one or more professionals from both nursing education and nursing practice. All evaluation team members are required to participate in CCNE training programs prior to participating on evaluation teams. Prior to the on-site evaluation, programs must provide the evaluation team access to the program's resource materials in a *Virtual Resource Room* (CCNE, 2021). Following the on-site visit, the evaluation team prepares a *Team Report* describing the program's compliance with CCNE accreditation standards and key elements. CCNE staff review the team report and send it to the program administrator, who is provided an opportunity to submit a written response offering corrections of fact, comments, and documents demonstrating progress made toward compliance with accreditation standards.

The CCNE Accreditation Review Committee (ARC) reviews the self-study, the report of the evaluation team, and the response of the program to the team report. The ARC makes a recommendation to the CCNE Board of Commissioners regarding accreditation. The CCNE Board of Commissioners reviews the ARC's recommendation and makes the final accreditation decision. Accreditation decisions include granting initial or continuing accreditation and denial or withdrawal of program accreditation. The Board of Commissioners monitors continued compliance with accreditation standards through submission of a *Mid-Cycle Report* required by all programs granted initial and continuing accreditation approval. Documents and resources regarding accreditation and on-site evaluations are located on the AACN website (AACN, n.d.).

Initial and Continuing Accreditation

Programs seeking initial CCNE accreditation approval must first request new applicant status. A letter signed by the institution's Chief Executive Officer, the chief academic officer, and the chief nurse administrator is submitted to CCNE requesting initiation of the accreditation process. A written application must include information regarding institutional accreditation, program approval by the state's board of nursing, and a summary of the program's ability to meet CCNE's accreditation standards. Following acceptance as a new applicant, the nursing program has 2 years to submit the self-study document and host an on-site evaluation. A maximum accreditation term of 5 years may be granted to programs receiving initial accreditation approval. For postgraduate APRN certificate programs, initial accreditation may be granted for a term consistent with the degree program being evaluated. A *Continuous Improvement Progress Report* is required to be submitted by the program at the midpoint of the initial accreditation term.

Nursing programs seeking reaffirmation of their CCNE accreditation are required to contact CCNE 12 to 18 months before the on-site evaluation is to be scheduled. The chief nurse administrator submits a letter of intent for reevaluation and possible dates for the on-site visit. Following the on-site visit, CCNE's ARC considers the team report, self-study, and supporting documents and information, submitting an accreditation recommendation to the CCNE Board of Commissioners. For programs found to be in compliance with CCNE standards, continuing accreditation may be granted for periods of up to 10 years. A *Continuous Improvement Progress Report* is due at the midpoint of the accreditation term.

Accreditation decisions include continued accreditation and denial or withdrawal of accreditation. Accreditation is withdrawn by the CCNE Board for programs who do not demonstrate substantial compliance with CCNE standards, key elements, and/or procedures. CCNE may issue a directive to show cause when substantive questions and concerns are raised regarding a program's compliance with accreditations standards, key elements, and/or procedures. Programs have the opportunity to appeal CCNE's decision to deny or withdraw accreditation within a specified timeframe. CCNE accreditation decisions are communicated to USDE and other appropriate accrediting agencies.

National League for Nursing Commission for Nursing Education Accreditation

In September 2013, the NLN created the CNEA, in response to requests for additional accreditation options for nursing education programs. The NLN CNEA is recognized by the USDE and accredits all types of nursing programs including practical/vocational, diploma (RN), associate, bachelor's, master's, postgraduate certificates, and doctor of nursing practice programs. The NLN CNEA does not provide Title IV gatekeeping functions. Information about the NLN CNEA can be found on their website at https://cnea.nln.org/.

As stated in its mission, the NLN CNEA "promotes excellence and integrity in nursing education globally through an accreditation process that respects the diversity of program mission, curricula, students, and faculty; emphasizes a culture of continuous quality improvement; and influences the preparation of a caring and competent nursing workforce" (NLN CNEA, n.d.-a). NLN CNEA is governed by a 15-member Board of Commissioners representing nursing education (10), practice (3), and the public (2). The NLN CNEA Executive Director reports to the NLN CNEA Board of Commissioners. NLN CNEA staff report to the executive director and provide support for all board and standing committee activities and administration of accreditation processes and procedures. Standing committees include the Evaluation, Nominations, Policies and Procedures, Program Review, and Standards Committees. Subcommittees include the Initial Program Application and Mid-Cycle Review subcommittees.

Professionals representing nursing education and practice serve as on-site program evaluators and committee members. All on-site program evaluators must meet required criteria to be eligible for appointment as an on-site program evaluator.

NLN CNEA Standards, Quality Indicators, and Interpretive Guidelines

In October 2021, the NLN CNEA published the revised *Accreditation Standards for Nursing Education Programs* (NLN CNEA, 2021). The five NLN CNEA standards are based upon a model of continuous quality improvement guided by the NLN's core values of caring, diversity, integrity, and excellence. The five standards are:

- Culture of Excellence—Program Outcomes;
- Culture of Integrity and Accountability—Mission, Governance, and Resources;
- Culture of Excellence and Caring—Faculty;
- Culture of Excellence and Caring—Students; and
- Culture of Learning and Diversity—Curriculum and Evaluation Processes

Quality Indicators and accompanying *Interpretive Guidelines* further define each standard, while *Supporting Evidence Exemplars* provide examples of documentation and information programs may use as evidence that the quality indicator has been met. The standards, policies, and process for accreditation can be found on the NLN CNEA website at https://cnea.nln.org/.

Initial and Continuing Accreditation

The accreditation process consists of three stages: preaccreditation, initial accreditation, and continuing accreditation. Preaccreditation candidacy applications are reviewed by the Program Review Committee's Initial Program Application Subcommittee (IPASC). Approved preaccreditation status indicates that the program(s) demonstrates the potential to meet the NLN CNE standards and eligibility to submit an application for initial accreditation. Programs granted preaccreditation status have a maximum of 3 years to complete a self-study report, host an on-site evaluation, and achieve initial accreditation (NLN CNEA, 2019). Programs with preaccreditation approval may request an NLN CNEA process navigator to assist in preparation for the initial accreditation on-site evaluation visit.

Completed applications for initial accreditation require a preliminary review and recommendation from the NLN CNEA Program Review Committee (PRC) or one of its subcommittees and a final accreditation decision by the NLN CNEA Board of Commissioners. Steps in the initial accreditation process include:

1. formal notification of intent to proceed with the accreditation process;
2. submission of the self-study report;
3. participation in an on-site program evaluation visit; and
4. the committee review and board decision-making process (NLN CNEA, 2019, pp. 8–11).

Compliance with the *NLN CNEA Standards of Accreditation* must be demonstrated for the Board of Commissioners to grant initial accreditation. The length of initial accreditation is maximum of 6 years, with a required midcycle report due in the third year of the initial accreditation term.

Written requests for continuing NLN CNEA accreditation are submitted by the chief academic nurse administrator no later than 6 to 12 months prior to expiration of initial accreditation. Following submission of the program's self-study report and completion of the on-site program evaluation, the NLN CNEA Program Review Committee reviews all reports and supporting evidence and submits a recommendation to Board of Commissioners. All final accreditation decisions are the responsibility of the NLN CNEA Board of Commissioners. Continuing accreditation may be awarded up to a maximum of 10 years, with a required midcycle report due halfway through the continuing accreditation period. Information regarding continuing education is located in the online NLN CNEA accreditation handbook located on their website at https://cnea.nln.org/programs. (See Case Study 27.1.)

CASE STUDY 27.1 Seeking Accreditation for a New BSN Program

A new baccalaureate degree nursing (BSN) program with both traditional and an online accelerated BSN track is seeking initial program accreditation approval. The program is part of a private, nonprofit university approved by the Higher Learning Commission (HLC). State board of nursing approval for the BSN program (including both tracks) was granted 3 months prior to program initiation in December 2020. Initial cohorts of 10 traditional and 10 accelerated BSN students started in January 2021. Most students commute to campus, are 25 and older, and rely on financial aid programs to fund their education. The chief nurse administrator and faculty are working to identify an accrediting agency for the BSN program and the steps for initial accreditation approval.

1. How does institutional accreditation differ from programmatic accreditation?
2. What is the benefit of institutional recognition by the US Department of Education (USDE) on student eligibility for federally funded financial aid programs?
3. How do the nursing accrediting agencies differ regarding Category 3 and Category 2 recognition by the USDE? For this scenario, which nursing accrediting agency(s) would be possibilities for the program to consider when seeking program accreditation?

GENERAL INFORMATION: PREPARING FOR PROGRAM ACCREDITATION

Preparation for the programmatic accreditation process should begin 1 to 3 years prior to the anticipated on-site program evaluation visit to allow sufficient time for completion of all accreditation processes. Preparation time may vary based on the number of programs to be accredited. For example, a nursing program may have baccalaureate, MSN, and DNP degree options to be reviewed for accreditation. Other institutions may have only one nursing program, such as an associate or baccalaureate degree program.

Program evaluation is facilitated through ongoing, systematic assessment and analysis of all elements of the nursing program(s) through evaluation strategies developed to measure and improve program quality and effectiveness. The evaluation process determines the extent to which the mission, goals, and program outcomes are met. A *Program Evaluation Plan* serves as the written blueprint for collecting, analyzing, and organizing data in a systematic manner. The evaluation plan includes specified measurable performance indicators and benchmarks, appropriate measurement tools, timelines and individuals responsible for data collection and analysis, and dissemination of findings (see Chapter 26).

Professional Standards and Guidelines

Professional standards and guidelines need to be reflected in the program and its components. These standards and guidelines serve as building blocks for the nursing curriculum and must be consistent with the mission, goals, and expected outcomes of the program. Professional standards and guidelines are developed by professional nursing and specialty organizations, state regulatory agencies, and nationally recognized accreditation organizations. ACEN, CCNE, and NLN CNEA support the use of professional nursing standards and guidelines appropriate to the legal requirements and scope of practice for the degree program(s) seeking initial and continued accreditation. Nursing accrediting agencies expect programs' incorporation of professional standards and guidelines in the curriculum and their alignment with overall program outcomes. Although CCNE requires certain AACN professional standards (*Essentials*) based on program type, nursing programs have the opportunity to use other professional standards and guidelines in addition to those required. Examples of professional standards and guidelines are provided in Box 27.1.

Preparing the Self-Study Report

Information in the self-study report is used by the on-site program evaluators to guide review of the nursing program. Accrediting agencies establish the format for the self-study report and expect it to be organized by standards and associated criteria. The self-study narrative should address each standard and associated criteria systematically. A summary of the program's strengths and areas for improvement should be noted at the end of each

---

BOX 27.1 Examples of Professional Standards

- Accreditation Standards for Nursing Education Programs (NLN CNEA, 2021).
- Adult-Gerontology Acute Care Nurse Practitioner Competencies (AACN, 2012).
- Adult-Gerontology Acute Care and Primary Care NP Competencies (NONPF, 2016).
- CNS Statement for Clinical Nurse Specialist Practice and Education (National Association of Clinical Nurse Specialists [NACNS], 2019).
- Core Competencies for Interprofessional Collaborative Practice (Interprofessional Education Collaborative, 2016).
- Criteria for Evaluation of Clinical Nurse Specialist Master's, Practice Doctorate, and Post-Graduate Certificate Educational Programs (AACN, 2011).
- Education Standards and Curriculum Guidelines for Neonatal Nurse Practitioner Programs (National Association of Neonatal Nurses [NANN], 2017).
- Guidelines for Distance Education and Enhanced Technologies in Nurse Practitioner Education (NONPF, 2011).
- National Association of Neonatal Nurses (NANN, 2022).

- National Patient Safety Goals (The Joint Commission, 2022).
- NLN Core Competencies for Nurse Educators, a Decade of Influence (NLN, 2019).
- NLN Core Competencies for Nurse Educators: A Decade of Influence (NLN, 2019).
- NLN Hallmarks of Excellence (NLN, 2020).
- NLN Outcomes and Competencies for Graduates of Practical/Vocational, Diploma, Baccalaureate, Master's, Practice Doctorate and Research Doctorate Programs in Nursing (NLN, 2012).
- Outcomes and Competencies for Graduates of Practical/Vocational, Diploma, Associate Degree, Baccalaureate, Master's, Practice Doctorate and Research Doctorate Programs in Nursing (NLN, 2012).
- Standards for Accreditation of Entry-to-Practice Nurse Residency Programs (CCNE, 2021).
- The Updated National Task Force Criteria for Evaluation of Nurse Practitioner Programs (NCSBN, 2021).

---

standard. Accreditation decisions are based on the program's ability to demonstrate that the standards have been met.

The first step in preparing the self-study report is to identify the individual(s) responsible for coordinating all self-study activities and key individuals involved in drafting each standard. It is important to also identify individuals who have critical information needed for the report. Individuals providing specific information should be informed on specific formatting requirements and due dates for submission of the requested documentation. Programs may choose to create a representative *Steering Committee,* composed of the identified key individuals who lead writing teams of faculty for each standard. The Steering Committee members work with specific teams and guide development of the self-study by:

- identifying documents/materials/information needed to address each standard and quality indicator;
- detecting information gaps and strategies for filling the gaps;

- making team assignments and identifying any additional support needed;
- establishing a timeline for completion of written drafts;
- identifying and reviewing supporting evidence to include in the self-study; and
- developing plans for engaging faculty in the self-study process.

Faculty with expertise in writing and editing and strategic placement of these individuals on specific teams will facilitate timely completion of the self-study report. Faculty members who serve as on-site accreditation reviewers will be useful as internal consultants during the creation of the self-study. These individuals can provide valuable insights into the development and organization of the self-study document. Examples of additional approaches which may be utilized to develop the self-study report include: matching individual standards to specific standing committees for creation of the first draft; for development of first drafts, assignment of one or two faculty members to write the self-study, assignment of faculty teams to write each standard; hiring a professional writer; or developing a self-study steering committee composed of individuals who represent all internal programs and administration.

A timeline for completion of the self-study document should be created by working backward, starting with the dates for the on-site evaluation visit. Items to be represented on the self-study timeline include:

- due dates for completion of initial and final drafts of each standard;
- dates for faculty meetings to discuss standards throughout development of the self-study;
- logistics related to preparation for the on-site visit;
- documentation of program improvement and program outcomes;
- completion and final review of the self-study report;
- dates for a mock site visit with an external consultant;
- dates for printing and binding self-study copies for faculty, administration, and visitors;
- preparation of the resource room; and
- finalizing the agenda for the site visit.

Faculty members should be knowledgeable about information contained within the self-study report and familiar with how accreditation standards and criteria have been addressed. If outside consultants have been involved in development of the self-study, it is especially important for faculty to familiarize themselves with its content so that they can respond accurately to questions from on-site reviewers, providing clarification where necessary. All faculty are expected to be involved in development of the self-study report. Examples of faculty activities include: collecting and assembling supporting evidence documents; drafting narratives related to the standards and quality indicators; identifying program strengths and areas for improvement; gathering student work demonstrating student's ability to meet the course and program outcomes; preparing students for the on-site evaluation; and facilitating on-site program evaluator visits to clinical practice settings. Faculty members who serve as on-site accreditation reviewers may be utilized as internal consultants during the creation of the self-study, providing valuable insights into the development and organization of the self-study document.

Developing the Self-Study Narrative

Accurate interpretation of the accreditation standards and associated criteria is crucial for development of the self-study document and sets the stage for a successful on-site review. Each nursing accrediting agency provides self-study workshops, webinars, and forums for faculty to attend that provide important information related to interpretation of each standard, clarifications, and examples of supporting evidence related to each standard and associated criteria. The self-study narrative should highlight how the standards and associated criteria contribute to program quality and achievement of the program's mission, goals, and outcomes. Program identification of strengths, challenges, and areas for improvement provides evidence of the program's overall commitment to continuous quality improvement.

Faculty members developing the self-study need to understand the importance of providing a clear, concise narrative for each standard and its criteria and the importance of supporting documentation in assessing the degree to which each standard and criteria is being met. A sample narrative response to CCNE Standard I-A is presented in Box 27.2. This example is conceptual and not prescriptive, because various strategies may be employed to address the compliance of a program with accreditation criteria.

During development of the self-study report, team members should identify areas where additional supporting evidence (e.g., pictures, tables) would be useful. Working drafts should be reviewed to ensure they address each standard and criteria and include references to supporting documents in the narrative. Supporting documents demonstrating how the program meets and/or exceeds accreditation standards and criteria are an important aspect of the self-study report. Supporting documents should be discussed in the self-study narrative and/or organized in the appendix according to the specific standard and criteria. Examples of documents that reflect compliance with specific criteria include: committee, course, and faculty organization meeting minutes; course syllabi; the program evaluation plan; charts and tables with aggregate, trended data; evaluations of clinical facilities; faculty license verifications and certifications; approvals by state Boards of Nursing; course evaluations; and aggregate graduate and employer survey results.

Use of Assessment Data for Continuous Program Improvement

Assessment data should be analyzed by faculty and used to make evidence-based program improvement decisions as part of the continuous improvement process. Use of data for quality improvement helps self-study authors maintain their focus on quality while performing a thorough programmatic assessment. The self-study team must demonstrate in the self-study document collection and use of assessment data to close "feedback loops." Narrative statements in the self-study report require supporting, documented evidence demonstrating how criteria are met. Supporting documents may be provided in the appendices or on-site based on guidelines accrediting agency guidelines.

Accrediting agencies require nursing programs to provide information reflecting the use of outcomes data for program improvement. Providing tangible examples of how accreditation criteria are met through analysis and use of outcomes data strengthens the self-study report and demonstrates the program's commitment to continuous quality improvement efforts. For example, evaluations for a particular course may not consistently meet a program-established benchmark (e.g., 90% of students will rate satisfaction with courses at ≥ 3.5 on a 5.0 scale). Faculty use of evaluation data for course revisions, such as modified teaching strategies or content delivery methods, demonstrates closure of the feedback loop. Collection of evaluation data without faculty analysis and use (if indicated) is ineffective in ensuring appropriate program improvement strategies are developed and implemented. Examples of data-based programmatic decision making and supporting documentation should be reflected in self-study narrative and/or appendices.

Formatting the Self-Study Report

The self-study report should be neatly formatted and easily accessible. The self-study narrative and supporting documents should be printed and available on-site and/or available electronically according to the accrediting agencies' policies. The ability of readers to move easily from standard to standard and from standard to specific supporting tables and appendices is important to on-site evaluators and reviewers. The use of printed tab dividers between each standard and for each appendix helps ensure accessibility of printed materials. Providing a detailed table of contents and list of all tables and appendices facilitates review of the report and supporting documents by the on-site evaluators and decreases the time needed to search for specific information.

Required documents and information should be addressed in relation to the appropriate standard and criteria. References to institutional documents and catalogs should include page numbers, URLs, and other source locations to facilitate a concise programmatic review. The use of tables, charts, and graphs is recommended wherever possible. Essential tables and figures should be placed in the body of the self-study. Documents such as the strategic plan, curriculum evaluation system, and organizational chart should be appropriately referenced and placed in the appendices, where page limitations are not as much of an issue. If the self-study and supporting documents are provided in digital format to the on-site reviewers, the program can use hyperlinks in the narrative (if approved by the accrediting agency), providing readers with easy online access to reference documents. Program files such as course and faculty evaluations and faculty CVs can also be provided in electronic format for reviewers. An example of a response to CCNE Standard I-A is presented in Box 27.2. This example is conceptual and not prescriptive, because various strategies may be employed to address the compliance of a program with accreditation criteria.

External Consultants

An external consultant who is knowledgeable about the specific accrediting agency and its standards, policies, and procedures can be

BOX 27.2   Example of a Commission on Collegiate Nursing Education Self-Study Response

Standard I: Key Element I-A

I-A. The mission, goals, and expected program outcomes are:
- congruent with those of the parent institution; and
- reviewed periodically and revised as appropriate.

Elaboration: The program's mission, goals, and expected program outcomes are written and accessible to current and prospective students, faculty, and other constituents. Program outcomes include student outcomes, faculty outcomes, and other outcomes identified by the program. The mission may relate to all nursing programs offered by the nursing unit, or specific programs may have separate mission statements. Program goals are clearly differentiated by level when multiple degree/certificate programs exist. Expected program outcomes may be expressed as competencies, objectives, benchmarks, or other terminology congruent with institutional and program norms.

Program Response
Mission and Vision

The School of Nursing's (SON's) mission is to *promote and protect the health of the public by preparing future leaders in nursing practice, education, and research.* This mission is consistent with that of the University and shares the common themes of education, research, and quality health care. The SON's mission is written and publicly accessible to current and prospective students and faculty through the SON Handbook (available in the Resource Room) and to other constituents through the SON website under Facts About the School. The mission statement was revised earlier this year to more accurately describe the direction of the SON.

Central to our mission is the vision that the SON will be an academic leader in nursing education through innovation and excellence in nursing practice, education, and research. The strategic priorities of the SON include:
- Develop future generations of leaders in education, practice, research, and policy.
- Create new knowledge and apply it to practice.
- Lead in the transformation of the health care system so that nurses will practice to the fullest extent of their education and training.
- Understand and participate in health care policy development.
- Collaborate effectively with other health care professions in learning and practice.

- Ensure that SON activities are aligned with University goals.
- Engage with community partners to improve health care.

Differentiation Among Program Goals

The SON *prepares future leaders in nursing practice* by educating nurse leaders and practitioners whose practice is client centered and evidence based. Program goals describe our graduates and clearly differentiate among each of the program levels.
- The Clinical Nurse Leader (MSN) program prepares graduates as generalist nurses with a focus on practice and clinical leadership at the microsystem level.
- The Doctor of Nursing Practice (DNP) program prepares graduates to effect change through evidence-based decision making, outcomes management, and health policy improvements for diverse populations in a variety of settings. The DNP program includes BSN to DNP and MSN to DNP options that include preparation as APRNs (nurse anesthetists, clinical nurse specialists, nurse practitioners) in one of five population foci (adult-gerontology, family/individual across the lifespan, neonatal, pediatrics, and psychiatric-mental health), Advanced Public Health Nurses (APHNs), Systems Leaders, and Leaders to Enhance Population Health Outcomes.
- The postgraduate certificate program prepares graduates who seek advanced knowledge and skills and acquire certification to function as APRNs in one of four population foci: adult-gerontology, pediatrics, neonatal, or psych/mental health.
- The Doctor of Philosophy in Nursing Sciences (PhD) prepares clinical researchers who contribute to the scientific basis of care provided to individuals across the lifespan.

Expected student outcomes are described as terminal objectives that are specific to each program level. Cognitive outcomes that are common to all programs include knowledge of core concepts, analytic thinking, evidence-based decisions, outcomes assessment, and nursing roles. Psychomotor outcomes are reflected in the clinical evaluation tools and are role specific. Affective outcomes include advocacy, autonomy, human dignity, and integrity. The DNP terminal objectives were revised in 2021 in concert with the transition of advanced specialty programs to the DNP level.

instrumental in completion of the self-study document and preparation for the on-site visit. External consultants complete a detailed review of the self-study document and conduct interviews during a *mock visit*, providing an additional perspective and offering objective recommendations for improvement. During the mock visit, students, faculty, and administrators are provided opportunities to engage in a simulated accreditation visit, practice responses to potential on-site evaluator questions, and share concerns and suggestions for improvement.

The external consultant can assist faculty in revealing gaps in information and unnoticed strengths. If organized early, the program has time to update the self-study report with additional information and narrative as identified by the external consultant providing time to address identified areas for improvement. The mock on-site visit can assist in identifying faculty members who may be better suited for responding to certain types of questions. The mock visit highlights for faculty the importance of preparation, knowledge of the accreditation standards and program responses, and how to engage with the on-site program evaluators during the site visit. During the mock visit, faculty members should be reminded to respond with short answers and use examples to further clarify their points.

The On-Site Evaluation Visit

The purpose of the on-site visit is to provide the evaluation team with the opportunity to verify, clarify, and amplify information provided in the self-study document. During the on-site visit, accreditation reviewers assess the compliance of the program with accreditation standards and learn how the nursing program uses assessment data for quality improvement purposes. The evaluation team accomplishes its purpose by conducting interviews with the communities of interest, including faculty members, students, central administration, clinical agency representatives, alumni, employers, and any other program stakeholders. The leader of the evaluation team and nursing program administrator jointly determine the agenda for the on-site accreditation visit. Throughout the visit, the evaluation team is

provided a designated or "resource room" where a hard copy of the self-study and supporting documents is made available. This area will serve as the "home base" for the evaluation team during the on-site visit. Programs undergoing virtual site evaluations will provide prepared documents and information in an online portal or via flash drives.

Preparing for the On-Site Visit

Careful preparation for the on-site visit helps to ensure that the evaluation team has access to necessary documents and to create a positive and pleasant climate for the evaluation team members and the nursing program. The nursing program administrators will develop a draft agenda that will be sent to the team leader or chair of the evaluation team for their final approval. It is not unusual for this approval process to go through multiple iterations before finalization. During the development of the agenda, time needs to be designated for evaluation interviews with various institutional and program administrators, academic support staff and individuals and groups including the president, provost, clinical agencies, students, faculty, and alumni. It is important to inform the communities of interest in the program about the accreditation visit in a timely manner so that scheduling will be manageable. Letters are sent by the chief nurse administrator to the communities of interest that include the on-site visit dates and agenda and an invitation for these individuals or groups to submit comments about the nursing program. Notices are placed on websites and in college publications, are announced in class, and are distributed electronically through learning management systems and e-mail lists. Information about public meetings related to the accreditation visit can be placed in local media, including newspapers and radio.

The on-site visit agenda should reflect meeting times for the following individuals, groups, and sites to be visited: central administration, including the president and provost; key individuals on campus, such as the deans of the graduate school, libraries, and distance education, if applicable, as well as the registrar and chief financial officer; students, faculty, alumni, and clinical agency representatives; and clinical and classroom sites.

Transportation to and from meetings and clinical sites needs to be finalized based on the agenda.

Faculty members and clinical site leadership need to be notified if the evaluation team will be visiting their clinical sites. Finally, there need to be ample blocks of time designated for the evaluation team to spend in the resource room. Time for breaks between meetings should be included in the agenda for the on-site review. Although planning the agenda events may occur several months in advance, it is a good practice to confirm the agenda with all stakeholders a week or two before the actual visit.

Preparing the Resource Room

The resource room should be equipped in a manner sufficient to meet the needs of the evaluation team. Because the resource room serves as the dedicated space for evaluators to review documents and information, it is important to have available tables and chairs; a phone; computer resources; office supplies such as pens, pencils, and sticky notes; and a listing of all exhibits available for review. It is also helpful to have water, soft drinks, and snacks available for the team. Everything should be easily accessible to the evaluation team including individuals available to obtain any additional information requested by the team.

When preparing the resource room, one approach is to assign specific faculty who are responsible for ensuring that all documents are labeled and correctly placed in the resource room files. Resource files should be categorized by standards and criteria or key elements.

For example, multiple copies of documents such as faculty meeting minutes can be made in highlighted areas indicating specific information as cited in the self-study. A copy of the minutes could then be placed in the folders for each criterion where the minutes show support within the self-study. This provides simultaneous access to information by more than one evaluation team member.

The resource file should contain documents including (but not limited to) examples of student work, course syllabi, course schedules, faculty teaching assignments, faculty vitae and accomplishments, evaluation responses from all sources, minutes cited in the self-study that demonstrate utilization of data, student handbooks, and other

information as indicated in the accrediting agency standards. Sample student and faculty files should be available for review if requested by the evaluation team. The team may want to review the files of students who have submitted complaints and/or grievances to evaluate the program's application of the due process procedure. Evidence of trended aggregate data including NCLEX and certification examination pass rates and employment rates should be available in the resource room for review. The resource room should also contain documents related to the most recent reviews by other external agencies, including the regional accreditor and the state board of nursing.

Many nursing programs use information technology, including learning management systems, for document management and delivery of course content. Resource rooms may incorporate digital resources. For example, on-site reviewers may be provided with access to internal data sources such as a password-protected shared drive where accreditation documents are housed. External services such as Dropbox and Google Drive are web-supported file-sharing options. Document management systems such as Dokmee and FileHold allow users to centralize documents securely online and ensure that current versions of software are used (Capterra, n.d.; Thompson & Bovril, 2011).

Some programs may elect to use a hybrid approach to providing documents to the team. Items such as the self-study and college and university catalogs may be made available in both hard copy and electronic formats, and other files, such as course and instructor evaluations, may be provided digitally. The on-site evaluation team may be provided with flash drives that contain all accreditation-related documents or temporary access to password-protected shared drives or learning management systems where accreditation-related documents are stored. The self-study narrative can provide direct links to online supporting documentation through the use of hyperlinks. Providing information in digital format for the evaluation team lessens the amount of hard copy documentation required. Digitally prepared documents save time by eliminating the need to copy and bind documents and reports. Digital documents, including the self-study and supporting evidence, are advantageous to reviewers because the need to transport weighty hard copy documents is obviated, and accreditation-related documents can be viewed from any computer workstation (Thompson & Bovril, 2011).

Information about documents that should be available to the team during accreditation visits is provided by all nursing accrediting agencies in policy and procedure manuals located on their respective websites. (See Case Study 27.2.)

Decision-Making Process by the Accreditation Organization

All accrediting agencies follow similar steps in their decision-making processes, which are in part regulated by the USDE. The processes of these agencies include the following steps:

- The on-site peer evaluation team submits a report to the accreditation agency based on their assessment of the program's compliance with the accreditation standards as demonstrated in the self-study document and verified through the on-site visit.
- The chief nursing administrator of the nursing program has the opportunity to respond to the report of the evaluation team.
- The report of the evaluation team, the program's response, and the self-study document are sent to the review panel of the accreditation agency. The review panel makes a recommendation(s) to the Board of Commissioners regarding the accreditation decision.
- The review panel's recommendation(s) and all relevant materials are sent to the Board of

---

CASE STUDY 27.2   Preparing for an Accreditation Visit

A school of nursing at a large midwestern university has a graduate Doctor of Nursing Practice (DNP)–Family Nurse Practitioner (FNP) program. The program utilizes a hybrid (face-to-face and online) competency-based curriculum model. The graduate nursing program was granted 5-year initial accreditation approval in 2010. In 2015, the school hosted an on-site evaluation and the graduate program was subsequently awarded a full 10-year accreditation. In the last year, four doctorally prepared graduate faculty have left the program. The graduate program is due for an on-site evaluation for continued accreditation approval in 2 years.

1. What should be the priorities for action?
2. How should the faculty organize the self-study report?
3. What preparations should be made to accommodate the on-site evaluator team?

Commissioners, which makes the final decision on whether to grant, reaffirm, deny, or withdraw program accreditation.
- The final accreditation decision is communicated to the USDE, the parent institution, and appropriate accreditation and regulatory agencies.

Each nursing accrediting agency has an appeals process that programs may choose to pursue based on an adverse accreditation decision. Accreditation appeals must be generated within required timeframes. Additional fees may be incurred by the program associated with submission of an appeal.

▊ CHAPTER SUMMARY: KEY POINTS

- Accreditation is a voluntary, peer-reviewed, quality assurance process provided by private, nongovernmental agencies that involves granting public recognition to an institution or specialized program, with a history spanning over 100 years in the United States and globally.
- Numerous benefits to institutional and program accreditation have been identified for the public, students, programs, and the profession.

- Recognition by the CHEA and/or the USDE confirms that standards and processes utilized by US accrediting agencies are effective in "assuring and improving quality in higher education" (CHEA, n.d.-a).
  - Regional accrediting bodies and the USDE provide accreditation services to higher education institutions across the United States.

- Programmatic accreditation is designed for individual, professional programs at colleges, universities, or independent institutions.
- Individual state regulatory boards and agencies approve a variety of programs and require compliance with a specific set of rules and regulations.
- Higher education institutions and programs granted public recognition through accreditation demonstrate a commitment to quality educational practices and ongoing quality improvement efforts.
- Accreditation does not ensure the quality of individual graduates but provides reasonable assurance of the context and quality of the education that is offered.
- Accrediting agencies recognized by the USDE may serve as "gatekeepers" for accredited programs and institutions that wish to participate in Title IV federal student aid programs.
- Nursing accreditation agencies:
  - Baccalaureate and higher degree programs may seek program accreditation from ACEN, CCNE, or NLN CNEA.
  - Associate degree, diploma, and practical/vocational nursing programs seeking accreditation may seek accreditation from ACEN or NLN CNEA.
  - Each nursing accrediting agency provides detailed guidelines for programs in pursuit of initial and continuing accreditation.
  - Additional accrediting agencies also grant accreditation to specialized programs.
- The components of self-review and self-assessment should be viewed as ongoing rather than sporadic; achievement of accreditation demonstrates the program's commitment to quality assessment and quality improvement.
- The on-site evaluation visit provides the evaluation team with the opportunity to verify, clarify, and amplify information provided in the self-study document.
- Final accreditation decisions are the responsibility of the accrediting agency's Board of Commissioners.

REFLECTING ON THE EVIDENCE

1. Describe the purpose and importance of nursing program accreditation and list three nursing accrediting agencies.
2. Identify the benefits of accreditation for the public, student programs, and the nursing profession.
3. Discuss the steps for obtaining initial and continued accreditation by ACEN, CCNE, or NLN CNEA.
4. Define the accreditation review cycle utilized by ACEN, CCNE, and NLN CNEA for programs granted continued accreditation.
5. Explain the process of developing the self-study report, steps for preparation of the on-site resource room, and the role of faculty in the accreditation process.
6. Describe the process and information utilized by accrediting agencies related to final accreditation decisions.

REFERENCES

Abdelhadi, A. (2020). Effect of COVID-19 pandemic on academic accreditation. *Journal of Public Health Research, 9*(S1). https://www.ncbi.nlm.nih.gov/pmc/articles/PMC7771022/.

Accreditation Commission for Education in Nursing. (2020, July). *ACEN accreditation manual: 2017 Standards and Criteria*. https://www.acenursing.org/acen-accreditation-manual/

American Association of Colleges of Nursing. (2021). *AACN essentials*. https://www.aacnnursing.org/AACN-Essentials

American Association of Colleges of Nursing. (n.d.). *Accreditation resources*. https://www.aacnnursing.org/CCNE-Accreditation/Accreditation-Resources

Capterra. (n.d.). *Document management software*. https://www.capterra.com/document-management-software/

Commission on Collegiate Nursing Education. (2021, September 17). *Procedures for accreditation of baccalaureate and graduate nursing programs.* https://www.aacnnursing.org/Portals/42/CCNE/PDF/Procedures.pdf

Council for Higher Education Accreditation (CHEA). (n.d.-a). *About accreditation.* https://www.chea.org/about-accreditation

Council for Higher Education Accreditation (CHEA). (n.d.-b). *CHEA-recognized accrediting organizations.* https://www.chea.org/chea-recognized-accrediting-organizations

Council for Higher Education Accreditation (CHEA). (2021, December 3). *CHEA standards and procedures for recognition.* https://www.chea.org/chea-standards-and-procedures-recognition

Eaton, J. (2017, March). *Disruption in the U.S. accreditation space.* Council for Higher Education Accreditation. https://www.chea.org/disruption-us-accreditation-space

Federal Student Aid. (n.d.). *Financial aid toolkit.* U.S. Department of Education. https://financialaidtoolkit.ed.gov/tk/learn/types.jsp

Hegji, A. (2019, February 14). *Institutional eligibility for participation in Title IV student financial aid programs.* Congressional Research Service. https://sgp.fas.org/crs/misc/R43159.pdf.

Hegji, A. (2020, October). *An overview of accreditation of higher education in the United States.* Congressional Research Service. https://sgp.fas.org/crs/misc/R43826.pdf.

National League for Nursing Commission for Nursing Education Accreditation. (2019). *Accreditation handbook: Policies and procedures.* https://cnea.nln.org/resources

National League for Nursing Commission for Nursing Education Accreditation. (2021). *Accreditation standards for nursing education programs.* https://cnea.nln.org/standards-of-accreditation

Thompson, C., & Bevil, C. (2011). Information technology as a tool to facilitate the academic accreditation process. *Nurse Educator, 36*(5), 192–196. https://pubmed.ncbi.nlm.nih.gov/21857336/.

U.S. Department of Education. (n.d.). *Accreditation in the United States.* https://www2.ed.gov/admins/finaid/accred/index.html

INDEX

Note: Page numbers followed by *f* indicate figures, *t* indicate tables, and *b* indicate boxes.

A

AACN. *See* American Association of Colleges of Nursing

AAUP. *See* American Association of University Professors

Abbreviated form, of syllabus, 223–225

Ability, in microaggressions, 367–368

Abroad programs, roles of faculty leading study, 278*b*

Absolute scale, 559, 559*t*

Academia, faculty rights and responsibilities in, 9–10

Academia–service partnerships, 413–414

Academic achievement variables, 37

Academic advising, 623

Academic dishonesty, 69–71
   factors that contribute to, 484*t*
   in online environment, 71

Academic failure
   in classroom settings, 66–67
   in clinical settings, 62–65

Academic framework, 277

Academic freedom, 15

Academic institutions, inclusive excellence in, 371–382

Academic issues, due process for, 57–59

Academic nurse educators (ANEs)
   role
      future of, 8–9
   workforce, 1
      characteristics of, 1–2

Academic performance
   in classroom settings, 62–68
   in clinical settings, 62–68
      assisting student in, 65–66
   ethical issues related to, 68–72
   of students, 51

Academic-practice partnerships, 394

Academic preparation, lack of, 32

Academic programs, in multicultural education, 373–376

Academic progression in Nursing (APIN) program, 178–179

Academic progression models, 178–179, 197–199
   for licensed practical/vocational nurses, 179–180

Academic success
   social class differences and, 31–33
   students' characteristics on, 37–38
      academic achievement variables, 37
      circumstance variables, 38
      personal variables, 38

Academic support programs, 36

Accountability, 173
   for program evaluation, 631–632

Accreditation
   benefits of, 636–637
   components, 639
   COVID-19 impact on, 638
   definition of, 635
      ACEN, 640
   description of, 635
   evaluation plan based on criteria from, 632*b*
   history of, 636
   for new BSN program, 646*b*
   nursing programmatic agencies, 640–646
   on-site visit and, 651–653
   preparation for programmatic, 646–653
   process, 635
      ACEN, 640–641
      CCNE, 643–644
      initial and continuing, 645
      NLN CNEA, 645
      overview of, 639
   regulation *vs.*, 635
   self-study report preparation and, 646–651
   in United States, 636–638

Accreditation Commission for Education in Nursing (ACEN), 489, 600, 635, 640–642
   accreditation process of, 640–641
   initial and continuing accreditation and, 641–642
   standards and criteria of, 640

Accreditation Commission for Midwifery Education (ACME), 635, 639

Accreditation organization, decision-making process by, 653

Accreditation Review Committee (ARC), 643–644

Accreditation teams, 618

Accrediting agencies, 592
   categories of, 638–639
   decision-making process of, 653
   institutional and programmatic, 638–639
   nursing programmatic, 640–646

Accrediting bodies. *See also* Commission on Collegiate Nursing Education
   program evaluation and, 588

ACEN. *See* Accreditation Commission for Education in Nursing

Achieving Competency-Based, Time-Variable Health Professions Education, 124

Achieving Diversity and Meaningful Inclusion in Nursing Education, 79

ACME. *See* Accreditation Commission for Midwifery Education

Active learning, 216
   benefits of, 216
   overview, 216
   in simulation scale, 440*t*

Papers, 524–525
  advantages of, 524
  description and uses of, 524, 524b
  disadvantages of, 525
  issues of, 525
Partial task trainers, 423–424
Partnerships
  development, in education
      abroad experiences, 278
  evaluation of, 622, 622b
  models, 180–181
  value of, 205b
Passive learning, 216–217
  overview of, 216
Patient care
  assignments, 406–408, 407b,
      408b
  preparing students for, 406–409
Patient outcomes, in IPE and CP,
      238–239
Patient progress notes, 572
Patient Protection and Affordable
      Care Act (PPACA), 8, 110
Patients
  clinical performance evaluation
      and, 567–568
  standardized, 424
Patient simulation, 531–533. *See also*
      Simulations
  advantages of, 531–532
  description and uses of, 531
  disadvantages of, 532
  issues of, 532–533
Pedagogical innovations, 450–451
Pedagogy, 293–294
Peer active learning, 216
Peer, definition of, 601–602
Peer evaluation, 3
  accreditation and, 635–637
  clinical performance evaluation
      and, 567
  distance education and, 489
  of faculty performance, 614
  of teaching strategies, 601–602
Peer evaluators, 567
Peer learning, 331–332
  advantages of, 331
  disadvantages of, 331
  teaching tips for, 331
PEPS. *See* Productivity
      Environmental Preference
      Survey

Performance, teaching, evaluation
      of, 17–18
Personal variables, 38
Personnel salaries, 619
PhD program
  design, 196–197
  graduate of, 196–197
  in nursing degree, 192
Philosophical approaches, to
      evaluation, 495–496
Philosophical perspectives,
      summary of, 158t
Philosophies
  concepts of, 159–161
  curricular elements and, 157f
  description of, 155–156
  nursing education and, 158–159,
      158t
  statements of
    curricula and, 156–158, 157f
    developing or refining,
        163–165, 166t
    examples of, 162b
    purpose of, 161–163
Physical disabilities, students with,
      85–87
Physical fidelity, 423
Physical learning space for
      technology-enhanced
      classroom, 454
Plagiarism, 70, 482
Planning
  for arrival, in education abroad
      experiences, 281
  development, for faculty, 260–261
  goal of, 258–259
  learning activities, 262
  phase, 220
  test, 540–542
Podcasts, 458–459, 459b, 468t,
      475
  creation tools, 476
  enhanced, 475–476
Point-of-care technology, 411–412
Policies, 618–619
Portfolios, 346, 500, 516–521, 577
  advantages of, 346, 521
  description and uses of, 516–521
  disadvantages of, 346, 521
  issues of, 521
  teaching tips for, 346
Positive education, 38

Positive/friendly language, in
      warm syllabus, 223t
Positive learning practices, 42b
Positive psychology, 38
Postclinical conferences, 409–410
Poster, 343–344
  advantages of, 343–344
  disadvantages of, 344
  teaching tips for, 343
Postexperience debriefing,
      in education abroad
      experiences, 281
Postgraduate certificate programs,
      198
Postmaster's certificate programs,
      198
Postmodernism, 158t
Posttenure review, 15–16
Power relationships, 228
PPACA. *See* Patient Protection and
      Affordable Care Act
Practice learning environment,
      388–395
  acute and transitional care
      environments, 393–394
  for advanced practice nursing,
      395
  clinical cases, unfolding case
      studies, scenarios, and
      simulations, 394
  clinical learning resource centers,
      389–390
  community-based environments,
      394–395
  evaluating, 397
  health care agency environments,
      building relationship within,
      396–397
  learner-centered clinical
      education environment, 395
  selecting health care
      environments, 395–397
  simulation, 391–392
  telehealth, 392–393
  understanding, 388–389
  virtual clinical learning
      environments, 392
Practice model of nursing, 10
Practice tests, 541–542
Practice, transition to, 375–376
Practicum experiences, 398
Pragmatism, 158t

T